BRITISH
NATIONAL
FORMULARY
1985

BRITISH NATIONAL FORMULARY

Number 10 (1985)

British Medical Association
and
The Pharmaceutical Society of Great Britain

Copies may be obtained through any bookseller or, in any case of difficulty, direct from the publishers:

British Medical Association
Tavistock Square
London WC1H 9JP, England

The Pharmaceutical Press
1 Lambeth High Street
London SE1 7JN, England

ISBN: 0 85369 149 5. ISSN: 0260–535X

Typeset in Great Britain by Page Bros (Norwich) Ltd, Norwich, Norfolk, and printed and bound by The Bath Press, Bath, Avon.

Joint Formulary Committee
1985–86

Contents

Arrangement of Information

Arrangement of the text

The main text consists of classified notes on drugs and preparations used in the treatment of diseases and conditions. These notes are split into 15 chapters, each of which is related to a particular system of the human body or to another main subject (infections, vaccines etc.). Each chapter is divided into sections which begin with appropriate *notes for prescribers*. These notes are intended to provide information to doctors, pharmacists, nurses etc. to facilitate the selection of suitable treatment. The notes are followed by details of relevant drugs and preparations.

Guidance on prescribing

This chapter includes information on prescription writing, prescribing for children and elderly patients, prescribing in terminal care, and prescribing for patients with liver or kidney disease and in pregnancy or lactation. Information is also given on adverse reactions, controlled drugs, and dependence.

Emergency treatment of poisoning

The main intention of this chapter is to provide information on the management of acute poisoning when first seen in the home, although certain aspects of hospital-based treatment are mentioned.

Drugs

Drugs appear under pharmacopoeial or other non-proprietary titles. When there is an *appropriate current monograph* (Medicines Act 1968, Section 65) preference is given to a name at the head of that monograph; otherwise a British Approved Name, if available, is used. If there is an acknowledged reference drug, information on it is usually given first; otherwise the drugs are arranged alphabetically.

Preparations

These usually follow immediately after the drug which is their main ingredient. They are printed in text-sized type but those considered by the Committee to be less suitable for prescribing are described in smaller type. Small type is also used for the entries describing foods for special diets and preparations for stoma care. Preparations are included under a non-proprietary title only if (a) they are marketed under such a title, (b) various proprietary products are available that comply with the non-proprietary description, (c) they are not otherwise prescribable under the NHS, or (d) they may be prepared extemporaneously. If proprietary preparations are of a distinctive colour this is stated, but flavour is not usually mentioned.

Formulated preparations that are commonly prepared extemporaneously are described briefly in the relevant chapter and full formulae are given in the Formulary section.

Cautionary and advisory labels that are recommended for application by pharmacists to dispensed medicines have been noted against the relevant preparations. A detailed description of the labels and their rationale will be found in Appendix 4. A reference list of the label wordings appears inside the back cover.

Compound preparations

The indications, cautions, contra-indications, side-effects, and drug inter-actions of all constituents should be taken into account in prescribing; usually the ingredients should be looked up separately, or other sources consulted. It should be remembered that compound preparations may contain ingredients not suggested by the name or title; e.g. Sandocal® contains potassium ions.

Preparations not available for NHS prescription

The symbol NHS has been placed against those preparations included in the BNF that are not prescribable under the NHS. Those prescribable for specific disorders only have a foot-note specifying the condition(s) for which the preparation remains available. Prescribers are reminded that although some proprietary preparations are not *prescribable* under the NHS they can nevertheless be *dispensed* if no non-proprietary preparation is marketed.

Prescription-only medicines

The symbol PoM has been placed against those preparations that are available only on medical or dental prescription. The symbol applies when the item is ordered in the usual strength or dosage; for more detailed information and exceptions see *Medicines and Poisons Guide*, 4th edition, London, Pharmaceutical Press, 1984. The symbol **CD** indicates that the preparation is subject to control of the Misuse of Drugs Act. For regulations governing prescriptions for such preparations see pages 26–7.

Drug interactions

The Table in Appendix 1 contains section numbers which correspond with those used in the chapters.

These section numbers have been added to the Drug Interactions cross-reference in relevant monographs—a number in roman type indicates 'drug affected' (column 1 of the Table) and a number in italic type a 'drug interacting' (column 2).

For example the reference given in the paragraph headed 'cautions' under Latamoxef Sodium reads 'Drug interactions: see Appendix 1 (sections *2.8B*, 5.1).' In Appendix 1, under 2.8B, in column 2 is the information that latamoxef (drug interacting) potentiates the action of warfarin (drug affected); under 5.1 in column 1 is the information that latamoxef (drug affected) taken with alcohol (drug interacting) produces an 'Antabuse' reaction.

Prices

The relative price bands (see inside front cover) have been calculated whenever possible from the basic cost used in pricing NHS prescriptions dispensed in February 1985; these prices are based on the largest pack size of the preparation in use in general practice pharmacies or, in the case of an extemporaneous preparation, on the net cost of the ingredients used to make it.

Diluents

The diluents indicated in the entries for certain creams, ointments, elixirs, and mixtures are intended to be used when lower strengths or doses are ordered, as indicated under 'General Information'.

Preface

A new type of British National Formulary was introduced in February 1981, and the scope of the book was considerably increased although it still remained a pocket book for those concerned with the prescribing, dispensing and administration of medicines. Earlier editions of the BNF included only those products that had the confidence of the Joint Formulary Committee, and consequently only a limited selection of the many drugs and preparations available were described in the book.

From 1981, the basis of selection has been changed and information is included on most products available to prescribers in the United Kingdom. The entries, coupled with the relevant notes for prescribers, are intended to help in the choice of appropriate treatment of each patient.

Most of the preparations now follow immediately after the notes for prescribers with which they are associated. It is considered that this arrangement will help in the selection process. A small formulary section has been retained for convenience in dispensing those formulated preparations that are commonly prepared extemporaneously.

Following the publication of the first nine editions of the new book, numerous comments and suggestions for improvement have been received from doctors, pharmacists, nurses, and others and the Joint Formulary Committee would like to thank all those who have sent notes and suggestions. As a result, many changes have been made throughout the text, which has also been updated to include new products that have become available.

In preparing the tenth edition the notes have been considerably revised in the following sections of chapter 1: antacids, antispasmodics, and ulcer-healing drugs; some minor amendments have been made to the classification and the table of antacids has been replaced by a list. Significant amendments have also been made in chapter 7: drugs used in urinary-tract disorders; ammonium chloride mixture has been moved to this section.

This is the first BNF to be published since limitations were introduced on the prescribing and dispensing of drugs under the NHS. A symbol (NHS) has been used to identify those preparations in the BNF that have ceased to be prescribable.

The indications of relative cost introduced in 1981 were generally welcomed but numerous suggestions for improvement have been made. The bands represent the relative basic cost of a typical prescription and enable prescribers to take into account the need to make the best use of available resources. Good prescribing requires careful consideration of the needs of the patient and the condition being treated; these factors may result in a limitation of choice. However, where there is a choice of a number of suitable preparations to treat a particular disease or condition the price bands may be used in making a selection on a basis of cost. The Committee has investigated some alternative methods of indicating relative prices and has concluded that weekly treatment costs or prices based on a course of treatment are of limited application in a work of this nature and do not offer any real advantage over the present method.

It should be emphasised that cost-effective prescribing must take into account other factors such as dose frequency and duration of treatment that affect the total cost. The use of more expensive drugs is also justified if it will result in better treatment of the patient or a reduction of the length of an illness or the time spent in hospital.

The BNF is revised twice yearly and numerous changes are made between issues. All copies of BNF Number 9 (1985) should therefore be withdrawn and replaced by BNF Number 10 (1985). Changes after the preparation of the main text are included in a late changes section, page 451.

The Committee has received numerous requests to include information on the presence of excipients that may give rise to hypersensitivity, particularly tartrazine. In commercial formulations the presence of such ingredients is confidential. Most manufacturers will supply information to prescribers in response to individual requests related to the treatment of particular patients, but not all are willing to supply it for publication. The Committee is therefore unable to provide this information in the BNF. A number of formulated preparations included in the British Pharmacopoeia or the British Pharmaceutical Codex contain tartrazine, and these are included in the formulary section, so that they can be prepared specially, omitting the dye, if so ordered for tartrazine-sensitive patients.

The BNF is intended to be a pocket book for rapid reference and so cannot contain all the information necessary for prescribing and dispensing. It should be supplemented as necessary from specialised publications. Manufacturers' data sheets prepared in accordance with the Medicines (Data Sheet) Regulations 1972 are available for most proprietary medicines and these should also be consulted. Less detail is given in the chapters on malignant disease and immunosuppression, and anaesthesia, as it is expected that those undertaking treatment will have specialised knowledge and will consult specialist literature. Supplementary information may be available from local drug information services.

The Joint Formulary Committee acknowledges the help of individuals and organisations that provided information or advised on specific matters. The principal contributors for this edition were J. M. Aitken, R. S. Atkinson, L. Beeley, D. G. Beevers, D. A. Chamberlain, R. Dinwiddie, J. A. Dudgeon, H. M. Elliston, A. M. Geddes, A. H. Ghodse, H. M. Gilles, C. H. Hawkes, A. V. Hoffbrand, M. J. S. Langman, R. Marks, N. E. Miller, R. G. Penn, A. T. Proudfoot, J. R. Robson, M. C. Sheppard, N. K. Shinton, S. D. Shorvon, C. W. Smith, E. R. Tallett, V. R. Tindall, M. E. Turner-Warwick, P. Watkins, J. M. A. Whitehouse, J. Williamson. The Committee also wishes to express its thanks to correspondents in the pharmaceutical industry who provided information and made numerous comments on points of detail, to colleagues who have advised members of the committee and the editorial staff on specific matters, and to S. E. Wallace for clerical assistance.

Comments and constructive criticism will be welcome, and should be sent to the Executive Editor, British National Formulary, 1 Lambeth High Street, London SE1 7JN.

Drug Information Services

Information on any aspect of drug therapy can be obtained, free of charge, from Regional and District Drug Information Services. Details regarding the *local* services provided within your Region can be obtained by telephoning the following numbers.

England

Bristol	0272 20256	Direct Line
Guildford	0483 504312	Direct Line
Ipswich	0473 712233	Extn 4322/4323
Leeds	0532 430715	Direct Line
Leicester	0533 555779	Direct Line
Liverpool	051-236 4620	Extn 2126/2127/2128
London (Guy's Hospital)	01-407 7600	Extn 2568
London (London Hospital)	01-247 5454	Extn 147/62
London (Northwick Park)	01-423 4535	Direct Line
Manchester	061-276 1234	Extn 6270/6110
Newcastle	0632 321525	Direct Line
Reading	0734 875111	Extn 302
Southampton	0703 780323	Direct Line
Sutton Coldfield	021-378 2211	Extn 3565

Northern Ireland

Belfast	0232 240503	Extn 2032

Scotland

Aberdeen	0224 681818	Extn 2316
Dundee	0382 60111	Extn 2351
Edinburgh	031-229 2477	Extn 2234
Glasgow	041-552 3535	Extn 4407/4486
Inverness	0463 234151	Extn 288

Wales

Cardiff	0222 759541	Direct Line

Guidance on Prescribing

General Information

Medicines should be prescribed only when they are essential, and in all cases the benefit of administering the medicine should be considered in relation to the risk involved. This is particularly important with pregnant patients where the risk to both patient and fetus must be considered, as there are many drugs for which there is not sufficient evidence to ensure that they are entirely harmless to the fetus, especially during the first trimester of pregnancy.

TITLES AND ABBREVIATIONS. In general, titles of drugs and preparations should be written *in full*. Unofficial abbreviations should not be used as they may be misinterpreted; obsolete titles, such as Mist. Expect. and Mist. Tussis should not be used.

NON-PROPRIETARY TITLES. It is recommended that where non-proprietary ('generic') titles are given, they should be used in prescribing. This will enable any suitable product to be dispensed, thereby saving delay to the patient and sometimes expense to the health service. The only exceptional circumstance is in those few instances (such as lithium carbonate tablets) where bioavailability problems are so important that it is desirable that, once treatment has been started, the patient should continue to be treated with the product of the same manufacturer; in such cases, the brand name should be used or the manufacturer should be stated.

Titles used as headings for monographs included in the formulary section may be used freely in Great Britain and Northern Ireland but in other countries may be subject to restriction.

Many of the non-proprietary titles used in this book are titles of monographs in the European Pharmacopoeia, British Pharmacopoeia 1980 or British Pharmaceutical Codex 1973. In such cases the preparations must comply with the standard (if any) in the appropriate publication, as required by the Medicines Act (section 65).

PROPRIETARY TITLES. Names followed by the symbol® are or have been used as proprietary names in the United Kingdom. These names may in general be applied only to products supplied by the owners of the trade marks.

DOSES. The doses stated in the BNF are intended for general guidance and represent, unless otherwise stated, the usual range of doses that are generally regarded as being suitable for adults; unless otherwise indicated the quantities are those generally suitable for administration on one occasion.

DILUTION. When fractional doses are prescribed *liquid preparations* for oral use will be diluted with a suitable vehicle to dose-volumes of 5 ml or a multiple thereof, unless otherwise directed in the text. Dilution should be effected at the time of dispensing and such diluted preparations may be less stable than the original undiluted prep-

arations. Where a complete recipe is given in the formulary section the diluent is the specified vehicle, otherwise the diluent specified in the text should be used.

In the case of *creams, ointments etc.*, where a complete recipe is available the diluent is the specified vehicle, otherwise only diluents specified in the text should be used.

STRENGTHS AND QUANTITIES. The strength or quantity to be contained in capsules, lozenges, tablets, etc. should be stated by the prescriber.

If a pharmacist receives an incomplete prescription for a systemically administered preparation other than a prescription for a controlled drug and he considers it would not be appropriate for the patient to return to the doctor, the following procedures will apply:

(a) an attempt must always be made to contact the prescriber to ascertain his intention;

(b) if the attempt is successful the pharmacist must, where practicable, subsequently arrange for details of quantity, strength where applicable, and dosage to be inserted by the prescriber on the incomplete form;

(c) where, although the prescriber has been contacted, it has not proved possible to obtain his written intention regarding an incomplete prescription, the pharmacist may endorse the form 'p.c.' (prescriber contacted) and add details of the quantity and strength where applicable of the preparation supplied, and of the dose indicated. The endorsement should be initialled and dated by the pharmacist;

(d) where the prescriber cannot be contacted and the pharmacist has sufficient information to make a professional judgment he may dispense a sufficient quantity of the preparation to complete up to 5 days' treatment; except that where a combination pack (i.e., a proprietary pack containing more than one medicinal product) or oral contraceptive is prescribed by name only, the smallest pack shall be dispensed. In all cases he must endorse the prescription 'p.n.c.' (prescriber not contacted) and indicate the quantity, the strength, where applicable, of the preparation supplied, and the dose, and initial and date the endorsement;

(e) if the pharmacist has any doubt about exercising discretion, an incomplete prescription must be referred back to the prescriber.

CONTROLLED DRUGS. A prescription for a controlled drug may not be dispensed by a pharmacist unless the requirements of Regulation 15 of the Misuse of Drugs Regulations, 1973 are met. He may not add to the prescription or otherwise exercise discretion on the quantity, dosage, or strength of the drug which is to be dispensed. All incomplete prescriptions must therefore be referred back to the prescriber.

APPLIANCES AND CHEMICAL REAGENTS. A limited selection of appliances (including dressings, elastic hosiery, and trusses) and chemical reagents is available for prescribing by general medical practitioners in the National Health Service. For details the appropriate edition of the Drug Tariff should be consulted.

DRUGS AND DRIVING. Prescribers should advise patients if treatment is likely to affect their ability to drive motor vehicles. This applies particularly to drugs with sedative or anticholinergic effects and patients should be warned that these effects are increased by alcohol. See also Appendix 4.

NOTICE CONCERNING PATENTS. In the British National Formulary certain drugs have been included notwithstanding the existence of actual or potential patent rights. In so far as such substances are protected by Letters Patent, their inclusion in this Formulary neither conveys, nor implies, licence to manufacture.

HEALTH AND SAFETY. The British National Formulary is intended for the guidance of medical practitioners, pharmacists, dentists, nurses, and other workers who have the necessary training and experience to interpret the information it provides. It is intended as a reference book for the pocket, and should be supplemented by a study of more detailed publications when required.

When handling chemical or biological materials particular attention should be given to the possibility of allergy, fire, explosion, radiation, or poisoning. Some substances, including corticosteroids, antibiotics, phenothiazine derivatives, and many cytotoxic substances, are irritant or very potent and should be handled with caution. Contact with the skin and inhalation of dust should be avoided.

SAFETY IN THE HOME. Patients must be warned to keep all medicines out of the reach of children in a safe locked place. As an additional precaution certain medicines may be supplied in child-resistant containers or strip packaging. Arthritic or infirm patients should be advised to ask the pharmacist to replace child-resistant closures by suitable ordinary closures. All patients should be advised to dispose of unwanted medicines by flushing them down a WC or returning them to the supplier for destruction.

LABELLING OF CONTAINERS WITH THE NAME OF THE PREPARATION. The Councils of the British Medical Association and the Pharmaceutical Society have agreed that the name of the preparation should appear on the label unless the prescriber indicates otherwise.
1. Subject to the conditions of paragraphs 4 and 6 below, the name of the prescribed preparation is stated on the label of dispensed medicines unless the prescriber deletes the letters 'NP' which appear on National Health Service prescription forms.
2. The strength is also stated on the label in the case of tablets, capsules, and similar preparations that are available in different strengths.
3. If it is the wish of the prescriber that a description of the preparation such as 'The Sedative Tablets' should appear on the label, he should write the desired description on the prescription form.
4. The arrangement will extend to approved names, proprietary names or titles given in the BP, BPC, BNF, or DPF. The arrangement does not apply when a prescription is written so that several ingredients are given.
5. The name written on the label is that used by the prescriber on the prescription.
6. If more than one item is prescribed on one form and the prescriber does not delete the letters 'NP', each dispensed medicine is named on the label, subject to the conditions given above in paragraph 4. If the prescriber wants only selected items on such a prescription to be so labelled he will indicate this by deleting the letters 'NP' on the form and writing 'NP' alongside the medicines to be labelled.
7. When a prescription is written other than on a National Health Service prescription form the name of the prescribed preparation will be stated on the label of the dispensed medicine unless the prescriber indicates otherwise.

Prescription Writing

Prescriptions should be written legibly in ink or typewritten, dated and signed by the prescriber, and the full name and address of the individual patient added. The age of the patient should preferably be stated, and is essential for children[1].

The following recommendations should be observed:
(a) For solids, quantities of 1 gram or more should be written as 1 g etc. Quantities less than 1 gram should be written in milligrams, for example 500 mg, not 0.5 g. Similar quantities less than 1 mg should be written in micrograms, for example 100 micrograms, not 0.1 mg. 'Micrograms' and 'nanograms' should **not** be abbreviated.

---

1. This is a legal requirement in the case of prescription-only medicines.

(b) When decimals are unavoidable a zero should be written in front of the decimal point where there is no other figure, for example 0.5 ml, not .5 ml.

(c) The term 'millilitre' (ml) is used in medicine and pharmacy, and cubic centimetre, c.c., or cm³ should not be used.

(d) Dose and dose frequency should be stated. For liquid medicines, doses should preferably be stated in terms of 5-ml spoonfuls for the linctus or elixir type and for preparations for children, and 10-ml quantities for mixtures for adults. In the case of mixtures with a dose of 10 ml or more, the patient will be directed to take the dose with water unless the prescription states the contrary.

When doses other than 5 or 10 ml are prescribed, the liquid medicine will be diluted to provide a dose of 5 or 10 ml or a multiple thereof. Exception is made with certain preparations, which are measured by means of a pipette. The volume of liquid preparation prescribed should normally be 50, 100, 150, 200, 300, or 500 ml.

(e) Total quantities of solids prescribed should normally be selected from the range 25, 50, 100, 200, 300, and 500 grams.

(f) Because of the large number of drug names in use care should be taken to avoid misinterpretation. Names should be written clearly and the use of abbreviations for names of drugs and preparations should be avoided.

(g) Ensure that the prescription contains the symbol 'NP' if the medicine is to be labelled with the name of the prescribed preparations. The symbol 'NP' is printed on National Health Service prescription forms. It should be deleted by the prescriber if labelling with the name of the prescribed preparation is not required. For full details see under General Information.

(h) The quantity to be supplied may be stated by indicating the *length of treatment required*. The number of days' treatment should be inserted in the box provided on National Health forms, and in most cases the exact amount will be supplied. This does not apply to items directed to be used as required, as it is not then possible to calculate the exact amount; unless the dose and frequency are given the quantity to be supplied should be stated on the prescription. When several items are ordered on one form the box can be marked with the number of days and the quantity added for any item for which the amount cannot be calculated.

(i) Dose frequency and other directions should preferably be stated in English without abbreviation.

(j) Prescriptions written in accordance with these recommendations are acceptable for prescription-only medicines (PoM). For items marked **CD** refer to the instructions for writing prescriptions for controlled drugs.

(k) A prescription for a preparation that has been withdrawn from the market or needs to be specially imported for a named patient should be handwritten and signed by the doctor. The name of the preparation should be endorsed with his signature and the letters 'WD' (withdrawn or specially-imported drug); this will be a valuable indication to the pharmacist of the prescriber's intentions. There may be a considerable delay in obtaining a withdrawn medicine.

In hospitals the following should also be noted:

(a) There should be a prescription sheet on which prescriptions and a record of dispensing and administration *only* are written.

(b) Not more than one prescription sheet should be in use at any one time for any one patient.

(c) Frequency of administration of 'as required' medicines should be indicated by clear and definitely stated intervals.

(d) The route of administration should be clearly shown.

(e) The prescription sheet should show signed and dated cancellations of any prescriptions no longer current.

Arrangements should be made for doses to be given at special times when intervals are critical.

Quantities of Preparations

The following list indicates the quantities of preparations suitable for various purposes.

Liquid Preparations

Adult Mixtures (10-ml dose)	200 ml (20 doses)
	300 ml (30 doses)
Elixirs, Linctuses, and Paediatric Mixtures (5-ml dose)	50 ml (10 doses)
	100 ml (20 doses)
	150 ml (30 doses)
Ear-drops, Eye-drops, and Nasal Drops	10 ml
Eye Lotions, Gargles, and Mouth-washes	200 ml
Inhalations and Sprays	25 ml
Liniments	100 ml

Dermatological Preparations

	Creams and Ointments	Lotions
Face	5 to 15 g	100 ml
Both hands	25 to 50 g	200 ml
Scalp	50 to 100 g	200 ml
Both arms or both legs	100 to 200 g	200 ml
Body	200 g	500 ml
Groins and genitalia	15 to 25 g	100 ml
Dusting-powders	50 to 100 g	
Paints	10 to 25 ml	

Approximate Conversions and Units

lb	kg	stones	kg	ml	fl. oz (approx)
1	0.45	1	6.35	50	1.8
2	0.91	2	12.70	100	3.5
3	1.36	3	19.05	150	5.3
4	1.81	4	25.40	200	7.0
5	2.27	5	31.75	500	17.6
6	2.72	6	38.10	1000	35.2
7	3.18	7	44.45		
8	3.63	8	50.80		
9	4.08	9	57.15		
10	4.54	10	63.50		
11	4.99	11	69.85		
12	5.44	12	76.20		
13	5.90	13	82.55		
14	6.35	14	88.90		
		15	95.25		

Mass

1 kilogram (kg)	= 1000 grams (g)
1 gram (g)	= 1000 milligrams (mg)
1 milligram (mg)	= 1000 micrograms
1 microgram	= 1000 nanograms
1 nanogram	= 1000 picograms

Volume

1 litre	= 1000 millilitres (ml)
1 millilitre	= 1000 microlitres
1 pint	≈ 568 ml

Other units

1 kilocalorie (kcal)	= 4186.8 joules (J)
1000 kilocalories (kcal)	= 4.1868 megajoules (MJ)
1 megajoule (MJ)	= 238.8 kilocalories (kcal)
1 millimetre of mercury (mmHg)	= 133.3 pascals (Pa)
1 kilopascal (kPa)	= 7.5 mmHg (pressure)

Emergency Supply of Prescription-only Medicines

The Medicines (Prescription Only) Order 1977, as amended, allows exemptions from the Prescription Only requirements for emergency supply to be made by a person lawfully conducting a retail pharmacy business provided:

(a) that the pharmacist has interviewed the person requesting the prescription-only medicine and has satisfied himself that: (i) there is immediate need for the prescription-only medicine and that it is impracticable in the circumstances to obtain a prescription without undue delay; (ii) that the treatment with the prescription-only medicine has on a previous occasion been prescribed by a doctor for the person requesting it; and (iii) as to the dose which it would be appropriate for the person to take;

(b) that no greater quantity shall be supplied than will provide five days' treatment except when the prescription-only medicine is: (i) an ointment, cream or preparation for the relief of asthma in an aerosol dispenser when the smallest pack can be supplied; (ii) an oral contraceptive when a full cycle may be supplied; or (iii) an antibiotic in liquid form for oral adminstration when the smallest quantity that will provide a full course of treatment can be supplied;

(c) that an entry shall be made in the prescription book stating: (i) the date of supply; (ii) the name, quantity and, where appropriate, the pharmaceutical form and strength; (iii) the name and address of the patient; and (iv) the nature of the emergency;

(d) that the container or package must be labelled to show: (i) the date of supply; (ii) the name, quantity and, where appropriate, the pharmaceutical form and strength; (iii) the name of the patient; (iv) the name and address of the pharmacy; and (v) the words "Emergency supply".

(e) that the prescription-only medicine does not contain a Controlled Drug or other substance specifically excluded from the emergency supply provision: for details see *Medicines and Poisons Guide*, 4th Edition, London, Pharmaceutical Press, 1984.

THE PHARMACEUTICAL SOCIETY'S GUIDELINES

(1) The pharmacist should consider the medical consequences, if any, of **not** supplying.

(2) The pharmacist should identify the patient through means of documentary evidence and/or personal knowledge.

(3) The doctor who prescribed on a previous occasion should preferably be identified and contacted, if possible.

(4) The question should be asked of the patient as to whether the doctor has stopped the treatment.

(5) Inquiries should be made as to whether any other medicine is being taken at the same time to check any drug interactions.

(6) An emergency supply should not be made if the item requested was prescribed previously more than six months prior to the request. Variations may be made in the case of those illnesses which occur infrequently, for example, hay fever, asthma attack, or migraine.

(7) Consideration should be given to providing less than five days' quantity if this is justified in the circumstances.

(8) Labelling should be clear and legible and there should be some suitable identification of emergency supply entries in the prescription book.

Prescribing for Children

All children, and particularly neonates, differ from adults in their response to drugs. Special care is needed in the neonatal period (first 30 days of life) and doses should always be calculated according to weight. At this age, the risk of toxicity is increased by inefficient renal filtration, relative enzyme deficiencies, differing target organ sensitivity, and inadequate detoxifying systems causing delayed excretion. In childhood dosage should be adjusted for weight until 50 kg or puberty is reached.

Prescriptions must state the age of the child, the dose, frequency and route of drug administration, and length of treatment. A statement of the patient's body-weight is helpful.

It is particularly important to state the strengths of capsules or tablets. Although liquid preparations are particularly suitable for children, most contain sucrose which encourages dental decay. When taken over a long period, sugar-free tablets, liquid medicines, and diluents should be used when possible.

When a prescription for a liquid oral preparation is written and the dose ordered is smaller than 5 ml, the preparation will normally be diluted with a suitable vehicle so that the required dose is contained in 5 ml. Parents must be instructed to use the standard 5-ml spoon to measure the dose and not to heap up a viscous preparation. They should also be advised not to add any medicines to the contents of the infant's feeding bottle, since the drug may interact with the milk or other liquid in it, or the ingested dosage may be reduced, because the patient may not drink all of the contents.

See also General Information, Safety in the home, p. 3.

Dosage in Children

Doses for children are stated in the individual drug entries as far as possible, except where paediatric use is not recommended, as with tetracyclines, or where there are special hazards.

Doses are generally based on body-weight (in kilograms) or the following age ranges:

first month (neonate)
up to 1 year (infant)
1–5 years
6–12 years

Where a single dose is quoted for a given range, it applies to the middle of the age range and some extrapolation may be necessary to obtain doses for ages at the lower and upper limits of the stated range.

DOSE CALCULATION. If no dose is stated in the BNF, children's doses may be calculated from adult doses by using age, body-weight, or body-surface area or by a combination of these factors. The most reliable methods are those based on body-surface area.

Body-weight may be used to calculate doses expressed in mg/kg, and some children's doses in

the BNF are stated in this way. Young children may require a higher dose per kilogram body-weight than adults because of their higher metabolic rates. Calculation of approximate dose from the following formulas may underestimate dosage in the infant:

$$\frac{\text{Patient's weight in kg}}{70} \times \text{adult dose}$$

or

$$\frac{\text{Patient's weight in lb}}{150} \times \text{adult dose}$$

Other problems need to be considered. For example, calculation by body-weight in the obese child would result in much higher doses being administered than necessary. In such cases, dose should be calculated from an ideal weight, related to height and age. Where new or potentially toxic drugs are used, the manufacturers' recommended doses should be carefully followed.

Body-surface estimates are more accurate for calculation of paediatric doses than body-weight since many physical phenomena are more closely related to body-surface area. The average body-surface area of a 70-kilogram human is about 1.8 m^2. Thus, to calculate the dose for a child the following formula may be used:

Approximate dose for patient =

$$\frac{\text{surface area of patient } (m^2)}{1.8} \times \text{adult dose}$$

Approximate values of body-surface for average children of different ages are shown in the Table, together with an approximate percentage of the adult dose. This percentage may be conveniently used to calculate children's doses of commonly prescribed drugs with a high therapeutic index. The most appropriate combination of age, weight, and height should be used in determining the percentage to use.

	Ideal body-weight		Height		Body-surface	Percentage of adult
Age	kg	lb	mm	in	m^2	dose
Newborn*	3.4	7.5	500	20	0.23	12.5
1 month*	4.2	9	550	22	0.26	14.5
3 months*	5.6	12	590	23	0.32	18
6 months	7.7	17	670	26	0.40	22
1 year	10	22	760	30	0.47	25
3 years	14	31	940	37	0.62	33
5 years	18	40	1080	42	0.73	40
7 years	23	51	1200	47	0.88	50
12 years	37	81	1480	58	1.25	75
Adult						
Male	68	150	1727	68	1.8	100
Female	56	123	1626	64	1.6	100

* The figures relate to full term and not preterm infants who may need reduced dosage according to their clinical condition.

More precise body-surface values may be calculated from height and weight by means of a table (for example *The Pharmaceutical Codex*, 11th Edition, London, Pharmaceutical Press, 1979) or a nomogram (for example, J. Insley and B. Wood, *A Paediatric Vademecum*, 10th Edition, London, Lloyd Luke, 1982).

Prescribing for the Elderly

As a group, old people are the largest consumers of medicines. While being potentially the greatest beneficiaries from modern drugs, carefully and rationally prescribed, they are also highly vulnerable to adverse reactions.

Elderly patients are apt to receive multiple drugs for their multiple diseases. They also commonly present with vague symptoms such as headache, sleeplessness, and lightheadedness which may be associated with social stress, as in widowhood, loneliness, and family dispersal. The use of drugs for such psychosomatic conditions can at best be a poor substitute for effective social measures and at worst pose a serious threat from adverse reactions.

In very old subjects, manifestations of normal ageing may be mistaken for disease and inappropriate drugs prescribed. A common misuse of drugs occurs where old people are prescribed drugs such as prochlorperazine, which are effective in Ménière's disease, because they complain of vague giddiness as their postural control is impaired. There is no possibility of benefit from such treatment and the patient may experience serious side-effects such as drug-induced parkinsonism, postural hypotension (with falls and fractures), and mental confusion.

Further difficulties may arise in old people who take non-prescribed medicines such as aspirin-containing mixtures and an often bewildering variety of laxatives. It may be quite difficult to establish exactly what the patient is taking unless the patient is visited in the home where medicine bottles can be viewed whilst directly questioning the patient and relatives.

PHARMACOLOGICAL CONSIDERATIONS. The ageing nervous system shows increased *sensitivity* to many commonly used drugs, for example opium alkaloids, many sedatives and tranquillisers, and antiparkinsonian drugs.

The speed and degree of drug absorption, as well as drug metabolism and excretion, may all be altered in old age. This will often prolong the retention of a drug in the body and may increase plasma half-life by as much as 50%.

By far the most important factor affecting *drug concentration* in the body is the decrease in renal clearance which declines from early adulthood onwards. This must inevitably reduce the rate of drug elimination since most drugs are excreted via the kidney. There is also evidence that the liver's ability to metabolise drugs decreases with old age.

Reduction in plasma albumin concentrations (and reduced plasma binding) occurs commonly in sick old people and may increase the concentration of unbound bioavailable drug. There is little evidence to suggest that drug absorption is significantly altered in old age but drug distribution may be altered by the reduction in body water and increased fat which occurs with ageing.

The net result of all these changes is that a given dose in an aged patient will produce higher plasma or tissue concentrations over longer periods of time. Old people are more likely to receive several drugs simultaneously and the dangers of drug interactions are increased.

DOSAGE. First one must always pose the question of whether a drug is indicated at all. Where a placebo effect is necessary, it is essential to use a genuinely inert substance and the temptation to prescribe a 'mild psychotropic' in the vague hope that it might provide additional symptomatic relief must be resisted.

When prescribing drugs in the elderly, it is a sensible policy to limit the range of drugs used to a minimum so that the prescriber may familiarise himself more thoroughly with their doses and side-effects in elderly patients.

It is good practice to initiate treatment in aged patients with doses of little more than half that recommended for younger subjects. Paediatric formulations may be useful in allowing greater flexibility of dose.

A system of regular review should be instituted in patients on repeat prescriptions since they may no longer require the medicine or their needs may change from time to time. The correct maintenance dose of a drug may be difficult to establish but is generally significantly lower than for younger patients. It should also be remembered that episodes of acute intercurrent illness, such as myocardial infarction or respiratory-tract infection, may lead to rapid reduction in renal clearance, especially when dehydration supervenes. In these circumstances continuing the usual therapeutic dose of a drug such as digoxin may constitute a toxicity hazard.

COMMON ADVERSE REACTIONS. Adverse reactions often present in the elderly in a vague and non-specific fashion. *Mental confusion* is often the presenting symptom. Other common manifestations are *constipation* (as with anticholinergics and many tranquillisers) and postural *hypotension* (as with diuretics and many psychotropics).

Hypnotics in common use are responsible for many adverse reactions in the elderly as many of them have plasma half-lives of 30 or more hours. Hence patients may have marked hangover effects throughout the day, with drowsiness, unsteady gait, and sometimes slurred speech and confusion. Prescribers should therefore ascertain the half-lives of the hypnotics they use and should be prepared to switch to those with a shorter action (see section 4.1.1).

Diuretics cause the greatest absolute number of adverse reactions because they are so widely prescribed. They are often used in conditions where drug treatment is unnecessary. For example, they are commonly used to treat simple gravitational oedema and this, in most instances, may be relieved in a more physiological manner by encouraging movement, raising the legs, and supplying support stockings.

The following groups are associated with the greatest risk of adverse reactions in old age; drugs used in parkinsonism, antihypertensives, psychotropics, digoxin, hypnotics, and diuretics.

PATIENT COMPLIANCE. At all ages poor compliance with the prescriber's instructions presents a threat to safe treatment and it is obvious that this danger is greater in old patients who have memory impairment, poor eyesight, and difficulty in coping with complex drug regimens. Several rules apply:
(a) determine whether the patient is capable of understanding and remembering the prescriber's instructions. If not, the help of a third party is essential. This person is usually a relative but may be a neighbour, home help, the warden (in sheltered housing), or occasionally a district nurse;
(b) ensure that prescriptions and containers are clearly and explicitly marked with the prescriber's instructions and dose, even for repeat prescriptions. Avoid expressions like 'as directed'. Containers must also be capable of being opened by the patient and it may be necessary to ask the pharmacist to avoid dispensing drugs in child-resistant containers;
(c) simplify drug regimens as far as possible.

Problems associated with imperfect compliance are already formidable and bound to increase. A recent study showed that 25% of old people were taking drugs which had not been recorded as 'current medication' by their general practitioner. Members of primary health care teams should recognise this problem and seek to reduce the dangers including those associated with the uncritical use of repeat prescriptions.

Prescribing in Terminal Care

In recent years there has been increased interest in providing better treatment and support for patients with terminal illness. The aim is to keep the patient as comfortable, sensibly conscious, and free of pain as possible. If the patient is to end his days in serenity it may also be necessary to direct attention to his financial, social, or family problems. The patient's minister or the hospital chaplain may give invaluable help.

DOMICILIARY TREATMENT. Whenever possible patients should end their days in their own homes with their families. Although families may at first be resistant to, or perhaps frightened of, taking care of the patient at home, they will usually do so if they can be assured that the patient will be readily admitted to hospital when the family can no longer manage. Support from the social services and district nursing service may be required.

HOSPITAL TREATMENT. The most important lesson to be drawn from the experience of hospices is that both doctors and nurses must give time to listen to the patient. This, in itself, is a major therapeutic measure that gives great support and comfort to a patient who may otherwise suffer intolerable loneliness. Often problems come to light that can easily be dealt with—adjusting a blind in the late afternoon, an irritating noise to be avoided, drinks to be placed in easier reach, someone to read the newspaper, or the TV to be replaced by radio. The staff should not exclude the family from contributing to the patient's care; if prevented they may be resentful or subsequently suffer a feeling of guilt.

DRUG TREATMENT. The number of drugs used to control symptoms in an individual patient should be as few as possible, for even the taking of medicine may be an effort.

PAIN. Analgesics are always more effective in preventing the development of pain than in the relief of established pain. Of the non-narcotic analgesics (see section 4.7.1.1), aspirin 600 mg every 4 hours or paracetamol 1 g every 4 hours will often make the use of more potent analgesics unnecessary. Other anti-inflammatory analgesics (see section 10.1.1.2) may control the pain of bone secondaries if aspirin is inadequate. Typical regimens include naproxen 250 mg every 6–8 hours, ibuprofen 400 mg every 4–8 hours, or indomethacin 100 mg rectally every 12 hours.

NARCOTIC ANALGESICS. Morphine is the most useful strong analgesic. It may be prescribed as a simple elixir (morphine hydrochloride dissolved in chloroform water) by writing the formula as described under 'Analgesic elixirs of diamorphine and morphine', section 4.7.2. The dose and time interval can be adjusted. The dose should be the lowest compatible with pain control. With regular administration every 4 hours small doses of 5 to 20 mg are surprisingly effective but there need be no hesitation in increasing to 30 to 60 mg, or occasionally 90 to 150 mg, to control pain. If the patient cannot swallow, morphine suppositories may be prescribed, or diamorphine (more soluble than morphine) may be given by injection. One mg of diamorphine hydrochloride by injection is generally considered to be approximately as effective as 3 or 4 mg of morphine hydrochloride or sulphate by mouth. Sustained-release oral and parenteral preparations of morphine may be useful.

Some patients are nauseated on starting morphine. Prochlorperazine mesylate 5 to 10 mg (as elixir) may be given in conjunction with morphine elixir. It is usually only needed for 4 to 5 days.

MISCELLANEOUS CONDITIONS. *Headache due to intracranial pressure* often responds to corticosteroids in high dosage, for example, dexamethasone 16 mg daily for 4 to 5 days, reduced if possible to 4 to 6 mg daily. *Intractable cough* may be relieved by inhalations or by diamorphine linctus 2.5 to 10 ml every 4 hours or methadone linctus 5 ml every 4 hours; extemporaneously prepared solutions of morphine hydrochloride, in an initial dose of 5 mg every 4 hours, may, however, be preferable (particularly in relation to methadone which, with its long duration of action, tends to accumulate). *Excessive respiratory secretion*

(death rattle) may be reduced by subcutaneous injection of hyoscine hydrobromide 200 to 600 micrograms. *Restlessness and confusion* may require treatment with drugs described in section 4.2.1, for example, chlorpromazine hydrochloride 50 to 100 mg by mouth initially, followed by 25 to 50 mg every 8 hours, or haloperidol 5 to 10 mg by injection initially, followed by 3 to 5 mg by mouth every 8 hours. *Hiccup* may be treated with chlorpromazine, or perphenazine by mouth or by intramuscular injection. *Fungating growth* may be treated by cleansing with a mixture of 1 part of 4% povidone-iodine skin cleanser solution and 4 parts of liquid paraffin. *Capillary bleeding* may be reduced by applying gauze soaked in adrenaline solution (1 in 1000).

Prescribing in Liver Disease

Liver disease may alter the response to drugs in several ways as indicated below, and drug prescribing should be kept to a minimum in all patients with severe liver disease. The Table may be used as a guide to treatment of patients with impaired liver function but is not exhaustive as drugs are included only when there is sufficient information available to provide treatment guidelines.

IMPAIRED DRUG METABOLISM. Metabolism by the liver is the main route of elimination for many drugs, but the hepatic reserve appears to be large and liver disease has to be severe before important changes in drug metabolism occur. Routine liver-function tests are a poor guide to the capacity of the liver to metabolise drugs, and in the individual patient it is not possible to predict the extent to which the metabolism of a particular drug may be impaired.

A few drugs, for example rifampicin and fusidic acid, are excreted in the bile unchanged and may accumulate in patients with intrahepatic or extrahepatic obstructive jaundice.

HYPOPROTEINAEMIA. The hypoalbuminaemia in severe liver disease is associated with reduced protein binding and increased toxicity of some

highly protein-bound drugs such as phenytoin and prednisone.

REDUCED CLOTTING. Reduced hepatic synthesis of blood-clotting factors, indicated by a prolonged prothrombin time, increases the sensitivity to oral anticoagulants such as warfarin and phenindione.

HEPATIC ENCEPHALOPATHY. In severe liver disease many drugs can further impair cerebral function and may precipitate hepatic encephalopathy. These include all sedative drugs, narcotic analgesics, those diuretics that produce hypokalaemia, and drugs that cause constipation.

FLUID OVERLOAD. Oedema and ascites in chronic liver disease may be exacerbated by drugs that give rise to fluid retention. These include anti-inflammatory analgesics such as indomethacin, corticosteroids and corticotrophin, and carbenoxolone.

HEPATOTOXIC DRUGS. Hepatotoxicity is either dose-related or unpredictable (idiosyncratic). Drugs causing dose-related toxicity may do so at lower doses than in patients with normal liver function, and some drugs producing reactions of the idiosyncratic kind do so more frequently in patients with liver disease. These drugs should be avoided.

Table: Drugs to be avoided or used with caution in liver disease

Drugs	Comment	Drugs	Comment
1: Gastro-intestinal system			
1.1 Antacids	In patients with fluid retention, avoid those containing large amounts of sodium, e.g. magnesium trisilicate mixture, Gaviscon®. Avoid those causing constipation, e.g. calcium compounds, as this can precipitate coma		
		1.3 Ulcer-healing drugs	
		Carbenoxolone	Produces fluid retention and hypokalaemia
		Cimetidine	Occasional risk of confusional states
		1.4 Antidiarrhoeal drugs	
		Diphenoxylate	May precipitate coma

Table: Drugs to be avoided or used with caution in liver disease (*continued*)

Drugs	Comment	Drugs	Comment
1.9 Drugs affecting intestinal secretions			be reduced. Chlorpromazine is hepatotoxic
Chenodeoxycholic acid,	Avoid in patients with chronic liver disease.		
Ursodeoxycholic acid	Patients with a non-functioning gall-bladder do not respond	*4.3 Antidepressants*	Tricyclics are preferable to monoamine-oxidase inhibitors but sedative effects are increased. Iprindole and MAOIs may cause idiosyncratic hepatotoxicity
Dehydrocholic acid	Avoid in patients with intra-hepatic cholestasis or complete biliary obstruction		
2: Cardiovascular system		*4.6 Drugs used in nausea*	Avoid antihistamines and phenothiazines—may precipitate coma. Chlorpromazine is hepatotoxic
2.2 Diuretics	Hypokalaemia may precipitate coma. A potassium-sparing diuretic should be used to prevent this.		
Bumetanide, Ethacrynic acid, Frusemide, Piretanide,			
Thiazides	Increased risk of hypomagnesaemia in alcoholic cirrhosis	*4.7 Analgesics*	
		Anti-inflammatory analgesics, Ibuprofen, Phenylbutazone, etc.	Increased risk of gastro-intestinal bleeding and can cause fluid retention
2.3 Anti-arrhythmic drugs			
Lignocaine, Mexiletine, Tocainide	Avoid—or reduce dose in severe liver disease	Aspirin	Increased risk of gastro-intestinal bleeding—avoid
Verapamil	Reduce dose	Narcotic analgesics	Avoid—may precipitate coma
2.4 Beta-adrenoceptor blocking drugs			
Labetalol, Propranolol	Reduce oral dose	Paracetamol	Dose-related toxicity—avoid large doses
2.5 Antihypertensive drugs		*Antimigraine drugs*	
Methyldopa	Avoid—increased risk of hepatotoxicity	Ergotamine	Avoid in severe liver disease—the risk of toxicity may be increased
Sodium nitroprusside	Avoid in severe liver disease		
2.8 Anticoagulants, oral	Avoid, especially if prothrombin time is already prolonged	*4.8 Antiepileptics*	Phenobarbitone and primidone may precipitate coma. Phenytoin dose should be reduced to avoid toxicity. Sodium valproate should be avoided if possible—hepatotoxicity and liver failure may occasionally occur, usually within the first 6 months of treatment
2.12 Drugs used in hyperlipidaemia			
Bezafibrate, Clofibrate	Avoid in severe liver disease		
Cholestyramine	Interferes with absorption of fat-soluble vitamins and may aggravate the malabsorption associated with primary biliary cirrhosis		
3: Respiratory system		**5: Infections**	
Aminophylline	Reduce dose	*5.1 Antibacterial drugs*	
Antihistamines—see *4.6*		Chloramphenicol	Increased risk of bone-marrow depression—avoid
Antitussives	Avoid those containing opiates, e.g. codeine, pholcodine	Clindamycin	Reduce dose
		Erythromycin estolate	May cause idiosyncratic hepatotoxicity
4: Central nervous system		Fusidic acid	Impaired biliary excretion. May be increased risk of hepatotoxicity. Avoid or reduce dose
4.1 Hypnotics and sedatives *4.2 Antipsychotics*	All can precipitate coma. A small dose of lorazepam or oxazepam is probably the safest. The oral dose of chlormethiazole must		

Table: Drugs to be avoided or used with caution in liver disease (*continued*)

Drugs	Comment	Drugs	Comment
Isoniazid, Pyrazinamide	Idiosyncratic hepatotoxicity more common in patients with liver disease—avoid	**6.4 *Sex hormones*** Androgens and anabolic steroids (17α-alkyl derivatives)—Methyltestosterone, Oxymetholone, Stanozolol	Dose-related toxicity—avoid
Metronidazole	Reduce dose in decompensated liver disease	**6.5 *Hypothalamic hormones***	
Penicillins Bacampicillin, Pivampicillin, Talampicillin	Avoid in severe liver disease—potentially toxic products of hydrolysis of ester may accumulate	Clomiphene	Avoid in severe liver disease
		7: Obstetrics, gynaecology, and urinary-tract disorders	
Rifampicin	Impaired elimination. May be increased risk of hepatotoxicity. Avoid or reduce dose	Oral contraceptives	Increased risk in cholestatic liver disease and in patients with a history of pruritus or cholestasis during pregnancy—avoid
Tetracyclines	Dose-related toxicity by i/v route—avoid		
5.2 *Antifungal drugs*			
Ketoconazole	Induces a hepatitis-like reaction; may accumulate in hepatic failure. Avoid if possible	**8: Malignant disease and immunosuppression**	
		Doxorubicin	Reduce dose according to bilirubin concentration
5.5 *Anthelmintics* Niridazole	Increased CNS toxicity in patients with cirrhosis or portal-systemic shunts	Methotrexate	Dose-related toxicity—avoid in treatment of non-malignant conditions such as psoriasis
6: Endocrine system		**10: Musculoskeletal and joint disease**	
6.1 *Antidiabetic drugs*		Analgesics—see *4.7*	
Metformin	Avoid—increased risk of lactic acidosis	Dantrolene	Avoid in active or chronic liver disease—may cause severe liver damage
Sulphonylureas—Chlorpropamide, Tolbutamide	Avoid—increased risk of hypoglycaemia and can produce jaundice	Gold (sodium aurothiomalate)	Avoid in severe liver disease—hepatotoxicity may occur
6.3 *Corticosteroids*			
Prednisolone, Prednisone	Side-effects are more common. Prednisolone is preferable to prednisone which has to be converted to prednisolone by the liver before it is active	**13: Skin** Etretinate	Avoid—further impairment of liver function may occur

Prescribing in Renal Impairment

The use of drugs in patients with reduced renal function can give rise to problems for several reasons. Failure to excrete a drug or its metabolites may produce toxicity; sensitivity to some drugs is increased even if elimination is unimpaired; many side-effects are tolerated poorly by patients in renal failure; and some drugs cease to be effective when renal function is reduced. Many of these problems can be avoided by reducing the dose or by using alternative drugs.

Principles of dose adjustment in renal impairment

The level of renal function below which the dose of a drug must be reduced depends on whether the drug is eliminated entirely by renal excretion or is partly metabolised, and on how toxic it is.

For many drugs with only minor or no dose-related side-effects very precise modification of the dose regimen is unnecessary and a simple scheme for dose reduction is sufficient.

For more toxic drugs with a small safety margin dose schedules based on glomerular filtration rate should be used. For drugs where both efficacy and toxicity are closely related to plasma concentrations the recommended schedules should be seen only as a guide to initial treatment, and subsequent treatment must be adjusted according to the clinical response and the plasma concentration achieved.

The total daily maintenance dose of a drug can be reduced either by reducing the size of the individual doses or by increasing the interval between doses. For some drugs, if the size of the maintenance dose is reduced it will be important to give a loading dose if an immediate effect is required. This is because when a patient is given a regular dose of any drug it takes more than five times the half-life to achieve steady-state plasma concentrations. As the plasma half-life of drugs excreted by the kidney is prolonged in renal failure it may take many days for the reduced dosage to achieve a therapeutic plasma concentration. The loading dose should usually be the same size as the initial dose for a patient with normal renal function.

Nephrotoxic drugs should, if possible, be avoided in patients with renal disease because the consequences of nephrotoxicity are likely to be more serious when the renal reserve is already reduced.

Use of dosage table

Dose recommendations are based on the severity of renal impairment. This is expressed in terms of glomerular filtration rate (GFR), also known as the **creatinine clearance**. The serum-creatinine concentration can be used instead as a measure of renal function but is only a rough guide unless corrected for age, weight, and sex. Nomograms are available for making the correction and should be used where accuracy is important.

Renal impairment is arbitrarily divided into 3 grades:

Grade	GFR	Serum creatinine (approx.)
Mild	20–50 ml/min	150–300 μmol/litre
Moderate	10–20 ml/min	300–700 μmol/litre
Severe	< 10 ml/min	> 700 μmol/litre

Renal function declines with age, and many elderly patients have a glomerular filtration rate less than 50 ml/minute which may not be indicated by a change in serum creatinine. It is probably wise to assume at least mild impairment of renal function when prescribing for the elderly.

In the Table, drugs are listed under the same body systems as the chapters and only those which are known to require a reduction in dose, which are potentially harmful, or which are ineffective are mentioned. Nevertheless drug prescribing should be kept to the minimum in all patients with severe renal disease.

Renal function should be checked before prescribing any drug which requires dose modification even when renal impairment is mild.

Table: Drugs to be avoided or used with caution in renal impairment

Drugs	GFR ml/minute	Dosage recommendations	Comments
1: Gastro-intestinal system			
1.1 Antacids			
Gaviscon®	<10	Avoid	High sodium content
Magnesium carbonate, Magnesium trisilicate	<10	Avoid	Risk of magnesium toxicity. Magnesium carbonate mixture and magnesium trisilicate mixture also have high sodium content
Sodium bicarbonate	<10	Avoid	High sodium content
1.2 Antispasmodics and other drugs altering gut motility			
Colven®	<10	Avoid	High sodium content
Metoclopramide	<10	Avoid or use small dose	Increased risk of extrapyramidal reactions
1.3 Ulcer-healing drugs			
Carbenoxolone	<10	Avoid	Causes fluid retention
Cimetidine	10–20	400–600 mg daily	Occasional risk of confusional states
	<10	400 mg daily	
De-Nol®, De-Noltab®	<10	Avoid	
Ranitidine	<10	Use half normal dose	

Table: Drugs to be avoided or used with caution in renal impairment (*continued*)

Drugs	GFR ml/minute	Dosage recommendations	Comments
1.5 Treatment of chronic diarrhoeas			
Sulphasalazine	<10	Ensure high fluid intake	Rashes and blood dyscrasias. Crystalluria is a risk
1.6 Laxatives			
Fybogel®	<10	Avoid	High sodium content
2: Cardiovascular system			
2.1 Cardiac glycosides			
Digitoxin	<10	Max. 100 micrograms daily	Toxicity may be increased by electrolyte disturbances in severe renal impairment
Digoxin	20–50	250 micrograms daily	As digitoxin
	10–20	125–250 micrograms daily	
	<10	Up to 125 micrograms daily	
Medigoxin	<50	Reduce by similar amount as for digoxin	As digitoxin
2.2 Diuretics			
Aldosterone antagonists,	20–50	Monitor plasma K⁺	High risk of hyperkalaemia in renal impairment
Amiloride, Triamterene	<20	Avoid	
Bumetanide	<20	May need high doses	
Ethacrynic acid	<10	Avoid	Ototoxic
Frusemide	<20	May need high doses	Deafness may follow rapid i/v injection
Thiazides and related diuretics (except metolazone)	<20	Avoid	Ineffective (metolazone remains effective at low GFR)
2.3 Anti-arrhythmic drugs			
Disopyramide	20–50	100 mg every 8 hours *or* 150 mg every 12 hours	
	10–20	100 mg every 12 hours	
	<10	150 mg every 24 hours	
Flecainide, Tocainide	<50	Reduce dose	
Procainamide	<50	Avoid or reduce dose	
2.4 Beta-adrenoceptor blocking drugs			
Acebutolol	<10	Start with small dose	Active metabolite accumulates
Atenolol, Nadolol, Pindolol, Sotalol	<20	Reduce dose or use another beta-blocker	Excreted unchanged
Betaxolol	<10	Start with small dose	
Metoprolol, Propranolol	<10	Start with small dose	Higher plasma concentrations after oral administration. May reduce renal blood flow and adversely affect renal function in severe renal impairment
2.5 Antihypertensive drugs			
Bethanidine, Debrisoquine, Guanethidine	<20	Avoid	Increased postural hypotension and decrease in renal blood flow

Table: Drugs to be avoided or used with caution in renal impairment (*continued*)

Drugs	GFR ml/minute	Dosage recommendations	Comments
Captopril	20–50	Max. daily dose 150 mg	Increased risk of hyperkalaemia
	10–20	Max. daily dose 75 mg	
	<10	Max. daily dose 37·5 mg	
Diazoxide	<10	75–150 mg i/v	Increased sensitivity to hypotensive effect
Enalapril	20–50	Initial daily dose 10 mg	Increased risk of hyperkalaemia
	10–20	Initial daily dose 5 mg	
	<10	Initial daily dose 2·5 mg	
Hydralazine	<10	Start with small dose	Increased hypotensive effect
Methyldopa	<10	Start with small dose	Increased sensitivity to hypotensive effect
Prazosin	<10	Start with small dose	Increased sensitivity to hypotensive effect
Sodium nitroprusside	<20	Avoid prolonged use	
2.12 Drugs used in hyperlipidaemia			
Bezafibrate, Clofibrate	10–50	Reduce dose	Further deterioration in renal function; myopathy with clofibrate
	<10	Avoid	
4: Central nervous system			
4.1 Hypnotics and sedatives	<10	Start with small doses	Increased cerebral sensitivity
Amylobarbitone	<10	Reduce dose	Active metabolite accumulates
4.2 Antipsychotics	<10	Start with small doses	Increased cerebral sensitivity
Lithium	20–50	Avoid if possible or reduce dose and monitor carefully	
	<20	Avoid	
Sulpiride	<20	Avoid if possible, or reduce dose	
4.3 Antidepressants			
Nomifensine	<20	Avoid	Excreted by kidney
4.7 Analgesics			
Anti-inflammatory analgesics	<10	Avoid if possible	Fluid retention and deterioration in renal function
Aspirin	<10	Avoid	As above. Also increased risk of gastro-intestinal bleeding
Azapropazone, Sulindac	<20	Avoid	Excreted by kidney
Diflunisal	<10	Avoid	Excreted by kidney
Compound analgesics			
Solpadeine®, Solpadeine Forte®	<10	Avoid	High sodium content
Narcotic analgesics			
Codeine, Dihydrocodeine, Morphine	<20	Avoid	Increased and prolonged effect
Dextropropoxyphene, Pethidine	<10	Avoid	Increased CNS toxicity
Antimigraine drugs			
Ergotamine	<20	Avoid	Nausea and vomiting; risk of renal vasoconstriction

Table: Drugs to be avoided or used with caution in renal impairment (*continued*)

Drugs	GFR ml/minute	Dosage recommendations	Comments
4.8 Antiepileptics			
Phenobarbitone, Primidone	<10	Avoid large doses	
Sulthiame	<20	Avoid	Produces a metabolic acidosis
4.9 Drugs for parkinsonism			
Amantadine	<50	Avoid	
5: Infections			
5.1 Antibacterial drugs			
Aminoglycosides			
Amikacin, Gentamicin, Kanamycin, Netilmicin, Streptomycin, Tobramycin	<50	Reduce dose. Monitor plasma concentrations	Ototoxic and nephrotoxic
Neomycin	<50	Avoid	Ototoxic and nephrotoxic
Antituberculous drugs			
Capreomycin	<50	Reduce dose	Neurotoxic and ototoxic
Cycloserine	<50	Avoid	
Ethambutol	<50	Reduce dose	Optic nerve damage
Isoniazid	<10	Max. 200 mg daily	Peripheral neuropathy
Cephalosporins			
Cefadroxil	<20	Reduce dose	
Cefotaxime	<5	Use half dose	
Cefoxitin, Ceftazidime, Ceftizoxime, Cefuroxime, Cephamandole, Cephazolin, Cephradine	<50	Reduce dose	
Cefsulodin	<20	Reduce dose	
Cephalexin	<10	Max. 500 mg daily	
Cephaloridine, Cephalothin	<50	Avoid	Nephrotoxic
Latamoxef	<50	Reduce dose	
Penicillins			
Amoxycillin	<10	Reduce dose	Rashes more common
Ampicillin	<10	Reduce dose	Rashes more common
Azlocillin	<20	Reduce dose	
Bacampicillin, Pivampicillin, Talampicillin	<10	Avoid	Potentially toxic products of hydrolysis of ester may accumulate
Benzylpenicillin	<10	Max. 6 g daily	Neurotoxicity
Carbenicillin	<20	Reduce dose	Neurotoxic. May produce bleeding diathesis. 1 g contains 5.4 mmol sodium
Ciclacillin	<50	Reduce dose	
Mezlocillin	<10	Reduce dose	
Piperacillin	<20	Reduce dose	
Urinary antimicrobial drugs			
Cinoxacin	<20	Avoid	Nausea, rashes
Hexamine	<20	Avoid	Ineffective
Nalidixic acid	<20	Avoid	Increased risk of nausea, vomiting, rashes, photosensitivity
Nitrofurantoin	<50	Avoid	Peripheral neuropathy

Table: Drugs to be avoided or used with caution in renal impairment (*continued*)

Drugs	GFR ml/minute	Dosage recommendations	Comments
Other antibacterial drugs			
Chloramphenicol	<10	Avoid unless no alternative	Dose-related depression of haemopoiesis
Colistin sulphomethate sodium	<50	Reduce dose	Nephrotoxic and neuro-toxic
Co-trimoxazole	<10	Max. 960 mg daily	Rashes and blood dyscrasias
Lincomycin	<20	Use clindamycin instead	
Sulphadiazine	<10	Avoid	High risk of crystalluria
Other sulphonamides	<10	Ensure high fluid intake	Rashes and blood dyscrasias. Crystalluria is a risk
Tetracyclines (except doxycy-cline and minocycline)	<50	Avoid—use doxycy-cline or minocycline if necessary	Anti-anabolic effect, increased plasma urea, further deterioration in renal function
Trimethoprim	<10	Reduce dose	Possible deterioration in renal function
Vancomycin	<50	Avoid parenteral use if possible	Ototoxic and nephro-toxic
5.2 Antifungal drugs			
Amphotericin	<50	Use only if no alter-native	Nephrotoxic
Flucytosine	<50	Reduce dose	
5.3 Antiviral drugs			
Acyclovir	<50	Reduce dose	May produce transient increase in plasma urea
Inosine pranobex	<50	Avoid	Metabolised to uric acid
5.5 Anthelmintics			
Piperazine	<10	Reduce dose	Neurotoxic
6: Endocrine system			
6.1 Antidiabetic drugs			
Acetohexamide, Chlorpropamide	<50	Avoid	Tolbutamide and gliqui-done are suitable alter-natives
Other sulphonylureas	<10	May need dose reduction	Increased risk of pro-longed hypoglycaemia
Insulin	<10	May need dose reduction	Insulin requirements fall, and compensatory response to hypo-glycaemia is impaired
Metformin	<50	Avoid	Increased risk of lactic acidosis
6.2 Thyroid and antithyroid drugs			
Propylthiouracil	<50	Reduce dose	
6.6 Drugs affecting bone metabolism			
Disodium etidronate	20–50	Max. 5 mg/kg daily	Excreted by kidney
	<20	Avoid	
7: Obstetrics, gynaecology, and urinary-tract disorders			
Phenazopyridine	<50	Avoid	Crystalluria, methaemo-globinaemia
Potassium citrate	<20	Avoid	Risk of hyperkalaemia

Table: Drugs to be avoided or used with caution in renal impairment (*continued*)

Drugs	GFR ml/minute	Dosage recommendations	Comments
8: Malignant disease and immunosuppression			
Azathioprine	<10	Reduce dose	
Bleomycin, Cyclophosphamide, Melphalan, Mercaptopurine, Procarbazine, Thioguanine	<20	Reduce dose	
Cisplatin	<10	Avoid	Nephrotoxic
Methotrexate	20–50	Reduce dose	Accumulates. Also
	<20	Avoid	nephrotoxic
9: Nutrition and blood			
Potassium supplements	<20	Avoid routine use	High risk of hyperkalaemia
Sandocal®	<10	Avoid	High potassium content
10: Musculoskeletal and joint disease			
10.1 Drugs used in rheumatic disease Anti-inflammatory analgesics—see *4.7*			
Chloroquine	20–50	Max. 75 mg daily	Applies only to pro-
	10–20	Max. 50 mg daily	longed use
	<10	Avoid	
Gold (sodium aurothio-malate)	<50	Avoid	Nephrotoxic
Penicillamine	<50	Avoid if possible or reduce dose	Nephrotoxic
10.1 Drugs used in gout			
Allopurinol	10–20	Max. 200 mg daily	Increased toxicity;
	<10	Max. 100mg daily	rashes
Colchicine	<10	Avoid or reduce dose if no alternative	
Probenecid	<20	Avoid	Ineffective and toxicity increased
Sulphinpyrazone	<20	Avoid	Ineffective as a urico-suric
10.2 Drugs for musculoskeletal disorders			
Baclofen	<50	Use smaller doses	Excreted by kidney
11: Eye			
Acetazolamide	<10	Avoid	Causes metabolic acidosis
15: Anaesthetics			
Neuromuscular blocking drugs Gallamine	<20	Avoid	Prolonged paralysis
Alcuronium, Pancuronium, Tubocurarine	<20	Reduce dose	Large or repeated doses can produce prolonged paralysis

Prescribing in Pregnancy

Drugs can have harmful effects on the fetus at any time during pregnancy. During the *first trimester* they may produce congenital malformations (teratogenesis), and the period of greatest risk is from the third to the eleventh week of pregnancy. Few drugs have been shown conclusively to be teratogenic in man but no drug is safe beyond all doubt in early pregnancy. During the *second* and *third trimesters* drugs may affect the growth and functional development of the fetus or have toxic effects on fetal tissues; and drugs given shortly before term or during labour may have adverse effects on the neonate after delivery.

Drugs should be prescribed in pregnancy only if the expected benefit to the mother is thought to be greater than the risk to the fetus, and all drugs should be avoided if possible during the first trimester. Drugs which have been extensively used in pregnancy and appear to be usually safe should be prescribed in preference to new or untried drugs; and the smallest effective dose should be used.

The Table below lists drugs which may have harmful effects in pregnancy and indicates the trimester in which these effects occur.

Experience with many drugs in pregnancy is limited. The Table is based on human data and *animal* toxicological studies have been excluded. Therefore it should be noted that the absence of a drug from the list does not imply safety.

Table: Drugs to be avoided or used with caution in pregnancy

Drugs	Trimester of risk	Adverse effects
1: Gastro-intestinal system		
Chenodeoxycholic acid	1, 2, 3	Theoretical risk of effects on fetal metabolism
Stimulant laxatives	1, 2, 3	Best avoided during pregnancy as they may increase uterine activity in susceptible patients
Sulphasalazine	3	Theoretical risk of neonatal haemolysis and of kernicterus in jaundiced neonates
2: Cardiovascular system		
2.2 Diuretics	3	Reduce plasma volume and placental perfusion and should not be used to treat hypertension in pregnancy
Thiazides	3	May cause neonatal thrombocytopenia
2.3 Anti-arrhythmic drugs		
Amiodarone	2, 3	Releases iodine with possible risk of neonatal goitre. Use only if no effective alternative
2.4 Beta-adrenoceptor blocking drugs	3	Neonatal hypoglycaemia and bradycardia. The risk is greater in women with severe hypertension
2.5 Antihypertensive drugs		
Bethanidine, Debrisoquine, Guanethidine	3	Postural hypotension and reduced uteroplacental perfusion. Should not be used to treat hypertension in pregnancy
Captopril	1, 2, 3	May adversely affect fetal and neonatal blood pressure control and renal function
Diazoxide	2, 3	Prolonged use may produce alopecia and impaired glucose tolerance in the neonate. Inhibits uterine activity during labour
Reserpine	3	Neonatal bradycardia, drowsiness, and nasal stuffiness
2.6 Vasodilators		
Nifedipine	3	Calcium antagonists may inhibit labour
2.7 Vasoconstrictors		
Metaraminol, Noradrenaline, etc.	1, 2, 3	Avoid—may reduce placental perfusion
2.8 Anticoagulants		
Heparin	1, 2, 3	Osteoporosis has been reported after prolonged use
Oral anticoagulants	1, 2, 3	Congenital malformations. Fetal and neonatal haemorrhage. Subcutaneous heparin should be substituted in the last few weeks of pregnancy in deep-vein thrombosis
2.10 Fibrinolytic drugs		
Streptokinase, Urokinase	1, 2, 3	Possibility of premature separation of placenta in first 18 weeks. Theoretical possibility of fetal haemorrhage throughout pregnancy. Avoid postpartum use—maternal haemorrhage

Table: Drugs to be avoided or used with caution in pregnancy (*continued*)

Drugs	Trimester of risk	Adverse effects
2.11 Antifibrinolytic drugs		
Aminocaproic acid	1, 2, 3	Avoid—may increase the risk of thrombosis
2.12 Drugs used in hyperlipidaemia		
Clofibrate, Probucol	1, 2, 3	Avoid—theoretical possibility of interference with embryonic growth and development due to anticholesterol effect
3: Respiratory system		
Aminophylline	3	Neonatal irritability and apnoea have been reported
Iodides (in preparations for cough)	2, 3	Neonatal goitre and hypothyroidism
Selective beta-adrenoceptor stimulants (such as salbutamol)	3	Large parenteral doses given for asthma at term could delay the onset of labour
4: Central nervous system		
4.1 Hypnotics and sedatives	3	Depress neonatal respiration
Alcohol	1, 2 3	Teratogenic and may cause growth retardation. Withdrawal syndrome may occur in babies of alcoholic mothers
Barbiturates	3	Withdrawal effects in neonate
Benzodiazepines	3	Neonatal drowsiness, hypotonia, and withdrawal symptoms. Avoid large doses and regular use. Oxazepam and temazepam may be safer than longer-acting benzodiazepines
4.2 Antipsychotic drugs		
Lithium salts	1, 2, 3	Congenital malformations. Neonatal goitre has been reported. Lithium toxicity (hypotonia and cyanosis) in the neonate if maternal therapy poorly controlled. Maternal dose requirement increased during pregnancy
Phenothiazine derivatives	3	Extrapyramidal effects in neonate occasionally reported
4.3 Antidepressants		
Tricyclic antidepressants	3	Tachycardia, irritability, muscle spasms, and convulsions in the neonate reported occasionally
4.7 Analgesics *Anti-inflammatory analgesics*		
Aspirin	3	Impaired platelet function and risk of haemorrhage. Kernicterus in jaundiced neonates. With regular use of high doses, closure of fetal ductus arteriosus *in utero* and possibly persistent pulmonary hypertension of the newborn. Delayed onset and increased duration of labour with increased blood loss. Avoid if possible in last week of pregnancy
Indomethacin, Naproxen etc.	3	With regular use closure of fetal ductus arteriosus *in utero* and possibly persistent pulmonary hypertension of the newborn. Delayed onset and increased duration of labour
Narcotic analgesics Dextropropoxyphene, Diamorphine, Pentazocine etc.	3	Depress neonatal respiration. Withdrawal effects in neonates of dependent mothers. Gastric stasis and risk of inhalation pneumonia in mother during labour
Antimigraine drugs Ergotamine	1, 2, 3	Oxytocic effects on the pregnant uterus

Table: Drugs to be avoided or used with caution in pregnancy (*continued*)

Drugs	Trimester of risk	Adverse effects
4.8 Antiepileptics		Benefit of treatment outweighs risk to the fetus
Ethosuximide	1	May possibly be teratogenic
Phenytoin, Phenobarbitone	1, 3	Congenital malformations. Neonatal bleeding tendency— prophylactic vitamin K_1 should be given. Caution in interpreting maternal plasma phenytoin concentrations which may be reduced without a fall in the effective (free) phenytoin concentration
Sodium valproate	1	Increased risk of neural tube defects reported

5:   Infections
5.1 Antibacterial drugs

Drugs	Trimester of risk	Adverse effects
Aminoglycosides	2, 3	Auditory or vestibular nerve damage. Risk greatest with streptomycin and kanamycin; probably small with gentamicin and tobramycin
Chloramphenicol	3	Neonatal grey syndrome
Dapsone	3	Neonatal haemolysis and methaemoglobinaemia
Rifampicin	3	Risk of neonatal bleeding may be increased
Sulphonamides (and co-trimoxazole)	3	Neonatal haemolysis and methaemoglobinaemia. Increased risk of kernicterus in jaundiced neonates
Tetracyclines	2, 3	Dental discoloration. Maternal hepatotoxicity with large parenteral doses
Trimethoprim (and co-trimoxazole)	1	Possible teratogenic risk (folate antagonist)
5.2 Antifungals		
Flucytosine	1	Possible teratogenic risk
5.4 Antimalarials	1, 3	Benefit of prophylaxis and treatment in malaria outweighs risk
Primaquine	3	Neonatal haemolysis and methaemoglobinaemia
Pyrimethamine	1	Possible teratogenic risk (folate antagonist)
Quinine	1	High doses are teratogenic

6:   Endocrine system
6.1 Oral hypoglycaemic drugs

Drugs	Trimester of risk	Adverse effects
Sulphonylureas	3	Neonatal hypoglycaemia. Insulin is normally substituted in all diabetics. If oral drugs are used therapy should be stopped at least 2 days before delivery
6.2 Antithyroid drugs		
Carbimazole, Iodine, Propylthiouracil	2, 3	Neonatal goitre and hypothyroidism
Radioactive iodine	1, 2, 3	Permanent hypothyroidism—avoid
6.3 Corticosteroids	2, 3	High doses (>10 mg prednisolone daily) may produce fetal and neonatal adrenal suppression. Corticosteroid cover will be required by the mother during labour
6.4 Sex hormones		
Androgens, Oestrogens, Progestogens (high doses)	1, 2, 3	Virilisation of female fetus
Progestogens used to prevent abortion	1	May possibly be teratogenic
Stilboestrol	1	High doses associated with vaginal carcinoma in female offspring

Table: Drugs to be avoided or used with caution in pregnancy (*continued*)

Drugs	Trimester of risk	Adverse effects
6.7 *Other endocrine drugs*		
Danazol	1, 2, 3	Has weak androgenic effects and virilisation of female fetus has been reported
Trilostane	1, 2, 3	Interferes with placental sex hormone production
7: Obstetrics, gynaecology, and urinary-tract disorders		
Oral contraceptives	1	May possibly be a small risk of congenital malformations
8: Malignant disease and immunosuppression		
Cytotoxic drugs		
Alkylating drugs, Methotrexate	1	Teratogenic—high risk
Others	1	Teratogenic—lower risk
Immunosuppressants		
Azathioprine	1	The risk of teratogenicity appears to be small
9: Nutrition and blood		
Vitamin A	1	Excessive doses may possibly be teratogenic
Vitamin K		
Menadiol sodium diphosphate	3	Neonatal haemolysis. Increased risk of kernicterus in jaundiced neonates
10: Musculoskeletal and joint diseases		
Gold (sodium aurothiomalate)	1, 2, 3	No good evidence of harm but avoid if possible
Penicillamine	1, 2, 3	Fetal abnormalities have been reported rarely. Avoid if possible
13: Skin		
Etretinate	1, 2, 3	Teratogenic. Effective contraception must be continued for one year after stopping treatment
Isotretinoin	1, 2, 3	Teratogenic. Causes serious CNS malformations. Effective contraception must be continued for at least 4 weeks after stopping treatment
Podophyllum resin	1, 2, 3	Avoid application to large areas or in the treatment of anogenital warts. Neonatal death and teratogenesis have been reported
Povidone-iodine	2, 3	Sufficient iodine may be absorbed to affect the fetal thyroid
14: Vaccines		
Live vaccines	1	Theoretical risk of congenital malformations
15: Anaesthesia		
Inhalational and intravenous anaesthetics	3	Depress neonatal respiration
Local anaesthetics	3	With large doses, neonatal respiratory depression, hypotonia, and bradycardia after paracervical or epidural block
Prilocaine, Procaine	3	Neonatal methaemoglobinaemia
Neostigmine, Pyridostigmine etc.	3	Neonatal myasthenia with large doses
Treatment of alcoholism		
Disulfiram	1	It is possible that the high levels of acetaldehyde which occur in the presence of alcohol may be teratogenic

Prescribing during Breast-feeding

Administration of some drugs to nursing mothers may cause toxicity in the infant, for example diazepam, barbiturates, and ergotamine (see Table 1), whereas administration of other drugs, for example digoxin, has little effect on the neonate (see Table 2). For many drugs there is insufficient information available and it is advisable to administer only essential drugs to the mother during breast-feeding.

Toxicity to the infant can occur if the drug enters the milk in pharmacologically significant quantities. Milk concentrations of some drugs, for example iodides, may exceed those in the maternal plasma and cause toxicity to the infant but not the mother. Some drugs inhibit the infant's sucking reflex, for example phenobarbitone, or inhibit lactation, for example, bromocriptine and oestrogens. Drugs may, at least theoretically,

cause hypersensitivity in the infant even when concentrations are too low for a pharmacological effect.

Table 1 lists drugs which should be used with caution or which are contra-indicated in breast-feeding for the reasons given above.

Table 2 lists drugs which, on present evidence, may be given to the mother during breast-feeding, because they are excreted in milk in amounts which are too small to be harmful to the infant.

Table 3 lists drugs which are not known to be harmful to the infant although they are present in milk in significant amounts.

These Tables should be used only as a guide because of the inadequacy of currently available information on drugs in breast milk and absence from the Tables does not imply safety.

Table 1:   Drugs to be avoided or used with caution in breast-feeding

Drugs	Comments
1: Gastro-intestinal system	
Atropine	May possibly have anticholinergic effects in infants
Laxatives	
Anthraquinones	Avoid; large doses may cause increased gastric motility and diarrhoea, particularly cascara and danthron
Phenolphthalein	Avoid; increased gastric motility, diarrhoea, and possibly rashes
Sulphasalazine—see 5 (sulphonamides)	
2: Cardiovascular system	
Amiodarone	Avoid. Present in milk in significant amounts. Theoretical risk from release of iodine—see *6.2*
Beta-adrenoceptor blocking drugs	Monitor infant; possible toxicity due to beta-blockade but amount of most beta-blockers excreted in milk is too small to affect infant
Oral anticoagulants	Risk of haemorrhage; increased by vitamin-K deficiency. Warfarin appears safe but some authorities consider breast-feeding is contra-indicated during therapy. Phenindione should be avoided
3: Respiratory system	
Aminophylline	Irritability in infant has been reported
Clemastine	Drowsiness in infant has been reported
Cough mixtures containing iodides—see *6.2*	Use alternative cough mixtures
Ephedrine, Pseudoephedrine	Irritability and disturbed sleep reported with ephedrine. Significant amounts of pseudophedrine in milk
4: Central nervous system	
4.1 Hypnotics and sedatives	
Alcohol	Large amounts may affect infant
Barbiturates	Avoid if possible (see also *4.8*—phenobarbitone). Large doses may produce drowsiness
Benzodiazepines	Avoid repeated doses; lethargy and weight loss may occur in infant
Bromide salts	Avoid; sedation and rash in infant
Chloral hydrate, Dichloralphenazone	Sedation in infant
Meprobamate	Concentration in milk may exceed maternal plasma concentrations fourfold and may cause drowsiness in infant

Table 1:   Drugs to be avoided or used with caution in breast-feeding (*continued*)

Drugs	Comments
4.2 Antipsychotic drugs	
Haloperidol	Amount excreted in milk probably too small to be harmful
Lithium salts	Monitor infant for possible intoxication; low incidence of adverse effects but increased by continuous ingestion. Good control of maternal plasma concentrations minimises the risk
Phenothiazine derivatives	As for haloperidol, but drowsiness has been reported with chlorpromazine
4.7 Analgesics	
Narcotic analgesics	
Diamorphine, Morphine	Therapeutic doses are unlikely to affect infant. Withdrawal symptoms occur in infants of dependent mothers. Breast-feeding is no longer considered best method of treating dependence in offspring of dependent mothers and should be stopped
Methadone	Withdrawal symptoms in infant; breast-feeding permissible during maintenance dosage
Antimigraine drugs	
Ergotamine	Avoid where possible; ergotism may occur in infant. Repeated doses may inhibit lactation
4.8 Antiepileptics	
Phenobarbitone, Primidone	Avoid when possible; drowsiness may occur but risk probably small. One case of methaemoglobinaemia reported with phenobarbitone and phenytoin
5: Infections	
Chloramphenicol	Stop breast-feeding; may cause bone-marrow toxicity in infant. Concentration in milk usually insufficient to cause grey syndrome
Dapsone	Haemolytic anaemia. Risk to infant very small
Isoniazid	Monitor infant for possible toxicity; theoretical risk of convulsions and neuropathy. Prophylactic pyridoxine advisable in mother and infant
Metronidazole	May give a bitter taste to the milk
Nalidixic acid	Risk to infant very small but one case of haemolytic anaemia reported
Penicillins	Possibility of hypersensitivity in infant
Sulphonamides and co-trimoxazole	Monitor infant, especially in first few weeks of life. Small risk of kernicterus in jaundiced infants and, in G6PD-deficient infants, haemolytic anaemia, particularly with long-acting sulphonamides
Tetracyclines	Some authorities recommend avoidance but absorption and therefore discoloration of teeth in infant probably prevented by chelation with calcium in milk
6: Endocrine system	
6.1 Antidiabetic drugs	
Oral hypoglycaemic drugs	Caution; theoretical possibility of hypoglycaemia in infant
6.2 Antithyroid drugs	
Carbimazole, Iodine	Stop breast-feeding; danger of neonatal hypothyroidism or goitre. Iodine appears to be concentrated in the milk
Propylthiouracil	Monitor infant's thyroid status but amounts in milk probably too small to affect infant
Radioactive iodine	Breast-feeding contra-indicated after therapeutic doses. With diagnostic doses withhold breast-feeding for at least 24 hours
6.2 Thyroid hormones	
Liothyronine, Thyroxine	May interfere with neonatal screening for hypothyroidism

Table 1:   Drugs to be avoided or used with caution in breast-feeding (*continued*)

Drugs	Comments
6.3 *Corticosteroids*	Continuous therapy with high doses (>10 mg prednisolone daily) could possibly affect the infant's adrenal function—monitor carefully
6.4 *Sex hormones*	High doses of oestrogens, progestogens, and androgens suppress lactation—see also 7
Androgens	Avoid breast-feeding; may cause masculinisation in the female infant or precocious development in the male infant
Cyproterone	Caution; possibility of anti-androgen effects in neonate
6.7 *Other endocrine drugs* Bromocriptine	Suppresses lactation
7: Obstetrics, gynaecology, and urinary-tract disorders	
Oestrogen/progestogen contraceptives	Usually have little effect on milk flow. In some women, usually when lactation is not well established, suppression of milk flow may occur. Progestogen-only contraceptives do not appear to adversely affect established milk flow but may alter milk composition
Povidone-iodine	Iodine absorbed from vaginal preparations is concentrated in milk. Avoid
8: Malignant disease and immunosuppression	
Cytotoxics and immunosuppressants	Discontinue breast-feeding
Cyclosporin	Caution—excreted in milk
9: Nutrition and blood	
Calciferol (vitamin D)	Caution with high doses; may cause hypercalcaemia in infant
Thiamine	Severely thiamine-deficient mothers should avoid breast-feeding as the toxic methylglyoxal is excreted in milk
Vitamin A	Theoretical risk of toxicity in infants of mothers taking large doses
10: Musculoskeletal and joint diseases	
Carisoprodol	Concentrated in milk. No adverse effects reported but best avoided
Colchicine	Caution because of its cytotoxicity
Gold (sodium aurothiomalate)	Caution—excreted in milk. Theoretical possibility of rashes and idiosyncratic reactions
Phenylbutazone	Caution, theoretical possibility of blood dyscrasias in infant but amounts excreted in milk are very small
Salicylates	Occasional doses are safe (preferably taken after feeding) but caution with continuous therapy, as rashes and hypoprothrombinaemia (with inadequate neonatal vitamin K stores) may occur in infant
13: Skin Idoxuridine	May possibly make milk taste unpleasant

Table 2:   Drugs present in milk in amounts too small to be harmful

The list of drugs given below is not comprehensive and is based on current information concerning the use of these drugs in therapeutic dosage

Acetazolamide	Corticotrophin	Flupenthixol
Antidepressants, tricyclic	Cycloserine	Frusemide
Azathioprine	Dextropropoxyphene	Heparin
Baclofen	Diclofenac	Hyoscine
Captopril	Digoxin	Ibuprofen
Cephalosporins	Disopyramide	Insulin
Chlormethiazole	Domperidone	Labetalol
Chlorprothixene	Ethambutol	Loprazolam
Codeine	Fenbufen	Mebeverine

Table 2: Drugs present in milk in amounts too small to be harmful (*continued*)

Mefenamic acid	Phenytoin	Sodium valproate
Methyldopa	Pirenzepine	Suprofen
Metoclopramide	Piroxicam	Terbutaline
Mexiletine	Procainamide	Thiazides
Mianserin	Pyrazinamide	Tolmetin
Naproxen	Pyridostigmine	Verapamil
Nitrazepam	Rifampicin	Warfarin (see also Table 1)
Nomifensine		

Table 3: Drugs present in milk in significant amounts but not known to be harmful
The list of drugs given below is not comprehensive and is based on current information concerning the use of these drugs in therapeutic dosage

Antihistamines	Hydroxychloroquine	Ranitidine
Cimetidine	Minoxidil	Spironolactone
Erythromycin	Paracetamol	Trimethoprim
Ethamsylate	Pyrimethamine	
Ethosuximide	Quinidine	

Adverse Reactions to Drugs

Any drug may produce unwanted or unexpected adverse reactions. The detection and recording of these reactions is of vital importance, as has been shown for practolol and benoxaprofen.

Doctors are urged to help by reporting adverse reactions to The Medical Assessor, The Committee on Safety of Medicines, Market Towers, 1 Nine Elms Lane, London SW8 5NQ. Telephone: 01-720 2188. A supply of yellow prepaid postcards for reporting suspected adverse reactions is available from the above address. A 24-hour Freefone service is now available to all parts of the United Kingdom, for doctors seeking advice and information on adverse reactions. To use the service, the enquirer dials the operator and asks for 'Freefone Committee on Safety of Medicines'. Outside office hours a telephone-answering machine will take messages. When, on rare occasions, it is considered essential to report particularly serious and unexpected adverse reactions immediately, a doctor may use the Freefone service. Written confirmation will be requested, however, and this method does not supersede the normal system.

In addition to the national scheme there are some regional schemes for collecting data on adverse reactions.

Suspected adverse reactions to *any* therapeutic agent should be reported. This includes drugs, blood products, vaccines, X-ray contrast media, dental or surgical materials, intra-uterine contraceptive devices, absorbable sutures, and contact lens fluids.

Newer drugs

These are indicated by the sign ▼ in the BNF, MIMS, and ABPI Data Sheet Compendium. Doctors are asked to report any adverse or any unexpected event, however minor, which could conceivably be attributed to the drug. Reports should be made despite uncertainty in the doctor's mind about a causal relationship, irrespective of whether the reaction is well recognized, and even if other drugs have been given concurrently.

Established drugs

Doctors are asked to report any suspected adverse drug reaction which was potentially dangerous, incapacitating, or lethal; they should be reported even though the toxic effect is well recognised. Examples include anaphylaxis, blood dyscrasias, endocrine disturbances, effects on fertility, haemorrhage from any site, renal impairment, jaundice, ophthalmic disorders, severe CNS effects, severe skin reactions, reactions in pregnant women, and any drug interactions. Reports of serious adverse reactions are required to enable risk/benefit ratios to be compared with other drugs of a similar class. For established drugs doctors are asked not to report well-known, relatively minor side-effects, such as dry mouth with tricyclic antidepressants, constipation with opiates, or nausea with digoxin.

Special problems

Delayed drug effects. Doctors are reminded that some reactions (e.g. the development of cancers, chloroquine retinopathy, and retroperitoneal fibrosis) may become manifest months or years after drug exposure. Any suspicion of such an association should be reported.
Drugs in the elderly. Doctors are asked to be particularly alert to the possibility of adverse reactions when drugs are given to the elderly.
Congenital abnormalities. When an infant is born with a congenital abnormality or there is a malformed aborted fetus doctors are asked to consider the possibility that this might be an adverse reaction to a drug and to report all drugs (includ-

ing self-medication) taken by the mother during pregnancy.

Vaccines. Doctors are asked to report all suspected reactions to both new and established vaccines. The balance between risks and benefits from vaccines is liable to change and needs to be kept under continuous review.

Prevention of adverse reactions

1. Never use any drug unless there is a good indication. If the patient is pregnant do not use a drug unless the need for it is imperative.
2. It is very important to recognise allergy and idiosyncrasy as causes of adverse drug reactions. Ask the patient if he has had previous reactions.
3. Ask the patient if he is already taking other drugs *including self-medication* and remember that drug interactions may occur.
4. Remember that age, hepatic disease, or renal disease may alter the metabolism or excretion of drugs, so that they may need to be prescribed in much smaller doses than usual. Pharmacogenetic factors may also be responsible for variations in the rate of metabolism of drugs, notably isoniazid and the tricyclic antidepressants. Appropriate dose adjustments may be necessary to compensate for these variations.
5. Prescribe as few drugs as possible and give very clear instructions to the elderly or any patient likely to misunderstand complicated instructions.
6. When possible use a drug with which you are familiar. If you use a new drug be particularly alert for adverse reactions or unexpected events.
7. If serious adverse reactions are liable to occur warn the patient.

It is often wise to ask the patient to carry a card with information about his treatment, especially if it is to be long continued. Standard cards are available for oral anticoagulant treatment (section 2.8.2), monoamine-oxidase inhibitors (section 4.3.2), and corticosteroids (section 6.3.4).

Controlled Drugs and Drug Dependence

Prescriptions for controlled drugs

Preparations which are subject to the prescription requirements of the Misuse of Drugs Regulations 1973 are distinguished throughout the British National Formulary by the symbol CD (Controlled Drugs). The principal legal requirements relating to medical prescriptions are listed below.

Prescriptions ordering Controlled Drugs subject to prescription requirements must be *signed* and *dated*[1] by the prescriber and give his *address*. The prescription must always state *in the prescriber's own handwriting* (unless the prescriber has been specially exempted from this requirement) in ink or otherwise so as to be indelible:
1. The name and address of the patient
2. In the case of a preparation, the form and where appropriate the strength of the preparation
3. The total quantity of the drug or preparation, or the number of dose units, *in both words and figures*
4. The dose

A prescription may order a Controlled Drug to be dispensed by instalments; the amount of the instalments and the intervals to be observed must be specified.[2] 'Repeat' prescriptions are **not** permitted.

It is an offence for a doctor to issue an incomplete prescription and a pharmacist is **not** allowed to dispense a Controlled Drug unless all the information required by law is given on the prescription. Failure to comply with the regulations concerning the writing of prescriptions will result in inconvenience to patients and delay in supplying the necessary medicine.

Drug dependence related to misuse of drugs

The prevalence of drug dependence and misuse in Great Britain, particularly amongst young people, continues to give cause for concern to teachers, social workers, and the police, as well as doctors.

The most serious drugs of addiction are **diamorphine** (heroin), **morphine**, and the **synthetic narcotics.** The likelihood that the dose will be increased is considerable, psychic dependence is common, and the withdrawal syndrome may be severe.

Dependence on **amphetamine** is less serious and now less common than it used to be. It has been shown that the incidence of dependence and misuse of the amphetamines was related to the extent to which they were prescribed. As a result of the campaign run by doctors with the intention of reducing the prescribing of amphetamines, their use has fallen very markedly and many combination products containing amphetamines have been withdrawn from the market.

The principal **barbiturates** are now Controlled Drugs (class B), but phenobarbitone and phenobarbitone sodium are exempt from the handwriting requirement, and because of their use in

---

1. A prescription is valid for 13 weeks from the date stated thereon
2. A special form, FP10HP(ad), in Scotland HBP(A), is available to certain doctors in the National Health Service for prescribing cocaine, dextromoramide, diamorphine, dipipanone, methadone, morphine, or pethidine by instalments. Forms FP10 and FP10HP, in Scotland GP10 and HBP, are valid for supply on only **one** occasion

epilepsy are available under the emergency supply regulations (p. 5).

Cannabis (Indian hemp) has no approved medicinal use and cannot be prescribed by doctors (except under licence from the Home Secretary). Its use is illegal but has become widespread in certain sections of society. Cannabis is a mild hallucinogen. It is seldom accompanied by a desire to increase the dose and withdrawal symptoms are unusual. **Lysergide** (lysergic acid diethylamide, LSD) is a much more potent hallucinogen. Its use can lead to severe psychotic states in which life may be at risk.

The Misuse of Drugs Act, 1971

This Act was passed in 1971 to provide more flexible and more comprehensive control over the misuse of drugs of all kinds than was possible under the earlier Dangerous Drugs Act. The Act prohibits certain activities in relation to 'Controlled Drugs', in particular their manufacture, supply, and possession. The penalties applicable to offences involving the different drugs are graded broadly according to the *harmfulness attributable to a drug when it is misused* and for this purpose the drugs are defined in the following three classes:

Class A includes: alfentanil, cocaine, dextromoramide, diamorphine (heroin), dipipanone, lysergide (LSD), methadone, morphine, opium, pethidine, phencyclidine, and class B substances when prepared for injection

Class B includes: oral amphetamines, barbiturates, cannabis, cannabis resin, codeine, ethylmorphine, phenmetrazine, and pholcodine

Class C includes: certain drugs related to the amphetamines such as benzphetamine and chlorphentermine, diethylpropion, and pipradrol

The Misuse of Drugs Regulations 1973 define the classes of person who are authorised to supply and possess controlled drugs while acting in their professional capacities and lay down the conditions under which these activities may be carried out. In the regulations drugs are divided into four schedules each specifying the requirements governing such activities as import, export, production, supply, possession, prescribing, and record keeping which apply to them.

Notification of Addicts

The Misuse of Drugs (Notification of and Supply to Addicts) Regulations 1973 require that a medical practitioner must notify in writing the Chief Medical Officer, Drugs Branch, Queen Anne's Gate, London SW1H 9AT of any person he considers, or has reasonable grounds to suspect, is addicted to any of the following substances:

Cocaine	Hydromorphone
Dextromoramide	Levorphanol
Diamorphine	Methadone
Dipipanone	Morphine
Hydrocodone	Opium

Oxycodone	Phenazocine
Pethidine	

Dipipanone is only legally available as Diconal® Tablets. These have been much misused by opiate addicts in recent years; only medical practitioners with a special licence may now prescribe them for addicts to treat addiction. Doctors and others should be suspicious of young people who ask for them, especially as temporary residents.

Particulars to be notified to the Chief Medical Officer are:

Name and address
Sex
Date of birth
National Health Service number
Date of first attendance
Name or names of drug or drugs to which the patient is or is suspected of being addicted
Whether or not the medical practitioner making the notification is prescribing for the patient

Written notification must be made within seven days of first becoming aware that the patient may be an addict and only the particulars of which the practitioner has knowledge need be notified immediately; the remainder may be notified at a later date. Notification should be confirmed annually in writing if the patient is still being treated by the practitioner. Notified information is incorporated in an Index which is maintained in the Home Office and any doctor may refer to this Index for information about a person under his care; in fact, it is good medical practice to check all new cases of addiction or suspected addiction with the Index before prescribing or supplying controlled drugs since this is a safeguard against addicts obtaining supplies simultaneously from two or more doctors. Enquiries can be made either in writing to the Chief Medical Officer or, preferably, by telephone 01-213 5141 (surnames A–F), 01-213 4274 (G–L), 01-213 6083 (M–P and S), 01-213 7352 (Q–R, T–Z). To keep notified information confidential, such enquiries are normally answered by means of a return telephone call. The reply will come from lay staff who are not qualified to give guidance on the clinical handling of cases.

The preceding paragraph applies only to medical practitioners in England, Scotland, and Wales. In Northern Ireland notification should be sent to the Chief Medical Officer, Department of Health and Social Services, Dundonald House, Belfast BT4 3SF, and any enquiries about the Northern Ireland Regulations or addicts should be made to that Department, also at Dundonald House, telephone number 0232 63939 extension 2874.

Prescribing of diamorphine (heroin), dipipanone, and cocaine for addicts

The Misuse of Drugs (Notification of and Supply to Addicts) Regulations also provide that only medical practitioners who hold a special licence issued by the Home Secretary may prescribe diamorphine, dipipanone (Diconal®), or cocaine for addicts; other practitioners must refer any addict who requires these drugs to a treatment centre. General practitioners and other doctors may still prescribe diamorphine and cocaine for patients (including addicts) for relief of pain due to organic disease or injury without a special licence. Whenever possible the addict will be introduced by a member of staff from the treatment centre to a pharmacist whose agreement has been obtained and whose pharmacy is conveniently sited for the patient. Prescriptions for weekly supplies will be sent to the pharmacy by post and will be dispensed on a daily basis as indicated by the doctor. If any alterations of the arrangements are requested by the addict, the pharmacist **must** contact the treatment centre to ensure that such alteration is acceptable.

Prescribing drugs likely to cause dependence or misuse

The prescriber has three main responsibilities. The first is to see that he does not create dependence by introducing drugs to patients without sufficient reason. In this context, the proper use of the morphine-like drugs is well understood. The dangers of other controlled drugs are less clear because recognition of dependence is not easy and its effects, and those of withdrawal, are less obvious. Consequently, divergent views are held. Perhaps the most notable result of uninhibited prescribing is that there is a very large number of patients in the country taking tablets which do them neither much good nor much harm, but who are committed to them indefinitely because they cannot readily be stopped.

The second is to see that the patient does not gradually increase the dose of a drug, given for good medical reasons, to the point where dependence becomes more likely. This tendency is seen especially with the barbiturates and also with other hypnotics and tranquillisers, including the benzodiazepines. The prescriber should keep a close eye on the amount he prescribes to prevent patients from accumulating stocks that would enable them to arrange their own dosage or even that of their families and friends. A minimal amount should be prescribed in the first instance, or when seeing a new patient for the first time.

The third is for the prescriber to see that he is not being used as an unwitting source of supply for addicts. This manoeuvre is often attempted by addicts to narcotic analgesics and they may be very skilled, plausible, and persistent in attaining their ends.

The methods include visiting more than one doctor, fabricating stories to substantiate demands, and forging prescriptions. A doctor should therefore be wary of prescribing for strangers and he may be able to get information about suspected opiate addicts from the Drugs Branch of the Home Office or in Northern Ireland from the Drugs Branch, Department of Health and Social Services (see above).

Patients under temporary care should be given only small supplies of drugs unless they present an unequivocal letter from their own doctors. Doctors should remember that their own patients may be doing a collecting round with other doctors, especially in hospitals. It is sensible to decrease dosages steadily or to issue weekly or even daily prescriptions for small amounts if it is apparent that dependence is occurring.

The stealing and misuse of prescription forms could be minimised by the following precautions:
(a) lock up prescription pads whenever possible and avoid leaving them unattended if called away from the consulting room;
(b) draw a diagonal line across the blank part of the form under the prescription;
(c) write the quantity in words and figures when prescribing drugs prone to abuse; this is obligatory for controlled drugs (see Prescriptions for Controlled Drugs, above);
(d) alterations are best avoided but if any are made they should be clear and unambiguous; add initials against altered items;
(e) if prescriptions are left for collection they should be left in a safe place in a sealed envelope.

Preparations used in the treatment of drug dependence

CD **Methadone Mixture 1 mg /ml,** methadone hydrochloride 1 mg/ml (see Formulary). Price 100 ml = **C.** Used in replacement and maintenance treatment
Note: this preparation is 2½ times the strength of methadone linctus

Preparations used in the treatment of alcoholism

Disulfiram (Antabuse®) is used as an adjunct to the treatment of alcoholism. It gives rise to extremely unpleasant systemic reactions after the ingestion of even small amounts of alcohol because it leads to accumulation of acetaldehyde in the body. Reactions include flushing of the face, throbbing headache, palpitations, tachycardia, nausea, vomiting, and, with large doses of alcohol, arrhythmias, hypotension, and collapse. Even the small amounts of alcohol included in many oral medicines may be sufficient to precipitate a reaction. It may be advisable for patients to carry a card warning of the danger of administration of alcohol. For drug interactions of disulfiram see Appendix 1 (sections *2.8B, 4.1, 4.3, 4.8, 5.1*).

For use of chlormethiazole in withdrawal treatment see section 4.1.1 and for use of benzodiazepines see section 4.1.2.

PoM **Antabuse 200®** (CP)
Tablets, scored, disulfiram 200 mg. Price 20 tabs = **F.** Label: 2
Dose: 800 mg on the first day, reducing over 5 days to 100–200 mg daily

Emergency Treatment of Poisoning

These notes deal with the management of acute poisoning when first seen in the home and although brief mention is given to certain aspects of hospital-based treatment, it is recommended that the reader refers to other sources for further information. The notes are divided into the following subsections.

General measures
1 Respiratory function
2 Hypotension
3 Hypothermia
4 Arrhythmias
5 Convulsions
6 Removal of poison from the stomach
7 Oral adsorbents
8 Active elimination techniques
9 Hospital admission
Notes on some common poisons
10 Amphetamine and related drugs
11 Aspirin and other Salicylates
12 Barbiturates and other Sedatives
13 Iron salts
14 Lithium salts
15 Morphine and other Narcotic Analgesics
16 Non-steroidal anti-inflammatory drugs
17 Paracetamol
18 Co-proxamol (Dextropropoxyphene and Paracetamol)
19 Phenothiazine derivatives
20 Theophylline and related drugs
21 Tricyclic and related Antidepressants
22 Carbon Monoxide
23 Sulphur Dioxide, Chlorine, Phosgene, Ammonia
24 Snake and Insect Bites
25 Paraquat
26 Organophosphorus insecticides
27 Antidotes to other poisons

General measures

1.   Respiratory function

Respiration is often impaired in unconscious patients. An obstructed airway requires immediate attention. Pull the tongue forward, remove dentures and oral secretions, hold the jaw forward, insert an oropharyngeal airway if one is available, and turn the patient semiprone. The risk of inhaling vomit is minimised with the patient positioned semiprone and head down.

Most poisons that impair consciousness also depress respiration. Assisted ventilation by mouth to mouth or Ambu bag inflation may be needed according to circumstances. Oxygen is not a substitute for adequate ventilation, though it should be given in the highest concentration possible in poisoning with carbon monoxide and irritant gases.

Respiratory stimulants do not help and are **potentially dangerous**.

2.   Hypotension

Hypotension is most common in severe barbiturate poisoning. A systolic blood pressure of less than 80 mmHg may lead to irreversible brain damage or renal tubular necrosis. The patient should be carried head downwards on a stretcher and nursed in this position in the ambulance. Oxygen should be given to correct hypoxia and an intravenous infusion should be set up if at all practicable. Vasopressor drugs should **not** be used.

Fluid depletion without hypotension is common after prolonged coma and after aspirin poisoning on account of vomiting, sweating, and hyperpnoea.

3.   Hypothermia

Hypothermia may develop in patients of any age who have been deeply unconscious for some hours particularly following barbiturates or phenothiazines. It may be missed unless temperature is measured rectally using a low-reading rectal thermometer. It is best treated by wrapping the patient in blankets to conserve his own heat. Hot-water bottles are of little value and may cause burns.

4.   Arrhythmias

Cardiac conduction defects and arrhythmias may occur in acute poisoning, notably with tricyclic antidepressants. Arrhythmias often respond to correction of underlying hypoxia or acidosis. Ventricular arrhythmias that have been confirmed by emergency electrocardiography and which are causing serious hypotension may require treatment with lignocaine hydrochloride 50–100 mg intravenously. Supraventricular arrhythmias are seldom immediately life-threatening and drug treatment is best withheld until the patient reaches hospital.

5.   Convulsions

Single short-lived convulsions do not require treatment. Diazepam, up to 10 mg by slow intravenous injection, preferably in emulsion form, should be given if convulsions are protracted or recur frequently; it should not be given intramuscularly.

6.   Removal of poison from the stomach

The dangers of attempting to empty the stomach have to be balanced against the toxicity of the ingested poison, as assessed by the quantity ingested, the severity of poisoning likely to result, and the time that has elapsed since ingestion. Gastric emptying is clearly unnecessary if the risk of toxicity is small or the patient presents too late. Emptying the stomach by **gastric lavage** or **emesis** is of doubtful value if attempted more than 4 hours after ingestion. However, a worthwhile recovery of salicylates can be achieved up to 24 hours after ingestion and of tricyclic antidepressants (which delay gastric emptying) up to 8 hours after ingestion. The chief danger of gastric aspiration and lavage is inhalation of stomach contents, and it should **not** be attempted in drowsy or comatose patients unless there is a good enough cough reflex or the airway can be protected by a cuffed endotracheal tube. Stomach tubes should **not** be passed after corrosive poisoning.

Petroleum products are more dangerous in the lungs than in the stomach and therefore removal from the stomach is **not** advised because of the risk of inhalation.

On balance gastric lavage is seldom practical or desirable before the patient reaches hospital.

Emesis induced by using **ipecacuanha** (Paediatric Ipecacuanha Emetic Mixture, equivalent in strength to ipecacuanha syrup USP or Adelaide Children's Hospital formula) is favoured in children and is also effective in adults. It may be given safely in the home providing that the patient is fully conscious and that the poison ingested is neither a corrosive nor a petroleum distillate.

Salt solutions, copper sulphate, apomorphine, and mustard are dangerous and should **not** be used.

Ipecacuanha Emetic Mixture, Paediatric, total alkaloids (as emetine) 14 mg/10 ml (see Formulary). Price 100 ml = **C**
Dose: ADULT 30 ml; CHILD 6–18 months 10 ml, older children 15 ml; the dose is followed by a tumblerful of water and repeated after 20 minutes if necessary

7. Oral adsorbents

Absorption of some poisons from the gut may be reduced by adsorption on to other substances taken by mouth. **Activated charcoal** is safe and is particularly useful for the prevention of absorption of poisons which are toxic in small amounts, e.g. antidepressants. It may also be useful in treating poisoning by phenobarbitone and phenytoin. The usual adult dose is 50 g in water, repeated at intervals. An effervescent formulation is available.

CHARCOAL, ACTIVATED
(Charcoal)
Indications; Dose: see notes above

Charcoal Powder. Price 50 g = **C**
Carbomix® (Penn)
Powder, charcoal. Price 50-g bottle = **H**. Label: 13
Medicoal® (Lundbeck)
Granules, effervescent, charcoal 5 g/sachet. Price 10 sachets = **G**. Label: 13
Dose: as for activated charcoal (above)

8. Active elimination techniques

Techniques which are intended to enhance the elimination of poisons that have already been absorbed are only practicable in hospital. They are suitable for only a small number of patients who are severely poisoned with a limited number of poisons. Examples include:

Forced alkaline diuresis for salicylates and phenobarbitone
Haemodialysis for salicylates, phenobarbitone, methyl alcohol (methanol), ethylene glycol, and lithium
Charcoal haemoperfusion for medium- and short-acting barbiturates, meprobamate, glutethimide, ethchlorvynol, and methaqualone

9. Hospital admission

Hospital admission is generally advisable for all patients who show symptoms of poisoning. Patients who appear well should also be referred if they have taken poisons with delayed actions such as salicylates, iron, paracetamol, tricyclic antidepressants, paraquat, and diphenoxylate with atropine, or sustained-release capsules or tablets. A note should be sent of what is known and what treatment has been given.

The identity of the poison and the size of the dose is often impossible to establish with certainty. Fortunately this is not usually important because there are few poisonings for which there are specific antidotes, e.g. narcotic analgesics and iron, and few patients require active removal of the drug. All others are dealt with by treating the clinical state as it presents. Nevertheless, knowledge of the type of poisoning does help in anticipating the course of events. Patients' reports may be little help, as they are confused or can only say they have taken an undefined amount, possibly of mixed drugs. Parents may think a child has taken something which might be poisonous and may exaggerate or underplay the risks out of anxiety or guilt. Sometimes symptoms are due to an illness such as appendicitis. Accidents may arise from a large number of domestic and industrial products the contents of which are not generally known. Information can be obtained from the poisons information services at the following telephone numbers.

National Poisons Information Service

Belfast	0232 240503
Cardiff	0222 569200
Dublin	0001 745588
Edinburgh	031-229 2477
	031-228 2441
	(Viewdata)
London	01-635 9191
	or 01-407 7600

Other Centres

Birmingham	021-554 3801
Leeds	0532 430715
	or 0532 432799
Newcastle	0632 325131

Laboratory analysis may help in the diagnosis and management of a small number of cases. Information on the available services can be obtained from the National Poisons Information Service in London.

C = 51-100p, **D** = 101-180p, **E** = 181-300p, **F** = 301-450p, **G** = 451-650p, **H** = 651-900p, **I** = 901-1200p, **J** = over 1200p.

Notes on some common poisons

10.   Amphetamine and related drugs

These cause wakefulness, excessive activity, paranoia, hallucinations, and hypertension followed by exhaustion, convulsions, hyperthermia, and coma. The early stages can be controlled by chlorpromazine or beta-adrenoceptor blocking drugs. Later, tepid sponging, anticonvulsants, and artificial respiration may be needed. Amphetamine excretion can be increased by forced acid diuresis.

11.   Aspirin and other Salicylates

Absorption of aspirin and other salicylates may be delayed, especially if enteric-coated tablets have been taken. The chief features of poisoning are hyperventilation, tinnitus, deafness, vasodilatation, and sweating. Coma is uncommon but indicates very severe poisoning. The associated acid-base disturbances are complex and determine the distribution of salicylates to tissues. Gastric aspiration and lavage should be performed in all cases. Treatment must be in hospital where plasma salicylate, pH, and electrolytes can be measured. Fluid losses are replaced and forced alkaline diuresis should be considered when the plasma-salicylate concentration is greater than 50 mg/100 ml (500 mg/litre) in adults or 30 mg/100 ml (300 mg/litre) in children.

12.   Barbiturates and other Sedatives

These cause drowsiness, coma, respiratory depression, hypotension, and hypothermia. The duration and depth of cerebral depression vary greatly with the drug, the dose, and the tolerance of the patient. The severity of poisoning is often greater with a large dose of barbiturate hypnotics than with the longer-acting phenobarbitone. The majority of patients survive with supportive measures alone. Forced alkaline diuresis may be considered in severe phenobarbitone poisoning. Charcoal haemoperfusion is the treatment of choice for the small minority of patients with very severe barbiturate poisoning who fail to improve, or who deteriorate despite good supportive care.

Benzodiazepines taken alone cause drowsiness, ataxia, dysarthria, and occasionally minor and short-lived depression of consciousness. They potentiate the effects of other central nervous system depressants taken concomitantly.

13.   Iron salts

Iron poisoning is commonest in childhood and is usually accidental. The symptoms are nausea, vomiting, abdominal pain, diarrhoea, haematemesis, and rectal bleeding. Hypotension, coma, and hepatocellular necrosis occur later. Mortality is reduced with intensive and specific therapy. The effective antidote is **desferrioxamine**, which chelates iron. The stomach should be emptied at once, preferably by inducing vomiting, as this is

quickest. Gastric lavage in hospital should follow as soon as possible, using desferrioxamine mesylate solution 2 g in 1 litre of water. A solution of 10 g of desferrioxamine mesylate in 50 ml water should be left in the stomach. Absorbed iron can also be chelated by an intramuscular injection of 2 g of desferrioxamine mesylate in 10 ml of water.

DESFERRIOXAMINE MESYLATE

Indications: removal of iron from the body in poisoning

Side-effects: pain at site of intramuscular injection, anaphylactic reactions, and hypotension when given too rapidly by intravenous injection

Dose: by mouth after gastric lavage, 5–10 g in 50–100 ml of liquid

By intramuscular injection, 1–2 g in 10–20 ml of water for injections every 3–12 hours

By continuous intravenous infusion, up to 15 mg/kg/hour with a max. in 24 hours of 80 mg/kg

PoM **Desferal**® (Ciba)

Injection, powder for reconstitution, desferrioxamine mesylate. Price 500-mg vial = **D**

14.   Lithium salts

Most cases of lithium intoxication occur as a complication of long-term therapy and are caused by reduced excretion of the drug due to a variety of factors including deterioration of renal function, infections, dehydration, and co-administration of diuretics. Acute deliberate overdoses may also occur with delayed onset of symptoms (12 hours or more) due to slow entry of lithium into the tissues and continuing absorption from sustained-release formulations.

The early clinical features are non-specific and may include apathy and restlessness which could be confused with mental changes due to the patient's depressive illness. Vomiting, diarrhoea, ataxia, weakness, dysarthria, muscle twitching, and tremor may follow. Severe poisoning is associated with convulsions, coma, renal failure, electrolyte imbalance, and hypotension.

Therapeutic lithium concentrations are within the range of 0.6–1.2 mmol/litre. Higher concentrations are likely to cause toxicity. Plasma lithium concentrations in excess of 2.2–2.5 mmol/litre are usually associated with serious toxicity and such cases may need treatment with forced diuresis or dialysis (if there is renal failure). Otherwise treatment is supportive with special regard to electrolyte balance, renal function, and control of convulsions.

15.   Morphine and other Narcotic Analgesics

These cause varying degrees of coma, reduction of the respiratory rate, and pinpoint pupils. The specific antidote naloxone is indicated if there is coma or bradypnoea. **Naloxone** is short-acting and 0.8–2 mg is given subcutaneously, intramuscularly, or intravenously, and repeated as required according to the respiratory rate and depth of

---

Relative prices: **A** = up to 20p, **B** = 21-50p,

coma. Alternatively, it may be given by continuous intravenous infusion, the rate of administration being adjusted according to response.

NALOXONE HYDROCHLORIDE

Indications: overdosage with morphine-like compounds

Cautions: physical dependence on narcotics

Dose: by subcutaneous, intramuscular, or intravenous injection, 0.8–2 mg repeated at intervals of 2–3 minutes to a max. of 10 mg if respiratory function does not improve; CHILD 10 micrograms/kg

By continuous intravenous infusion, 2 mg diluted in 500 ml intravenous infusion solution at a rate adjusted to the response

PoM **Narcan**® (Du Pont)
Injection, naloxone hydrochloride 400 micrograms/ml. Price 1-ml amp = G

16. Non-steroidal anti-inflammatory drugs

Mefenamic acid is the most common member of this group encountered in overdosage. Convulsions are the only important feature of toxicity and should be managed as indicated above.

Ibuprofen may cause nausea, vomiting, and tinnitus, but more serious toxicity is very uncommon. Gastric lavage is indicated if more than 10 tablets have been ingested within the preceding 4 hours, followed by symptomatic measures.

17. Paracetamol

As little as 10–15 g of paracetamol may cause severe hepatocellular necrosis and, less frequently, renal tubular necrosis. Nausea and vomiting, the only early features of poisoning, usually settle within 24 hours. Persistence beyond this time, often associated with the onset of right subcostal pain and tenderness, usually indicates the development of hepatic necrosis. Liver damage is maximal 3–4 days after ingestion and may lead to encephalopathy, haemorrhage, hypoglycaemia, cerebral oedema, and death.

Antidotes such as **acetylcysteine** and **methionine** protect the liver if given within 10–12 hours of ingestion. Patients at risk of liver damage and therefore requiring treatment can be identified from a single measurement of the plasma-paracetamol concentration related to the time from ingestion, provided the time interval is not less than 4 hours. Those whose concentrations are above a line joining plots of 200 mg/litre at 4 hours and 30 mg/litre at 15 hours on a semilogarithmic graph should be given an antidote. The patient should be referred to hospital urgently.

In remote geographic areas emesis should be induced if the patient presents within 4 hours of ingestion of the tablets, and methionine (2.5 g) should be given by mouth once vomiting has occurred. It will seldom be practicable to give acetylcysteine outside hospital. The need for continuation of treatment can be decided from the plasma-paracetamol concentration related to the time interval since ingestion, once the patient reaches hospital.

ACETYLCYSTEINE

Indications: paracetamol overdosage

Side-effects: bronchoconstriction, rashes

Dose: by intravenous infusion, initially 150 mg/kg in 200 ml glucose intravenous infusion 5% over 15 minutes, followed by 50 mg/kg in 500 ml glucose intravenous infusion 5% over 4 hours and 100 mg/kg in 1000 ml glucose intravenous infusion 5% over 16 hours

PoM **Parvolex**® (DF)
Injection, acetylcysteine 200 mg/ml. Price 10-ml amp = E

METHIONINE

Indications: paracetamol overdosage

Dose: by mouth, 2.5 g initially, followed by 3 further doses of 2.5 g every 4 hours depending on the plasma-paracetamol concentration

Methionine Tablets, methionine 250 mg. Price 20 tabs = C

18. Co-proxamol (Dextropropoxyphene and Paracetamol)

Combinations of dextropropoxyphene and paracetamol (in Distalgesic® etc.) are frequently taken in overdosage. The initial features are those of acute narcotic overdosage with coma, respiratory depression, and pinpoint pupils. Patients may die of acute cardiovascular collapse before reaching hospital (particularly if alcohol has also been consumed) unless adequately resuscitated or given **naloxone** as antidote to the dextropropoxyphene. Paracetamol hepatotoxicity may develop later and should be anticipated and treated as indicated above.

19. Phenothiazine derivatives

Phenothiazine derivatives cause less depression of consciousness and respiration than other sedatives. Hypotension, hypothermia, sinus tachycardia, and arrhythmias (particularly with thioridazine) may complicate poisoning. Dystonic reactions can occur with therapeutic doses, (particularly with prochlorperazine and trifluoperazine) and convulsions may occur in severe cases. Drugs to control arrhythmias and convulsions may be needed. Dystonic reactions are rapidly abolished by injection of orphenadrine hydrochloride or procyclidine hydrochloride (see section 4.9.2).

20. Theophylline and related drugs

Theophylline and related drugs are often prescribed as sustained-release formulations and toxicity may therefore be delayed. They cause vomiting (which may be severe and intractable), agitation, restlessness, dilated pupils, and sinus tachycardia. More serious effects are haematemesis, convulsions, and supraventricular and

---

C = 51-100p, **D** = 101-180p, **E** = 181-300p, **F** = 301-450p, **G** = 451-650p, **H** = 651-900p, **I** = 901-1200p, **J** = over 1200p.

ventricular arrhythmias. Profound hypokalaemia may develop rapidly.

The stomach should be emptied as early as possible and hypokalaemia corrected by intravenous infusion of potassium chloride (up to 60 mmol/hour in sodium chloride 0.9% or glucose 5% solutions). Convulsions should be controlled by intravenous administration of diazepam (see above). Sedation with chlorpromazine or diazepam may be necessary in agitated patients. In non-asthmatic patients extreme tachycardia, hypokalaemia, and hyperglycaemia may be reversed by intravenous administration of propranolol.

21. Tricyclic and related Antidepressants

Tricyclic and related antidepressants cause dry mouth, coma of varying degree, hypotension, hypothermia, hyperreflexia, extensor plantar responses, convulsions, respiratory failure, cardiac conduction defects, and arrhythmias. Dilated pupils and urinary retention also occur. Metabolic acidosis may complicate severe poisoning, and delirium with confusion, agitation, and visual and auditory hallucinations, are common during recovery.

Hospital admission is strongly advised and supportive measures to ensure a patent airway and adequate ventilation during transfer are mandatory. Diazepam may be required for control of convulsions (see above). Although arrhythmias are worrying, the use of anti-arrhythmic drugs is best avoided. Diazepam given by mouth is usually adequate to sedate delirious patients but large doses may be required. Symptomatic treatment and activated charcoal by mouth may reasonably be given in the home before transfer.

22. Carbon Monoxide

Carbon monoxide poisoning is now usually due to inhalation of smoke, car exhaust, or fumes caused by blocked flues or incomplete combustion of fuel gases in confined spaces. Its toxic effects are entirely due to hypoxia.

Immediate treatment is essential. The person should be removed into the fresh air, the airway cleared, and artificial ventilation given. **Oxygen** 100% should be administered as soon as available. Artificial respiration should be given as necessary and continued until adequate spontaneous breathing starts, or stopped only after persistent and efficient treatment of cardiac arrest has failed. Admission to hospital is desirable because complications may arise after a delay of hours or days. Cerebral oedema should be anticipated in severe poisoning and should be treated with an intravenous infusion of mannitol (see section 2.2.5) and intramuscular injections of dexamethasone, 4 mg every 6 hours (see section 6.3.4).

23. Sulphur Dioxide, Chlorine, Phosgene, Ammonia

The immediate effect of all except phosgene is coughing and choking. Pulmonary oedema, with severe breathlessness and cyanosis may develop suddenly up to 36 hours after exposure. Death may occur. Patients should be kept under observation and those who develop pulmonary oedema should be given corticosteroids and oxygen. Assisted ventilation may be necessary in the most serious cases.

24. Snake and Insect Bites

SNAKE BITE. Acute poisoning due to venomous snakes is extremely rare in the United Kingdom and the only indigenous venomous snake is the adder. The bite may cause local and systemic effects. The local effects include pain and swelling. Systemic effects include agitation, restlessness, abdominal colic, diarrhoea, and vomiting. Death is unlikely except in the case of a very weak debilitated person who receives a large amount of venom.

Only patients with persistent or recurrent hypotension, polymorphonuclear leucocytosis, electrocardiographic abnormalities, or extensive limb swelling within 4 hours of the bite should be given antivenom. Two ampoules of Zagreb antivenom (the dose is the same for adults and children) diluted with 2–3 volumes of sodium chloride intravenous infusion 0.9% are given intravenously and repeated in 1–2 hours if there is no clinical improvement. Adrenaline injection should be immediately to hand for treatment of serum hypersensitivity reactions.

For slight or moderate poisoning (local pain and swelling, possibly vomiting and diarrhoea), symptomatic treatment only is required. The site should be cleaned, covered with a dry dressing, and immobilised. Antibiotics and antitetanus immunoglobulin are of no value. An antihistamine may be given by injection for its sedative effects.

Antivenom is available for certain foreign snakes. Information is available from poisons information centres (see subsection 9 above).

INSECT BITES. Stings from ants, wasps, bees, and hornets cause local pain and swelling but seldom cause severe toxicity. If the bite is in the mouth or on the tongue marked swelling may cause respiratory distress. The stings from these insects are usually treated by cleansing the area, applying a cooling lotion (such as a calamine preparation), and giving an antihistamine by mouth. Bee stings should be removed by scraping them off with a finger nail or knife before cleansing the area. Anaphylactic reactions require treatment with **adrenaline**. Inhalation of adrenaline (1–3 puffs of Medihaler-epi®, see section 3.1.1.2) is sufficient for mild attacks and is convenient for patients at risk to carry. A dose of 0.5 ml of adrenaline injection 1 in 1000 should be given subcutaneously for moderate reactions and intramuscularly in more severe cases (see section 3.4.3).

25. Paraquat

Gramoxone®, the liquid paraquat formulation

which is available only to farmers and horticulturists, contains 20% paraquat and is extremely toxic. The granular preparations available for garden use contain only 2.5% of paraquat. There have been few deaths following ingestion of the granular material but poisoning with the concentrated liquid is much more serious.

Paraquat has local and systemic effects. Splashes in the eyes irritate and ulcerate the cornea and conjunctiva. Copious washing of the eye and instillation of antibacterial eye-drops, should aid healing but it may be a long process. Skin irritation, blistering, and ulceration can occur from contact both with the concentrated and dilute forms. Inhalation of spray, mist, or dust containing paraquat may cause nose bleeding and sore throat.

Ingestion of concentrated paraquat solutions is followed by nausea, vomiting, and diarrhoea. Painful ulceration of the tongue, lips, and fauces may appear after 36–48 hours together with renal failure. Some days later there may be dyspnoea with pulmonary fibrosis due to proliferative alveolitis and bronchiolitis.

Treatment should be started immediately. The single most useful measure is to give **Fuller's earth** or **bentonite** orally to adsorb paraquat and reduce absorption. The stomach should then be emptied by careful gastric lavage and 300 ml of a suspension containing 30 g of Fuller's earth and 5 g of magnesium sulphate in each 100 ml of water left in the stomach. Further quantities of 300 ml of a 30% Fuller's earth suspension should be given after 2 and 4 hours and magnesium sulphate or mannitol given as required to produce diarrhoea and empty the gut. Intravenous fluids and analgesics as necessary are also required. Oxygen therapy should be avoided if possible since this may exacerbate damage to the lungs. Measures to enhance elimination of absorbed paraquat are probably valueless but should be discussed with the Poisons Information Services.

A simple qualitative urine test will confirm paraquat absorption. The likely outcome of poisoning may be predicted from the plasma-paraquat concentrations related to the time since ingestion. This can be arranged through the National Poisons Information Service (see subsection 9 above).

26. Organophosphorus insecticides

Organophosphorus insecticides are usually supplied as powders or dissolved in hydrocarbon solvents. All are absorbed through the bronchi and intact skin as well as through the gut and act by inhibiting cholinesterase at nerve endings and ganglia, as well as in the brain. However there is considerable variation in toxicity between different organophosphorus compounds. The onset of toxic features may be delayed after skin exposure.

Anxiety, restlessness, dizziness, headache, miosis, nausea, hypersalivation, vomiting, abdominal colic, diarrhoea, bradycardia, and sweating are common. Muscle weakness and fasci-

culation may develop and progress to generalised flaccid paralysis including the ocular and respiratory muscles. Convulsions, coma, pulmonary oedema with copious bronchial secretions, hypoxia, and arrhythmias occur in severe cases. Hyperglycaemia and glycosuria without ketonuria may also be present.

Further absorption should be prevented by emptying the stomach, removing the patient to fresh air, or removing soiled clothing and washing contaminated skin as appropriate. In severe poisoning it is vital to ensure a clear airway, frequent removal of bronchial secretions, and adequate ventilation and oxygenation. **Atropine** reverses the muscarinic effects of cholinesterase inhibitors. The dose is 2 mg as atropine sulphate injection (intramuscularly or intravenously according to the severity of poisoning) every 20 to 30 minutes until the skin becomes flushed and dry, the pupils dilate, and a tachycardia develops.

Pralidoxime mesylate (P2S), a cholinesterase reactivator, is indicated in moderate or severe poisoning but is only effective if given within 24 hours. It may be obtained from designated centres, the names of which are held by the National Poisons Information Service (see subsection 9 above). A dose of 1 g by slow intravenous infusion should produce improvement in muscle power within 30 minutes but repeated doses or, in severe cases, an intravenous infusion of up to 500 mg/hour may be required.

27. Antidotes to other poisons

A number of antidotes other than those mentioned above are available i.e. for **cyanides** (dicobalt edetate, or alternatively sodium nitrite and thiosulphate) and for **heavy metals** (dimercaprol, disodium edetate, penicillamine).

DICOBALT EDETATE

Indications: acute poisoning with cyanides
Cautions: toxic in absence of cyanides
Side-effects: transient hypotension, tachycardia, and vomiting
Dose: by intravenous injection, 300 mg (20 ml) over 1 minute, followed by 50 ml of glucose intravenous infusion 50%, both repeated once or twice if necessary

PoM **Kelocyanor®** (Lipha)
Injection, dicobalt edetate 300 mg/20 ml. Price 20-ml amp = E

DIMERCAPROL
(BAL)
Indications: poisoning by antimony, arsenic, bismuth, gold, mercury, thallium
Side-effects: hypertension, tachycardia, malaise, nausea, vomiting, lachrymation, sweating, burning sensation, constriction of throat and chest, muscle spasm; rarely serious in normal dosage; pyrexia in children
Dose: by intramuscular injection, 2.5–3 mg/kg every 4 hours for 2 days, 2–4 times on the 3rd

day, then 1–2 times daily for 10 days or until recovery

PoM **Dimercaprol Injection,** dimercaprol 50 mg/ ml. Price 2-ml amp = **B**

PENICILLAMINE
Indications: poisoning, particularly by copper and lead
Cautions; Contra-indications; Side-effects: see section 10.1.3
Dose: 0.5–2 g daily; CHILD 20 mg/kg daily, in divided doses

Preparations
See section 10.1.3

SODIUM CALCIUMEDETATE
Indications: poisoning by heavy metals, especially lead
Cautions: impaired renal function
Side-effects: nausea, cramp; in overdosage renal damage
Dose: by intravenous infusion, adults and children, up to 40 mg/kg twice daily in sodium chloride intravenous infusion 0.9% or glucose intravenous infusion 5% for up to 5 days, repeated if necessary after 48 hours

PoM **Ledclair**® (Sinclair)
Injection, sodium calciumedetate 200 mg/ml. Price 5-ml amp = **E**
Cream, sodium calciumedetate 10%. Price 50 g = **E**; 100 g = **G**. For lesions and skin sensitivity due to contact with heavy metals

SODIUM NITRITE
Indications: poisoning with cyanides
Side-effects: flushing and headache due to vasodilatation

PoM **Sodium Nitrite Injection,** sodium nitrite 3% (30 mg/ml) in water for injections
Dose: 10 ml by intravenous injection over 3 minutes, followed by 25 ml of sodium thiosulphate injection 50%, given over 10 minutes

SODIUM THIOSULPHATE
Indications: poisoning with cyanides

PoM **Sodium Thiosulphate Injection,** sodium thiosulphate 50% (500 mg/ml) in water for injections
Dose: see above under Sodium Nitrite Injection

Classified Notes on Drugs and Preparations

1: Drugs acting on the
GASTRO-INTESTINAL SYSTEM

The drugs and preparations in this chapter are described under the following sections:

1.1 Antacids
1.2 Antispasmodics and other drugs altering gut motility
1.3 Ulcer-healing drugs
1.4 Antidiarrhoeal drugs
1.5 Treatment of chronic diarrhoeas
1.6 Laxatives
1.7 Rectal and colonic drugs
1.8 Stoma care
1.9 Drugs affecting intestinal secretions

For antibacterial prophylaxis in abdominal surgery see section 5.1, Table 2.

1.1 Antacids

1.1.1 Official antacids and simple proprietaries
1.1.2 Compound proprietary antacids and proprietary complexes
1.1.3 Calcium- and bismuth-containing antacids

Antacids are still useful for treating gastro-intestinal disease; they can often relieve symptoms in both ulcer and non-ulcer dyspepsia, and in reflux oesophagitis. They are best given when symptoms occur or are expected, usually between meals and at bedtime, four or more times daily; additional doses may be required up to once an hour. High doses of magnesium- or aluminium-containing antacids, such as 200 to 300 ml of aluminium hydroxide mixture daily, to give a neutralising capacity of about 150 to 1000 mmol daily, will promote duodenal ulcer healing, but possibly less well than antisecretory agents (section 1.3); proof of a relationship between healing and neutralising capacity is lacking. Liquid preparations are more effective than solids.

Magnesium- and aluminium-containing antacids, such as magnesium carbonate, hydroxide and trisilicate, and aluminium glycinate and hydroxide, being relatively insoluble in water, are long-acting if retained in the stomach. They are suitable for most antacid purposes, and aluminium-containing antacids are also used as phosphate-binding agents in renal impairment. Magnesium-containing antacids tend to be laxative whereas aluminium-containing antacids may be constipating.

Sodium bicarbonate, being soluble in water, is rapid-acting, but absorbed bicarbonate can cause alkalosis in excessive doses. Like other carbonate-containing antacids it liberates carbon dioxide which causes belching. Sodium bicarbonate and antacid preparations with a high sodium content, such as magnesium trisilicate mixture, should be avoided in patients on salt-restricted diets (in heart failure, hepatic and renal impairment, and during pregnancy).

Bismuth-containing antacids (section 1.1.3) are best avoided because absorbed bismuth can be neurotoxic, causing encephalopathy; they tend to be constipating. Calcium-containing antacids (section 1.1.3) should be avoided since they can induce rebound acid hypersecretion, and absorbed calcium can cause hypercalcaemia and precipitate the milk-alkali syndrome; they also cause alkalosis on prolonged use.

Antacids should not be taken at the same time as other drugs as they may impair their absorption. Antacids may also damage enteric coatings designed to prevent dissolution in the stomach. Drug interactions: see Appendix 1 (sections *1*, *2.3*, *4.2*, *4.7*, *5.1*, *5.2*, *10*).

LABELS. If additional advisory labelling is indicated for antacids guidance is given in the dosage statement.

1.1.1 Official antacids and simple proprietaries

ALUMINIUM HYDROXIDE
Indications: dyspepsia; hyperphosphataemia
Cautions: see notes above
Aluminium Hydroxide Tablets, dried aluminium hydroxide 500 mg (low Na⁺). Price 20 tabs = **B**
Dose: 1–2 tablets chewed when required
Aluminium Hydroxide Mixture (gel), about 4% w/w Al_2O_3 in water (low Na⁺). Diluent water for preparations, life of diluted mixture 14 days. Price 100 ml = **A**
Dose: 5–15 ml when required
Alu-Cap® (Riker)
Capsules, green/red, dried aluminium hydroxide 475 mg (low Na⁺). Price 20 caps = **C**
Dose: hyperphosphataemia, 4–20 capsules daily; dyspepsia, 1 capsule 4 times daily and at bedtime
NHS **Aludrox®** (Wyeth)
Gel, aluminium hydroxide mixture (see above). Price 100 ml = **A**

MAGNESIUM SALTS (ANTACID)
Indications: dyspepsia
Cautions: renal impairment; see also notes above. Drug interactions: see Appendix 1 (sections *9*, *15*)
Side-effects: diarrhoea; carbonate—belching due to liberated carbon dioxide
Magaldrate Suspension (= mixture), magaldrate 800 mg/5 ml. Low Na⁺. Price 100 ml = **C**
Dose: 5–10 ml when required
Magnesium Carbonate Mixture (see Formulary). Contains about 9 mmol Na⁺/10 ml. Price 200 ml = **B**
Dose: 10–20 ml when required
Magnesium Carbonate Mixture, Aromatic, (see Formulary). Contains about 6 mmol Na⁺/10 ml. Price 200 ml = **B**
Dose: 10–20 ml when required

Magnesium Hydroxide Mixture, magnesium oxide (hydrated) about 550 mg/10 ml (low Na$^+$). Do not store in a cold place. Price 100 ml = **A**
Dose: 5–10 ml when required
Magnesium Trisilicate Tablets, Compound, magnesium trisilicate 250 mg, dried aluminium hydroxide 120 mg (low Na$^+$). Price 20 tabs = **A**
Dose: 1–2 tablets chewed when required
Magnesium Trisilicate Mixture (see Formulary). Contains about 6 mmol Na$^+$/10 ml. Price 200 ml = **A**
Dose: 10–20 ml when required
Magnesium Trisilicate (powder). (Low Na$^+$). Price 20 g = **A.** Label: 13
Dose: 0.5–2 g in liquid when required
Magnesium Trisilicate Oral Powder, Compound, magnesium trisilicate 250 mg, chalk 250 mg, heavy magnesium carbonate 250 mg, sodium bicarbonate 250 mg/g. Contains about 3 mmol Na$^+$/g. Price 20 g = **A.** Label: 13
Dose: 1–5 g in liquid when required

SODIUM BICARBONATE

Indications: rapid relief of dyspepsia
Cautions: renal impairment; patients on a sodium-restricted diet; avoid prolonged use. Drug interactions: see Appendix 1 (section *4.2*)
Side-effects: belching due to liberated carbon dioxide and, with prolonged use, alkalosis
Dose: 1–5 g in water when required

Sodium Bicarbonate (powder). Price 50 g = **A.** Label: 13
Sodium Bicarbonate Mixture, Paediatric (see Formulary). Price 100 ml = **A**
Dose: CHILD up to 1 year 5 ml, 1–5 years 10 ml
Sodium Bicarbonate Tablets, Compound (Soda Mint Tablets), sodium bicarbonate 300 mg. Contains about 4 mmol Na$^+$/tab. Price 20 tabs = **A**
Dose: 2–6 tablets sucked when required

1.1.2 Compound proprietary antacids and proprietary complexes

Compound proprietary preparations have no clear advantages over simpler preparations: neutralising capacity may be the same. Those containing readily dissociated complexes, such as alexitol sodium, almasilate, and hydrotalcite, are not especially useful. Dimethicone added as an antifoaming agent to relieve flatulence is of uncertain value. Alginates added as protectants against reflux oesophagitis in Gastrocote®, Gaviscon® and Topal® may be useful, but the antacid content of all three is relatively low; Gastrocote® and Gaviscon® both contain sodium as the bicarbonate. Surface anaesthetics (oxethazaine in Mucaine®) may be included in antacids to relieve the discomfort in oesophagitis but they are of doubtful efficacy. For preparations containing an antispasmodic with an antacid see section 1.2.1.

NHS **Actal®** (Winthrop)
Tablets, alexitol sodium 360 mg. Low Na$^+$. Price 20 tabs = **B**

Dose: 1–2 tablets chewed or sucked when required
Suspension (= mixture), alexitol sodium 360 mg/5 ml. Diluent syrup, life of diluted mixture 14 days. Low Na$^+$. Price 100 ml = **B**
Dose: 5–10 ml when required
Actonorm® (Wallace Mfg)
Gel (= mixture), dried aluminium hydroxide 220 mg, activated dimethicone 25 mg, magnesium hydroxide 200 mg/5 ml. Price 100 ml = **C**
Dose: 5–20 ml when required
NHS **Altacaps®** (Roussel)
Capsules, activated dimethicone 125 mg, hydrotalcite 500 mg. Price 20 caps = **D**
Dose: 2 capsules sucked or chewed between meals and at bedtime
NHS **Altacite®** (Roussel)
Tablets, hydrotalcite 500 mg. Low Na$^+$. Price 20 tabs = **C**
Dose: 2 tablets chewed when required; CHILD 6–12 years 1 tablet
Suspension (= mixture), hydrotalcite 500 mg/5 ml. Low Na$^+$. Do not dilute. Price 100 ml = **D**
Dose: 10 ml when required; CHILD 6–12 years 5 ml
NHS **Altacite Plus®** (Roussel)
Tablets, activated dimethicone 250 mg, hydrotalcite 500 mg. Low Na$^+$. Price 20 tabs = **D**
Dose: 2 tablets chewed when required; CHILD 8–12 years 1 tablet
Suspension (= mixture), activated dimethicone 125 mg, hydrotalcite 500 mg/5 ml. Low Na$^+$. Do not dilute. Price 100 ml = **D**
Dose: 10 ml when required; CHILD 8–12 years 5 ml
NHS **Aludrox®** (Wyeth)
Tablets, aluminium hydroxide-magnesium carbonate co-dried gel 282 mg, magnesium hydroxide 85 mg. Low Na$^+$. Price 20 tabs = **B**
Dose: 2 tablets chewed when required
NHS **Andursil®** (Ciba Consumer)
Tablets, aluminium hydroxide-magnesium carbonate co-dried gel 750 mg, activated dimethicone 250 mg. Contains about 1 mmol Na$^+$/tablet. Price 20 tabs = **C**
Dose: 1–2 tablets when required
Suspension (= mixture), Al$_2$O$_3$ 200 mg (as aluminium hydroxide mixture), magnesium hydroxide 200 mg, aluminium hydroxide-magnesium carbonate co-dried gel 200 mg, activated dimethicone 150 mg/5 ml. Low Na$^+$. Do not dilute. Price 100 ml = **B**
Dose: 5–10 ml when required
NHS **Antasil®** (Stuart)
Tablets, dried aluminium hydroxide 400 mg, activated dimethicone 250 mg, magnesium hydroxide 400 mg. Low Na$^+$. Price 20 tabs = **C**
Dose: 1–2 tablets chewed or sucked when required
Liquid (= mixture), dried aluminium hydroxide 400 mg, activated dimethicone 150 mg, magnesium hydroxide 400 mg/5 ml. Low Na$^+$. Price 100 ml = **C**
Dose: 5–30 ml when required

NHS **Asilone®** (Berk)

Tablets or *Orange Tablets*, dried aluminium hydroxide 500 mg, activated dimethicone 270 mg. Low Na⁺. Price 20 tabs (both) = **C**
Dose: 1–2 tablets chewed or sucked when required
Gel and *Suspension* (=mixture), dried aluminium hydroxide 420 mg, activated dimethicone 135 mg, light magnesium oxide 70 mg/5 ml. Low Na⁺. Diluent purified water, freshly boiled and cooled, life of diluted mixture 14 days. Price 100 ml (both) = **C**
Dose: 5–10 ml when required

NHS **Asilone for Infants®** (Berk)

Paediatric mixture, dried aluminium hydroxide 84 mg, activated dimethicone 27 mg, light magnesium oxide 14 mg/5 ml. Diluent as above. Price 100 ml = **D**
Dose: CHILD 1–3 months 2.5 ml, over 3 months 5 ml when required, before or with feeds

NHS **Dijex®** (Crookes Products)

Tablets, pink, aluminium hydroxide-magnesium carbonate co-dried gel 400 mg. Price 20 tabs = **B**
Dose: 1–2 tablets chewed 2–4 hourly
Liquid (=mixture), aluminium hydroxide mixture 98%, magnesium hydroxide 1.7%. Price 100 ml = **B**
Dose: 5–10 ml 2–4 hourly

NHS **Diovol®** (Pharmax)

Tablets, white/yellow, aluminium hydroxide-magnesium carbonate co-dried gel 300 mg, dimethicone 25 mg, magnesium hydroxide 100 mg. Low Na⁺. Price 20 tabs = **B**
Dose: 1–2 tablets chewed or sucked when required; CHILD 6–12 years ½–1 tablet
Suspension (=mixture), white (mint-flavoured) or yellow (fruit-flavoured), aluminium hydroxide 200 mg, dimethicone 25 mg, magnesium hydroxide 200 mg/5 ml. Low Na⁺. Diluent water for preparations, life of diluted mixture 14 days. Price 100 ml (both) = **B**
Dose: 10–20 ml when required; CHILD 6–12 years 5–10 ml

NHS **Droxalin®** (Sterling Health)

Tablets, alexitol sodium 200 mg, magnesium trisilicate 162 mg. Low Na⁺. Price 20 tabs = **B**
Dose: 1–2 or more tablets chewed when required

NHS **Dynese®** (Galen)

Suspension (=mixture), magaldrate 800 mg/5 ml. Low Na⁺. Price 100 ml = **C**
Dose: 5–10 ml when required; CHILD 6–12 years 2.5–5 ml

NHS **Gastrils®** (Jackson)

Pastilles, green (mint-flavoured) or yellow (fruit-flavoured), s/c, aluminium hydroxide-magnesium carbonate co-dried gel 500 mg. Price 90 g (22) = **B**
Dose: 1–2 pastilles sucked when required; CHILD 1 pastille 3 times daily

Gastrocote® (MCP)

Tablets, alginic acid 200 mg, dried aluminium hydroxide 80 mg, magnesium trisilicate 40 mg, sodium bicarbonate 70 mg. Contains about 1 mmol Na⁺/tablet. Price 20 tabs = **C**

Dose: 1–3 tablets chewed when required. Not recommended for children under 6 years

Gaviscon® (R&C)

Tablets, alginic acid 500 mg, dried aluminium hydroxide 100 mg, magnesium trisilicate 25 mg, sodium bicarbonate 170 mg, with mannitol and sucrose. Contains 2 mmol Na⁺/tablet. Price 20 tabs = **C**
Dose: 1–2 tablets chewed when required and followed by liquid; CHILD 1 tablet

NHS **Granules**, brown, alginic acid 481 mg, dried aluminium hydroxide 208 mg, magnesium trisilicate 52 mg, sodium alginate 521 mg, sodium bicarbonate 177 mg, with sucrose/5-g sachet. Contains about 5 mmol Na⁺/sachet. Price 10 sachets = **D**
Dose: 1 sachet chewed when required and followed by liquid; CHILD ½ sachet (1 level 5-ml spoonful)

Liquid (=mixture), pink, sodium alginate 250 mg, sodium bicarbonate 133.5 mg, with saccharin/5 ml. Contains about 3 mmol Na⁺/5 ml. Price 100 ml = **C**
Dose: 10–20 ml when required; CHILD 5–10 ml

Infant Gaviscon® (R&C)

Oral powder, alginic acid 924 mg, dried aluminium hydroxide 200 mg, magnesium trisilicate 50 mg, sodium bicarbonate 340 mg, with mannitol and colloidal silica/2-g sachet. Contains 4 mmol Na⁺/sachet. Price 10 sachets = **D**
Dose: INFANT ½–1 sachet mixed with feeds when required; CHILD 1 sachet after food

Gelusil® (Warner)

NHS *Tablets*, dried aluminium hydroxide 250 mg, magnesium trisilicate 500 mg. Low Na⁺. Price 20 tabs = **A**
Dose: 1–2 tablets chewed or sucked when required; CHILD half adult dose
Suspension (=mixture), dried aluminium hydroxide 310 mg, magnesium trisilicate 620 mg/5 ml. Diluent water for preparations, life of diluted mixture 28 days. Price 100 ml = **C**
Dose: 5–20 ml with water when required; CHILD 6–12 years half adult dose

Maalox® (Rorer)

NHS *Tablets*, dried aluminium hydroxide 400 mg, magnesium hydroxide 400 mg. Low Na⁺. Price 20 tabs = **C**
Dose: 1–2 tablets chewed when required
Suspension (=mixture), dried aluminium hydroxide 220 mg, magnesium hydroxide 195 mg/5 ml. Low Na⁺. Price 100 ml = **C**; 20 × 10-ml sachets = **D**
Dose: 10–20 ml when required

Maalox Concentrate® (Rorer)

Tablets, dried aluminium hydroxide 600 mg, magnesium hydroxide 300 mg. Low Na⁺. Price 20 tabs = **C**
Dose: 1–2 tablets chewed when required
NHS *Suspension* (=mixture), dried aluminium hydroxide 600 mg, magnesium hydroxide 300 mg/5 ml. Low Na⁺. Price 100 ml = **C**; 20 × 10-ml sachets = **E**
Dose: 5–10 ml when required

NHS Maalox Plus® (Rorer)
Tablets, white/yellow, dried aluminium hydroxide 200 mg, activated dimethicone 25 mg, magnesium hydroxide 200 mg. Low Na⁺. Price 20 tabs = **C**
Dose: 2–4 tablets chewed when required
Suspension (= mixture), dried aluminium hydroxide 220 mg, activated dimethicone 25 mg, magnesium hydroxide 195 mg/5 ml. Low Na⁺. Price 100 ml = **C**
Dose: 10–20 ml when required

NHS Malinal® (Robins)
Tablets, scored, almasilate 500 mg. Low Na⁺. Price 20 tabs = **C**
Dose: 2 tablets chewed when required
Suspension (= mixture), almasilate 500 mg/5 ml. Low Na⁺. Price 100 ml = **C**
Dose: 10 ml when required

PoM Mucaine® (Wyeth)
Suspension (= mixture), aluminium hydroxide mixture 4.75 ml, magnesium hydroxide 100 mg, oxethazaine 10 mg/5 ml. Diluent water for preparations, life of diluted mixture 14 days. Price 100 ml = **A**. Label: 22, see dose
Dose: 5–10 ml (without fluid) 3–4 times daily 15 minutes before meals and at bedtime

Mucogel® (Pharmax)
Suspension (= mixture), dried aluminium hydroxide 220 mg, magnesium hydroxide 195 mg/5 ml. Price 100 ml = **B**
Dose: 10–20 ml when required

Phazyme® (Stafford-Miller)
Tablets, pink, s/c, activated dimethicone 20 mg outer layer, 40 mg core. Price 20 tabs = **C**
Dose: 1–2 tablets when required

Polyalk® (Galen)
NHS *Tablets*, dried aluminium hydroxide 500 mg, activated dimethicone 250 mg. Price 20 tabs = **C**
Dose: 1–2 tablets chewed or sucked when required
NHS *Gel* (viscous suspension = mixture), dried aluminium hydroxide 440 mg, dimethicone 125 mg, light magnesium oxide 70 mg/5 ml. Low Na⁺. Price 100 ml = **C**
Dose: 5–10 ml when required
Suspension (= mixture), ingredients, price, and dose, as for gel

NHS Polycrol® (Nicholas)
Tablets, green/white, aluminium hydroxide-magnesium carbonate co-dried gel 275 mg, activated dimethicone 25 mg, magnesium hydroxide 100 mg. Low Na⁺. Price 20 tabs = **B**
Dose: 1–2 tablets chewed or sucked when required; CHILD 6–12 years 1 tablet 2–3 times daily
Gel (= mixture), aluminium hydroxide mixture 4.75 ml, activated dimethicone 25 mg, magnesium hydroxide 100 mg/5 ml. Low Na⁺. Price 100 ml = **C**
Dose: 5–10 ml when required; CHILD 6–12 years 5 ml up to six times daily

NHS Polycrol Forte® (Nicholas)
Tablets, aluminium hydroxide-magnesium carbonate co-dried gel 275 mg, activated dimethicone 250 mg, magnesium hydroxide 100 mg. Low Na⁺. Price 20 tabs = **B**

Dose: 1–2 tablets chewed or sucked when required
Gel (= mixture), aluminium hydroxide mixture 4.75 ml, activated dimethicone 125 mg, magnesium hydroxide 100 mg/5 ml. Low Na⁺. Price 100 ml = **C**
Dose: 5–10 ml when required; CHILD 5–12 years 5 ml, up to six times daily

NHS Prodexin® (Bencard)
Tablets, aluminium glycinate 900 mg, magnesium carbonate 100 mg. Low Na⁺. Price 20 tabs = **B**
Dose: 1 or more tablets chewed or sucked when required

NHS Siloxyl® (Martindale)
Tablets, dried aluminium hydroxide 500 mg, activated dimethicone 250 mg. Price 20 tabs = **C**
Dose: 1–2 tablets chewed or sucked when required
Suspension (= mixture), dried aluminium hydroxide 420 mg, activated dimethicone 125 mg, light magnesium oxide 70 mg/5 ml. Price 100 ml = **C**
Dose: 5–10 ml when required; CHILD 6–12 years 5 ml

NHS Sylopal® (Norton)
Suspension (= mixture), dimethicone 125 mg, light magnesium oxide 70 mg, aluminium hydroxide mixture to 5 ml. Price 100 ml = **C**
Dose: 5–10 ml when required

NHS Synergel® (Servier)
Gel (= mixture), aluminium phosphate mixture 55%, pectin-agar gel 45%. Contains about 8 mmol Na⁺/15 ml. Price 10 × 15-ml sachet = **C**
Dose: 1 sachet when required; CHILD 5 ml/4.5 kg daily in divided doses

Topal® (Concept)
Tablets, alginic acid 200 mg, dried aluminium hydroxide 30 mg, light magnesium carbonate 40 mg. Price 20 tabs = **B**
Dose: 1–3 tablets chewed between meals and at bedtime

NHS Unigest® (Unigreg)
Tablets, dried aluminium hydroxide 450 mg, dimethicone 400 mg. Low Na⁺. Price 12 tabs = **C**
Dose: 1–2 tablets chewed or sucked when required

1.1.3 Calcium- and bismuth-containing antacids

These should generally be avoided (see introductory notes).

Calcium Carbonate Mixture, Compound, Paediatric (see Formulary). Price 100 ml = **A**
Dose: CHILD up to 1 year 5 ml, 1–5 years 10 ml

Calcium Carbonate Powder, Compound, calcium carbonate 375 mg, light kaolin 125 mg, heavy magnesium carbonate 125 mg, sodium bicarbonate 375 mg. Price 100 g = **A**. Label: 13
Dose: 1–5 g in liquid when required

Chalk Mixture, Paediatric (see Formulary). Price 100 ml = **A**
Dose: CHILD up to 1 year 5 ml, 1–5 years 10 ml, when required

---

Magnesium Carbonate Tablets, Compound, heavy magnesium carbonate 200 mg, light kaolin 60 mg, sodium bicarbonate 120 mg, calcium carbonate 200 mg. Price 20 tabs = **A**
Dose: 1–2 tablets chewed when required

Magnesium Carbonate Powder, Compound, heavy magnesium carbonate 333 mg, light kaolin 83 mg, sodium bicarbonate 250 mg, calcium carbonate 333 mg. Price 100 g = **B**. Label: 13
Dose: 1–5 g in liquid when required

NHS **Nulacin®** (Bencard)
Tablets, calcium carbonate 130 mg, heavy magnesium carbonate 30 mg, heavy magnesium oxide 130 mg, magnesium trisilicate 230 mg, with milk solids, dextrins and maltose. Price 25 tabs = **C**
Dose: 1–2 tablets chewed or sucked when required

NHS **Roter®** (Roterpharma)
Tablets, pink, bismuth subnitrate 300 mg, frangula 25 mg, magnesium carbonate 400 mg, sodium bicarbonate 200 mg. Price 20 tabs = **B**. Label: 13, 21
Dose: 1–2 tablets dispersed in warm water 3 times daily after meals

NHS **Titralac®** (Riker)
Tablets, calcium carbonate 420 mg, glycine 180 mg. Price 20 tabs = **A**
Dose: 1–2 tablets chewed, sucked, or swallowed when required

1.2   Antispasmodics and other drugs altering gut motility

The smooth muscle relaxant properties of anticholinergic and other antispasmodic drugs may be useful as adjunctive treatment in non-ulcer dyspepsia, in the irritable bowel syndrome, and in diverticular disease. The gastric antisecretory effects of conventional anticholinergic drugs are of little practical importance since dosage is limited by atropine-like side-effects. Moreover, they have been superseded by more powerful and specific antisecretory drugs, including the histamine H_2-receptor antagonists and the selective anticholinergic pirenzepine.

The dopamine-receptor antagonists metoclopramide and domperidone have different properties, tending to stimulate transit in the gut, but are nevertheless of value in non-ulcer dyspepsia.

ANTICHOLINERGICS. The anticholinergics (more correctly termed 'antimuscarinics') can be divided into atropine and its related alkaloids (including the belladonna alkaloids), and synthetic anticholinergics. The synthetic anticholinergics can, in turn, be divided into tertiary amines (dicyclomine hydrochloride and piperidolate hydrochloride) and quaternary ammonium compounds (ambutonium bromide, glycopyrronium bromide, mepenzolate bromide, penthienate methobromide, pipenzolate bromide, poldine methylsulphate, and propantheline bromide). The tertiary amine **dicyclomine hydrochloride** has a much less marked anticholinergic action than atropine and may also have some direct action on smooth muscle.

Quaternary ammonium compounds are less lipid soluble than atropine and so may be less likely to cross the blood–brain barrier; they are also less well absorbed. Although central atropine-like side-effects, such as confusion, are thereby reduced, peripheral atropine-like side-effects remain common with dry mouth, difficult visual accommodation, hesitant micturition, and constipation at doses which act as gut neuromuscular relaxants or inhibitors of acid secretion. The elderly are particularly susceptible; glaucoma and urinary retention may occur.

Anticholinergics tend to relax the oesophageal sphincter and should be avoided in patients with symptomatic reflux; all antispasmodics should be avoided in paralytic ileus. Despite these side-effects anticholinergics are nevertheless useful in some dyspeptics, in the irritable bowel syndrome, and in diverticular disease. A dose at night will delay gastric emptying and prolong the gastric retention of antacids, thus helping to reduce nocturnal acidity; side-effects are also better tolerated then.

The quaternary ammonium compound, **hyoscine butylbromide** is advocated as a gastro-intestinal antispasmodic, but it is poorly absorbed and its action is brief. Another quaternary ammonium compound **atropine methonitrate** (as Eumydrin®) is occasionally used to treat pylorospasm in infants and congenital hypertrophic pyloric stenosis but its value in these conditions is very doubtful.

OTHER ANTISPASMODICS. Alverine citrate (Spasmonal®), mebeverine hydrochloride (Colofac®), and peppermint oil (Colpermin®) are believed to be direct relaxants of intestinal smooth muscle and may relieve pain in the irritable bowel syndrome and diverticular disease. They have no serious adverse effects but, like all antispasmodics, should be avoided in paralytic ileus. Peppermint oil occasionally causes heartburn.

DOPAMINE ANTAGONIST MOTILITY STIMULANTS. Metoclopramide hydrochloride (Maxolon® etc.) and domperidone (Motilium®) stimulate gastric emptying and small intestinal transit, and enhance the strength of oesophageal sphincter contraction. They are useful in some patients with non-ulcer dyspepsia, in speeding the transit of barium in an intestinal follow-through examination, as accessory treatments for oesophageal reflux, and in treating nonspecific or cytotoxic-induced nausea and vomiting (see section 4.6).

Metoclopramide and, occasionally, domperidone induce extrapyramidal reactions with facial and skeletal muscle spasms and oculogyric crises. These are more common in the young (including young adults) and the very old, usually occur shortly after starting treatment, and subside within 24 hours of stopping the drug. Injection of an anti-parkinsonian agent such as procyclidine (see section 4.9.2) will abort attacks. Other side-effects are rare, but gynaecomastia and galactorrhoea can occur. Dosage of both drugs should be reduced in renal impairment and both drugs should be avoided in the period immediately after abdominal surgery.

ALVERINE CITRATE

Indications: irritable bowel syndrome
Cautions: paralytic ileus
Dose: 60–120 mg 1–3 times daily

NHS Normacol Antispasmodic® (Norgine)
Granules, orange, coated, sterculia 62%, alverine citrate 0.5% (for the treatment of spastic colon). Price 100 g = **D**. Label: 25, 27, see dose below
Dose: for constipation, 1–2 heaped 5-ml spoonfuls swallowed without chewing with water once or twice daily after meals; CHILD half the adult dose

Spasmonal® (Norgine)
Capsules, blue/grey, alverine citrate 60 mg. Price 20 caps = **D**

AMBUTONIUM BROMIDE

Indications: adjunct in gastro-intestinal disorders characterised by smooth muscle spasm
Cautions; Contra-indications; Side-effects: see under Atropine Sulphate

NHS PoM Aludrox SA® (Wyeth)
Suspension (= mixture), green, ambutonium bromide 2.5 mg, aluminium hydroxide mixture 4.75 ml, magnesium hydroxide 100 mg/5 ml. Diluent water for preparations, life of diluted mixture 14 days. Price 100 ml = **A**
Dose: 5–10 ml 3–4 times daily between meals and at bedtime

ATROPINE METHONITRATE

Indications: pylorospasm in infants; congenital hypertrophic pyloric stenosis
Cautions; Contra-indications; Side-effects: see under Atropine Sulphate. Dehydration and alkalosis should first be treated

PoM Eumydrin® (Winthrop)
Oral solution, atropine methonitrate 0.6% (approx. 200 micrograms/drop) in 90% alcohol. Price 15-ml dropper bottle = **E**. Store in a cool place, tightly closed to prevent concentration by evaporation. Counselling advised, use of dropper, storage
Dose: INFANT 1–2 drops (200–400 micrograms) 20 minutes before each feed, gradually increased over several days to 3-4 drops (600–800 micrograms)/feed

ATROPINE SULPHATE

Indications: adjunct in gastro-intestinal disorders characterised by smooth muscle spasm
Cautions: in the elderly, urinary retention, prostatic enlargement, tachycardia, cardiac insufficiency, paralytic ileus, ulcerative colitis, and pyloric stenosis; may aggravate gastro-oesophageal reflux; breast-feeding. Drug interactions of anticholinergic drugs: see Appendix 1 (sections *1*, *2.3*, 4.9, 5.2)
Contra-indications: glaucoma
Side-effects: peripheral anticholinergic side-effects include dry mouth with difficulty in swallowing and thirst, dilatation of the pupils with loss of accommodation and sensitivity to light, increased intra-ocular pressure, flushing, dry skin, bradycardia followed by tachycardia, palpitations and arrhythmias, difficulty with micturition, and constipation; rarely fever, confusional states and rashes
Dose: by mouth, 0.25–2 mg daily in single or divided doses; dosage should be gradually increased to the max. tolerated
By intravenous injection, diagnosis of colicky pain, 0.4–1 mg (usually 600 micrograms)

PoM Atropine Sulphate Tablets, atropine sulphate 600 micrograms. Price 20 tabs = **B**
Atropine Sulphate Injection—see section 2.3.2

BELLADONNA ALKALOIDS

Indications: adjunct in gastro-intestinal disorders characterised by smooth muscle spasm
Cautions; Contra-indications; Side-effects: see under Atropine Sulphate

Aluminium Hydroxide and Belladonna Mixture, belladonna alkaloids 300 micrograms/10 ml (see Formulary). Low Na+. Price 100 ml = **A**
Dose: 5 ml between meals
Belladonna Mixture, Paediatric, belladonna alkaloids 45 micrograms/5 ml (see Formulary). Price 100 ml = **A**
Dose: CHILD up to 1 year 5 ml, 1–5 years 10 ml half an hour before meals
Magnesium Trisilicate and Belladonna Mixture, belladonna alkaloids 150 micrograms/10 ml (see Formulary). Contains about 6 mmol Na+/10 ml. Price 200 ml = **A**
Dose: 10–20 ml between meals when necessary
NHS Alka-Donna® (Carlton)
Tablets, belladonna alkaloids 80 micrograms (calc. as hyoscyamine), dried aluminium hydroxide 250 mg, magnesium trisilicate 500 mg. Price 20 tabs = **A**
Dose: 1–2 tablets, sucked 3 times daily before meals
Suspension (=mixture), belladonna alkaloids 60 micrograms (calc. as hyoscyamine), aluminium hydroxide mixture 2.15 ml, magnesium trisilicate 342.5 mg/5 ml. Price 100 ml = **A**
Dose: 5–10 ml 3 times daily between meals
NHS Aluhyde® (Sinclair)
Tablets, scored, belladonna liquid extract 7.8 mg, dried aluminium hydroxide 245 mg, magnesium trisilicate 245 mg. Price 20 tabs = **C**
Dose: 2 tablets 3 times daily
NHS Bellocarb® (Sinclair)
Tablets, beige, scored, belladonna dry extract 10 mg (equivalent to 100 micrograms of hyoscyamine), magnesium carbonate 300 mg, magnesium trisilicate 300 mg. Price 20 tabs = **C**
Dose: 1–2 tablets 4 times daily
NHS Carbellon® (Medo)
Tablets, black, belladonna dry extract 6 mg (equivalent to 60 micrograms hyoscyamine), charcoal 100 mg, magnesium hydroxide 100 mg, peppermint oil 0.003 ml. Price 20 tabs = **B**
Dose: flatulence and abdominal distension, 2–4 tablets 3 times daily; CHILD 1–5 years 1½ tablets, 6–12 years 2 tablets

NHS **Neutradonna**® (Nicholas)
Tablets, belladonna alkaloids 48 micrograms (calc. as hyoscyamine), aluminium sodium silicate 650 mg. Price 20 tabs = **B**
Dose: 2–3 tablets, preferably chewed, up to 4 times daily; CHILD 2–5 years ½–1 tablet, 6–12 years 1–1½ tablets
Powder, belladonna alkaloids 75 micrograms (calc. as hyoscyamine), aluminium sodium silicate 989.6 mg/g. Price 25 g = **B**. Label: 13
Dose: 5–10 ml, in liquid, up to 4 times daily after meals; CHILD 2–5 years 2.5 ml, 6–12 years 2.5–5 ml

PoM **Peptard**® (Riker)
Tablets, s/r, hyoscyamine sulphate 200 micrograms. Price 20 tabs = **D**. Label: 13
Dose: 2–3 tablets twice daily; CHILD over 10 years 1–2 tablets

DICYCLOMINE HYDROCHLORIDE

Indications: adjunct in gastro-intestinal disorders characterised by smooth muscle spasm
Cautions; Contra-indications; Side-effects: see under Atropine Sulphate. Contra-indicated in infants under 6 months
Dose: 10–20 mg 3 times daily; CHILD 6–24 months 5–10 mg up to 3–4 times daily, 15 minutes before feeds, 2–12 years 10 mg 3 times daily

NHS **Kolanticon**® (Merrell)
Gel (= mixture), dicyclomine hydrochloride 2.5 mg, dried aluminium hydroxide 200 mg, light magnesium oxide 100 mg, dimethicone 20 mg/5 ml. Diluent purified water, freshly boiled and cooled, life of diluted mixture 14 days. Price 125 ml = **B**
Dose: 10–20 ml every 4 hours when required
NHS **Kolantyl**® (Merrell)
Gel (= mixture), dicyclomine hydrochloride 2.5 mg, dried aluminium hydroxide 200 mg, light magnesium oxide 100 mg/5 ml. Diluent purified water, freshly boiled and cooled, life of diluted mixture 14 days. Price 125 ml = **B**
Dose: 10–20 ml 4 hourly when required
PoM **Merbentyl**® (Merrell)
Tablets, dicyclomine hydrochloride 10 mg. Price 20 tabs = **C**
Syrup (= elixir), dicyclomine hydrochloride 10 mg/5 ml. Diluent syrup, life of diluted elixir 14 days. Price 100 ml = **C**

DOMPERIDONE

Indications: see notes above; for use in nausea and vomiting, see section 4.6
Cautions; Side-effects; Dose: see notes above and section 4.6

Preparations
See section 4.6

GLYCOPYRRONIUM BROMIDE

Indications: adjunct in gastro-intestinal disorders characterised by smooth muscle spasm

Cautions; Contra-indications; Side-effects: see under Atropine Sulphate
Dose: 1–4 mg 2–3 times daily

PoM **Robinul**® (Robins)
Tablets, pink, scored, glycopyrronium bromide 2 mg. Price 20 tabs = **D**

HYOSCINE BUTYLBROMIDE

Indications: adjunct in gastro-intestinal disorders characterised by smooth muscle spasm
Cautions; Contra-indications; Side-effects: see under Atropine Sulphate
Dose: by mouth, 20 mg 4 times daily; CHILD 6–12 years, 10 mg 3 times daily
By intramuscular or intravenous injection (acute spasm), 20 mg, repeated after 30 minutes if necessary

PoM **Buscopan**® (Boehringer Ingelheim)
Tablets, s/c, hyoscine butylbromide 10 mg. Price 20 tabs = **C**
Injection, hyoscine butylbromide 20 mg/ml. Price 1-ml amp = **A**

MEBEVERINE HYDROCHLORIDE

Indications: irritable bowel syndrome
Cautions: paralytic ileus
Dose: 135 mg 3 times daily preferably 20 minutes before meals

PoM **Colofac**® (Duphar)
Tablets, s/c, mebeverine hydrochloride 135 mg. Price 20 tabs = **D**. Label: 22
▼ PoM **Colven**® (R&C)
Granules, yellowish-brown, effervescent, ispaghula husk 3.5 g, mebeverine hydrochloride 135 mg/sachet. Contains 6.1 mmol Na$^+$/sachet; caution in renal impairment. Price 20 sachets = **G**. Label: 13, 22
Dose: irritable bowel syndrome, 1 sachet in water twice daily 30 minutes before food

MEPENZOLATE BROMIDE

Indications: adjunct in gastro-intestinal disorders characterised by smooth muscle spasm
Cautions; Contra-indications; Side-effects: see under Atropine Sulphate
Dose: 25–50 mg 3–4 times daily; CHILD 6–12 years 12.5 mg

PoM **Cantil**® (MCP)
Tablets, yellow, scored, mepenzolate bromide 25 mg. Price 20 tabs = **C**
Elixir, red, mepenzolate bromide 12.5 mg/5 ml. Diluent water for preparations, life of diluted elixir 7 days. Price 100 ml = **D**

METOCLOPRAMIDE HYDROCHLORIDE

Indications: see notes above; for use in nausea and vomiting, see section 4.6
Cautions: treatment should begin with a low dose and gradually increase. Avoid doses exceeding 500 micrograms/kg/day. Reduce dose in renal

---

failure. Caution in elderly patients and in children; measure dose accurately, preferably with a pipette. May mask underlying disorders such as cerebral irritation; avoid for 3–4 days following gastro-intestinal surgery. Drug interactions: see Appendix 1 (sections 1, 2.5, 4.2, 4.7, 4.9, 6.7)

Side-effects: extrapyramidal effects, especially in patients under 15 years of age, rarely drowsiness, constipation, hyperprolactinaemia, galactorrhoea

Dose: by mouth, or by intramuscular or intravenous injection, 10 mg (5–10 mg in young adults 15–20 years) 3 times daily; CHILD up to 1 year 1 mg twice daily, 1–2 years 1 mg 2–3 times daily, 3–5 years 2 mg 2–3 times daily, 6–14 years 2.5–5 mg 3 times daily

For radiological examinations, as a single dose *by mouth* 10–15 minutes before examination or *by intramuscular or intravenous injection* 5–10 minutes before examination, 10–20 mg; CHILD under 3 years 1 mg, 3–5 years 2 mg, 6–14 years 2.5–5 mg

PoM **Metoclopramide Tablets,** metoclopramide hydrochloride (anhydrous) 10 mg. Price 20 tabs = **C**

PoM **Metoclopramide Elixir,** metoclopramide hydrochloride (anhydrous) 5 mg/5 ml. Price 100 ml = **D**

PoM **Metoclopramide Injection,** metoclopramide hydrochloride (anhydrous) 5 mg/ml. Price 2-ml amp = **A**

PoM **Maxolon**® (Beecham)
Tablets, scored, metoclopramide hydrochloride (anhydrous) 10 mg. Price 20 tabs = **E**
Syrup (=elixir), yellow, metoclopramide hydrochloride (anhydrous) 5 mg/5 ml. Diluent purified water, freshly boiled and cooled, life of diluted elixir 14 days. Price 100 ml = **D**
Paediatric liquid, yellow, metoclopramide hydrochloride (anhydrous) 1 mg/ml. Diluent as above. Price 15 ml with pipette = **D**. Counselling advised, use of pipette
Injection, metoclopramide hydrochloride (anhydrous) 5 mg/ml. Price 2-ml amp = **B**

Maxolon High Dose: see section 4.6

PoM **Metox**® (Steinhard)
Tablets, scored, metoclopramide hydrochloride (anhydrous) 10 mg. Price 20 tabs = **D**

PoM **Mygdalon**® (DDSA)
Tablets, scored, metoclopramide hydrochloride (anhydrous) 10 mg. Price 20 tabs = **C**

PoM **Parmid**® (Lagap)
Tablets, scored, metoclopramide hydrochloride (anhydrous) 10 mg. Price 20 tabs = **C**
Syrup (=elixir), metoclopramide hydrochloride (anhydrous) 5 mg/5 ml. Price 100 ml = **D**
Injection, metoclopramide hydrochloride (anhydrous) 5 mg/ml. Price 2-ml amp = **A**

PoM **Primperan**® (Berk)
Tablets, scored, metoclopramide hydrochloride (anhydrous) 10 mg. Price 20 tabs = **C**
Syrup (=elixir), lime, metoclopramide hydrochloride (anhydrous) 5 mg/5 ml. Diluent syrup, life of diluted elixir 14 days. Price 100 ml = **D**

Injection, metoclopramide hydrochloride (anhydrous) 5 mg/ml. Price 2-ml amp = **A**

PENTHIENATE METHOBROMIDE

Indications: adjunct in gastro-intestinal disorders characterised by smooth muscle spasm
Cautions; Contra-indications; Side-effects: see under Atropine Sulphate
Dose: 2.5–10 mg 3–4 times daily; max. 40 mg daily

PoM **Monodral**® (Sterling Research)
Tablets, yellow, scored, penthienate methobromide 5 mg. Price 20 tabs = **D**

PEPPERMINT OIL

Indications: relief of abdominal colic and distension, particularly in irritable bowel syndrome
Cautions: ulcerative colitis, paralytic ileus, rarely sensitivity to menthol
Side-effects: heartburn, local irritation

Colpermin® (Tillotts)
Capsules, light blue/dark blue, green band, e/c, peppermint oil 0.2 ml. Price 20 caps = **E**. Label: 5, 22, 25
Dose: 1–2 capsules, swallowed whole with water, 3 times daily before meals for up to 2–3 months if necessary

PIPENZOLATE BROMIDE

Indications: adjunct in gastro-intestinal disorders characterised by smooth muscle spasm
Cautions; Contra-indications; Side-effects: see under Atropine Sulphate
Dose: 5 mg 3 times daily 15 minutes before meals and 5–10 mg at night

PoM **Piptal**® (MCP)
Tablets, peach, pipenzolate bromide 5 mg. Price 20 tabs = **B**

PoM **Piptalin**® (MCP)
Suspension (=mixture), orange, pipenzolate bromide 4 mg, activated dimethicone 40 mg/5 ml. Diluent syrup or water for preparations, life of diluted mixture 14 days. Price 100 ml = **D**
Dose: 10 ml 3–4 times daily before meals; CHILD up to 10 kg 2.5 ml 15 minutes before feeds, 10–20 kg 2.5–5 ml, 20–40 kg 5 ml, 3–4 times daily

PIPERIDOLATE HYDROCHLORIDE

Indications: adjunct in gastro-intestinal disorders characterised by smooth muscle spasm
Cautions; Contra-indications; Side-effects: see under Atropine Sulphate
Dose: 50 mg 4 times daily before meals

PoM **Dactil**® (MCP)
Tablets, piperidolate hydrochloride 50 mg. Price 20 tabs = **C**

POLDINE METHYLSULPHATE

Indications: adjunct in gastro-intestinal disorders characterised by smooth muscle spasm

Cautions; Contra-indications; Side-effects: see under Atropine Sulphate

Dose: 2–4 mg, gradually increased to max. tolerated, 3 times daily and at bedtime

PoM **Nacton**® (Bencard)
Tablets, scored, poldine methylsulphate 2 mg. Price 20 tabs = **B**
Tablets forte, orange, scored, poldine methylsulphate 4 mg. Price 20 tabs = **C**

PROPANTHELINE BROMIDE

Indications: adjunct in gastro-intestinal disorders characterised by smooth muscle spasm; for use with retention enemas see section 1.7.2 (for use in nocturnal enuresis see section 7.4.2)

Cautions; Contra-indications; Side-effects: see under Atropine Sulphate. Drug interactions: see Appendix 1 (section *1*)

Dose: 15 mg 3 times daily 1 hour before meals and 30 mg at night, max. 120 mg daily
Diagnostic procedures, 30 mg 45 minutes before the procedure

PoM **Propantheline Tablets**, s/c, propantheline bromide 15 mg. Price 20 tabs = **A**. Label: 22
PoM **Pro-Banthine**® (Gold Cross)
Tablets, pink, s/c, propantheline bromide 15 mg. Price 20 tabs = **B**. Label: 22

1.2.1   Compound antispasmodic preparations

These preparations, which may contain an antispasmodic and a sedative, should be **avoided**; in particular, those containing a barbiturate are to be deprecated. The dosage of individual agents cannot be properly titrated in compound preparations.

Actonorm® (Wallace Mfg)
NHS *Tablets*, atropine sulphate 50 micrograms, papaverine hydrochloride 200 micrograms, dried aluminium hydroxide 25 mg, calcium carbonate 109 mg, light kaolin 75 mg, magnesium carbonate 225 mg, magnesium trisilicate 50 mg, thiamine hydrochloride 500 micrograms. Price 20 tabs = **B**
Dose: 1–2 tablets chewed or swallowed 3 times daily after meals and at bedtime
NHS *Powder*, atropine sulphate 100 micrograms, papaverine hydrochloride 400 micrograms, dried aluminium hydroxide 50 mg, calcium carbonate 145 mg, light kaolin 50 mg, magnesium carbonate 300 mg, magnesium trisilicate 50 mg, sodium bicarbonate 373 mg, thiamine hydrochloride 1 mg/g. Price 85 g = **D**. Label: 13
Dose: 5-ml spoonful in liquid 3 times daily after meals and at bedtime
NHS CD **Alka-Donna-P**® (Carlton)
Tablets, belladonna dry extract 8 mg, phenobarbitone 8 mg, dried aluminium hydroxide 250 mg, magnesium trisilicate 500 mg. Price 20 tabs = **A**
Dose: 1–2 tablets sucked before meals when required
Mixture, belladonna tincture 0.2 ml, phenobarbitone

8 mg, aluminium hydroxide mixture 2.15 ml, magnesium trisilicate 342.5 mg/5 ml. Price 100 ml = **A**
Dose: 5–10 ml 3 times daily
NHS PoM **APP Stomach Tablets**® (Consolidated)
Tablets, homatropine methylbromide 1.5 mg, papaverine hydrochloride 3 mg, aluminium hydroxide mixture 15 mg, bismuth carbonate 12.5 mg, calcium carbonate 180.5 mg, magnesium carbonate 195 mg, magnesium trisilicate 92.5 mg. Price 20 tabs = **B**
Dose: 1–2 tablets 3–4 times daily after meals
NHS PoM **APP Stomach Powder**® (Consolidated)
Powder, homatropine methylbromide 1 mg, papaverine hydrochloride 1 mg, aluminium hydroxide mixture 30 mg, bismuth carbonate 20 mg, calcium carbonate 378 mg, magnesium carbonate 375 mg, magnesium trisilicate 195 mg/g. Price 100 g = **C**. Label: 13
Dose: 5-ml spoonful in liquid 3–4 times daily
CD **Cantil with Phenobarbitone**® (MCP)
Tablets, brown, scored, mepenzolate bromide 25 mg, phenobarbitone 15 mg. Price 20 tabs = **D**. Label: 2
Dose: 1–2 tablets 3 times daily
Emetrol® (Rorer)
Oral solution, yellow, fructose 1.87 g, glucose 1.87 g, phosphoric acid 21.5 mg/5 ml. Price 100 ml = **C**
Dose: nausea, 15–30 ml every 15 minutes; prevention of morning sickness 15–30 ml every 3 hours; avoid fluids within 15 minutes; CHILD, nausea, 5–10 ml every 15 minutes or, to prevent regurgitation, 15 minutes before feeds
NHS PoM **Libraxin**® (Sauter)
Tablets, green, f/c, chlordiazepoxide 5 mg, clidinium bromide 2.5 mg. Price 20 tabs = **C**. Label: 2
Dose: 1–2 tablets 3–4 times daily (elderly patients 1 tablet twice daily) before meals and at bedtime
PoM **Stelabid**® (SK&F)
Tablets, yellow, s/c, isopropamide 5 mg (as iodide), trifluoperazine 1 mg (as hydrochloride). Price 20 tabs = **C**. Label: 2
Dose: 1 tablet in the morning and 1–2 tablets at night
Tablets forte, yellow, s/c, isopropamide 7.5 mg (as iodide), trifluoperazine 2 mg (as hydrochloride). Price 20 tabs = **D**. Label: 2
Dose: 1 tablet twice daily

1.3   Ulcer-healing drugs

Peptic ulceration is a common condition involving the stomach, duodenum, oesophagus, and, after gastric surgery, the gastro-enterostomy stoma. Duodenal ulcers occur about four times more commonly than gastric ulcers and each type of ulcer has a distinct pathogenesis with differing complications and management problems.

Ulcer healing may often be accelerated by simple measures such as short periods of bedrest and the avoidance of smoking whilst regular meals and antacids may provide symptomatic relief. Antacids may be effective in healing duodenal ulcers but the large regular doses that are required are inconvenient to the patient (section 1.1). It is only in the last two decades that potent ulcer-healing drugs have emerged. Originally **carbenoxolone** (Biogastrone®, Duogastrone®), and **tripotassium dicitratobismuthate** (De-Nol®) were introduced and were later followed by **cimetidine** (Tagamet®), **ranitidine** (Zantac®) and, more recently, **sucralfate** (Antepsin®) and **pirenzepine** (Gastrozepin®). The main problem with all these drugs is the high rate of relapse after treatment is discontinued; surgery may be necessary in such cases.

Tripotassium dicitratobismuthate (De-Nol®) is a bismuth chelate which promotes healing of gastric and duodenal ulcers. It is claimed that healing is longer lasting than with the other drugs. Encephalopathy has followed the use of older bismuth preparations and therefore, although it has not been demonstrated with this preparation, its use should be restricted to short courses. It may act by coating the ulcer and so protecting its surface. As the elixir, which has a pungent ammoniacal odour, is likely to adhere to food rather than to the surface of the ulcer, patients should be advised to avoid food and large quantities of drink for half an hour before and two hours after each dose. Tablets (De-Noltab®) are as effective as the elixir and more palatable.

Carbenoxolone, a synthetic derivative of glycyrrhizic acid (a constituent of liquorice) is effective in gastric ulcer; it is also effective in duodenal ulcer if released at the site of the lesion. It is better suited to younger rather than older patients because of the nature of its side-effects, which include sodium retention and hypokalaemia and which may aggravate conditions such as oedema, hypertension, cardiac failure, and muscle weakness. For these reasons regular monitoring of weight, blood pressure, and electrolytes is advisable during treatment. Carbenoxolone may act by protecting the mucosal barrier from acid–pepsin attack and increasing mucosal mucin production. **Deglycyrrhizinised liquorice** is free from these side-effects but is of doubtful efficacy.

Sucralfate (Antepsin®) has been recently introduced for the treatment of gastric and duodenal ulcers and may act by protecting the gastric mucosa from acid-pepsin attack. It has shown promise in initial trials but still requires long-term assessment. It is a complex of aluminium hydroxide and sulphated sucrose but has minimal antacid properties.

Cimetidine and **ranitidine** heal peptic ulcers, by a reduction in gastric acid output, as a result of their H_2-receptor blocking action. They may also relieve heartburn in peptic oesophagitis, in high doses reduce gastric acid output in the Zollinger-Ellison syndrome, and inhibit acid peptic breakdown of pancreatic enzyme supplements. Given prophylactically they reduce the frequency of bleeding from gastroduodenal erosions in patients with fulminating hepatic coma and possibly in others undergoing intensive care, but there is no substantial evidence that they arrest haemorrhage or prevent rebleeding in haematemesis and melaena. Cimetidine may be used in the treatment of persistent dyspeptic symptoms with or without ulceration. Both drugs, by ameliorating symptoms and inducing surface healing, can delay the diagnosis of gastric cancer.

Both drugs are well tolerated and symptomatic side-effects are rare. Cimetidine binds to androgen receptors, occasionally causes gynaecomastia and may, rarely, cause impotence. Cimetidine also retards the oxidative phase of hepatic drug metabolism by binding to microsomal cytochrome P450. Clinical effects due to the potentiation of drugs such as benzodiazepines and some beta-adrenoceptor blocking agents are unlikely to be noticed but may be important where drugs, such as phenytoin, warfarin, and aminophylline are in use where the margin between toxic and therapeutic concentrations is small. Confusion which rapidly reverses on stopping treatment is also described, particularly in elderly and severely ill patients. Acute pancreatitis or thrombocytopenia may occur rarely and interstitial nephritis is another well described but rare effect.

Ranitidine does not have anti-androgenic effects, does not inhibit the metabolism of phenytoin, warfarin, theophyllines, or, probably, that of other drugs. Ranitidine, like cimetidine, may cause reversible confusion. Headache, constipation, and nausea have been reported occasionally. In addition, some temporary increases in serum transaminases and gamma glutamyl transpeptidases have occurred. Anaphylactoid reactions have occurred rarely. In a few patients decreases in white blood cell counts and thrombocytopenia have occurred.

Reports of diarrhoea, rash, and photosensitivity with either drug are of doubtful significance. Evidence that hypochlorhydria induced by H_2-receptor blockade allows nitrosamine formation in the stomach and so could predispose to gastric cancer has been contested, and no coherent evidence exists to show that any clinical hazard arises.

Maintenance treatment with 400 mg of cimetidine or 150 mg of ranitidine at night will prevent ulcer relapse, but does not seem to modify natural history once treatment has stopped.

Treatment is probably best given in courses of 4–8 weeks, with further short courses if symptoms recur. Maintenance treatment is likely to be particularly appropriate where recurrences are severe and frequent and where, because of age or concomitant disease, surgery is likely to be hazardous.

Pirenzepine (Gastrozepin®) is a selective anticholinergic drug. It specifically inhibits gastric acid and pepsin secretion and may have fewer peripheral side-effects than the drugs in section 1.2; as it does not cross the blood-brain barrier it is unlikely to have central effects. It still requires long-term assessment and may be as effective as cimetidine but side-effects, although minor, are more frequent. It has also been used in conjunction with cimetidine in resistant cases.

BISMUTH CHELATE

Indications: peptic ulceration
Cautions: renal impairment; see also notes above
Side-effects: constipation, may blacken faeces

De-Nol® (Brocades)

Liquid (=elixir), red, tripotassium dicitratobismuthate 120 mg/5 ml. Price 100 ml = **D**; 560 ml = **I**. Counselling advised, see notes above
Dose: adults and children, 5 ml 4 times daily, in 15 ml of water 30 minutes before the 3 main

---

meals and 2 hours after the last meal for complete course of 28 days

De-Noltab® (Brocades)
Tablets, pink, tripotassium dicitratobismuthate 120 mg. Price 20 tabs = E. Counselling advised, see dose
Dose: adults and children, 1 tablet chewed and swallowed with water as for De-Nol (above)

CARBENOXOLONE SODIUM

Indications: gastric and duodenal ulceration in young and middle-aged patients
Cautions: elderly patients, cardiac disease, hypertension, impaired hepatic and renal function. See also notes above. Potassium supplements and thiazide diuretics may be necessary. Drug interactions: see Appendix 1 (sections 1, *2.1*, *2.2*, *2.5*, *6.3*)
Contra-indications: avoid use with spironolactone and amiloride
Side-effects: sodium and water retention leading to oedema, alkalosis, hypertension, hypokalaemia

PoM **Biogastrone**® (Winthrop)
Tablets, scored, carbenoxolone sodium 50 mg. Price 20 tabs = F. Label: 21
Dose: for gastric ulceration, 2 tablets 3 times daily after meals for 1 week, then 1 tablet 3 times daily until the ulcer is healed (4–6 weeks)

PoM **Duogastrone**® (Winthrop)
Capsules (for duodenal release), carbenoxolone sodium 50 mg. Price 28 caps = I. Label: 22, 25
Dose: for duodenal ulceration, 1 capsule with liquid 4 times daily 15–30 minutes before meals for 6–12 weeks

PoM **Pyrogastrone**® (Winthrop)
Tablets, chewable, carbenoxolone sodium 20 mg, alginic acid 600 mg, dried aluminium hydroxide 240 mg, magnesium trisilicate 60 mg, sodium bicarbonate 210 mg. Price 20 tabs = F. Label: 21, 24
Dose: for oesophageal inflammation and ulceration, 1 tablet, chewed, 3 times daily immediately after meals, and 2 at night, for 6–12 weeks
Liquid (= mixture), carbenoxolone sodium 10 mg, dried aluminium hydroxide 150 mg (Na⁺ 0.97 mmol, K⁺ 1.5 mmol)/5 ml when reconstituted with water for preparations. Price 100 ml = E. Label: 21
Dose: 10 ml 3 times daily after meals and 20 ml at night, for 6–12 weeks

CIMETIDINE

Indications: benign gastric and duodenal ulceration, stomal ulcer, reflux oesophagitis, Zollinger-Ellison syndrome, other conditions where gastric acid reduction is beneficial (see notes above and section 1.9.4)
Cautions: see notes above. Renal and hepatic impairment. Avoid intravenous injection in high dosage (may rarely cause arrhythmias) or in cardiovascular impairment. Drug interactions: see Appendix 1 (sections 1, *2.3*, *2.4*, *2.6*, *2.8B*, *3*, *4.1*, *4.3*, *4.7*, *4.8*, *5.1*, *5.2*)

Side-effects: see notes above
Dose: by mouth, 400 mg twice daily (with breakfast and at night) *or* 200 mg 3 times daily and 400 mg at night *or* 800 mg as a single daily dose at night. Doses should be taken for at least 4 weeks (6 weeks in gastric ulceration); when necessary the dose may be increased to 400 mg 4 times daily or rarely to a max. of 2.4 g daily in divided doses to maintain intragastric pH above 4; CHILD 20–40 mg/kg daily in divided doses
Maintenance, 400 mg at night *or* 400 mg morning and night
Reflux oesophagitis, Zollinger-Ellison syndrome, 400 mg 4 times daily (continued in reflux oesophagitis for 8 weeks)
Gastric acid reduction (prophylaxis of acid aspiration), obstetrics 400 mg at start of labour, then 200 mg every 2 hours to a max. of 1.6 g; surgical procedures 400 mg 90–120 minutes before induction, supplemented when necessary
Short-bowel syndrome, 1 g daily in divided doses to reduce malabsorption and fluid loss
By intramuscular or slow intravenous injection, 200 mg every 4–6 hours; max. 2.4 g daily
By intravenous infusion, 100–200 mg/hour for 2 hours repeated after an interval of 4–6 hours *or* 400 mg in 100 ml of sodium chloride 0.9% intravenous infusion infused over ½–1 hour repeated after an interval of 4–6 hours *or* by continuous infusion at an average rate of 50–100 mg/hour over 24 hours, max. 2.4 g daily; CHILD, *by slow intravenous injection or infusion*, 20–40 mg/kg daily in divided doses

PoM **Tagamet**® (SK&F)
Tablets, green, f/c, cimetidine 200 mg. Price 20 tabs = E
Tablets, green, f/c, cimetidine 400 mg. Price 14 tabs = F
Tablets, green, f/c, cimetidine 800 mg. Price 28-tab calendar pack = J
Syrup (= elixir), orange, cimetidine 200 mg/5 ml. Diluent syrup, life of diluted elixir 28 days. Price 100 ml = F
Injection, cimetidine 100 mg/ml. Price 2-ml amp = B
Intravenous infusion, cimetidine 4 mg/ml in sodium chloride intravenous infusion 0.9%. Price 100-ml infusion bag = F

LIQUORICE, DEGLYCYRRHIZINISED
Indications: peptic ulceration

Caved-S® (Tillotts)
Tablets, brown, deglycyrrhizinised liquorice 380 mg, aluminium hydroxide mixture 100 mg, magnesium carbonate 200 mg, sodium bicarbonate 100 mg. Price 20 tabs = C. Label: 24
Dose: 1–2 tablets chewed 3–6 times daily; CHILD over 10 years half adult dose
Rabro® (Sinclair)
Tablets, brown, deglycyrrhizinised liquorice 400 mg, calcium carbonate 500 mg, frangula 25 mg, magnesium oxide 100 mg. Price 20 tabs = C. Label: 21, 24

Dose: 1–2 tablets chewed and swallowed with liquid 3 times daily after meals for 1–2 months

PIRENZEPINE

Indications: gastric and duodenal ulceration
Side-effects: occasionally dry mouth and visual disturbances
Dose: 50 mg twice daily, increased if necessary to a max. of 150 mg daily in 3 divided doses, for 4–6 weeks, or in resistant cases for up to 3 months. Doses should preferably be taken 30 minutes before meals

▼ PoM **Gastrozepin®** (Boots)
Tablets, scored, pirenzepine 50 mg (as hydrochloride). Price 20 tabs = **H**. Label: 22

RANITIDINE

Indications: benign gastric and duodenal ulceration, stomal ulcer, reflux oesophagitis, Zollinger–Ellison syndrome, other conditions where reduction of gastric acidity is beneficial (see notes above and section 1.9.4)
Cautions: see notes above. Reduce dosage in impaired renal function. Drug interactions: see Appendix 1 (section 5.2)
Side-effects: see notes above
Dose: by mouth, 150 mg twice daily with breakfast and at night, or for patients with duodenal ulceration 300 mg as a single daily dose at night, for 4 weeks, or up to 8 weeks in reflux oesophagitis; Zollinger–Ellison syndrome, 150 mg 3 times daily increased if necessary to 6 g daily in divided doses
Maintenance, 150 mg at night
CHILD 8–18 years up to 150 mg twice daily
Gastric acid reduction (prophylaxis of acid aspiration in obstetrics), *by mouth*, 150 mg at onset of labour, then every 6 hours; surgical procedures, *by intramuscular or slow intravenous injection*, 50 mg 45–60 minutes before induction, or *by mouth*, 150 mg 2 hours before induction, and also, when possible on the preceding evening, supplemented when necessary
By slow intravenous injection, 50 mg every 6–8 hours
By intravenous infusion, 25 mg/hour for 2 hours, repeated if necessary after an interval of 6–8 hours

▼ PoM **Zantac®** (Glaxo)
Tablets, f/c, ranitidine 150 mg (as hydrochloride). Price 20 tabs = **I**
Dispersible tablets, f/c, scored, ranitidine 150 mg (as hydrochloride). Price 20 tabs = **I**. Label: 13
Tablets, f/c, ranitidine 300 mg (as hydrochloride). Price 10 tabs = **I**
Injection, ranitidine 25 mg (as hydrochloride)/ml. Price 2-ml amp = **C**

SUCRALFATE

Indications: gastric and duodenal ulceration; chronic gastritis
Cautions: renal disease. Drug interactions: see Appendix 1 (sections 2.8A, 5.1)
Side-effects: constipation

Dose: 1 g 4 times daily 1 hour before meals and at night, increased if necessary to a max. of 8 g daily in divided doses, for 4–6 weeks or in resistant cases 12 weeks

▼ PoM **Antepsin®** (Ayerst)
Tablets, scored, sucralfate 1 g. Price 20 tabs = **E**. Label: 5, 22

1.4 Antidiarrhoeal drugs

1.4.1 Antidiarrhoeal adsorbent mixtures
1.4.2 Antidiarrhoeal drugs which reduce motility
1.4.3 Other antidiarrhoeal preparations

The first line of treatment in acute diarrhoea, as in gastro-enteritis, is prevention or treatment of fluid and electrolyte depletion. This is particularly important in infants and in frail and elderly patients. Milder symptoms are managed by the frequent administration of small volumes of fluid in proportion to the quantity of watery stools passed. Home-made solutions containing sugar and small amounts of salt may be used for one or two days. However, one of the oral electrolyte replacement preparations, such as **Sodium Chloride and Glucose Oral Powder, Compound** (see section 9.2.1.1), is usually preferred since home-made solutions are not adequate to replace potassium and bicarbonate, which may be depleted in gastro-enteritis. Solids or whole milk are usually withdrawn during the acute phase and gradually reintroduced as the patient recovers. Clinical signs of severe dehydration require immediate admission to hospital for intravenous therapy and urgent replacement of fluid, sodium, potassium, and chloride deficits (see section 9.2.2).

Antidiarrhoeal drugs are of secondary value in the treatment of diarrhoea, may have undesirable side-effects, and may distract from giving fluids. The symptomatic remedies below may be of value if diarrhoea is inconvenient or has lasted for longer than 24 hours. It is rarely necessary to use antidiarrhoeals in infants and children but if considered appropriate they may be given as an adjunct to fluid and electrolyte replacement.

Antispasmodics (section 1.2) are occasionally of value in treating abdominal cramp associated with diarrhoea but they should not be used for primary treatment. Antispasmodics and anti-emetics should generally be **avoided** in young children with gastro-enteritis as they are rarely effective and have troublesome side-effects.

Antibiotics and sulphonamides are generally unnecessary in simple gastro-enteritis, even when a bacterial cause is suspected, because the complaint will usually resolve quickly without such treatment, and most infective diarrhoeas in this country are caused by viral infections. Systemic bacterial infection does, however, need appropriate systemic treatment. **Erythromycin** (see section 5.1.5) is the drug of choice for treating enteritis caused by *Campylobacter* spp. **Co-trimoxazole** (see section 5.1.8) is used to treat shigella infec-

C = 51-100p, **D** = 101-180p, **E** = 181-300p, **F** = 301-450p, **G** = 451-650p, **H** = 651-900p, **I** = 901-1200p, **J** = over 1200p.

tions with severe systemic involvement and sal-monella gastro-enteritis with suspected or confirmed septicaemia and is effective in both these conditions. Co-trimoxazole is also effective in ameliorating the symptoms of traveller's diarrhoea but prophylactic use is not advisable.

For treatment of diarrhoea associated with chronic disease see section 1.5; for antibacterial treatment in gastro-intestinal infections see Table 1, section 5.1; for amoebicides see section 5.4.2; for anthelmintic treatment see section 5.5.

1.4.1   Antidiarrhoeal adsorbent mixtures

Mixtures of **chalk** (Paediatric Chalk Mixture, Aromatic Chalk Powder) and **kaolin** (Kaolin Mixture, Paediatric Kaolin Mixture) may be effective in controlling diarrhoea. **Methylcellulose** is used in diarrhoea and is also specially useful in controlling faecal consistency in ileostomy and colostomy.

KAOLIN, LIGHT
Indications: diarrhoea
Cautions: drug interactions: see Appendix 1 (section *5.1*)

Kaolin   Mixture (see Formulary).   Price 200 ml = **B**
Dose: 10–20 ml every 4 hours
Kaolin Mixture, Paediatric (see Formulary). Price 100 ml = **B**
Dose: CHILD up to 1 year 5 ml, 1–5 years 10 ml every 4 hours
Kaopectate® (Upjohn)
Mixture, kaolin 1.03 g/5 ml. Diluent water for preparations, life of diluted mixture 14 days. Price 100 ml = **C**
Dose: 30–120 ml after each bowel movement; CHILD 5–60 ml according to age
KLN® (Ashe)
Mixture, kaolin 1.15 g, pectin 57.5 mg, sodium citrate 17.25 mg/5 ml. Price 100 ml = **C**
Dose: CHILD 6 months–1 year 5 ml, 1–3 years 10 ml, 3–10 years 20 ml every 4 hours

CERATONIA
Indications: diarrhoea

Arobon® (Nestlé)
Powder, ceratonia 80%, starch 15%, cocoa 5%. Price 150 g (with measure) = **D**
Dose: adults and children 20–40 g, in liquid, daily; infants 2–10%, premature infants 1%, added to feeds

CHALK
Indications: diarrhoea

Chalk Mixture, Paediatric (see Formulary). Price 100 ml = **A**
Dose: CHILD up to 1 year 5 ml, 1–5 years 10 ml, every 4 hours
Chalk Powder, Aromatic, chalk 250 mg, carda-mom seed 30 mg, clove 40 mg, nutmeg 80 mg, cinnamon 100 mg, sucrose 500 mg/g. Price 100 g = **C**. Label: 13
Dose: 0.5–5 g in liquid, every 4 hours

ISPAGHULA HUSK
Indications: diarrhoea (also constipation, section 1.6.1)
Side-effects: flatulence, abdominal distension
    Note: for diarrhoea the dose given in section 1.6.1 should be taken with a minimum of water

Preparations
Section 1.6.1

METHYLCELLULOSE
Indications: diarrhoea (also ileostomy, colos-tomy control, and constipation, section 1.6.1)
    Note: for diarrhoea the dose given in section 1.6.1 should be taken with a minimum of water

Preparations
Section 1.6.1

STERCULIA
Indications: diarrhoea (also ileostomy and colos-tomy control and constipation, section 1.6.1)
    Note: for diarrhoea the dose given in section 1.6.1 should be taken with a minimum of water

Preparations
Section 1.6.1

1.4.2   Antidiarrhoeal drugs which reduce motility

These are used for the symptomatic relief of diarrhoeas not controlled by adsorbent mixtures. **Codeine, diphenoxylate** (Lomotil®), **loperamide** (Imodium®), **morphine** (Kaolin and Morphine Mixture), and **opium** (Aromatic Chalk with Opium Mixture) are useful. In chronic diarrhoeas (section 1.5) loperamide may be preferable to the centrally acting opiates (morphine, codeine, and diphenoxylate) as it is unlikely to cause dependence.

There are few side-effects associated with these drugs but, except in the case of loperamide, excessive sedation may occur in children and in patients with chronic liver disease. They should be used with caution in colitic attacks as they may possibly increase the risk of toxic megacolon. Prolonged use could possibly aggravate irritable bowel syndrome. Drug interactions: see Appendix 1 (sections *1, 2.3, 4.1, 4.3*).

They should be used with caution in the elderly as they may induce faecal impaction, producing incontinence, spurious diarrhoea, abdominal pain, and rarely colonic obstruction. They are seldom necessary in children where fluid and electrolyte replacement in gastro-enteritis and the specific treatment of other diseases causing diarrhoea is usually more appropriate, and they are potentially harmful if used to treat infective diarrhoeas as they may delay the passage of liquid faeces, encourage proliferation of pathogens, and cause the severity of the diarrhoea to be underestimated.

CODEINE PHOSPHATE

Indications; Cautions; Contra-indications; Side-effects: see notes above
Dose: 10–60 mg every 4–6 hours; CHILD over 4 years 1–3 mg/kg daily in divided doses

PoM **Codeine Phosphate Tablets,** codeine phosphate 15 and 30 mg, price 20 tabs (both) = **B**; 60 mg, price 20 tabs = **D**
Codeine Phosphate Syrup, codeine phosphate 25 mg/5 ml. Price 100 ml = **C**
PoM **Diarrest**® (Galen)
Liquid (= elixir), yellow, codeine phosphate 5 mg, dicyclomine hydrochloride 2.5 mg, potassium chloride 40 mg, sodium chloride 50 mg, sodium citrate 50 mg/5 ml. For diarrhoea, vomiting, and cramp. Price 100 ml = **D**
Dose: 20 ml; CHILD 4–5 years 5 ml, 6–9 years 10 ml, 10–13 years 15 ml. Doses should be taken with water 4 times daily
Kaodene® (Boots)
Mixture, codeine phosphate 10 mg, light kaolin 3 g/10 ml. Price 250 ml = **C**
Dose: 20 ml 3–4 times daily; CHILD over 5 years 10 ml

DIPHENOXYLATE HYDROCHLORIDE

Indications; Cautions; Contra-indications; Side-effects: see under Codeine Phosphate
Dose: initially 10 mg, followed by 5 mg every 6 hours until diarrhoea is controlled; CHILD 4–8 years 2.5 mg 3 times daily, 9–12 years 2.5 mg 4 times daily, 13–16 years 5 mg 3 times daily

PoM **Lomotil**® (Gold Cross)
Tablets, diphenoxylate hydrochloride 2.5 mg, atropine sulphate 25 micrograms. Price 20 tabs = **E**
Liquid (= mixture), red, diphenoxylate hydrochloride 2.5 mg, atropine sulphate 25 micrograms/5 ml. Diluent glycerol, life of diluted elixir 14 days. Price 100 ml = **F**

LOPERAMIDE HYDROCHLORIDE

Indications; Contra-indications: see notes above
Side-effects: occasional rashes
Dose: 4 mg initially followed by 2 mg after each loose stool up to a max. of 16 mg daily; CHILD 4–8 years 1 mg 4 times daily, 9–12 years 2 mg 4 times daily
Chronic diarrhoea, 4–8 mg daily in divided doses initially and then if necessary adjusted according to response and given twice daily for maintenance

Imodium® (Janssen)
Capsules, green/grey, loperamide hydrochloride 2 mg. Price 20 caps = **E**
Syrup (= elixir), red, loperamide hydrochloride 1 mg/5 ml (sugar-free). Diluent water for preparations, life of diluted elixir 14 days. Price 100 ml = **E**
Note: a proprietary brand of loperamide hydrochloride capsules 2 mg (Arret®) is on sale to the public

OPIUM AND MORPHINE

Indications: diarrhoea
Cautions; Contra-indications; Side-effects: see under Codeine Phosphate. Sedation and the risk of dependence are greater

PoM **Aromatic Chalk with Opium Mixture,** morphine 5 mg/10 ml (see Formulary). Price 200 ml = **C**
Dose: 10–20 ml every 4 hours; CHILD 4–5 years 5 ml, 6–12 years 5–10 ml
Kaolin and Morphine Mixture, morphine hydrochloride 916 micrograms/10 ml (see Formulary). Price 200 ml = **B**
Dose: 10 ml every 4 hours

1.4.3 Other antidiarrhoeal preparations

Poorly-absorbed drugs such as phthalylsulphathiazole, dihydrostreptomycin, neomycin, and sulphaguanidine should be **avoided** altogether in gastro-intestinal infection. They prolong rather than shorten the time taken to control diarrhoea by causing masked bacterial diarrhoea, carrier states, or pseudomembranous colitis. Clioquinol should be avoided as it is neurotoxic and of doubtful efficacy and the lactobacillus preparations are probably valueless.

NHS **Flar**® (Consolidated)
Capsules, lactic acid bacilli resistant to most common antibacterial drugs 5×10^9 cells, with vitamins. Price 20 caps = **C**
Dose: 1–4 capsules before meals; CHILD 1–2 capsules
PoM **Guanimycin**® (A&H)
Suspension forte (= mixture), orange, dihydrostreptomycin sulphate 250 mg, light kaolin 4.25 g, sulphaguanidine 1.985 g/15 ml. Price 150 ml = **D**
Dose: 15 ml 4 hourly before meals; CHILD 1–4 years 5 ml, 5–9 years 5–10 ml, 10–15 years 10 ml

1.5 Treatment of chronic diarrhoeas

When diarrhoea is persistent and the presence of a tumour has been ruled out, the following should be considered. Manipulation of diet or exclusion of certain foods as well as drug treatment is important in the management of such disorders. It is also important to maintain adequate fluid intake (see section 9.2). See also section 9.4, foods for special diets.

IRRITABLE BOWEL SYNDROME. This can present with pain, constipation, or diarrhoea, all of which may benefit from a high-fibre diet with bran or other agents which increase stool bulk (section 1.6.1) if necessary. In some patients there may be important psychological aggravating factors which respond to reassurance. Antidiarrhoeal drugs such as **loperamide** (Imodium®) may sometimes be necessary but prolonged use may aggravate the condition (section 1.4.2). Antispasmodics such as **mebeverine** (Colofac®), section 1.2, may be necessary.

C = 51-100p, **D** = 101-180p, **E** = 181-300p, **F** = 301-450p, **G** = 451-650p, **H** = 651-900p, **I** = 901-1200p, **J** = over 1200p.

MALABSORPTION SYNDROMES. The most common cause in this country is *coeliac disease* (intolerance to gluten) and is usually treated with a gluten-free diet (see section 9.4.1). Pancreatic deficiency states are treated with **pancreatin** supplements (section 1.9.4).

ULCERATIVE COLITIS. For mild disease, topical treatment with **corticosteroids** such as prednisolone enemas or suppositories (section 1.7.2) is used to control symptoms. More extensive disease is treated with **sulphasalazine** (Salazopyrin®) by mouth both in the acute attack and also on a long-term maintenance basis where it has been shown to reduce the frequency of relapse. More serious cases may need additional treatment with **oral corticosteroids**, usually prednisolone, while in fulminating attacks prednisolone or other corticosteroids are given intravenously or intramuscularly. In resistant cases immunosuppressants, usually **azathioprine** (Imuran®) may be given under careful supervision and may reduce the frequency of relapse.

Laxatives are required to facilitate bowel movement when proctitis is present but a high-fibre diet and bulk-forming drugs such as **methylcellulose** are more useful in adjusting faecal consistency (section 1.6.1).

Symptoms of mild ulcerative colitis may be relieved with antidiarrhoeal drugs such as **codeine** or **loperamide** (Imodium®) but they should be used with caution in severe cases as paralytic ileus and toxic megacolon may be precipitated. For similar reasons antispasmodics should **not** be used in ulcerative colitis.

See also sections 1.7.2 and 1.7.3 for preparations containing corticosteroids.

CROHN'S DISEASE. Treatment is similar to that of ulcerative colitis. Oral **sulphasalazine** may relieve symptoms in colonic Crohn's disease but is of no value in small bowel disease. **Azathioprine**, given on a long-term maintenance basis, may reduce the recurrence rate of quiescent Crohn's disease. **Metronidazole** has been used with benefit in acute and chronic cases. In certain circumstances **oral corticosteroids** (see section 6.3.2), **corticotrophin**, and **tetracosactrin** (see section 6.5.1) are also used. Antibiotics are not recommended in Crohn's disease except when hospital investigation has revealed definite evidence of the overgrowth of bacteria in the small intestine or when a large inflammatory mass or abscess is present.

Cholestyramine (Questran®) and **aluminium hydroxide mixture** (section 1.1.1), bind unabsorbed bile salts and provide symptomatic relief of diarrhoea following ileal disease or resection, in bacterial colonisation of the small bowel, and in post-vagotomy diarrhoea.

PSEUDOMEMBRANOUS COLITIS. This is due to colonisation of the colon with *Clostridium difficile* which may develop after antibiotic therapy. It is usually of acute onset, but may run a chronic course. Ampicillin, clindamycin, and lincomycin have been implicated most frequently but few antibiotics are free of this side-effect. Oral **vancomycin** (see section 5.1.7) or **metronidazole** (see section 5.1.11.1) have been advocated as specific treatment.

DIVERTICULAR DISEASE. This is treated with a high-fibre diet, **bran supplements** and **bulk-forming laxatives. Antispasmodics** may provide symptomatic relief when colic is a problem (section 1.2). **Antibiotics** should be used only when the diverticula in the intestinal wall become infected. **Antidiarrhoeal** drugs which slow intestinal motility, for example codeine, diphenoxylate, and loperamide (Imodium®) could possibly exacerbate the symptoms of diverticular disease and are therefore **contra-indicated**.

AZATHIOPRINE

Indications: induction and maintenance of remission in ulcerative colitis and Crohn's disease
Cautions; Side-effects: see section 8.2.1
Dose: 1–3 mg/kg daily

Preparations
See section 8.2.1

CHOLESTYRAMINE

Indications: diarrhoea associated with ileal disease, ileal resection and post-vagotomy diarrhoea; pruritus in liver disease
Cautions; Contra-indications; Side-effects: see section 2.12
Dose: diarrhoea, initially 12–24 g in liquid daily, in single or divided doses, subsequently adjusted as required
Pruritus, 4–8 g in liquid daily

PoM **Questran**® (Bristol-Myers)
Powder, cholestyramine (anhydrous) 4 g/sachet. Price 10 sachets = **F**. Label: 13, counselling advised, avoid other drugs at same time

PREDNISOLONE

Indications: induction and maintenance of remission in ulcerative colitis, and Crohn's disease
Cautions; Contra-indications; Side-effects: see section 6.3.3
Dose: by mouth, initial dose 40 mg daily, in single or divided doses, until remission occurs, followed by reducing doses
By intravenous injection, for emergency treatment (under hospital supervision only), the equivalent of 20 mg of prednisolone (as prednisolone sodium phosphate) every 8 hours

Preparations
Oral and parenteral, see section 6.3.4; rectal, sections 1.7.2 and 1.7.3

SODIUM CROMOGLYCATE

Indications: food allergy (in conjunction with dietary restriction)

Side-effects: occasional nausea, rashes, and joint pain
Dose: 200 mg 4 times daily before meals; CHILD 2–14 years 100 mg; capsules may be swallowed whole or the contents dissolved in hot water and diluted with cold water before taking. May be increased if necessary after 2–3 weeks to a max. of 40 mg/kg daily and then reduced according to the response

PoM **Nalcrom**® (Fisons)
Capsules, sodium cromoglycate 100 mg. Price 20 caps = E. Label: 22, counselling advised, see dose above

SULPHASALAZINE

Indications: induction and maintenance of remission in ulcerative colitis and colonic Crohn's disease
Cautions: maintain adequate fluid intake to prevent crystalluria; pregnancy; hepatic and renal disease; glucose-6-phosphate dehydrogenase deficiency. Blood counts and urine analysis necessary during prolonged treatment; withdraw treatment if blood dyscrasias or hypersensitivity reactions develop
Contra-indications: salicylate and sulphonamide hypersensitivity
Side-effects: nausea, vomiting, epigastric discomfort, headache, vertigo, tinnitus, rashes, fever, minor haematological abnormalities such as Heinz-body anaemia, reversible neutropenia, folate malabsorption; rarely frank haemolytic anaemias, pancreatitis, agranulocytosis, Stevens–Johnson syndrome, neurotoxicity, photosensitisation, polyarteritis nodosa, allergic myocarditis, pulmonary fibrosis, reversible azoospermia. Urine may be coloured orange
Dose: by mouth, acute attack 1–2 g 4 times daily until remission occurs (if necessary corticosteroids may also be given), reducing to a maintenance dose of 500 mg 3–4 times daily; CHILD, acute attack 40–60 mg/kg daily, maintenance dose 20–30 mg/kg daily
By rectum, in suppositories, alone or in conjunction with oral treatment 0.5–1 g morning and night after defaecation. As an enema, 3 g at night, retained for at least 1 hour

PoM **Salazopyrin**® (Pharmacia)
Tablets, orange-brown, scored, sulphasalazine 500 mg. Price 20 tabs = D. Label: 14
EN-tablets® (= tablets e/c), orange-brown, f/c, sulphasalazine 500 mg. Price 20 tabs = D. Label: 5, 14, 25
Suppositories, brown, sulphasalazine 500 mg. Price 10 suppos = E
Retention enema, sulphasalazine 3 g in 100-ml single-dose disposable packs fitted with a nozzle. Price 100 ml = D

1.6   Laxatives
1.6.1 Bulk-forming drugs

1.6.2 Stimulant laxatives
1.6.3 Faecal softeners
1.6.4 Osmotic laxatives
1.6.5 Rectally administered laxatives
1.6.6 Other laxatives

Misconceptions about bowel habits have led to excessive laxative use. Abuse may lead to hypokalaemia and an atonic non-functioning colon. Simple constipation is usually relieved by increasing the intake of dietary fibre. The use of laxatives in children is undesirable but the introduction of fruit purée into the diet may be sufficient to regulate bowel action. In infants constipation is often remedied by adjustment of the diet.

Laxatives should generally be **avoided** except where straining will exacerbate a condition (such as angina) or increase the risk of rectal bleeding as in haemorrhoids. Laxatives are also of value in drug-induced constipation, for the expulsion of parasites after anthelmintic treatment, and to clear the alimentary tract before surgery and radiological procedures.

The laxatives that follow have been divided into 4 main groups (sections 1.6.1–1.6.4). This simple classification disguises the fact that some laxatives have a complex action. For example **dioctyl sodium sulphosuccinate** (docusate sodium) has been classified as a faecal softener but it also increases intestinal secretions by stimulating adenyl cyclase. This has an important effect on intestinal motility.

The laxatives in section 1.6.6 should preferably be avoided in prescribing.

1.6.1   Bulk-forming drugs

These relieve constipation by increasing faecal mass which stimulates peristalsis, but patients should be told that the full effect may take some days to develop. They are useful in the management of patients with colostomy, ileostomy, haemorrhoids, anal fissure, chronic diarrhoea associated with diverticular disease, irritable bowel syndrome, and ulcerative colitis (section 1.5). Adequate fluid intake must be maintained to avoid intestinal obstruction. Unprocessed wheat **bran**, taken with food or fruit juice, is a most effective bulk-forming preparation. Finely ground bran, though more palatable, has poorer water-retaining properties, but can be taken as bran bread or biscuits in appropriately increased quantities. Oat bran is also used.

Methylcellulose, **ispaghula**, and **sterculia** are useful in patients who cannot tolerate bran. Methylcellulose also acts as a faecal softener.

BRAN
Indications: constipation caused by inadequate fibre intake, diverticular disease, chronic diarrhoea (section 1.5)
Cautions; Contra-indications; Side-effects: see under Ispaghula Husk. Calcium and iron absorption may be impaired. Avoid in gluten enteropathies and coeliac disease
Dose: 8–24 g or more daily in divided doses

C = 51-100p, D = 101-180p, E = 181-300p, F = 301-450p, G = 451-650p, H = 651-900p, I = 901-1200p, J = over 1200p.

NHS **Fybranta**® (Norgine)

Tablets, brown, bran 2 g. Price 20 tabs = **B**. Label: 24, 27

Dose: 1–3 tablets chewed and swallowed with water 3–4 times daily, preferably with meals

NHS **Lejfibre**® (Britannia)

Biscuits, bran (oat) 40%. Price 25 × 10 g biscuit = **E**. Label: 24, 27

Dose: 2 biscuits with fluid

NHS **Proctofibe**® (Roussel)

Tablets, beige, f/c, fibrous grain extract 375 mg, fibrous citrus extract 94 mg. Price 20 tabs = **C**. Label: see dose below

Dose: adults and children over 3 years 4–12 tablets daily in divided doses chewed, swallowed, or dispersed in water

NHS **Trifyba**® (Labaz)

Powder (= oral powder), bran (80% fibre) 3.5 g sachet. Price 30 sachets = **E**; 250 g = **G**. Label: 21

Dose: 2–3 sachets daily mixed with food

ISPAGHULA HUSK

Indications: constipation caused by inadequate fibre intake, diverticular disease, chronic diarrhoea (section 1.5), haemorrhoids, anal fissure, colostomy control

Cautions: adequate fluid intake should be maintained; ulcerative colitis

Contra-indications: intestinal obstruction, colonic atony, faecal impaction

Side-effects: flatulence, abdominal distension, and intestinal obstruction

Fybogel® (R&C)

Granules, buff, effervescent, ispaghula husk 3.5 g/sachet. Contains 6 mmol Na+/sachet; caution in renal impairment. Price 10 sachets (plain or orange flavoured) = **C**. Label: 13

Dose: 1 sachet in water twice daily preferably after meals; CHILD ½–1 level 5-ml spoonful

Isogel® (A&H)

Granules, pink, ispaghula husk 90%. Price 200 g = **C**. Label: 13

Dose: constipation, 2 teaspoonfuls in water once or twice daily, preferably after meals; CHILD 1 teaspoonful

Diarrhoea (section 1.4.1), 1 teaspoonful 3 times daily

Metamucil® (Searle)

Powder, buff, ispaghula husk 49% (3.4 g/7-g sachet), gluten-free. Price 10 sachets = **C**; 100 g = **C**. Label: 13

Dose: one 5-ml spoonful or 1 sachet 1–3 times daily in 150 ml water; CHILD 6–12 years 2.5–5 ml

Regulan® (Gold Cross)

Powder, beige, effervescent, ispaghula husk 3.6 g/6.4-g sachet (gluten-free). Price 10 sachets = **C**. Label: 13

Dose: 1 sachet in 150 ml water 1–3 times daily; CHILD 6–12 years 2.5–5 ml

Vi-Siblin® (P-D)

Granules, brown, ispaghula husk 66%. Price 250 g = **E**. Label: 27

Dose: two 5-ml spoonfuls with a tumblerful of water one or more times daily

METHYLCELLULOSE

Indications: constipation caused by inadequate fibre intake; diverticular disease, chronic diarrhoea (section 1.5); haemorrhoids, anal fissure, colostomy, and ileostomy control

Cautions; Contra-indications; Side-effects: see under Ispaghula Husk

Methylcellulose Granules, pink, methylcellulose '450', '2500', or '4500' 64%. Price 100 g = **D**. Label: 27

Dose: 1.5–6 g (2.5–10 ml) with water

Celevac® (WBP)

Tablets, pink, methylcellulose '450' 500 mg. Price 20 tabs = **A**. Label: see dose below

NHS *Granules*, pink, methylcellulose '450' 64%. Price 100 g = **C**. Label: see dose below

Dose: 3–6 tablets (5–10 ml granules) twice daily. In constipation the dose should be taken with at least 300 ml of water. In diarrhoea, ileostomy, and colostomy control, minimise liquid intake for 30 minutes before and after the dose. Liquid and intragastric feeding, 5 ml granules per litre

Cellucon® (Medo)

Tablets, brown, methylcellulose '2500' 500 mg. Price 20 tabs = **A**. Label: see dose below

Dose: constipation, 1–4 tablets, chewed 3 times daily; CHILD 1–2 tablets 3–4 times daily. Doses should be followed by a tumblerful of liquid. Colostomy control 3 tablets chewed 2–3 times daily, adjusted according to response; minimise liquid intake for 30 minutes before and after the dose

NHS **Cologel**® (Lilly)

Mixture, yellow, methylcellulose '450' 900 mg/10 ml. Diluent water for preparations, life of diluted mixture 14 days. Price 100 ml = **C**. Label: see dose below

Dose: constipation, 5–15 ml taken with a tumblerful of water preferably after meals 3 times daily initially, reducing to a maintenance dose of 5–15 ml daily

STERCULIA

Indications: constipation caused by inadequate fibre intake; diverticular disease, chronic diarrhoea (section 1.5); haemorrhoids, anal fissure, colostomy and ileostomy control

Cautions; Contra-indications; Side-effects: see under Ispaghula Husk

Normacol Special® (Norgine)

Granules, coated, sterculia 62% (for the treatment of diverticular disease, constipation in pregnancy, and in colostomy and ileostomy control). Price 100 g = **C**. Label: 25, 27, see dose below

Dose: 1–2 heaped 5-ml spoonfuls swallowed without chewing with water once or twice daily after meals; CHILD half the adult dose

Compound preparations

NHS **Normacol Standard**® (Norgine)

Granules, brown, coated, sterculia 62%, fran-

gula (standardised) 8%. Price 100 g = C. Label: 25, 27, see dose above
Dose: see under Normacol Special

NHS **Normacol Standard Sugar-free Formula®** (Norgine)
As for Normacol Standard (above). Contains no sugar. Price 100 g = D. Label: 25, 27, see dose above

1.6.2 Stimulant laxatives

The most commonly used stimulant laxatives include **bisacodyl** and some of the anthraquinone group such as **danthron** and **senna**. These act by increasing intestinal motility and often cause abdominal cramp. These preparations should not be used in intestinal obstruction, and prolonged use should be avoided as they can eventually precipitate the onset of an atonic non-functioning colon and hypokalaemia. They should preferably be avoided in children. Other laxatives should preferably be used during pregnancy.

Stimulant laxatives which should be avoided in prescribing are indicated in section 1.6.6.

The **anticholinesterases** bethanechol, distigmine, neostigmine, and pyridostigmine (see sections 7.4.1 and 10.2.1) enhance parasympathetic activity in the gut and increase intestinal motility. They are rarely used for their gastro-intestinal effects but may be needed in cases of paralytic ileus, for example postoperatively. Organic obstruction of the gut must first be excluded and they should be used with caution in bowel anastomosis.

BISACODYL
Indications: constipation, bowel evacuation before radiological procedures, endoscopy, and surgery. Tablets act within 10–12 hours; suppositories act within 1 hour (see also section 1.6.5)
Cautions; Contra-indications; Side-effects: see general notes on stimulant laxatives. The tablets may cause gastro-intestinal disturbances. The suppositories may cause local irritation
Dose: by mouth for constipation, 10 mg after food, usually at night. Avoid taking with antacids
By rectum in suppositories for constipation, 10 mg usually in the morning; CHILD 5 mg
Before radiological procedures etc., 10 mg by mouth at bedtime for 2 days before examination and, if necessary, a 10-mg suppository 1 hour before examination. An enema may also be used immediately before the investigation (section 1.6.5)

Oral preparations
Bisacodyl Tablets, e/c, s/c, bisacodyl 5 mg. Price 20 tabs = A. Label: 5, 25
NHS **Dulcodos®** (Boehringer Ingelheim)
Tablets, e/c, s/c, bisacodyl 5 mg, dioctyl sodium sulphosuccinate 100 mg. Price 20 tabs = C. Label: 5, 25
Dose: 2 tablets, usually at bedtime; avoid taking with antacids

Dulcolax® (Boehringer Ingelheim)
NHS *Tablets,* yellow, e/c, s/c, bisacodyl 5 mg. Price 20 tabs = A. Label: 5, 25

Rectal preparations
Section 1.6.5

CASCARA
Indications: constipation. Acts within 6–8 hours
Cautions; Contra-indications; Side-effects: see notes on stimulant laxatives. The urine may be coloured red. Caution in nursing mothers

NHS **Cascara Tablets,** s/c unless otherwise indicated, 20 mg total hydroxyanthracene derivatives of which not less than 40% consists of cascarosides. Price 20 tabs (s/c) = A. Label: 14
Dose: 1–2 tablets, usually at bedtime

CASTOR OIL
Indications: constipation; bowel evacuation before radiological procedures, endoscopy, surgery. Acts within 2–8 hours
Cautions: menstruation. See also notes on stimulant laxatives
Contra-indications: intestinal obstruction
Side-effects: nausea, vomiting
Dose: 5–20 ml when required; CHILD up to 1 year 1–5 ml, 1–12 years 5–15 ml, in milk or fruit juice before breakfast or on an empty stomach
Price 100 ml = B

DANTHRON
Indications: constipation, bowel evacuation before radiological procedures, endoscopy, and surgery. Acts within 6–12 hours
Cautions; Contra-indications; Side-effects: see notes on stimulant laxatives. The urine may be coloured red. Avoid prolonged contact with skin (as in infants with napkins and in incontinent patients) since irritation and excoriation may occur. Caution in nursing mothers
Dose: constipation, 25–75 mg usually at bedtime; CHILD 12.5–25 mg
Before radiological procedures etc., 50–100 mg

Co-danthramer Capsules (Danthron and Poloxamer Capsules). When co-danthramer capsules are prescribed and no strength is stated capsules containing danthron 25 mg and poloxamer '188' 200 mg should be dispensed. Price 20 caps = C. Label: 14
Dose: constipation 1–2 capsules, usually at bedtime; CHILD 1 capsule
Before radiological procedures etc., 2–4 capsules
Co-danthramer Mixture (Danthron and Poloxamer Mixture). When co-danthramer mixture is prescribed and no strength is stated a mixture containing danthron 25 mg and poloxamer '188' 200 mg/5 ml should be dispensed. When strong co-danthramer mixture is prescribed a mixture containing danthron 75 mg and poloxamer '188' 1 g/5 ml should be dispensed. Diluent tragacanth mucilage or syrup, life of diluted mixture 14

days. Price, 100 ml (mixture) = **C**; 100 ml (strong mixture) = **D**. Label: 14
Dose: mixture, constipation, 5–10 ml, usually at bedtime; CHILD 2.5 ml.
Before radiological procedures etc. 10–20 ml.
Strong mixture, constipation, 5 ml, usually at bedtime
Co-danthrusate Capsules (Danthron and Dioctyl Sodium Sulphosuccinate Capsules). When co-danthrusate capsules are prescribed and no strength is stated capsules containing danthron 50 mg and dioctyl sodium sulphosuccinate 60 mg should be dispensed. Price 20 caps = **B**. Label: 14
Dose: 1–3 capsules, usually at bedtime; CHILD 6–12 years 1 capsule
Dorbanex® (Riker)
Capsules, yellow, danthron 25 mg, poloxamer '188' 200 mg. Price 20 caps = **C**. Label: 14
Dose: constipation 1–2 capsules, usually at bedtime; CHILD 1 capsule
Before radiological procedures etc., 2–4 capsules
Liquid (=mixture), orange, danthron 25 mg, poloxamer '188' 200 mg/5 ml. Diluent tragacanth mucilage or syrup, life of diluted elixir 14 days. Price 100 ml = **C**. Label: 14
Dose: constipation, 5–10 ml, usually at bedtime; CHILD 2.5 ml
Before radiological procedures etc., 10–20 ml
Liquid forte (=strong mixture), orange, danthron 75 mg, poloxamer '188' 1 g/5 ml. Diluent as above. Price 100 ml = **D**. Label: 14
Dose: constipation, 5 ml usually at bedtime
Normax® (Bencard)
Capsules, brown, danthron 50 mg, dioctyl sodium sulphosuccinate 60 mg. Price 20 caps = **B**. Label: 14
Dose: 1–3 capsules, usually at bedtime; CHILD 6–12 years 1 capsule

FIG
Indications: mild constipation (also has demulcent properties)

NHS **Figs Elixir, Compound** (figs syrup, compound), fig 3.2 g, cascara elixir 0.5 ml, compound rhubarb tincture 0.5 ml, senna liquid extract 1 ml/10 ml. Price 100 ml = **C**
Dose: 2.5–10 ml when required

SENNA
Indications: constipation; bowel evacuation before abdominal radiological procedures, endoscopy, and surgery. Acts in 8–12 hours
Cautions; Contra-indications; Side-effects: see introduction to stimulant laxatives. The urine may be coloured red

Senna Tablets, ≡ total sennosides 7.5 mg. Price 20 tabs = **A**. Label: 14

Dose: 2–4 tablets, usually at night; initial dose should be low then gradually increased; CHILD over 6 years, half adult dose
NHS **Agiolax®** (Rorer)
Granules, brown, s/c, sennoside B 0.31%, ispaghula seed 54.2%. Price 100 g = **D**; 250 g = **E**. Label: 14, 25, 27
Dose: 1–2 level 5 ml spoonfuls with water after supper and, if necessary, before breakfast or every 6 hours in resistant cases for 1–3 days; CHILD 5–12 years half the adult dose
Senokot® (R&C)
NHS Tablets, brown, ≡ sennoside B 7.5 mg. Price 20 tabs = **A**. Label: 14
Dose: 2–4 tablets, usually at bedtime; initial dose should be low then gradually increased; CHILD over 6 years, half adult dose
Granules, brown, sennoside B 14.9 mg/5 ml or 5.5 mg/g (one 5-ml spoonful = 2.7 g). Price 100 g = **D**. Label: 14
Dose: 5–10 ml, usually at bedtime; CHILD over 6 years 2.5–5 ml
Syrup (=elixir), brown, ≡ sennoside B 7.5 mg/5 ml. Diluent syrup, life of diluted elixir 14 days. Price 100 ml = **C**. Label: 14
Dose: 10–20 ml, usually at bedtime; CHILD 2–6 years 2.5–5 ml, over 6 years 5–10 ml
X-Prep® (Napp)
Liquid (=mixture), brown, total sennosides 72 mg/72 ml (for bowel evacuation before radiological procedures). Price 72-ml bottle = **B**
Dose: 72 ml with at least 2 tumblerfuls of water late in the afternoon of the day before the procedure; CHILD and underweight adult 1 ml/kg

SODIUM PICOSULPHATE
Indications: constipation, bowel evacuation before abdominal radiological procedures, endoscopy, and surgery
Cautions; Contra-indications; Side-effects: see general notes on stimulant laxatives
Dose: 5–15 mg, usually at bedtime; CHILD up to 5 years 2.5 mg, 6–12 years 2.5–5 mg

NHS **Laxoberal®** (WBP)
Elixir, yellow, sodium picosulphate 5 mg/5 ml. Diluent purified water, freshly boiled and cooled, life of diluted elixir 14 days. Acts within 10–14 hours. Price 100 ml = **C**
Picolax® (Nordic)
Oral powder, sodium picosulphate 10 mg/sachet, with magnesium citrate. For bowel evacuation before radiological procedures, surgery, colonoscopy, etc. Price 2 sachets = **C**
Dose: 1 sachet in water in the morning and a second in the afternoon of the day preceding investigatory or surgical procedures. Acts within 3 hours

1.6.3 Faecal softeners

These act by lubricating the faeces (for example liquid paraffin or poloxamer 188) or by softening the faeces (for example dioctyl sodium sulphosuccinate). This may cause sufficient rectal stimulation to promote a bowel action. These drugs are useful in the management of haemorrhoids and anal fissure. See also drugs administered rectally to relieve constipation (section 1.6.5).

DIOCTYL SODIUM SULPHOSUCCINATE
(Docusate Sodium)
Indications: constipation (acts within 1–2 days); aid in abdominal radiological procedures
Dose: constipation, up to 500 mg daily in divided doses; CHILD 12.5–25 mg 3 times daily. Initial doses should be large and gradually reduced
With barium meal, 400 mg

Dioctyl® (Medo)
Tablets, yellow, s/c, dioctyl sodium sulphosuccinate 100 mg. Price 20 tabs = C
Paediatric syrup (=elixir), yellow, dioctyl sodium sulphosuccinate 12.5 mg/5 ml (see section 1.6.5 for use as an enema). Diluent syrup, life of diluted elixir 14 days. Price 100 ml = B
Syrup (=elixir), dioctyl sodium sulphosuccinate 50 mg/5 ml (see section 1.6.5 for use as an enema). Diluent as above. Price 100 ml = C

LIQUID PARAFFIN
Indications: constipation
Cautions: avoid prolonged use
Side-effects: anal seepage of paraffin and consequent anal irritation after prolonged use, granulomatous reactions caused by absorption of small quantities of liquid paraffin (especially from the emulsion), lipoid pneumonia, and interference with the absorption of fat-soluble vitamins
Dose: 10–30 ml when required

Liquid Paraffin Mixture, liquid paraffin 5 ml/ 10 ml. Price 100 ml = A
Dose: 10–30 ml when required
NHS **Petrolagar No. 1®** (Wyeth)
Mixture, liquid paraffin 7%, light liquid paraffin 18%. Price 100 ml = B
Dose: 10 ml morning and night or after meals

1.6.4 Osmotic laxatives

These act by maintaining a volume of fluid in the bowel by osmosis.

Saline purgatives are commonly abused but are satisfactory for occasional use. Adequate fluid intake should be maintained. Magnesium sulphate is useful where rapid bowel evacuation is required; a dose taken before breakfast or on an empty stomach and followed by a tumblerful of warm fluid usually causes evacuation within 2 hours. Sodium salts should be avoided as they may give rise to sodium and water retention in susceptible individuals.

Lactulose is a semi-synthetic disaccharide which is not absorbed from the gastro-intestinal tract. It produces an osmotic diarrhoea of low faecal pH, and discourages the proliferation of ammonia-producing organisms. It is therefore useful in the treatment of hepatic encephalopathy.

LACTULOSE
Indications: constipation (acts within 2 days), hepatic encephalopathy
Contra-indications: galactosaemia, intestinal obstruction
Side-effects: occasional nausea and vomiting
Dose: expressed in terms of the elixir containing lactulose 3.35 g/5 ml
Constipation, initially 15 ml twice daily, gradually reduced according to patient's needs; CHILD under 1 year 2.5 ml, 1–5 years 5 ml, 6–12 years 10 ml twice daily, gradually reduced
Hepatic encephalopathy, 30–50 ml 3 times daily, subsequently adjusted to produce 2–3 soft stools daily

Lactulose Solution, lactulose 3.35 g/5 ml with other ketoses. Price 100 ml = C
NHS **Duphalac®** (Duphar)
Syrup (=elixir), pale yellow, lactulose 3.35 g/ 5 ml with other ketoses. Price 100 ml = C

MAGNESIUM CARBONATE
Indications: mild constipation (acts within 2–4 hours)
Cautions: use only occasionally; the elderly, in renal impairment. Drug interactions: see Appendix 1 (section *15*)
Contra-indications: intestinal obstruction
Side-effects: eructation due to liberated carbon dioxide
Dose: 2–5 g followed by a tumblerful of water when required

Preparations
Section 1.1.1

MAGNESIUM HYDROXIDE
Indications: mild constipation (acts within 2–4 hours)
Cautions; Contra-indications: see under Magnesium Carbonate
Dose: 2–4 g followed by a tumblerful of water, when required

Liquid Paraffin and Magnesium Hydroxide Mixture, magnesium hydroxide mixture 7.35 ml, liquid paraffin 2.5 ml, chloroform spirit 0.15 ml/ 10 ml. Price 100 ml = A
Dose: 5–20 ml when required
Magnesium Hydroxide Mixture, magnesium oxide (hydrated) about 550 mg/10 ml. Do not store in a cold place. Price 100 ml = A
Dose: 25–50 ml when required

MAGNESIUM SULPHATE
Indications: rapid bowel evacuation (acts within 2–4 hours)
Cautions; Contra-indications: see under Magnesium Carbonate

C = 51-100p, D = 101-180p, E = 181-300p, F = 301-450p, G = 451-650p, H = 651-900p, I = 901-1200p, J = over 1200p.

Side-effects: colic
Dose: 5–15 g with 100–200 ml of water before breakfast or on an empty stomach; CHILD 100–250 mg/kg when required

Magnesium Sulphate (Epsom salts). Price 20 g = **A**. Label: 13, 23
Magnesium Sulphate Mixture, magnesium sulphate 4 g/10 ml (see Formulary). Price 200 ml = **B**. Label: 23
Dose: 10–20 ml with water or on an empty stomach; CHILD 5–10 ml

1.6.5   Rectally administered laxatives

Enemas containing **arachis oil** or **dioctyl sodium sulphosuccinate**, and **glycerol** suppositories lubricate and soften impacted faeces and promote a bowel movement.

Bisacodyl (Dulcolax®), **dioctyl sodium sulphosuccinate** and **phosphate enemas** are useful in bowel clearance before radiological procedures, endoscopy, and surgery.

The use of soft soap enema should be **avoided**, especially in pregnancy as it may inflame the colonic mucosa.

Bisacodyl Suppositories, bisacodyl 10 mg. Price 12 suppos = **C**
Bisacodyl Suppositories, Paediatric, bisacodyl 5 mg. Price 12 suppos = **C**
Glycerol Suppositories, gelatin 140 mg, glycerol 700 mg, purified water to 1 g. Price 12 suppos, child and infant (both) = **B**; adult = **C**
Dose: 1 suppository moistened with water before use. The usual sizes are for *infants* small (1-g mould), *children* medium (2-g mould), *adults* large (4-g mould)
Phosphates Enema Formula B, sodium acid phosphate 12.8 g, sodium phosphate 10.24 g, purified water, freshly boiled and cooled, to 128 ml. Price 128 ml = **B**
Dose: adults and children over 6 years 128 ml; CHILD 3–6 years 50 ml
NHS **Beogex®** (Pharmax)
Adult suppositories, sodium acid phosphate 1.72 g in an effervescent basis. Price 6 suppos = **B**
Dose: 1 suppository, inserted 30 .ninutes before evacuation is required. Moisten with water before use
Dioctyl® (Medo)—see section 1.6.3 for oral preparations used by rectum
Paediatric syrup (= elixir, used also as enema). Price 100 ml = **B**
Dose: by rectum, 15–40 ml; CHILD up to 1 year 5–10 ml, over 1 year 7.5–15 ml
Syrup (= elixir), dilute with 3 parts of water for use instead of the paediatric syrup, as an enema. Price 100 ml = **C**
Dulcolax® (Boehringer Ingelheim)
NHS *Suppositories,* bisacodyl 10 mg. Price 12 suppos = **B**
Dose: 1 suppository inserted 20–60 minutes before evacuation is required. For use in radiological procedures see section 1.6.2

Paediatric suppositories, bisacodyl 5 mg. Price 12 suppos = **C**
Dose: CHILD up to 10 years 1 suppository inserted 20–60 minutes before evacuation is required
Rectal solution (= enema), bisacodyl 2.74 mg/ml in macrogol basis. Price 100 ml = **C**
Dose: for bowel evacuation before radiological procedures, endoscopy, and surgery, 2–3 ml; CHILD 1–2 ml
Mixed with barium sulphate enema, 2–5 ml for every 1–3 litres of barium sulphate enema

Fletchers' Arachis Oil Retention Enema® (Pharmax)
Enema, arachis oil in 130-ml single-dose disposable packs. Price 130 ml = **D**
Dose: 130 ml; the enema should be warmed before use

Fletchers' Enemette® (Pharmax)
Enema, dioctyl sodium sulphosuccinate 90 mg, glycerol 3.78 g, macrogol 2.25 g, sorbic acid 5 mg/5 ml. Price 5-ml unit = **B**
Dose: adults and children over 3 years, 5 ml when required

Fletchers' Magnesium Sulphate Retention Enema® (Pharmax)
Enema, magnesium sulphate 50%, in 130-ml single-dose disposable packs. Price 130 ml = **C** (Hosp. only)
Dose: as an aid in neurosurgery, 130 ml

Fletchers' Phosphate Enema® (Pharmax)
Enema, phosphates enema formula B (see above). Price 128 ml with a standard tube = **B**; with long rectal tube = **C**
Dose: 128 ml when required

Klyx® (Ferring)
Enema, dioctyl sodium sulphosuccinate 0.1%, sorbitol 25% in single-dose disposable packs (with a plastic sleeve). Price 120 and 240 ml (both) = **B**
Dose: 120 or 240 ml; preferably retained for 5 minutes

Micralax Micro-enema® (SK&F)
Enema, sodium citrate 450 mg, sodium alkylsulphoacetate 45 mg, sorbic acid 5 mg in a viscous solution in 5-ml single-dose disposable packs with nozzle. Price 5 ml = **B**
Dose: adults and children over 3 years, 5 ml when required

Micolette Micro-enema® (Ayerst)
Enema, sodium citrate 450 mg, sodium lauryl sulphoacetate 45 mg, glycerol 625 mg in a viscous solution, in 5-ml single-dose disposable packs with nozzle. Price 5 ml = **B**
Dose: 5–10 ml

Relaxit Micro-enema® (Pharmacia)
Enema, sodium citrate 450 mg, sodium lauryl sulphate 75 mg, sorbic acid 5 mg, in a viscous solution in 5-ml single-dose disposable packs with nozzle. Price 5 ml = **B**
Dose: 5 ml

Veripaque® (Sterling Research)
Enema, powder for reconstitution, oxyphenisatin 50 mg in 3 g. Price 1 vial = **D**
Dose: before diagnostic procedures or surgery, oxyphenisatin 50 mg in 2 litres of water (or *pro*

---

rata) given over 5–8 minutes

Mixed with barium sulphate enema, oxyphenisatin 50 mg for every 2 litres of barium sulphate enema (or *pro rata*)

1.6.6 Other laxatives

Unstandardised preparations of cascara, frangula, rhubarb, and senna should be **avoided** as their laxative action is unpredictable.

Aloes, colocynth, and jalap should be **avoided** as they have a drastic purgative action.

Phenolphthalein should be **avoided** as it may cause rashes, albuminuria, and haemoglobinuria. Its laxative effects may continue for several days because of enterohepatic recycling.

NHS **Liquid Paraffin and Phenolphthalein Mixture,** phenolphthalein 30 mg/10 ml in liquid paraffin mixture. Price 100 ml = **A**. Label: 14
Dose: 5–20 ml, usually at bedtime
NHS **Phenolphthalein Tablets,** phenolphthalein 125 mg. Price 20 tabs = **C**. Label: 14
Dose: 125 mg, usually at bedtime
NHS **Rhubarb Mixture, Compound** (see Formulary). Price 100 ml = **A**
Dose: 10–20 ml, usually at bedtime
NHS **Rhubarb and Soda Mixture, Ammoniated** (see Formulary). Price 100 ml = **A**
Dose: 10–20 ml, usually at bedtime
NHS **Agarol**® (Warner)
Mixture, phenolphthalein 66 mg, liquid paraffin 1.6 ml, agar 10 mg/5 ml. Diluent water for preparations, life of diluted mixture 28 days. Price 100 ml = **B**. Label: 14
Dose: 5–15 ml, usually at bedtime
NHS **Alophen**® (P-D)
Pills, brown, f/c, aloin 15 mg, belladonna dry extract 5 mg, ipecacuanha 4 mg, phenolphthalein 30 mg. Price 20 pills = **B**. Label: 14
Dose: 1–3 pills, usually at bedtime
NHS **Kest**® (Berk)
Tablets, magnesium sulphate 300 mg, phenolphthalein 50 mg. Price 20 tabs = **A**. Label: 14
Dose: 1 tablet with water at bedtime and 2 tablets in the morning
NHS PoM **Opobyl**® (Bengué)
Pills, blue, aloes 20 mg, bile salts 50 mg, boldo extract 10 mg, euonymus 2 mg, desiccated liver 50 mg, podophyllin 2 mg. Price 20 pills = **B**
Dose: 1–2 pills when required
NHS **Petrolagar No. 2**® (Wyeth)
Mixture, phenolphthalein 17.5 mg, liquid paraffin 0.35 ml, light liquid paraffin 0.9 ml/5 ml. Price 100 ml = **B**. Label: 14
Dose: 10 ml morning and night

1.7 Rectal and colonic drugs

1.7.1 Soothing agents
1.7.2 Rectal corticosteroids
1.7.3 Compound preparations with corticosteroids
1.7.4 Other rectal preparations

Anal and perianal pruritus, soreness, and excoriation are best treated by application of bland ointments, suppositories, and dusting-powders (section 1.7.1). These conditions occur commonly in patients suffering from haemorrhoids, fistulas, and proctitis. Careful local toilet as well as adjustment of the diet to avoid hard stools, and bulk-forming materials such as bran (section 1.6.1) and

a high residue diet are also helpful. In proctitis these measures may supplement treatment with corticosteroids or sulphasalazine.

When necessary topical preparations containing **local anaesthetics** (section 1.7.1) or **corticosteroids** (section 1.7.3) are used provided perianal thrush has been excluded. This infection is best treated with **nystatin** by mouth and by local application (see sections 5.2 and 13.10.2).

Proctitis may be treated with suppositories or enemas containing **corticosteroids** (section 1.7.2) or **sulphasalazine** (section 1.5).

Glycerol suppositories and phosphates enemas are occasionally used for their local action in severe constipation (section 1.6.5).

See also sections 13.2.1 and 13.10.5 for preparations used in napkin rash.

1.7.1 Soothing agents

Bland soothing preparations may contain mild astringents such as bismuth subgallate, zinc oxide, and hamamelis. Many proprietary preparations also contain lubricants (such as lauromacrogol 400 and sodium oleate); vasoconstrictors (adrenaline, ephedrine, phenylephrine); or mild antiseptics (chlorothymol, Peru balsam, bronopol, and resorcinol). Prolonged application of preparations containing **resorcinol** should be **avoided** because they may interfere with thyroid function. Heparinoids are used to promote the resorption of local oedema and extravasated blood.

Soothing agents such as **hamamelis suppositories** may give symptomatic relief in haemorrhoids.

Local anaesthetics are used to relieve pain associated with haemorrhoids, anal fissure, and pruritus ani. They are added to many proprietary preparations. They should be used only for short periods (no longer than 2 weeks) as they may cause sensitisation of the anal skin.

Lignocaine gel and ointment (see section 15.2) may be useful for application to anal fissures and are best applied on a plastic dilator. This ensures that the ointment comes into contact with the base of the fissure and encourages healing.

Alternative local anaesthetics include amethocaine, cinchocaine, and pramoxine, but they are more irritant.

ADMINISTRATION. Unless otherwise indicated a suppository is usually inserted into the rectum night and morning and after defaecation. Rectal ointments and creams are applied night and morning and after defaecation, externally or by rectum using a rectal nozzle.

Bismuth Subgallate Suppositories, Compound, bismuth subgallate 200 mg, castor oil 60 mg, resorcinol 60 mg, zinc oxide 120 mg, in theobroma oil or other suitable basis. Price 12 suppos = **D**
Hamamelis Suppositories, hamamelis dry extract, usual strength 200 mg in theobroma oil or other suitable basis. Price 12 suppos = **D**
Hamamelis and Zinc Oxide Suppositories. Usual strength hamamelis dry extract 200 mg, zinc oxide 600 mg. Price 12 suppos = **E**

C = 51–100p, **D** = 101–180p, **E** = 181–300p, **F** = 301–450p, **G** = 451–650p, **H** = 651–900p, **I** = 901–1200p, **J** = over 1200p.

Alcos-Anal® (Norgine)
Ointment, sodium oleate 10%, lauromacrogol
'400' 2%, chlorothymol 0.1%. Price 20 g (with
applicator) = **D**
Suppositories, sodium oleate 200 mg, lauro-
macrogol '400' 20 mg, chlorothymol 700 micrograms. Price 10 suppos = **D**
Anodesyn® (Crookes Products)
Ointment, ephedrine hydrochloride 0.25%, lignocaine hydrochloride 0.5%, allantoin 0.5%.
Price 25 g = **C**
Prolonged use should be avoided
Suppositories, ephedrine hydrochloride 5.1 mg,
lignocaine hydrochloride 10.25 mg, allantoin
10.25 mg, bronopol 4.1 mg. Price 12
suppos = **C**
Prolonged use should be avoided
Anusol® (Warner)
Cream, bismuth oxide 2.14%, Peru balsam
1.8%, zinc oxide 10.75%. Price 23 g (with rectal
nozzle) = **C**
Ointment, bismuth oxide 0.875%, bismuth
subgallate 2.25%, zinc oxide 10.75%, Peru
balsam 1.875%. Price 25 g (with rectal
nozzle) = **C**
Suppositories, bismuth oxide 24 mg, bismuth
subgallate 59 mg, Peru balsam 49 mg, zinc oxide
296 mg. Price 12 suppos = **C**
Bismodyne® (Loveridge)
Ointment, bismuth subgallate 2%, hexachloro-
phane 0.5%, lignocaine 0.5%, zinc oxide 7.5%.
Price 25 g (with applicator) = **C**
Prolonged use should be avoided
Suppositories, bismuth subgallate 150 mg, hexa-
chlorophane 2.5 mg, lignocaine 10 mg, zinc
oxide 120 mg. Price 12 suppos = **C**
Prolonged use should be avoided
Lasonil® (Bayer)
Ointment, hyaluronidase 150 units, heparinoids
equivalent to 50 units of heparin/g. Price
14 g = **B**; 40 g = **D** (both with applicator)
Nestosyl® (Bengué)
Ointment, benzocaine 2%, butyl aminobenzoate 2%,
hexachlorophane 0.1%, resorcinol 2%, zinc oxide 10%.
Price 30 g (with rectal nozzle) = **C**
Prolonged use should be avoided

1.7.2   Rectal corticosteroids

Corticosteroids are used to relieve inflammation
but should only be used for limited periods and
when the presence of infection has been excluded.
Hydrocortisone cream and ointment are useful
for treating the perianal regions. **Hydrocortisone
suppositories** and, for larger areas, the corticosteroid **retention enemas** are used to relieve
the inflammation of ulcerative colitis and proctitis.
Corticosteroid retention enemas are best administered by laying the patient on the left side with
the knees drawn up and buttock elevated on a
small pillow. The tip of the rectal catheter or unit,
lubricated with soft paraffin, is then inserted into
the anal orifice. The contents are slowly injected,
the unit removed, and the patient instructed to
roll over to lie face downwards for 3–5 minutes.
The patient then sleeps in the most comfortable
position, retaining the enema for as long as

possible. In patients with diarrhoea the administration of propantheline bromide 30 mg, given
30 minutes before the enema is administered, will
facilitate retention. Corticosteroid foam preparations such as **Colifoam**® may be a useful alternative for patients with difficulty in retaining corticosteroid enemas.
    In hospitalised patients, hydrocortisone may be
administered by slow rectal drip and this method
achieves deepest penetration into the colon. It
is given over approximately 30 minutes using a
transfusion set attached to a rectal catheter. See
section 6.3.4 for hydrocortisone injections.
    Oral **sulphasalazine** (section 1.5) may sup-
plement these treatments if necessary.
    For compound rectal preparations with cor-
ticosteroids see section 1.7.3.

HYDROCORTISONE

Indications: inflammation associated with colitis,
    proctitis, haemorrhoids, and related conditions
Cautions; Contra-indications; Side-effects: see
    section 6.3.3. Prolonged use should be avoided.
    Avoid use of enemas and rectal foams in
    obstruction, bowel perforation, and extensive
    fistulas. Contra-indicated in untreated infection

PoM **Hydrocortisone Cream,** hydrocortisone or
hydrocortisone acetate 1%—see section 13.4
Apply sparingly to perianal area 2–4 times daily
when required
PoM **Hydrocortisone Ointment,** hydrocortisone
0.5, 1, or 2.5%—see section 13.4
Apply sparingly to perianal area 2–4 times daily
when required

PoM **Hydrocortisone Suppositories,** hydrocortisone or hydrocortisone acetate 25 mg in theobroma oil or other suitable basis. Price 6
suppos = **D**
Dose: 1 suppository inserted night and morning
and after defaecation
PoM **Colifoam**® (Stafford-Miller)
Foam in aerosol pack, hydrocortisone acetate
10%. Price 25 g (14 applications) with applicator = **H**
    Dose: initially 1 applicatorful (125 mg hydro-
    cortisone acetate) inserted into the rectum once
    or twice daily for 2–3 weeks, then once on
    alternate days
PoM **Cortenema**® (Bengué)
Retention enema, hydrocortisone (partially solu-
bilised) 100 mg/60 ml in viscous suspension, in
single-dose disposable packs with nozzle. Price
7 × 60-ml enemas = **G**
    Dose: initially 1 enema at bedtime for 2–3
    weeks; then alternate days. The enema should
    be retained for at least 1 hour

BETAMETHASONE VALERATE

Indications: inflammation of the anus and peri-
    anal regions
Cautions; Contra-indications; Side-effects: see
    under Hydrocortisone

Betnovate rectal preparations: section 1.7.3
Betnovate cream and ointment: section 13.4

Relative prices: **A** = up to 20p, **B** = 21-50p,

PREDNISOLONE
Indications; Cautions; Contra-indications; Side-effects: see under Hydrocortisone

PoM **Predenema**® (Pharmax)
Retention enema, prednisolone 20 mg (as the sodium metasulphobenzoate salt) in 100-ml single-dose disposable pack. Price 7 × 100-ml enemas, standard tube = **G**; long tube = **H**
Dose: initially 1 enema at bedtime for 2–4 weeks; then on alternate days. The enema should be retained for at least 1 hour

PoM **Predsol**® (Glaxo)
Retention enema, prednisolone 20 mg (as the sodium phosphate salt) in 100-ml single-dose disposable packs fitted with a nozzle. Price 7 × 100-ml enemas = **G**
Dose: initially 1 enema at bedtime for 2–4 weeks then reduced. The enema should be retained for at least 1 hour
Suppositories, prednisolone 5 mg (as the sodium phosphate salt). Price 10 suppos = **C**
Dose: 1 suppository inserted night and morning and after defaecation

1.7.3 Compound preparations with corticosteroids

See section 1.7.2 for discussion of corticosteroids used locally in diseases of the colon and rectum and section 1.7.1 for other ingredients of rectal preparations.

Rectal preparations which contain **antibiotics** should be **avoided** because they are generally ineffective owing to the large bacterial population in the bowel and the development of resistance; hypersensitivity may also occur.

ADMINISTRATION. Unless otherwise indicated a suppository is inserted into the rectum night and morning and after defaecation. Rectal ointments and creams are applied night and morning and after defaecation, externally or by rectum using a rectal nozzle. Prolonged use should be avoided.

PoM **Anacal**® (Luitpold)
Rectal ointment, hexachlorophane 0.5%, lauromacrogol '400' 5%, heparinoid 0.2%, prednisolone 0.15%. Price 30 g (with rectal nozzle) = **F**
Apply 1–4 times daily
Suppositories, hexachlorophane 5 mg, lauromacrogol '400' 50 mg, a heparinoid 4 mg, prednisolone 1 mg. Price 10 suppos = **D**
PoM **Anugesic-HC**® (Warner)
Cream, benzyl benzoate 1.2%, bismuth oxide 0.875%, hydrocortisone acetate 0.5%, Peru balsam 1.85%, pramoxine hydrochloride 1%, resorcinol 0.875%, zinc oxide 12.35%. Price 15 g (with rectal nozzle) = **E**
PoM **Anugesic-HC**® (Warner)
Suppositories, benzyl benzoate 33 mg, bismuth oxide 24 mg, bismuth subgallate 59 mg, hydrocortisone acetate 5 mg, Peru balsam 49 mg, pramoxine hydrochloride 27 mg, zinc oxide 296 mg. Price 12 suppos = **E**
PoM **Anusol-HC**© (Warner)
Ointment, benzyl benzoate 1.25%, bismuth oxide

0.875%, bismuth subgallate 2.25%, hydrocortisone acetate 0.25%, Peru balsam 1.875%, resorcinol 0.875%, zinc oxide 10.75%. Price 15 g (with rectal nozzle) = **E**
Suppositories, benzyl benzoate 33 mg, bismuth oxide 24 mg, bismuth subgallate 59 mg, hydrocortisone acetate 10 mg, Peru balsam 49 mg, resorcinol 24 mg, zinc oxide 296 mg. Price 12 suppos = **D**

PoM **Betnovate**® (Glaxo)
Rectal ointment, betamethasone valerate 0.05%, lignocaine hydrochloride 2.5%, phenylephrine hydrochloride 0.1%. Price 25 g (with applicator) = **C**
Apply 2–3 times daily until inflammation subsides then once daily, externally or by rectum, max. 25 g weekly
Compound suppositories, betamethasone valerate 500 micrograms, lignocaine hydrochloride 40 mg, phenylephrine hydrochloride 2 mg. Price 10 suppos = **C**
PoM **Proctofoam HC**® (Stafford-Miller)
Foam in aerosol pack, hydrocortisone acetate 1%, pramoxine hydrochloride 1%. Price 24-g pack (approx. 40 applications) with applicator = **G**
Insert 1 applicatorful (4–6 mg hydrocortisone acetate, 4–6 mg pramoxine hydrochloride) by rectum 2–3 times daily and after defaecation or apply perianally as required

PoM **Proctosedyl**® (Roussel)
Ointment, aesculin 1%, cinchocaine hydrochloride 0.5%, framycetin sulphate 1%, hydrocortisone 0.5%. Price 30 g = **G** (with cannula)
Suppositories, aesculin 10 mg, cinchocaine hydrochloride 5 mg, framycetin sulphate 10 mg, hydrocortisone 5 mg. Price 12 suppos = **E**
PoM **Scheriproct**® (Schering)
Ointment, cinchocaine hydrochloride 0.5%, clemizole undecenoate 1%, prednisolone hexanoate 0.19%. Price 30 g = **F**
In severe cases use 3–4 times daily on first day then once or twice daily, externally or by rectum
Suppositories, cinchocaine hydrochloride 1 mg, clemizole undecenoate 5 mg, prednisolone hexanoate 1.3 mg. Price 12 suppos = **E**
Dose: in severe cases insert 1 suppository 2–3 times daily and then once daily after defaecation
PoM **Ultraproct**® (Schering)
Ointment, cinchocaine hydrochloride 0.5%, clemizole undecenoate 1%, fluocortolone hexanoate 0.095%, fluocortolone pivalate 0.092%. Price 10 g (with rectal nozzle) = **D**
In severe cases apply 3–4 times on the first day then once or twice daily
Suppositories, cinchocaine hydrochloride 1 mg, clemizole undecenoate 5 mg, fluocortolone hexanoate 630 micrograms, fluocortolone pivalate 610 micrograms. Price 12 suppos = **E**
Dose: in severe cases insert 1 suppository 2–3 times daily then once daily or on alternate days after defaecation
PoM **Uniroid**® (Unigreg)
Ointment, cinchocaine hydrochloride 0.5%, hydrocortisone 0.5%, neomycin sulphate 0.5%, polymyxin B sulphate 6250 units/g. Price 15 g (with applicator) = **D**
Suppositories, cinchocaine hydrochloride 5 mg, hydrocortisone 5 mg, neomycin sulphate 10 mg, polymyxin B sulphate 12500 units. Price 10 suppos = **D**

C = 51-100p, **D** = 101-180p, **E** = 181-300p, **F** = 301-450p, **G** = 451-650p, **H** = 651-900p, **I** = 901-1200p, **J** = over 1200p.

PoM **Xyloproct**® (Astra)
Ointment (=cream), aluminium acetate 3.5%, hydrocortisone acetate 0.275%, lignocaine 5%, zinc oxide 18%. Price 30 g (with applicator) = **F**
  Apply several times daily
Suppositories, aluminium acetate 50 mg, hydrocortisone acetate 5 mg, lignocaine 60 mg, zinc oxide 400 mg. Price 10 suppos = **D**
  Dose: 1 suppository at night and after defaecation

1.7.4   Other rectal preparations

Oily phenol injection is used to inject haemorrhoids particularly when unprolapsed.

Sulphasalazine enemas and suppositories are available for use in proctitis (section 1.5), but are generally not employed except in patients who cannot tolerate the side-effects of oral administration.

PHENOL
Indications: injection of haemorrhoidal veins
Side-effects: irritation, tissue necrosis
Dose: 2–3 ml of oily phenol injection into the submucosal layer at the base of the pile; several injections may be given at different sites, max. total injected 10 ml at any one time

PoM **Oily Phenol Injection,** phenol 5% in almond oil or other suitable oil. Price 2- and 5-ml amp (both) = **B**; 25-ml vial = **D**

1.8   Stoma care

1.8.1 Local care of stoma
1.8.2 Prescribing for patients with stoma

1.8.1   Local care of stoma

Patients are usually given advice about the use of cleansing agents, protective creams, lotions, deodorants, or sealants whilst in hospital, either by the surgeon or by the health authority stoma care nurses. Voluntary organisations offer help and support to patients with stoma.

Items in the following list are prescribable as drugs or as accessories to stoma appliances (see Drug Tariff).

Adhesives
Aquadry® (Raymed)
  Medical adhesive. Price 20 ml (with brush) = **E**
Chiron® (Downs)
  Skin adhesive. Price 52-g tube = **F**
Dow Corning DC 355® (Dow Corning)
  Medical adhesive brushable. Price 20-ml bottle (with brush) = **E**
Dow Corning Medical Adhesive B Spray® (Dow Corning)
  Spray adhesive. Price 170-g aerosol spray = **H**
Hollister® (Abbott)
  Medical adhesive spray (with silicones). Price per aerosol spray = **I**
Saltair® (Salt)
  Ostomy adhesive solution. Price per tube = **C**
  Caution: flammable

Adhesive removers
Dow Corning Remover® (Dow Corning)
  Adhesive remover spray. For removal of Medical Adhesive B Spray. Price 170-g aerosol spray = **G**
Hollister® (Abbott)
  Adhesive remover spray. Price per aerosol spray = **I**
Raymed Plaster Remover® (Raymed)
  Adhesive remover spray. Price per unit = **D**
Salts 'SPR' Plaster Remover® (Salt)
  Adhesive remover spray. Price 150-g aerosol spray = **D**
  Caution: flammable

Deodorants
Atmocol® is used as a deodorising spray when emptying the appliance. The other deodorants listed are placed in the appliance.

Atmocol® (Raymed)
  Aerosol deodorant. Price 1 unit (400 sprays) = **D**
Chironair Odour Control Liquid® (Downs)
  Deodorant solution. Price 115 ml = **F**
Dor® (Simpla)
  Deodorant solution. Price 7 ml = **C**
Nilodor® (Loxley)
  Deodorant solution. Price (with dropper) 7.5 ml = **D**; 15 ml = **E**
Ostobon® (Coloplast)
  Deodorant powder. Price 22 g = **E**
Saltair No-Roma® (Salt)
  Deodorant solution. Price 30 ml = **C**; 300 ml = **E**
Stomogel® (Raymed)
  Deodorant gel. Price 50 g = **E**
Translet Plus One® (Franklin)
  Deodorant solution for men. Price 7 ml = **E**
Translet Plus Two® (Franklin)
  Deodorant solution for women. Price 7 ml = **E**

Skin protectives, fillers, and cleansers
Chiron® (Downs)
  Barrier cream (with antiseptic). Price 52 g = **E**
Comfeel® (Coloplast)
  Elastic ostomy paste. Price 60 g = **E**
Downs Karaya Gel® (Downs)
  Gel. Price 35 g = **F**
Downs Karaya Gum Powder® (Downs)
  Powder. Price 100 g = **F**
Downs Ostomy Seal Protective Paste® (Downs)
  Paste. Price 52 g = **F**
Hollister® (Abbott)
  Karaya paste. Price 128 g = **F**
  Do not apply to severely excoriated skin
  Karaya powder. Price 71 g = **F**
  Skin gel. Price 28 g = **F**
  Caution: flammable
  Do not apply to severely excoriated skin
Orabase® (Squibb)
  Paste, see section 12.3.1
Orahesive® (Squibb)
  Powder (with adherent properties), see section 12.3.1
Saltair® (Salt)
  Karaya gum powder. Price 115 g = **E**
  Lotion. Price 110 g = **D**. For sore or excoriated skin
  Ostomy cleansing soap (soap spirit). Price per bottle = **D**
  'Protect' Friar's Balsam Spray (compound benzoin tincture). Price 150 g aerosol spray = **E**
Simpla Sassco® (Simpla)
  Gel. Price 95 g = **B**
Stomahesive® (Squibb)
  Paste. Price 60 g = **F**. For filling and sealing skin creases
Stomobar® (Raymed)
  Barrier cream. Price per unit = **D**
Stomosol® (Raymed)
  Antiseptic liquid. Dilute before use. Price 200 ml = **F**

Translet® (Franklin)
Barrier cream. Price 51 g = **D**

1.8.2 Prescribing for patients with stoma

Enteric-coated and *sustained-release* preparations are **unsuitable**, particularly in patients with ileostomies, as there may not be sufficient release of the active ingredient.

Laxatives. Enemas and washouts should **not** be prescribed for patients with ileostomies as they may cause rapid and severe dehydration.

Colostomy patients may suffer from constipation and whenever possible should be treated by increasing fluid intake or dietary fibre. **Bulk-forming laxatives** (section 1.6.1) should be tried. If they are insufficient, as small a dose as possible of danthron or senna (section 1.6.2) should be used. Preparations such as X-Prep® should be avoided when preparing patients for radiological procedures as they may cause severe dehydration with nausea, vomiting, and griping.

Antidiarrhoeals. Intestinal sedatives such as **loperamide**, **codeine phosphate**, or **diphenoxylate** (with atropine) are effective. Bulk-forming drugs (section 1.6.1) may be tried but it is often difficult to adjust the dose appropriately.

Antibiotics should **not** be given for an episode of acute diarrhoea.

Antacids. The tendency to diarrhoea from magnesium salts or constipation from aluminium salts may be increased in these patients.

Diuretics should be used with caution in patients with ileostomies as they may become excessively dehydrated and potassium depletion may easily occur. It is usually advisable to use a **potassium-sparing** diuretic (see section 2.2.3).

Digoxin. Patients with a stoma are particularly susceptible to hypokalaemia whilst on digoxin therapy and potassium supplements may be advisable (see section 9.2.1.1).

Potassium supplements. Liquid formulations are preferred to sustained-release formulations.

Analgesics. Narcotic analgesics (see sections 4.7.1.2 and 4.7.2) may cause troublesome constipation in colostomy patients. When a non-narcotic analgesic is required **paracetamol** is usually suitable but anti-inflammatory analgesics may cause gastric irritation and bleeding.

Iron preparations may cause loose stools and sore skin in these patients. If this is troublesome and if iron is definitely indicated one of the intramuscular iron preparations (see section 9.1.1.2) should be used. Sustained-release preparations should be **avoided** for the reasons given above.

1.9 Drugs affecting intestinal secretions

1.9.1 Drugs acting on the gall bladder
1.9.2 Drugs which increase gastric acidity
1.9.3 Aprotinin
1.9.4 Pancreatin supplements
1.9.5 Other pancreatin preparations

For electrolyte content of gastro-intestinal secretions see section 9.2.4, Table 4.

1.9.1 Drugs acting on the gall bladder

Oral **chenodeoxycholic** or **ursodeoxycholic acid** therapy is used in certain patients to dissolve cholesterol gallstones. It is used in selected patients as an alternative to elective surgery where surgery is inadvisable or the patient expresses preference for medical treatment. Chenodeoxycholic and ursodeoxycholic acid therapy is used in patients who have mild symptoms, unimpaired gall bladder function, and small or medium sized radiolucent stones; the treatment is not suitable for patients with radio-opaque stones, which are unlikely to be dissolved. Treatment is longer and less effective in patients with large stones. Patients should preferably be hospital supervised because radiological monitoring is required. Long-term prophylaxis may be needed after complete dissolution of the gallstones has been confirmed (preferably with cholecystograms and ultrasound on two separate occasions) as gallstones may recur in up to 25% of patients within one year of stopping treatment. A **terpene** mixture (Rowachol®) also raises biliary cholesterol solubility. It is less effective than the bile acids but may be a useful adjunct.

Ursodeoxycholic acid (Destolit®) has a similar action to chenodeoxycholic acid. It rarely causes diarrhoea, a side-effect that limits the value of chenodeoxycholic acid.

Dehydrocholic acid is used to improve biliary drainage by stimulating the secretion of thin watery bile. It is given after surgery of the biliary tract to flush the common duct and drainage tube and wash away small calculi obstructing flow through the common bile duct but its value has not been established.

CHENODEOXYCHOLIC ACID

Indications: dissolution of cholesterol gallstones (see notes above)
Cautions: see notes above
Contra-indications: do not use when stones are radio-opaque, in pregnancy, in non-functioning gall bladders, in chronic liver disease, and inflammatory diseases of the small intestine and colon
Side-effects: diarrhoea particularly initially with high dosage (reduce dose for few days), pruritus, minor hepatic abnormalities and transient rise in serum transaminases
Dose: 10–15 mg/kg daily as a single dose at bedtime *or* in divided doses for 3–24 months, depending on size of stone; treatment is continued for 3 months after stones dissolve

PoM **Chenodeoxycholic Acid Capsules,** chenodeoxycholic acid 125 and 250 mg, price 20 caps (both) = **F**
PoM **Chendol**® (CP)
Capsules, orange/white, chenodeoxycholic acid 125 mg. Price 20 caps = **F**
Tablets, orange, f/c, scored, chenodeoxycholic acid 250 mg. Price 20 tabs = **H**

C = 51-100p, **D** = 101-180p, **E** = 181-300p, **F** = 301-450p, **G** = 451-650p, **H** = 651-900p, **I** = 901-1200p, **J** = over 1200p.

PoM **Chenocedon**® (Tillotts)
Capsules, green/blue, chenodeoxycholic acid 250 mg. Price 20 caps = **F**

PoM **Chenofalk**® (Thames)
Capsules, chenodeoxycholic acid 250 mg. Price 20 caps = **G**

DEHYDROCHOLIC ACID

Indications: (improves biliary drainage) biliary tract surgery; to flush away small calculi in the bile duct; to accelerate visualisation and aid elimination of contrast media in the gall bladder

Contra-indications: complete mechanical biliary obstruction and occlusive hepatitis, chronic liver disease

Dose: 250–750 mg, 3 times daily
Cholecystography, 500–750 mg every 4 hours for 12 hours before and after the examination

Dehydrocholic Acid Tablets, dehydrocholic acid 250 mg. Price 20 tabs = **E**

URSODEOXYCHOLIC ACID

Indications; Cautions; Contra-indications: see under Chenodeoxycholic Acid

Side-effects: see under Chenodeoxycholic Acid; diarrhoea occurs rarely; liver changes have not been reported

Dose: 8–12 mg/kg (obese patients up to 15 mg/kg) daily as a single dose at bedtime or in divided doses, for up to 2 years; treatment is continued for 3–4 months after stones dissolve

▼ PoM **Destolit**® (Merrell)
Tablets, scored, ursodeoxycholic acid 150 mg. Price 20 tabs = **G**. Label: 21

▼ PoM **Ursofalk**® (Thames)
Capsules, ursodeoxycholic acid 250 mg. Price 20 caps = **I**. Label: 21

OTHER PREPARATIONS FOR BILIARY DISORDERS

Rowachol® (Tillotts)
Capsules, green, e/c, borneol 5 mg, camphene 5 mg, cineole 2 mg, menthol 32 mg, menthone 6 mg, pinene 17 mg in olive oil. Price 20 caps = **E**. Label: 22
Dose: 1–2 capsules 3 times daily before food
Liquid, yellow, borneol 50 mg, camphene 50 mg, cineole 20 mg, menthol 320 mg, menthone 60 mg, pinene 170 mg/g in olive oil. Price 10-ml dropper bottle = **G**. Label: 22
Dose: 3–5 drops 4–5 times daily before food

1.9.2 Drugs which increase gastric acidity

Acidol-Pepsin® and Muripsin® used in achlorhydria and hypochlorhydria but are of uncertain value. They have replaced dilute hydrochloric acid for these conditions.

Acidol-Pepsin® (Sterling Research)
Tablets, pepsin 97 mg, betaine hydrochloride 388 mg: 1 tablet ≈ 1 ml dilute hydrochloric acid. Price 20 tabs = **C**. Label: see dose below

Dose: 1–3 tablets crushed and dissolved in water 3 times daily after meals; to be taken through a straw or glass tube

Muripsin® (Norgine)
Tablets, orange, f/c, glutamic acid hydrochloride 500 mg, pepsin 35 mg: 1 tablet ≈ 1 ml dilute hydrochloric acid. Price 20 tabs = **C**. Label: 21
Dose: 1–2 tablets with meals

1.9.3 Aprotinin

Aprotinin is a proteolytic enzyme inhibitor used in the treatment of acute pancreatitis. Its value has not been substantiated.

APROTININ

Indications: prevention of pancreatitis after abdominal surgery; acute pancreatitis; disseminated intravascular coagulation

Side-effects: occasional hypersensitivity reactions

Dose: therapeutic, *by slow intravenous injection*, 500000 kallidinogenase (kallikrein) inactivator units, then 200000 units *by intravenous infusion* every 4 hours. In disseminated intravascular coagulation dosage may be increased to 1000000 units

Prophylactic, *by slow intravenous injection*, 200000 kallidinogenase (kallikrein) inactivator units pre-operatively, repeated postoperatively every 4 hours by slow intravenous injection or continuous infusion for 2 days

PoM **Trasylol**® (Bayer)
Injection, aprotinin 20000 kallidinogenase (kallikrein) inactivator units/ml. Price 5-ml amp = **F**; 10-ml amp = **H**

1.9.4 Pancreatin supplements

Pancreatin preparations may be administered by mouth to compensate for the reduced or absent exocrine secretion in children with cystic fibrosis and in adults following pancreatectomy, total gastrectomy or chronic pancreatitis. They assist the digestion of starch, fat, and protein. As pancreatic enzymes are inactivated by gastric acid, pancreatin supplements are more effective when gastric acid secretion is temporarily inhibited by antacids, or cimetidine, or ranitidine given before the pancreatin preparation.

ENZYME ACTIVITY. For practical purposes, the minimum enzyme activity specified in the *British Pharmacopoeia 1980* for each component is approximately 1½ times the potency originally specified in the *British Pharmacopoeia 1973* and 5 times the minimum potency required by the *British Pharmacopoeia 1968*.

Note. The BP 1980 also includes Pancreatic Extract which has half the potency of Pancreatin.

UNITS. Potencies in the table are expressed in BP units or NF = United States National Formulary, now known as USP units.

One BP unit of protease activity = approximately 62.5 NF (USP) units

One BP unit of lipase activity = approximately 1 NF (USP) unit

---

Table 1: Pancreatin Supplements

Preparation and Price	Presentation	Dose	Minimum activity in BP units (approx.)		
			Protease	Amylase	Lipase
Pancreatin BP 1980 Price 100 g = **F**. Label: see dose above	Powder	See notes above	1400/g	24000/g	20000/g
Cotazym® (Organon) Price 50 caps = **D**. Counselling advised, see dose	Capsules, green, to be opened before use	1–2 capsules sprinkled on food or with milk 3–4 times daily	500	10000	14000
Creon® (Duphar) Price 50 caps = **H**. Label: 21, 25	Capsules, brown/yellow, enclosing buff-coloured e/c granules, to be swallowed whole	5–15 capsules daily with meals	210	9000	8000
Nutrizym® (Merck) Price 50 tabs = **F**. Label: 5, 21, 25	Tablets, s/c, outer layer bromelains 50 mg; inner core e/c, pancreatin 400 mg, ox bile 30 mg	1–2 (max. 6) tablets during or after each meal CHILD 1–2 (or more) tablets with meals	560	10000	10000
Pancrex® (Paines & Byrne) Price 100 g = **F**. Label: 5, 22, 25	Granules, e/c	5–10 g 4 times daily before meals swallowed dry or with liquid	300/g	4000/g	5000/g
Pancrex V® (Paines & Byrne) Price 100 g = **G**. Counselling advised, see dose	Powder	0.5–2 g 4 times daily with meals swallowed dry or with liquid	1400/g	30000/g	25000/g
Price 50 caps = **D**. Counselling advised, see dose	Capsules, to be opened before use or swallowed whole	Up to 1 year 1–2 capsules mixed with feeds. Adults and children over 1 year 2–3 capsules 4 times daily with meals or sprinkled on food	430	9000	8000
Price 50 tabs = **B**. Label: 5, 22, 25	Tablets, e/c, s/c	5–15 tablets 4 times daily before food	110	1700	1900
Price 50 tabs = **D**. Label: 5, 22, 25	Tablets forte, e/c, s/c	2–6 tablets 4 times daily before food	330	5000	5600

Notes: Pancreatin BP 1980 is equivalent to Strong Pancreatin Powder BNF 1976–78.
When mixing pancreatin with food or liquid, excessive heat should be avoided.

One BP unit of amylase activity = approximately 4.15 NF (USP) units

One BP unit of protease, lipase, and amylase activity = approximately 1 FIP unit

PANCREATIN

Indications: see notes above

Cautions: if mixed with liquids or feeds the resulting mixture should not be allowed to stand for longer than 1 hour

Side-effects: it may irritate the skin surrounding the mouth and anus

Dose: 2–4 g of Pancreatin BP with each meal using the larger dose for main meals; CHILD up to 1 year 500–750 mg with each feed, 1–12 years 0.75–1 g before each meal.

Dosage is adjusted according to the size, number, and consistency of stools so that the patient thrives. It is given immediately before or with the main meals and extra allowance may be needed if snacks are taken between meals

Preparations

The preparations available for replacement therapy are shown in Table 1. The activity of pancreatin as powder or from capsules is destroyed by the acidity of the stomach. Such preparations are best taken with food, or in divided doses immediately before, with, or after food. **Antacids** (section 1.1) or **cimetidine** or **ranitidine** (section 1.3) may be given 30 to 45 minutes before the pancreatin preparation to reduce gastric acid secretion and potentiate the action of the enzyme. **Pancreatin Granules** and **Pancreatin Tablets** are enteric-coated and may be taken before meals but concurrent use of antacids may dissolve the enteric coating.

1.9.5   Other pancreatin preparations

The following preparations containing pancreatin are claimed to relieve discomfort caused by dietary imbalance. They are of doubtful value.

Combizym® (Luitpold)

Tablets, yellow, f/c, inner layer, pancreatin 220 mg; outer layer mixture of amylase, cellulase, hemicellulase, and protease 120 mg. Price 50 tabs = **E**. Label: 21, 25

Dose: adults and children, 1–2 tablets with meals

Combizym Compositum® (Luitpold)

Tablets, orange, inner layer, ox bile extract 60 mg, pancreatin 400 mg; outer layer, mixture of amylase, cellulase, hemicellulase, and protease 120 mg. Price 50 tabs = **E**. Label: 21, 25

Dose: adults and children, 1 tablet with or after meals

2: Drugs used in the treatment of diseases of the
CARDIOVASCULAR SYSTEM

In this chapter, drug treatment is discussed under the following headings:

2.1   Cardiac glycosides

These are used in the treatment of heart failure and supraventricular tachycardias, especially atrial fibrillation. The cardiac stimulant action is probably due to an alteration of the intracellular environment with increased accumulation and availability of calcium ions. The glycosides decrease the rate of conduction through the atrioventricular node and this slows the ventricular response in atrial fibrillation.

Loss of appetite, nausea, and vomiting are common toxic effects. Sinus bradycardia, atrioventricular block, ventricular extrasystoles, and sometimes ventricular tachycardia or atrial tachycardia with block also occur—especially in the presence of underlying conducting-system defects or myocardial disease. These unwanted effects depend on both the plasma concentrations of the drugs and the sensitivity of the conducting system or myocardium, which is often increased in patients with heart disease. Thus, no one plasma concentration can indicate toxicity reliably but the likelihood increases progressively through the range 1.5 to 3.0 micrograms/litre. Higher steady-state concentrations must certainly be avoided. Measurements of plasma concentration are not necessary, however, unless problems occur during maintenance treatment. Hypokalaemia predisposes to toxicity.

Renal function is the most important determinant of digoxin dosage, whereas elimination of digitoxin depends on metabolism by the liver. Manifestations of toxicity can often be managed by discontinuing therapy and correcting hypokalaemia if appropriate. Serious manifestations require urgent specialist management.

Digoxin (Lanoxin® etc.) is the glycoside most commonly used. In patients with mild failure a loading dose is not required, and a satisfactory plasma concentration can be achieved over a period of about a week, using a dose of 125 to 250 micrograms twice a day which may then be reduced having special regard to renal function. For management of atrial fibrillation, the most common indication, the maintenance dose can usually be governed by ventricular response which should not be allowed to fall below 50 beats per minute.

When very rapid control is needed, digoxin may be given intravenously in a digitalising dose of 0.75 to 1.25 mg, preferably as an infusion (suggested volume 50 ml) over two or more hours, followed by normal maintenance therapy. The intramuscular route is not recommended, except when other methods of administration are not available.

Lanatoside C (Cedilanid®) is less well absorbed than digoxin. Most is converted to digoxin after ingestion. The maintenance dose is about twice that of digoxin, and depends in part on renal function.

Ouabain has a relatively short half-life and may be used intravenously in some emergency situations.

Digitoxin has a long half-life and consequently maintenance doses need only be given once daily.

It is often possible to withdraw cardiac glycosides without any clinical deterioration once the heart failure has been controlled—clearly desirable in elderly patients; a diuretic may need to be continued.

CHILDREN. The dose is based on body-weight; they require a relatively larger dose of digoxin than adults.

DIGOXIN

Indications: heart failure, supraventricular arrhythmias (particularly atrial fibrillation)
Cautions: recent infarction, hypothyroidism; reduce dose in the elderly and in renal impairment; avoid hypokalaemia. Drug interactions: see Appendix 1 (sections 2.1, *15*)
Side-effects: anorexia, nausea, vomiting, visual disturbances, arrhythmias, heart block
Dose: by mouth, for rapid digitalisation, 1–1.5 mg in divided doses over 24 hours; less urgent digitalisation, 125–250 micrograms twice daily for up to 1 week
For maintenance and intravenous doses, see notes above

PoM **Digoxin Tablets,** digoxin 62.5, 125, and 250 micrograms. Price 20 tabs (all) = **A**
PoM **Lanoxin®** (Wellcome)
Tablets, digoxin 125 micrograms. Price 20 tabs = **A**
Tablets, scored, digoxin 250 micrograms. Price 20 tabs = **A**
Injection, digoxin 250 micrograms/ml. Price 2-ml amp = **B**

C = 51-100p, D = 101-180p, E = 181-300p, F = 301-450p, G = 451-650p, H = 651-900p, I = 901-1200p, J = over 1200p.

PoM **Lanoxin-PG**® (Wellcome)
Tablets, blue, digoxin 62.5 micrograms. Price 20 tabs = **A**
Elixir, yellow, digoxin 50 micrograms/ml. Do not dilute, measure with pipette. Price 60 ml = **E**. Counselling advised, use of pipette

DIGITOXIN

Indications: heart failure, supraventricular arrhythmias (particularly atrial fibrillation)
Cautions; Side-effects: see under Digoxin
Dose: 50–200 micrograms daily

PoM **Digitoxin Tablets,** digitoxin 100 micrograms. Price 20 tabs = **B**
PoM **Digitaline Nativelle**® (Lewis)
Tablets, pink, digitoxin 100 micrograms. Price 20 tabs = **B**
Solution (=elixir), digitoxin 1 mg/ml (5 drops ≈ 100 micrograms). Price 10 ml = **D**. Counselling advised, use of pipette

LANATOSIDE C

Indications: heart failure, supraventricular arrhythmias (particularly atrial fibrillation)
Cautions; Side-effects: see under Digoxin
Dose: slow digitalisation 1.5–2 mg daily for 3–5 days; maintenance 0.25–1 mg daily

PoM **Cedilanid**® (Sandoz)
Tablets, scored, lanatoside C 250 micrograms. Price 20 tabs = **B**

MEDIGOXIN

Indications: heart failure, supraventricular arrhythmias (particularly atrial fibrillation)
Cautions; Side-effects: see under Digoxin
Dose: digitalisation 200 micrograms twice daily for 3–5 days; maintenance 100 micrograms 2–3 times daily

PoM **Lanitop**® (Roussel)
Tablets, yellow, scored, medigoxin 100 micrograms. Price 20 tabs = **C**

OUABAIN

Indications: acute heart failure, supraventricular arrhythmias
Cautions; Side-effects: see under Digoxin
Dose: by slow intravenous injection, up to 1 mg

PoM **Ouabaine Arnaud**® (Lewis)
Injection, ouabain 250 micrograms/ml. Price 1-ml amp = **C**

2.2   Diuretics

2.2.1 Thiazides and related diuretics
2.2.2 Loop diuretics
2.2.3 Potassium-sparing diuretics
2.2.4 Aldosterone antagonists
2.2.5 Osmotic diuretics
2.2.6 Mercurial diuretics
2.2.7 Carbonic anhydrase inhibitors

2.2.8 Combined diuretics and potassium supplements

For potassium supplements, see section 9.2.1.1.
For drug interactions of diuretics see Appendix 1 (sections 2.2, *4.2*).

Thiazide diuretics (section 2.2.1) are used to relieve oedema due to heart failure, a condition characterised by reduced glomerular filtration, increased reabsorption of sodium from the renal tubules, and an increased production of aldosterone contributing to fluid retention. They are also used in lower doses to reduce blood pressure.

The more potent **'loop' diuretics** such as frusemide or bumetanide (section 2.2.2) are used in patients with pulmonary oedema due to left ventricular failure and in patients with long-standing heart failure who no longer respond to the thiazide diuretics.

Diuretics are usually administered early in the day so that the diuresis does not interfere with sleep.

Hypokalaemia may occur with both thiazide and loop diuretics; potassium supplements (see section 9.2.1.1) may be unnecessary when thiazides are used to lower blood pressure in the absence of heart failure. Often the use of potassium-sparing diuretics (section 2.2.3) avoids the need to take potassium supplements. Intermittent diuretic therapy is less likely to induce hypokalaemia than continuous treatment.

In patients with oedema resistant to treatment with one diuretic, combination treatment may be effective. For example, a loop diuretic may be combined with a potassium-sparing diuretic (section 2.2.3) or with spironolactone (section 2.2.4).

The combination of a thiazide diuretic with spironolactone is of value in less severe heart failure when hypokalaemia is difficult to counter or when any degree of hypokalaemia should be avoided, as in patients with a continuing tendency to life-threatening ventricular arrhythmias.

In hepatic failure hypokalaemia caused by diuretics can precipitate encephalopathy. Diuretics may also increase the risk of hypomagnesaemia in alcoholic cirrhosis.

2.2.1   Thiazides and related diuretics

Thiazides and related compounds act at the beginning of the distal convoluted tubule and are moderately potent diuretics. Side-effects include hypokalaemia, hypochloraemic alkalosis, hyperuricaemia, hyperglycaemia, and increases in plasma cholesterol concentrations. Hypokalaemia is dangerous in severe coronary artery disease and in patients being treated with cardiac glycosides. Less common side-effects include rashes and thrombocytopenia, and when given in late pregnancy thiazides have been reported to cause neonatal thrombocytopenia.

All thiazides are active by mouth with an onset of action within 1 to 2 hours and duration of 12 to 24 hours.

Small doses of the thiazides are used long-term to control hypertension—often alone in mild hypertension, but also with other drugs in more severe hypertension. They act in part by reducing peripheral vascular resistance. Increasing the dose has little additional antihypertensive effect, yet augments the long-term effects on glucose tolerance and plasma lipids, which are cause for concern. Optimum doses for the control of heart failure may be larger, and long-term effects are of less importance.

Bendrofluazide is an appropriate drug for mild or moderate cardiac failure when the patient is not desperately ill and severe pulmonary oedema is not present. This drug is also effective either alone in the treatment of mild hypertension or with other drugs in more severe hypertension. Combined preparations of thiazide diuretics and potassium chloride are available; they may be useful when there is a compliance problem but have no other advantage over bendrofluazide or other thiazide diuretics prescribed in conjunction with potassium supplements (see section 9.2.1.1). Combined preparations and potassium-sparing diuretics should **not** usually be given together.

Chlorthalidone (Hygroton®), a thiazide-related compound, has a longer duration of action than the thiazides and may be given on alternate days to control hypertension. It is also useful if acute retention may be precipitated by a more rapid diuresis or if patients dislike the altered pattern of micturition promoted by diuretics.

There are many thiazide and thiazide-related compounds available but none offer any significant advantage over the ones mentioned.

NEWER COMPOUNDS. **Xipamide** (Diurexan®) resembles chlorthalidone structurally, and is more potent than the other thiazides. **Indapamide** (Natrilix®) is chemically related to chlorthalidone. It is claimed to lower blood pressure with less metabolic disturbance, particularly less aggravation of diabetes mellitus. The advantages of these newer agents over longer-established thiazides need further evaluation.

BENDROFLUAZIDE

Indications: oedema, hypertension
Cautions: may cause hypokalaemia, aggravates diabetes and gout; pregnancy; renal and hepatic impairment. Drug interactions: see Appendix 1 (sections *2.1*, 2.2, *2.2*, *2.3*, *2.4*, *6.1*, *6.3*, *9*)
Contra-indications: renal failure
Side-effects: rashes, thrombocytopenia; impotence (reversible on withdrawal of treatment)
Dose: oedema, initially 5–10 mg in the morning daily *or* on alternate days; maintenance 2.5–10 mg 1–3 times weekly
Hypertension, 2.5–5 mg in the morning

PoM **Bendrofluazide Tablets,** bendrofluazide 2.5 and 5 mg. Price 20 tabs (both) = **A**
PoM **Aprinox®** (Boots)
Tablets, bendrofluazide 2.5 and 5 mg. Price 20 tabs (both) = **A**
PoM **Berkozide®** (Berk)
Tablets, bendrofluazide 2.5 mg. Price 20 tabs = **A**

Tablets, scored, bendrofluazide 5 mg. Price 20 tabs = **A**
PoM **Centyl®** (Burgess)
Tablets, bendrofluazide 2.5 mg. Price 20 tabs = **B**
Tablets, scored, bendrofluazide 5 mg. Price 20 tabs = **C**
PoM **Neo-NaClex®** (DF)
Tablets, scored, bendrofluazide 5 mg. Price 20 tabs = **A**
PoM **Urizide®** (DDSA)
Tablets, bendrofluazide 5 mg. Price 20 tabs = **A**

CHLOROTHIAZIDE

Indications: oedema, hypertension
Cautions; Contra-indications; Side-effects: see under Bendrofluazide
Dose: oedema, initially 0.5–1 g 1–2 times daily; maintenance 0.5–1 g daily, on alternate days, or less frequently
Hypertension, 0.5–1 g daily in single or divided doses

PoM **Saluric®** (MSD)
Tablets, scored, chlorothiazide 500 mg. Price 20 tabs = **B**

CHLORTHALIDONE

Indications: oedema, hypertension, diabetes insipidus (see section 6.5.2)
Cautions; Contra-indications; Side-effects: see under Bendrofluazide
Dose: oedema, initially 50 mg in the morning *or* 100–200 mg on alternate days, reduced for maintenance if possible
Hypertension, 25 mg, increased to 50 mg if necessary, in the morning

PoM **Hygroton®** (Geigy)
Tablets, yellow, scored, chlorthalidone 50 mg. Price 20 tabs = **C**
Tablets, scored, chlorthalidone 100 mg. Price 20 tabs = **D**

CLOPAMIDE

Indications: oedema, hypertension
Cautions; Contra-indications; Side-effects: see under Bendrofluazide
Dose: oedema, initially 40–60 mg in the morning; maintenance 20–60 mg daily or less frequently
Hypertension, 20–40 mg in the morning

Preparations
Section 2.2.8

CYCLOPENTHIAZIDE

Indications: oedema, hypertension
Cautions; Contra-indications; Side-effects: see under Bendrofluazide
Dose: oedema, initially 0.5–1 mg in the morning; maintenance 500 micrograms on alternate days
Hypertension, 250–500 micrograms in the morning
Max. 1.5 mg daily

PoM **Navidrex**® (Ciba)
Tablets, scored, cyclopenthiazide 500 micrograms. Price 20 tabs = **B**

HYDROCHLOROTHIAZIDE

Indications: oedema, hypertension
Cautions; Contra-indications; Side-effects: see under Bendrofluazide; also photosensitivity
Dose: oedema, initially 50–100 mg 1–2 times daily; maintenance 25–50 mg on alternate days
Hypertension, 25–100 mg daily in single or divided doses

PoM **Hydrochlorothiazide Tablets**, hydrochlorothiazide 25 mg, price 20 tabs = **B**; 50 mg, price 20 tabs = **C**
PoM **Esidrex**® (Ciba)
Tablets, scored, hydrochlorothiazide 25 mg. Price 20 tabs = **B**
Tablets, scored, hydrochlorothiazide 50 mg. Price 20 tabs = **C**
PoM **HydroSaluric**® (MSD)
Tablets, scored, hydrochlorothiazide 25 mg. Price 20 tabs = **B**
Tablets, scored, hydrochlorothiazide 50 mg. Price 20 tabs = **C**

HYDROFLUMETHIAZIDE

Indications: oedema, hypertension
Cautions; Contra-indications; Side-effects: see under Bendrofluazide
Dose: oedema, initially 50–200 mg in the morning; maintenance 25–50 mg on alternate days
Hypertension, 25–50 mg daily

PoM **Hydrenox**® (Boots)
Tablets, hydroflumethiazide 50 mg. Price 20 tabs = **B**

INDAPAMIDE

Indications: hypertension
Cautions: severe hepatic or renal impairment. Drug interactions: see Appendix 1 (section 2.2)
Side-effects: nausea, headache, slight weight loss; diuresis with doses above 2.5 mg daily
Dose: 2.5 mg in the morning

▼ PoM **Natrilix**® (Servier)
Tablets, pink, s/c, indapamide 2.5 mg. Price 20 tabs = **F**

MEFRUSIDE

Indications: oedema, hypertension
Cautions; Contra-indications; Side-effects: see under Bendrofluazide
Dose: initially 25–50 mg in the morning, increased to 75–100 mg for oedema; maintenance 25 mg daily *or* on alternate days

PoM **Baycaron**® (Bayer)
Tablets, scored, mefruside 25 mg. Price 20 tabs = **D**

METHYCLOTHIAZIDE

Indications: oedema, hypertension
Cautions; Contra-indications; Side-effects: see under Bendrofluazide
Dose: 2.5–5 mg in the morning, increased to 10 mg daily if required

PoM **Enduron**® (Abbott)
Tablets, pink, scored, methyclothiazide 5 mg. Price 20 tabs = **B**

METOLAZONE

Indications: oedema, hypertension
Cautions; Contra-indications; Side-effects: see under Bendrofluazide
Dose: oedema, 5–10 mg in the morning, increased if necessary; max. 80 mg daily
Hypertension, initially 5 mg in the morning; maintenance 5 mg on alternate days

PoM **Metenix 5**® (Hoechst)
Tablets, blue, metolazone 5 mg. Price 20 tabs = **D**

POLYTHIAZIDE

Indications: oedema, hypertension
Cautions; Contra-indications; Side-effects: see under Bendrofluazide
Dose: usually 1–4 mg daily; in hypertension 500 micrograms daily may be adequate

PoM **Nephril**® (Pfizer)
Tablets, scored, polythiazide 1 mg. Price 20 tabs = **C**

XIPAMIDE

Indications: oedema, hypertension
Cautions; Contra-indications: see under Bendrofluazide. Drug interactions: see Appendix 1 (section 2.2)
Side-effects: slight gastro-intestinal disturbances; mild dizziness
Dose: oedema, initially 40 mg in the morning, increased to 80 mg in resistant cases; maintenance 20 mg in the morning
Hypertension, 20–40 mg in the morning

PoM **Diurexan**® (Merck)
Tablets, scored, xipamide 20 mg. Price 20 tabs = **E**

2.2.2   Loop diuretics

These drugs inhibit resorption from the ascending loop of Henle in the renal tubule and are powerful diuretics. Hypokalaemia frequently develops, and care is needed to avoid hypotension. If there is an enlarged prostate, urinary retention may occur; this is less likely if small doses and less potent diuretics are used initially.

Frusemide (Lasix® etc.) and **bumetanide** (Burinex®) have similar activity. Oral administration is effective within 1 hour and diuresis is complete within 6 hours, so that the drugs can be given twice daily without interfering with sleep. Given intravenously they act rapidly, the peak

---

effect occurring within 30 minutes. The diuresis is related to the size of dose, and in patients with impaired renal function very large doses may occasionally have to be given. In such doses both drugs can cause deafness and bumetanide can cause myalgia.

Ethacrynic acid (Edecrin®) has a similar onset and duration of action and may be useful in patients who have become refractory to frusemide and bumetanide. Deafness may occur in patients with renal failure, especially when ethacrynic acid is given intravenously.

Piretanide (Arelix®) is the newest member of this group, and has properties similar to those of frusemide and bumetanide, but is promoted for the treatment of hypertension.

For the use of potassium supplements with loop diuretics, see section 9.2.1.1.

FRUSEMIDE

Indications: oedema, oliguria due to renal failure
Cautions: pregnancy; causes hypokalaemia and hyponatraemia, aggravates diabetes and gout, liver failure, prostatism. Drug interactions: see Appendix 1 (sections *2.1, 2.2, 2.2, 2.3, 2.4, 5.1, 6.1, 6.3*)
Contra-indications: liver cirrhosis
Side-effects: rashes; tinnitus and deafness in impaired renal function
Dose: by mouth, oedema, initially 40 mg in the morning; maintenance 20 mg daily *or* 40 mg on alternate days, increased in resistant oedema to 80 mg daily
Oliguria, initially 250 mg daily; if necessary larger doses, increasing in steps of 250 mg, may be given every 4–6 hours to a max. of a single dose of 2 g
CHILD 1–3 mg/kg daily
By intramuscular or slow intravenous injection, initially 20–50 mg; CHILD 0.5–1.5 mg/kg
By intravenous infusion, in oliguria, 0.25–1 g at a rate not exceeding 4 mg/minute

PoM **Frusemide Tablets**, frusemide 20 mg, price 20 tabs = **B**; 40 mg, price 20 tabs = **A**; 500 mg, price 20 tabs = **G**
PoM **Frusemide Injection**, frusemide 10 mg/ml. Price 2-ml amp = **A**; 5-ml amp = **C**; 25-ml amp = **D**
PoM **Aluzine**® (Steinhard)
Tablets, scored, frusemide 20 mg. Price 20 tabs = **C**
Tablets, scored, frusemide 40 mg. Price 20 tabs = **C**
Tablets, yellow, scored, frusemide 500 mg. Price 20 tabs = **I**
PoM **Diuresal**® (Lagap)
Tablets, frusemide 40 mg. Price 20 tabs = **B**
Injection, frusemide 10 mg/ml. Price 2- and 5-ml amp (both) = **B**
PoM **Dryptal**® (Berk)
Tablets, scored, frusemide 40 mg. Price 20 tabs = **B**
Tablets, yellow, scored, frusemide 500 mg. Price 20 tabs = **I**

Injection, frusemide 10 mg/ml. Price 2- and 5-ml amp (both) = **B**; 25-ml amp = **E** (Hosp. only)
PoM **Frusetic**® (Unimed)
Tablets, scored, frusemide 40 mg. Price 20 tabs = **C**
PoM **Frusid**® (DDSA)
Tablets, scored, frusemide 40 mg. Price 20 tabs = **B**
PoM **Lasix**® (Hoechst)
Tablets, scored, frusemide 20 mg. Price 20 tabs = **C**
Tablets, scored, frusemide 40 mg. Price 20 tabs = **C**
Tablets, yellow, scored, frusemide 500 mg. Price 20 tabs = **I**
Paediatric liquid (= mixture), frusemide 1 mg/ml when reconstituted with water for preparations. Price 150 ml = **D**
Injection, frusemide 10 mg/ml. Price 2-ml amp = **B**; 5-ml amp = **C**; 25-ml amp = **E**

BUMETANIDE

Indications: oedema, oliguria due to renal failure
Cautions; Contra-indications: see under Frusemide. Drug interactions: see Appendix 1 (sections *2.1, 2.2, 2.2, 2.3, 2.4, 6.1, 6.3*)
Side-effects: see under Frusemide; also myalgia
Dose: by mouth, 1 mg daily, increased if required; 5 mg in oliguria, increased if required
By intramuscular or intravenous injection, 1–2 mg, repeated after 20 minutes
By intravenous infusion, 2–5 mg over 30–60 minutes

PoM **Burinex**® (Leo)
Tablets, yellow, scored, bumetanide 1 mg. Price 20 tabs = **D**
Tablets, scored, bumetanide 5 mg. Price 20 tabs = **G**
Liquid (= mixture), green, bumetanide 1 mg/5 ml. Price 150 ml = **E**
Injection, bumetanide 500 micrograms/ml. Price 2-ml amp = **B**; 4-ml amp = **C**; 10-ml amp = **D**

ETHACRYNIC ACID

Indications: oedema, oliguria due to renal failure
Cautions; Contra-indications; Side-effects: see under Frusemide; also pain on injection. Drug interactions: see Appendix 1 (sections *2.1, 2.3, 2.4, 5.1, 6.3*)
Dose: by mouth, initially 50 mg daily, maintenance 50–150 mg daily or on alternate days; max. 400 mg daily
By slow intravenous injection or infusion, 50 mg, increased to 100 mg if necessary

PoM **Edecrin**® (MSD)
Tablets, scored, ethacrynic acid 50 mg. Price 20 tabs = **C**. Label: 21
Injection, powder for reconstitution, ethacrynic acid (as sodium salt). Price 50-mg vial = **D**

PIRETANIDE

Indications: hypertension

C = 51-100p, D = 101-180p, E = 181-300p, F = 301-450p, G = 451-650p, H = 651-900p, I = 901-1200p, J = over 1200p.

Cautions: causes hypokalaemia, monitor plasma electrolytes in hepatic and renal impairment; prostatism. Drug interactions: see Appendix 1 (sections *2.1*, 2.2, *2.2*, *2.3*, *2.4*, *5.1*, *6.3*)
Contra-indications: severe electrolyte imbalance, hypovolaemia
Side-effects: rarely nausea, vomiting, diarrhoea, rashes; myalgia after high doses
Dose: 6–12 mg in the morning with food

▼ PoM **Arelix®** (Hoechst)
Capsules, s/r, green/orange, enclosing yellow pellets, piretanide 6 mg. Price 28 caps = **F**. Label: 21

2.2.3   Potassium-sparing diuretics

Amiloride (Midamor®) and **triamterene** (Dytac®) on their own are weak diuretics. They cause retention of potassium and are therefore used as an alternative to giving potassium supplements with thiazide or loop diuretics. Although it is preferable to prescribe the two types of diuretic separately, the use of fixed combinations of a thiazide with triamterene or amiloride may be justified if compliance is a problem (see section 2.2.4 for preparations); there is an increased risk of hyponatraemia if they are given with chlorpropamide (see Appendix 1, section 2.2).

AMILORIDE HYDROCHLORIDE
Indications: oedema, potassium conservation with thiazide and loop diuretics
Cautions: pregnancy; diabetes mellitus, hepatic cirrhosis. Drug interactions: see Appendix 1 (sections *1*, 2.2, *2.5*, *4.2*)
Contra-indications: hyperkalaemia, renal failure
Side-effects: rashes, mental confusion
Dose: initially 10 mg daily alone, or 5–10 mg daily with other diuretics; max. 20 mg daily

PoM **Midamor®** (Morson)
Tablets, yellow, amiloride hydrochloride 5 mg. Price 20 tabs = **D**

TRIAMTERENE
Indications: oedema, potassium conservation with thiazide and loop diuretics
Cautions; Contra-indications: see under Amiloride Hydrochloride; monitor plasma urea and potassium, particularly in the elderly and in renal impairment; also may cause blue fluorescence of urine. Drug interactions: see Appendix 1 (sections 2.2, *2.5*)
Side-effects: gastro-intestinal disturbances, dry mouth, rashes
Dose: initially 150–250 mg daily, reducing to alternate days after 1 week; lower initial dose when given with other diuretics

PoM **Dytac®** (SK&F)
Capsules, maroon, triamterene 50 mg. Price 20 caps = **D**. Label: 14, 21

2.2.4   Aldosterone antagonists

Spironolactone (Aldactone® etc.) is a weak di-

uretic but it potentiates thiazide or loop diuretics by antagonising aldosterone. It is of value in the treatment of the oedema of cirrhosis of the liver and occasionally may help in oedema of cardiac failure that is resistant to therapy, particularly when congestion has caused hepatic engorgement. Spironolactone is potassium sparing, so potassium supplements must **not** be given.

Spironolactone is also used in Conn's syndrome (primary hyperaldosteronism), and has a limited role in the treatment of hypertension when there is a tendency to hypokalaemia.

Potassium canrenoate (Spiroctan-M®) has similar uses to spironolactone, but can be given parenterally. It is metabolised to canrenone, which is also a metabolite of spironolactone.

POTASSIUM CANRENOATE
Indications: oedema associated with cardiac dysfunction, secondary aldosteronism, liver failure, nephrotic syndrome
Cautions; Contra-indications: see under Spironolactone; also contra-indicated in hyponatraemia
Side-effects: nausea and vomiting, particularly after high doses; pain and irritation at injection site
Dose: by slow intravenous injection or intravenous infusion, up to 800 mg daily, in single or divided doses

▼ PoM **Spiroctan-M®** (MCP)
Injection, potassium canrenoate 20 mg/ml. Price 10-ml amp = **C**

SPIRONOLACTONE
Indications: oedema in cirrhosis of the liver, nephrotic syndrome, congestive heart failure, potentiation of thiazide and loop diuretics, hypertension, Conn's syndrome
Cautions: pregnancy. Drug interactions: see Appendix 1 (sections *1*, *2.1*, 2.2, *2.5*)
Contra-indications: hyperkalaemia, renal failure
Side-effects: gastro-intestinal disturbances, gynaecomastia
Dose: 100–200 mg daily, increased to 400 mg if required; CHILD 3 mg/kg daily in divided doses
Hypertension, 50–100 mg daily; max. 200 mg daily

PoM **Spironolactone Tablets,** spironolactone 25 mg, price 20 tabs = **D**; 50 mg, price 20 tabs = **E**; 100 mg, price 20 tabs = **G**
PoM **Aldactone®** (Searle)
Tablets, buff, f/c, spironolactone 25 mg. Price 20 tabs = **D**
Tablets, off-white, f/c, spironolactone 50 mg. Price 20 tabs = **F**
Tablets, buff, f/c, spironolactone 100 mg. Price 20 tabs = **H**
PoM **Diatensec®** (Gold Cross)
Tablets, f/c, spironolactone 50 mg. Price 20 tabs = **F**
PoM **Laractone®** (Lagap)
Tablets, f/c, spironolactone 25 mg. Price 20 tabs = **D**

Tablets, f/c, spironolactone 100 mg. Price 20 tabs = **G**

PoM **Spiretic**® (DDSA)

Tablets, yellow, spironolactone 25 mg. Price 20 tabs = **D**

Tablets, yellow, spironolactone 100 mg. Price 20 tabs = **G**

PoM **Spiroctan**® (MCP)

Tablets, blue, s/c, spironolactone 25 mg. Price 20 tabs = **D**

Tablets, green, s/c, spironolactone 50 mg. Price 20 tabs = **E**

Capsules, green, spironolactone 100 mg. Price 20 caps = **G**

PoM **Spirolone**® (Berk)

Tablets, s/c, spironolactone 25 mg. Price 20 tabs = **D**

Tablets, s/c, spironolactone 50 mg. Price 20 tabs = **E**

Tablets, s/c, spironolactone 100 mg. Price 20 tabs = **G**

COMPOUND PREPARATIONS OF POTASSIUM-SPARING DIURETICS

PoM **Aldactide 25**® (Gold Cross)

Tablets, buff, f/c, scored, spironolactone 25 mg, hydroflumethiazide 25 mg. Price 20 tabs = **F**

Dose: 1–4 tablets in the morning

PoM **Aldactide 50**® (Gold Cross)

Tablets, buff, f/c, scored, spironolactone 50 mg, hydroflumethiazide 50 mg. Price 20 tabs = **G**

Dose: 1–2 tablets in the morning

PoM **Amilco**® (Norton)

Tablets, peach, scored, amiloride hydrochloride 5 mg, hydrochlorothiazide 50 mg. Price 20 tabs = **D**

Dose: 1–2 tablets, increased if necessary to a max. of 4, daily

PoM **Dyazide**® (SK&F)

Tablets, peach, scored, triamterene 50 mg, hydrochlorothiazide 25 mg. Price 20 tabs = **D**. Label: 14, 21

Dose: 1–2 tablets daily; max. 4 tablets daily

PoM **Dytide**® (SK&F)

Capsules, clear/maroon, triamterene 50 mg, benzthiazide 25 mg. Price 20 caps = **D**. Label: 14, 21

Dose: 1–3 capsules daily, reducing to alternate days after 1 week

▼ PoM **Frumil**® (Berk)

Tablets, orange, scored, amiloride hydrochloride 5 mg, frusemide 40 mg. Price 28 tabs = **F**

Dose: 1–2 tablets in the morning

PoM **Frusene**® (Rorer)

Tablets, yellow, scored, triamterene 50 mg, frusemide 40 mg. Price 20 tabs = **D**. Label: 14, 21

Dose: 1–2 tablets daily

▼ PoM **Kalspare**® (Armour)

Tablets, orange, f/c, scored, triamterene 50 mg, chlorthalidone 50 mg. Price 28 tabs = **E**. Label: 14, 21

Dose: 1–2 tablets in the morning

▼ PoM **Lasilactone**® (Hoechst)

Capsules, blue/white, spironolactone 50 mg, frusemide 20 mg. Price 20 caps = **F**

Dose: 1–4 capsules daily

PoM **Moduret 25**® (Morson)

Tablets, off-white, amiloride hydrochloride 2.5 mg, hydrochlorothiazide 25 mg. Price 28 tabs = **E**

Dose: 1–4 tablets daily

PoM **Moduretic**® (MSD)

Tablets, peach, scored, amiloride hydrochloride 5 mg, hydrochlorothiazide 50 mg. Price 20 tabs = **D**

Dose: 1–2 tablets, increased if necessary to a max. of 4, daily

Oral solution (= mixture), amiloride hydrochloride 5 mg, hydrochlorothiazide 50 mg/5 ml. Do not dilute. Price 200 ml = **G**

Dose: as for tablets above (5 ml = 1 tablet)

PoM **Synuretic**® (DDSA)

Tablets, peach, amiloride hydrochloride 5 mg, hydrochlorothiazide 50 mg. Price 20 tabs = **D**

Dose: 1–2 tablets, increased if necessary to a max. of 4, daily

---

2.2.5 Osmotic diuretics

They are rarely used in heart failure as they may acutely expand the blood volume. **Mannitol** is the most commonly used—in forced diuresis in cases of drug overdose, and in cerebral oedema.

MANNITOL

Indications: cerebral oedema, forced diuresis

Cautions: extravasation causes inflammation and thrombophlebitis

Contra-indications: congestive cardiac failure, pulmonary oedema

Side-effects: chills, fever

Dose: *by intravenous infusion*, 50–200 g over 24 hours, preceded by a test dose of 200 mg/kg by slow intravenous injection

PoM **Mannitol Intravenous Infusion**

10% solution. Price 500-ml container = **D**

20% solution. Price 250- and 500-ml containers (both) = **D**

25% solution. Price 50-ml amp = **D**

PoM **Osmitrol**® (Travenol)

Intravenous infusion, mannitol 10%. Price 500-ml container = **D**

Intravenous infusion, mannitol 15%. Price 500-ml container = **E**

Intravenous infusion, mannitol 20%. Price 200- and 500-ml container (both) = **E**

UREA

Indications: cerebral oedema

Cautions: see under Mannitol

Contra-indications: renal failure, hepatic failure, intracerebral haemorrhage

Side-effects: headache, mental confusion

Dose: *by intravenous infusion*, 40–80 g as a 30% solution in glucose intravenous infusion 5 or 10%, at a rate not exceeding 3–4 ml/minute

---

C = 51-100p, **D** = 101-180p, **E** = 181-300p, **F** = 301-450p, **G** = 451-650p, **H** = 651-900p, **I** = 901-1200p, **J** = over 1200p.

PoM **Ureaphil**® (Abbott)
Intravenous infusion, powder for reconstitution, urea. Price 40-g vial = **J**

2.2.6   Mercurial diuretics

They are effective diuretics but are now little used because of their nephrotoxicity. Mersalyl **must** be given by intramuscular injection; intravenous use may cause severe hypotension and sudden death.

MERSALYL

Indications: oedema unresponsive to other diuretics
Cautions: recent myocardial infarction, treatment with cardiac glycosides, frequent extrasystoles; pregnancy
Contra-indications: renal impairment
Side-effects: gastro-intestinal disturbances, allergic reactions

PoM **Mersalyl Injection**, mersalyl sodium 100 mg, theophylline 50 mg/ml. Price 2-ml amp = **D**
Dose: by deep intramuscular injection, 0.5–2 ml

2.2.7   Carbonic anhydrase inhibitors

Acetazolamide and dichlorphenamide are weak diuretics, and are little used for their diuretic effect. They inhibit the formation of aqueous fluid, and are used in glaucoma (see section 11.6). Although acetazolamide is used as a prophylactic measure for mountain sickness it is not a substitute for acclimatisation.

2.2.8   Combined diuretics and potassium supplements

Many patients on diuretics do not need potassium supplements (see section 9.2.1.1). For many of those who do, the amount of potassium ion in combined preparations may not be enough, and for this reason their use is to be discouraged.

PoM **Brinaldix K**® (Sandoz)
Tablets, effervescent, clopamide 20 mg, potassium 12 mmol. Price 20 tabs = **D**. Label: 13
PoM **Burinex K**® (Leo)
Tablets, bumetanide 500 micrograms, potassium 7.7 mmol for sustained release. Price 20 tabs = **C**. Label: 25
PoM **Centyl K**® (Burgess)
Tablets, green, bendrofluazide 2.5 mg, potassium 7.7 mmol for sustained release. Price 20 tabs = **C**. Label: 25
PoM **Diumide-K Continus**® (Napp)
Tablets, white/orange, frusemide 40 mg, potassium 8 mmol for sustained release. Price 20 tabs = **D**. Label: 25
PoM **Esidrex-K**® (Ciba)
Tablets, s/c, hydrochlorothiazide 12.5 mg, potassium 8.1 mmol for sustained release. Price 20 tabs = **B**. Label: 25
PoM **Hygroton-K**® (Geigy)
Tablets, red, s/c, chlorthalidone 25 mg, potassium 6.7 mmol for sustained release. Price 20 tabs = **B**. Label: 25
PoM **Lasikal**® (Hoechst)
Tablets, white/yellow, f/c, frusemide 20 mg, potassium 10 mmol for sustained release. Price 20 tabs = **D**. Label: 25

PoM **Lasix + K**® (Hoechst)
Tablets, scored, frusemide 40 mg, with *tablets*, s/r, yellow, potassium chloride (potassium 10 mmol). Price 30 + 60 tabs = **F**. Label: 25
PoM **Navidrex-K**® (Ciba)
Tablets, yellow, s/c, cyclopenthiazide 250 micrograms, potassium 8.1 mmol for sustained release. Price 20 tabs = **B**. Label: 25
PoM **Neo-NaClex-K**® (DF)
Tablets, pink/white, f/c, bendrofluazide 2.5 mg, potassium 8.4 mmol for sustained release. Price 20 tabs = **B**. Label: 25

2.3   Anti-arrhythmic drugs

2.3.1 Treatment of individual arrhythmias
2.3.2 Drugs used in supraventricular tachycardias
2.3.3 Drugs used in ventricular arrhythmias

2.3.1   Treatment of individual arrhythmias

Management of an arrhythmia, apart from the treatment of associated heart failure, requires precise diagnosis of the type of arrhythmia, and electrocardiography is essential.
Atrial fibrillation. The ventricular rate can be controlled by digoxin (section 2.1).
Ectopic beats. If spontaneous with a normal heart, these rarely require treatment beyond reassurance. If they are particularly troublesome, beta-adrenoceptor blocking drugs are sometimes effective and may be safer than other suppressant drugs.
Atrial flutter. The ventricular rate can often be controlled with digoxin. Reversion to sinus rhythm (if indicated) is best achieved by appropriately synchronised d.c. shock, rather than by drug therapy.
Paroxysmal supraventricular tachycardia. In most patients this remits spontaneously or can be returned to sinus rhythm by reflex vagal stimulation, respiratory manoeuvres, prompt squatting, or pressure over one carotid sinus. If this fails, digitalisation or a beta-adrenoceptor blocking drug such as intravenous practolol may be effective. Intravenous verapamil is useful for patients without myocardial or valvular disease. For arrhythmias that are poorly tolerated, synchronised d.c. shock usually provides rapid relief.

In cases of paroxysmal atrial tachycardia with block, digitalis toxicity should be suspected, especially if the patient is hypokalaemic. Apart from stopping administration of the cardiac glycoside and giving potassium supplements, phenytoin or practolol given intravenously may be useful in controlling the tachycardia.
Acute arrhythmias after myocardial infarction. It is best to do nothing in patients with a paroxysmal tachycardia or rapid irregularity of the pulse until an ECG record is obtainable. If the condition of the patient is such that death due to the arrhythmia seems possible, 100 mg of lignocaine should be given intravenously. Bradycardia, particularly if complicated by hypotension, should be treated

---

by atropine sulphate in an initial dose of 300 micrograms, increasing to 1 mg if necessary
Ventricular tachycardia. In an emergency with a severely ill patient reversion is best achieved by d.c. shock. Alternatively, lignocaine (section 2.3.3) is at present the preferred drug. Other drugs are best administered under specialist supervision.

2.3.2   Drugs used in supraventricular tachycardias

Digoxin (section 2.1) by mouth is the treatment of choice in slowing ventricular response in cases of atrial fibrillation and atrial flutter. Intravenous digoxin, preferably infused slowly, is occasionally required if the ventricular rate needs rapid control.

Beta-adrenoceptor blocking drugs (section 2.4) prolong atrioventricular nodal conduction and may be used in conjunction with digoxin to control the ventricular response, especially in patients with thyrotoxicosis. Beta-adrenoceptor blocking drugs are also useful in the management of supraventricular tachycardias. See section 2.4 for potential problems associated with this use.

Verapamil (Cordilox®) is usually effective for supraventricular tachycardias, including those associated with the Wolff-Parkinson-White syndrome; an initial intravenous dose may be followed by oral treatment. Hypotension may occur with larger doses. Verapamil should not be injected into patients recently treated with beta-adrenoceptor blocking drugs because of the risk of causing hypotension and asystole. It has been suggested, however, that when verapamil injection has been given first, an interval of 30 minutes before giving a beta-adrenoceptor blocking drug is sufficient but this too is open to doubt. (For use in angina see section 2.6.1.)

Amiodarone (Cordarone X®) is used in the treatment of the Wolff-Parkinson-White syndrome. It may only be used for the treatment of other arrhythmias when they have proved refractory to conventional therapy. These include supraventricular and ventricular tachycardias, atrial fibrillation and flutter, and recurrent ventricular fibrillation. Amiodarone has a very long half-life and need only be given once daily; patients should be monitored to ensure the lowest effective dose is used. Most patients develop corneal microdeposits; these rarely interfere with vision and are reversible on withdrawal of treatment. Because of the possibility of phototoxic reactions, patients should be advised to shield the skin from light and to use a sunscreen to protect against long ultraviolet and visible light.

Amiodarone contains iodine which can be released and cause disorders of thyroid function. Both hypothyroidism and hyperthyroidism can occur. Thyroid function tests which rely on plasma concentrations of thyroxine alone rather than thyroxine plus triiodothyronine may also be spuriously elevated, but where concern about thyroid function exists amiodarone should be withdrawn.

Quinidine (section 2.3.3) may be effective in

suppressing supraventricular and ventricular arrhythmias. The drug itself may precipitate rhythm disorders, and is best used on specialist advice.

AMIODARONE HYDROCHLORIDE

Indications: see notes above
Cautions: heart failure; liver-function and thyroid-function tests required in long-term therapy; interferes with tests of thyroid function; regular eye examinations during long-term treatment. Drug interactions: see Appendix 1 (sections *2.1*, 2.3, *2.3*, *2.8B*, *4.8*)
Contra-indications: sinus bradycardia, atrioventricular block, thyroid dysfunction; pregnancy and breast-feeding; iodine sensitivity
Side-effects: corneal microdeposits, peripheral neuropathy, phototoxicity and rarely persistent slate-grey skin discoloration (see also notes above); hypothyroidism, hyperthyroidism, diffuse pulmonary alveolitis, hepatitis; rarely nausea, vomiting, metallic taste, tremor, nightmares, vertigo, headache, sleeplessness, fatigue
Dose: by mouth, 200 mg 3 times daily for 1 week reduced to 200 mg twice daily for a further week; maintenance, usually 200 mg daily or the minimum required to control the arrhythmia
By intravenous infusion via caval catheter, up to 5 mg/kg over 20–120 minutes with ECG monitoring; max. 1.2 g in 24 hours

▼ PoM **Cordarone X®** (Labaz)
Tablets, scored, amiodarone hydrochloride 100 mg. Price 20 tabs = **F**. Label: 11
Tablets, scored, amiodarone hydrochloride 200 mg. Price 20 tabs = **G**. Label: 11
Injection, amiodarone hydrochloride 50 mg/ml. Price 3-ml amp = **D**

ATROPINE SULPHATE

Indications: bradycardia after myocardial infarction, bradycardia caused by beta-adrenoceptor blocking drugs
Cautions: glaucoma, paralytic ileus, enlarged prostate. Drug interactions: see Appendix 1 (sections *1*, *2.3*)
Side-effects: dry mouth, confusion, tachycardia
Dose: by intravenous injection, 0.3–1 mg; max. 3 mg in 24 hours

PoM **Atropine Sulphate Injection**
400 micrograms/ml. Price 1-ml amp = **B**
600 micrograms/ml. Price 1-ml amp = **B**; 25-ml vial = **C**
800 micrograms/ml. Price 1-ml amp = **B**
1 mg/ml. Price 1-ml amp = **B**
1.2 mg/ml. Price 0.5-ml amp = **A**
1.25 mg/ml. Price 1-ml amp = **B**

VERAPAMIL HYDROCHLORIDE

Indications: supraventricular   arrhythmias, angina pectoris, hypertension
Cautions: do not administer intravenously to a patient taking beta-adrenoceptor blocking drugs. May be given by mouth concurrently

C = 51-100p, **D** = 101-180p, **E** = 181-300p, **F** = 301-450p, **G** = 451-650p, **H** = 651-900p, **I** = 901-1200p, **J** = over 1200p.

with beta-adrenoceptor blocking drugs only if myocardial function is well preserved; reduce dose in hepatic impairment. Drug interactions: see Appendix 1 (sections *2.1*, 2.3, 2.5)

Contra-indications: bradycardia, heart block, heart failure

Side-effects: nausea, vomiting, constipation; hypotension, bradycardia, heart block, and asystole after intravenous administration

Dose: by mouth, arrhythmias, 40–120 mg 3 times daily; angina, 80–120 mg 3 times daily; hypertension, 120–240 mg twice daily

By slow intravenous injection, 5 mg, repeated after 5–10 minutes if necessary

By intravenous infusion, 5–10 mg over 1 hour; max. 100 mg in 24 hours

PoM **Verapamil Hydrochloride Tablets,** verapamil hydrochloride 40 mg, price 20 tabs = C; 80 mg, price 20 tabs = E; 120 mg, price 20 tabs = **F**

PoM **Berkatens**® (Berk)
Tablets, yellow, f/c, verapamil hydrochloride 40 mg. Price 20 tabs = C
Tablets, yellow, f/c, verapamil hydrochloride 80 mg. Price 20 tabs = D
Tablets, yellow, f/c, verapamil hydrochloride 120 mg. Price 20 tabs = E

PoM **Cordilox**® (Abbott)
Tablets, yellow, f/c, verapamil hydrochloride 40 mg. Price 20 tabs = D
Tablets, yellow, f/c, verapamil hydrochloride 80 mg. Price 20 tabs = E
Tablets, yellow, f/c, verapamil hydrochloride 120 mg. Price 20 tabs = F
▼ *Tablets*, yellow, f/c, verapamil hydrochloride 160 mg. Price 20 tabs = F
Injection, verapamil hydrochloride 2.5 mg/ml. Price 2-ml amp = C
▼ PoM **Securon**® (Knoll)
Tablets, yellow, s/c, verapamil hydrochloride 120 mg. Price 28-tab calendar pack = F
▼ PoM **Securon MID**® (Knoll)
Tablets, yellow, s/c, verapamil hydrochloride 80 mg. Price 28-tab calendar pack = E

2.3.3   Drugs used in ventricular arrhythmias

Lignocaine is the treatment of choice to suppress ventricular extrasystoles and ventricular tachycardia following an acute myocardial infarction. It has not been shown convincingly to reduce mortality when used prophylactically. In patients with cardiac or hepatic failure doses may need to be reduced to avoid convulsions, depression of the central nervous system, or depression of the cardiovascular system.

If lignocaine is ineffective **mexiletine** (Mexitil®) which has a similar action, can be given as a slow intravenous injection followed by infusion at a decreasing rate until the arrhythmia is controlled. Adverse cardiovascular and central

nervous system effects may limit the dose which can be tolerated.

Tocainide (Tonocard®) is an analogue of lignocaine with similar activity, and can be given by mouth or intravenous injection. **Flecainide** (Tambocor®) is a newer agent in the same general class which can also be given by mouth or intravenously, but its role in relation to older agents remains to be established.

Other drugs that may be given by slow intravenous injection to control arrhythmias include **procainamide** (Pronestyl®), which should be used cautiously if lignocaine has already been given, as the cumulative negative inotropic effect severely depresses the myocardium; **disopyramide** (Dirythmin®, Rythmodan®) and **practolol** (Eraldin®), both of which may impair cardiac contractility; and **phenytoin** (Epanutin®), which is particularly useful in digitalis-induced arrhythmias.

Evidence is now available that at least some beta-adrenocepter blocking drugs (such as metoprolol) can reduce the incidence of life-threatening arrhythmias in the acute stage of myocardial infarction, but their influence on mortality when given at this stage remains to be determined (see also section 2.4).

Bretylium (Bretylate®) has been given by intramuscular injection, but can cause severe hypotension.

Once the arrhythmias have been controlled by parenteral therapy, treatment by mouth may be considered. However, the likelihood of life-threatening arrhythmias occurring diminishes sharply over the first 24 hours after infarction, especially in patients without heart failure or shock. Moreover, most or all drugs which are effective in countering arrhythmias can also provoke them in some circumstances, and this so-called pro-arrhythmic effect has to be taken into account when their safety is considered. Hypokalaemia enhances the pro-arrhythmic effect of many drugs. Nausea and vomiting associated with mexiletine may prevent an effective dose being given; prolonged use of procainamide can cause a syndrome resembling lupus erythematosus; disopyramide has an anticholinergic effect which limits its use in patients with glaucoma or urinary retention; and quinidine can cause hypersensitivity reactions and gastro-intestinal upsets. Amiodarone (section 2.3.2) is also used.

BRETYLIUM TOSYLATE

Indications: ventricular arrhythmias resistant to other treatment

Cautions: do not give noradrenaline or other sympathomimetic amines

Side-effects: hypotension, nausea

Dose: by intramuscular injection, 5 mg/kg repeated after 6–8 hours if necessary

PoM **Bretylate**® (Wellcome)
Injection, bretylium tosylate 50 mg/ml. Price 2-ml amp = E

DISOPYRAMIDE

Indications: ventricular arrhythmias, especially after myocardial infarction

Cautions: glaucoma; heart failure or diminished cardiac output; reduce dose in renal impairment. Drug interactions: see Appendix 1 (sections 2.3, *4.9*)

Side-effects: myocardial depression, hypotension, atrioventricular block; anticholinergic effects include dry mouth, blurred vision, urinary retention

Dose: by mouth, 300–800 mg daily in divided doses

By slow intravenous injection, 2 mg/kg over at least 5 minutes to a max. of 150 mg, with ECG monitoring; maintenance, 400 micrograms/kg/hour *by intravenous infusion;* max. 300 mg in 1 hour and 800 mg daily

PoM **Disopyramide Capsules,** disopyramide 100 mg, price 20 caps = **D**; 150 mg, price 20 caps = **E**

PoM **Dirythmin**® (Astra)
Capsules, orange/white, disopyramide 100 mg (as phosphate). Price 20 caps = **D**
Injection, disopyramide 20 mg (as phosphate)/ml. Price 5-ml amp = **D**

PoM **Dirythmin SA**® (Astra)
Durules® (=tablets, s/r), f/c, disopyramide 150 mg (as phosphate). Price 20 tabs = **E**. Label: 25
Dose: 300 mg every 12 hours; max. 900 mg daily

PoM **Rythmodan**® (Roussel)
Capsules, green/yellow, disopyramide 100 mg. Price 20 caps = **D**
Capsules, disopyramide 150 mg. Price 20 caps = **E**
Injection, disopyramide 10 mg (as phosphate)/ml. Price 5-ml amp = **C**

PoM **Rythmodan Retard**® (Roussel)
Tablets, s/r, scored, f/c, disopyramide 250 mg (as phosphate). Price 20 tabs = **G**. Label: 25
Dose: 250–375 mg every 12 hours

FLECAINIDE ACETATE

Indications: ventricular and supraventricular arrhythmias

Cautions: patients with pacemakers; reduce dose in renal impairment; pregnancy (toxicity in *animal* studies). Drug interactions: see Appendix 1 (section 2.3)

Contra-indications: heart failure, sino-atrial disorders, atrioventricular block

Side-effects: dizziness, visual disturbances; rarely nausea and vomiting

Dose: by mouth, 100–200 mg twice daily; max. 400 mg daily, reduced after 3–5 days if possible; elderly patients 100 mg twice daily, reduced after 1 week if possible

By slow intravenous injection, 2 mg/kg over 10–30 minutes, max. 150 mg; followed if required by *infusion* at a rate of 1.5 mg/kg/hour for 1 hour, then 250 micrograms/kg/hour; transfer to *oral* treatment, 100-mg tablet, then withdraw

infusion over 4 hours by hourly decrements of 20%, and continue oral treatment as above

▼ PoM **Tambocor**® (Riker)
Tablets, scored, flecainide acetate 100 mg. Price 20 tabs = **G**
Injection, flecainide acetate 10 mg/ml. Price 15-ml amp = **F**

LIGNOCAINE HYDROCHLORIDE

Indications: ventricular arrhythmias, especially after myocardial infarction

Cautions: lower doses in congestive cardiac failure, in hepatic failure, and following cardiac surgery. Drug interactions: see Appendix 1 (section 2.3, *2.4*)

Contra-indications: sino-atrial disorders, all grades of atrioventricular block, severe myocardial depression

Side-effects: confusion, convulsions

Dose: by intravenous injection, in patients without gross circulatory impairment, 100 mg as a bolus over a few minutes, followed by *infusion* of 4 mg/minute for 30 minutes, 2 mg/minute for 2 hours, then 1 mg/minute

PoM **Lignocaine 0.1% in Glucose Injection,** lignocaine hydrochloride 1 mg/ml in glucose intravenous infusion 5%. Price 500-ml container = **D**; 1-litre container = **D**

PoM **Lignocaine 0.2% in Glucose Injection,** lignocaine hydrochloride 2 mg/ml in glucose intravenous infusion 5%. Price 500-ml container = **D**; 1-litre container = **D**

PoM **Xylocard**® (Astra)
Injection 100 mg, lignocaine hydrochloride (anhydrous) 20 mg/ml. Price 5-ml syringe = **D**
Intravenous infusion, lignocaine hydrochloride (anhydrous) 200 mg/ml. To be diluted before use. Price 5-ml syringe (1 g) = **E**; 10-ml syringe (2 g) = **E**

MEXILETINE HYDROCHLORIDE

Indications: ventricular arrhythmias, especially after myocardial infarction

Cautions: drug interactions: see Appendix 1 (section 2.3)

Contra-indications: bradycardia, heart block

Side-effects: bradycardia, hypotension, confusion, dysarthria, nystagmus, tremor

Dose: by mouth, initial dose 400 mg, followed after 2 hours by 200–250 mg 3–4 times daily

By intravenous injection, 100–250 mg at a rate of 25 mg/minute followed by *infusion* of 250 mg as a 0.1% solution over 1 hour, 125 mg/hour for 2 hours, then 500 micrograms/minute

PoM **Mexitil**® (Boehringer Ingelheim)
Capsules, purple/red, mexiletine hydrochloride 50 mg. Price 20 caps = **C**
Capsules, red, mexiletine hydrochloride 200 mg. Price 20 caps = **E**
Injection, mexiletine hydrochloride 25 mg/ml. Price 10-ml amp = **D**

C = 51-100p, **D** = 101-180p, **E** = 181-300p, **F** = 301-450p. **G** = 451-650p, **H** = 651-900p, **I** = 901-1200p, **J** = over 1200p.

PoM **Mexitil PL**® (Boehringer Ingelheim)
Perlongets® (=capsules, s/r, each enclosing 5 miniature tablets), turquoise/scarlet, mexiletine hydrochloride 360 mg. Price 20 caps = **F**. Label: 25
Dose: 1 capsule twice daily

PHENYTOIN SODIUM
Indications: ventricular arrhythmias, especially those caused by cardiac glycosides (for use in epilepsy, see section 4.8.1)
Cautions: do not give with lignocaine hydrochloride
Contra-indications: supraventricular tachycardias (except those induced by digitalis), heart block
Side-effects: bradycardia, hypotension, asystole, confusion
Dose: by intravenous injection via caval catheter, 3.5–5 mg/kg at a rate not exceeding 50 mg/minute. Repeat after 10 minutes if necessary

PoM **Epanutin Ready Mixed Parenteral**® (P-D)
Injection, phenytoin sodium 50 mg/ml. Price 5-ml amp = **F**

PRACTOLOL
Indications: supraventricular tachycardias; ventricular tachycardias, especially after myocardial infarction
Cautions: chronic obstructive airways disease; for cautions with verapamil see notes (section 2.3.2). Drug interactions: see Appendix 1 (sections 2.3, 2.4, 2.5, 2.7, 6.1, 15)
Side-effects: bradycardia, hypotension, heart failure, bronchospasm
Dose: by slow intravenous injection, 5 mg, repeated if required

PoM **Eraldin**® (ICI)
Injection, practolol 2 mg/ml. Price 5-ml amp = **C** (Hosp. only)

PROCAINAMIDE HYDROCHLORIDE
Indications: ventricular arrhythmias, especially after myocardial infarction
Cautions: renal impairment, asthma, myasthenia gravis. Drug interactions: see Appendix 1 (section 2.3)
Contra-indications: heart block, heart failure, hypotension
Side-effects: nausea, diarrhoea, rashes, fever, myocardial depression, heart failure, lupus erythematosus-like syndrome, agranulocytosis after prolonged treatment
Dose: by mouth, 250 mg every 4–6 hours, preferably controlled by measurement of plasma concentration
By slow intravenous injection, 25–50 mg/minute with ECG monitoring, until arrhythmia is controlled; max. 1 g
Maintenance, *by mouth* as above or *by intramuscular injection*, 100–250 mg every 4–6 hours, preferably controlled by measurement of plasma concentration

PoM **Procainamide Durules**® (Astra)
Tablets, s/r, yellow, procainamide hydrochloride 500 mg. Price 20 tabs = **D**. Label: 25
Dose: 1–1.5 g every 8 hours
PoM **Pronestyl**® (Squibb)
Tablets, scored, procainamide hydrochloride 250 mg. Price 20 tabs = **C**
Injection, procainamide hydrochloride 100 mg/ml. Price 10-ml vial = **E**

QUINIDINE
Indications: prevention of supraventricular tachycardias, ventricular arrhythmias
Cautions: 200-mg test dose to detect hypersensitivity reactions. Drug interactions: see Appendix 1 (sections 2.1, 2.3, 15)
Contra-indications: heart block
Side-effects: see under Procainamide Hydrochloride; also ventricular arrhythmias, thrombocytopenia, haemolytic anaemia; rarely granulomatous hepatitis
Dose: by mouth, quinidine sulphate 200–400 mg 3–4 times daily
Note: quinidine sulphate 200 mg ≡ quinidine bisulphate 250 mg

PoM **Quinidine Sulphate Tablets,** quinidine sulphate 200 and 300 mg. Price 20 tabs (both) = **D**
PoM **Kiditard**® (Delandale)
Capsules, s/r, blue, quinidine bisulphate 250 mg. Price 20 caps = **E**. Label: 25
Dose: 500 mg every 12 hours, adjusted as required
PoM **Kinidin Durules**® (Astra)
Tablets, s/r, f/c, quinidine bisulphate 250 mg. Price 20 tabs = **E**. Label: 25
Dose: 500 mg every 12 hours, adjusted as required
PoM **Quinicardine**® (Lewis)
Tablets, scored, quinidine sulphate 200 mg. Price 20 tabs = **F**

TOCAINIDE HYDROCHLORIDE
Indications: ventricular arrhythmias, especially after myocardial infarction
Cautions: severe hepatic or renal impairment, uncompensated heart failure, pregnancy (toxicity in *animal* studies). Drug interactions: see Appendix 1 (section 2.3)
Contra-indications: see under Lignocaine Hydrochloride
Side-effects: CNS effects including tremor, dizziness, convulsions, paraesthesia; gastro-intestinal effects including nausea and vomiting; bradycardia and hypotension after injection; rash and fever; rarely lupus erythematosus-like syndrome, fibrosing alveolitis, agranulocytosis, transient neutropenia
Dose: chronic arrhythmias, *by mouth*, 1.2 g daily in 2–3 divided doses; max. 2.4 g daily
Acute treatment, *by slow intravenous injection or infusion*, 500–750 mg over 15–30 minutes, followed immediately by 600–800 mg by mouth
Maintenance, *by mouth*, 1.2 g daily, in 2–3 divided doses

▼ PoM **Tonocard**® (Astra)

Tablets, yellow, f/c, tocainide hydrochloride
400 mg. Price 20 tabs = **F**

Tablets, yellow, f/c, tocainide hydrochloride
600 mg. Price 20 tabs = **F**

Injection, tocainide hydrochloride 50 mg/ml.
Price 15-ml vial = **G**

Intravenous infusion, tocainide hydrochloride
10 mg/ml. Price 75-ml bottle = **G**

2.4 Beta-adrenoceptor blocking drugs

This group of drugs blocks the beta-adreno-receptors in the heart, peripheral vasculature, bronchi, pancreas, and liver. Beta-blockers are used in the treatment of hypertension, they relieve the symptoms of angina, and are beneficial in the secondary prevention of myocardial infarction. In addition beta-blockers have been employed in the treatment of migraine, anxiety states, essential tremor, thyrotoxicosis, glaucoma (used topically), and hypertrophic obstructive cardiomyopathy. Many beta-blockers are now available and in general they are all equally effective. There are, how-ever, differences between them which may affect choice in treating individual diseases or patients. Intrinsic sympathomimetic activity (ISA, partial agonist activity) represents the capacity of beta-blockers to stimulate as well as to block adrenergic receptors. Oxprenolol, pindolol, and acebutolol have ISA and they tend to cause less bradycardia than the other beta-blockers and may also cause less coldness of the extremities.

Some beta-blockers are lipid soluble and some are water soluble. Atenolol, nadolol, and sotalol are the most water-soluble; they are less likely to enter the brain, and may therefore cause less sleep disturbance and nightmares. Water-soluble beta-blockers are excreted by the kidneys and may accumulate in renal impairment; smaller doses are often necessary.

Some beta-blockers have a relatively short dur-ation of action and have to be given twice or three times daily. Many of these are, however, available in slow-release formulations so that in general it is not necessary to give beta-blockers more often than once daily.

All beta-blockers slow the heart and may induce myocardial depression and precipitate heart fail-ure. They should not therefore be given to patients who have incipient cardiac failure or those with second or third degree heart block.

Beta-blockers may precipitate asthma and this effect can be dangerous. Some beta-blockers tend to have less effect on the beta$_2$ (bronchial) recep-tors and are therefore relatively cardioselective. Metoprolol, atenolol, and acebutolol are cardio-selective but they are not cardiospecific. They have a lesser effect on airways resistance but are not free of this side-effect. Patients who have a tendency towards obstructive airways disease should be treated with caution and may require to take increased doses of their beta$_2$ agonists (e.g.

salbutamol) to overcome the effect of blockade of the bronchial adrenoceptors. Beta-blockers may induce or aggravate intermittent claudication. Beta-blockers can lead to a small deterioration of glucose tolerance in diabetics. They also interfere with the metabolic and autonomic response of diabetics to hypoglycaemia. Their use is not contra-indicated in diabetics, but cardioselective beta-blockers may be preferable. However they should be avoided in diabetics who have frequent episodes of hypoglycaemia.

Practolol (section 2.3.3) which is now used by injection for treatment of arrhythmias was with-drawn from general use as it caused the oculo-mucocutaneous syndrome with conjunctival scar-ring, psoriasiform rash, and peritoneal fibrosis when taken by mouth. It is doubtful whether this toxic effect occurs with the other beta-blockers.

Labetalol (Trandate®) combines alpha- and beta-receptor blocking activity. Alpha-blocking activity in the peripheral vessels lowers peripheral resistance. There is no evidence that labetalol is more effective than pure beta-blockers. The alpha-blocking properties tend to offset the lack of cardioselectivity of the beta blockade, with the net effect that labetalol and atenolol have roughly similar effects on airways resistance.

HYPERTENSION

Beta-blockers are effective antihypertensive drugs but their mode of action is not understood; they reduce cardiac output, alter baroceptor reflex sensitivity, and block peripheral adrenoceptors. Some beta-blockers depress plasma renin secretion. It is possible that a central effect may also explain their mode of action. Despite the many contra-indications blood pressure can be usually controlled with relatively few side-effects. In general the dose of beta-blocker does not have to be as high as originally thought. The maximum dose of oxprenolol and propranolol is probably 320 mg daily. Atenolol can usually be given in a dose of 50 mg daily and it is only rarely necessary to increase to 100 mg.

While beta-blockers are expensive their use is justified on the grounds of their fewer clinical and biochemical side-effects. There is also some uncontrolled evidence to suggest that beta-block-ers prevent more complications than other anti-hypertensive drugs. Where beta-blockers have proved insufficient to control blood pressure it is conventional to add a thiazide diuretic. Combined thiazide/beta-blocker tablet formulations are now available and these may help compliance' with treatment regimens.

Beta-blockers can be used to control the pulse rate in patients with *phaeochromocytoma*. How-ever, they should never be used alone as beta-blockade without concurrent alpha-blockade may lead to a hypertensive crisis. For this reason phenoxybenzamine should always be used together with the beta-blocker.

ANGINA

Beta-blockers improve exercise tolerance and relieve symptoms in patients with angina; this effect is caused by their reduction of cardiac work. As with hypertension there is no good evidence of the superiority of any one drug, although occasionally a patient will respond better to one beta-blocker than to another. There is some doubtful evidence that sudden withdrawal may cause an exacerbation of angina although this is not proved. As doubt remains, gradual reduction of dose is preferable when beta-blockers are to be stopped. There is a risk of precipitating heart failure when beta-blockers and calcium-channel blockers are used together in patients with established ischaemic heart disease.

MYOCARDIAL INFARCTION

Several studies have now shown that beta-blockers can cause a reduction in the recurrence rate of myocardial infarction. However, pre-existing heart failure, hypotension, bradyarrhythmias, and obstructive airways disease render this group of drugs unsuitable in some patients who have recovered from a myocardial infarction. There is some doubt whether beta-blockers should be started immediately after a myocardial infarction or after some weeks. It is also not known whether the protective effect of beta-blockers continues after two years; it is possible that sudden cessation may cause a rebound worsening of myocardial ischaemia.

ARRHYTHMIAS

Beta-blockers are used to control supraventricular tachycardia following myocardial infarction. They can be given intravenously and practolol is still the favoured drug. (See also section 2.3.)

THYROTOXICOSIS

Beta-blockers are used in pre-operative preparation for thyroidectomy. Doses of 40 to 200 mg daily of propranolol given six-hourly can reverse clinical features of thyrotoxicosis within 4 days. Routine tests of increased thyroid function remain unaltered. The thyroid gland is rendered less vascular thus making surgery easier (see section 6.2.2).

OTHER USES

Beta-blockers have been used to alleviate some symptoms of anxiety; probably patients with palpitations, tremor, and tachycardia respond best. (See also sections 4.1.2 and 4.9.3.) Beta-blockers are also used in the prophylaxis of migraine (see section 4.7.4.2).

PROPRANOLOL HYDROCHLORIDE

Indications: hypertension, angina, arrhythmias, thyrotoxicosis, secondary prevention after acute myocardial infarction

Cautions: late pregnancy; breast-feeding; avoid abrupt withdrawal in angina. Reduce oral dose of propranolol in liver disease; reduce initial dose in renal impairment. See also notes above. Drug interactions: see Appendix 1 (sections 2.3, 2.4, 2.5, 2.7, 4.2, 6.1, 15)

Contra-indications: asthma, heart failure, second or third degree heart block, intermittent claudication

Side-effects: bradycardia, heart failure, bronchospasm, peripheral vasoconstriction, gastrointestinal disturbances

Dose: by mouth, hypertension, initially 80 mg twice daily, increased at weekly intervals as required; maintenance 160–320 mg daily

Angina, initially 40 mg 2–3 times daily; maintenance 120–240 mg daily

Arrhythmias and thyrotoxicosis, 10–40 mg 3–4 times daily

Prophylaxis after infarction, 40 mg 4 times daily for 2–3 days, then 80 mg twice daily, beginning 5 to 21 days after infarction

By intravenous injection, 1 mg over 1 minute, preceded by atropine sulphate 1–2 mg; if necessary repeat at 2-minute intervals; max. 10 mg (5 mg in anaesthesia)

PoM **Propranolol Tablets,** propranolol hydrochloride 10, 40, and 80 mg, price 20 tabs (all) = **A**; 160 mg, price 20 tabs = **B**. Label: 8

PoM **Angilol**® (DDSA)
Tablets, pink, f/c, propranolol hydrochloride 10 mg. Price 20 tabs = **B**. Label: 8
Tablets, pink, f/c, propranolol hydrochloride 40 mg. Price 20 tabs = **B**. Label: 8
Tablets, pink, f/c, propranolol hydrochloride 80 mg. Price 20 tabs = **C**. Label: 8
Tablets, pink, f/c, propranolol hydrochloride 160 mg. Price 20 tabs = **D**. Label: 8

PoM **Apsolol**® (APS)
Tablets, pink, f/c, scored, propranolol hydrochloride 10 mg. Price 20 tabs = **A**. Label: 8
Tablets, pink, f/c, scored, propranolol hydrochloride 40 mg. Price 20 tabs = **A**. Label: 8
Tablets, pink, f/c, scored, propranolol hydrochloride 80 mg. Price 20 tabs = **A**. Label: 8
Tablets, pink, f/c, scored, propranolol hydrochloride 160 mg. Price 20 tabs = **B**. Label: 8

PoM **Bedranol**® (Lagap)
Tablets, pink, f/c, propranolol hydrochloride 10 mg. Price 20 tabs = **B**. Label: 8
Tablets, pink, f/c, propranolol hydrochloride 40 mg. Price 20 tabs = **C**. Label: 8
Tablets, pink, f/c, propranolol hydrochloride 80 mg. Price 20 tabs = **C**. Label: 8
Tablets, pink, f/c, propranolol hydrochloride 160 mg. Price 20 tabs = **D**. Label: 8

PoM **Berkolol**® (Berk)
Tablets, pink, f/c, scored, propranolol hydrochloride 10 mg. Price 20 tabs = **B**. Label: 8
Tablets, pink, f/c, scored, propranolol hydrochloride 40 mg. Price 20 tabs = **C**. Label: 8

Tablets, pink, f/c, scored, propranolol hydrochloride 80 mg. Price 20 tabs = **C**. Label: 8
Tablets, pink, f/c, scored, propranolol hydrochloride 160 mg. Price 20 tabs = **D**. Label: 8

PoM **Half-Inderal LA**® (ICI)
Capsules, s/r, lavender/pink, propranolol hydrochloride 80 mg. Price 28 caps = **F**. Label: 8, 25

PoM **Inderal**® (ICI)
Tablets, pink, f/c, propranolol hydrochloride 10 mg. Price 20 tabs = **B**. Label: 8
Tablets, pink, f/c, propranolol hydrochloride 40 mg. Price 20 tabs = **C**. Label: 8
Tablets, pink, f/c, propranolol hydrochloride 80 mg. Price 20 tabs = **D**. Label: 8
Tablets, pink, f/c, propranolol hydrochloride 160 mg. Price 20 tabs = **E**. Label: 8
Injection, propranolol hydrochloride 1 mg/ml. Price 1-ml amp = **B**

PoM **Inderal-LA**® (ICI)
Capsules, s/r, lavender/pink, propranolol hydrochloride 160 mg. Price 28 caps = **H**. Label: 8, 25

PoM **Sloprolol**® (CP)
Capsules, s/r, green/clear enclosing off-white pellets, propranolol hydrochloride 160 mg. Price 20 caps = **F**. Label: 8, 25

ACEBUTOLOL

Indications: hypertension, angina, arrhythmias
Cautions; Contra-indications; Side-effects: see under Propranolol Hydrochloride
Dose: by mouth, hypertension, initially 400 mg once daily *or* 200 mg twice daily, increased as required; maintenance up to 1.2 g daily
Angina, initially 400 mg once daily *or* 200 mg twice daily; 300 mg 3 times daily in severe angina; maintenance up to 1.2 g daily
Arrhythmias, initially 200 mg, then 100–200 mg 2–3 times daily
By intravenous injection, 5–25 mg over 3–5 minutes; further doses by slow intravenous injection or infusion

PoM **Sectral**® (M&B)
Capsules, buff/white, acebutolol 100 mg (as hydrochloride). Price 20 caps = **D**. Label: 8
Capsules, buff/pink, acebutolol 200 mg (as hydrochloride). Price 20 caps = **E**. Label: 8
Tablets, f/c, acebutolol 400 mg (as hydrochloride). Price 28 tabs = **H**. Label: 8
Injection, acebutolol 5 mg (as hydrochloride)/ml. Price 2-ml amp = **C**

ATENOLOL

Indications: hypertension, angina, arrhythmias, early intervention in acute myocardial infarction
Cautions; Contra-indications; Side-effects: see under Propranolol Hydrochloride; reduce dose in renal impairment
Dose: by mouth, hypertension, 50–100 mg daily; angina, 100 mg daily in 1 or 2 doses; arrhythmias, 50–100 mg daily
By intravenous injection, 2.5 mg at a rate of 1 mg/minute, repeated at 5-minute intervals to a max. of 10 mg

By intravenous infusion, 150 micrograms/kg over 20 minutes, repeated every 12 hours if required
Early intervention within 12 hours of infarction, 5 mg *by slow intravenous injection*, then *by mouth* 50 mg after 15 minutes, 50 mg after 12 hours, then 100 mg daily for up to 10 days

PoM **Tenormin**® (Stuart)
Tablets, orange, f/c, atenolol 100 mg. Price 28 tabs = **H**. Label: 8
▼ *Injection*, atenolol 500 micrograms/ml. Price 10-ml amp = **C** (Hosp. only)

PoM **Tenormin LS**® (Stuart)
Tablets, orange, f/c, atenolol 50 mg. Price 28 tabs = **G**. Label: 8

BETAXOLOL HYDROCHLORIDE

Indications: hypertension
Cautions; Contra-indications; Side-effects: see under Propranolol Hydrochloride; reduce dose in renal impairment
Dose: 20 mg daily (elderly patients 10 mg), increased to 40 mg if required

▼ PoM **Kerlone**® (Lorex)
Tablets, f/c, scored, betaxolol hydrochloride 20 mg. Price 28 tabs = **H**. Label: 8

LABETALOL HYDROCHLORIDE

Indications: hypertension (including hypertension in pregnancy, hypertension with angina, and hypertension following acute myocardial infarction); hypertensive crisis; controlled hypotension in surgery
Cautions: heart block, heart failure, asthma, late pregnancy, breast-feeding; avoid abrupt withdrawal; reduce oral dose in liver disease; interferes with laboratory tests for catecholamines. Drug interactions: see Appendix 1 (see under Propranolol Hydrochloride)
Side-effects: postural hypotension, tiredness, weakness, headache, rashes, scalp tingling, difficulty in micturition, epigastric pain, nausea, vomiting; rarely lichenoid rash
Dose: by mouth, initially 100–200 mg twice daily with food, increased at 14-day intervals; max. 2.4 g daily
By intravenous injection, 50 mg over 1 minute, repeated after 5 minutes if necessary; max. 200 mg
By intravenous infusion, 2 mg/minute to a max. of 200 mg
Hypertension of pregnancy, 20 mg/hour, doubled every 30 minutes; max. 160 mg/hour
Hypertension following infarction, 15 mg/hour, gradually increased to max. 120 mg/hour

PoM **Trandate**® (DF)
Tablets, orange, f/c, labetalol hydrochloride 100 mg. Price 20 tabs = **D**. Label: 8, 21
Tablets, orange, f/c, labetalol hydrochloride 200 mg. Price 20 tabs = **E**. Label: 8, 21
Tablets, orange, f/c, labetalol hydrochloride 400 mg. Price 20 tabs = **F**. Label: 8, 21

C = 51-100p, **D** = 101-180p, **E** = 181-300p, **F** = 301-450p, **G** = 451-650p, **H** = 651-900p, **I** = 901-1200p, **J** = over 1200p.

Injection, labetalol hydrochloride 5 mg/ml. Price 20-ml amp = **E**

METOPROLOL TARTRATE

Indications: hypertension, angina, arrhythmias (including arrhythmias during anaesthesia), thyrotoxicosis, early intervention in acute myocardial infarction

Cautions; Contra-indications; Side-effects: see under Propranolol Hydrochloride. Reduce initial dose in renal impairment

Dose: by mouth, hypertension, initially 100 mg daily, maintenance 100–400 mg daily in 1–2 doses

Angina, 50–100 mg 2–3 times daily

Arrhythmias, usually 50 mg 2–3 times daily, up to 300 mg daily in divided doses if necessary

Thyrotoxicosis, 50 mg 4 times daily

By intravenous injection, up to 5 mg at rate 1–2 mg/minute, repeated after 5 minutes if necessary, total dose 10–15 mg

In surgery, 2–4 mg *by slow intravenous injection* at induction or to control arrhythmias developing during anaesthesia; 2-mg doses may be repeated to a max. of 10 mg

Early intervention within 12 hours of infarction, 5 mg *by intravenous injection* every 2 minutes to a max. of 15 mg, then 50 mg *by mouth* every 6 hours for 48 hours; maintenance 200 mg daily

PoM **Metoprolol Tartrate Tablets,** metoprolol tartrate 50 mg, price 20 tabs = **C**; 100 mg, price 20 tabs = **D**. Label: 8

PoM **Metoprolol Tartrate Injection,** metoprolol tartrate 1 mg/ml. Price 5-ml amp = **A**

PoM **Betaloc®** (Astra)

Tablets, scored, metoprolol tartrate 50 mg. Price 20 tabs = **C**. Label: 8

Tablets, scored, metoprolol tartrate 100 mg. Price 20 tabs = **D**. Label: 8

Injection, metoprolol tartrate 1 mg/ml. Price 5-ml amp = **B**

PoM **Betaloc-SA®** (Astra)

Durules® (= tablets, s/r), metoprolol tartrate 200 mg. Price 20 tabs = **G**. Label: 8, 25

Dose: 200–400 mg daily

PoM **Lopresor®** (Geigy)

Tablets, pink, f/c, scored, metoprolol tartrate 50 mg. Price 20 tabs = **C**. Label: 8

Tablets, blue, f/c, scored, metoprolol tartrate 100 mg. Price 20 tabs = **D**. Label: 8

Injection, metoprolol tartrate 1 mg/ml. Price 5-ml amp = **A** (Hosp. only)

PoM **Lopresor SR®** (Geigy)

Tablets, s/r, yellow, f/c, metoprolol tartrate 200 mg. Price 28 tabs = **H**. Label: 8, 25

Dose: 200–400 mg daily

NADOLOL

Indications: hypertension, angina, arrhythmias, thyrotoxicosis

Cautions; Contra-indications; Side-effects: see under Propranolol Hydrochloride; reduce dose in renal impairment

Dose: hypertension, 80 mg daily, increased at weekly intervals; angina and arrhythmias, initially 40 mg daily; thyrotoxicosis 80–160 mg daily. Max. 240 mg daily

PoM **Corgard®** (Squibb)

Tablets, blue, nadolol 40 mg. Price 28 tabs = **G**. Label: 8

Tablets, blue, scored, nadolol 80 mg. Price 28 tabs = **H**. Label: 8

OXPRENOLOL HYDROCHLORIDE

Indications: hypertension, angina, arrhythmias, thyrotoxicosis

Cautions; Contra-indications; Side-effects: see under Propranolol Hydrochloride

Dose: by mouth, hypertension, initially 80 mg twice daily, increased as required at weekly intervals

Angina, 40–160 mg 3 times daily

Arrhythmias, initially 20–40 mg 3 times daily

Thyrotoxicosis, 40–120 mg daily in 2–3 divided doses

Max. 480 mg daily

By slow intravenous injection, 1–2 mg, repeated after 5 minutes if required; max. 16 mg

PoM **Oxprenolol Tablets,** f/c, oxprenolol hydrochloride 20 mg = **B**; 40 mg, price 20 tabs = **C**; 80 mg, price 20 tabs = **D**; 160 mg, price 20 tabs = **E**. Label: 8

PoM **Apsolox®** (APS)

Tablets, f/c, oxprenolol hydrochloride 20 mg. Price 20 tabs = **B**. Label: 8

Tablets, f/c, oxprenolol hydrochloride 40 mg. Price 20 tabs = **C**. Label: 8

Tablets, yellow, f/c, oxprenolol hydrochloride 80 mg. Price 20 tabs = **C**. Label: 8

Tablets, orange, f/c, oxprenolol hydrochloride 160 mg. Price 20 tabs = **E**. Label: 8

PoM **Laracor®** (Lagap)

Tablets, f/c, oxprenolol hydrochloride 20 mg. Price 20 tabs = **C**. Label: 8

Tablets, f/c, oxprenolol hydrochloride 40 mg. Price 20 tabs = **C**. Label: 8

Tablets, f/c, oxprenolol hydrochloride 80 mg. Price 20 tabs = **D**. Label: 8

Tablets, f/c, oxprenolol hydrochloride 160 mg. Price 20 tabs = **E**. Label: 8

▼ PoM **Slow-Pren®** (Norton)

Tablets, s/r, f/c, oxprenolol hydrochloride 160 mg. Price 28 tabs = **G**. Label: 8, 25

Dose: 160–480 mg daily

PoM **Slow-Trasicor®** (Ciba)

Tablets, s/r, f/c, oxprenolol hydrochloride 160 mg. Price 28 tabs = **H**. Label: 8, 25

Dose: 160–480 mg daily

PoM **Trasicor®** (Ciba)

Tablets, f/c, oxprenolol hydrochloride 20 mg. Price 20 tabs = **C**. Label: 8

Tablets, f/c, oxprenolol hydrochloride 40 mg. Price 20 tabs = **D**. Label: 8

Tablets, yellow, f/c, oxprenolol hydrochloride 80 mg. Price 20 tabs = **D**. Label: 8

Tablets, orange, f/c, oxprenolol hydrochloride 160 mg. Price 20 tabs = **E**. Label: 8

Injection, powder for reconstitution, oxprenolol hydrochloride. Price 2-mg amp = **B**

PENBUTOLOL SULPHATE

Indications: hypertension
Cautions; Contra-indications; Side-effects: see under Propranolol Hydrochloride
Dose: 40 mg daily, increased to twice daily if required

Preparations
See under Compound Preparations

PINDOLOL

Indications: hypertension, angina
Cautions; Contra-indications; Side-effects: see under Propranolol Hydrochloride; reduce dose in renal impairment
Dose: hypertension, initially 5 mg 2–3 times daily *or* 15 mg once daily, increased as required at weekly intervals, max. 45 mg daily
Angina, 2.5–5 mg up to 3 times daily

PoM **Visken**® (Sandoz)
Tablets, scored, pindolol 5 mg. Price 20 tabs = E. Label: 8
Tablets, scored, pindolol 15 mg. Price 20 tabs = G. Label: 8

PRACTOLOL
See section 2.3.3

SOTALOL HYDROCHLORIDE

Indications: hypertension, angina, arrhythmias, thyrotoxicosis, secondary prevention after acute myocardial infarction
Cautions; Contra-indications; Side-effects: see under Propranolol Hydrochloride; reduce dose in renal impairment
Dose: by mouth, hypertension and angina, initially 80 mg twice daily *or* 160 mg once daily; maintenance 200–600 mg daily
Arrhythmias, 120–240 mg daily in single or divided doses
Thyrotoxicosis, 120–240 mg daily in single or divided doses
Prophylaxis after infarction, 320 mg daily, starting 5–14 days after infarction
By slow intravenous injection, 10–20 mg, repeated if necessary

PoM **Sotalol Hydrochloride Tablets**, sotalol hydrochloride 40 mg, price 20 tabs = C; 80 mg, price 20 tabs = E; 160 mg, price 14 tabs = E; 200 mg, price 30 tabs = G. Label: 8
PoM **Beta-Cardone**® (DF)
Tablets, green, scored, sotalol hydrochloride 40 mg. Price 20 tabs = C. Label: 8
Tablets, red, scored, sotalol hydrochloride 80 mg. Price 20 tabs = D. Label: 8
Tablets, scored, sotalol hydrochloride 200 mg. Price 30 tabs = F. Label: 8
PoM **Sotacor**® (Bristol-Myers)
Tablets, pink, sotalol hydrochloride 80 mg. Price 28 tabs = E. Label: 8

Tablets, blue, sotalol hydrochloride 160 mg. Price 14 tabs = E. Label: 8
Injection, sotalol hydrochloride 2 mg/ml. Price 5-ml amp = **B**

TIMOLOL MALEATE

Indications: hypertension, angina, secondary prevention after acute myocardial infarction
Cautions; Contra-indications; Side-effects: see under Propranolol Hydrochloride
Dose: hypertension, initially 5 mg twice daily *or* 10 mg once daily; max. 60 mg daily
Angina, initially 5 mg 2–3 times daily, maintenance 15–45 mg daily
Prophylaxis after infarction, initially 5 mg twice daily, increased after 2 days to 10 mg twice daily, starting 7 to 28 days after infarction

PoM **Timolol Maleate Tablets,** timolol maleate 10 mg. Price 20 tabs = D. Label: 8
PoM **Betim**® (Burgess)
Tablets, scored, timolol maleate 10 mg. Price 20 tabs = D. Label: 8
PoM **Blocadren**® (MSD)
Tablets, blue, scored, timolol maleate 10 mg. Price 20 tabs = E. Label: 8

COMPOUND PREPARATIONS

Where both diuretic and beta-blocking drugs are required to control hypertension in combination, they can be prescribed together in a single tablet. There is good evidence that this improves compliance but patients should only be changed to this once their blood pressure is under reasonable control. There is also evidence that beta-blockers reduce the hypokalaemia caused by thiazide diuretics.

PoM **Co-Betaloc**® (Astra)
Tablets, scored, metoprolol tartrate 100 mg, hydrochlorothiazide 12.5 mg. Price 20 tabs = G. Label: 8
PoM **Co-Betaloc SA**® (Astra)
Tablets, yellow, f/c, metoprolol tartrate 200 mg (for sustained release), hydrochlorothiazide 25 mg. Price 28 tabs = H. Label: 8, 25
▼ PoM **Corgaretic 40**® (Squibb)
Tablets, scored, nadolol 40 mg, bendrofluazide 5 mg. Price 28 tabs = G. Label: 8
▼ PoM **Corgaretic 80**® (Squibb)
Tablets, scored, nadolol 80 mg, bendrofluazide 5 mg. Price 28 tabs = H. Label: 8
PoM **Inderetic**® (ICI)
Capsules, propranolol hydrochloride 80 mg, bendrofluazide 2.5 mg. Price 20 caps = E. Label: 8
PoM **Inderex**® (ICI)
Capsules, pink/grey, propranolol hydrochloride 160 mg (for sustained release), bendrofluazide 5 mg. Price 28 caps = H. Label: 8, 25
▼ PoM **Lasipressin**® (Hoechst)
Tablets, yellow-white, f/c, scored, penbutolol sulphate 40 mg, frusemide 20 mg. Price 20 tabs = G. Label: 8

C = 51-100p, D = 101-180p, E = 181-300p, F = 301-450p, G = 451-650p, H = 651-900p, I = 901-1200p, J = over 1200p.

PoM **Lopresoretic**® (Geigy)
Tablets, f/c, scored, metoprolol tartrate 100 mg, chlorthalidone 12.5 mg. Price 28 tabs = **F**. Label: 8

PoM **Moducren**® (Morson)
Tablets, blue, scored, timolol maleate 10 mg, amiloride hydrochloride 2.5 mg, hydrochlorothiazide 25 mg. Price 28 tabs = **H**. Label: 8

PoM **Prestim**® (Leo)
Tablets, scored, timolol maleate 10 mg, bendrofluazide 2.5 mg. Price 20 tabs = **E**. Label: 8

PoM **Prestim Forte**® (Leo)
Tablets, scored, timolol maleate 20 mg, bendrofluazide 5 mg. Price 20 tabs = **G**. Label: 8

▼ PoM **Secadrex**® (M&B)
Tablets, f/c, acebutolol 200 mg (as hydrochloride), hydrochlorothiazide 12.5 mg. Price 28 tabs = **H**. Label: 8

PoM **Sotazide**® (Bristol-Myers)
Tablets, blue, sotalol hydrochloride 160 mg, hydrochlorothiazide 25 mg. Price 28 tabs = **H**. Label: 8

▼ PoM **Spioprop**® (Searle)
Tablets, pink, f/c, propranolol hydrochloride 80 mg, spironolactone 50 mg. Price 28 tabs = **H**. Label: 8

▼ PoM **Tenoret 50**® (Stuart)
Tablets, brown, f/c, atenolol 50 mg, chlorthalidone 12.5 mg. Price 28 tabs = **G**. Label: 8

PoM **Tenoretic**® (Stuart)
Tablets, brown, f/c, atenolol 100 mg, chlorthalidone 25 mg. Price 28 tabs = **H**. Label: 8

▼ PoM **Tolerzide**® (Bristol-Myers)
Tablets, lilac, sotalol hydrochloride 80 mg, hydrochlorothiazide 12.5 mg. Price 28 tabs = **F**. Label: 8

PoM **Trasidrex**® (Ciba)
Tablets, red, s/c, oxprenolol hydrochloride 160 mg for sustained release, cyclopenthiazide 250 micrograms. Price 28 tabs = **H**. Label: 8

PoM **Viskaldix**® (Sandoz)
Tablets, scored, pindolol 10 mg, clopamide 5 mg. Price 28 tabs = **H**. Label: 8

2.5   Antihypertensive drugs

2.5.1 Vasodilator antihypertensive drugs
2.5.2 Centrally acting antihypertensive drugs
2.5.3 Adrenergic neurone blocking drugs
2.5.4 Alpha-adrenoceptor blocking drugs
2.5.5 Angiotensin-converting enzyme inhibitors
2.5.6 Ganglion blocking drugs
2.5.7 Other antihypertensive drugs

Antihypertensive therapy has improved the outlook for patients with high blood pressure by decreasing the frequency of stroke, heart failure, and renal failure. There is some evidence that it may also reduce the number of myocardial infarctions. The aim should be to reduce the blood pressure preferably to below 90 mmHg and certainly to below 100 mmHg. In patients over the age of 65 years blood pressure should not be reduced to such a low level. The quality of control

of blood pressure at follow-up is an important predictor of outcome, and efficient long-term care is necessary.

In general, patients whose average diastolic pressure exceeds 100 mmHg should receive antihypertensive therapy. Below that level the benefits of therapy are unproven.

Malignant (or accelerated) hypertension or very severe hypertension (diastolic blood pressure > 140 mmHg) is not an indication for parenteral antihypertensive therapy. Normally treatment should be by mouth with a beta-blocker (atenolol or labetalol), a calcium-channel blocker (nifedipine), or a vasodilator (hydralazine). Within the first 24 hours the diastolic blood pressure should not be reduced to below 110 mmHg. Over the next two or three days blood pressure should be normalised by using beta-blockers, calcium-channel blockers, diuretics, vasodilators, or angiotensin-converting enzyme inhibitors. Very rapid falls in blood pressure can cause reduced cerebral perfusion leading to cerebral infarction, a reduction in renal perfusion causing a deterioration in renal function, and myocardial ischaemia. Parenteral antihypertensive drugs are, therefore, hardly ever necessary.

Sodium nitroprusside by infusion is the parenteral antihypertensive drug of choice. Small doses of diazoxide by slow intravenous injection, labetalol by infusion, or hydralazine by slow intravenous injection may also be used, but again precipitate falls in blood pressure should be carefully avoided.

In hypertension, the practitioner has the choice of using one or more of the following classes of drugs:
thiazide diuretics—section 2.2.1
beta-adrenoceptor blocking drugs—section 2.4
vasodilator antihypertensive drugs—2.5.1
centrally acting antihypertensive drugs—2.5.2
adrenergic neurone blocking drugs—2.5.3

The **thiazides** or **beta-adrenoceptor** blocking drugs alone may be adequate to control blood pressure and where either is inadequate they are best used together.

The strategy for reducing blood pressure is probably best as follows:
1. *Non-drug treatment*—high salt intake, obesity, and high alcohol intake may elevate blood pressure and these should be corrected.
2. *Diuretic therapy*—any thiazide diuretic will be effective, e.g. bendrofluazide 2.5 mg/day (section 2.2.1). The optimum dose of a thiazide used to treat hypertension is the lowest possible dose; higher doses do not have a major additional antihypertensive effect, but do cause more metabolic side-effects. Potassium supplements are seldom necessary but plasma-potassium concentration should be checked regularly. Potassium-sparing diuretics (spironolactone, amiloride, or triamterene) are usually not necessary in the routine treatment of hypertension, unless hypokalaemia develops.
3. *Beta-adrenoceptor blocking drugs* (section 2.4) are all antihypertensive, where these are not effec-

tive alone they should be used in combination with a thiazide.

4. *Vasodilator therapy*—patients are usually maintained on a thiazide with a beta-blocker and a vasodilator is added to this regimen. Hydralazine (section 2.5.1) 25 to 50 mg may be given twice daily; higher doses can cause a lupus erythematosus-like syndrome. Nifedipine (section 2.6.1) is an alternative; 20 to 40 mg as a sustained-release preparation being given twice daily. About 10% of patients, however, cannot tolerate nifedipine because of headaches, flushing, or ankle swelling.

Captopril (section 2.5.5) is a potent vasodilator; if the dose is kept below 50 mg daily, few side-effects are encountered. Above this dose, proteinuria, rashes, and leucopenia have been described. Captopril may cause a precipitate drop in blood pressure in patients with renal damage and/or receiving diuretic therapy. In such patients, a test dose of 6.25 mg orally should be administered on an in-patient basis. In essential hypertension captopril is very potent if used in conjunction with high doses of frusemide. Enalapril (section 2.5.5) is a new angiotensin-converting enzyme inhibitor given once daily in a dose of 10 to 20 mg. It is uncertain whether enalapril has any major advantages over captopril.

Diazoxide and minoxidil (section 2.5.1) are extremely potent vasodilator antihypertensive drugs, with many side-effects. They should only be used where other vasodilators have failed. Minoxidil causes fluid retention (necessitating frusemide), tachycardia (necessitating beta-blockers), and hypertrichosis (rendering it unsuitable for women). Diazoxide may precipitate diabetes mellitus.

The addition of either methyldopa or prazosin to beta-blocker/thiazide/hydralazine therapy is sometimes effective.

SYSTOLIC HYPERTENSION. High systolic blood pressure carries a poor prognosis. This may be because the height of the systolic blood pressure reflects evidence of end-organ damage caused by the hypertension itself. The quality of control of systolic blood pressure over-rides the quality of control of diastolic blood pressure in the prediction of the outcome of patients with antihypertensive treatment.

HYPERTENSION IN PREGNANCY. It is important to control blood pressure in pregnancy. High blood pressure may be due to pre-existing essential hypertension or to pre-eclampsia. Oral methyldopa or atenolol or labetalol are safe in pregnancy. Thiazides and other diuretics are best avoided as they may reduce placental blood flow. Hydralazine by mouth is useful as second line therapy, and by intravenous injection can be used to control hypertensive crises associated with eclampsia.

HYPERTENSION IN THE ELDERLY. There is some evidence that treating hypertension in patients up to the age of 80 years is worthwhile. Pending the

publication of more information it seems reasonable to reduce blood pressure in these patients to below 100 mmHg if the untreated diastolic pressure is above this level.

DRUG INTERACTIONS. The effects of antihypertensive drugs are modified by a number of other drugs. See Appendix 1 (sections 2.5 and 15), and also under individual entries.

2.5.1 Vasodilator antihypertensive drugs

These are potent drugs, especially when used in combination with a beta-blocking drug and a thiazide. **Diazoxide** (Eudemine®) is diabetogenic and is not used by mouth, except in very severe hypertension. Diazoxide by intravenous injection however, can be used in hypertensive emergencies. **Hydralazine** (Apresoline®) given by mouth is a useful adjunct to other treatment, but when used alone causes tachycardia and fluid retention. Side-effects can be few if the dose is kept below 100 mg daily. **Sodium nitroprusside** (Nipride®) is given by intravenous infusion to control severe hypertensive crises. **Minoxidil** (Loniten®) should be reserved for the treatment of severe hypertension resistant to other drugs. Vasodilatation is accompanied by increased cardiac output and tachycardia and the patients develop fluid retention. For this reason a beta-blocker and a diuretic (usually frusemide) are mandatory. Hypertrichosis is troublesome and renders this drug unsuitable for women. Prazosin (section 2.5.4) has alpha-blocking and vasodilator properties.

DIAZOXIDE

Indications: hypertensive crisis, (for use in hypoglycaemia, see section 6.1.4)

Cautions: ischaemic heart disease, pregnancy, labour, impaired renal function. Drug interactions: see Appendix 1 (section 6.1)

Side-effects: tachycardia, hyperglycaemia, fluid retention

Dose: by rapid intravenous injection, 300 mg, repeated up to 3 times in 24 hours

PoM **Eudemine®** (A&H)
Injection, diazoxide 15 mg/ml. Price 20-ml amp = **E**

HYDRALAZINE HYDROCHLORIDE

Indications: moderate to severe hypertension, in addition to a beta-adrenoceptor blocking drug or diuretic; hypertensive crisis

Cautions: reduce initial dose in renal impairment; over-rapid blood pressure reduction is occasionally encountered even with low parenteral doses

Side-effects: postural hypotension, tachycardia, fluid retention, nausea, and vomiting; systemic lupus erythematosus-like syndrome after long-term therapy with more than 100 mg daily

Dose: by mouth, 25 mg twice daily, increased to a max. of 50 mg twice daily

C = 51-100p, D = 101-180p, E = 181-300p, F = 301-450p, G = 451-650p, H = 651-900p, I = 901-1200p, J = over 1200p.

By slow intravenous injection, 5–20 mg over 20 minutes; 40 mg over 20 minutes is occasionally needed in resistant cases (see Cautions)
By intravenous infusion, 20–40 mg, repeated if necessary

PoM **Apresoline®** (Ciba)
Tablets, yellow, s/c, hydralazine hydrochloride 25 mg. Price 20 tabs = **B**
Tablets, violet, s/c, hydralazine hydrochloride 50 mg. Price 20 tabs = **C**
Injection, powder for reconstitution, hydralazine hydrochloride. Price 20-mg amp = **B**

MINOXIDIL
Indications: severe hypertension, in addition to a diuretic and a beta-adrenoceptor blocking drug
Cautions: avoid oedema, may aggravate heart failure and angina, lower doses in dialysis patients
Contra-indications: phaeochromocytoma
Side-effects: gastro-intestinal disturbances, weight gain, peripheral oedema, tachycardia, hypertrichosis, breast tenderness
Dose: initially 5 mg daily, in 1–2 doses, increased by 5–10 mg every 3 or more days; max. usually 50 mg daily

PoM **Loniten®** (Upjohn)
Tablets, scored, minoxidil 2.5 mg. Price 20 tabs = **D**
Tablets, scored, minoxidil 5 mg. Price 20 tabs = **E**
Tablets, scored, minoxidil 10 mg. Price 20 tabs = **G**

SODIUM NITROPRUSSIDE
Indications: hypertensive crisis; controlled hypotension in surgery; acute or chronic heart failure
Cautions: hypothyroidism, severe renal impairment
Contra-indications: hepatic failure; vitamin B_{12} deficiency; Leber's optic atrophy; compensatory hypertension
Side-effects: headache, dizziness, nausea, and vomiting; palpitations and retrosternal pain— reduce infusion rate
Dose: hypertensive crisis, *by intravenous infusion*, 0.5–1.5 micrograms/kg/minute initially, then adjusted; usual range 0.5–8 micrograms/kg/minute (usual range 20–400 micrograms/minute; max. 800 micrograms/minute)
Heart failure, *by intravenous infusion*, initially 10–15 micrograms/minute, increased every 5–10 minutes as necessary; usual range 10–200 micrograms/minute; max. 400 micrograms/minute

PoM **Nipride®** (Roche)
Infusion, powder for reconstitution, sodium nitroprusside. Price 50-mg amp (with solvent) = **F** (Hosp. only)

2.5.2   Centrally acting antihypertensive drugs
This group includes methyldopa and clonidine and is largely falling from use. **Methyldopa** (Aldomet®), however, has the advantage of being safe in asthmatics, in heart failure, and in pregnancy. Side-effects are minimised if the daily dose is kept below 1 g. Sudden withdrawal of clonidine (Catapres®) may cause a hypertensive crisis. Rauwolfia and reserpine are not used much in Britain but if their dose is kept low and tablets are taken at night, blood pressure control can be achieved in mild hypertensives with few side-effects.

CLONIDINE HYDROCHLORIDE
Indications: moderate to severe hypertension (for use in migraine, see section 4.7.4.2)
Cautions: must be withdrawn gradually to avoid hypertensive crisis. Drug interactions: see Appendix 1 (section 2.5)
Contra-indications: history of depression
Side-effects: dry mouth, sedation, depression, fluid retention, bradycardia, Raynaud's phenomenon
Dose: by mouth, 50–100 micrograms 3 times daily, increased every 3rd day; max. daily dose usually 1.2 mg
By slow intravenous injection, 150–300 micrograms; max. 750 micrograms in 24 hours

PoM **Catapres®** (Boehringer Ingelheim)
Tablets, scored, clonidine hydrochloride 100 micrograms. Price 20 tabs = **D**. Label: 2, 8
Tablets, scored, clonidine hydrochloride 300 micrograms. Price 20 tabs = **E**. Label: 2, 8
Perlongets® (= capsules s/r), red/yellow, clonidine hydrochloride 250 micrograms. Price 14 caps = **F**. Label: 2, 8, 25
Dose: initially 250 micrograms in the evening; maintenance usually 250–750 micrograms daily in divided doses
Injection, clonidine hydrochloride 150 micrograms/ml. Price 1-ml amp = **B**

METHYLDOPA
Indications: moderate to severe hypertension, in conjunction with a diuretic; hypertensive crisis
Cautions: positive direct Coombs' test in 20% of patients (may affect blood cross-matching); interference with laboratory tests; reduce initial dose in renal impairment; blood counts and liver-function tests advised. Drug interactions: see Appendix 1 (section 4.9)
Contra-indications: history of depression, active liver disease, phaeochromocytoma
Side-effects: dry mouth, sedation, depression, drowsiness, diarrhoea, fluid retention, failure of ejaculation, liver damage, haemolytic anaemia, systemic lupus erythematosus-like syndrome
Dose: by mouth, 250 mg 3 times daily, gradually increased; max. daily dose 3 g
By intravenous infusion, methyldopate hydrochloride 250–500 mg, repeated after 6 hours if required

PoM **Methyldopa Tablets,** f/c, methyldopa (anhydrous) 125 mg, price 20 tabs = **B**; 250 mg, price 20 tabs = **C**; 500 mg, price 20 tabs = **D**. Label: 3, 8

PoM **Aldomet**® (MSD)
Tablets, yellow, f/c, methyldopa (anhydrous) 125 mg. Price 20 tabs = **C**. Label: 3, 8
Tablets, yellow, f/c, methyldopa (anhydrous) 250 mg. Price 20 tabs = **D**. Label: 3, 8
Tablets, yellow, f/c, methyldopa (anhydrous) 500 mg. Price 20 tabs = **E**. Label: 3, 8
Suspension (= mixture), methyldopa 250 mg/5 ml. Do not dilute. Price 200 ml = **F**. Label: 3, 8
Injection, methyldopate hydrochloride 50 mg/ml. Price 5-ml amp = **E**

PoM **Dopamet**® (Berk)
Tablets, yellow, f/c, methyldopa (anhydrous) 125 mg. Price 20 tabs = **B**. Label: 3, 8
Tablets, yellow, f/c, methyldopa (anhydrous) 250 mg. Price 20 tabs = **C**. Label: 3, 8
Tablets, yellow, f/c, methyldopa (anhydrous) 500 mg. Price 20 tabs = **D**. Label: 3, 8

PoM **Hydromet**® (MSD)
Tablets, pink, f/c, methyldopa (anhydrous) 250 mg, hydrochlorothiazide 15 mg. Price 20 tabs = **D**. Label: 3, 8

PoM **Medomet**® (DDSA)
Capsules, yellow, methyldopa (anhydrous) 250 mg. Price 20 caps = **C**. Label: 3, 8
Capsules, yellow, methyldopa (anhydrous) 500 mg. Price 20 caps = **C**. Label: 3, 8
Tablets, yellow, f/c, methyldopa (anhydrous) 250 mg. Price 20 tabs = **C**. Label: 3, 8
Tablets, yellow, f/c, methyldopa (anhydrous) 500 mg. Price 20 tabs = **D**. Label: 3, 8

RESERPINE AND RAUWOLFIA ALKALOIDS

Indications: hypertension
Cautions: late pregnancy, breast-feeding. Drug interactions: see Appendix 1 (sections *4.3*, *4.9*)
Contra-indications: history of depression, phaeochromocytoma, peptic ulcer, Parkinson's disease
Side-effects: dry mouth, nasal congestion, sedation, depression, postural hypotension, bradycardia, fluid retention

PoM **Reserpine Tablets,** reserpine 100 and 250 micrograms. Price 20 tabs (both) = **A**. Label: 2
PoM **Abicol**® (Boots)
Tablets, pink, scored, reserpine 150 micrograms, bendrofluazide 2.5 mg. Price 20 tabs = **A**. Label: 2
PoM **Decaserpyl**® (Roussel)
Tablets, scored, methoserpidine 5 mg. Price 20 tabs = **D**. Label: 2
Tablets, pink, scored, methoserpidine 10 mg. Price 20 tabs = **E**. Label: 2
PoM **Decaserpyl Plus**® (Roussel)
Tablets, scored, methoserpidine 10 mg, benzthiazide 20 mg. Price 20 tabs = **E**. Label: 2
PoM **Harmonyl**® (Abbott)
Tablets, pink, scored, deserpidine 250 micrograms. Price 20 tabs = **B**. Label: 2
PoM **Hypercal**® (Carlton)
Tablets, rauwolfia alkaloids 2 mg. Price 20 tabs = **A**. Label: 2

PoM **Rautrax**® (Squibb)
Tablets, red, s/c, rauwolfia serpentina 50 mg, hydroflumethiazide 50 mg, potassium chloride 625 mg (8.4 mmol K⁺). Price 20 tabs = **D**. Label: 2, 25
PoM **Rauwiloid**® (Riker)
Tablets, cream, alseroxylon 2 mg. Price 20 tabs = **B**. Label: 2
PoM **Serpasil**® (Ciba)
Tablets, blue, reserpine 100 micrograms. Price 20 tabs = **A**. Label: 2
Tablets, blue, scored, reserpine 250 micrograms. Price 20 tabs = **A**. Label: 2
PoM **Serpasil-Esidrex**® (Ciba)
Tablets, scored, reserpine 150 micrograms, hydrochlorothiazide 10 mg. Price 20 tabs = **B**. Label: 2

2.5.3 Adrenergic neurone blocking drugs

These drugs prevent the release of noradrenaline from postganglionic adrenergic neurones. Guanethidine (Ismelin®) also depletes the nerve endings of noradrenaline. These drugs do not control supine blood pressure and may cause postural hypotension, for this reason they have largely fallen from use, but may be necessary in combination with other therapy in resistant hypertension.

BETHANIDINE SULPHATE

Indications: moderate to severe hypertension, in conjunction with a diuretic or beta-adrenoceptor blocking drug
Cautions; Contra-indications; Side-effects: see under Guanethidine Monosulphate (except diarrhoea)
Dose: 10 mg 3 times daily after food, increased by 5 mg at intervals; max. daily dose 200 mg

PoM **Bethanidine Tablets,** bethanidine sulphate 10 mg, price 20 tabs = **C**; 50 mg, price 20 tabs = **F**. Label: 21
PoM **Bendogen**® (Lagap)
Tablets, scored, bethanidine sulphate 10 mg. Price 20 tabs = **C**. Label: 21
Tablets, scored, bethanidine sulphate 50 mg. Price 20 tabs = **G**. Label: 21
PoM **Esbatal**® (Calmic)
Tablets, peach, scored, bethanidine sulphate 10 mg. Price 20 tabs = **D**. Label: 21
Tablets, peach, scored, bethanidine sulphate 50 mg. Price 20 tabs = **G**. Label: 21

DEBRISOQUINE

Indications: moderate to severe hypertension, in conjunction with a diuretic or beta-adrenoceptor blocking drug
Cautions; Contra-indications; Side-effects: see under Guanethidine Monosulphate (except diarrhoea)
Dose: 10 mg 1–2 times daily, increased by 10 mg every 3 days; max. daily dose usually 120 mg

PoM **Declinax**® (Roche)
Tablets, scored, debrisoquine 10 mg (as sulphate). Price 20 tabs = **C**
Tablets, blue, scored, debrisoquine 20 mg (as sulphate). Price 20 tabs = **C**

C = 51-100p, **D** = 101-180p, **E** = 181-300p, **F** = 301-450p, **G** = 451-650p, **H** = 651-900p, **I** = 901-1200p, **J** = over 1200p.

GUANETHIDINE MONOSULPHATE

Indications: moderate to severe hypertension, in conjunction with a diuretic or beta-adrenoceptor blocking drug

Cautions: postural hypotension may cause falls in elderly patients; pregnancy. Drug interactions: see Appendix 1 (section 2.5)

Contra-indications: phaeochromocytoma, renal failure

Side-effects: postural hypotension, failure of ejaculation, fluid retention, nasal congestion, diarrhoea

Dose: by mouth, 20 mg daily, increased by 10 mg at weekly intervals; max. daily dose usually 100 mg

By intramuscular injection, 10–20 mg, repeated after 3 hours if required

PoM **Ismelin**® (Ciba)
Tablets, guanethidine monosulphate 10 mg. Price 20 tabs = **B**
Tablets, pink, guanethidine monosulphate 25 mg. Price 20 tabs = **D**
Injection, guanethidine monosulphate 10 mg/ml. Price 1-ml amp = **B**

2.5.4   Alpha-adrenoceptor blocking drugs

Prazosin (Hypovase®) has alpha-blocking and vasodilator properties and rarely causes tachycardia. It does, however, cause a rapid reduction in blood pressure after the first dose and should be used with caution.

Phenoxybenzamine (Dibenyline®) and **indoramin** (Baratol®) are alpha-blockers which are effective agents, but have many side-effects. They can be used in conjunction with beta-blockers and/or diuretics.

Phenoxybenzamine (with a beta-blocker) is used in resistant hypertension and in the preoperative preparation of patients with phaeochromocytoma, for clonidine withdrawal, and for treatment of pressor responses to monoamine-oxidase inhibitors and foods containing pressor amines. **Phentolamine** (Rogitine®) is only rarely used as a suppression test for phaeochromocytoma.

INDORAMIN

Indications: hypertension, usually in conjunction with a diuretic or a beta-adrenoceptor blocking drug

Cautions: patient's ability to drive or operate machinery may be impaired; control incipient heart failure with diuretics and digoxin; hepatic or renal impairment; Parkinson's disease

Contra-indications: established heart failure; patients being treated with monoamine-oxidase inhibitors

Side-effects: sedation; dizziness, depression, failure of ejaculation, dry mouth, nasal congestion occur less frequently

Dose: initially 25 mg twice daily, increased by 25–50 mg daily at intervals of 2 weeks; max. daily dose 200 mg in 2–3 divided doses

▼ PoM **Baratol**® (Wyeth)
Tablets, blue, f/c, indoramin 25 mg (as hydrochloride). Price 20 tabs = **E**. Label: 2
Tablets, green, scored, f/c, indoramin 50 mg (as hydrochloride). Price 20 tabs = **F**. Label: 2

PHENOXYBENZAMINE HYDROCHLORIDE

Indications: hypertension (see notes above), (for use in urinary retention see section 7.4.1)

Cautions: elderly patients; ischaemic heart disease, marked arteriosclerosis, renal impairment; carcinogenic in *animals*

Contra-indications: congestive heart failure

Side-effects: marked tachycardia and postural hypotension; dizziness, lassitude, nasal congestion, miosis, retrograde ejaculation; rarely gastro-intestinal disturbances

Dose: by mouth, phaeochromocytoma, 10 mg twice daily, increased by 10 mg daily; usual dose 1–2 mg/kg daily in 2 divided doses

PoM **Dibenyline**® (SK&F)
Capsules, red/white, phenoxybenzamine hydrochloride 10 mg. Price 20 caps = **E**
Injection, phenoxybenzamine hydrochloride 50 mg/ml. To be diluted before use. 2-ml amp (Hosp. only)

PHENTOLAMINE MESYLATE

Indications: hypertensive crises due to phaeochromocytoma, clonidine withdrawal, reaction between monoamine-oxidase inhibitors and foods containing pressor amines; acute left ventricular failure

Side-effects: hypotension, tachycardia, dizziness; nausea, diarrhoea, nasal congestion after high doses

Dose: by intravenous injection, 5–10 mg repeated as necessary

By intravenous infusion, 5–60 mg over 10–30 minutes at a rate of 0.1–2 mg/minute

PoM **Rogitine**® (Ciba)
Injection, phentolamine mesylate 10 mg/ml. Price 1-ml amp = **B**; 5-ml amp = **D**

PRAZOSIN HYDROCHLORIDE

Indications: hypertension; congestive heart failure

Cautions: first dose may cause collapse due to hypotension; reduce initial dose in renal failure. Avoid abrupt withdrawal in heart failure

Side-effects: postural hypotension, drowsiness, weakness

Dose: hypertension, 500 micrograms 2–3 times daily, the initial dose being taken after retiring to bed at night; increased to a max. of 20 mg daily

Heart failure, 500 micrograms initially, then 1 mg 3–4 times daily; maintenance 4–20 mg daily

Raynaud's syndrome, initially 500 micrograms twice daily; maintenance 1–2 mg twice daily

---

PoM **Hypovase**® (Pfizer)
Tablets, prazosin hydrochloride 500 micrograms.
Price 20 tabs = **C**. Label: 3, 8
Tablets, orange, scored, prazosin hydrochloride
1 mg. Price 20 tabs = **D**. Label: 3, 8
Tablets, scored, prazosin hydrochloride 2 mg.
Price 20 tabs = **D**. Label: 3, 8
Tablets, scored, prazosin hydrochloride 5 mg.
Price 20 tabs = **F**. Label: 3, 8
B.d. starter pack, 8 tablets, prazosin hydro-
chloride 500 micrograms; 32 orange tablets,
prazosin hydrochloride 1 mg. Price per pack =
E. Label: 3, 8

2.5.5   Angiotensin-converting enzyme inhibitors

Captopril (Capoten®) and **enalapril** (Innovace®)
inhibit the conversion of angiotensin I to angiotensin II; they are used in the treatment of hypertension refractory to other treatment or where
other drugs are specifically contra-indicated. Captopril has also been used in the treatment of heart
failure. A thiazide or more usually a loop diuretic
may also be required. Serious side-effects may be
avoided with captopril if the dose is kept below
50 mg daily. Both may cause very rapid falls of
blood pressure in some patients (see Cautions).

CAPTOPRIL
Indications: see notes above
Cautions: first dose may cause marked hypotension within 3 hours in patients taking diuretics, on a low-sodium diet, or on dialysis (may
recur with next 1 or 2 doses); reduce dose in
renal impairment; white blood cell counts (in
renal impairment or autoimmune disease) and
urinary protein estimations (in renal impairment) before and during treatment; pregnancy.
Drug interactions: see Appendix 1 (sections
2.2, 2.5)
Side-effects: loss of taste, stomatosis, abdominal
pain, rashes, hypotension (see Cautions); proteinuria, agranulocytosis, neutropenia, hyperkalaemia (all more common in renal
impairment)
Dose: 25 mg twice daily (6.25 mg in patients
already taking a diuretic) 1 hour before food;
higher doses of up to 50 mg 3 times daily are
rarely necessary; a diuretic (usually frusemide)
is often needed in essential hypertension. The
dose of frusemide should be gradually increased
to 120 mg daily

▼ PoM **Captopril Tablets,** captopril 25 mg, price
20 tabs = **F**; 50 mg, price 20 tabs = **H**. Label: 22
▼ PoM **Acepril**® (DF)
Tablets, scored, captopril 25 mg. Price 20
tabs = **G**. Label: 22
Tablets, scored, captopril 50 mg. Price 20
tabs = **H**. Label: 22
▼ PoM **Capoten**® (Squibb)
Tablets, scored, captopril 12.5 mg. Price 20
tabs = **F**. Label: 22
Tablets, captopril 25 mg. Price 20 tabs = **G**; 56-
tab calendar pack = **J**. Label: 22

Tablets, scored, captopril 50 mg. Price 20
tabs = **H**; 56-tab calendar pack = **J**. Label: 22

ENALAPRIL MALEATE
Indications: see notes above
Cautions: first dose may rarely cause hypotension
especially in patients taking diuretics, on a low-
sodium diet, on dialysis, or dehydrated; reduce
dose in renal impairment; pregnancy (toxicity
in *animal* studies). Drug interactions: see
Appendix 1 (sections 2.5)
Side-effects: dizziness, headache, fatigue, and
weakness; hypotension (see also Cautions),
alteration of taste, nausea, diarrhoea, muscle
cramps, cough, rash, and angioedema occur
less frequently; increases in blood urea and
plasma creatinine more common in renal
impairment
Dose: initially 10 mg daily in mild hypertension,
renovascular hypertension, elderly patients,
and when added to existing antihypertensive
therapy; initially 20 mg daily for other grades
of hypertension and as usual maintenance dose;
max. 40 mg daily

▼ PoM **Innovace**® (MSD)
Tablets, scored, enalapril maleate 5 mg. Price 20
tabs = **G**
Tablets, red, enalapril maleate 10 mg. Price 20
tabs = **H**
Tablets, peach, enalapril maleate 20 mg. Price
20 tabs = **I**

2.5.6   Ganglion-blocking drugs
Trimetaphan (Arfonad®) is used to provide hypotension in surgery.

TRIMETAPHAN CAMSYLATE
Indications: see notes above
Cautions: hepatic or renal impairment, diabetes
mellitus, Addison's disease, CNS degenerative
disease
Contra-indications: severe arteriosclerosis or cardiac disease
Side-effects: tachycardia and respiratory depression (particularly with muscle relaxants); pupil-
lary dilatation
Dose: by intravenous infusion, 3–4 mg/minute
initially, then adjusted according to response

PoM **Arfonad**® (Roche)
Injection, trimetaphan camsylate 50 mg/ml.
Price 5-ml amp = **E**

2.5.7   Other antihypertensive drugs
Metirosine (Demser®) inhibits the enzyme tyro-
sine hydroxylase, and consequently the synthesis
of catecholamines. It is used in the pre-operative
treatment of phaeochromocytoma, and long term
in patients unsuitable for surgery; an alpha-
adrenoceptor blocking drug may also be required.
Metirosine should **not** be used to treat essential
hypertension.

C = 51-100p, **D** = 101-180p, **E** = 181-300p, **F** = 301-450p, **G** = 451-650p, **H** = 651-900p, **I** = 901-1200p, **J** = over 1200p.

Veratrum alkaloids have a very low therapeutic index and should no longer be used in the treatment of hypertension.

There is no justification for the use of barbiturates in the treatment of hypertension.

METIROSINE

Indications: see notes above

Cautions: maintain high fluid intake and adequate blood volume; may impair ability to drive or operate machinery. Drug interactions: see Appendix 1 (sections 2.5, *4.9*)

Side-effects: sedation; extrapyramidal symptoms; diarrhoea (may be severe); hypersensitivity reactions

Dose: initially 250 mg 4 times daily, increased to max. of 4 g daily in divided doses; doses of 2–3 g daily should be given for 5–7 days before surgery

▼ PoM **Demser**® (MSD)
Capsules, blue, metirosine 250 mg (Hosp. only). Label: 2

VERATRUM ALKALOIDS
(Alkavervir)

Indications: see notes above

Contra-indications: cardiovascular disease, phaeochromocytoma

Side-effects: postural hypotension, bradycardia, arrhythmias, nausea, vomiting, epigastric pain, respiratory depression

PoM **Rauwiloid + Veriloid**® (Riker)
Tablets, brown, alkavervir 3 mg, alseroxylon 1 mg. Price 20 tabs = **D**
PoM **Thiaver**® (Riker)
Tablets, blue, scored, alkavervir 4 mg, epithiazide 4 mg. Price 20 tabs = **D**
PoM **Veriloid**® (Riker)
Tablets, yellow, scored, alkavervir 2 mg. Price 20 tabs = **C**

COMPOUND PREPARATIONS CONTAINING BARBITURATES

CD **Hypercal-B** ® (Carlton)
Tablets, rauwolfia alkaloids 2 mg, amylobarbitone 15 mg. Price 20 tabs = **A**. Label: 2
CD **Seominal** ® (Winthrop)
Tablets, yellow, scored, reserpine 200 micrograms, phenobarbitone 10 mg, theobromine 325 mg. Price 20 tabs = **E**. Label: 2

2.6   Vasodilators

2.6.1 Vasodilators used in angina pectoris
2.6.2 Vasodilators used in heart failure
2.6.3 Peripheral vasodilators
2.6.4 Cerebral vasodilators

For the use of vasodilators in hypertension, see section 2.5.1.

2.6.1   Vasodilators used in angina pectoris

Most patients with angina pectoris will be treated with maintenance beta-adrenoceptor blocking drugs (section 2.4) or calcium-channel blockers. However, short-acting nitrates retain an important role both for prophylactic use before exertion and for chest pain occurring at rest. Nitrates are sometimes used appropriately as sole therapy, especially in elderly patients with infrequent symptoms.

NITRATES. Sublingual **glyceryl trinitrate** is one of the most effective drugs for providing rapid symptomatic relief, but its effect lasts only for 20 to 30 minutes. Though a potent coronary vasodilator, its principal benefit follows from a reduction in venous return which reduces left ventricular work. Unwanted effects such as flushing, headache, and postural hypotension may limit therapy, especially when angina is severe or when patients are unusually sensitive to the effects of nitrates. The 300-microgram tablet is often appropriate when glyceryl trinitrate is first used and tolerance to the unwanted effects has not developed. Duration of action may be prolonged by slow-release preparations. The aerosol spray (Coro-Nitro®, Nitrolingual®) provides an alternative method of rapid relief of symptoms for those who find difficulty in dissolving sublingual preparations. The percutaneous preparations (Percutol®, Transiderm-Nitro®) are useful in the prophylaxis of angina for patients who suffer attacks at rest, especially at night.

Isosorbide dinitrate is active sublingually and is a more stable preparation for those who only require nitrates infrequently. It is also effective by mouth for prophylaxis; although the effect is slower in onset, it may persist for several hours. Duration of action of up to 12 hours is claimed for sustained-release preparations. The activity of isosorbide dinitrate may depend on the production of active metabolites, the most important of which is isosorbide 5-mononitrate. **Isosorbide mononitrate** is available for angina prophylaxis, though the advantages over isosorbide dinitrate have not yet been firmly established.

Glyceryl trinitrate injection (Tridil®) or isosorbide dinitrate injection (Cedocard IV®, Isoket®) may be tried when the sublingual form is ineffective in patients with chest pain due to myocardial infarction or severe ischaemia. The intravenous preparations are also useful in the treatment of acute left ventricular failure.

CALCIUM-CHANNEL BLOCKERS. **Verapamil** is used for the treatment of angina as well as arrhythmias (section 2.3.2). It interferes with the inward displacement of calcium ions across cardiac cell membranes (and thereby inhibits excitation-contraction coupling), decreases cardiac contractility, decreases oxygen requirements of the heart, and does not block beta-adrenoceptors. It may precipitate heart failure, exacerbate conduction disorders, and cause hypotension at high doses and should be used with caution with beta-adrenoceptor blocking drugs.

Nifedipine (Adalat®) is a more potent peripheral and coronary vasodilator than verapamil but does not have anti-arrhythmic activity. It is particularly valuable in forms of angina associated with coronary constriction, and is useful as an adjunct to beta-blockers for patients with severe symptoms and for those who are intolerant of beta-blockers. Like verapamil and beta-blockers, nifedipine has a negative inotropic effect but it rarely precipitates heart failure because of its concomitant reduction in left ventricular work. Minor side-effects associated with vasodilatation such as flushing and headache (which become less obtrusive after a few days), and ankle swelling are common.

Nifedipine in a dose of 20 mg as a sustained-release preparation twice daily, increasing to 40 mg twice daily, is very useful in managing hypertensive patients, especially in conjunction with beta-blockers.

Diltiazem (Tildiem®) is effective in most forms of angina. It may be used in patients for whom beta-blockers are contra-indicated or ineffective, but because of the risk of bradycardia, should be used with caution with beta-blockers. Significant myocardial depression occurs rarely.

Lidoflazine (Clinium®) is a long-acting coronary vasodilator and inhibits influx of calcium ions across cardiac cell membranes. Increased exercise tolerance develops gradually over several weeks.

There is some evidence that sudden withdrawal of calcium-channel blockers may be associated with an exacerbation of angina.

GLYCERYL TRINITRATE

Indications: prophylaxis and treatment of angina; left ventricular failure
Cautions: hypotensive conditions. Drug interactions: see Appendix 1 (section 2.5)
Side-effects: throbbing headache, flushing, dizziness, postural hypotension, tachycardia
Dose: sublingually, 0.3–1 mg, repeated as required
By mouth, 2.6–6.4 mg as sustained-release tablets, 2–3 times daily
By intravenous infusion, 10–200 micrograms/minute

Glyceryl Trinitrate Tablets, glyceryl trinitrate 300, 500, and 600 micrograms. Price 20 tabs (all) = **A**. Label: 16
Note: glyceryl trinitrate tablets should be supplied in glass containers of not more than 100 tablets, closed with a foil-lined cap, and containing no cotton wool wadding: they should be discarded after 8 weeks in use
▼ **Coro-Nitro Spray®** (MCP)
Aerosol spray, glyceryl trinitrate 400 micrograms/metered dose. Price 200-dose unit = **G**
Dose: treatment or prophylaxis of angina, 1–2 metered doses sprayed on the oral mucosa (preferably on or under the tongue) and the mouth then closed
Caution: flammable
GTN 300 mcg (Martindale)
Tablets, glyceryl trinitrate 300 micrograms. Price 20 tabs = **A**. Label: 16

PoM **Natirose®** (Lewis)
Tablets, pink, s/c, glyceryl trinitrate 750 micrograms, ethylmorphine hydrochloride 3 mg, hyoscamine hydrobromide 50 micrograms. Price 20 tabs = **C**
▼ PoM **Nitrocine®** (Sanol Schwarz)
Injection, glyceryl trinitrate 1 mg/ml. To be diluted before use. Price 10-ml amp = **I**; 50-ml bottle = **J**
Glass or polyethylene apparatus is preferable; loss of potency will occur if PVC is used
Nitrocontin Continus® (Napp)
Tablets, s/r, pink, glyceryl trinitrate 2.6 mg. Price 20 tabs = **C**. Label: 25
Tablets, s/r, pink, glyceryl trinitrate 6.4 mg. Price 20 tabs = **C**. Label: 25
▼ **Nitrolingual Spray®** (Lipha)
Aerosol spray, glyceryl trinitrate 400 micrograms/metered dose. Price 200-dose unit = **G**
Dose: treatment or prophylaxis of angina, 1–2 metered doses sprayed on the oral mucosa (preferably on or under the tongue) and the mouth then closed
Note: do not shake canister
Caution: flammable
▼ **Percutol®** (R&C)
Ointment, glyceryl trinitrate 2%. Price 30 g = **F**. Counselling advised, see administration below
Administration: prophylaxis of angina, ½–2 inches of ointment measured on to Applirule, which is applied to body (usually chest, arm, or thigh) without rubbing in, and secured with a dressing; repeat every 3–4 hours or as required
Note: 1 inch of ointment contains glyceryl trinitrate 16.64 mg
Suscard Buccal® (Pharmax)
Tablets, s/r, glyceryl trinitrate 1 mg. Price 20 tabs = **D**. Counselling advised, see administration below
Tablets, s/r, glyceryl trinitrate 2 mg. Price 20 tabs = **E**. Counselling advised, see administration below
Tablets, s/r, glyceryl trinitrate 3 mg. Price 20 tabs = **F**. Counselling advised, see administration below
Tablets, s/r, glyceryl trinitrate 5 mg. Price 20 tabs = **G**. Counselling advised, see administration below
Dose: treatment of angina, 1–2 mg as required; prophylaxis 1–2 mg 3 times daily; 5 mg in severe angina. Congestive heart failure, 5 mg 3 times daily, increased to 10 mg 3 times daily in severe cases. Tablets are placed between upper lip and gum, and left to dissolve
Sustac® (Pharmax)
Tablets, s/r, pink, glyceryl trinitrate 2.6 mg. Price 20 tabs = **D**. Label: 25
Tablets, s/r, pink, glyceryl trinitrate 6.4 mg. Price 20 tabs = **D**. Label: 25
Tablets, s/r, pink, glyceryl trinitrate 10 mg. Price 20 tabs = **E**. Label: 25
Dose: severe angina, 10 mg 3 times daily
▼ **Transiderm-Nitro®** (Geigy)
5 dressing, self-adhesive, pink, containing glyceryl trinitrate 25 mg, and releasing approx.

C = 51-100p, **D** = 101-180p, **E** = 181-300p, **F** = 301-450p, **G** = 451-650p, **H** = 651-900p, **I** = 901-1200p, **J** = over 1200p.

5 mg/24 hours when in contact with skin. Price 30 dressings = **J**. Counselling advised, see administration below

10 dressing, self-adhesive, pink, containing glyceryl trinitrate 50 mg, and releasing approx. 10 mg/24 hours when in contact with skin. Price 30 dressings = **J**. Counselling advised, see administration below

Administration: prophylaxis of angina, 1 dressing applied to the lateral chest wall, and replaced with a further dressing every 24 hours, siting the replacement dressing on a different area of skin

▼ PoM **Tridil**® (American Hospital Supply)
Injection, glyceryl trinitrate 500 micrograms/ml. To be diluted before use. Price 10-ml amp = **G**

Injection, glyceryl trinitrate 5 mg/ml. To be diluted before use. Price 10-ml amp = **J**; 10-ml amp with polyethylene giving set = **J**
Glass or polyethylene infusion apparatus is preferable; loss of potency will occur if PVC apparatus is used

DILTIAZEM HYDROCHLORIDE

Indications: prophylaxis and treatment of angina
Cautions: reduce dose in hepatic and renal impairment. Drug interactions: see Appendix 1 (section *2.1*)
Contra-indications: bradycardia, second or third degree heart block, sick sinus syndrome
Side-effects: bradycardia, ankle oedema; rarely headache, nausea, rashes
Dose: initially 60 mg 3 times daily (elderly patients twice daily); max. 360 mg daily

▼ PoM **Tildiem**® (Lorex)
Tablets, s/r, off-white, diltiazem hydrochloride 60 mg. Price 20 tabs = **F**. Label: 25

ISOSORBIDE DINITRATE

Indications: prophylaxis and treatment of angina; left ventricular failure
Cautions; Side-effects: see under Glyceryl Trinitrate
Dose: sublingually, 5–10 mg
By mouth, daily in divided doses, angina 30–120 mg, congestive heart failure 40–160 mg, up to 240 mg if required
By intravenous infusion, 2–10 mg/hour

Isosorbide Dinitrate Tablets, isosorbide dinitrate 10 and 20 mg, price 20 tabs (both) = **B**; 30 mg, price 20 tabs = **C**
Cedocard-5® (Tillotts)
Tablets (sublingual), scored, isosorbide dinitrate 5 mg. Price 20 tabs = **B**
Cedocard-10® (Tillotts)
Tablets, pink, scored, isosorbide dinitrate 10 mg. Price 20 tabs = **B**
PoM **Cedocard-20**® (Tillotts)
Tablets, blue, scored, isosorbide dinitrate 20 mg. Price 20 tabs = **C**

Cedocard Retard® (Tillotts)
Tablets, s/r, yellow, scored, isosorbide dinitrate 20 mg. Price 20 tabs = **D**. Label: 25
Dose: prophylaxis of angina, 20 mg every 12 hours
PoM **Cedocard IV**® (Tillotts)
Injection, isosorbide dinitrate 1 mg/ml. To be diluted before use. Price 10-ml amp = **F**; 50- and 100-ml infusion bottle (both) = **J**
Glass or polyethylene infusion apparatus is preferable; loss of potency will occur if PVC apparatus is used
Isoket 5® (Sanol Schwarz)
Tablets, scored, isosorbide dinitrate 5 mg. Price 20 tabs = **B**
Isoket 10® (Sanol Schwarz)
Tablets, scored, isosorbide dinitrate 10 mg. Price 20 tabs = **B**
Isoket 20® (Sanol Schwarz)
Tablets, scored, isosorbide dinitrate 20 mg. Price 20 tabs = **B**
Isoket Retard® (Sanol Schwarz)
Tablets, s/r, yellow, scored, isosorbide dinitrate 20 mg. Price 20 tabs = **D**. Label: 25
Dose: prophylaxis of angina, 20 mg every 12 hours
PoM **Isoket IV**® (Sanol Schwarz)
Injection, isosorbide dinitrate 1 mg/ml. To be diluted before use. Price 10-ml amp = **F**; 50- and 100-ml bottle (both) = **J**
Glass or polyethylene infusion apparatus is preferable; loss of potency will occur if PVC apparatus is used
Isordil® (Ayerst)
Tablets (sublingual), pink, isosorbide dinitrate 5 mg. Price 20 tabs = **B**. Label: 26
Tablets, scored, isosorbide dinitrate 10 mg. Price 20 tabs = **B**
Tablets, scored, isosorbide dinitrate 30 mg. Price 20 tabs = **C**
Tembids®(= capsules s/r), blue/clear, isosorbide dinitrate 40 mg. Price 20 caps = **D**. Label: 25
Dose: prophylaxis of angina, 40 mg 2–3 times daily
▼ **Soni-Slo**® (Lipha)
Capsules, s/r, pink/clear, enclosing off-white pellets, isosorbide dinitrate 20 mg. Price 20 caps = **D**. Label: 25
Capsules, s/r, red/clear, enclosing off-white pellets, isosorbide dinitrate 40 mg. Price 20 caps = **D**. Label: 25
Dose: prophylaxis of angina, 40–80 mg daily in divided doses
Sorbichew® (Stuart)
Tablets (chewable), green, scored, isosorbide dinitrate 5 mg. Price 20 tabs = **B**. Label: 24
Sorbid SA® (Stuart)
Tablets, s/r, yellow, isosorbide dinitrate 40 mg. Price 20 tabs = **E**. Label: 25
Dose: prophylaxis of angina, 1–2 tablets twice daily
Sorbitrate® (Stuart)
Tablets, yellow, scored, isosorbide dinitrate 10 mg. Price 20 tabs = **B**
Tablets, blue, scored, isosorbide dinitrate 20 mg.

Price 20 tabs = **B**

Vascardin® (Nicholas)

Tablets, scored, isosorbide dinitrate 10 mg. Price 20 tabs = **B**

ISOSORBIDE MONONITRATE

Indications: prophylaxis and treatment of angina

Cautions; Side-effects: see under Glyceryl Trinitrate

Dose: initially 20 mg 2–3 times daily; up to 120 mg daily in divided doses if required

▼ PoM **Isosorbide Mononitrate Tablets,** isosorbide mononitrate 20 mg, price 20 tabs = **D**. Label: 25

▼ PoM **Elantan 20**® (Sanol Schwarz)

Tablets, scored, isosorbide mononitrate 20 mg. Price 20 tabs = **D**. Label: 25

▼ PoM **Elantan 40**® (Sanol Schwarz)

Tablets, scored, isosorbide mononitrate 40 mg. Price 20 tabs = **E**. Label: 25

Dose: prophylaxis of angina, 40 mg twice daily

▼ PoM **Ismo 20**® (MCP)

Tablets, scored, isosorbide mononitrate 20 mg. Price 20 tabs = **D**. Label: 25

▼ PoM **Monit**® (Stuart)

Tablets, scored, isosorbide mononitrate 20 mg. Price 28 tabs = **E**. Label: 25

▼ PoM **Mono-Cedocard 20**® (Tillotts)

Tablets, scored, isosorbide mononitrate 20 mg. Price 20 tabs = **D**. Label: 25

▼ **Mono-Cedocard 40**® (Tillots)

Tablets, scored, isosorbide mononitrate 40 mg. Price 20 tabs = **E**. Label: 25

LIDOFLAZINE

Indications: prophylaxis of angina

Cautions: may precipitate ventricular tachycardia

Side-effects: gastro-intestinal disturbances, dizziness, tinnitus, headaches

Dose: 1st week, 120 mg once daily; 2nd week, 120 mg twice daily; 3rd and subsequent weeks, 120 mg 3 times daily

▼ PoM **Clinium**® (Janssen)

Tablets, lidoflazine 120 mg. Price 20 tabs = **E**

NIFEDIPINE

Indications: prophylaxis and treatment of angina; hypertension; Raynaud's phenomenon

Cautions: withdraw the drug if ischaemic pain occurs or existing pain worsens shortly after initiating treatment; may inhibit labour. Drug interactions: see Appendix 1 (sections *2.1*, *2.4*, *2.5*, *2.6*, *6.1*)

Side-effects: see under Glyceryl Trinitrate; peripheral oedema may also occur and can sometimes be severe and relatively refractory to diuretics

Dose: angina, initially 10 mg 3 times daily with food, increased to 20 mg 3 times daily if necessary; in elderly patients, initially 5 mg 3 times daily; for immediate effect bite into capsule and retain liquid in mouth

Raynaud's phenomenon, 10 mg 3 times daily; max. 60 mg daily

PoM **Adalat**® (Bayer)

Capsules, orange, nifedipine 5 mg. Price 20 caps = **D**. Label: 21, counselling advised, see above

Capsules, orange, nifedipine 10 mg. Price 20 caps = **E**. Label: 21, counselling advised, see above

▼ PoM **Adalat Retard**® (Bayer)

Tablets, s/r, pink, nifedipine 20 mg. Price 20 tabs = **F**. Label: 21, 25

Dose: hypertension, initially 20 mg twice daily after food, increased to 40 mg twice daily if necessary

PENTAERYTHRITOL TETRANITRATE

Indications: prophylaxis of angina; left ventricular failure

Cautions; Side-effects: see under Glyceryl Trinitrate

Dose: 20–60 mg 3–4 times daily

Cardiacap® (Consolidated)

Capsules, s/r, blue/yellow, pentaerithrol tetranitrate 30 mg. Price 20 caps = **C**. Label: 22, 25

Dose: prophylaxis of angina, 30 mg every 12 hours

Mycardol® (Winthrop)

Tablets, scored, pentaerythrol tetranitrate 30 mg. Price 20 tabs = **C**. Label: 22

PoM **Pentoxylon**® (Riker)

Tablets, brown, pentaerythrol tetranitrate 10 mg, alseroxylon 1 mg. Price 20 tabs = **B**. Label: 22

Peritrate® (Warner)

Tablets, green, pentaerythrol tetranitrate 10 mg. Price 20 tabs = **A**. Label: 22

Peritrate SA® (Warner)

Tablets, s/r, green, pentaerythrol tetranitrate 80 mg. Price 20 tabs = **B**. Label: 22, 25

Dose: 80 mg every 12 hours

PRENYLAMINE

Indications: prophylaxis of angina

Cautions: avoid hypokalaemia. Drug interactions: see Appendix 1 (section *2.4*)

Contra-indications: severe hepatic or renal impairment, cardiac conduction defects, severe uncompensated heart failure

Side-effects: nausea, vomiting, diarrhoea, myocardial depression, syncope due to ventricular tachycardia (especially with hypokalaemia)

Dose: 60 mg 3 times daily, increased to 4 or 5 times daily if response is inadequate after 14 days; reduce to lowest effective dose after response occurs

PoM **Synadrin**® (Hoechst)

Tablets, pink, s/c, prenylamine 60 mg (as lactate). Price 20 tabs = **E**. Label: 25

2.6.2 Vasodilators used in heart failure

Until recently, treatment of heart failure was restricted to restoring contractility with cardiac glycosides and relieving congestion with diuretics.

C = 51-100p, D = 101-180p, E = 181-300p, F = 301-450p, G = 451-650p, H = 651-900p, I = 901-1200p, J = over 1200p.

Cardiac glycosides have been shown to have limited inotropic potential in long-term treatment and it now appears that vasodilators may produce improvement in cardiac performance comparable with that achieved by the most potent inotropic drugs.

Vasodilators act in heart failure by one of two methods: by arteriolar dilatation which reduces both peripheral vascular resistance and left ventricular pressure at systole and results in improved cardiac output, or by venous dilatation which results in a dilatation of capacitance vessels, an increase of venous pooling, and diminution of venous return to the heart thus decreasing left ventricular end-diastolic pressure. Symptoms of heart failure are therefore relieved. Three groups of drugs should be considered—nitrates (glyceryl trinitrate, isosorbide dinitrate, pentaerythritol tetranitrate) which act predominantly by venous dilatation; captopril and enalapril and hydralazine which act predominantly by arteriolar dilatation; and phentolamine, prazosin, and sodium nitroprusside which produce both arteriolar and venous dilatation. Combinations of drugs with different effects can be tried.

Captopril and enalapril—section 2.5.5
Glyceryl trinitrate and other nitrates—section 2.6.1
Hydralazine hydrochloride—section 2.5.1
Phentolamine mesylate—section 2.5.4
Prazosin hydrochloride—section 2.5.4
Sodium nitroprusside—section 2.5.1

2.6.3   Peripheral vasodilators

Most serious peripheral disorders are now known to be due to occlusion of vessels, either by spasm or sclerotic plaques; use of vasodilators may increase blood flow at rest, but no controlled studies have shown any improvement in walking distance or sustained increase in muscle blood flow during exercise. Rest pain is rarely affected.

BAMETHAN SULPHATE

Indications: Raynaud's disease, poor peripheral circulation
Cautions: angina
Contra-indications: recent myocardial infarction
Side-effects: postural hypotension, tachycardia, flushing
Dose: 25 mg 4 times daily

Vasculit® (Boehringer Ingelheim)
Tablets, bamethan sulphate 12.5 mg. Price 20 tabs = **B**

CINNARIZINE

Indications: peripheral vascular disease, Raynaud's disease
Cautions; Side-effects: see under Cyclizine (section 4.6); also hypersensitivity reactions, caution in hypotension
Dose: initially, 75 mg 3 times daily; maintenance, 75 mg 2–3 times daily

Stugeron Forte® (Janssen)
Capsules, orange/cream, cinnarizine 75 mg. Price 20 caps = **E**. Label: 2
Stugeron: see section 4.6

NICOTINIC ACID DERIVATIVES

Indications: peripheral vascular disease (for the use of nicotinic acid and nicofuranose in hyperlipidaemia, see section 2.12)
Cautions: diabetes mellitus
Side-effects: flushing, dizziness, nausea, vomiting, hypotension (more frequent with nicotinic acid than derivatives)

Bradilan® (Napp)
Tablets, e/c and s/c, nicofuranose 250 mg. Price 20 tabs = **D**. Label: 5, 25
Dose: 500 mg 3 times daily, increased if required
Hexopal® (Winthrop)
Tablets, scored, inositol nicotinate 500 mg. Price 20 tabs = **E**
Dose: 0.5–1 g 3 times daily, increased to 4 g daily if required
Tablets forte, scored, inositol nicotinate 750 mg. Price 20 tabs = **F**
Dose: 1.5–3 g daily
Suspension (=mixture), inositol nicotinate 1 g/5 ml. Diluent syrup, life of diluted mixture 14 days. Price 100 ml = **G**
Dose: as for tablets (above)
NHS **Pernivit**® (DF)
Tablets, pink, s/c, nicotinic acid 25 mg, acetomenaphthone 7 mg. Price 20 tabs = **A**
Ronicol® (Roche)
Tablets, scored, nicotinyl alcohol 25 mg (as tartrate). Price 20 tabs = **B**
Dose: 25–50 mg 4 times daily
Timespan® (=tablets s/r), red, s/c, nicotinyl alcohol 150 mg (as tartrate). Price 20 tabs = **D**. Label: 25
Dose: 150–300 mg twice daily

OXPENTIFYLLINE

Indications: peripheral vascular disease
Cautions: hypotension
Side-effects: nausea, dizziness, flushing
Dose: by mouth, 400 mg 2–3 times daily
By slow intravenous injection or infusion, 100 mg; max. 400 mg daily

PoM **Trental**® (Hoechst)
Tablets, s/r, pink, s/c, oxpentifylline 400 mg. Price 20 tabs = **F**. Label: 21, 25
Injection, oxpentifylline 20 mg/ml. Price 5-ml amp = **C**

THYMOXAMINE

Indications: Raynaud's disease, peripheral vascular disease, vascular spasm
Cautions: coronary artery disease, diabetes mellitus
Side-effects: nausea, diarrhoea, flushing, headache, dizziness
Dose: by mouth, 40 mg 4 times daily

By intravenous injection, 100 micrograms/kg; may be repeated 4 times daily or followed by oral administration
By intra-arterial injection, 5 mg

PoM **Opilon**® (Warner)
Tablets, yellow, scored, thymoxamine 40 mg (as hydrochloride). Price 20 tabs = E. Label: 21
Injection, thymoxamine 5 mg (as hydrochloride)/ml. Price 1-ml amp = C
Injection forte, thymoxamine 15 mg (as hydrochloride)/ml. Price 2-ml amp = C

OTHER PREPARATION USED IN PERIPHERAL VASCULAR DISEASE

Rutosides (oxerutins, Paroven®) are not vasodilators and are not generally regarded as effective preparations as capillary sealants or for the treatment of cramps.

Paroven® (Zyma)
Capsules, yellow, oxerutins 250 mg. Price 20 caps = E. Label: 21

2.6.4 Cerebral vasodilators

These drugs are claimed to improve mental function. Some improvements in performance of psychological tests have been reported but the drugs have not been shown clinically to be of much benefit in senile dementia.

CO-DERGOCRINE MESYLATE

Indications: adjunct in the management of senile dementia
Cautions: severe bradycardia
Side-effects: nausea, vomiting, flushing, rashes, nasal congestion, postural hypotension in hypertensive patients
Dose: 1.5 mg 3 times daily *or* 4.5 mg once daily

PoM **Hydergine**® (Sandoz)
Tablets, scored, co-dergocrine mesylate 1.5 mg. Price 20 tabs = F. Label: 22
Tablets, co-dergocrine mesylate 4.5 mg. Price 28 tabs = J. Label: 22

CYCLANDELATE

Indications: peripheral vascular disease; adjunct in the management of senile dementia
Contra-indications: acute phase of cerebrovascular accident
Side-effects: nausea, flushing, dizziness with high doses
Dose: 1.2–1.6 g daily in 2–4 divided doses

Cyclobral® (Norgine)
Capsules, pink/brown, cyclandelate 400 mg. Price 20 caps = D
Cyclospasmol® (Brocades)
Capsules, pink/grey, cyclandelate 400 mg. Price 20 caps = E
Tablets, pink, s/c, cyclandelate 400 mg. Price 28 tabs = F

Suspension (= mixture), cyclandelate 400 mg/5 ml when reconstituted with freshly boiled and cooled purified water. Diluent syrup, life of diluted mixture 14 days. Price 100 ml = E

ISOXSUPRINE HYDROCHLORIDE

Indications: cerebral and peripheral vascular disease
Contra-indications: recent arterial haemorrhage
Side-effects: flushing, tachycardia, palpitations, nausea, vomiting
Dose: by mouth, 20 mg 4 times daily *or* 40 mg (in sustained-release form) every 12 hours
By intramuscular injection, 5–10 mg up to 4 times daily
By intravenous infusion, initially 100 micrograms/minute, increased to 500 micrograms/minute if required

Defencin CP® (Bristol-Myers)
Capsules, s/r, pink/red, isoxsuprine hydrochloride (as resinate) 40 mg. Price 28 caps = F. Label: 25
Duvadilan® (Duphar)
Tablets, pink, scored, isoxsuprine hydrochloride 20 mg. Price 20 tabs = C
PoM *Injection*, isoxsuprine hydrochloride 5 mg/ml. Price 2-ml amp = B; 10-ml amp = D
Duvadilan Retard® (Duphar)
Capsules, s/r, red/white, isoxsuprine hydrochloride (as resinate) 40 mg. Price 28 caps = F. Label: 25

NAFTIDROFURYL OXALATE

Indications: cerebral and peripheral vascular disease
Contra-indications: parenteral administration in atrioventricular block
Side-effects: nausea, epigastric pain
Dose: by mouth, 100 mg 3 times daily, increased to 200 mg 3 times daily if necessary

PoM **Praxilene**® (Lipha)
Capsules, pink, naftidrofuryl oxalate 100 mg. Price 20 caps = E
Injection forte, naftidrofuryl oxalate 20 mg/ml. Price 10-ml amp = D
Dose: peripheral vascular disease, by intravenous or intra-arterial infusion, 200 mg over at least 90 minutes, twice daily

2.7 Sympathomimetics

2.7.1 Sympathomimetics with inotropic activity
2.7.2 Sympathomimetics causing vasoconstriction

Xanthine derivatives such as aminophylline are also used as cardiac stimulants, particularly in congestive heart failure. For details of preparations, see section 3.1.3.

For drug interactions of sympathomimetic amines see Appendix 1 (sections 2.4, 2.5, 4.3) and under individual entries.

C = 51-100p, D = 101-180p, E = 181-300p, F = 301-450p, G = 451-650p, H = 651-900p, I = 901-1200p, J = over 1200p.

2.7.1 Sympathomimetics with inotropic activity

The cardiac stimulants **dobutamine** (Dobutrex®) and **dopamine** (Intropin®) act on sympathetic receptors in cardiac muscle, and increase contractility with little effect on rate; they are used in cardiogenic shock.

Prenalterol (Hyprenan®) has similar cardiac stimulant activity but has a more selective action on beta$_1$ receptors, so may also be used to reverse the cardiac effects of beta-adrenoceptor blocking drugs.

Isoprenaline also acts on sympathetic receptors and increases both heart rate and contractility; it may prevent Stokes-Adams attacks, but insertion of a pacemaker is preferable.

DOBUTAMINE HYDROCHLORIDE

Indications: inotropic support in infarction, cardiac surgery, septic shock, and cardiogenic shock

Cautions: severe hypotension complicating cardiogenic shock

Side-effects: tachycardia and marked increase in systolic blood pressure indicate overdosage

Dose: by intravenous infusion, 2.5–10 micrograms/kg/minute, adjusted according to response

PoM **Dobutrex**® (Lilly)
Injection, powder for preparation of an infusion, dobutamine hydrochloride. Price 250-mg vial = **I**

DOPAMINE HYDROCHLORIDE

Indications: cardiogenic shock in infarction or cardiac surgery

Cautions: correct hypovolaemia; low dose in shock due to acute myocardial infarction

Contra-indications: tachyarrhythmia, phaeochromocytoma

Side-effects: nausea and vomiting, peripheral vasoconstriction, hypotension, hypertension, tachycardia

Dose: by intravenous infusion, 2–5 micrograms/kg/minute initially, increased if necessary

PoM **Intropin**® (American Hospital Supply)
Injection, dopamine hydrochloride 40 mg/ml. For dilution and use as an infusion. Price 5-ml amp or syringe = **G**
Injection, dopamine hydrochloride 160 mg/ml. For dilution and use as an infusion. Price 5-ml amp = **J**

PoM **Select-A-Jet Dopamine**® (IMS)
Injection, dopamine hydrochloride 40 mg/ml. For dilution and use as an infusion. Price 5-ml vial = **F**; 10-ml vial = **H**; 20-ml vial = **J**

ISOPRENALINE HYDROCHLORIDE

Indications: heart block, severe bradycardia

Cautions: ischaemic heart disease, diabetes mellitus, hyperthyroidism. Drug interactions: see Appendix 1 (section *15*)

Side-effects: tachycardia, arrhythmias, hypotension, sweating, tremor, headache

Dose: by mouth, 30 mg every 8 hours, then increased; max. daily dose usually 840 mg

By intravenous infusion, 0.5–10 micrograms/minute

PoM **Isuprel**® (Winthrop)
Injection, isoprenaline hydrochloride 200 micrograms/ml. Price 1-ml amp = **F**; 5-ml amp = **J**

PoM **Saventrine**® (Pharmax)
Tablets, s/r, isoprenaline hydrochloride 30 mg. Price 20 tabs = **D**. Label: 25

PoM **Saventrine IV**® (Pharmax)
Injection, isoprenaline hydrochloride 1 mg/ml. For dilution and use as an infusion. Price 2-ml amp = **B**

PoM **Select-A-Jet Isoprenaline**® (IMS)
Injection, isoprenaline hydrochloride 200 micrograms/ml. For dilution and use as an infusion. Price 5-ml vial = **E**; 10-ml vial = **F**

PRENALTEROL HYDROCHLORIDE

Indications: inotropic support in infarction, cardiac surgery or shock; reversal of the cardiac effect of beta-blockers

Cautions: correct hypovolaemia; angina pectoris and recent myocardial infarction, obstructive subvalvular cardiomyopathy, diabetes mellitus, hypokalaemia, pregnancy (toxicity in *animal* studies)

Contra-indications: serious ventricular arrhythmias

Side-effects: palpitations, nervousness; isolated ventricular ectopic beats, increase in attack rate in patients with angina pectoris, excessive increase in blood pressure or heart rate (may be counteracted by intravenous injection of beta-blocker)

Dose: inotropic support, *by intravenous infusion*, 500 micrograms/minute, adjusted according to response; max. total dose 20 mg

Reversal of beta-blockade, *by intravenous injection*, 2–5 mg over 5 minutes, repeated if necessary to a max. of 20 mg

▼ PoM **Hyprenan**® (Astra)
Product discontinued

2.7.2 Sympathomimetics causing vasoconstriction

Vasoconstrictors raise blood pressure transiently by constricting peripheral vessels. They are sometimes used as an emergency method of elevating blood pressure while preparations are being made for more effective therapy such as transfusion. They may also be used in general and spinal anaesthesia to control blood pressure.

The danger of vasoconstrictors is that although they raise blood pressure they do so at the expense of perfusion of vital organs such as the kidney. Further, in many patients with shock the peripheral resistance is already high, and to raise it further is unhelpful. Thus the use of vaso-constrictors in the treatment of shock is to be generally **deprecated**. The use of volume expanders such as blood or plasma, or the inotropic agents dopamine, dobutamine, or iso-prenaline is more appropriate (section 2.7.1). Treatment of the underlying condition, e.g. with antibiotics, in septic shock, is obviously impor-tant, and, in addition high doses of corticosteroids may be helpful.

METARAMINOL

Indications: acute hypotension
Cautions; Contra-indications: see under Nor-adrenaline Acid Tartrate
Side-effects: tachycardia, arrhythmias, reduced renal blood flow
Dose: by subcutaneous or intramuscular injec-tion, 2–10 mg
By intravenous infusion, 15–100 mg

PoM **Aramine**® (MSD)
Injection, metaraminol 10 mg (as tartrate)/ml. Price 1-ml amp = **B**

METHOXAMINE HYDROCHLORIDE

Indications: hypotension in anaesthesia
Cautions: hyperthyroidism; pregnancy. Drug interactions: see Appendix 1 (section 2.7)
Contra-indications: severe coronary or cardio-vascular disease
Side-effects: headache, hypertension, brady-cardia
Dose: by intramuscular injection, 5–20 mg
By slow intravenous injection, 5–10 mg

PoM **Vasoxine**® (Calmic)
Injection, methoxamine hydrochloride 20 mg/ml. Price 1-ml amp = **B**

NORADRENALINE ACID TARTRATE

Indications: acute hypotension, cardiac arrest
Cautions: extravasation at injection site may cause necrosis. Drug interactions: see Appen-dix 1 (section 2.7)
Contra-indications: myocardial infarction, pregnancy
Side-effects: headache, palpitations, bradycardia
Dose: by intravenous infusion, 8–12 micrograms/minute, adjusted as required
By rapid intravenous or intracardiac injection, 100–150 micrograms
Note: noradrenaline acid tartrate 2 mg ≡ noradrenaline 1 mg

PoM **Levophed**® (Winthrop)
Injection, noradrenaline acid tartrate 2 mg/ml. For dilution and use as an infusion. Price 2- and 4-ml amp (both) = **C**
Special injection, noradrenaline acid tartrate 200 micrograms/ml. Price 2-ml amp = **C**

OXEDRINE TARTRATE

Indications: hypotension

Cautions; Contra-indications; Side-effects: see under Phenylephrine Hydrochloride

PoM **Sympatol**® (Lewis)
Liquid (oral), oxedrine tartrate 10%. Price 20 ml = **D**; 100 ml = **H**
Dose: 20–30 drops 3 times daily
Injection, oxedrine tartrate 60 mg/ml. Price 1-ml amp = **A**
Dose: by subcutaneous, intramuscular, or intra-venous injection, 60–120 mg every 1–2 hours

PHENYLEPHRINE HYDROCHLORIDE

Indications: acute hypotension
Cautions; Contra-indications: see under Nor-adrenaline Acid Tartrate; also contra-indicated in severe hypertension and hyperthyroidism
Side-effects: hypertension with headache, pal-pitations, vomiting; tachycardia or reflex bradycardia; tingling and coolness of skin
Dose: by subcutaneous or intramuscular injec-tion, 5 mg
By slow intravenous injection, 100–500 micrograms
By intravenous infusion, 5–20 mg

PoM **Phenylephrine Injection 1%**, phenylephrine hydrochloride 10 mg/ml. Price 1-ml amp = **B**

2.8 Anticoagulants and Protamine

2.8.1 Parenteral anticoagulants
2.8.2 Oral anticoagulants
2.8.3 Protamine sulphate

The main use of anticoagulants is to prevent thrombus formation or the extension of an existing thrombus in the slower-moving venous side of the circulation, where the thrombus consists of a fibrin web enmeshed with platelets and red cells. Anti-coagulants are therefore widely used in the pre-vention and treatment of deep-vein thrombosis in the legs.

Anticoagulants are of less use in preventing thrombus formation in arteries, for in faster-flowing vessels thrombi are composed mainly of platelets with little fibrin. Anticoagulants are used to prevent thrombi forming on prosthetic heart valves. Any success anticoagulants have had in reducing mortality after myocardial infarction is probably due to the decreased incidence of deep-vein thrombosis in recumbent patients.

2.8.1 Parenteral anticoagulants

Heparin is given to initiate anticoagulation and is rapidly effective. As its effects are short-lived it is best given by continuous infusion; if given by intermittent intravenous injection, the interval between doses must not exceed 6 hours. Oral anticoagulants are started at the same time, and the heparin infusion withdrawn after 3 days.

If oral anticoagulants cannot be given and hep-arin is continued, its dose is adjusted after deter-

---

C = 51-100p, D = 101-180p, E = 181-300p, F = 301-450p, G = 451-650p, H = 651-900p, I = 901-1200p, J = over 1200p.

mination of the activated partial thromboplastin time.

If haemorrhage occurs it is usually sufficient to withdraw heparin, but if rapid reversal of the effects of heparin is required, protamine sulphate is a specific antidote (section 2.8.3).

For the prophylaxis of thrombosis in patients undergoing heart surgery or renal dialysis full therapeutic doses of heparin are given for the duration of the procedure. Low-dose heparin by subcutaneous injection is used to prevent postoperative deep-vein thrombosis and pulmonary embolism. Laboratory monitoring is not required with this regimen.

Ancrod (Arvin®) has been shown to be as effective as heparin in the resolution of deep-vein thromboses, but some patients develop resistance. The initial infusion must be given slowly, as there is a risk of massive intravascular formation of unstable fibrin. The response can be monitored by observing clot size after blood has been allowed to stand for about 2 hours, the aim being to predict a dose that produces a 2–3 mm clot. Alternatively, plasma-fibrinogen concentrations can be measured directly.

The major complication is haemorrhage. Since it takes 12–24 hours to reach haemostatic fibrinogen concentrations after administration has ceased it may be necessary to give ancrod antivenom (0.2-ml test dose subcutaneously followed by 0.8 ml intramuscularly, and 30 minutes later 1 ml intravenously). Anaphylaxis may occur and adrenaline and hydrocortisone should be available. As an alternative to antiserum, reconstituted freeze-dried fibrinogen may be given. Subcutaneous injection of ancrod has been used for prophylaxis in patients likely to develop deepvein thrombosis.

HEPARIN

Indications: deep-vein thrombosis, disseminated intravascular coagulation, prevention of postoperative thrombosis

Cautions: pregnancy. Drug interactions: see Appendix 1 (section 2.8)

Contra-indications: haemophilia and other haemorrhagic disorders, peptic ulcer, cerebral aneurysm, severe hypertension, severe liver disease, recent surgery of eye or nervous system, hypersensitivity to heparin

Side-effects: haemorrhage, thrombocytopenia, hypersensitivity reactions; osteoporosis after prolonged use, alopecia

Dose: by intravenous injection, loading dose of 5000 units followed by continuous *infusion* of 40 000 units over 24 hours *or* 10 000 units by *intravenous injection* every 6 hours

By subcutaneous injection, 5000 units before surgery, then every 12 hours until patient is ambulant

Intravenous preparations

PoM **Heparin Injection** (heparin sodium)
1000 units/ml. Price 5-ml amp = C; 5-ml vial = C

5000 units/ml. Price 5-ml amp = C; 5-ml vial = D

PoM **Monoparin**® (CP)
Injection, heparin sodium (mucous) 1000 units/ml. Price 1-ml amp = A; 5-ml amp = B
Injection, heparin sodium (mucous) 5000 units/ml. Price 1-ml amp = B
Injection, heparin sodium (mucous) 25 000 units/ml. Price 1-ml amp = D

PoM **Multiparin**® (CP)
Injection, heparin sodium (mucous) 1000 units/ml. Price 5-ml vial = B
Injection, heparin sodium (mucous) 5000 units/ml. Price 5-ml vial = D
Injection, heparin sodium (mucous) 25 000 units/ml. Price 5-ml vial = G

PoM **Pump-Hep**® (Burgess)
Intravenous infusion, heparin sodium (mucous) 1000 units/ml. Price 20-ml amp = D
Dose: by continuous infusion pump, 20 000–40 000 units daily

PoM **Unihep**® (Leo)
Injection, heparin sodium (mucous) 1000 units/ml. Price 1-ml amp = A
Injection, heparin sodium (mucous) 5000 units/ml. Price 1-ml amp = B
Injection, heparin sodium (mucous) 10 000 units/ml. Price 1-ml amp = B
Injection, heparin sodium (mucous) 25 000 units/ml. Price 1-ml amp = D

Subcutaneous preparations

PoM **Heparin Injection** (heparin sodium or heparin calcium)
25 000 units/ml (subcutaneous). Price 0.2-ml amp and syringe (both) = C

PoM **Calciparine**® (Labaz)
Injection (subcutaneous), heparin calcium 25 000 units/ml. Price 0.2-ml syringe = C; 0.5- and 0.8-ml amp (both) = D

PoM **Heparin Retard**® (Boots)
Injection (intramuscular or subcutaneous), heparin sodium 10 000 units/ml. Price 2-ml amp = E

PoM **Minihep**® (Leo)
Darts (= subcutaneous injection), heparin sodium 10 000 units/ml. Price 0.5-ml injector system = C
Injection (subcutaneous), heparin sodium 25 000 units/ml. Price 0.2-ml amp = B

PoM **Minihep Calcium**® (Leo)
Darts (= subcutaneous injection), heparin calcium 10 000 units/ml. Price 0.5-ml injector system = B
Injection (subcutaneous), heparin calcium 25 000 units/ml. Price 0.2-ml amp = B

PoM **Monoparin**® (CP)
Injection (subcutaneous), heparin sodium (mucous) 25 000 units/ml. Price 0.2-ml amp = B

PoM **Uniparin**® (CP)
Injection (subcutaneous), heparin sodium 25 000 units/ml. Price 0.2-ml syringe = C

Sterile solutions
PoM **Hep-Flush**® (Burgess)

Solution, heparin sodium 100 units/ml. Price 2-ml amp = **B**

To maintain patency of catheters, cannulas, etc., 200 units flushed through every 4–8 hours. Not for therapeutic use

PoM **Hepsal**® (CP)

Solution (sterile), heparin sodium 10 units/ml. Price 5-ml amp = **B**

To maintain patency of catheters, cannulas, etc., 50 units flushed through every 4 hours. Not for therapeutic use

ANCROD

Indications: deep-vein thrombosis, prevention of postoperative thrombosis

Cautions; Contra-indications; Side-effects: see under Heparin; resistance may develop; avoid administration with dextrans

Dose: by intravenous infusion, 2–3 units/kg over 4–12 hours (usually 6–8 hours), then *by infusion or slow intravenous injection*, 2 units/kg every 12 hours

PoM **Arvin**® (Armour)

Injection, ancrod 70 units/ml. Price 1-ml amp = **I** (Hosp. only)

Note: Arvin Antidote is available from Armour

2.8.2 Oral anticoagulants

They antagonise the effects of vitamin K, and take at least 36 to 48 hours for the anticoagulant effect to develop; if an immediate effect is required, heparin must be given concomitantly.

The main indication for oral anticoagulant therapy is deep-vein thrombosis. Patients with poorly controlled atrial fibrillation who are at risk of embolisation should also be treated, as should patients with heart valve prostheses, to prevent emboli developing on the valves; antiplatelet drugs may also be useful in these patients.

Oral anticoagulants should not be used in cerebral thrombosis or peripheral arterial occlusion, but may be of value in patients with transient brain ischaemic attacks whether due to carotid or vertebrobasilar arterial disease; if these patients also have severe hypertension anticoagulants are contra-indicated, and antiplatelet drugs are an alternative (section 2.9).

Warfarin and other coumarins are the drugs of choice, as they are less likely to cause sensitivity reactions than phenindione.

Whenever possible, the base-line prothrombin time should be determined before the initial dose is given. A typical induction dose is 10 mg daily for 3 days but this should be reduced if the base-line prothrombin time is prolonged, the liver-function tests are abnormal, or the patient is in cardiac failure, is on parenteral feeding, is less than average weight, or is over 80 years of age. The subsequent maintenance dose must depend upon the prothrombin time reported by the laboratory as the British Ratio (BR). The currently recommended therapeutic ranges are 2–2.5 for prophylactic therapy of deep-vein thrombosis including high-risk surgery; 2–3 for prophylactic therapy in hip surgery and fractured femur operations, for treatment of deep-vein thrombosis, pulmonary embolism, and transient ischaemic attacks; 3–4.5 for recurrent deep-vein thrombosis and pulmonary embolism, arterial disease including myocardial infarction, arterial grafts, and prosthetic heart valves and grafts.

It is essential that the BR be determined on the second and third days of treatment, then on alternate days with longer intervals once stability of dosage has been achieved. The daily maintenance dose is usually 3 to 9 mg and should be taken at the same time each day.

Change in the patient's clinical condition, particularly associated with liver disease or drug administration, necessitates more frequent testing. Patients taking a fixed dose of warfarin and a microsomal enzyme-inducing agent such as phenobarbitone or phenytoin are at risk of haemorrhage if the agent is withdrawn and the anticoagulant dose maintained. There is an increased risk of haemorrhage if patients on warfarin are prescribed drugs such as phenylbutazone, aspirin, or clofibrate. [See Appendix 1 (section 2.8) for further interactions with warfarin.] Patients may be given regular doses of aspirin for its antiplatelet effect, providing this is taken into account in assessing the dosage of warfarin required.

The main adverse effect of all oral anti-coagulants is haemorrhage. Omission of dosage with checking of the BR is essential. The following recommendations are based on the result of the BR and the clinical state:

BR 4.5–7 without haemorrhage—withhold warfarin for 1 or more days, according to BR

BR >7 without haemorrhage—withhold warfarin and consider giving phytomenadione (vitamin K_1) 1–2 mg by mouth or intravenous injection

BR < 4.5 with haemorrhage—give fresh frozen plasma and investigate cause

BR > 2 with life-threatening haemorrhage—phytomenadione 2.5–10 mg by slow intravenous injection with factors II, IX, and X (or fresh frozen plasma) and investigate cause.

Phytomenadione will take up to 12 hours to act and will prevent oral anticoagulants from acting for several days or even weeks (see section 9.6.6.). Cerebral haemorrhage should be treated similarly but is often fatal.

PREGNANCY. Oral anticoagulants are weakly teratogenic and should not be given in the first trimester of pregnancy. Women at risk of pregnancy should be warned of this danger. Also, oral anticoagulants cross the placenta with risk of placental or fetal haemorrhage; they should therefore not be given during the last few weeks of pregnancy.

Anticoagulant treatment cards must be carried by patients, and cards are available from:

DHSS Store
No. 2 Site
Manchester Rd
Heywood
Lancs OL10 2PZ

In Scotland the cards are available from:
SHHD (Div IIID)
Room 9
St. Andrew's House
Edinburgh EH1 3DE
Cards giving advice for patients on anti-coagulant treatment may be given to patients at the discretion of the doctor or pharmacist.

WARFARIN SODIUM

Indications: deep-vein thrombosis, transient brain ischaemic attacks, prophylaxis with prosthetic heart valves

Cautions: hepatic or renal disease, recent surgery. Drug interactions: see Appendix 1 (section 2.8)

Contra-indications: pregnancy, peptic ulcer, severe hypertension, bacterial endocarditis

Side-effects: haemorrhage

Dose: see notes above

PoM **Marevan**® (DF)
Tablets, brown, scored, warfarin sodium 1 mg. Price 20 tabs = **A**. Label: 10 anticoagulant card
Tablets, blue, scored, warfarin sodium 3 mg. Price 20 tabs = **A**. Label: 10 anticoagulant card
Tablets, pink, scored, warfarin sodium 5 mg. Price 20 tabs = **A**. Label: 10 anticoagulant card

PoM **Warfarin WBP** (Boehringer Ingelheim)
Tablets, brown, scored, warfarin sodium 1 mg. Price 20 tabs = **A**. Label: 10 anticoagulant card
Tablets, blue, scored, warfarin sodium 3 mg. Price 20 tabs = **A**. Label: 10 anticoagulant card
Tablets, pink, scored, warfarin sodium 5 mg. Price 20 tabs = **A**. Label: 10 anticoagulant card

NICOUMALONE

Indications: deep-vein thrombosis, transient brain ischaemic attacks, prophylaxis with prosthetic heart valves

Cautions; Contra-indications; Side-effects: see under Warfarin Sodium; avoid breast-feeding

Dose: 8–12 mg on 1st day; 4–8 mg on 2nd day; maintenance dose usually 1–8 mg daily

PoM **Sinthrome**® (Geigy)
Tablets, pink, nicoumalone 1 mg. Price 20 tabs = **A**. Label: 10 anticoagulant card
Tablets, scored, nicoumalone 4 mg. Price 20 tabs = **B**. Label: 10 anticoagulant card

PHENINDIONE

Indications: deep-vein thrombosis

Cautions; Contra-indications; Side-effects: see under Warfarin Sodium; also hypersensitivity reactions including rashes, fever, leucopenia, agranulocytosis, diarrhoea, renal and hepatic damage; urine coloured pink; avoid breast-feeding. Drug interactions: see Appendix 1 (section 2.8)

Dose: 200 mg on 1st day; 100 mg on 2nd day; maintenance dose usually 50–150 mg daily

PoM **Dindevan**® (DF)
Tablets, phenindione 10 mg. Price 20 tabs = **A**.

Label: 10 anticoagulant card, 14
Tablets, green, phenindione 25 mg. Price 20 tabs = **B**. Label: 10 anticoagulant card, 14
Tablets, phenindione 50 mg. Price 20 tabs = **B**. Label: 10 anticoagulant card, 14

2.8.3 Protamine sulphate

Although protamine sulphate is used to counteract overdosage with heparin, if used in excess protamine has an anticoagulant effect.

PROTAMINE SULPHATE

Indications: neutralisation of the anticoagulant effect of heparin

Cautions: overdose of protamine sulphate has an anticoagulant effect

Side-effects: flushing, hypotension, bradycardia

Dose: by slow intravenous injection, 1 mg neutralises 100 units heparin (mucous) or 80 units heparin (lung) when given within 15 minutes; if a longer time has elapsed, less protamine is required as heparin is rapidly excreted; max. dose 50 mg

PoM **Protamine Sulphate Injection,** protamine sulphate 10 mg/ml. Price 5- and 10-ml amp (both) = **C**

2.9   Antiplatelet drugs

By decreasing platelet adhesiveness, these drugs may inhibit thrombus formation on the arterial side of the circulation, where thrombi are formed by platelet aggregation and anticoagulants have little effect. Antiplatelet drugs have little effect in venous thromboembolism.

Dipyridamole (Persantin®) is used with anticoagulants to prevent thrombus formation on prosthetic valves, and its use in diabetic retinopathy is under investigation. **Aspirin** (see section 10.1.1.1) and **sulphinpyrazone** (Anturan®) are under investigation for prophylactic use in coronary disease including infarction, and transient brain ischaemic attacks.

DIPYRIDAMOLE

Indications: thromboembolism, angina

Cautions: may exacerbate migraine, hypotension. Drug interactions: see Appendix 1 (sections *2.8, 2.8E*)

Side-effects: nausea, diarrhoea, throbbing headache, hypotension

Dose: angina, *by mouth,* 50 mg 3 times daily
By slow intravenous injection, 10–20 mg 2–3 times daily
Thromboembolism, *by mouth,* 100 mg 3–4 times daily before food increased to 600 mg daily if required

PoM **Persantin**® (Boehringer Ingelheim)
Tablets, orange, s/c, dipyridamole 25 mg. Price 20 tabs = **C**. Label: 22
Tablets, s/c, dipyridamole 100 mg. Price 20 tabs = **E**. Label: 22

For all abbreviations and symbols see inside cover.   Relative prices: **A** = up to 20p, **B** = 21-50p,

Injection, dipyridamole 5 mg/ml. Price 2-ml amp = **A**

SULPHINPYRAZONE

Indications: prophylaxis after myocardial infarction (for use in gout, see section 10.1.4)
Cautions; Contra-indications; Side-effects: see section 10.1.4
Dose: 200 mg 4 times daily with food, starting 1 month after infarction

PoM **Anturan**® (Geigy)
Tablets, yellow, s/c, sulphinpyrazone 200 mg. Price 28 tabs = **E**. Label: 12, 21

2.10 Fibrinolytic drugs

These activate plasminogen to form plasmin, which degrades fibrin and so breaks up thrombi. **Streptokinase** is used in the treatment of life-threatening venous thrombosis, and in pulmonary embolism. Treatment must be started rapidly, within an hour of the event, and controlled by measurement of the thrombin clotting time. Corticosteroids or antihistamines may be required to control allergic reactions.

Urokinase is currently used for thrombolysis in the eye and in arteriovenous shunts. It has the advantage of being non-antigenic.

Stanozolol (see section 6.4.3) in a dosage of 10 mg daily has a fibrinolytic effect, and is used in the treatment of Raynaud's disease and lipodermatosclerosis.

STREPTOKINASE

Indications: venous thrombosis, pulmonary embolism, thrombosed arteriovenous shunts; thrombolysis in the eye
Cautions: atrial fibrillation, recovery from streptococcal infection
Contra-indications: recent haemorrhage, coagulation defects, severe hypertension, streptococcal infections, surgery in previous 72 hours, menstruation, pregnancy
Side-effects: allergic reactions, fever, rashes, haemorrhage (if due to overdose, can give aminocaproic acid or tranexamic acid)
Dose: by intravenous infusion, 250 000–600 000 units over 30 minutes, then 100 000 units every hour for up to 1 week

PoM **Kabikinase**® (KabiVitrum)
Injection, powder for reconstitution, streptokinase 100 000 units, price per vial = **I**; 600 000 units, price per vial = **J**
PoM **Streptase**® (Hoechst)
Injection, powder for reconstitution, streptokinase 100 000 units, price per vial = **H**; 250 000 and 750 000 units, price per vial (both) = **J**

UROKINASE

Indications: thrombosed arteriovenous shunts; thrombolysis in the eye
Contra-indications: recent haemorrhage, surgery in previous 72 hours, pregnancy

Side-effects: haemorrhage (if due to overdose, give tranexamic acid), fever
Dose: by instillation into arteriovenous shunt, 5000–37 500 International units in 2–3 ml sodium chloride intravenous infusion 0.9%
Intra-ocular administration, 5000–37 500 International units in 2 ml sodium chloride intravenous infusion 0.9%
Note: 1.5 International units ≈ 1 Ploug unit

PoM **Ukidan**® (Serono)
Injection, powder for reconstitution, urokinase 5000 International units, price per vial = **G**; 25 000 International units, price per vial = **J**
PoM **Urokinase** (Leo)
Injection, powder for reconstitution, urokinase 7500 International units (5000 Ploug units), price per amp = **I**; 37 500 International units (25 000 Ploug units), price per amp = **J**

2.11 Antifibrinolytic drugs and haemostatics

Fibrin stabilisation can be encouraged by the administration of **aminocaproic acid** (Epsikapron®) or **tranexamic acid** (Cyklokapron®), which inhibit plasminogen activation and interfere with fibrinolysis. They may be useful when haemorrhage cannot be staunched, for example in prostatectomy, dental extraction in haemophiliacs, or menorrhagia associated with intra-uterine contraceptive devices; they may also be used in streptokinase overdose.

Aprotinin (see section 1.9.3) is a proteolytic enzyme inhibitor acting on plasmin and kallidinogenase. Its value in the treatment of disseminated intravascular coagulation has not been substantiated.

Ethamsylate (Dicynene®) reduces capillary bleeding in the presence of a normal number of platelets. It does not act by fibrin stabilisation, but probably by correcting abnormal platelet adhesion.

AMINOCAPROIC ACID

Indications: haemorrhage after surgery, particularly prostatectomy; menorrhagia
Cautions: lower dose in renal impairment, haemophilia
Contra-indications: history of thromboembolic disease; pregnancy
Side-effects: nausea, diarrhoea, dizziness; rarely myalgia (discontinue treatment)
Dose: 3 g 4–6 times daily

PoM **Epsikapron**® (KabiVitrum)
Powder, effervescent, aminocaproic acid 3 g in sachet. Price 10 sachets = **E**. Label: 13
Syrup (= mixture), aminocaproic acid 1.5 g/ 5 ml. Price 100 ml = **E**

ETHAMSYLATE

Indications: haemorrhage from small blood vessels; menorrhagia
Side-effects: nausea, headache, rashes

C = 51-100p, D = 101-180p, E = 181-300p, F = 301-450p, G = 451-650p, H = 651-900p, I = 901-1200p, J = over 1200p.

Dose: by mouth, 500 mg 4 times daily
By intramuscular or intravenous injection, 1 g;
maintenance 500 mg every 4–6 hours

PoM **Dicynene**® (Delandale)
Tablets, ethamsylate 250 mg. Price 20 tabs = **E**
Tablets, ethamsylate 500 mg. Price 20 tabs = **F**
Injection, ethamsylate 125 mg/ml. Price 2-ml
  amp = **C**
Injection, ethamsylate 500 mg/ml. Price 2-ml
  amp = **D**

TRANEXAMIC ACID
Indications: see under Aminocaproic Acid
Cautions; Contra-indications; Side-effects: see
  under Aminocaproic Acid
Dose: by mouth, 1–1.5 g 2–4 times daily
By slow intravenous injection, 1 g 3 times daily

PoM **Cyklokapron**® (KabiVitrum)
Tablets, tranexamic acid 500 mg. Price 20
  tabs = **F**
Syrup (= elixir), tranexamic acid 500 mg/5 ml.
  Diluent syrup, life of diluted elixir 14 days.
  Price 100 ml = **G**
Injection, tranexamic acid 100 mg/ml. Price
  5-ml amp = **D**

2.12   Drugs used in the treatment of hyperlipidaemia

There are a number of common conditions, some
familial, in which there are very high plasma concentrations of cholesterol, or triglycerides, or
both. There is evidence that therapy which lowers
the lipid concentration reduces the progression
of premature atherosclerosis. Young patients are
likely to benefit more than old. Lipid-lowering
drugs should be reserved for patients in whom
severe hyperlipidaemia is inadequately controlled
by weight reduction. Any drug therapy must be
combined with strict adherence to diet, maintenance of near-ideal body weight and, if appropriate, reduction of blood pressure and cessation
of smoking.

Clofibrate (Atromid-S®), **bezafibrate**
(Bezalip®), **nicotinic acid**, and **nicofuranose** (Bra-
dilan®) lower plasma cholesterol and plasma triglyceride concentrations, probably in part by
reducing hepatic secretion of lipoproteins.
Cholestyramine (Questran®) and **colestipol** (Cole-
stid®), both of which are resins, bind bile salts,
decrease the absorption of cholesterol in the gut,
and lower plasma cholesterol concentrations. **Probucol** (Lurselle®) lowers plasma cholesterol concentrations by increasing the catabolism of low-
density lipoproteins.

Dextrothyroxine (Choloxin®) is no longer recommended as a lipid-lowering drug. It lowers the
plasma cholesterol concentration but may cause
tachycardia and, in patients with ischaemic heart
disease, angina.

BEZAFIBRATE
Indications: see notes above
Cautions: reduce dose in moderate renal impairment. Drug interactions: see Appendix 1 (sections *2.8, 2.8B, 6.1*)
Contra-indications: severe renal or hepatic
impairment, hypoalbuminaemia, primary biliary cirrhosis, gall bladder disease, nephrotic
syndrome, pregnancy
Side-effects: nausea, abdominal discomfort;
rarely myositis-like syndrome, pruritus, urticaria, impotence
Dose: 200 mg 3 times daily with or after food;
may be reduced to 200 mg twice daily in
hypertriglyceridaemia

▼ PoM **Bezalip**® (MCP)
Tablets, f/c, bezafibrate 200 mg. Price 20 tabs =
E. Label: 21

CHOLESTYRAMINE
Indications: see notes above
Cautions: supplements of fat-soluble vitamins
and of folic acid may be required with high
doses, particularly in children. Drug interactions: see Appendix 1 (sections *2.1, 2.8, 2.8C,
4.7, 5.1, 6.2, 10*)
Contra-indications: complete biliary obstruction,
pregnancy
Side-effects: nausea, constipation or diarrhoea,
heartburn, flatulence, abdominal discomfort,
rashes; rarely steatorrhoea (with large doses)
Dose: usually 4–8 g 2–3 times daily in liquid; up
to 36 g daily in resistant cases

PoM **Questran**® (Bristol-Myers)
Powder, sachets, cholestyramine (anhydrous)
4 g. Price 10 sachets = **F**. Label: 13, counselling
advised, avoid other drugs at same time

CLOFIBRATE
Indications: see notes above
Cautions; Contra-indications: see under Beza-
fibrate. Drug interactions: see Appendix 1 (sec-
tions *2.8, 2.8B, 6.1*)
Side-effects: see under Bezafibrate; also chol-
esterol cholelithiasis
Dose: 500 mg 2–3 times daily after meals

PoM **Atromid-S**® (ICI)
Capsules, red, clofibrate 500 mg. Price 20 caps =
C. Label: 21

COLESTIPOL HYDROCHLORIDE
Indications: see notes above
Cautions; Contra-indications; Side-effects: see
under Cholestyramine. Drug interactions: see
Appendix 1 (section *2.1*)
Dose: 5–10 g 2–3 times daily in liquid

▼ PoM **Colestid**® (Upjohn)
Granules, yellow, colestipol hydrochloride.
Price 10 × 5-g sachets = **F**. Label: 13, coun-
selling advised, avoid other drugs at same time

DEXTROTHYROXINE SODIUM
Indications: see notes above

Cautions: drug interactions: see Appendix 1 (section *2.8B*)

Contra-indications: severe kidney or liver disease; ischaemic heart disease

Side-effects: tachycardia, angina in patients with pre-existing subclinical coronary artery disease

Dose: 1–2 mg daily, increased by 1–2 mg at monthly intervals; max. dose 8 mg daily

PoM **Choloxin**® (Travenol)
Tablets, yellow, scored, dextrothyroxine sodium 2 mg. Price 20 tabs = **F**

NICOFURANOSE

Indications: see notes above (for use in peripheral vascular disease, see section 2.6.3)

Cautions; Side-effects: see under Nicotinic Acid, but prostaglandin-mediated symptoms less severe

Dose: 0.5–1 g 3 times daily

Bradilan® (Napp)
Tablets, e/c and s/c, nicofuranose 250 mg. Price 20 tabs = **D**. Label: 5, 25

NICOTINIC ACID

Indications: see notes above

Cautions: diabetes mellitus, gout, liver disease, peptic ulcer

Contra-indications: pregnancy, breast-feeding

Side-effects: flushing, dizziness, palpitations, pruritus (prostaglandin-mediated symptoms can be reduced by low initial doses taken with meals, or by taking aspirin 300 mg 30 minutes before the dose); nausea, vomiting; rarely impaired liver function and rashes

Dose: initially 100–200 mg 3 times daily (see above), gradually increased over 2–4 weeks to 1–2 g 3 times daily

Nicotinic Acid Tablets, nicotinic acid 25, 50, and 100 mg. Price 20 tabs (all) = **A**. Label: 21

PROBUCOL

Indications: see notes above

Cautions: avoid pregnancy during and for 6 months after stopping treatment

Contra-indications: breast-feeding

Side-effects: nausea, vomiting, flatulence, diarrhoea, abdominal pain; rarely angioedema, hypersensitivity reactions

Dose: 500 mg twice daily with food

PoM **Lurselle** (Merrell)
Tablets, probucol 250 mg. Price 20 tabs = **E**. Label: 21

2.13 Local sclerosants

Ethanolamine oleate and sodium tetradecyl sulphate are used in sclerotherapy of varicose veins, and phenol is used in thrombosed haemorrhoids (see section 1.7.4).

ETHANOLAMINE OLEATE

Indications: sclerotherapy of varicose veins

Cautions: extravasation may cause necrosis of tissues

Contra-indications: inability to walk, acute phlebitis, oral contraceptive use, obese legs

Side-effects: allergic reactions

PoM **Ethanolamine Oleate Injection,** ethanolamine oleate 5%. Price 2- and 5-ml amp (both) = **B**
Dose: by intravenous injection, 2–5 ml divided between 3–4 sites; repeated at weekly intervals

---

SODIUM TETRADECYL SULPHATE

Indications: sclerotherapy of varicose veins

Cautions; Contra-indications; Side-effects: see under Ethanolamine Oleate

PoM **STD**® (STD Pharmaceutical)
Injection, sodium tetradecyl sulphate 3%. Price 1-ml amp = **B**; 30-ml vial = **G**
Dose: by intravenous injection, 0.5–1 ml at up to 4 sites

C = 51-100p, **D** = 101-180p, **E** = 181-300p, **F** = 301-450p, **G** = 451-650p, **H** = 651-900p, **I** = 901-1200p, **J** = over 1200p.

3: Drugs used in the treatment of diseases of the
RESPIRATORY SYSTEM

In this chapter, drug treatment is described under the following headings:

The initial treatment of upper respiratory tract infections leading to exacerbation of chronic bronchitis and bacterial pneumonia is indicated in section 5.1 (Table 1) and the treatment of tuberculosis is discussed in section 5.1.9.

3.1 Bronchodilators

3.1.1 Adrenoceptor stimulants (sympathomimetics)

Most mild to moderate attacks of asthma respond rapidly to aerosol administration of a selective beta₂-adrenoceptor stimulant such as salbutamol or terbutaline (section 3.1.1.1). In frequently occurring moderate asthma the introduction of sodium cromoglycate (section 3.3), oral theophylline (section 3.1.3), or corticosteroid aerosol inhalation (section 3.2) may stabilise the asthma and avoid the use of oral corticosteroids. However in more severe attacks a short course of an oral corticosteroid may be necessary to bring the asthma under control (see section 6.3.4).

Treatment of patients with severe airways obstruction or status asthmaticus (see also below) is safer in hospital where oxygen and resuscitation facilities are immediately available.

Many patients with chronic bronchitis and emphysema are generally considered to have irreversible airways obstruction, but they nevertheless often respond partially to the beta₂-adrenoceptor stimulant drugs or to the anticholinergic drug ipratropium (section 3.1.2).

CHOICE OF DRUG. The **selective beta₂-adrenoceptor stimulants** (section 3.1.1.1) such as salbutamol or terbutaline (preferably given by aerosol inhalation) are the safest and most effective preparations. The drugs described in section 3.1.1.2 should be avoided whenever possible.

There is little difference between the various selective beta₂-adrenoceptor stimulant drugs. **Salbutamol** (Ventolin®) and **terbutaline** (Bricanyl®) are available in the widest range of formulations. **Rimiterol** (Pulmadil®) is shorter-acting than salbutamol whilst **fenoterol** (Berotec®) and terbutaline may have a longer duration of action. **Pirbuterol** (Exirel®), which has recently been introduced, is similar to the others. In many instances the dose or frequency of administration of beta₂-adrenoceptor stimulants can be reduced by concurrent treatment with xanthine derivatives (section 3.1.3) or corticosteroid aerosol inhalations (section 3.2), or by the use of sodium cromoglycate (section 3.3).

CHOICE OF FORMULATION. The *pressurised aerosol inhaler* is an effective and convenient method of administration for mild to moderate airways obstruction. Aerosol inhalers usually act for about 3 to 5 hours (rimiterol less than the others) but this depends to some extent on the severity of the asthma. Aerosol inhalation is preferred because it provides relief more rapidly and causes fewer side-effects (such as tremor and nervous tension) than tablets; the drug is delivered directly to the bronchi and is therefore effective in smaller doses.

Patients should be given careful instruction on the use of their pressurised aerosol inhalers and it is important to check that they continue to use them correctly as inadequate technique may be mistaken for drug failure. Most patients, including some young children (under parental supervision), can be successfully taught to use pressurised aerosol inhalers but some patients, particularly the elderly, the arthritic, and small children are unable to use them; some patients are unable to synchronise their breathing with the administration of aerosol.

Patients should be warned against excessive use of aerosol inhalers. The dose should be stated explicitly in terms of the number of inhalations at one time, the frequency, and the maximum number of inhalations allowed in 24 hours. Patients should be advised to seek medical advice when they fail to obtain their usual degree of symptomatic relief as this usually indicates a worsening of the asthma and may require alternative medication.

Modified inhalers such as Pulmadil Auto® (rimiterol) or *dry powder inhalers* (insufflation cartridges; Ventolin Rotacaps®) may help some patients with poor inhaler technique. These devices are actuated by the patient's inspiration, and by ensuring that more drug is inhaled, they are of particular value in subjects who cannot use pressurised aerosol inhalers correctly. Insufflation cartridges are particularly useful in young children though the dry powder may cause coughing and the units are bulky to carry. The Bricanyl Spacer® (terbutaline) incorporates a collapsible extended mouth-piece which acts as a drug reservoir and this is intended to give greater flexibility with the timing of inspiration than conventional aerosols. The Nebuhaler® incorporates a plastic cone and one-way valve and is used with a refill canister. There is recent evidence that it is helpful to patients with poor inhalation technique.

Oral preparations are commonly used in children and in patients who cannot tolerate the aerosol inhalation. They have a slower onset but slightly more prolonged action than the aerosol inhalers. The *sustained-release* preparations (Ventolin Spandets®; Bricanyl SA®) may be of value in patients with nocturnal asthma as an alternative to the sustained-release theophylline preparations (section 3.1.3).

Intravenous, and occasionally *subcutaneous*, injections of salbutamol and terbutaline are given in severe bronchospasm when bronchial narrowing prevents delivery of the aerosol to the airways.

Aqueous aerosols (respirator solutions) of salbutamol and terbutaline, and more recently fenoterol and reproterol are increasingly used for the treatment of acute asthma both in hospital and in general practice but whether they will eventually replace intravenous administration as the treatment of choice is contentious. Aqueous aerosols are easy to inhale and are administered over a period of about 15 minutes from a nebuliser or delivered by intermittent positive-pressure ventilation through a tightly fitted mask. Domiciliary use is limited by the need to provide patients with costly units which are not currently prescribable under the NHS. If respirator solutions are used unsupervised, patients must be given meticulous instructions on their use, as the nebuliser delivers substantial doses of beta$_2$-adrenoceptor stimulant. For example, a 2.5-ml Ventolin Nebule® contains 2.5 mg of salbutamol, which is equivalent to 25 puffs from the aerosol inhaler.

EMERGENCY TREATMENT OF SEVERE ACUTE ASTHMA. Severe asthma can be fatal and **must** be treated promptly and energetically. It is characterised by persistent dyspnoea poorly relieved by bronchodilators, restlessness, exhaustion, a high pulse rate (usually over 110/minute), often pulsus paradoxus of over 10 mmHg, and a very low peak expiratory flow. The respiration is so shallow that wheezing may be absent. Such patients should be given **salbutamol** or **terbutaline** by subcutaneous or intravenous injection, or **aminophylline** by slow intravenous injection (section 3.1.3). They must also be given a large dose of a **corticosteroid**, see section 6.3.4, adults 200 mg of hydrocortisone (as sodium phosphate or succinate) intravenously or 40 mg of prednisolone orally, children half these doses (see also section 3.2).

Further treatment of these patients is safer in hospital where oxygen therapy and resuscitation facilities are immediately available. Treatment should **never** be delayed for investigations, patients should **never** be sedated, and the possibility of a pneumothorax should also be remembered.

3.1.1.1 SELECTIVE BETA$_2$-ADRENOCEPTOR STIMULANTS

SALBUTAMOL

Indications: reversible airways obstruction, status asthmaticus

Cautions: hyperthyroidism, ischaemic heart disease, hypertension, pregnancy, elderly patients (reduce dose); intravenous administration to diabetics (blood sugar estimates required). See also notes above

Side-effects: fine tremor (usually hands), nervous tension, headache, peripheral vasodilatation, tachycardia (seldom troublesome when given by aerosol inhalation); hypokalaemia after intravenous injection; slight pain on intramuscular injection

Dose: by mouth, 3–4 times daily, 4 mg (increased if necessary to 8 mg, elderly and sensitive patients 2 mg); CHILD 2–5 years 1–2 mg, 6–12 years 2 mg

By subcutaneous or intramuscular injection, 500 micrograms every 4 hours

By slow intravenous injection, 250 micrograms, repeated if necessary

By continuous intravenous infusion, initially 5 micrograms/minute, adjusted to 3–20 micrograms/minute or more if necessary

By aerosol inhalation, intermittent episodes, prophylaxis in exercise-induced bronchospasm, 100–200 micrograms (1–2 puffs) repeated after 4 hours if necessary; CHILD 100 micrograms (1 puff)
Chronic maintenance therapy, 200 micrograms (2 puffs) 3–4 times daily, or in severe bronchospasm every 4 hours; CHILD 100 micrograms (1 puff) 3–4 times daily

By inhalation of a powder (insufflation cartridges), intermittent episodes, prophylaxis in exercise-induced bronchospasm, 200–400 micrograms, repeated after 4 hours if necessary; CHILD 200 micrograms
Chronic maintenance therapy, 400 micrograms 3–4 times daily or in severe bronchospasm every 4 hours; CHILD 200 micrograms 3–4 times daily

By inhalation of nebulised solution (respirator solution), 2.5–5 mg, increased if necessary to 10 mg (usually as 0.1% or 0.2% solution) up to 4 times daily *or* by continuous inhalation, 1–2 mg/hour (as 0.005–0.01% solution). Dilution of nebulised solution is adjusted according to equipment and length of administration; CHILD, 2.5–5 mg (usually as 0.1% or 0.2% solution) up to 4 times daily

Oral preparations
PoM **Asmaven®** (APS)
Tablets, pink, salbutamol 2 mg (as sulphate). Price 20 tabs = **A**
Tablets, pink, salbutamol 4 mg (as sulphate). Price 20 tabs = **B**
PoM **Cobutolin®** (Cox Pharmaceuticals)
Tablets, pink, salbutamol 2 mg (as sulphate). Price 20 tabs = **A**

C = 51-100p, **D** = 101-180p, **E** = 181-300p, **F** = 301-450p, **G** = 451-650p, **H** = 651-900p, **I** = 901-1200p, **J** = over 1200p.

Tablets, pink, salbutamol 4 mg (as sulphate). Price 20 tabs = **B**

PoM **Salbulin**® (Riker)
Tablets, salbutamol 2 mg (as sulphate). Price 20 tabs = **A**
Tablets, salbutamol 4 mg (as sulphate). Price 20 tabs = **B**
Liquid (= elixir), orange, sugar-free, salbutamol 2 mg (as sulphate)/5 ml. Diluent purified water, freshly boiled and cooled, life of diluted elixir 28 days. Price 150 ml = **C**

PoM **Ventolin**® (A&H)
Tablets, pink, scored, salbutamol 2 mg (as sulphate). Price 20 tabs = **B**
Tablets, pink, scored, salbutamol 4 mg (as sulphate). Price 20 tabs = **B**
Spandets® (= tablets s/r), pink/white, salbutamol 8 mg (as sulphate). Price 20 tabs = **C**. Label: 25
Dose: 8 mg twice daily, increased if necessary to a max. of 32 mg daily; CHILD over 12 years 8 mg twice daily
Syrup (= elixir), sugar-free, salbutamol 2 mg (as sulphate)/5 ml. Diluent purified water, freshly boiled and cooled, life of diluted elixir 28 days. Price 100 ml = **B**

Parenteral preparations
PoM **Ventolin**® (A&H)
Injection, salbutamol 50 micrograms (as sulphate)/ml. Price 5-ml amp = **C**
Injection, salbutamol 500 micrograms (as sulphate)/ml. Price 1-ml amp = **B**
Solution for intravenous infusion, salbutamol 1 mg (as sulphate)/ml. Dilute before use. Price 5-ml amp = **F**

Inhalation preparations
PoM **Asmaven**® (APS)
Inhaler (= aerosol inhalation), salbutamol 100 micrograms/metered inhalation. Price 200-dose unit = **E**
Advise patients not to exceed prescribed dose and to follow manufacturer's directions

PoM **Cobutolin**® (Cox Pharmaceuticals)
Inhaler (= aerosol inhalation), salbutamol 100 micrograms/metered inhalation. Price 200-dose unit = **E**
Advise patients not to exceed prescribed dose and to follow manufacturer's directions

PoM **Salbulin**® (Riker)
Inhaler (= aerosol inhalation), salbutamol 100 micrograms/metered inhalation. Price 200-dose unit = **E**
Advise patients not to exceed prescribed dose and to follow manufacturer's directions

PoM **Ventolin**® (A&H)
Inhaler (= aerosol inhalation), salbutamol 100 micrograms/metered inhalation, 200-dose unit. Price (complete unit) = **E**
Advise patients not to exceed prescribed dose and to follow manufacturer's directions
Nebules® (= respirator solution in single-dose ampoules), salbutamol 0.1% (1 mg/ml, as sulphate). Price 2.5-ml amp = **A**. For use undiluted with nebuliser

Rotacaps® (= insufflation cartridges), light blue/clear, salbutamol 200 micrograms (as sulphate). Price 20 cartridges = **D**
Rotacaps® (= insufflation cartridges), dark blue/clear, salbutamol 400 micrograms (as sulphate). Price 20 cartridges = **D**
Rotahaler® (for use with Rotacaps). Price per unit = **C**
Respirator solution (for use with a nebuliser or ventilator), salbutamol 0.5% (5 mg/ml, as sulphate). Price 20 ml = **E**. Before use dilute 0.5–1 ml with sterile sodium chloride solution or sterile purified water to 2–2.5 ml or according to length of administration

TERBUTALINE SULPHATE

Indications; Cautions; Side-effects: see under Salbutamol
Dose: by mouth, 5 mg 2–3 times daily; CHILD 2–5 years 0.75–1.5 mg 3 times daily, 6–12 years 2.5 mg 2–3 times daily
By subcutaneous, intramuscular, or slow intravenous injection, 250–500 micrograms 2–4 times daily; CHILD 2–15 years 10 micrograms/kg to a max. of 300 micrograms
By continuous intravenous infusion as a solution containing 3–5 micrograms/ml, 1.5–5 micrograms/minute for 8–10 hours; reduce dose for children
By aerosol inhalation, intermittent episodes, prophylaxis in exercise-induced bronchospasm, adults and children 250–500 micrograms (1–2 puffs) repeated after 4 hours if necessary
Chronic maintenance therapy, 250–500 micrograms (1–2 puffs) 3–4 times daily, or in severe bronchospasm every 4 hours, max. 2 mg (8 puffs) daily; CHILD 250 micrograms (1 puff) 3–4 times daily
By inhalation of nebulised solution (respirator solution), 2–5 mg increasing if necessary to 10 mg 2–3 times daily *or* by continuous inhalation 1–2 mg/hour (as a solution containing 100 micrograms/ml). Dilution of nebulised solution is adjusted according to equipment and length of administration; CHILD, up to 200 micrograms/kg 2–3 times daily

PoM **Bricanyl**® (Astra)
Tablets, scored, terbutaline sulphate 5 mg. Price 20 tabs = **C**
Syrup (= elixir), terbutaline sulphate 1.5 mg/5 ml (sugar-free). Diluent water for preparations, life of diluted elixir 14 days. Price 100 ml = **C**
Injection, terbutaline sulphate 500 micrograms/ml. Price 1-ml amp = **B**
Inhaler (= aerosol inhalation), terbutaline sulphate 250 micrograms/metered inhalation, 400-dose unit. Price (complete unit) = **G**
Advise patients not to exceed prescribed dose and to follow manufacturer's directions
Refill canister (= aerosol inhalation), terbutaline sulphate 250 micrograms/metered inhalation, 400-dose unit. Price = **G**
For use with Nebuhaler or Spacer inhaler
Advise patients as above

Spacer inhaler (= aerosol inhalation), terbutaline sulphate 250 micrograms/metered inhalation with 'spacer' tube (collapsible extended mouthpiece), 400-dose unit. Price (complete unit) = **H**

Advise patients as above

Respirator solution (for use with nebuliser or ventilator), terbutaline sulphate 2.5 mg/ml. Price 2-ml single-dose amp = **A**

Respirator solution (for use with a nebuliser or ventilator), terbutaline sulphate 10 mg/ml. Price 10 ml = **D**. Before use dilute with sterile sodium chloride solution or sterile purified water

PoM **Bricanyl SA**® (Astra)

Tablets, s/r, terbutaline sulphate 7.5 mg. Price 20 tabs = **D**. Label: 25

Dose: 7.5 mg twice daily

Nebuhaler® (Astra)

Inhaler, fitted with plastic cone and one-way valve. For use with Bricanyl and Pulmicort refill canisters. Price = **F**

FENOTEROL HYDROBROMIDE

Indications; Cautions; Side-effects: see under Salbutamol

Dose: by aerosol inhalation, intermittent episodes and prophylaxis in exercise-induced bronchospasm, 180–360 micrograms (1–2 puffs) repeated after 6–8 hours if necessary; CHILD 180 micrograms (1 puff)

Chronic maintenance therapy, 180–360 micrograms (1–2 puffs) 3–4 times daily, or in severe bronchospasm every 4 hours; CHILD 6–12 years 180 micrograms (1 puff)

By inhalation of nebulised solution (respirator solution), 0.5–2.5 mg (increased in severe cases to a max. of 5 mg) up to 4 times daily, usually as a 0.025–0.125% solution; dilution adjusted to equipment and length of administration; CHILD 6–14 years, up to 1 mg up to 3 times daily

PoM **Berotec**® (WBP)

Inhaler (= aerosol inhalation), fenoterol hydrobromide 180 micrograms/metered inhalation, 200-dose unit. Price (complete unit) = **E**

Advise patients not to exceed prescribed dose and to follow manufacturer's directions

Nebuliser solution (= respirator solution), fenoterol hydrobromide 0.5% (5 mg/ml, 20 drops ≈1 ml). Price 20 ml (with dropper) = **D**. For use with nebuliser or ventilator

ISOETHARINE HYDROCHLORIDE

Indications: reversible airways obstruction

Cautions; Side-effects: see under Salbutamol

PoM **Numotac**® (Riker)

Tablets, s/r, isoetharine hydrochloride 10 mg. Price 20 tabs = **C**. Label: 25

Dose: 10–20 mg 3–4 times daily

PIRBUTEROL

Indications: reversible airways obstruction

Cautions; Side-effects: see under Salbutamol

Dose: by mouth, 10–15 mg 3–4 times daily; CHILD 6–12 years 7.5 mg up to 4 times daily

By aerosol inhalation, intermittent episodes, prophylaxis in exercise-induced bronchospasm, 200–400 micrograms (1–2 puffs) repeated after 4 hours if necessary; max. 2.4 mg (12 puffs) daily

Chronic maintenance therapy, 400 micrograms (2 puffs) 3–4 times daily or in severe bronchospasm every 4 hours; max. 2.4 mg (12 puffs) daily

▼ PoM **Exirel**® (Pfizer)

Capsules, turquoise/olive, pirbuterol 10 mg (as hydrochloride). Price 20 caps = **B**

Capsules, turquoise/beige, pirbuterol 15 mg (as hydrochloride). Price 20 caps = **C**

Syrup (= elixir), pirbuterol 7.5 mg (as hydrochloride)/5 ml. Price 150 ml = **D**

Aerosol inhalation, pirbuterol 200 micrograms (as acetate)/metered inhalation, 200-dose unit. Price (complete unit) = **F**

Advise patients not to exceed prescribed dose and to follow manufacturer's directions

REPROTEROL HYDROCHLORIDE

Indications: reversible airways obstruction

Cautions; Side-effects: see under Salbutamol

Dose: by mouth, 10–20 mg 3 times daily; CHILD 6–12 years 10 mg 3 times daily

By aerosol inhalation, intermittent episodes and prophylaxis in exercise-induced bronchospasm, 0.5–1 mg (1–2 puffs) repeated after 3–6 hours if necessary; CHILD 6–12 years 500 micrograms (1 puff)

Chronic maintenance therapy, 1 mg (2 puffs) 3 times daily or in severe bronchospasm every 3–6 hours; CHILD 6–12 years 500 micrograms (1 puff) 3 times daily

By inhalation of nebulised solution (respirator solution), 10–20 mg diluted to 3 ml with sterile sodium chloride solution, over 10 minutes, when required. Dilution may be adjusted to equipment and length of administration

▼ PoM **Bronchodil**® (Schering)

Tablets, scored, reproterol hydrochloride 20 mg. Price 20 tabs = **C**

Elixir, red, reproterol hydrochloride 10 mg/5 ml (sugar-free). Diluent purified water, freshly boiled and cooled, life of diluted elixir 14 days. Price 100 ml = **C**

Aerosol inhalation, reproterol hydrochloride 500 micrograms/metered inhalation, 400-dose unit. Price (complete unit) = **H**

Advise patients not to exceed prescribed dose and to follow manufacturer's directions

Respirator solution, reproterol hydrochloride 10 mg/ml. Price 50 ml = **G**

RIMITEROL HYDROBROMIDE

Indications: reversible airways obstruction; status asthmaticus (short acting)

Cautions; Side-effects: see under Salbutamol

Dose: by aerosol inhalation, intermittent epi-

C = 51-100p, **D** = 101-180p, **E** = 181-300p, **F** = 301-450p, **G** = 451-650p, **H** = 651-900p, **I** = 901-1200p, **J** = over 1200p.

sodes and prophylaxis in exercise-induced bronchospasm, adults and children 200–600 micrograms (1–3 puffs) repeated after 30 minutes if
necessary; max. 8 doses daily

PoM **Pulmadil®** (Riker)
Inhaler (= aerosol inhalation), rimiterol hydrobromide 200 micrograms/metered inhalation,
300-dose unit. Price (complete unit) = **H**
Advise patients not to exceed prescribed dose
and to follow manufacturer's directions

PoM **Pulmadil Auto®** (Riker)
Inhaler (= aerosol inhalation), rimiterol hydrobromide 200 micrograms/metered inhalation,
300-dose cartridge in breath-actuated unit.
Price (complete unit) = **H**; replacement cartridge = **H**
Advise patients as above

3.1.1.2   OTHER ADRENOCEPTOR STIMULANTS

These preparations (including the partially selective orciprenaline) are now regarded as less suitable and less safe for use as bronchodilators than
the selective beta₂-adrenoceptor stimulants, as
they are more likely to cause arrhythmias and
other side-effects. For use as nasal decongestants
see section 3.10.

Adrenaline injection (1 in 1000) is used in the
emergency treatment of acute allergic and anaphylactic reactions (section 3.4.3).

ADRENALINE

Indications: reversible airways obstruction,
emergency treatment of acute anaphylaxis
Cautions: hyperthyroidism, diabetes, ischaemic
heart disease, hypertension, elderly patients.
Tolerance to bronchodilator effect may
develop. Avoid intravenous use with tricyclic
antidepressants, digoxin, or quinidine because
of increased risk of arrhythmias. Drug interactions: see Appendix 1 (sections *2.4*, 2.7, *15*)
Side-effects: anxiety, tremor, tachycardia,
arrhythmias, dry mouth, cold extremities (seldom troublesome when given by aerosol inhalation, but tolerance and increased viscosity of
bronchial secretions occur)
Dose: acute airways obstruction, as a single dose,
by subcutaneous or intramuscular injection,
200–500 micrograms, repeated at intervals of
15–30 minutes; CHILD 10 micrograms/kg; max.
500 micrograms as a single dose
By aerosol inhalation, adrenaline acid tartrate
280–840 micrograms (1–3 puffs) repeated if necessary after not less than 30 minutes, up to 8
times daily
Acute anaphylaxis, *by intramuscular injection*,
0.5–1 mg repeated as necessary; CHILD, 10
micrograms/kg by small repeated doses of 100
micrograms to a max. of 500 micrograms usually
given as a single dose over 5 minutes

PoM **Adrenaline Injection**, adrenaline 1 in 1000

(adrenaline 1 mg/ml as acid tartrate). Price 0.5-
and 1-ml amp (both) = **A**
PoM **Medihaler-epi®** (Riker)
Aerosol inhalation, adrenaline acid tartrate 280
micrograms/metered inhalation, 400-dose unit. Price
(complete unit) = **E**. Advise patients not to exceed prescribed dose and to follow manufacturer's directions
PoM **Min-i-Jet Adrenaline®** (IMS)
Injection, adrenaline 1 in 1000 (1 mg/ml as hydrochloride). Price 0.5- and 1-ml disposable syringe
(both) = **D**

EPHEDRINE HYDROCHLORIDE

Indications: reversible airways obstruction
Cautions; Side-effects: see under Adrenaline, but
incidence of tachycardia is lower and anxiety,
restlessness, and insomnia are common. May
cause acute retention in prostatic hypertrophy.
Drug interactions: see Appendix 1 (section *4.3*)
Dose: 3 times daily, 15–60 mg; CHILD 3 times
daily, up to 1 year 7.5 mg, 1–5 years 15 mg, 6–
12 years 30 mg

PoM **Ephedrine Hydrochloride Tablets**, ephedrine
hydrochloride 15, 30, and 60 mg. Price 20 tabs (all) = **A**
PoM **Ephedrine Elixir**, yellow, ephedrine hydrochloride
15 mg/5 ml. Price 100 ml = **B**

ISOPRENALINE SULPHATE

Indications: reversible airways obstruction
Cautions; Side-effects: see under Salbutamol
(section 3.1.1.1) and notes above. Drug interactions: see Appendix 1 (section *15*)
Dose: sublingually, 10–20 mg 1–3 times daily;
CHILD 5–10 mg 1–3 times daily
By aerosol inhalation, adults and children 80–
240 micrograms (1–3 puffs of iso-autohaler or
medihaler-iso), or up to 1.2 mg (3 puffs of
medihaler-iso forte); the dose should not be
repeated within 30 minutes and not more than
8 times in 24 hours
By inhalation of a nebulised solution containing
1%, 1 ml when necessary

PoM **Aleudrin®** (Lewis)
Tablets (sublingual), scored, isoprenaline sulphate
20 mg. Price 20 tabs = **B**. Label: 26
Spray solution, isoprenaline sulphate 1% (for use with
nebuliser). Price 10 ml = **B**
PoM **Iso-Autohaler®** (Riker)
Aerosol inhalation, isoprenaline sulphate
80 micrograms/metered inhalation, 400-dose vial in
breath-actuated unit. Price (complete unit) = **F**; 400-
dose refill vial = **E**. Advise patients not to exceed prescribed dose and to follow manufacturer's directions
PoM **Medihaler-Iso®** (Riker)
Aerosol inhalation, isoprenaline sulphate 80 micrograms/
metered inhalation, 400-dose vial. Price (complete
unit) = **E**. Advise patients as above
PoM **Medihaler-Iso Forte®** (Riker)
Aerosol inhalation, isoprenaline sulphate 400
micrograms/metered inhalation, 400-dose vial. Price
(complete unit) = **F**. Advise patients as above

METHOXYPHENAMINE HYDROCHLORIDE

Indications: reversible airways obstruction; see
also section 3.10

Cautions; Side-effects: see under Salbutamol (section 3.1.1.1) and notes above
Dose: 50–100 mg every 3–4 hours; CHILD 25–50 mg every 4–6 hours

Orthoxine Hydrochloride® (Upjohn)
Tablets, scored, methoxyphenamine hydrochloride 100 mg. Price 20 tabs = C. Label: 2

ORCIPRENALINE SULPHATE

Indications: reversible airways obstruction
Cautions; Side-effects: see under Salbutamol (section 3.1.1.1) and notes above
Dose: by mouth, 20 mg 4 times daily; CHILD up to 1 year 5–10 mg 3 times daily, 1–5 years 5–10 mg 4 times daily, 6–12 years 40–60 mg daily in divided doses
By deep intramuscular injection, 500 micrograms, repeated if necessary after 30 minutes; CHILD up to 5 years 250 micrograms, over 5 years 500 micrograms
By aerosol inhalation, 670–1340 micrograms (1–2 puffs) repeated if necessary after not less than 30 minutes to a max. of 8.04 mg (12 puffs) daily; CHILD up to 6 years 670 micrograms (1 puff) up to 4 times daily, 6–12 years 670–1340 micrograms (1–2 puffs) up to 4 times daily

PoM **Alupent®** (Boehringer Ingelheim)
Tablets, scored, orciprenaline sulphate 20 mg. Price 20 tabs = C
Syrup (= elixir), orciprenaline sulphate 10 mg/5 ml (sugar-free). Diluents syrup or sorbitol solution, life of diluted elixir 14 days. Price 100 ml = C
Injection, orciprenaline sulphate 500 micrograms/ml. Price 1-ml amp = A
Metered aerosol (= aerosol inhalation), orciprenaline sulphate 670 micrograms/metered inhalation, 300-dose vial with mouthpiece. Price complete unit (15 ml) = F; 300-dose refill vial (15 ml) = E. Advise patients not to exceed prescribed dose and to follow manufacturer's directions

3.1.2 Anticholinergic bronchodilators

These drugs have traditionally been regarded as more effective in relieving bronchoconstriction associated with chronic bronchitis. Of this group, **ipratropium** (Atrovent®) may provide some bronchodilation in patients with chronic bronchitis who fail to respond to the selective beta$_2$-adrenoceptor stimulants (section 3.1.1.1). Unlike the other anticholinergic drugs, side-effects are rare and it does not increase sputum viscosity or affect mucociliary clearance of sputum. The aerosol inhalation has a slower onset, with a maximum action 30–60 minutes after administration. Its duration of action is variable but may last several hours; it is therefore more useful in preventing than controlling attacks.

The other atropine-like bronchodilators are now rarely used and often have unpleasant side-effects which limit their usefulness. They should be avoided, particularly in children, because although they reduce bronchial secretions, sputum viscosity may be increased and this can lead to blockage of the smaller airways.

IPRATROPIUM BROMIDE

Indications: reversible airways obstruction, particularly in chronic bronchitis
Cautions: glaucoma; prostatic hypertrophy
Side-effects: dry mouth; rarely urinary retention, constipation
Dose: by aerosol inhalation, 18–36 micrograms (1–2 puffs) increased if necessary to 72 micrograms (4 puffs) 3–4 times daily; CHILD up to 5 years 18 micrograms (1 puff), 6–12 years 18–36 micrograms (1–2 puffs) 3 times daily
By inhalation of nebulised solution, 100–500 micrograms up to 4 times daily; single dose, max. 2 mg; CHILD 3–14 years 100–500 micrograms up to 3 times daily; single dose, max. 1 mg. Dilution of solution is adjusted according to equipment and length of administration

PoM **Atrovent®** (Boehringer Ingelheim)
Aerosol inhalation, ipratropium bromide 18 micrograms/metered inhalation, 200-dose unit. Price (complete unit) = F
Advise patient not to exceed prescribed dose and to follow manufacturer's directions
Nebuliser solution, isotonic, ipratropium bromide 250 micrograms/ml (0.025%); 20 drops ≡ 1 ml. Price 20 ml (with dropper) = D. If necessary dilute with sterile sodium chloride solution
Because paradoxical bronchospasm may occur, treatment should always be initiated in hospital under close supervision during the first week

OTHER ANTICHOLINERGIC BRONCHODILATORS

PoM **Eumydrin®** (Winthrop)
Oral solution, atropine methonitrate 0.6% (approx. 200 micrograms/drop) in 90% alcohol. Price 15-ml dropper bottle = E. Counselling advised, use of dropper, storage
Note: store in a cool place, tightly closed to prevent concentration by evaporation
Dose: 5–15 drops; CHILD, every 4 hours, up to 6 months 2–4 drops, 6 months–2 years 3–6 drops, 3–5 years 4–8 drops, over 6 years 6–12 drops

3.1.3 Xanthine bronchodilators

With the introduction of the beta$_2$-adrenoceptor stimulants (section 3.1.1.1), the use of *rapid-release* oral aminophylline and theophylline preparations has declined because of the high incidence of side-effects. However, there has been a revival of interest in these drugs since the introduction of *sustained-release* preparations which have the advantage of producing adequate plasma concentrations for up to 12 hours; they are all equally effective.

Aminophilline and **theophylline** sustained release preparations are used in less severe and more chronic asthma as an alternative to prophylactic drugs such as sodium cromoglycate (section 3.3); and are administered every 12 hours. They are often effective when given as a single dose at night for controlling nocturnal asthma and early

---

C = 51-100p, D = 101-180p, E = 181-300p, F = 301-450p, G = 451-650p, H = 651-900p, I = 901-1200p, J = over 1200p.

morning wheezing, and have replaced amino-phylline suppositories (which may show an unpredictable response and cause proctitis) for this purpose. Recent studies have suggested that the xanthine derivatives have an additive effect when used in conjunction with the beta$_2$-adrenoceptor stimulants though such combinations may increase the risk of arrhythmias if the beta$_2$-adrenoceptor stimulant is given in high doses. The side-effects commonly associated with the xanthine derivatives are reduced with the sustained-release preparations but include gastric irritation, headache, and caffeine-like stimulation, and usually occur with plasma-theophylline concentrations above 20 micrograms/ml. Treatment should be initiated with small doses which are then gradually increased, because patient response to the xanthine preparations may be unpredictable, as patients show widely differing rates of metabolism and absorption.

Various modifications such as choline theophyllinate are available which are claimed to be better tolerated. Acepifylline and diprophylline are theophylline derivatives which are better tolerated but their efficacy is doubtful and their use is not widespread.

The use of aminophylline *injection*, given intravenously, is of established value in the treatment of severe attacks of asthma and is still preferred by many prescribers to intravenous treatment with the selective beta$_2$-adrenoceptor stimulants (section 3.1.1.1). Plasma concentrations should be monitored, particularly if patients have previously been taking oral xanthine preparations, as serious side-effects such as convulsions and arrhythmias can occasionally occur before the appearance of other symptoms of toxicity.

Aminophylline injection is also effective in the treatment of left ventricular failure though diuretics (see sections 2.2.1 and 2.2.2) and the narcotic analgesics (see section 4.7.2) are used more frequently for this purpose. However, aminophylline is useful in those patients who are also suffering from asthma and bronchitis because it may have a dual action in relieving airways obstruction as well as increasing myocardial contractility. Morphine is contra-indicated in such patients because of its respiratory depressant effects.

AMINOPHYLLINE

Indications: reversible airways obstruction, status asthmaticus, left ventricular failure
Cautions: see notes above; also liver disease (reduce dose), epilepsy, breast-feeding, cardiac disease, elderly patients, fever
Side-effects: (minimised by sustained-release preparations) tachycardia, palpitations, nausea, gastro-intestinal disturbances, insomnia, arrhythmias, and convulsions especially if given rapidly by intravenous injection; use of suppositories for more than a few days may cause proctitis; intramuscular injection is painful (this route is therefore not used)
Dose: by mouth, 100–300 mg, 3–4 times daily, after food

By slow intravenous injection over a period of at least 10–15 minutes, 250–500 mg (5 mg/kg) when necessary; maintenance if required, in patients not previously treated with xanthines, 500 micrograms/kg/hour *by slow intravenous infusion*
CHILD, *by slow intravenous injection*, 5 mg/kg; maintenance, if required, in patients not previously treated with xanthines, 6 months–9 years 1.2 mg/kg/hour, reduced to 1 mg/kg/hour, 10–16 years 1 mg/kg/hour, reduced to 800 micrograms/kg/hour *by slow intravenous infusion*
By rectum in suppositories, 360 mg once or twice daily; CHILD, once or twice daily, up to 1 year 12.5–25 mg, 1–5 years 50–100 mg, 6–12 years 100–200 mg

Aminophylline Tablets, aminophylline 100 mg. Price 20 tabs = **B**. Label: 21
PoM **Aminophylline Injection,** aminophylline 25 mg/ml, price 10-ml amp = **B**; 250 mg/ml, price 2-ml amp = **B**
Aminophylline Suppositories, aminophylline 50, 100, 150, 180, and 360 mg. Price 12 suppos (all) = **D**

Theodrox® (Riker)
Tablets, aminophylline 195 mg, dried aluminium hydroxide gel 260 mg. Price 20 tabs = **B**. Label: 21
Dose: 1 tablet 3 times daily and at night, after food

Sustained-release preparations
Phyllocontin Continus® (Napp)
Tablets, s/r, yellow, f/c, aminophylline 225 mg. Price 20 tabs = **D**. Label: 25
Forte tablets, s/r, yellow, scored, f/c, aminophylline 350 mg. Price 20 tabs = **E**. Label: 25
Dose: every 12 hours, 225–350 mg, increased after 1 week to 450–700 mg if required; nocturnal attacks, 225–700 mg at night
Tablets, paediatric, s/r, pale orange, aminophylline 100 mg. Price 20 tabs = **C**. Label: 25
Dose: 6 mg/kg every 12 hours, increased after 1 week to 12 mg/kg

---

CHOLINE THEOPHYLLINATE

Indications: reversible airways obstruction
Cautions; Side-effects: see under Aminophylline
Dose: by mouth, 100–400 mg 2–4 times daily preferably after food; CHILD, 3 times daily, 3–5 years 62.5–125 mg, 6–12 years 100 mg

Choledyl® (Warner)
Tablets, pink, compression coated, choline theophyllinate 100 mg. Price 20 tabs = **B**
Tablets, yellow, compression coated, choline theophyllinate 200 mg. Price 20 tabs = **C**
Syrup (= elixir), yellow, choline theophyllinate 62.5 mg/5 ml. Diluent syrup (without preservative), life of diluted elixir 14 days. Price 100 ml = **D**
Sabidal Retention Enema® (Zyma)
Retention enema, choline theophyllinate 78.5 mg

Relative prices: **A** = up to 20p, **B** = 21-50p,

(= theophylline 50 mg) in 3-ml disposable flexible tube. Price 5 × 3-ml tube = **F**

Retention enema, choline theophyllinate 157 mg (= theophylline 100 mg) in 3-ml disposable flexible tube. Price 5 × 3-ml tube = **F**

Dose: as theophylline, adults and children over 9 years 9–16 mg/kg daily in 3–4 divided doses; CHILD up to 2 years 16–24 mg/kg daily, 2–9 years 13–17 mg/kg daily; acute attacks, up to 2 years 4–6 mg/kg, over 2 years 3–4 mg/kg, as a single dose

Sustained-release preparations

Sabidal SR 90® (Zyma)

Tablets, s/r yellow, choline theophyllinate 142 mg (= 90 mg theophylline). Price 20 tabs = **C**. Label: 25

Dose: CHILD 2–5 years 1 tablet in the morning and 1 at night, 6–9 years 1 tablet in the morning and 2 at night, 10–15 years 2 tablets in the morning and 2 at night, then adjusted

Sabidal SR 270® (Zyma)

Tablets, s/r, light yellow, choline theophyllinate 424 mg (= 270 mg theophylline). Price 20 tabs = **D**. Label: 25

Dose: 1 tablet in the morning and 2 at night; sensitive patients 1 tablet twice daily for 3 days, then adjusted

THEOPHYLLINE

Indication: reversible airways obstruction

Cautions; Side-effects: see under Aminophylline. Drug interactions: see Appendix 1 (sections 3, 4.2)

Dose: 60–250 mg 3–4 times daily after food; CHILD, 3–4 times daily, up to 2 years 4–5 mg/kg, 2–6 years 60–90 mg, 7–12 years 62.5–125 mg

Labophylline® (LAB)

Tablets, yellow, theophylline 100 mg, lysine 81 mg. Price 20 tabs = **B**. Label: 21

Dose: 1–2 tablets 3–4 times daily; CHILD over 6 years ½–1 tablet 3 times daily

Nuelin® (Riker)

Tablets, scored, theophylline 125 mg. Price 20 tabs = **C**. Label: 21

Liquid (= elixir), brown, theophylline 60 mg (as sodium glycinate)/5 ml. Diluent syrup, life of diluted elixir 14 days. Price 100 ml = **D**. Label: 21

Sustained-release preparations

Lasma® (Pharmax)

Tablets, s/r, scored, theophylline 300 mg. Price 20 tabs = **E**. Label: 25, 27

Dose: 300 mg every 12 hours *or* 600 mg every 24 hours (increased to 900 mg after 1 week in patients over 70 kg); adjust dose by 150-mg increments as required

Nuelin SA® (Riker)

Tablets, s/r, theophylline 175 mg. Price 20 tabs = **D**. Label: 25, 27

Dose: 175–350 mg every 12 hours; nocturnal attacks 175–350 mg at night; CHILD over 6 years 175 mg every 12 hours or at night

Nuelin SA 250® (Riker)

Tablets, s/r, scored, theophylline 250 mg. Price 20 tabs = **D**. Label: 25, 27

Dose: 250–500 mg every 12 hours; nocturnal attacks 250–500 mg at night; CHILD over 6 years 125–250 mg every 12 hours or at night

Pro-Vent® (Wellcome)

Capsules, s/r, white/clear, theophylline 300 mg. Price 20 caps = **D**. Label: 25, 27

Dose: 300 mg every 12 hours, adjusted according to response; max. 900 mg daily in divided doses; nocturnal attacks 300 mg at night

Slo-Phyllin® (Lipha)

Capsules, s/r, white/clear, enclosing white pellets, theophylline 60 mg. Price 20 caps = **C**. Label: 25, 27

Capsules, s/r, brown/clear, enclosing brown and white pellets, theophylline 125 mg. Price 20 caps = **D**. Label: 25, 27

Capsules, s/r, blue/clear, enclosing blue and white pellets, theophylline 250 mg. Price 20 caps = **D**. Label: 25, 27

Dose: 250–500 mg every 12 hours; CHILD, every 12 hours, 2–6 years 60–120 mg, 7–12 years 125–250 mg. Max. in adults and children over 9 years 13 mg/kg daily, children up to 9 years 24 mg/kg daily

Theo-Dur® (Fisons)

Tablets, s/r, scored, theophylline 200 mg. Price 20 tabs = **D**. Label: 25, 27

Tablets, s/r, scored, theophylline 300 mg. Price 20 tabs = **D**. Label: 25, 27

Dose: 200–300 mg every 12 hours, increased if necessary by 100–150 mg increments; nocturnal attacks 200–300 mg at night; CHILD up to 35 kg 100 mg, over 35 kg 200 mg, every 12 hours, increased or decreased as necessary by 100 mg

Theograd® (Abbott)

Tablets, s/r, f/c, theophylline 350 mg. Price 20 tabs = **B**. Label: 25, 27

Dose: 350 mg every 12 hours; initial dose in severe cases 700 mg; nocturnal attacks 350 mg at night

Uniphyllin Continus® (Napp)

Tablets, s/r, scored, theophylline 400 mg. Price 20 tabs = **E**. Label: 25, 27

Dose: initially 400 mg daily, increased after 1 week to 600–800 mg daily

Paediatric tablets, s/r, scored, theophylline 200 mg. Price 20 tabs = **D**. Label: 25, 27

Dose: 9 mg/kg every 24 hours, increased after 1 week to 18 mg/kg every 24 hours

ACEPIFYLLINE

Indications: reversible airways obstruction

Cautions; Side-effects: see under Aminophylline and notes above

Dose: 0.5–1 g 3 times daily preferably after food; CHILD, 3–4 times daily, up to 1 year 62.5 mg, 1–5 years 125 mg, 6–12 years 250 mg

Etophylate® (Delandale)

Tablets, acepifylline 250 mg. Price 20 tabs = **B**

Tablets forte, scored, acepifylline 500 mg. Price 20 tabs = **C**

C = 51-100p, **D** = 101-180p, **E** = 181-300p, **F** = 301-450p, **G** = 451-650p, **H** = 651-900p, **I** = 901-1200p, **J** = over 1200p.

Syrup (= elixir), yellow, acepifylline 125 mg/5 ml. Diluent syrup (without preservative), life of diluted elixir 14 days. Price 100 ml = **C**
Syrup forte (= strong elixir), orange, acepifylline 500 mg/5 ml. Diluent as above. Price 100 ml = **D**

DIPROPHYLLINE

Indications; Cautions; Side-effects: see under Aminophylline and notes above; intramuscular injection is less painful
Dose: by mouth, acute conditions, 400 mg every 6 hours, preferably after food, reducing to a maintenance dose of 200–400 mg 3 times daily; CHILD, every 6 hours, up to 1 year 10–30 mg, 1–2 years 40 mg, 3–5 years 60 mg, 6–12 years 100 mg
By intramuscular or slow intravenous injection, 500 mg 2–3 times daily; CHILD, up to 1 year 5 mg/kg, 1–5 years 50–100 mg, 6–12 years 100–200 mg
By rectum in suppositories, 400 mg at bedtime or twice daily

Silbephylline® (Berk)
Tablets, scored, diprophylline 200 mg. Price 20 tabs = **B**
Syrup (= elixir), red, diprophylline 100 mg/5 ml. Diluent syrup, life of diluted elixir 14 days. Price 100 ml = **D**
PoM *Injection,* diprophylline 250 mg/ml. Price 2-ml amp = **B**
Suppositories, diprophylline 400 mg. Price 10 suppos = **E**

PROXYPHYLLINE

Indications: reversible airways obstruction
Cautions; Side-effects: see under Aminophylline and notes above
Dose: 300 mg 3 times daily and 600 mg at night

Thean® (Lagap)
Tablets, scored, proxyphylline 300 mg. Price 20 tabs = **C**

3.1.4 Compound bronchodilator preparations

Compound bronchodilator preparations have no place in the management of patients with airways obstruction. Patients are best treated with a single ingredient preparation such as a selective beta$_2$-adrenoceptor stimulant (section 3.1.1.1). Some compound preparations also include sedatives which are intended to allay the anxiety associated with severe bronchospasm but such preparations, particularly those containing barbiturates, should be **avoided** as they depress respiration.

Solutions of adrenaline deteriorate rapidly on exposure to air.

Adrenaline and Atropine Spray, Compound, adrenaline acid tartrate 0.8%, atropine methonitrate 0.1%, papaverine hydrochloride 0.8%. Price 100 ml = **F**. For use in hand spray
NHS PoM **Alupent Expectorant®** (Boehringer Ingelheim)
Tablets, scored, bromhexine hydrochloride 8 mg, orciprenaline sulphate 20 mg. Price 20 tabs = **D**
Dose: 1 tablet = 10 ml mixture
Mixture, bromhexine hydrochloride 4 mg, orciprenaline sulphate 10 mg/5 ml. Diluents sorbitol solution or syrup, life of diluted mixture 14 days. Price 100 ml = **D**

Dose: 10 ml 4 times daily; CHILD up to 5 years 5 ml twice daily, 6–10 years 5 ml 3–4 times daily
PoM **Amesec®** (Lilly)
Capsules, blue/orange, aminophylline 130 mg, ephedrine hydrochloride 25 mg. Price 20 caps = **B**. Label: 21
Dose: 1 capsule 1–3 times daily
PoM **Asmapax®** (Nicholas)
Tablets, buff, scored, ephedrine hydrochloride 50 mg (as resinate), theophylline 65 mg. Price 20 tabs = **C**. Label: 21
Dose: 1–2 tablets 2–3 times daily; CHILD 5–12 years ½ tablet
Asma-Vydrin® (Lewis)
Spray, adrenaline 0.55%, atropine methonitrate 0.14%, papaverine hydrochloride 0.88%, chlorbutol 0.5%. Price 30 ml = **D**; 120 ml = **G**. For use in hand nebuliser
NHS PoM **Bricanyl Compound®** (Astra)
Tablets, guaiphenesin 100 mg, terbutaline sulphate 2.5 mg. Price 20 tabs = **D**
Dose: 2 tablets 3 times daily
NHS PoM **Bricanyl Expectorant®** (Astra)
Elixir, guaiphenesin 66.5 mg, terbutaline sulphate 1.5 mg/5 ml. Diluent water for preparations, life of diluted elixir 14 days. Price 100 ml = **C**
Dose: 10–15 ml 3 times daily
PoM **Bronchilator®** (Sterling Research)
Aerosol inhalation, isoetharine mesylate 350 micrograms, phenylephrine hydrochloride 70 micrograms/metered dose. Price 250-dose unit = **H**
Dose: 1–2 puffs repeated after 30 minutes if necessary; max. 16 puffs daily
Brovon® (Napp)
Inhalant spray, adrenaline 0.5%, atropine methonitrate 0.14%, papaverine hydrochloride 0.88%. Price 20-ml bottle = **C**; 50-ml bottle = **E**; midget inhaler = **E**; reservoir and closure = **D**; rubber bulb = **C**
Dose: 1–2 puffs twice daily and at night
PoM **Brovon Pressurised®** (Napp)
Aerosol inhalation, adrenaline 250 micrograms, atropine methonitrate 500 micrograms/metered inhalation, 330-dose unit. Price 17 ml (complete unit) = **E**
Dose: 1 puff, repeated after 30 minutes if necessary every 4–6 hours
CAM® (Rybar)
Syrup (= elixir), green, butethamate citrate 4 mg, ephedrine hydrochloride 4 mg/5 ml. Diluent syrup or water for preparations, life of diluted elixir 14 days. Price 150 ml = **C**
Dose: 20 ml 3–4 times daily; CHILD up to 2 years 2.5 ml, 3–4 years 5 ml, over 4 years 10 ml, 3 times daily
PoM **Duo-Autohaler®** (Riker)
Aerosol inhalation, isoprenaline hydrochloride 160 micrograms, phenylephrine bitartrate 240 micrograms/metered inhalation, breath-actuated 400-dose unit. Price (complete unit) = **G**; refill = **F**
Dose: adults and children, 1–3 puffs repeated after 30 minutes if necessary; max. 24 puffs daily
PoM **Duovent®** (WBP)
Aerosol inhalation, fenoterol hydrobromide 90 micrograms, ipratropium bromide 36 micrograms/metered inhalation, 200-dose unit with mouthpiece. Price (complete unit) = **G**
Dose: 1–2 puffs 3–4 times daily; CHILD over 6 years 1 puff 3 times daily
PoM **Iso-Brovon Pressurised (PIB)®** (Napp)
Aerosol inhalation, atropine methonitrate 50 micrograms, isoprenaline hydrochloride 180 micrograms/metered inhalation, 330-dose unit. Price 17 ml (complete unit) = **E**
Dose: 1–2 puffs, repeated after 30 minutes if necessary every 4–6 hours
PoM **Iso-Brovon Plus Pressurised (PIB Plus)®** (Napp)
Aerosol inhalation, atropine methonitrate 50 micrograms, isoprenaline hydrochloride 500 micrograms/metered inhalation. Price 17 ml (complete unit) = **E**

For all abbreviations and symbols see inside cover.   Relative prices: **A** = up to 20p, **B** = 21-50p,

Dose: 1–2 puffs, repeated after 30 minutes if necessary every 4–6 hours

PoM **Medihaler-duo**® (Riker)
Aerosol inhalation, isoprenaline hydrochloride 160 micrograms, phenylephrine bitartrate 240 micrograms/metered inhalation, 400-dose unit. Price (complete unit) = **F**
Dose: adults and children 1–3 puffs, repeated after 30 minutes if necessary; max. 24 puffs daily

PoM **Nethaprin Dospan**® (Merrell)
Tablets, s/r, scored, bufylline 180 mg, doxylamine succinate 25 mg, etafedrine hydrochloride 50 mg, phenylephrine hydrochloride 25 mg. Price 20 tabs = **D**. Label: 2, 25
Dose: 1 tablet twice daily; CHILD 6–12 years ½ tablet

Rybarvin Inhalant® (Rybar)
Spray solution, adrenaline 0.4%, atropine methonitrate 0.1%, benzocaine 0.08%, in saline vehicle. Price 30 ml = **D**. For use with Rybar no. 1 and no. 2 inhalers, price (both) = **H**

PoM **Taumasthman**® (Wallace Mfg)
Tablets, atropine sulphate 300 micrograms, caffeine 50 mg, ephedrine hydrochloride 10 mg, phenazone 100 mg, theophylline 100 mg. Price 20 tabs = **B**. Label: 21
Dose: 1–2 tablets 3 times daily or when required

PoM **Tedral**® (Warner)
Tablets, ephedrine hydrochloride 24 mg, theophylline 120 mg. Price 20 tabs = **B**. Label: 21
Dose: 1 tablet every 4 hours after food; CHILD 6–12 years ½ tablet
Elixir, yellow, ephedrine hydrochloride 6 mg, theophylline 30 mg/5 ml. Diluent syrup, life of diluted elixir 28 days. Price 200 ml = **C**. Label: 21
Dose: 20 ml every 4 hours, after food; CHILD 2–5 years 5 ml, 6–10 years 10 ml

PoM **Tedral SA**® (Warner)
Tablets, s/r, pink, ephedrine hydrochloride 48 mg, theophylline 180 mg. Price 20 tabs = **B**. Label: 21, 25, 27
Dose: 1 tablet twice daily after food; CHILD 6–12 years ½ tablet

BRONCHODILATORS WITH SEDATIVES

PoM **Expansyl**® (SK&F)
Spansule® (= capsules s/r), black/clear, enclosing blue, green, and white pellets, diphenylpyraline hydrochloride 5 mg, ephedrine sulphate 50 mg, trifluoperazine 2 mg (as hydrochloride). Price 20 caps = **D**. Label: 2, 25
Dose: 1 capsule twice daily; max. 3 capsules daily

CD **Franol**® (Winthrop)
Tablets, ephedrine hydrochloride 11 mg, phenobarbitone 8 mg, theophylline 120 mg. Price 20 tabs = **C**. Label: 21
Dose: 1 tablet 3–4 times daily after food

CD **Franol Plus**® (Winthrop)
Tablets, ephedrine sulphate 15 mg, phenobarbitone 8 mg, theophylline 120 mg, thenyldiamine hydrochloride 10 mg. Price 20 tabs = **F**. Label: 21
Dose: 1 tablet 3–4 times daily after food

NHS CD **Franol Expect**® (Winthrop)
Elixir, red, ephedrine 4.75 mg, guaiphenesin 25 mg, phenobarbitone 4 mg, theophylline 60 mg/5 ml. Diluent syrup, life of elixir diluted up to 50% 14 days. Price 100 ml = **D**. Label: 21
Dose: 10 ml 3–4 times daily after food

CD **Phyldrox**® (Carlton)
Tablets, ephedrine hydrochloride 12 mg, phenobarbitone 8 mg, theophylline 128 mg. Price 20 tabs = **A**. Label: 21
Dose: 1 tablet 3 times daily after food

Tablets, e/c, ingredients as above. Price 20 tabs = **A**. Label: 5, 25
Dose: 1 tablet at night

3.2 Corticosteroids

Corticosteroids have been used in the treatment of asthma for many years. In recent years, with the introduction of the corticosteroid aerosol inhalations, their use has increased and has been extended to the treatment of less severe and more chronic asthma, as the side-effects associated with systemic administration (see section 6.3.3) are much reduced. Corticosteroids are usually of no benefit in patients with chronic bronchitis and emphysema, although they may occasionally be tried in selected patients where asthma masquerades as chronic bronchitis, and in those who have shown a good response to the beta$_2$-adrenoceptor stimulants.

The action of corticosteroids is not fully understood but it is probable that they provide relief by reducing bronchial mucosal inflammatory reactions such as oedema and hypersecretion of mucus; they also modify allergic reactions. Corticosteroid *aerosol inhalations* must be used regularly to obtain maximum benefit, and alleviation of symptoms usually occurs 3 to 7 days after initiation of therapy. **Beclomethasone** (Becloforte®, Becotide®) is most commonly used. **Budesonide** (Pulmicort®), which has recently been introduced, is very similar to beclomethasone. *Insufflation cartridges* (Becotide Rotacaps®) may be tried in patients who are unable to use the pressurised aerosol inhalers (see section 3.1.1 for further description of insufflation cartridges). Beclomethasone suspension for nebulisation is useful for those patients who cannot manage the dry powder inhaler and pressurised aerosols. It is conveniently used when individuals already possess and use a home nebuliser for bronchodilator therapy. See also section 3.1.1. Maximum penetration of the corticosteroid to the bronchi is facilitated if a beta$_2$-adrenoceptor stimulant drug such as salbutamol is inhaled about 10 minutes before the corticosteroid inhalation and this is usual practice even in patients with only a mild degree of bronchospasm. Patients who have been taking long-term oral corticosteroids can often be successfully transferred to aerosol inhalers but the transfer must be done slowly, with gradual reduction in dose of oral corticosteroid, and at a time when the asthma is well controlled.

Patients with severe bronchospasm should be treated with short courses of oral corticosteroids given in high dosage, for example **prednisolone** 40 mg daily for a few days, gradually titrated down over a week as the attack subsides.

For use of corticosteroids in emergency treatment of severe acute asthma see section 3.1.1.

In chronic continuing asthma, when all other anti-asthma drugs have failed, continued administration of oral corticosteroids may be necessary. Some individuals may be adequately controlled on an alternate-day regimen taking the cor-

---

C = 51-100p, **D** = 101-180p, **E** = 181-300p, **F** = 301-450p, **G** = 451-650p, **H** = 651-900p, **I** = 901-1200p, **J** = over 1200p.

ticosteroid as a single dose in the morning, and this may reduce some of the side-effects. In others daily administration is necessary. Dosage should always be titrated to the lowest dose which controls symptoms. Regular monitored peak flow measurements often help both patient and doctor to adjust the dose optimally. Prednisolone is available as tablets of 1 mg as well as 5 mg, and the smaller tablets may conveniently be used to adjust the maintenance dosage to the minimum necessary. Prednisolone sodium phosphate tablets (Prednesol®) or prednisolone enteric-coated tablets (Deltacortril®) may be useful as they are thought to be less liable to cause or aggravate peptic ulceration.

Corticotrophin and **tetracosactrin** (see section 6.5.1) may occasionally be used instead of the corticosteroids. They may cause less growth inhibition in children and a small number of severe asthmatics who are apparently refractory to corticosteroids may respond to the corticotrophins.

BECLOMETHASONE DIPROPIONATE

Indications: chronic airways obstruction, especially in asthma not controlled by bronchodilators

Cautions: see notes above; also respiratory infection, active or quiescent tuberculosis

Side-effects: hoarseness; candidiasis of mouth or throat, usually only with large doses (responds to antifungal lozenges, see section 12.3.2, without discontinuation of therapy; rinsing the mouth with water after inhalation of a dose may also be helpful)

Dose: by aerosol inhalation, 100 micrograms (2 puffs Becotide®) 3–4 times daily or 200 micrograms (4 puffs Becotide®) twice daily (doubled initially if necessary in severe bronchospasm and subsequently reduced); in severe asthma maintenance dose may be increased if necessary to 500 micrograms (2 puffs Becloforte®) twice daily or 250–500 micrograms (1–2 puffs Becloforte®) 3–4 times daily; CHILD 50–100 micrograms (1–2 puffs Becotide®) 2–4 times daily, reduced to the minimum effective dose

By inhalation of powder (insufflation cartridges), 200 micrograms 3–4 times daily or 400 micrograms twice daily; max. 1 mg daily; CHILD 100 micrograms 2–4 times daily

By inhalation of nebulised suspension, 100 micrograms twice daily increased if necessary to max. 1 mg daily in divided doses; dilution is adjusted according to equipment and length of administration. CHILD up to 1 year 50 micrograms 2–4 times daily, over 1 year 100 micrograms 2–4 times daily, adjusted according to response

PoM **Becloforte®** (A&H)
Inhaler (= aerosol inhalation), beclomethasone dipropionate 250 micrograms/metered inhalation, 200-dose unit. Price (complete unit) = **J**. Label: 8, counselling advised, prescribed dose, manufacturer's directions

PoM **Becotide®** (A&H)
Inhaler (= aerosol inhalation), beclomethasone

dipropionate 50 micrograms/metered inhalation, 200-dose unit. Price (complete unit) = **G**. Label: 8, counselling advised, prescribed dose, manufacturer's directions

Rotacaps® (= insufflation cartridges), buff/clear, beclomethasone dipropionate 100 micrograms. Price 20 cartridges = **D**. Label: 8

Rotacaps® (= insufflation cartridges), brown/clear, beclomethasone dipropionate 200 micrograms. Price 20 cartridges = **E**. Label: 8

Rotahaler® (for use with Rotacaps). Price per unit = **C**

Suspension for nebulisation, beclomethasone dipropionate 50 micrograms/ml. Price 10 ml = **E**. For use with respirator or nebuliser. May be diluted up to 50% with sterile sodium chloride solution

Compound preparations
PoM **Ventide®** (A&H)
Inhaler (= aerosol inhalation), beclomethasone dipropionate 50 micrograms, salbutamol 100 micrograms/metered inhalation, 200-dose unit. Price (complete unit) = **H**. Label: 8, counselling advised, prescribed dose, manufacturer's directions
Dose: maintenance, 2 puffs 3–4 times daily; CHILD 1–2 puffs 2–4 times daily

---

BETAMETHASONE VALERATE

Indications; Cautions; Side-effects: see under Beclomethasone Dipropionate

Dose: by aerosol inhalation, initially 200 micrograms (2 puffs) 3–4 times daily; CHILD 100 micrograms (1 puff) 2–3 times daily, reduced to the minimum effective dose

PoM **Bextasol®** (Glaxo)
Inhaler (= aerosol inhalation), betamethasone valerate 100 micrograms/metered inhalation, 200-dose unit. Price (complete unit) = **G**. Label: 8, counselling advised, prescribed dose, manufacturer's directions

---

BUDESONIDE

Indications; Cautions; Side-effects: see under Beclomethasone Dipropionate

Dose: by aerosol inhalation, initially 200 micrograms (1 puff Pulmicort) twice daily, adjusted according to response to minimum effective dose but not less that 200 micrograms daily; in severe asthma dose may be increased to 1.2 mg (6 puffs Pulmicort) daily; CHILD 50–200 micrograms (1–4 puffs Pulmicort Paediatric) up to twice daily

▼ PoM **Pulmicort®** (Astra)
Inhaler (= aerosol inhalation), budesonide 200 micrograms/metered inhalation, 100-dose unit. Price (complete unit, with standard and collapsible spacer inhaler) = **I**; refill canister for use with Nebuhaler or Pulmicort Spacer Inhaler = **H**. Label: 8, counselling advised, prescribed dose, manufacturer's directions
Paediatric inhaler (= aerosol inhalation), budesonide 50 micrograms/metered inhalation, 200-dose unit. Price (complete unit, with collapsible

spacer) = **G**; refill canister for use with Nebu-haler or Pulmicort paediatric inhaler = **G**. Label: 8, counselling advised, prescribed dose, manufacturer's directions

Nebuhaler® (Astra)

Inhaler, fitted with plastic cone and one-way valve. For use with Bricanyl and Pulmicort refill canisters. Price = **F**

3.3   Prophylaxis of asthma

Regular administration of prophylactic drugs can reduce the incidence of attacks and often allow dosage reduction of concurrent corticosteroids and bronchodilators. Prophylactic drugs are of no value in the treatment of acute attacks as their effects take some time to develop.

Sodium cromoglycate (Intal®) is the main drug of this group and is administered by inhalation. Its mode of action is not completely understood but it prevents release of pharmacological mediators of bronchospasm by stabilising mast-cell membranes and is of particular value in patients whose asthma has an allergic basis, although it may also be useful in some patients in whom an allergic basis has not been demon-strated. It may also be of value in the prevention of exercise-induced asthma. Children seem to respond better than adults to sodium cromo-glycate but, as it is difficult to predict who will benefit, it is reasonable to try it in all patients whose asthma is poorly controlled with broncho-dilators. Patients, and particularly children, should be given careful instruction on the use of sodium cromoglycate inhalations and it should be emphasised that regular administration is necess-ary, whether symptoms are present or not. Dose frequency is adjusted according to the patient's response but is usually 4 times daily. As improve-ment occurs this may be reduced if possible. When used to prevent attacks in exercise-induced asthma, sodium cromoglycate is administered half an hour before exercise as a single dose. Sodium cromoglycate should be discontinued after 4 weeks if there is no response but should be con-tinued in patients who benefit.

Sodium cromoglycate has few side-effects. However, occasionally the dry powder inhalations may cause bronchospasm. In such patients, the best procedure is to use a selective beta$_2$-adreno-ceptor stimulant inhalation such as salbutamol or terbutaline a few minutes before the sodium cromoglycate inhalation is given. There is **no** advantage in using the compound inhalation of sodium cromoglycate which contains isoprenaline (Intal Compound®) as this has a less selective action; moreover, it may lead to the patient mis-using the preparation for relieving bronchospasm rather than for its prophylactic effect. Sodium cromoglycate nebuliser solution is useful for those patients who cannot manage the dry powder inhaler and pressurised aerosols. It is conveniently used when individuals already possess and use a home nebuliser for bronchodilator therapy. See also section 3.1.1.

Ketotifen (Zaditen®) is a newer drug with an action said to resemble that of sodium cro-moglycate. Although some studies have suggested that it has certain anti-asthma effects, in clinical practice it does not seem to have fulfilled its early promise in the majority of patients. It is given by mouth and, while this may be an advantage to patients who find inhalation difficult, ketotifen may have to be given for 4 weeks or more to achieve full prophylaxis. In addition, ketotifen is an antihistamine and as such may cause drow-siness. Doses for asthma prophylaxis and relief of allergy are similar.

There is some recent evidence that selective beta$_2$-adrenoceptor stimulants may be used on a regular basis for prophylaxis (as opposed to bronchodilator effects). As a consequence a num-ber of aerosols are being marketed which contain both a beta-agonist and a corticosteroid or an atropine derivative. While these are convenient and cheaper for the patient, they do not provide flexibility in dosage, and patient education is more difficult.

SODIUM CROMOGLYCATE

Indications: prophylaxis of asthma

Side-effects: coughing, transient bronchospasm, and throat irritation due to inhalation of powder (see also notes above)

Dose: by aerosol inhalation, adults and children, 2 mg (2 puffs) 4 times daily, increased in severe cases or during periods of risk to 6–8 times daily

By inhalation of powder (insufflation cartridges), adults and children, 20 mg 4 times daily, increased in severe cases to 8 times daily

By inhalation of nebulised solution, adults and children, 20 mg 4 times daily, increased in severe cases to 6 times daily

PoM **Intal**® (Fisons)

Halermatic insufflator® (automatic, for use with Intal and Intal Compound Spincaps). Price per unit = **D**

Inhaler (= aerosol inhalation), sodium cro-moglycate 1 mg/metered inhalation, 200-dose unit. Price (complete unit) = **I**. Label: 8

Spincaps® (= insufflation cartridges), yellow/clear, sodium cromoglycate 20 mg. Price 20 cartridges = **E**. Label: 8

Spinhaler insufflator® (for use with Intal and Intal Compound Spincaps). Price per unit = **D**

Nebuliser solution, sodium cromoglycate 10 mg/ml. Price 2-ml amp = **A**. For use with power-operated nebuliser

PoM **Intal Compound**® (Fisons)

Spincaps® (= insufflation cartridges), orange/clear, iso-prenaline sulphate 100 micrograms, sodium cromo-glycate 20 mg. Price 20 cartridges = **D**. Label: 8

Dose: see under sodium cromoglycate (above)

KETOTIFEN

Indications: see notes above

Cautions: may affect ability to drive or operate machinery and increase effects of alcohol; pre-vious anti-asthmatic treatment should be con-tinued for a minimum of 2 weeks after initiation of ketotifen treatment

---

C = 51-100p, **D** = 101-180p, **E** = 181-300p, **F** = 301-450p, **G** = 451-650p, **H** = 651-900p, **I** = 901-1200p, **J** = over 1200p.

Side-effects: dry mouth, sedation

Dose: 1–2 mg twice daily with food; initial treatment in readily sedated patients 0.5–1 mg at night; CHILD over 2 years 1 mg twice daily

PoM **Zaditen**® (Sandoz)

Capsules, ketotifen 1 mg (as hydrogen fumarate). Price 20 caps = **F**. Label: 2, 8, 21

Tablets, off-white, scored, ketotifen 1 mg (as hydrogen fumarate). Price 20 tabs = **F**. Label: 2, 8, 21

Elixir, ketotifen 1 mg (as hydrogen fumarate)/ 5 ml. Diluent syrup, life of diluted elixir 14 days. Price 150 ml = **H**. Label: 2, 8, 21

3.4   Allergic disorders

Drugs modifying allergic disorders are discussed under the following headings:

3.4.1 Antihistamines
3.4.2 Hyposensitisation
3.4.3 Allergic emergencies

For the treatment of asthma see sections 3.1.1 and 3.2. For the treatment of hay fever by nasal application of corticosteroids and prophylaxis with sodium cromoglycate see section 12.2. For eye preparations see section 11.4. For the treatment of allergic skin conditions with topical corticosteroid preparations see section 13.4.

3.4.1   Antihistamines

All antihistamines are of potential value in the treatment of nasal allergies, particularly the seasonal type (hay fever) and may be of some value in vasomotor rhinitis. They reduce rhinorrhoea and sneezing but are usually less effective in relieving nasal congestion.

Oral antihistamines are also of some value in preventing urticaria and are used to treat allergic rashes, pruritus, and insect bites and stings. They are also used in drug allergies. Chlorpheniramine or promethazine injections are used as adjuncts to adrenaline injection in the emergency treatment of angioedema and anaphylaxis (section 3.4.3).

There is no evidence that any one antihistamine is superior to another and patients vary widely in their response to them. They differ somewhat in their duration of action and incidence of side-effects (drowsiness and anticholinergic effects). Most of the antihistamines are relatively short-acting but some, such as **promethazine**, are active for up to 12 hours. They all cause sedation but promethazine, **trimeprazine**, and **dimenhydrinate** may be more sedating whilst **chlorpheniramine**, **cyclizine**, and **mequitazine** may be less so.

Astemizole (Hismanal®), **oxatomide** (Tinset®), and **terfenadine** (Triludan®) are recently introduced antihistamines which may have some advantages over the older antihistamines. Astemizole and terfenadine cause less sedation and do not cause psychomotor impairment because they only penetrate the blood brain barrier to a slight extent and for this reason the drug interactions described in Appendix 1 apply to a lesser extent and they do not appear to potentiate the effects of alcohol. Oxatomide may be more effective than the older antihistamines for relieving nasal allergies.

Several antihistamines are described in other chapters (see Index).

DISADVANTAGES OF ANTIHISTAMINES. A serious disadvantage is that they may frequently cause drowsiness; patients should be warned that their ability to drive or operate machinery may be impaired, and that the effects of alcohol may be increased. Other side-effects include headache, psychomotor impairment, anticholinergic effects such as urinary retention, dry mouth, blurred vision, and gastro-intestinal disturbances; paradoxical stimulation may rarely occur, especially in high dosage or in children. Antihistamines should be used with caution in epilepsy, prostatic hypertrophy, glaucoma, and hepatic disease. Drug interactions: see Appendix 1 (sections *4.1, 4.6, 4.9*).

ASTEMIZOLE

Indications: symptomatic relief of allergy such as hay fever, urticaria

Cautions: see notes above; pregnancy (toxicity at high doses in *animal* studies)

Side-effects: see notes above; weight gain occurs infrequently; incidence of sedation is low; anticholinergic effects and psychomotor impairment have not been reported

Dose: usually 10 mg daily before food, increased if necessary to 30 mg daily for up to 7 days; CHILD 6–12 years, half adult dose

▼ PoM **Hismanal**® (Janssen)

Tablets, scored, astemizole 10 mg. Price 20 tabs = **F**. Label: 23

AZATADINE MALEATE

Indications: symptomatic relief of allergy such as hay fever, urticaria

Cautions; Side-effects: see notes above

Dose: 1 mg, increased if necessary to 2 mg, twice daily; CHILD 1–5 years 250 micrograms twice daily, 6–12 years 0.5–1 mg twice daily

Optimine® (Kirby-Warrick)

Tablets, scored, azatadine maleate 1 mg. Price 20 tabs = **D**. Label: 2

Syrup (= elixir), azatadine maleate 500 micrograms/5 ml. Diluent syrup, life of diluted elixir 28 days. Price 120 ml = **D**. Label: 2

BROMPHENIRAMINE MALEATE

Indications: symptomatic relief of allergy such as hay fever, food allergy, urticaria

Cautions; Side-effects: see notes above

Dose: 4–8 mg 3–4 times daily; CHILD up to 3 years 0.4–1 mg/kg daily in 4 divided doses, 3–5 years 2 mg 3–4 times daily, 6–12 years 2–4 mg 3–4 times daily

Dimotane® (Robins)
Tablets, peach, scored, brompheniramine maleate 4 mg. Price 20 tabs = **B**. Label: 2
Elixir, yellow-green, brompheniramine maleate 2 mg/5 ml. Diluent syrup, life of diluted elixir 14 days. Price 100 ml = **C**. Label: 2

Dimotane LA® (Robins)
Tablets, s/r, peach, s/c, brompheniramine maleate 12 mg. Price 20 tabs = **C**. Label: 2, 25
Dose: 12–24 mg twice daily; CHILD 6–12 years 12 mg at bedtime, increased if necessary to 12 mg twice daily

CHLORPHENIRAMINE MALEATE

Indications: symptomatic relief of allergy such as hay fever, urticaria; emergency treatment of anaphylactic reactions
Cautions; Side-effects: see notes above. Injections may be irritant and cause transitory hypotension or CNS stimulation
Dose: by mouth, 4 mg 3–4 times daily; CHILD up to 1 year 1 mg twice daily, 1–5 years 1–2 mg three times daily, 6–12 years 2–4 mg 3–4 times daily
Allergic emergencies, *by subcutaneous, intramuscular, or slow intravenous injection*, 10–20 mg when necessary to a max. of 40 mg in 24 hours; CHILD, *by intravenous injection*, 200 micrograms/kg when necessary

Chlorpheniramine Tablets, chlorpheniramine maleate 4 mg. Price 20 tabs = **A**. Label: 2

Alunex® (Steinhard)
Tablets, yellow, scored, chlorpheniramine maleate 4 mg. Price 20 tabs = **A**. Label: 2

Piriton® (A&H)
Tablets, yellow, chlorpheniramine maleate 4 mg. Price 20 tabs = **A**. Label: 2
Duolets® (= tablets s/r), yellow, s/c, chlorpheniramine maleate 8 mg. Price 20 tabs = **B**. Label: 2, 25
Dose: 8 mg every 8–10 hours; CHILD over 12 years 8 mg daily
Spandets® (= tablets s/r), yellow/white, chlorpheniramine maleate 12 mg. Price 20 tabs = **C**. Label: 2, 25
Dose: 12 mg every 8–12 hours; CHILD over 12 years 12 mg daily
Syrup (= elixir), chlorpheniramine maleate 2 mg/5 ml. Diluent syrup (without preservative), life of diluted elixir 14 days. Price 150 ml = **B**. Label: 2
PoM *Injection*, chlorpheniramine maleate 10 mg/ml. Price 1-ml amp = **A**

CLEMASTINE

Indications: symptomatic relief of allergy such as hay fever, urticaria
Cautions; Side-effects: see notes above
Dose: 1 mg twice daily; CHILD up to 12 years 0.5–1 mg twice daily

Tavegil® (Sandoz)
Tablets, scored, clemastine 1 mg (as hydrogen fumarate). Price 20 tabs = **C**. Label: 2

Elixir, clemastine 500 micrograms (as hydrogen fumarate)/5 ml (sugar-free). Diluent syrup, life of diluted elixir 14 days. Price 100 ml = **B**. Label: 2

CYPROHEPTADINE HYDROCHLORIDE

Indications: symptomatic relief of allergy such as hay fever, urticaria; stimulation of appetite
Cautions; Side-effects: see notes above; also may inhibit lactation
Dose: allergy, 4–20 mg (max. 32 mg) daily in divided doses; CHILD 2–5 years 6 mg (max. 12 mg), 6–12 years 12 mg (max. 16 mg), daily in divided doses
Stimulation of appetite, 4 mg 3 times daily *or* 12 mg in the evening; CHILD 2–6 years up to 8 mg daily, 7–14 years up to 12 mg daily

Periactin® (MSD)
Tablets, scored, cyproheptadine hydrochloride 4 mg. Price 20 tabs = **C**. Label: 2
Syrup (= elixir), yellow, cyproheptadine hydrochloride 2 mg/5 ml. Diluent syrup, life of diluted elixir 14 days. Price 200 ml = **D**. Label: 2

DIMETHINDENE MALEATE

Indications: symptomatic relief of allergy such as hay fever, urticaria
Cautions; Side-effects: see notes above

Fenostil Retard® (Zyma)
Tablets, s/r, greyish-white, dimethindene maleate 2.5 mg. Price 20 tabs = **C**. Label: 2, 25
Dose: 2.5 mg twice daily

DIPHENHYDRAMINE HYDROCHLORIDE

Indications: symptomatic relief of allergy such as hay fever, urticaria
Cautions; Side-effects: see notes above
Dose: 25 mg 3 times daily and if necessary 50 mg at night

Benadryl® (P-D)
Capsules, pink, diphenhydramine hydrochloride 25 mg. Price 20 caps = **A**. Label: 2

DIPHENYLPYRALINE HYDROCHLORIDE

Indications: symptomatic relief of allergy such as hay fever, urticaria
Cautions; Side-effects: see notes above

Histryl® (SK&F)
Spansule® (= capsules s/r), pink/clear, enclosing pink and white pellets, diphenylpyraline hydrochloride 5 mg. Price 20 caps = **C**. Label: 2, 25
Dose: 5–10 mg twice daily
Paediatric Spansule® (= capsules s/r), pink/clear, enclosing pink and white pellets, diphenylpyraline hydrochloride 2.5 mg. Price 20 caps = **B**. Label: 1, 25
Dose: CHILD over 7 years 2.5 mg twice daily

Lergoban® (Riker)
Tablets, s/r, diphenylpyraline hydrochloride 5 mg. Price 20 tabs = **C**. Label: 2, 25
Dose: 5–10 mg twice daily; CHILD over 10 years 5 mg twice daily

KETOTIFEN
Section 3.3

MEBHYDROLIN
Indications: symptomatic relief of allergy such as hay fever, urticaria
Cautions: see notes above
Side-effects: see notes above; also reversible granulocytopenia occurs rarely
Dose: 50–100 mg 3 times daily; CHILD, daily in divided doses, up to 2 years 50–100 mg, 2–5 years 50–150 mg, 6–12 years 100–200 mg

PoM **Fabahistin®** (Bayer)
Tablets, orange, s/c, mebhydrolin 50 mg. Price 20 tabs = **C**. Label: 2
Suspension (= mixture), orange, mebhydrolin 50 mg (as napadisylate)/5 ml. Diluents tragacanth mucilage for 5 days storage, *or* carmellose sodium 0.5% and methyl hydroxybenzoate 0.07% in purified water, freshly boiled and cooled, for longer storage. Price 100 ml = **C**. Label: 2

MEPYRAMINE MALEATE
Indications: symptomatic relief of allergy such as hay fever, urticaria
Cautions; Side-effects: see notes above
Dose: 100 mg 3 times daily; CHILD 7–14 years 50 mg 3–4 times daily

Anthisan® (M&B)
Tablets, green, s/c, mepyramine maleate 50 mg. Price 20 tabs = **B**. Label: 2

MEQUITAZINE
Indications: symptomatic relief of allergy such as hay fever, urticaria
Cautions; Side-effects: see notes above
Dose: 5 mg twice daily

PoM **Primalan®** (M&B)
Tablets, mequitazine 5 mg. Price 20 tabs = **D**. Label: 2

OXATOMIDE
Indications: symptomatic relief of allergy such as hay fever, food allergy, urticaria
Cautions; Side-effects: see notes above but anticholinergic side-effects are absent. Drowsiness is most common side-effect. Weight gain may occur with doses above 120 mg daily
Dose: 30 mg twice daily after food, increased if necessary to 60 mg twice daily; CHILD 5–14 years 15–30 mg twice daily

▼ PoM **Tinset®** (Janssen)
Tablets, scored, oxatomide 30 mg. Price 20 tabs = **E**. Label: 2, 21

PHENINDAMINE TARTRATE
Indications: symptomatic relief of allergy such as hay fever, urticaria
Cautions; Side-effects: see notes above; may cause mild CNS stimulation
Dose: 25–50 mg up to 4 times daily; CHILD over 10 years 25 mg 1–3 times daily

Thephorin® (Sinclair)
Tablets, s/c, phenindamine tartrate 25 mg. Price 20 tabs = **C**. Label: 2

PHENIRAMINE MALEATE
Indications: symptomatic relief of allergy such as hay fever, urticaria
Cautions; Side-effects: see notes above

Daneral SA® (Hoechst)
Tablets, s/r, pink, s/c, pheniramine maleate 75 mg. Price 20 tabs = **D**. Label: 2, 25
Dose: 75–150 mg at night or 75 mg night and morning

PROMETHAZINE HYDROCHLORIDE
Indications: symptomatic relief of allergy such as hay fever, urticaria, emergency treatment of anaphylactic reactions
For use in premedication see section 15.1.4.2; sedation see section 4.1.1
Cautions; Side-effects: see notes above; intramuscular injection may be painful
Dose: by mouth, 20–75 mg daily in divided doses *or* as a single dose at night; CHILD 6–12 months 5–10 mg, 1–5 years 5–15 mg, 6–10 years 10–25 mg daily
By deep intramuscular injection, 25–50 mg; max. 100 mg; CHILD 5–10 years 6.25–12.5 mg
By slow intravenous injection in emergencies, 25–50 mg, max. 100 mg, as a solution containing 2.5 mg/ml in water for injections

Phenergan® (M&B)
Tablets, blue, s/c, promethazine hydrochloride 10 mg. Price 20 tabs = **B**. Label: 2
Tablets, blue, s/c, promethazine hydrochloride 25 mg. Price 20 tabs = **B**. Label: 2
Elixir, golden, promethazine hydrochloride 5 mg/5 ml. Diluent syrup, life of diluted elixir 14 days. Price 100 ml = **B**. Label: 2
PoM *Injection*, promethazine hydrochloride 25 mg/ml. Price 1- and 2-ml amp (both) = **B**
Note: a proprietary brand of promethazine hydrochloride tablets 20 mg (Sominex®) is on sale to the public for the treatment of occasional insomnia in adults

TERFENADINE
Indications: symptomatic relief of allergy such as hay fever, urticaria (see notes above)
Side-effects: see notes above; incidence of sedation is low; anticholinergic effects and psy-

---

Relative prices: **A** = up to 20p, **B** = 21-50p,

chomotor impairment have not been reported
Dose: 60 mg twice daily; CHILD 6–12 years 30 mg

▼ **Triludan**® (Merrell)
Tablets, scored, terfenadine 60 mg. Price 20
tabs = **D**
Suspension (= mixture), terfenadine 30 mg/5 ml.
Diluent syrup, life of diluted mixture 14 days
(in refrigerator). Price 120 ml = **E**

TRIMEPRAZINE TARTRATE

Indications: symptomatic relief of allergy, particularly pruritus
For use in premedication, see section 15.1.4.2;
sedation, see section 4.1.1
Cautions; Side-effects: see notes above
Dose: 10 mg 3–4 times daily, increased if necessary to max. 100 mg daily; CHILD 2.5–5 mg 3–4
times daily

PoM **Vallergan**® (M&B)
Tablets, blue, s/c, trimeprazine tartrate 10 mg.
Price 20 tabs = **B**. Label: 2
Syrup (= paediatric elixir), yellow, trimeprazine
tartrate 7.5 mg/5 ml. Diluent syrup, life of
diluted elixir 14 days. Price 125 ml = **C**.
Label: 2
Syrup forte (= strong paediatric elixir), pink,
trimeprazine tartrate 30 mg/5 ml. Diluent as
above. Price 125 ml = **D**. Label: 2

TRIPROLIDINE HYDROCHLORIDE

Indications: symptomatic relief of allergy such as
hay fever, urticaria
Cautions; Side-effects: see notes above
Dose: 2.5–5 mg 3 times daily (in severe allergy,
initial dose 5–7.5 mg, then 2.5–5 mg every 4
hours); CHILD, 3 times daily, up to 1 year 1 mg,
1–5 years 2 mg, 6–12 years 3 mg

Actidil® (Wellcome)
Tablets, scored, triprolidine hydrochloride
2.5 mg. Price 20 tabs = **C**. Label: 2
Elixir, orange, triprolidine hydrochloride
2 mg/5 ml. Diluent syrup, life of diluted elixir
14 days. Price 100 ml = **C**. Label: 2
Pro-Actidil® (Wellcome)
Tablets, s/r, white/pink/blue, triprolidine hydrochloride 10 mg. Price 20 tabs = **E**. Label: 2, 25
Dose: 10 mg early evening increased to 20 mg
daily when necessary; CHILD over 10 years 10 mg
daily

3.4.2 Hyposensitisation

Though commonly used, the value of specific
hyposensitisation is uncertain and only likely to
be beneficial in patients with specific allergy to
grass pollens, house dust mite (*Dermatophagoides
pteronyssinus*), or wasp and bee stings. Since the
majority of patients are also sensitive to a wide
range of other allergens (except wasp and bee
sting allergy), hyposensitisation with an extract of
a single allergen is, in most cases, no more than
partially successful. Patients should therefore be
carefully selected for treatment as the procedure
is unpleasant and risks precipitating allergic reactions which may be severe. Furthermore, the diagnostic skin tests are unreliable and can only be
used in conjunction with a detailed history of
allergen exposure. For example, many asthmatics
with positive skin tests for grass pollen have no
hay fever or summer exacerbations of asthma.

Patients with seasonal or perennial rhinitis due
to pollen or house dust mite seem to derive most
benefit from hyposensitisation and nose and eye
symptoms may be reduced by about half, though
the duration of benefit is unknown. The value of
hyposensitisation in patients with allergic asthma
and eczema is uncertain but it may benefit a small
proportion where pollen or house dust mite is
considered to be a major precipitating factor.

Where it is decided to undertake specific hyposensitisation, graded injections of increasing concentration are administered, usually every 1 to 2
weeks and usually over a period of about 10
weeks. Courses for pollen hyposensitisation (hay
fever) should be given preseasonally, usually
beginning in January to ensure the course is completed before commencement of the grass pollen
season. Courses are usually repeated for 2 to 3
consecutive years. *Maintenance courses* are also
available and are usually recommended for house
dust mite allergy. They consist of booster injections administered at gradually increasing time
intervals (4–6 weeks) after the initial treatment
course. The choice of preparation usually depends
on the prescriber's preference but the precipitated
or adsorbed extracts are probably safer and more
convenient than the soluble extracts. **Conjuvac**®
and **Spectralgen**® have been recently introduced
and are refined preparations that have been standardised immunologically. They are claimed to
reduce the incidence of allergic side-effects but
this has not been proved.

Wasp and bee venom hyposensitisation is effective and extracts of bee and wasp venom are
available. The procedure is not without risk of
precipitating severe reactions and the extract
should be administered with careful attention to
instructions or preferably under hospital
supervision.

Hyposensitisation with a mixture of several
allergens combined in a single solution is **not** recommended because there is no evidence that such
mixtures are effective. Their effects are unpredictable and they may precipitate dangerous
reactions.

Hyposensitisation may precipitate allergic reactions which may be severe and this is a particular
risk with children. Injections should therefore be
administered only when emergency resuscitation
equipment, including adrenaline injection, is at
hand. After each injection the patient should be
kept under observation for at least 30–60 minutes
and subcutaneous adrenaline given as soon as
symptoms appear and repeated until they subside
(section 3.1.1.2). Very sensitive patients may be
given an antihistamine tablet one hour before the

C = 51-100p, D = 101-180p, E = 181-300p, F = 301-450p, G = 451-650p, H = 651-900p, I = 901-1200p, J = over 1200p.

injection. Courses should be discontinued in the event of severe allergic reactions.

ALLERGEN EXTRACT VACCINES

Each set usually contains vials for the administration of graded amounts to patients undergoing hyposensitisation. Maintenance sets containing vials at the highest strength are also available

Indications: hypersensitivity to one or more common allergens (see notes above)

Cautions: see notes above; patients should be warned not to eat a heavy meal before the injection

Contra-indications: pregnancy, febrile conditions, acute asthma

Side-effects: allergic reactions, especially in small children

Dose: by subcutaneous injection, a volume appropriate to the needs of the patient, usually every 1–2 weeks, gradually increasing the amount of allergen

Note: PNU = protein nitrogen unit; BU = biological unit equivalent to one thousandth 'histamine-equivalent-prick'

Pollen allergy (hay fever) preparations

PoM **Alavac-P**® (Bencard)

Treatment set, alum precipitated extract of aqueous pyridine solutions, prepared from 12 varieties of common grass pollen, set of 3 × 5-ml vials containing 250, 2500, and 25000 Noon units/ml. Specially diluted extracts for very sensitive patients are supplied on request. Price (complete set) = **J**

PoM **Allpyral-G**® (Dome/Hollister-Stier)

Treatment set, alum precipitated extract of aqueous pyridine solutions, prepared from 5 varieties of common grass pollen, set of 3 × 5-ml vials containing 100, 1000, and 10000 PNU/ml. Vials containing 10 PNU/ml for very sensitive patients are supplied on request. Price (complete set) = **J**

Maintenance set, 1 × 5-ml vial containing 10000 PNU/ml. Price = **J**

▼ PoM **Conjuvac Two Grass**® (Dome/Hollister-Stier)

Treatment set, powder for reconstitution with water for injections, purified pollen extract in alginate carrier, prepared from Timothy (*Phleum pratense*) and Cocksfoot (*Dactylis glomerata*) for hyposensitisation in most common pollen allergies by cross-reactivity. Set of 12 single-dose vials for administration of 11 graded weekly doses; 4 vials of 10 units/ml for administration of 1, 2, 4, and 8 units doses; 3 vials of 100 units/ml (+ 1 spare vial) for administration of 15, 30, and 60 units doses; 3 vials of 500 units/ml for administration of 100, 200, and 400 units doses; and 1 vial of 1000 units/ml for administration of 800 units doses. Price (complete set with 12 × 2-ml amp water for injections) = **J**

Maintenance set, 4 vials of 1000 units/ml. Price (complete set with 4 × 2-ml amp water for injections) = **J**

▼ PoM **Norisen Grass**® (Merck)

Treatment set, aluminium-adsorbed extracts, prepared from 6 varieties of common grass pollen, set of 3 vials containing 100, 1000, and 10000 PNU/ml. Vials containing 10 PNU/ml for very sensitive patients are supplied on request. Price (complete set) = **J**

Maintenance set, 1 × 4.5-ml vial containing 10000 PNU/ml. Price = **J**

PoM **Pollinex**® (Bencard)

Treatment set, tyrosine-adsorbed extracts, prepared from 12 varieties of common grass pollen, set of 3 pre-filled syringes containing 300, 800, and 2000 Noon units/0.5 ml. Price (complete set) = **J**

▼ PoM **Spectralgen Single Species**® (Pharmacia)

Treatment set, powder for reconstitution as aqueous solution with NSA-diluent (normal serum albumin) or as aluminium-adsorbed extract with depot diluent (as specified), purified pollen extract prepared from any one of 7 varieties common grasses or trees, set of 4 vials containing 100, 1000, 10000, and 100000 BU/ml. Price (complete set with diluent) = **J**

Maintenance set, vial containing 10000 or 100000 BU/ml (as specified). Price with diluent = **J**

▼ PoM **Spectralgen 4 Grass Mix**® (Pharmacia)

Treatment set, powder for reconstitution as aqueous solution with NSA-diluent (normal serum albumin) or as aluminium-adsorbed extract with depot diluent (as specified), purified pollen extract prepared from 4 varieties common grasses, set of 4 vials containing 100, 1000, 10000, and 100000 BU/ml. Price (complete set with diluent) = **J**

Maintenance set, vial containing 10000 or 100000 BU/ml (as specified). Price with diluent = **J**

▼ PoM **Spectralgen 3 Tree Mix**® (Pharmacia)

Treatment set, powder for reconstitution as aqueous solution with NSA-diluent (normal serum albumin) or as aluminium-adsorbed extract with depot diluent (as specified), purified pollen extract prepared from 3 varieties of common trees, set of 4 vials containing 100, 1000, 10000, and 100000 BU/ml. Price (complete set with diluent) = **J**

Maintenance set, vial containing 10000 or 100000 BU/ml (as specified). Price with diluent = **J**

Note: Spectralgen® preparations are diluted with NSA-diluent (normal serum albumin 300 micrograms/ml) which is suitable for all forms of therapy and diagnostic tests *or* Depot diluent containing aluminium hydroxide which is suitable for use in the treatment and maintenance of ambulant patients

House dust mite allergy preparations

PoM **Allpyral D. pteronyssinus**® (Dome/Hollister-Stier)

Treatment set, alum precipitated extract of aqueous pyridine solution, prepared from *D. pteronyssinus*, set of 3 × 5-ml vials containing 100, 1000, and 4000 PNU/ml. Vials containing 10 PNU/ml for very sensitive patients are supplied on request. Price (complete set) = **J**

Maintenance set, 3 × 2-ml vials containing 4000 PNU/ml. Price (complete set) = **J**

PoM **Allpyral-Mite Fortified House Dust**® (Dome/Hollister-Stier)

Treatment set, alum precipitated extract of aqueous pyridine solution, prepared from fortified house dust mite (*Dermatophagoides* spp.), set of 3 × 5-ml vials containing 100, 1000, and 10000 PNU/ml. Vials containing 10 PNU/ml for very sensitive patients are supplied on request. Price (complete set) = **J**

Maintenance set, 1 × 10-ml vial containing 10000 PNU/ml. Price = **J**

PoM **Migen**® (Bencard)

Initial course, tyrosine-adsorbed extract, prepared from *D. pteronyssinus*, set of 6 pre-filled syringes containing 4, 10, 25, 60, 150, and 400 Noon units/0.5 ml. Price (complete set) = **J**

Maintenance set, 6 pre-filled syringes, containing 400 Noon units/0.5 ml. Price (complete set) = **J**

Specific allergy preparations

PoM **Alavac-S**® (Bencard)

Treatment set, alum-adsorbed extract of aqueous pyridine solutions, individually formulated and prepared from specific allergens to which patient is sensitive; max. 6 allergens in any one vaccine. Range of allergens includes dusts, epithelia, fabrics, fungi, house-dust mite, and pollens. Set of 3 × 5-ml vials; no. 1 and no. 2 are 1/100th and 1/10th dilutions of no. 3 vial. Price (complete set) = **J**

Maintenance set, 1 × 10-ml full strength vial. Price = **J**

PoM **Allpyral-Specific**® (Dome/Hollister-Stier)

Treatment set, alum precipitated extract of aqueous pyridine solutions, individually formulated and prepared from specific allergens to which patient is sensitive. Range of allergens includes dusts, epithelia, flour, fungi, pollens, and wasp and/or bee extracts. Set of 3 × 5-ml vials containing 100, 1000, and 10000 PNU/ml. Vials containing 10 PNU/ml for very sensitive patients are also available. Price (complete set) = **J**

Maintenance set, 1 × 5-ml vial containing 10000 PNU/ml. Price = **J**

▼ PoM **Norisen**® (Merck)

Treatment set, aluminium-adsorbed extracts, individually formulated and prepared from specific allergens to which patient is sensitive. Range of allergens includes dusts, epithelia, flour, fungi, house-dust mite, pollens, and wasp, hornet, and bee extracts. Allergens from stinging insects are not available in combination with other allergens. Set of 3 vials containing 100, 1000, and 10000 PNU/ml. Vials containing 10 PNU/ml for very sensitive patients are also available. Price (complete set) = **J**

Maintenance set, 1 × 10-ml vial containing 10000 PNU/ml. Price = **J**

PoM **SDV**® (Bencard)

Treatment set, aqueous solutions, individually formulated and prepared from a range of over 200 specific allergens to which patient is sensitive; max. 8 allergens in any one vaccine. Set of 3 × 10-ml vials. No. 1 and no. 2 vials are ₆₄th and ₈th dilutions of no. 3 vials. Alavac-S® (above) is usually preferred to SDV® in children. Price (complete set) = **J**

Maintenance set, 1 × 10-ml full strength vial. Price = **J**

Wasp and bee venom allergy preparations

▼ PoM **Albay Pure Venom**® (Dome/Hollister-Stier)

Treatment set, powder for reconstitution with diluent containing normal serum albumin, bee venom extract (*Apis mellifera*) 100 micrograms/ml. For administration of graded doses to a max. of 100 micrograms. Price 10-ml vial (with 1 × 10-ml vial and 3 × 2-ml vials diluent) = **J**. Also available containing wasp venom extract (*Vespula* spp.) 100 micrograms/ml

PoM **Pharmalgen**® (Pharmacia)

Treatment set, powder for reconstitution with NSA diluent, bee venom extract (*Apis mellifera*) 100 micrograms/ml. For administration of graded doses to a max. of 100 micrograms. Price 4 × 5-ml vials (with NSA diluent) = **J**. Also available containing wasp venom extract (*Vespula* spp.) 100 micrograms/ml

NSA-diluent, normal serum albumin 300 micrograms/ml. For reconstitution or dilution of Pharmalgen bee and wasp venom extracts. Price 10 × 4.5 ml = **H**

3.4.3 Allergic emergencies

Anaphylactic shock requires prompt energetic treatment. It is relatively uncommon but is usually precipitated by blood products, vaccines, insect stings, and certain drugs such as antibiotics, iron injections, anti-inflammatory analgesics, heparin, hyposensitising preparations, and neuromuscular blocking drugs. It is more likely to occur after parenteral administration and atopic individuals are particularly susceptible.

First-line treatment includes restoration of blood pressure, laying the patient flat, raising the feet, and administration of **adrenaline** injection (section 3.1.1.2). This is usually given intramuscularly in a dose of 0.5–1 mg (0.5–1 ml adrenaline injection 1 in 1000), repeated every 15 minutes until improvement occurs; several times the usual dose may be given if the patient is unconscious. Antihistamines, for example **chlorpheniramine**, given by slow intravenous injection (section 3.4.1), are a useful adjunctive treatment. This is given after adrenaline injection and continued for 24 to 48 hours to prevent relapse.

Intravenous **corticosteroids** are of secondary value in anaphylactic shock as their onset of action is delayed for several hours but they should be used to prevent further deterioration in severely affected patients (see section 6.3.4). Electrolyte solutions may also be required (see section 9.2.2). Some patients with severe allergy to insect stings are encouraged to carry adrenaline inhalations (Medihaler-epi®) or pre-filled adrenaline syringes (section 3.1.1.2) for emergency administration

---

C = 51-100p, **D** = 101-180p, **E** = 181-300p, **F** = 301-450p, **G** = 451-650p, **H** = 651-900p, **I** = 901-1200p, **J** = over 1200p.

during periods of risk. See also Emergency Treatment of Poisoning.

Angioedema is dangerous when it affects respiration. If obstruction is present, adrenaline injection as well as intravenous corticosteroids should be given as described above; antihistamine injections are also helpful. Tracheal intubation as well as other measures may also be necessary.

3.5   Respiratory stimulants

Respiratory stimulants (analeptic drugs) have a limited but useful place in the treatment of ventilatory failure in patients with chronic obstructive airways disease. They are effective only when given by intravenous injection or infusion and have a short duration of action. Respiratory stimulants should only be given under **expert supervision**, in hospital, except in a dire emergency and are best combined with active physiotherapy. There is no significant evidence that long-term use is of any value in chronic respiratory failure.

Nikethamide is the drug of choice and a bolus injection of 0.5–1 g (4–8 ml) will usually arouse patients with carbon dioxide narcosis. This will sometimes avoid recourse to tracheal intubation and artificial ventilation if used together with low-concentration oxygen therapy, supervised coughing, and antibacterial treatment.

Maintenance treatment with a respiratory stimulant may be required in those patients who are unable to tolerate even a 24% inspired oxygen concentration without becoming drowsy or comatose and in whom a long history of intolerable respiratory disability is a contra-indication to artificial ventilation. Choice of treatment lies between nikethamide and **doxapram** (Dopram®).

Nikethamide is given by regular bolus injection, in small doses, into the drip tubing of an intravenous infusion whereas doxapram may be given by continuous intravenous infusion. The effective dose of nikethamide is close to that causing toxic effects, especially convulsions. In this respect doxapram probably has a higher safety margin. Frequent arterial blood gas studies and pH measurements are necessary during treatment to ensure the correct dose, which should be carefully monitored. Epileptic patients should be treated with caution. Doxapram is also used postoperatively in anaesthetic practice (see section 15.1.7). **Ethamivan** (Clairvan®) has properties similar to those of nikethamide and is also given by repeated injection.

Respiratory stimulants are of no value, and may be harmful, in conditions where hypoxaemia is not associated with carbon dioxide retention, such as asthma, or in respiratory failure due to neurological or muscular disease and drug overdosage. They are only occasionally used in the asphyxiated newborn infant but clearing the airways is the first essential and valuable time may be wasted in giving respiratory stimulants. If they are used at all for this purpose, a few drops should be placed on the tongue.

NIKETHAMIDE

Indications: acute respiratory failure

Cautions: see notes above, severe hypertension, ischaemic heart disease

Contra-indications: respiratory failure due to neurological disease or drug overdose; status asthmaticus, coronary artery disease, thyrotoxicosis

Side-effects: nausea, restlessness, convulsions, dizziness, tremor, vasoconstriction, arrhythmias

Dose: by slow intravenous injection, 0.5–2 g repeated at intervals of 15–30 minutes as necessary

PoM **Nikethamide Injection,** nikethamide 250 mg/ ml. Price 2-ml amp = **B**; 5-ml amp = **C**

DOXAPRAM HYDROCHLORIDE

Indications: acute respiratory failure

Cautions: see notes above

Contra-indications: see under Nikethamide

Side-effects: see under Nikethamide; also perineal warmth

Dose: by intravenous infusion, 0.5–4 mg per minute according to patient's response

PoM **Dopram**® (Robins)
Intravenous infusion, doxapram hydrochloride 2 mg/ml in dextrose 5%. Price 500-ml bottle = **J**

ETHAMIVAN

Indications; Cautions; Contra-indications; Side-effects: see under Nikethamide and notes above

Dose: by mouth, PREMATURE INFANTS 12.5 mg (0.25 ml, 6 drops of 5% oral solution), FULL-TERM INFANTS 25 mg (0.5 ml, 12 drops of 5% oral solution)

By intravenous injection, 100 mg, repeated when necessary

PoM **Clairvan**® (Sinclair)
Oral solution, ethamivan 50 mg/ml (5%) in ethyl alcohol 25%. Price 5-ml dropper bottle = **G**
Injection, ethamivan 50 mg/ml (5%). Price 2-ml amp = **D**

3.6   Oxygen

Oxygen should be regarded as a drug. It is prescribed for hypoxaemic patients to increase alveolar oxygen tension and decrease the work of breathing necessary to maintain a given arterial oxygen tension. The concentration of inspired oxygen will depend on the condition being treated and an inappropriate concentration of inspired gas may have serious or even lethal effects.

High concentration oxygen therapy, given in concentrations of up to 60% for short periods, is both essential and safe in conditions such as pneumonia, pulmonary thromboembolism, and fibrosing alveolitis. In such conditions a low arterial plasma P_aO_2 is usually associated with low or normal arterial plasma P_aCO_2 and there is little risk of hypoventilation and carbon dioxide retention.

In severe acute asthma, the arterial plasma P_aCO_2 is subnormal initially but may later rise steeply (particularly in children) and arterial blood gas studies are essential to determine the concentration of oxygen to be delivered to the patient. Where facilities for blood gas measurements are not immediately available, for example while transferring the patient to hospital, the safest compromise would probably be to administer oxygen in concentrations of 24% or 28% with a Ventimask.

Low concentration oxygen therapy (controlled oxygen therapy) is reserved for use in patients with chronic obstructive airways disease. The concentration of inspired oxygen should not exceed 28% and in some patients even a concentration above 24% may be excessive. The aim of treatment is to provide the patient with just enough oxygen to correct hypoxaemia without worsening pre-existing carbon dioxide retention and respiratory acidosis. Such treatment should be initiated in hospital as repeated blood gas measurements are required to estimate the correct concentration of oxygen.

DOMICILIARY OXYGEN. Oxygen should be prescribed for patients in the home only after careful evaluation in hospital by respiratory experts and never on a placebo basis.

Oxygen may be prescribed for *intermittent* use in a variety of respiratory conditions. It is used in patients with hypoxaemia of short duration, for example asthma, when the condition is likely to recur over months or years. Such patients are usually supplied with oxygen in cylinders.

Alternatively, intermittent oxygen may be prescribed for patients with advanced irreversible respiratory disorders to increase mobility and capacity for exercise and ease discomfort, for example in chronic obstructive airways disease, emphysema, widespread fibrosis, and primary or thromboembolic pulmonary hypertension. These patients may be prescribed portable oxygen equipment through the hospital service, refillable from cylinders in the home.

Long-term administration of oxygen (at least 15 hours daily) may be prescribed on an elective basis to prolong survival in patients with severe chronic obstructive airways disease with cor pulmonale. Except during exacerbations, respiratory depression is seldom a problem once the disease has stabilised. At present there is no evidence of the benefits of such treatment in less severe forms of the disease and the possible damaging effects of long-term oxygen therapy have not yet been assessed completely. Such treatment obviously depends on patient acceptablity and is often difficult to put into practice because of the large number of cylinders required for effective therapy. For example, a patient receiving 15 hours of oxygen daily at 2 litres/minute will require 10 'F' size oxygen cylinders each week. Patients should also be advised of the fire risks when receiving therapy. Alternative equipment, particularly oxygen concentrators, has been developed. Oxygen concentrators are a more economical source of oxygen and overcome the difficulties of storage and delivery of cylinders. Changes in the supply of oxygen are likely to occur.

Under the National Health Service oxygen may be supplied only by chemist contractors as cylinders. Oxygen flow can be adjusted as the cylinders are equipped with an oxygen flow meter with 'medium' (2 litres/minute) and 'high' (4 litres/minute) settings. Patients are supplied with either constant or variable performance masks. The Intersurgical 010 28% or Ventimask Mk III 28% are constant performance masks and provide a nearly constant supply of oxygen (28%) over a wide range irrespective of the patient's breathing pattern. The variable performance masks include the Intersurgical 005 Mask and the MC Mask. With these, the concentration of oxygen supplied to the patient will vary with the rate of flow of supplied oxygen and also the patient's breathing pattern. They are generally used in patients who require oxygen concentrations below 28%. If any other type of equipment is required for domiciliary use, it must be supplied and serviced through the hospital service.

3.7   Mucolytics

Mucolytics are often prescribed to facilitate expectoration by reducing sputum viscosity in chronic asthma and bronchitis. Few patients, however, have been shown to derive much benefit from them although they do render sputum less viscid. The inhalational mucolytics, acetylcysteine (Airbron®) and tyloxapol (Alevaire®) are probably no more effective than water or steam inhalation, which in itself, with postural drainage, is good expectorant therapy in bronchiectasis and some chronic bronchitics. They are not commonly used as administration often causes febrile reactions.

Acetylcysteine (Fabrol®), **bromhexine** (Bisolvon®), **carbocisteine** (Mucodyne®), and **methylcysteine** (Visclair®) are given by mouth.

INHALATIONAL MUCOLYTICS

ACETYLCYSTEINE
Indications: reduction of sputum viscosity
Side-effects: bronchospasm, nausea, occasional febrile reactions; stomatitis
Dose: by inhalation of a nebulised solution, 0.4–1 g (2–5 ml of a 20% solution) through a mask or facepiece every 6–8 hours; may also be given *by direct instillation* into trachea, 200–400 mg (1–2 ml) every 1–4 hours, or nebulised into a tent, up to 50 g (250 ml)

PoM **Airbron®** (DF)
Solution, acetylcysteine 200 mg/ml (20%). Price 2-ml amp = **B**; 10-ml vial = **E**

Note: apparatus must be of glass or suitable plastic, not metal or rubber

TYLOXAPOL
Indications: reduction of sputum viscosity
Side-effects: occasional febrile reactions
Dose: by inhalation of a nebulised solution, continuous treatment using an Oxygenaire atomiser 144–360 ml (180–450 mg) over 24 hours *or* intermittent treatment 6–20 ml of a 0.125% solution (7.5–25 mg) over a period of 24 hours divided into 3–4 doses inhaled over 20 minutes; concentration adjusted to equipment and oxygen flow rate

Alevaire® (Winthrop)
Solution, tyloxapol 0.125% (1.25 mg/ml). Price 60 ml = **G**
Note: brass or copper apparatus should not be used

ORAL AND PARENTERAL MUCOLYTICS

ACETYLCYSTEINE
Indications: reduction of sputum viscosity
Side-effects: occasionally gastro-intestinal irritation, headache, urticaria, tinnitus, and sensitivity
Dose: adults and children over 6 years, 200 mg in water 3 times daily, usually for 5–10 days but if necessary may be extended to 6 months or longer; CHILD up to 2 years 200 mg daily, 2–6 years 200 mg twice daily

NHS ▼ PoM **Fabrol®** (Ciba)
Granules, yellow, acetylcysteine 200 mg/sachet. Price 30 sachets = **G**. Label: 13

BROMHEXINE HYDROCHLORIDE
Indications: reduction of sputum viscosity
Cautions: gastric ulceration
Side-effects: gastro-intestinal irritation, transient increased serum transaminase
Dose: by mouth, 8–16 mg 3–4 times daily; CHILD up to 1 year 2 mg twice daily, 1–5 years 4 mg twice daily, 6–10 years 4 mg 4 times daily
By slow intravenous or deep intramuscular injection, 8–24 mg daily
By intravenous infusion, 4–20 mg in 250–500 ml glucose intravenous infusion 5% or 4–40 mg in 450–500 ml of sodium chloride intravenous infusion 0.9%

PoM **Bisolvon®** (Boehringer Ingelheim)
NHS *Tablets*, yellow, bromhexine hydrochloride 8 mg. Price 20 tabs = **D**

NHS *Elixir*, yellow, bromhexine hydrochloride 4 mg, menthol 1 mg/5 ml. Diluent sorbitol solution or water for preparations, life of diluted elixir 14 days. Price 100 ml = **C**
Injection, bromhexine hydrochloride 2 mg/ml. Price 2-ml amp = **B**

CARBOCISTEINE
Indications: reduction of sputum viscosity
Side-effects: occasional gastro-intestinal irritation, rashes
Dose: 750 mg 3 times daily initially, then 1.5 g daily in divided doses; CHILD 2–5 years 62.5–125 mg 4 times daily, 6–12 years 250 mg 3 times daily

NHS PoM **Mucodyne®** (Berk)
Capsules, yellow, carbocisteine 375 mg. Price 20 caps = **F**
Syrup (= elixir), amber-coloured, carbocisteine 250 mg/5 ml. Diluent syrup (without preservative), life of diluted elixir 14 days. Price 100 ml = **E**
Syrup forte (= mixture), orange, carbocisteine 750 mg/5 ml. Diluent as above. Price 100 ml = **G**
Paediatric syrup (= elixir), red, carbocisteine 125 mg/5 ml. Diluent as above. Price 100 ml = **D**
NHS PoM **Mucolex®** (Warner)
Tablets, orange, carbocisteine 375 mg. Price 20 tabs = **E**
Syrup (= elixir), red, carbocisteine 250 mg/5 ml. Price 100 ml = **E**

METHYLCYSTEINE HYDROCHLORIDE
Indications: reduction of sputum viscosity
Dose: 100–200 mg 3–4 times daily before meals reduced to 200 mg twice daily after 6 weeks; CHILD over 5 years 100 mg 3 times daily
Prophylaxis, 100–200 mg 2–3 times every other day during winter months

NHS **Visclair®** (Sinclair)
Tablets, yellow, s/c, e/c, methylcysteine hydrochloride 100 mg. Price 20 tabs = **E**. Label: 5, 22, 25

3.8   Inhalations

Inhalations containing volatile substances such as eucalyptus oil are traditionally used and although the vapour may contain little of the additive it encourages deliberate inspiration of warm moist air which is often comforting in bronchitis. Inhalations are also used for the relief of nasal obstruction in acute rhinitis or sinusitis.

Benzoin Tincture, Compound, balsamic acids approx. 4.5%. Price 50 ml = **B**. Label: 15
Directions for use: add one teaspoonful to a pint of hot, not boiling, water and inhale the vapour

---

NHS **Menthol and Benzoin Inhalation,** menthol 2%, in benzoin inhalation (see Formulary). Price 50 ml = **B**. Label: 15
Directions for use: add one teaspoonful to a pint of hot, not boiling, water and inhale the vapour

Menthol and Eucalyptus Inhalation, (see Formulary). Price 50 ml = **A**
Directions for use: as above

NHS **Karvol®** (Crookes Products)
Inhalation capsules, menthol 35.9 mg, with chlorbutol, cinnamon oil, pine oil, terpineol, and thymol. Price 10 caps = **C**
Directions for use: inhale vapour from contents of 1 capsule expressed into handkerchief or a pint of hot, not boiling, water

3.9   Antitussives

3.9.1 Cough suppressants
3.9.2 Expectorant, demulcent, and compound cough preparations

3.9.1   Cough suppressants

The drawbacks of prescribing cough suppressants are rarely outweighed by the benefits of treatment and only occasionally are they useful, as, for example, if sleep is disturbed by a dry cough. Cough suppressants may cause sputum retention and this may be harmful in patients with chronic bronchitis and bronchiectasis. Though commonly used in acute bronchitis and pneumonia they are usually unnecessary and such conditions are best treated by prompt administration of antibacterial drugs (see section 5.1, Table 1).

Cough suppressants include codeine, dextromethorphan, isoaminile citrate (Dimyril®), noscapine, and pholcodine, sometimes prescribed in compound preparations (section 3.9.2); they are seldom sufficiently potent to be effective and all tend to cause constipation. Preparations containing opiates should be avoided in patients with liver disease.

Diamorphine and methadone are effective cough suppressants and are given in linctuses to control distressful cough in terminal lung cancer. In other circumstances they are contra-indicated because they induce sputum retention and ventilatory failure as well as causing narcotic dependence.

CODEINE PHOSPHATE

Indications: dry or painful cough
Cautions: asthma; see also notes above. Drug interactions: see Appendix 1 (sections *1*, *2.3*, *4.1*, *4.3*)
Contra-indications: liver disease
Side-effects: constipation, in large doses respiratory depression

Codeine Linctus, codeine phosphate 15 mg/5 ml. Price 100 ml = **B**
Dose: 5–10 ml 3–4 times daily

Codeine Linctus, Diabetic, codeine phosphate 15 mg/5 ml (see Formulary). Price 100 ml = **B**
Dose: 5–10 ml 3–4 times daily
Codeine Linctus, Paediatric, codeine phosphate 3 mg/5 ml (see Formulary). Price 100 ml = **A**
Dose: CHILD 1–5 years 10 ml

DEXTROMETHORPHAN HYDROBROMIDE

Indications: dry or painful cough
Cautions; Contra-indications; Side-effects: see under Codeine Phosphate and notes above

NHS **Cosylan®** (P-D)
Syrup (= elixir), dextromethorphan hydrobromide 13.5 mg/5 ml. Diluent syrup, life of diluted elixir 14 days. Price 100 ml = **C**
Dose: 5 ml 3–4 times daily; CHILD 1–5 years ¼ adult dose, 6–12 years ½ adult dose

DIAMORPHINE HYDROCHLORIDE

Indications: dry or painful cough in terminal disease
Cautions; Contra-indications; Side-effects: see under Codeine Phosphate and notes above
Dose: 1.5–6 mg every 4 hours when required

CD **Diamorphine Linctus,** diamorphine hydrochloride 3 mg/5 ml (see Formulary). Price 100 ml = **B**

ISOAMINILE CITRATE

Indications: dry or painful cough
Cautions: see notes above
Side-effects: rarely constipation, dizziness, nausea
Dose: 40 mg 3–5 times daily; CHILD, 20–40 mg 3–5 times daily

NHS PoM **Dimyril®** (Fisons)
Linctus, red, isoaminile citrate 40 mg/5 ml. Diluent syrup, life of diluted linctus 14 days. Price 150 ml = **E**

METHADONE HYDROCHLORIDE

Indications: dry or painful cough in terminal disease
Cautions; Contra-indications; Side-effects: see under Codeine Phosphate and notes above
Dose: 1–2 mg every 4 hours; CHILD 5–10 years 250 micrograms, 11–14 years 500 micrograms every 4 hours

CD **Methadone Linctus,** yellow, methadone hydrochloride 2 mg/5 ml (see Formulary). Price 100 ml = **C**
NHS CD **Physeptone®** (Calmic)
Linctus, brown, methadone hydrochloride 2 mg/5 ml. Diluent syrup, life of diluted linctus 14 days. Price 100 ml = **D**

C = 51-100p, D = 101-180p, E = 181-300p, F = 301-450p, G = 451-650p, H = 651-900p, I = 901-1200p, J = over 1200p.

NOSCAPINE

Indications: dry or painful cough

Cautions: see notes above

Dose: 15–30 mg 3–4 times daily; CHILD, 4 times daily, up to 1 year 1 mg, 2–5 years 2–5 mg, 6–12 years 6–12 mg

NHS **Noscapine Linctus,** noscapine 15 mg/5 ml (see Formulary). Price 100 ml = **B**

PHOLCODINE

Indications: dry or painful cough

Cautions; Contra-indications; Side-effects: see under Codeine Phosphate and notes above

Dose: 10 mg up to 6 times daily; CHILD 5 mg up to 6 times daily

Pholcodine Linctus, pholcodine 5 mg/5 ml. Price 100 ml = **B**

Pholcodine Linctus, Strong, pholcodine 10 mg/5 ml. Price 100 ml = **B**

Dia-tuss® (Lipha)

Syrup (= linctus), sugar-free, orange, pholcodine 10 mg/5 ml. Diluent sorbitol solution, life of diluted linctus 14 days. Price 100 ml = **C**

Dose: 5 ml 4 times daily; CHILD over 2 years half adult dose

NHS **Sancos®** (Sandoz)

Syrup (= linctus), pholcodine 5 mg/5 ml. Diluent syrup, life of diluted linctus 14 days. Price 100 ml = **B**

Dose: 10 ml every 3–4 hours; CHILD 2.5–5 ml

NHS **Triopaed®** (Sandoz)

Linctus, pholcodine 4 mg/5 ml. Diluent syrup, life of diluted linctus 14 days. Price 100 ml = **C**

Dose: CHILD 2–5 years 5 ml, 6–12 years 5–10 ml, every 6 hours

3.9.2 Expectorant, demulcent, and compound cough preparations

The prescriber is often called upon to prescribe such preparations for minor respiratory disorders. Although there is no scientific basis for prescribing any of the preparations listed in this section, it may be be that a harmless expectorant such as ammonia and ipecacuanha mixture or a demulcent such as simple linctus has a useful placebo role. Certainly this is preferable to the indiscriminate prescribing of antibiotics.

Expectorants are claimed to promote expulsion of bronchial secretions but there is no evidence that any drug, whether given by mouth, injection, or inhalation can specifically facilitate expectoration by stimulation or augmentation of the cough reflex.

Sub-emetic doses of expectorants such as ammonium chloride, ipecacuanha, and squill are commonly used to treat cough on the basis that emetic doses of these substances can without doubt expel mucus at the same time as provoking retching and vomiting by gastric irritation, but the assumption that sub-emetic doses can also promote expectoration is a myth. However, a simple expectorant mixture may serve a useful placebo function and has the advantage of being inexpensive. Expectorants are included in many compound preparations but the use of such mixtures should be avoided. Mucolytics (section 3.7) and inhalations (section 3.8) are also claimed to facilitate expectoration.

Demulcent cough preparations contain soothing substances such as syrup or glycerol and certainly some patients believe that such preparations relieve a dry irritating cough. Preparations such as **simple linctus** have the advantage of being harmless and inexpensive and **paediatric simple linctus** is particularly useful in children.

Compound cough preparations have no place in the treatment of respiratory disorders. Many of them contain an unnecessarily large number of ingredients, often in subtherapeutic doses, and often with similar therapeutic properties. Other preparations contain ingredients which have opposing effects, in particular the inclusion of expectorants together with antihistamines, sedatives, cough suppressants, bronchodilators, and sympathomimetics. Such preparations are to be **deprecated** not only as irrational but also for administering a large number of drugs to patients in inappropriate dosage and in excess of their needs; for example, the sedative effect of antihistamines may lead to carbon dioxide retention in patients with chronic bronchitis or emphysema. It is therefore best to prescribe one of the simple cough mixtures recommended above and if any other component is needed it may then be prescribed separately, tailored to the needs of the patient, and dosage adjusted accordingly.

NHS **Ammonia and Ipecacuanha Mixture** (see Formulary). Price 100 ml = **A**

Dose: 10–20 ml 3–4 times daily

NHS **Ammonium Chloride and Morphine Mixture** (see Formulary). Price 100 ml = **A**

Dose: 10–20 ml 3–4 times daily

NHS **Ipecacuanha and Morphine Mixture** (see Formulary). Price 100 ml = **A**

Dose: 10 ml 3–4 times daily

Simple Linctus (see Formulary). Price 100 ml = **A**

Dose: 5 ml 3–4 times daily

Simple Linctus, Paediatric (see Formulary). Price 100 ml = **A**

Dose: CHILD, 5–10 ml 3–4 times daily

NHS **Squill Linctus, Opiate,** Gee's Linctus (see Formulary). Price 100 ml = **A**

Dose: 5 ml 3–4 times daily

NHS **Squill Linctus, Opiate, Paediatric** (see Formulary). Price 100 ml = **B**

Dose: 5–10 ml 3–4 times daily

Squill Pastilles, Opiate (Gee's Pastilles), each = 2 ml opiate squill linctus. Price 20 pastilles = **B**

Dose: 1–2 pastilles sucked 3–4 times daily

NHS **Tolu Linctus, Compound, Paediatric** (see Formulary). Price 100 ml = **B**

Dose: CHILD, 5–10 ml 3–4 times daily

NHS **Actifed®** (Wellcome)

Compound linctus, red, dextromethorphan hydrobromide 10 mg, pseudoephedrine hydrochloride 30 mg, triprolidine hydrochloride 1.25 mg/5 ml. Diluent syrup,

---

Relative prices: **A** = up to 20p, **B** = 21–50p,

life of diluted linctus 14 days. Price 100 ml = **C**. Label: 2

Dose: 10 ml 3 times daily; CHILD 1–5 years 5 ml, 6–12 years 7.5 ml

NHS Actifed Expectorant® (Wellcome)

Elixir, orange, guaiphenesin 100 mg, pseudoephedrine hydrochloride 30 mg, triprolidine hydrochloride 1.25 mg/5 ml. Diluent syrup, life of diluted elixir 14 days. Price 100 ml = **C**. Label: 2

Dose: 10 ml 3 times daily; CHILD 1–5 years 2.5 ml, 6–12 years 5 ml

NHS Benylin Expectorant® (P-D)

Syrup (= elixir), red, ammonium chloride 135 mg, diphenhydramine hydrochloride 14 mg, sodium citrate 57 mg/5 ml. Diluent syrup, life of diluted elixir 14 days. Price 100 ml = **B**. Label: 2

Dose: 10 ml every 2–3 hours; CHILD 1–5 years 2.5 ml, 6–12 years 5 ml every 3–4 hours

NHS Benylin Paediatric® (P-D)

Syrup (= elixir), red, diphenhydramine hydrochloride 7 mg, menthol 550 micrograms, sodium citrate 28.5 mg/5 ml. Diluent syrup, life of diluted elixir 14 days. Price 100 ml = **B**. Label: 1

Dose: CHILD 1–5 years 5 ml, 6–12 years 10 ml every 3 hours

NHS Benylin with Codeine® (P-D)

Syrup (= elixir), red, codeine phosphate 5.7 mg, diphenhydramine hydrochloride 14 mg, menthol 1.1 mg, sodium citrate 57 mg/5 ml. Diluent syrup, life of diluted elixir 14 days. Price 100 ml = **C**. Label: 2

Dose: 10 ml every 3–4 hours; CHILD 1–5 years 2.5 ml, 6–12 years 5 ml

NHS Copholco® (Rorer)

Linctus, brown, pholcodine 5.63 mg, cineole 0.0026 ml, menthol 1.41 mg, terpin hydrate 2.82 mg/5 ml. Do not dilute. Price 100 ml = **C**

Dose: 10 ml 4–5 times daily; CHILD over 5 years 2.5–5 ml

Copholcoids® (Rorer)

Pastilles, black, pholcodine 4 mg, cineole 0.004 ml, menthol 2 mg, terpin hydrate 16 mg. Price 50 g = **C**

Dose: 1–2 pastilles sucked 3–4 times daily; CHILD over 5 years 1 pastille 3 times daily

NHS Davenol® (Wyeth)

Linctus, orange, carbinoxamine maleate 2 mg, ephedrine hydrochloride 7 mg, pholcodine 4 mg/5 ml. Diluent syrup (without preservative), life of diluted linctus 15 days. Price 100 ml = **B**. Label: 2

Dose: 5–10 ml 3–4 times daily; CHILD up to 5 ml

NHS Dimotane Expectorant® (Robins)

Elixir, pink, brompheniramine maleate 2 mg, guaiphenesin 100 mg, phenylephrine hydrochloride 5 mg, phenylpropanolamine hydrochloride 5 mg/5 ml. Diluent syrup, life of diluted elixir 14 days. Price 100 ml = **C**. Label: 2

Dose: 5–10 ml 3–4 times daily; CHILD up to 3 years 1–2.5 ml, 3–5 years 2.5–5 ml, 6–12 years 5 ml

NHS Dimotane with Codeine® (Robins)

Elixir, pink, sugar-free, brompheniramine maleate 2 mg, codeine phosphate 10 mg, pseudoephedrine hydrochloride 30 mg/5 ml. Diluent 70% glycerol, life of diluted elixir 14 days. Price 100 ml = **C**. Label: 2

Dose: 10 ml 3 times daily; CHILD 6–12 years 7.5 ml

NHS Dimotane with Codeine Paediatric® (Robins)

Elixir, pink, sugar-free, brompheniramine maleate 2 mg, codeine phosphate 3 mg, pseudoephedrine hydrochloride 15 mg/5 ml. Diluent as above. Price 100 ml = **C**. Label: 1

Dose: CHILD 2–3 years 5 ml, 4–6 years 10 ml, 7–12 years 15 ml, 3 times daily

NHS Expulin® (Galen)

Linctus, chlorpheniramine maleate 2 mg, ephedrine hydrochloride 8 mg, pholcodine 5 mg/5 ml. Diluent syrup, life of diluted linctus 14 days. Price 100 ml = **C**. Label: 2

Dose: 10–15 ml every 6 hours, max. 45 ml daily; CHILD 2–5 years 2.5–5 ml, 6–12 years 5–10 ml every 6 hours

Paediatric linctus, pink, chlorpheniramine maleate 1 mg, ephedrine hydrochloride 4 mg, pholcodine 2 mg/5 ml. Diluent syrup, life of diluted linctus 14 days. Price 100 ml = **C**. Label: 1

Dose: 3–12 months 2.5 ml, 1–5 years 5–10 ml, 6–12 years 10 ml 3 times daily

NHS PoM Extil Compound® (Evans)

Linctus, reddish-pink, carbinoxamine maleate 6 mg, noscapine 25 mg, pseudoephedrine 49.2 mg/10 ml. Do not dilute. Price 100 ml = **C**. Label: 2, counselling advised, do not shake

Dose: 10 ml 3–4 times daily; CHILD 2–12 years 2.5–5 ml

NHS Exyphen® (Norton)

Elixir, red, brompheniramine maleate 2 mg, guaiphenesin 80 mg, phenylephrine hydrochloride 4.75 mg, phenylpropanolamine hydrochloride 5 mg/5 ml. Diluent syrup, life of diluted elixir 14 days. Price 100 ml = **B**. Label: 2

Dose: 5–10 ml 4 times daily; CHILD 2.5–5 ml

NHS PoM Flavelix® (Pharmax)

Elixir, yellow, ammonium chloride 90 mg, ephedrine hydrochloride 10 mg, mepyramine maleate 12.5 mg, sodium citrate 40 mg/5 ml. Diluent syrup, life of diluted elixir 14 days. Price 100 ml = **B**. Label: 2

Dose: 10 ml 3–4 times daily; CHILD 1–5 years 2.5 ml, 6–10 years 5 ml, 3 times daily

NHS Guanor Expectorant® (RP Drugs)

Syrup (= elixir), red, ammonium chloride 135 mg, diphenhydramine hydrochloride 14 mg, menthol 1.1 mg, sodium citrate 57 mg/5 ml. Price 100 ml = **B**. Label: 2

Dose: 5–10 ml every 2–3 hours; CHILD 1–5 years 2.5 ml, 6–12 years 5 ml, every 3–4 hours

NHS Histalix® (Wallace Mfg)

Syrup (= elixir), ammonium chloride 135 mg, diphenhydramine hydrochloride 14 mg, menthol 1.1 mg, sodium citrate 57 mg/5 ml. Price 150 ml = **C**. Label: 2

Dose: 5–10 ml every 3 hours; CHILD 2.5–5 ml

NHS Linctifed Expectorant® (Wellcome)

Syrup (= elixir), orange, codeine phosphate 7.5 mg, guaiphenesin 100 mg, pseudoephedrine hydrochloride 20 mg, triprolidine hydrochloride 1.25 mg/5 ml. Diluent syrup, life of diluted elixir 14 days. Price 100 ml = **C**. Label: 2

Dose: 10 ml 3 times daily

NHS Linctifed Expectorant Paediatric® (Wellcome)

Syrup (= elixir), red, codeine phosphate 3 mg, guaiphenesin 50 mg, pseudoephedrine hydrochloride 12 mg, triprolidine hydrochloride 600 micrograms/5 ml. Diluent syrup, life of diluted elixir 14 days. Price 100 ml = **C**. Label: 1

Dose: CHILD 1–5 years 5 ml, 6–12 years 10 ml

NHS Lotussin® (Searle)

Linctus, amber, dextromethorphan hydrobromide 6.25 mg, diphenhydramine hydrochloride 5 mg, ephedrine hydrochloride 7.5 mg, guaiphenesin 50 mg/5 ml. Diluent syrup, life of diluted linctus 14 days. Price 100 ml = **C**. Label: 2

Dose: 10 ml 3 times daily; CHILD 1–5 years 2.5–5 ml, 6–12 years 5–10 ml

NHS PoM Nethaprin Expectorant® (Merrell)

Syrup (= elixir), orange, bufylline 60 mg, doxylamine succinate 6 mg, etafedrine hydrochloride 20 mg, guaiphenesin 100 mg/5 ml. Do not dilute. Price 100 ml = **C**. Label: 2

Dose: 5–10 ml every 3–4 hours; CHILD 6–12 years 5 ml

NHS Noradran® (Norma)

Syrup (= elixir), diphenhydramine hydrochloride 5 mg, diprophylline 50 mg, ephedrine hydrochloride 7.5 mg, guaiphenesin 25 mg/5 ml. Price 100 ml = **B**. Label: 2

Dose: 10 ml every 4 hours; CHILD over 5 years 5 ml

C = 51-100p, **D** = 101-180p, **E** = 181-300p, **F** = 301-450p, **G** = 451-650p, **H** = 651-900p, **I** = 901-1200p, **J** = over 1200p.

NHS **Organidin**® (WBP)

Elixir, yellow, iodinated glycerol 60 mg/5 ml. Diluent glycerol and water for preparations equal parts, life of diluted elixir 14 days. Price 100 ml = **D**

Dose: 5 ml 4 times daily

NHS **Orthoxicol**® (Upjohn)

Syrup (= elixir), red, codeine phosphate 10.95 mg, methoxyphenamine hydrochloride 16.9 mg, sodium citrate 325 mg/5 ml. Diluent syrup, life of diluted elixir 14 days. Price 100 ml = **C**

Dose: 5–10 ml every 3–4 hours; CHILD 6–12 years 2.5–5 ml every 4 hours

Pavacol-D® (WBP)

Mixture, brown, papaverine hydrochloride 1 mg, pholcodine 5 mg/5 ml, suitable for diabetics. Diluent sorbitol solution, life of diluted mixture 14 days. Price 100 ml = **B**

Dose: 5–10 ml when required; CHILD 1–2 years 2.5 ml 3–4 times daily, 3–5 years 5 ml 3 times daily, 6–12 years 5 ml 4–5 times daily

NHS **Phenergan Compound Expectorant**® (M&B)

Linctus, straw coloured, promethazine hydrochloride 5 mg, citric acid 65 mg, ipecacuanha liquid extract 0.01 ml, potassium guaiacolsulphonate 45 mg/5 ml. Diluent syrup, life of diluted linctus 14 days. Price 100 ml = **B**. Label: 2

Dose: 5–10 ml 2–3 times daily; CHILD up to 5 years 2.5 ml, 6–10 years 2.5–5 ml

NHS **Phensedyl**® (M&B)

Linctus, orange-brown, codeine phosphate 9 mg, ephedrine hydrochloride 7.2 mg, promethazine hydrochloride 3.6 mg/5 ml. Diluent syrup, life of diluted linctus 14 days. Price 100 ml = **B**. Label: 2

Dose: 5–10 ml 2–3 times daily; CHILD 2–5 years 2.5 ml, 6–10 years 2.5–5 ml

NHS **Pholcolix**® (P-D)

Syrup (= elixir), paracetamol 150 mg, phenylpropanolamine hydrochloride 12.5 mg, pholcodine 5 mg/5 ml. Diluent syrup, life of diluted elixir 14 days. Price 100 ml = **D**

Dose: 10 ml 4 times daily; CHILD 2–5 years 2.5 ml, 6–12 years 5 ml

Pholcomed® (Medo)

NHS *Linctus*, red, papaverine hydrochloride 1.25 mg, pholcodine 5 mg/5 ml. Diluent syrup, life of diluted linctus 14 days. Price 125 ml = **B**

Dose: 10–15 ml 3–4 times daily after food; CHILD up to 2 years 2.5 ml, over 2 years 5 ml

Pastilles, black, papaverine hydrochloride 1 mg, pholcodine 4 mg. Price 20 pastilles = **C**

Dose: 1–2 pastilles hourly, max. 15 daily; CHILD 1 pastille, max. 7 daily

Pholcomed Diabetic® (Medo)

Linctus, red, ingredients as for Pholcomed but without sugar. Diluent purified water, freshly boiled and cooled, life of diluted linctus 14 days. Price 125 ml = **C**

NHS **Pholcomed Expectorant**® (Medo)

Syrup (= elixir), red, guaiphenesin 62.5 mg, methylephedrine hydrochloride 625 micrograms/5 ml. Price 125 ml = **C**

Dose: 10–20 ml 3 times daily; CHILD 2.5–5 ml

NHS **Pholcomed Forte**® (Medo)

Linctus, red, papaverine hydrochloride 5 mg, pholcodine 19 mg/5 ml. Diluent syrup, life of diluted linctus 14 days. Price 125 ml = **D**

Dose: 5 ml 3 times daily

NHS **Pholcomed Forte Diabetic**® (Medo)

Linctus, red, ingredients as for Pholcomed Forte but without sugar. Diluent purified water, freshly boiled and cooled, life of diluted linctus 14 days. Price 125 ml = **D**

NHS **Pholtex**® (Riker)

Mixture, s/r, orange, sugar-free, phenyltoloxamine 10 mg, pholcodine 15 mg/5 ml, as resin complexes. Diluent syrup or tragacanth mucilage, life of diluted

mixture 14 days. Price 100 ml = **C**. Label: 2

Dose: 5 ml 2–3 times daily; CHILD 2.5–5 ml

NHS **Rinurel**® (Warner)

Linctus, yellow, paracetamol 150 mg, phenylpropanolamine hydrochloride 12.5 mg, phenyltoloxamine citrate 11 mg, pholcodine 5 mg/5 ml. Diluent syrup, life of diluted linctus 28 days. Price 100 ml = **C**. Label: 2

Dose: 10 ml 4 times daily; CHILD 2–5 years 2.5 ml, 6–12 years 5 ml

NHS **Rubelix**® (Pharmax)

Elixir, red, ephedrine hydrochloride 6 mg, pholcodine 4 mg/5 ml. Diluent syrup, life of diluted elixir 14 days. Price 150 ml = **B**

Dose: 10 ml 3–4 times daily; CHILD 1–5 years 2.5 ml, 6–10 years 5 ml, 3 times daily

NHS **Sancos Co**® (Sandoz)

Syrup (= linctus), chlorpheniramine maleate 2 mg, glycerol 600 mg, pholcodine 5 mg, pseudoephedrine hydrochloride 20 mg/5 ml. Diluent syrup, life of diluted linctus 14 days. Price 100 ml = **B**. Label: 2

Dose: 10–15 ml every 6 hours; CHILD 2–5 years 2.5–5 ml, 6–12 years 5–10 ml

NHS **Sudafed Expectorant**® (Calmic)

Syrup (= elixir), red, guaiphenesin 100 mg, pseudoephedrine hydrochloride 30 mg/5 ml. Diluent syrup, life of diluted elixir 14 days. Price 100 ml = **C**

Dose: 10 ml 3 times daily; CHILD 1–5 years 2.5 ml, 6–12 years 5 ml

NHS **Syrtussar**® (Armour)

Syrup (= elixir), red, dextromethorphan hydrobromide 10 mg, pheniramine maleate 7.5 mg/5 ml. Diluent syrup, life of diluted elixir 14 days. Price 150 ml = **D**. Label: 2

Dose: 5–10 ml 3–4 times daily; CHILD 2–5 years 2.5 ml 3 times daily, 6–12 years 5 ml 3–4 times daily

NHS **Tancolin**® (Ashe)

Linctus (paediatric), orange, ascorbic acid 12.35 mg, citric acid 45.85 mg, dextromethorphan hydrobromide 2.62 mg, glycerol 655 mg, sodium citrate 99.56 mg, theophylline 15 mg/5 ml. Price 100 ml = **C**

Dose: CHILD 1–3 years 5 ml, 4–5 years 10 ml, 6–12 years 15 ml, 3 times daily

NHS **Tercoda**® (Sinclair)

Elixir, yellow, codeine phosphate 8 mg, terpin hydrate 8 mg/5 ml. Price 100 ml = **C**

Dose: 5–10 ml 3 times daily

NHS **Tercolix**® (Norton)

Elixir, yellow, codeine phosphate 13 mg, cineole 0.002 ml, menthol 1.5 mg, terpin hydrate 6.5 mg/5 ml. Price 100 ml = **C**

Dose: 5–10 ml 3–4 times daily; CHILD 2.5–5 ml

NHS PoM **Terpoin**® (Hough)

Elixir, yellow, cineole 4.15 mg, codeine phosphate 15 mg, guaiphenesin 50 mg, menthol 18.3 mg, terpin hydrate 9.15 mg/5 ml. Price 100 ml = **D**

Dose: 5–10 ml every 3 hours; CHILD up to 5 ml

NHS **Tixylix**® (M&B)

Linctus, red, pholcodine 1.5 mg (as citrate), promethazine hydrochloride 1.5 mg/5 ml. Diluent syrup, life of diluted linctus 14 days. Price 100 ml = **B**. Label: 2

Dose: 10–20 ml 3 times daily; CHILD 1–2 years 2.5–5 ml, 3–5 years 5 ml, 6–10 years 5–10 ml, 2–3 times daily

NHS **Triocos**® (Sandoz)

Syrup (= elixir), chlorpheniramine maleate 2 mg, glycerol 600 mg, pholcodine 5 mg, pseudoephedrine hydrochloride 20 mg/5 ml. Diluent syrup, life of diluted elixir 14 days. Price 100 ml = **C**. Label: 2

Dose: 10–15 ml up to 3 times daily; CHILD 2–5 years 2.5–5 ml, 6–12 years 5–10 ml

NHS **Triotussic**® (Sandoz)

Suspension (= mixture), orange, paracetamol 250 mg, pheniramine maleate 12.5 mg, phenylpropanolamine hydrochloride 12.5 mg. Do not dilute. Price 100 ml = **C**. Label: 2

For all abbreviations and symbols see inside cover.   Relative prices: **A** = up to 20p, **B** = 21-50p,

Dose: 5–10 ml every 4 hours, max. 30 ml daily; CHILD 12–15 years 5 ml every 4 hours, max. 20 ml daily

NHS Tussifans® (Norton)

Syrup (= elixir), red, belladonna liquid extract 0.007 ml, ipecacuanha liquid extract 0.013 ml, potassium citrate 250 mg, squill syrup 0.3 ml, tolu syrup 0.4 ml/5 ml. Price 100 ml = A

Dose: CHILD 2.5–10 ml when required

3.10 Systemic nasal decongestants

These preparations are of doubtful value but unlike the preparations for local application (see section 12.2.2) they do not give rise to rebound nasal congestion. They contain sympatho-mimetics, and should therefore be **avoided** in patients with hypertension, hyperthyroidism, coronary heart disease, or diabetes, and in patients taking monoamine-oxidase inhibitors. Drug interactions: see Appendix 1 (sections *2.4*, *2.5*, *4.3*) Many of the preparations also contain antihistamines which may cause drowsiness and affect ability to drive or operate machinery.

Ephedrine Preparations
Section 3.1.1.2

NHS Actifed® (Wellcome)

Tablets, scored, pseudoephedrine hydrochloride 60 mg, triprolidine hydrochloride 2.5 mg. Price 20 tabs = C. Label: 2

Dose: 1 tablet 3 times daily

Syrup (= elixir), yellow, pseudoephedrine hydrochloride 30 mg, triprolidine hydrochloride 1.25 mg/5 ml. Diluent syrup, life of diluted elixir 14 days. Price 100 ml = C. Label: 2

Dose: 10 ml 3 times daily; CHILD 3–12 months 2.5 ml, 1–5 years 5 ml, 6–12 years 7.5 ml

NHS Benylin Decongestant® (P-D)

Syrup (= elixir), yellow, diphenhydramine hydrochloride 14 mg, menthol 1.1 mg, pseudoephedrine hydrochloride 10 mg, sodium citrate 57 mg/5 ml. Diluent syrup, life of diluted elixir 14 days. Price 100 ml = C. Label: 2

Dose: 10 ml 4 times daily; CHILD 1–5 years 2.5 ml, 6–12 years 5 ml

NHS Congesteze® (Kirby-Warrick)

PoM *Tablets*, s/c, azatadine maleate 1 mg, pseudoephedrine sulphate 60 mg in outer layer, pseudoephedrine sulphate 60 mg in s/r core. Price 20 tabs = E. Label: 2, 25

Dose: 1 tablet twice daily

PoM *Syrup* (= elixir), yellow, azatadine maleate 1 mg, pseudoephedrine sulphate 30 mg/5 ml. Diluent syrup, life of diluted elixir 28 days. Price 120 ml = F. Label: 2

Dose: 5–10 ml twice daily; CHILD 1–5 years 1.25 ml, 6–12 years 2.5–5 ml

Paediatric syrup (= elixir), azatadine maleate 250 micrograms, pseudoephedrine sulphate 7.5 mg/5 ml. Price 120 ml = D. Label: 1

Dose: CHILD 1–6 years 5 ml, 7–12 years 10–20 ml, twice daily

NHS Dimotapp® (Robins)

Elixir, red-brown, brompheniramine maleate 4 mg, phenylephrine hydrochloride 5 mg, phenylpropanolamine hydrochloride 5 mg/5 ml. Diluent syrup, life of diluted elixir 14 days. Price 100 ml = C. Label: 2

Dose: 5–10 ml 3–4 times daily; CHILD 6–12 years 5 ml

Elixir, paediatric, red-brown, brompheniramine maleate

1 mg, phenylephrine hydrochloride 2.5 mg, phenylpropanolamine hydrochloride 2.5 mg/5 ml. Diluent as above. Price 100 ml = C. Label: 1

Dose: CHILD up to 2 years 2.5 ml, 2–5 years 2.5–10 ml, 6–12 years 10 ml, 3–4 times daily

NHS Dimotapp LA® (Robins)

Tablets, s/r, brown, s/c, brompheniramine maleate 12 mg, phenylephrine hydrochloride 15 mg, phenylpropanolamine hydrochloride 15 mg. Price 20 tabs = D. Label: 2, 25, counselling advised, gluten

Dose: 1–2 tablets twice daily

NHS Eskornade® (SK&F)

Spansule® (= capsules s/r), grey/clear, enclosing red, grey, and white pellets, isopropamide 2.5 mg (as iodide), diphenylpyraline hydrochloride 5 mg, phenylpropanolamine hydrochloride 50 mg. Price 20 caps = D. Label: 2, 25

Dose: 1 capsule twice daily

Syrup (= elixir), green, diphenylpyraline hydrochloride 1.5 mg, isopropamide 750 micrograms (as iodide), phenylpropanolamine hydrochloride 15 mg/5 ml. Diluent syrup, life of diluted elixir 14 days. Price 150 ml = D. Label: 2

Dose: 10 ml 3 times daily; CHILD 2–6 years 2.5 ml, 7–12 years 5 ml

NHS Expurhin® (Galen)

Paediatric linctus, orange, sugar-free, chlorpheniramine maleate 1 mg, ephedrine hydrochloride 4 mg, menthol 1.1 mg/5 ml. Price 100 ml = C. Label: 1

Dose: CHILD 1–5 years 5–10 ml 3 times daily, 6–12 years 10–15 ml

NHS PoM Halin® (Nicholas)

Tablets, s/r, s/c, dexbrompheniramine maleate 6 mg, pseudoephedrine sulphate 120 mg. Price 20 tabs = D. Label: 2, 25

Dose: adults and children over 12 years, 1 tablet every 8–12 hours

NHS Haymine® (Pharmax)

Tablets, s/r, yellow, chlorpheniramine maleate 10 mg, ephedrine hydrochloride 15 mg. Price 30 tabs = E. Label: 2, 25

Dose: 1 tablet 1–2 times daily

NHS Nezcaam® (Rybar)

Syrup (= elixir), yellow, phenylpropanolamine hydrochloride 7.5 mg, guiaphenesin 30 mg/5 ml. Diluent syrup or water for preparations, life of diluted elixir 14 days. Price 150 ml = D

Dose: CHILD 2–5 years 5 ml, 6–12 years 10 ml, 2–3 times daily

Orthoxine®
Section 3.1.1.2

NHS Rinurel® (Warner)

Tablets, pink, scored, paracetamol 300 mg, phenylpropanolamine hydrochloride 25 mg, phenyltoloxamine citrate 22 mg. Price 20 tabs = C. Label: 2

Dose: 1 tablet every 4 hours, max. 6 daily; CHILD over 12 years half adult dose

Sudafed® (Calmic)

Tablets, pseudoephedrine hydrochloride 60 mg. Price 20 tabs = C

Dose: 1 tablet 3 times daily

Elixir, pink, pseudoephedrine hydrochloride 30 mg/5 ml. Diluent syrup, life of diluted elixir 14 days. Price 100 ml = C

Dose: 10 ml 3 times daily; CHILD 3–12 months 2.5 ml, 1–5 years 5 ml, 6–12 years 7.5 ml

NHS PoM Sudafed SA® (Calmic)

Capsules, s/r, red/clear, pseudoephredrine hydrochloride 120 mg. Price 20 caps = D. Label: 25

Dose: 1 capsule every 12 hours

NHS Sudafed-Co® (Calmic)

Tablets, scored, paracetamol 500 mg, pseudoephedrine hydrochloride 60 mg. Price 12 tabs = C

Dose: 1 tablet 3 times daily; CHILD 6–12 years, half tablet

C = 51-100p, D = 101-180p, E = 181-300p, F = 301-450p, G = 451-650p, H = 651-900p, I = 901-1200p, J = over 1200p.

NHS Triogesic® (Sandoz)

Tablets, pink, scored, paracetamol 500 mg, phenyl-propanolamine hydrochloride 12.5 mg. Price 20 tabs = **B**

Dose: 1–2 tablets every 4 hours, max. 8 daily; CHILD over 6 years ½ tablet every 4 hours, max. 4 daily

Elixir, red, paracetamol 125 mg, phenylpropanolamine hydrochloride 3 mg/5 ml. Diluent syrup, life of diluted elixir 14 days. Price 100 ml = **B**

Dose: 20 ml every 4 hours, max. 160 ml daily; CHILD 1–5 years 5–10 ml, 6–12 years 10 ml, up to 4 times daily

NHS Triominic® (Sandoz)

Tablets, yellow, pheniramine maleate 25 mg, phenyl-propanolamine hydrochloride 25 mg. Price 20 tabs = **B**. Label: 2

Dose: 1 tablet every 6–8 hours, max. 3 daily

Syrup (= elixir), orange, pheniramine maleate 12.5 mg, phenylpropanolamine hydrochloride 12.5 mg/5 ml. Diluent syrup, life of diluted elixir 14 days. Price 100 ml = **B**. Label: 2

Dose: 10 ml up to 3 times daily; CHILD over 12 years 5 ml

NHS Uniflu Plus Gregovite C® (Unigreg)

Tablets, composite pack of pairs of tablets: Uniflu *tablets*, mauve, s/c, caffeine 30 mg, codeine phosphate 10 mg, diphenhydramine hydrochloride 15 mg, paracetamol 500 mg, phenylephrine hydrochloride 10 mg; Gregovite C *tablets*, yellow, ascorbic acid 300 mg. Price 6 of each tab = **C**; or 12 of each tab = **C**. Label: 2

Dose: 1 of each tablet every 4 hours

For all abbreviations and symbols see inside cover.   Relative prices: **A** = up to 20p, **B** = 21-50p,

4: Drugs acting on the
CENTRAL NERVOUS SYSTEM

In this chapter, drug treatments are discussed under the following headings:

4.1 Hypnotics, sedatives, and anxiolytics
4.2 Drugs used in psychoses and related disorders
4.3 Antidepressant drugs
4.4 Central nervous stimulants
4.5 Appetite suppressants
4.6 Drugs used in nausea and vertigo
4.7 Analgesics
4.8 Antiepileptics
4.9 Drugs used in parkinsonism and related disorders

4.1 Hypnotics, sedatives, and anxiolytics

4.1.1 Hypnotics and sedatives
4.1.2 Anxiolytics
4.1.3 Barbiturates and methyprylone
For peri-operative sedation see section 15.1.4.

Most anxiolytics will induce sleep when given in large doses at night and most hypnotics will sedate when given in divided doses during the day. Prescribing of these drugs is widespread but dependence (either physical or psychological) and tolerance to their effects occurs, notably with the barbiturates, but also with the benzodiazepines. This may lead to difficulty in withdrawing the drug after the patient has been taking it regularly for more than a few weeks. A withdrawal syndrome (section 4.1.2) may occur if drug treatment is terminated too abruptly. Hypnotics, sedatives, and anxiolytics should therefore not be prescribed indiscriminately but be reserved for short courses to alleviate acute conditions after the causal factors have been established. Most hypnotics lose their sleep-promoting properties within 3 to 14 days of continuous use.

The increasing trend towards prescribing more than one of these drugs for the same indication is **not** recommended. It may constitute a hazard and there is no evidence that side-effects are minimised.

The **benzodiazepines** are the most common class of drugs used; they tend to have a hypnotic action in high dosage and an anxiolytic action in low dosage. They have replaced the barbiturates (section 4.1.3). There is little convincing evidence that they are efficacious in the treatment of anxiety after 4 months continuous treatment.

The advantages of the benzodiazepines over the barbiturates are that side-effects are less frequent and psychological and physical dependence less likely to occur; benzodiazepines are also much less dangerous in overdosage and are less likely to interact with other drugs because they do not induce liver microsomal enzymes. The benzodiazepine withdrawal syndrome lasts longer

than with other drugs of dependence (8 to 10 days) and is characterised by insomnia, anxiety, loss of appetite and body weight, tremor, perspiration, and perceptual disturbances.

Hypnotics and anxiolytics may impair judgement and increase reaction time, and so affect ability to drive or operate machinery. Moreover the hangover effects of a night-time dose may impair driving etc. on the following day.

4.1.1 Hypnotics and sedatives

Before a hypnotic is prescribed the cause of the insomnia should be established and, where possible, the underlying factors should be treated. However, it should be noted that some patients have unrealistic sleep expectations, and others understate their alcohol consumption which is often the cause of the insomnia.

Transient insomnia may occur in those who normally sleep well and may be due to extraneous factors such as noise, shift work, and jet lag. If a hypnotic is indicated a rapidly eliminated drug should be chosen and administered only once or twice.

Short-term insomnia is usually related to an emotional problem or serious medical illness, may last for a few weeks, and may recur. A hypnotic may be useful but should not be given for more than 3 weeks and preferably only one. Intermittent use is desirable with the omission of some nightly doses. A rapidly eliminated drug will generally be appropriate.

Chronic insomnia is rarely benefited by hypnotics and is more often due to injudicious prescribing causing mild dependence. Psychiatric disorders, especially depression, and abuse of drugs and alcohol are common causes. Other causes are daytime catnapping; physical causes such as pain, cough, pruritus, and dyspnoea; and such psychiatric causes as anxiety and depression. Sleep disturbance is very common in depressive illness and early wakening is often a useful pointer. The psychiatric complaint should therefore be treated, adapting the drug regimen to alleviate insomnia. For example, in the treatment of depressive illness, amitriptyline, given at night, will also help to promote sleep.

Hypnotics should **not** be prescribed indiscriminately and routine prescribing, especially in hospitals, is undesirable though commonplace. Ideally, they should be reserved for short courses of treatment in the acutely distressed. Tolerance to their effects develops within 3 to 14 days of continuous use and long-term efficacy cannot be assured. For drug interactions, see Appendix 1 (sections 2.5, 4.1).

The prescribing of hypnotics to children, except for occasional use such as for night terrors and somnambulism, is not justified. Hypnotics should also be avoided in the elderly who are at risk of becoming ataxic and confused and so liable to fall and injure themselves.

A major drawback of using hypnotics over prolonged periods is that they may cause rebound insomnia and precipitate a withdrawal syndrome (section 4.1.2) when the drug is discontinued.

Where prolonged administration cannot be avoided hypnotics should be discontinued as soon as possible and the patient should be warned that sleep may be disturbed for a few days before normal rhythm is re-established; broken sleep with vivid dreams and increased REM (rapid eye movement) may persist for several weeks. This must represent a mild form of dependence even if clinical doses are used.

The benzodiazepines used as hypnotics include **nitrazepam** (Mogadon® etc.), **flunitrazepam** (Rohypnol®), **loprazolam** (Dormonoct®), and **flurazepam** (Dalmane®) which have a prolonged action; this may give rise to residual effects on the following day and with repeated dosage tend to be cumulative.

Alprazolam (Xanax®), **bromazepam** (Lexotan®), **lormetazepam** (Loramet®, Nocta-mid®), **temazepam** (Euhypnos®, Normison®), and **triazolam** (Halcion®) act for a shorter time and have little or no hangover effect but are usually inappropriate for patients with early wakening. Withdrawal phenomena are more common with the short-acting benzodiazepines. Benzodiazepine anxiolytics such as **diazepam** (section 4.1.2) given as a single dose at night may also be used as hypnotics.

Chloral hydrate and chloral derivatives remain useful hypnotics. **Dichloralphenazone** (Welldorm®) and **triclofos sodium** cause fewer gastro-intestinal upsets than chloral hydrate. Elixirs of chloral hydrate and triclofos sodium have a place in treating children and elderly patients.

Chlormethiazole (Heminevrin®) may be a useful hypnotic for elderly patients because of its freedom from hangover but, as with all hypnotics, routine administration is undesirable and dependence occurs occasionally. It is used in the treatment of acute withdrawal symptoms in alcoholics but to minimise the risk of dependence administration should be limited to 9 days under inpatient supervision.

Promethazine (Phenergan®) and **trimeprazine** (Vallergan®) are popular for use in children. A proprietary brand of promethazine hydrochloride tablets 20 mg (Sominex®) is on sale to the public, for use by adults in the treatment of occasional insomnia.

Alcohol is a poor hypnotic as its diuretic action interferes with sleep during the latter part of the night. With chronic use, alcohol disturbs sleep patterns and causes insomnia. For drug interactions, see Appendix 1 (sections 2.5, 2.8B, 4.1, 4.3, 5.1, 6.1, 8, 13).

CHLORAL HYDRATE

Indications: insomnia, sedation in the elderly
Cautions; Side-effects: see under Nitrazepam; doses are taken well diluted to minimise gastro-intestinal disturbances. Rashes may occur. Contact with skin and mucous membranes should be avoided. Rarely excitement may occur

Contra-indications: severe cardiac disease, gastritis, marked hepatic or renal impairment
Dose: insomnia, 0.5–1 g (max. 2 g), 15–30 minutes before bedtime; CHILD 30–50 mg/kg up to a max. single dose of 1 g
Sedation, 250 mg 3 times daily

PoM **Chloral Mixture,** chloral hydrate 500 mg/5 ml (see Formulary). Price 100 ml = **A**. Label: 2, 27
Dose: insomnia, 5–20 ml; CHILD 1–5 years 2.5–5 ml, 6–12 years 5–10 ml, taken well diluted with water 15–30 minutes before bedtime
PoM **Chloral Elixir, Paediatric,** chloral hydrate 200 mg/5 ml (see Formulary). Price 100 ml = **B**. Label: 1, 27
Dose: up to 1 year 5 ml, well diluted with water
PoM **Noctec®** (Squibb)
Capsules, red, chloral hydrate 500 mg. Price 20 caps = **C**. Label: 2, 27. To be taken with water

CHLORMETHIAZOLE EDISYLATE

Indications: insomnia, agitation in elderly patients, acute alcohol withdrawal (under supervision)
Cautions: see under Nitrazepam, but hangover is less pronounced, doses less cumulative and fewer precautions are required in pregnancy, and in nursing mothers or elderly patients. Special precautions for intravenous infusion; see also section 4.8.2. Drug interactions: see Appendix 1 (section 4.1)
Side-effects: sneezing, conjunctival irritation, headache, gastro-intestinal disturbances; rarely, confusion. On intravenous infusion in high doses, cardiovascular and respiratory depression and localised thrombophlebitis
Dose: by mouth, insomnia, 1–2 capsules at bedtime
Sedation, 1 capsule 3 times daily
Alcohol withdrawal, initially 2–4 capsules, repeated if necessary; day 1, 9–12 capsules; day 2, 6–8 capsules; day 3, 4–6 capsules, then gradually reduced over days 4–6; capsules given in 3–4 divided doses; treatment for not more than 9 days
Note: for an equivalent therapeutic effect 1 capsule ≡ 5 ml elixir
By intravenous infusion, acute alcohol withdrawal, 40–100 ml (320–800 mg) initially as 0.8% solution over 5–10 minutes and the infusion rate then adjusted according to response *or* 30–50 ml (240–400 mg) initially as a 0.8% solution at a rate of about 60 drops (4 ml)/minute, until drowsy, reduced to 10–15 drops/minute, than adjusted according to the response

PoM **Heminevrin®** (Astra)
Capsules, grey/brown, chlormethiazole base 192 mg in an oily basis. Price 20 caps = **D**. Label: 2
Syrup (= elixir), chlormethiazole edisylate 250 mg/5 ml. Diluent water for preparations,

life of diluted elixir 14 days. Price 100 ml = **D**.
Label: 2

Intravenous infusion 0.8%, chlormethiazole
edisylate 8 mg/ml. Price 500-ml bottle = **G**

DICHLORALPHENAZONE

Indications: insomnia
Cautions; Contra-indications; Side-effects: see
under Chloral Hydrate, but fewer gastro-intestinal disturbances. Also contra-indicated in
acute intermittent porphyria. Drug interactions: see Appendix 1 (sections *2.8A, 7*)
Dose: insomnia, 1.3–1.95 g (2–3 tablets) with
water 20 minutes before bedtime; CHILD up to
1 year 112.5–225 mg (2.5–5 ml elixir), 1–5 years
225–450 mg (5–10 ml elixir), 6–12 years 450–
900 mg (10–20 ml elixir) taken well diluted with
water 20 minutes before bedtime

PoM **Welldorm**® (S&N Pharm.)
Tablets, purple, f/c, dichloralphenazone 650 mg.
Price 30 tabs = **D**. Label: 27
Elixir, red, dichloralphenazone 225 mg/5 ml.
Diluent syrup, life of diluted elixir 14 days.
Price 150 ml = **D**. Label: 27

FLUNITRAZEPAM

Indications: insomnia
Cautions; Contra-indications; Side-effects: see
under Nitrazepam
Dose: 0.5–1 mg (elderly patients 500
micrograms) 30 minutes before bedtime; severe
insomnia, 1–2 mg

NHS ▼ PoM **Rohypnol**® (Sauter)
Tablets, purple, f/c, scored, flunitrazepam 1mg.
Price 20 tabs = **D**. Label: 2

FLURAZEPAM

Indications: insomnia where daytime sedation is
acceptable
Cautions; Side-effects: see under Nitrazepam.
Drug interactions: see Appendix 1 (section 4.1)
Dose: 15–30 mg (elderly patients 15mg) half an
hour before bedtime

NHS PoM **Flurazepam Hydrochloride Capsules,**
flurazepam 15 mg (as monohydrochloride), price
20 caps = **C**; 30 mg, price 20 caps = **D**. Label: 2

NHS PoM **Dalmane**® (Roche)
Capsules, grey/yellow, flurazepam 15 mg (as
hydrochloride). Price 20 caps = **D**. Label: 2
Capsules, black/grey, flurazepam 30 mg (as
hydrochloride). Price 20 caps = **D**. Label: 2
NHS PoM **Paxane**® (Steinhard)
Capsules, green/grey, flurazepam 15 mg (as
hydrochloride). Price 20 caps = **C**. Label: 2
Capsules, green/black, flurazepam 30 mg (as
hydrochloride). Price 20 caps = **D**. Label: 2

LOPRAZOLAM

Indications: insomnia
Cautions; Side-effects: see under Nitrazepam

Contra-indications: acute pulmonary insufficiency, myasthenia gravis
Dose: 1 mg at bedtime, increased to 1.5 or 2 mg
if required (max. 1 mg in elderly or debilitated
patients)

NHS ▼ PoM **Dormonoct**® (Roussel)
Tablets, yellow, scored, loprazolam 1 mg (as
mesylate). Price 20 tabs = **E**. Label: 2

LORMETAZEPAM

Indications: insomnia (useful in the elderly)
Cautions; Side-effects: see under Nitrazepam but
hangover is uncommon; doses less cumulative.
Less appropriate in patients with early
wakening
Contra-indications: myasthenia gravis
Dose: 1 mg (elderly patients 500 micrograms) at
bedtime

NHS ▼ PoM **Loramet**® (Wyeth)
Capsules, orange, lormetazepam 1 mg. Price 20
caps = **D**. Label: 2
NHS ▼ PoM **Noctamid**® (Schering)
Tablets, scored, lormetazepam 500 micrograms.
Price 20 tabs = **D**. Label: 2
Tablets, scored, lormetazepam 1 mg. Price 20
tabs = **D**. Label: 2

NITRAZEPAM

Indications: insomnia where daytime sedation is
acceptable
Cautions: hangover may affect a patient's ability
to drive or operate machinery and increase the
effects of alcohol; avoid prolonged use and
abrupt withdrawal thereafter. Caution in
obstructive lung disease, respiratory depression, pregnancy, breast-feeding, patients with
a history of drug abuse; reduce dosage in elderly
and debilitated patients, liver disease, renal
impairment. Drug interactions: see Appendix
1 (section 4.1)
Side-effects: hangover with drowsiness, dizziness, ataxia (particularly in the elderly);
occasionally confusion, dry mouth, hypersensitivity reactions. Prolonged use may give
rise to cumulation, tolerance, rebound insomnia, and dependence
Dose: 5–10 mg (elderly patients 2.5–5 mg), 30
minutes before bedtime

NHS PoM **Nitrazepam Capsules,** nitrazepam 5 mg.
Price 20 caps = **B**. Label: 2
PoM **Nitrazepam Tablets,** nitrazepam 5 and
10 mg. Price 20 tabs (both) = **B**. Label: 2
PoM **Nitrazepam Mixture,** nitrazepam 2.5 mg/
5 ml. Diluent syrup, life of diluted mixture 14
days. Price 150 ml = **E**. Label: 2
NHS PoM **Mogadon**® (Roche)
Capsules, purple/black, nitrazepam 5 mg. Price
20 caps = **B**. Label: 2
Tablets, scored, nitrazepam 5 mg. Price 20
tabs = **B**. Label: 2
NHS PoM **Nitrados**® (Berk)
Tablets, scored, nitrazepam 5 mg. Price 20
tabs = **B**. Label: 2

C = 51-100p, **D** = 101-180p, **E** = 181-300p, **F** = 301-450p, **G** = 451-650p, **H** = 651-900p, **I** = 901-1200p, **J** = over 1200p.

NHS PoM **Noctesed®** (Unimed)
Tablets, scored, nitrazepam 5 mg. Price 20
tabs = **B**. Label: 2
NHS PoM **Remnos®** (DDSA)
Tablets, scored, nitrazepam 5 mg. Price 20
tabs = **C**. Label: 2
Tablets, yellow, scored, nitrazepam 10 mg. Price
20 tabs = **E**. Label: 2
NHS PoM **Somnite®** (Norgine)
Tablets, scored, nitrazepam 5 mg. Price 20
tabs = **B**. Label: 2
Suspension (= mixture), off-white, nitrazepam
2.5 mg/5 ml. Diluent syrup, life of diluted mix-
ture 14 days. Price 150 ml = **E**. Label: 2
NHS PoM **Surem®** (Galen)
Capsules, mauve/grey, nitrazepam 5 mg. Price
20 caps = **B**. Label: 2
NHS PoM **Unisomnia®** (Unigreg)
Tablets, scored, nitrazepam 5 mg. Price 20
tabs = **B**. Label: 2

PROMETHAZINE HYDROCHLORIDE
Indications: mild insomnia, sedation
Cautions; Side-effects: see section 3.4.1
Dose: by mouth, 25–75 mg at bedtime; CHILD 6–
12 months 10 mg, 1–5 years 15–20 mg, 6–10
years 20–25 mg, at bedtime *or*, for daytime sedation, once or twice daily using the lower dose

Preparations
See section 3.4.1

TEMAZEPAM
Indications: insomnia (useful in the elderly)
Cautions; Side-effects: see under Nitrazepam, but
except at high dosage hangover is uncommon
and doses less cumulative. Less appropriate in
patients with early wakening
Dose: 10–30 mg (elderly patients 5–15 mg),
increasing in severe insomnia to 60 mg, immediately before bedtime

PoM **Temazepam Capsules,** temazepam 10 mg,
price 20 caps = **C**; 15 and 20 mg (both), price 20
caps = **D**; 30 mg, price 20 caps = **E**. Label: 2
PoM **Temazepam Elixir,** temazepam 10 mg/5 ml.
Diluent glycerol, life of diluted elixir 14 days.
Price 100 ml = **D**. Label: 2
NHS PoM **Euhypnos®** (Farmitalia Carlo Erba)
Elixir, green, temazepam 10 mg/5 ml. Diluent
glycerol, life of diluted elixir 14 days. Price
100 ml = **D**. Label: 2
NHS PoM **Euhypnos 10®** (Farmitalia Carlo Erba)
Capsules, green, temazepam 10 mg. Price 20
caps = **C**. Label: 2
NHS PoM **Euhypnos 20®** (Farmitalia Carlo Erba)
Capsules, green, temazepam 20 mg. Price 20
caps = **D**. Label: 2
NHS PoM **Normison®** (Wyeth)
Capsules, yellow, temazepam 10 mg. Price 20
caps = **C**. Label: 2
Capsules, yellow, temazepam 20 mg. Price 20
caps = **D**. Label: 2

TRIAZOLAM
Indications: insomnia (useful in the elderly)
Cautions; Side-effects: see under Nitrazepam, but
hangover is uncommon and doses less cumulative. Less appropriate in patients with early
wakening. Drug interactions: see Appendix 1
(section 4.1)
Dose: 125–250 micrograms (elderly patients
125 micrograms) 15–30 minutes before bedtime

PoM **Triazolam   Tablets,**   triazolam
125 micrograms, price 20 tabs = **C**; 250 micro-
grams, price 20 tabs = **D**. Label: 2
NHS PoM **Halcion®** (Upjohn)
Tablets, lavender, scored, triazolam 125 micro-
grams. Price 20 tabs = **C**. Label: 2
Tablets, blue, scored, triazolam 250 micrograms.
Price 20 tabs = **D**. Label: 2

TRICLOFOS SODIUM
Indications: insomnia
Cautions; Contra-indications; Side-effects: see
under Chloral Hydrate, but gastro-intestinal
disturbances are less common and it is not irritant to skin and mucous membranes
Dose: 1–2 g 30 minutes before bedtime; CHILD up
to 1 year 100–250 mg, 1–5 years 250–500 mg, 6–
12 years 0.5–1 g

PoM **Triclofos Elixir,** triclofos sodium 500 mg/5 ml.
Price 100 ml = **E**. Label: 2

TRIMEPRAZINE TARTRATE
Indications: sedation in children
Cautions; Side-effects: see section 3.4.1
Dose: daytime sedation, CHILD 3–6 years 15–
60 mg, 7–12 years 60–90 mg, daily in divided
doses
Insomnia, CHILD, 3 mg/kg 1 hour before
bedtime

Preparations
See section 3.4.1

4.1.2 Anxiolytics
Benzodiazepine anxiolytics can be effective in
alleviating definite anxiety states and they are
widely prescribed. Although there is a tendency
to prescribe these drugs to almost anyone with
stress-related symptoms, unhappiness, or minor
physical disease, their use in many situations is
unjustified. They should be limited to patients
whose anxiety is clearly handicapping, as when
it interferes with their work, leisure, or family
relationships. In children anxiolytic treatment
should be used only to relieve acute anxiety (and
related insomnia) caused by fear.
  Anxiolytic treatment should be limited to the
lowest possible dose for the shortest possible time
since tolerance develops with continuous use and
because of the danger of insidious development
of dependence and subsequent difficulty in withdrawing the drug. Addiction is particularly likely
in patients with a history of alcoholism or drug
abuse and in patients with marked personality

disorders. Withdrawal of the drug following either high dosage or long-term administration should be gradual as abrupt withdrawal may produce confusion, toxic psychosis, convulsions, or a condition resembling delirium tremens. In milder cases, symptoms may be similar to the original complaint and encourage further prescribing.

Anxiolytics, particularly the benzodiazepines, have been termed 'minor tranquillisers'. This term is misleading because not only do they differ markedly from the antipsychotic drugs ('major tranquillisers') but their use is by no means minor. Antipsychotics, in low doses, are also sometimes used in severe anxiety for their sedative action (section 4.2.1).

Benzodiazepines are the most important anxiolytics. Diazepam, chlordiazepoxide, medazepam, clorazepate, clobazam, ketazolam, prazepam, and bromazepam are the most appropriate drugs for relieving chronic anxiety as they have a long half-life and consequently a sustained anxiolytic action. **Prazepam** (Centrax®) is long-acting and possibly less sedative. Shorter-acting compounds such as **oxazepam** and **lorazepam** may be more appropriate in acute anxiety or for relieving phobic panic attacks but may carry a greater risk of withdrawal symptoms; they may be preferred in patients with hepatic impairment. **Clobazam** (Frisium®) is claimed to produce less psychomotor impairment.

Diazepam or **lorazepam**, by intravenous injection or by mouth, may have a place in the control of severe panic attacks. The intravenous route is the most rapid but the procedure is not without risk (section 4.8.2) and should be used only when alternative measures have failed. The intramuscular route has no advantage over the oral route.

Benzodiazepines are also used in the treatment of alcohol withdrawal, beginning with a large dose which is gradually reduced.

Meprobamate is **less effective** than the benzodiazepines and also more hazardous in overdosage and more likely to induce dependence.

Propranolol (see section 2.4) is often very effective in alleviating the palpitations and tremor which accompany anxiety and apprehension; a daily dose in the range 80 to 160 mg is usually effective. Oxprenolol may also be used.

DIAZEPAM

Indications: anxiety, insomnia, adjunctive treatment of acute alcohol withdrawal

Cautions: may affect a patient's ability to drive or operate machinery and increase the effects of alcohol, avoid prolonged use and abrupt withdrawal thereafter. Caution in closed-angle glaucoma, respiratory disease, late pregnancy, breast-feeding, patients with a history of drug abuse: reduce dose in elderly and debilitated patients, liver disease, renal impairment. Special precautions are necessary when diazepam is given by intravenous injection (section 4.8.2). Drug interactions: see Appendix 1 (sections *2.5, 4.1, 4.8, 4.9*)

Side-effects: drowsiness, dizziness, ataxia (particularly in the elderly); occasionally confusion, dry mouth, headache, hypersensitivity reactions; respiratory depression; on intravenous injection, pain, thrombophlebitis

Dose: by mouth, anxiety, 2 mg 3 times daily increased in severe anxiety to 15–30 mg daily in divided doses (elderly patients half adult dose); CHILD 1–5 mg daily in divided doses
Insomnia, 5–30 mg at bedtime

By intramuscular injection or slow intravenous injection (at a rate of not more than 5 mg/minute), for severe anxiety, control of acute panic attacks, and acute alcohol withdrawal, 10 mg, repeated if necessary after 4 hours

*By intravenous infusion—*section 4.8.2

By rectum in suppositories, 5–10 mg when required

Rectal solution, for acute anxiety and agitation, adults and children over 3 years 10 mg; CHILD 1–3 years and elderly patients 5 mg; repeat after 5 minutes if necessary

PoM **Diazepam Capsules,** diazepam 2 and 5 mg. Price 20 caps (both) = **A**. Label: 2

PoM **Diazepam Tablets,** diazepam 2, 5, and 10 mg. Price 20 tabs (all)=**A**. Label: 2

PoM **Diazepam Elixir,** diazepam 2 mg/5 ml. Diluent syrup or sorbitol solution, life of diluted elixir 14 days. Price 100 ml = **C**. Label: 2

NHS PoM **Alupram®** (Steinhard)
Tablets, scored, diazepam 2 mg. Price 20 tabs = **A**. Label: 2
Tablets, yellow, scored, diazepam 5 mg. Price 20 tabs = **B**. Label: 2
Tablets, blue, scored, diazepam 10 mg. Price 20 tabs = **B**. Label: 2

NHS PoM **Atensine®** (Berk)
Tablets, scored, diazepam 2 mg. Price 20 tabs = **A**. Label: 2
Tablets, yellow, scored, diazepam 5 mg. Price 20 tabs = **A**. Label: 2
Tablets, blue, scored, diazepam 10 mg. Price 20 tabs = **B**. Label: 2

PoM **Diazemuls®** (KabiVitrum)
Injection (emulsion), diazepam 5 mg/ml. For intravenous injection or infusion. Price 2-ml amp = **B**

NHS PoM **Evacalm®** (Unimed)
Tablets, scored, diazepam 2 mg. Price 20 tabs = **A**. Label: 2
Tablets, yellow, scored, diazepam 5 mg. Price 20 tabs = **A**. Label: 2

NHS PoM **Solis®** (Galen)
Capsules, violet/turquoise, diazepam 2 mg. Price 20 caps = **A**. Label: 2
Capsules, violet/mauve, diazepam 5 mg. Price 20 caps = **A**. Label: 2

PoM **Stesolid®** (CP)
Injection, diazepam 5 mg/ml. Price 2- and 4-ml amp (both) = **B**
Rectal tubes (= rectal solution), diazepam 2 mg/ml. Price 5 × 2.5-ml tubes = **F**
Rectal tubes (= rectal solution), diazepam 4 mg/ml. Price 5 × 2.5-ml tubes = **G**

C = 51-100p, D = 101-180p, E = 181-300p, F = 301-450p, G = 451-650p, H = 651-900p, I = 901-1200p, J = over 1200p.

NHS PoM Tensium® (DDSA)

Tablets, scored, diazepam 2 mg. Price 20 tabs = **A**. Label: 2

Tablets, yellow, scored, diazepam 5 mg. Price 20 tabs = **A**. Label: 2

Tablets, blue, scored, diazepam 10 mg. Price 20 tabs = **B**. Label: 2

PoM Valium® (Roche)

NHS *Capsules*, blue/white, diazepam 2 mg. Price 20 caps = **A**. Label: 2

NHS *Capsules*, blue/yellow, diazepam 5 mg. Price 20 caps = **B**. Label: 2

NHS *Tablets*, scored, diazepam 2 mg. Price 20 tabs = **A**. Label: 2

NHS *Tablets*, yellow, scored, diazepam 5 mg. Price 20 tabs = **B**. Label: 2

NHS *Tablets*, blue, scored, diazepam 10 mg. Price 20 tabs = **B**. Label: 2

NHS *Syrup*(=elixir), pink, diazepam 2 mg/5 ml. Diluent syrup or sorbitol solution, life of diluted elixir 14 days. Price 100 ml = **D**. Label: 2

Injection, diazepam 5 mg/ml. Do not dilute (except for intravenous infusion). Price 2- and 4-ml amp (both) = **B**

Suppositories, diazepam 5 mg. Price 5 suppos = **C**. Label: 2

Suppositories, diazepam 10 mg. Price 5 suppos = **C**. Label: 2

NHS ▼ PoM Valrelease® (Roche)

Capsules, s/r, light blue/blue, diazepam 10 mg. Price 20 caps = **D**. Label: 2, 25

Dose: 1 capsule daily (usually early evening), equivalent to diazepam 5 mg 3 times daily

ALPRAZOLAM

Indications: short-term treatment of anxiety and anxiety associated with depression

Cautions; Side-effects: see under Diazepam. Drug interactions: see Appendix 1 (section 4.1)

Contra-indications: acute pulmonary insufficiency

Dose: 250–500 micrograms 3 times daily (elderly or debilitated patients 250 micrograms 2–3 times daily), increased if necessary to a total of 3 mg daily

NHS ▼ PoM Xanax® (Upjohn)

Tablets, scored, alprazolam 250 micrograms. Price 20 tabs = **C**. Label: 2

Tablets, peach, scored, alprazolam 500 micrograms. Price 20 tabs = **D**. Label: 2

BROMAZEPAM

Indications: short-term treatment of anxiety and associated states

Cautions; Side-effects: see under Diazepam

Contra-indications: acute pulmonary insufficiency, respiratory depression

Dose: 3–18 mg daily in divided doses; elderly patients half adult dose; max. (in hospitalised patients) 60 mg daily in divided doses

NHS ▼ PoM Lexotan® (Roche)

Tablets, lilac, scored, bromazepam 1.5 mg. Price 20 tabs = **C**. Label: 2

Tablets, pink, scored, bromazepam 3 mg. Price 20 tabs = **D**. Label: 2

CHLORDIAZEPOXIDE

Indications: anxiety, acute alcohol withdrawal

Cautions; Side-effects: see under Diazepam. Drug interactions: see Appendix 1 (sections 4.1, *4.9*)

Dose: by mouth, anxiety, 10 mg 3 times daily increased in severe anxiety to 100 mg daily in divided doses; elderly and debilitated patients initially 10 mg daily; CHILD 5–20 mg daily in divided doses

By slow deep intramuscular injection, control of acute panic attacks and acute alcohol withdrawal, 50–100 mg, followed, if necessary, by 25–100 mg 3–4 times daily

Note: chlordiazepoxide and its hydrochloride are used interchangeably

PoM Chlordiazepoxide Capsules, chlordiazepoxide hydrochloride 5 and 10 mg. Price 20 caps (both) = **A**. Label: 2

PoM Chlordiazepoxide Hydrochloride Tablets, chlordiazepoxide hydrochloride 5 and 10 mg, price 20 tabs (both) = **A**; 25 mg, price 20 tabs = **B**. Label: 2

PoM Chlordiazepoxide Tablets, chlordiazepoxide 5 and 10 mg, price 20 tabs (both) = **B**; 25 mg, price 20 tabs = **C**. Label: 2

PoM Librium® (Sauter)

NHS *Capsules*, green/yellow, chlordiazepoxide hydrochloride 5 mg. Price 20 caps = **B**. Label: 2

NHS *Capsules*, green/black, chlordiazepoxide hydrochloride 10 mg. Price 20 caps = **B**. Label: 2

NHS *Tablets*, blue/green, f/c, chlordiazepoxide 5 mg. Price 20 tabs = **B**. Label: 2

NHS *Tablets*, blue/green, f/c, chlordiazepoxide 10 mg. Price 20 tabs = **B**. Label: 2

NHS *Tablets*, blue/green, f/c, chlordiazepoxide 25 mg. Price 20 tabs = **C**. Label: 2

Injection, powder for reconstitution, chlordiazepoxide (as hydrochloride). Price 100-mg amp (with solvent) = **C**

NHS PoM Tropium® (DDSA)

Capsules, yellow/black, chlordiazepoxide hydrochloride 5 mg. Price 20 caps = **A**. Label: 2

Capsules, green/white, chlordiazepoxide hydrochloride 10 mg. Price 20 caps = **A**. Label: 2

Tablets, green, s/c, chlordiazepoxide hydrochloride 5 mg. Price 20 tabs = **A**. Label: 2

Tablets, green, s/c, chlordiazepoxide hydrochloride 10 mg. Price 20 tabs = **A**. Label: 2

Tablets, green, s/c, chlordiazepoxide hydrochloride 25 mg. Price 20 tabs = **B**. Label: 2

CHLORMEZANONE

Indications: anxiety, insomnia, muscle spasm

Cautions; Side-effects: see under Diazepam

Dose: 200 mg 3 times daily *or* 400 mg at bedtime; max. 800 mg daily; elderly patients half adult dose

PoM Trancopal® (Winthrop)

Tablets, yellow, chlormezanone 200 mg. Price 20 tabs = **D**. Label: 2

CLOBAZAM

Indications: anxiety; adjunctive treatment of epilepsy

Cautions; Side-effects: see under Diazepam but less sedating. Drug interactions: see Appendix 1 (section 4.1)

Dose: 20–30 mg daily in divided doses or as a single dose at bedtime, increased in severe anxiety (in hospitalised patients) to a max. of 60 mg daily in divided doses; elderly and debilitated patients 20 mg daily; CHILD over 3 years, up to half adult dose

NHS *PoM **Clobazam Capsules,** clobazam 10 mg. Price 20 caps = **D**. Label: 2

NHS PoM **Frisium**® (Hoechst)

Capsules, blue, clobazam 10 mg. Price 20 caps = **D**. Label: 2

* except for epilepsy and endorsed 'S3B' ('S2B' in Scotland)

CLORAZEPATE DIPOTASSIUM

Indications: anxiety

Cautions; Side-effects: see under Diazepam

Contra-indications: acute pulmonary insufficiency

Dose: 7.5–22.5 mg daily, at bedtime *or* in 2–3 divided doses; elderly patients half adult dose

NHS PoM **Tranxene**® (Boehringer Ingelheim)

Capsules, maroon/grey, clorazepate dipotassium 7.5 mg. Price 20 caps = **C**. Label: 2

Capsules, pink/grey, clorazepate dipotassium 15 mg. Price 20 caps = **D**. Label: 2

HYDROXYZINE HYDROCHLORIDE

Indications: anxiety, adjunctive treatment in stress-related urticaria and dermatoses

Cautions; Side-effects: see under Antihistamines (section 3.4.1); caution in liver disease

Dose: 50–100 mg 4 times daily; urticaria, 25 mg 3–4 times daily; CHILD up to 6 years 50 mg, over 6 years 50–100 mg, daily in divided doses

PoM **Atarax**® (Pfizer)

Tablets, orange, s/c, hydroxyzine hydrochloride 10 mg. Price 20 tabs = **B**. Label: 2

Tablets, green, s/c, hydroxyzine hydrochloride 25 mg. Price 20 tabs = **C**. Label: 2

Syrup (= elixir), hydroxyzine hydrochloride 10 mg/5 ml. Diluent syrup, life of diluted elixir 14 days. Price 150 ml = **D**. Label: 2

KETAZOLAM

Indications: anxiety

Cautions; Side-effects: see under Diazepam

Dose: initially 30 mg (elderly patients 15 mg) at bedtime, adjusted according to the response; usual range 15–60 mg daily

NHS PoM **Anxon**® (Beecham)

Capsules, dark pink/light pink, ketazolam 15 mg. Price 20 caps = **D**. Label: 2

Capsules, dark pink/light pink, ketazolam 30 mg. Price 20 caps = **F**. Label: 2

LORAZEPAM

Indications: anxiety, insomnia

Cautions; Side-effects: see under Diazepam. It is less cumulative and excessive drowsiness is therefore less likely. Drug interactions: see Appendix 1 (section *4.9*)

Dose: by mouth, anxiety, 1–4 mg, increased to 10 mg in severe anxiety, daily in divided doses; elderly patients half adult dose

Insomnia, 1–4 mg at bedtime

By slow intramuscular or slow intravenous injection, for the control of acute panic attacks, 25–30 micrograms/kg every 6 hours if necessary

PoM **Lorazepam Tablets,** lorazepam 1 mg, price 20 tabs = **B**; 2.5 mg, price 20 tabs = **C**. Label: 2

NHS PoM **Almazine**® (Steinhard)

Tablets, green, scored, lorazepam 1 mg. Price 20 tabs = **B**. Label: 2

Tablets, pink, scored, lorazepam 2.5 mg. Price 20 tabs = **C**. Label: 2

PoM **Ativan**® (Wyeth)

NHS Tablets, blue, scored, lorazepam 1 mg. Price 20 tabs = **B**. Label: 2

NHS *Tablets*, yellow, scored, lorazepam 2.5 mg. Price 20 tabs = **C**. Label: 2

▼ *Injection*, lorazepam 4 mg/ml. Price 1-ml amp = **B**. For intramuscular injection it should be diluted with an equal volume of water for injections or sodium chloride intravenous infusion 0.9%

MEDAZEPAM

Indications: anxiety, adjunctive treatment of acute alcohol withdrawal

Cautions; Side-effects: see under Diazepam. It is less cumulative and excessive drowsiness is therefore less likely

Dose: anxiety, 5 mg 2–3 times daily, increased in severe anxiety to a max. of 40 mg daily in divided doses (elderly patients not more than half adult dose)

NHS PoM **Nobrium**® (Roche)

Capsules, orange/yellow, medazepam 5 mg. Price 20 caps = **B**. Label: 2

Capsules, orange/black, medazepam 10 mg. Price 20 caps = **C**. Label: 2

MEPROBAMATE

Indications: anxiety, particularly with muscle spasm

Cautions: see under Diazepam, but the risk of dependence is higher; in epilepsy, abrupt withdrawal may precipitate convulsions

Contra-indications: acute intermittent porphyria

Side-effects: see under Diazepam, but the incidence is greater and drowsiness is the most common side-effect. Also gastro-intestinal disturbances, paraesthesia, weakness, CNS effects which include headache, paradoxical excitement, disturbances of vision; rarely agranulocytosis and rashes

Dose: 400 mg 3 times daily, increased when

C = 51-100p, D = 101-180p, E = 181-300p, F = 301-450p, G = 451-650p, H = 651-900p, I = 901-1200p, J = over 1200p.

necessary to a max. of 2.4 g daily in divided doses

PoM **Meprobamate Tablets,** meprobamate 200 and 400 mg, price 20 tabs (both) = **A.** Label: 2

PoM **Equanil**® (Wyeth)
Tablets, meprobamate 200 mg. Price 20 tabs = **A.** Label: 2
Tablets, scored, meprobamate 400 mg. Price 20 tabs = **A.** Label: 2

PoM **Meprate**® (DDSA)
Tablets, meprobamate 400 mg. Price 20 tabs = **A.** Label: 2

PoM **Tenavoid**® (Burgess)
Tablets, orange, f/c, meprobamate 200 mg, bendrofluazide 3 mg. Price 24 tabs = **E.** Label: 2
Dose: premenstrual syndrome, 1 tablet 3 times daily starting 5–7 days before menstruation

OXAZEPAM

Indications: anxiety, adjunctive treatment of acute alcohol withdrawal
Cautions; Side-effects: see under Diazepam but repeated doses are less cumulative; drowsiness is the most common side-effect
Dose: anxiety, 15–30 mg (elderly patients 10–20 mg) 3–4 times daily, increased in severe anxiety to a max. of 60 mg 3 times daily

PoM **Oxazepam Tablets,** oxazepam 10, 15, and 30 mg, price 20 tabs (all) = **B.** Label: 2

NHS PoM **Oxanid**® (Steinhard)
Tablets, oxazepam 10 mg. Price 20 tabs = **B.** Label: 2
Tablets, oxazepam 15 mg. Price 20 tabs = **B.** Label: 2
Tablets, oxazepam 30 mg. Price 20 tabs = **B.** Label: 2

NHS PoM **Serenid-D**® (Wyeth)
Tablets, oxazepam 10 mg. Price 20 tabs = **B.** Label: 2
Tablets, oxazepam 15 mg. Price 20 tabs = **B.** Label: 2

NHS PoM **Serenid Forte**® (Wyeth)
Capsules, red/green, oxazepam 30 mg. Price 20 caps = **B.** Label: 2

PRAZEPAM

Indications: anxiety
Cautions; Side-effects: see under Diazepam
Contra-indications: acute pulmonary insufficiency
Dose: 30 mg (elderly patients 15 mg), daily in divided doses; usual range 10–60 mg daily

NHS ▼ PoM **Centrax**® (Warner)
Tablets, blue, scored, prazepam 10 mg. Price 20 tabs = **C.** Label: 2

4.1.3   Barbiturates and methyprylone

The intermediate-acting **barbiturates** and **methyprylone** (Noludar®), given orally, may still have a place in the treatment of severe intractable insomnia, but they should be avoided in the elderly. The long-acting barbiturates phenobarbitone and methylphenobarbitone are of value

in epilepsy (section 4.8.1) but their use as sedatives is unjustified. The very short-acting barbiturates, methohexitone and thiopentone, are used in anaesthesia (see section 15.1.1).

BARBITURATES

Indications: severe intractable insomnia
Cautions: avoid use where possible. Dependence and tolerance readily occur. Abrupt withdrawal may precipitate a serious withdrawal syndrome (rebound insomnia, anxiety, tremor, dizziness, nausea, fits, and delirium). Repeated doses are cumulative and may lead to excessive sedation; may affect ability to drive or operate machinery and increase the effects of alcohol. Caution in respiratory disease, renal disease, hepatic impairment. Drug interactions: see Appendix 1 (sections *2.8A*, *5.1*, *6.3*, *7*) ,
Contra-indications: insomnia caused by pain, porphyria, pregnancy, breast-feeding; avoid in children, elderly and debilitated patients, also patients with a history of drug or alcohol abuse
Side-effects: hangover with drowsiness, dizziness, ataxia, respiratory depression, hypersensitivity reactions, headache, particularly with the elderly. Also paradoxical excitement and confusion occasionally precedes sleep

CD **Amytal**® (Lilly)
Tablets, amylobarbitone 15, 30, and 50 mg. Price 20 tabs (all) = **A.** Label: 2
Tablets, amylobarbitone 100 mg. Price 20 tabs = **B.** Label: 2
Tablets, scored, amylobarbitone 200 mg. Price 20 tabs = **C.** Label: 2
Dose: 100–200 mg 30 minutes before bedtime

CD **Nembutal**® (Abbott)
Capsules, yellow, pentobarbitone sodium 100 mg. Price 20 caps = **A.** Label: 2
Dose: 100–200 mg 30 minutes before bedtime

CD **Phanodorm**® (Winthrop)
Tablets, cyclobarbitone calcium 200 mg. Price 20 tabs = **D.** Label: 2
Dose: 100–400 mg 30 minutes before bedtime

CD **Seconal Sodium**® (Lilly)
Capsules, orange, quinalbarbitone sodium 50 mg. Price 20 caps = **C.** Label: 2
Capsules, orange, quinalbarbitone sodium 100 mg. Price 20 caps = **C.** Label: 2
Dose: 50–100 mg 30 minutes before bedtime

CD **Sodium Amytal**® (Lilly)
Capsules, blue, amylobarbitone sodium 60 mg. Price 20 caps = **B.** Label: 2
Capsules, blue, amylobarbitone sodium 200 mg. Price 20 caps = **C.** Label: 2
Tablets, amylobarbitone sodium 60 mg. Price 20 tabs = **B.** Label: 2
Tablets, amylobarbitone sodium 200 mg. Price 20 tabs = **C.** Label: 2
Dose: 60–200 mg 15–30 minutes before bedtime
Injection, powder for reconstitution, amylobarbitone sodium. Price 250- and 500-mg vial (both) = **E**
Dose: by intramuscular or slow intravenous injection, sedation in severely agitated patients, 0.25–1 g daily; max. single dose, intramuscular 500 mg, intravenous 1 g

CD **Soneryl**® (M&B)
Tablets, pink, scored, butobarbitone 100 mg. Price 20 tabs = **A.** Label: 2
Dose: 100–200 mg 30 minutes before bedtime

CD **Tuinal**® (Lilly)
Capsules, orange/blue, amylobarbitone sodium 50 mg,

quinalbarbitone sodium 50 mg. Price 20 caps = **B**.
Label: 2
Dose: 1–2 capsules 15–30 minutes before bedtime

METHYPRYLONE
Indications; Cautions; Contra-indications; Side-effects: see under Barbiturates, but side-effects occur less frequently. Rashes and gastro-intestinal disturbances may occur
Dose: 200–400 mg 15 minutes before bedtime

PoM **Noludar**® (Roche)
Tablets, scored, methyprylone 200 mg. Price 20 tabs = **C**. Label: 2

4.2   Drugs used in psychoses and related disorders

4.2.1 Antipsychotic drugs
4.2.2 Antipsychotic depot injections
4.2.3 Lithium salts

4.2.1   Antipsychotic drugs

Antipsychotic drugs are also known as 'neuroleptics' and (misleadingly) as 'major tranquillisers'. Antipsychotic drugs generally tranquillise without impairing consciousness and without causing paradoxical excitement but they should not be regarded merely as tranquillisers. For conditions such as schizophrenia the tranquillising effect is of secondary importance.

In the short-term they are used to quieten disturbed patients whatever the underlying psychopathology, which may be brain damage, mania, toxic delirium, agitated depression, or acute behavioural disturbance.

They are used to alleviate severe anxiety but this also should be a short-term treatment. In patients with anxiety and depression, caution is necessary as the symptoms of depression may be masked.
SCHIZOPHRENIA. Antipsychotic drugs relieve florid psychotic symptoms such as thought disorder, hallucinations, and delusions, and prevent relapse. They are usually less effective in apathetic withdrawn patients.

Sometimes they appear to have an activating influence. For example, large doses of chlorpromazine may restore the acutely ill schizophrenic to normal activity and social behaviour where previously he was withdrawn or even mute and akinetic. Patients with acute schizophrenia generally respond better than those with chronic symptoms.

Long-term treatment of patients with a definite diagnosis of schizophrenia may be necessary even after their first episode of illness in order to prevent the manifest illness from becoming chronic. Withdrawal of drug treatment requires careful surveillance because the patient who appears well on medication may suffer a disastrous relapse if treatment is withdrawn inappropriately. In addition the need for continuation of treatment may not become immediately evident because

relapse is often delayed for several weeks after cessation of treatment.

Antipsychotic drugs are considered to act by interfering with dopaminergic transmission in the brain by blocking dopamine receptors and may give rise to the extrapyramidal effects described below, and also to hyperprolactinaemia. The antipsychotic drugs also affect to varying degrees cholinergic, alpha-adrenergic, histaminergic, and tryptaminergic receptors.
SIDE-EFFECTS. Extrapyramidal symptoms are the most troublesome. They are caused most frequently by fluphenazine, haloperidol, and the depot preparations. They are easy to recognise but cannot be accurately predicted because they depend partly on the dose and partly on the type of drug, and on patient idiosyncrasy. They consist of dystonia (abnormal face and body movements) which may appear after only a few doses, akathisia (restlessness) which may resemble an exacerbation of the condition being treated, and a parkinsonism-like syndrome which usually takes longer to develop.

These symptoms remit if the drug is withdrawn. Parkinsonian effects may be suppressed by the administration of **anticholinergic** drugs (section 4.9.2), but routine administration of such drugs is **not** justified as not all patients are affected and because tardive dyskinesia is worsened by them. Tardive dyskinesia is of particular concern because it may be irreversible on withdrawing therapy and treatment may be ineffective. It occurs fairly frequently in patients (especially the elderly) on long-term therapy and with high dosage, and the treatment of such patients must be carefully and regularly reviewed. Tardive dyskinesia may also occur occasionally after short-term treatment with low dosage.

Hypotension and interference with temperature regulation are dose-related side-effects and are liable to cause dangerous falls and hypothermia in the elderly; very serious consideration should be given before prescribing these drugs for patients over 70 years of age.
SELECTION. The various drugs differ somewhat in predominant actions and side-effects. Selection is influenced by the degree of sedation required and the patient's susceptibility to extrapyramidal side-effects. The differences between the antipsychotic drugs are less important than the great variability in patient response, and tolerance to these secondary effects usually develops. The increasing trend towards prescribing more than one antipsychotic for the same indication is **not** recommended. It may constitute a hazard and there is no significant evidence that side-effects are minimised.

Chlorpromazine (Largactil® etc.) is widely used. It has a marked sedating effect and is particularly useful for treating violent patients without causing stupor. Agitated states in the elderly can be controlled without confusion, a dose of 25 mg usually being adequate.
Flupenthixol (Depixol®) and **pimozide** (Orap®) are less sedating than chlorpromazine. Pimozide is regarded by many psychiatrists as the current

drug of choice in schizophrenia particularly for apathetic withdrawn patients.

Fluphenazine, haloperidol, and **trifluoperazine** are also of value but their use is limited by the high incidence of extrapyramidal symptoms. **Haloperidol** may be preferred for the rapid control of hyperactive psychotic states.

Thioridazine (Melleril®) is popular for treating the elderly as there is a reduced incidence of extrapyramidal symptoms.

Promazine (Sparine®) is not sufficiently active to be used as an antipsychotic drug but may be of value in elderly patients with minor psychiatric problems.

OTHER USES. **Chlorpromazine** and **prochlorperazine** are effective drugs for the relief of nausea and vomiting (section 4.6), and hiccups. **Haloperidol** is used as adjunctive treatment in choreas and stuttering (section 4.9.3). **Benperidol** is used in deviant and antisocial sexual behaviour but its value is not established. For peri-operative use of antipsychotics, see section 15.1.4.

CLASSIFICATION OF ANTIPSYCHOTICS. The **phenothiazine** derivatives can be divided into 3 main groups.

Group 1: chlorpromazine, methotrimeprazine, and promazine, characterised by pronounced sedative effects and moderate anticholinergic and extrapyramidal side-effects.

Group 2: pericyazine, pipothiazine, and thioridazine, characterised by moderate sedative effects, marked anticholinergic effects, but fewer extrapyramidal side-effects than groups 1 or 3.

Group 3: fluphenazine, perphenazine, prochlorperazine, sulpiride, thiethylperazine, and trifluoperazine, characterised by fewer sedative effects, fewer anticholinergic effects, but more pronounced extrapyramidal side-effects than groups 1 and 2.

Drugs of other chemical groups tend to resemble the phenothiazines of *group 3*. They include the **butyrophenones** (benperidol, droperidol, haloperidol, and trifluperidol); **diphenylbutylpiperidines** (fluspirilene and pimozide); **thioxanthenes** (chlorprothixene, clopenthixol, and flupenthixol); and **oxypertine**.

CHLORPROMAZINE HYDROCHLORIDE

Indications: schizophrenia and related psychoses, tranquillisation and emergency control in behavioural disturbances; short-term adjunctive treatment of severe anxiety, terminal disease, intractable hiccup

Cautions: cardiovascular disease, respiratory disease, phaeochromocytoma, parkinsonism, epilepsy, acute infections, pregnancy, breastfeeding, renal and hepatic impairment, past history of jaundice, leucopenia; hypothyroidism, myasthenia gravis, prostatic hypertrophy; reduce dose in elderly and debilitated patients and with other drugs causing postural hypotension. Avoid drugs such as phenylbutazone that depress leucopoiesis. Initially, sedation may affect the ability to drive or operate machinery and increase the effects of alcohol. On prolonged use examinations for eye defects

and abnormal skin pigmentation are required. Avoid abrupt withdrawal. Patients should remain supine for 30 minutes after intramuscular injection. Drug interactions of phenothiazine derivatives: see Appendix 1 (sections 2.5, 4.2, *4.2, 4.3, 4.8, 4.9, 15*)

Contra-indications: coma caused by CNS depressants; bone-marrow depression; narrow-angle glaucoma

Side-effects: extrapyramidal symptoms (reversed by dose reduction or anticholinergic drugs) and, on prolonged administration, occasionally tardive dyskinesia; hypothermia (occasionally pyrexia), drowsiness, apathy, pallor, nightmares, insomnia, depression, and, more rarely, agitation. Anticholinergic symptoms such as dry mouth, nasal congestion, constipation, difficulty with micturition, and blurred vision; cardiovascular symptoms such as hypotension and arrhythmias; endocrine effects such as menstrual disturbances, galactorrhoea, and weight gain; sensitivity reactions such as agranulocytosis, leucopenia, leucocytosis, and haemolytic anaemia, photosensitisation, contact sensitisation, rashes, and jaundice. With prolonged high dosage, corneal and lens opacities and purplish pigmentation of the skin, cornea, conjunctiva, and retina. Intramuscular injection may be painful, cause hypotension and tachycardia (see Cautions), and give rise to nodule formation

Dose: by mouth, psychoses and severe anxiety, initially 25 mg 3 times daily (may be doubled in bedpatients), adjusted according to the response, to 1 g daily or more in psychoses; usual maintenance dose 75–300 mg daily; CHILD up to 5 years 5–10 mg up to 3 times daily, 6–12 years ⅓–½ adult dose

Intractable hiccup, 25–50 mg 3–4 times daily

Tablets should be swallowed whole

By deep intramuscular injection, (for relief of acute symptoms), 25–50 mg every 6–8 hours; CHILD, as dose by mouth

By rectum in suppositories, chlorpromazine 100 mg every 6–8 hours

Note: for equivalent therapeutic effect 100 mg chlorpromazine base given *rectally* as a suppository ≡ 20–25 mg chlorpromazine hydrochloride *by intramuscular injection* ≡ 40–50 mg of chlorpromazine base or hydrochloride *by mouth*

PoM **Chlorpromazine Tablets,** s/c, chlorpromazine hydrochloride 10 and 25 mg, price 20 tabs (both) = **A**; 50 and 100 mg, price 20 tabs (both) = **B**. Label: 2, 25

PoM **Chlorpromazine Elixir,** chlorpromazine hydrochloride 25 mg/5 ml. Price 100 ml = **B**. Label: 2

PoM **Chloractil**® (DDSA)
Tablets, s/c, chlorpromazine hydrochloride 25 and 50 mg, price 20 tabs (both) = **A**; 100 mg, price 20 tabs = **B**. Label: 2, 25

PoM **Dozine**® (RP Drugs)
Syrup (= elixir), brown, chlorpromazine hydrochloride 25 mg/5 ml. Diluent syrup, life of

diluted elixir 14 days. Price 100 ml = **A** (Hosp. only). Label: 2

PoM Largactil® (M&B)

Tablets, s/c, chlorpromazine hydrochloride 10 mg. Price 20 tabs = **A**; 25 mg, price 20 tabs = **A**; 50 mg, price 20 tabs = **B**; 100 mg, price 20 tabs = **C**. Label: 2, 25

Syrup (= elixir), brown, chlorpromazine hydrochloride 25 mg/5 ml. Diluent syrup (without preservative), life of diluted elixir 14 days. Price 100 ml = **B**. Label: 2

Suspension forte (= strong mixture), orange, chlorpromazine hydrochloride 100 mg (as embonate)/5 ml. Diluent syrup (without preservative), life of diluted mixture 14 days. Price 100 ml = **C**. Label: 2

Injection, chlorpromazine hydrochloride 25 mg/ml. Price 1-ml amp = **A**; 2-ml amp = **B**

Suppositories, chlorpromazine 100 mg. Price 10 suppos = **D**. Label: 2

BENPERIDOL

Indications: see notes above

Cautions; Contra-indications; Side-effects: see under Haloperidol

Dose: initially 0.25–1.5 mg daily in divided doses, adjusted according to the response

PoM Anquil® (Janssen)

Tablets, benperidol 250 micrograms. Price 20 tabs = **E**. Label: 2

CHLORPROTHIXENE

Indications: schizophrenia and related psychoses, tranquillisation in behavioural disturbances, short-term adjunctive treatment of severe anxiety

Cautions; Contra-indications; Side-effects: see under Chlorpromazine Hydrochloride. Possibly less effective than chlorpromazine but extrapyramidal symptoms are much less frequent and anticholinergic side-effects are more frequent

Dose: psychoses, up to 400 mg (in elderly patients up to 150 mg) daily in divided doses, adjusted according to the response

Severe anxiety, 30–45 mg daily in divided doses, adjusted according to the response; CHILD up to 6 years, 1–2 mg/kg daily in divided doses, over 6 years 15 mg 3–4 times daily

PoM Taractan® (Roche)

Tablets, pink, s/c, chlorprothixene 15 mg. Price 20 tabs = **C**. Label: 2

Tablets, red-brown, s/c, chlorprothixene 50 mg. Price 20 tabs = **D**. Label: 2

CLOPENTHIXOL DIHYDROCHLORIDE

Indications: schizophrenia and related psychoses, particularly when associated with agitated, aggressive, or hostile behaviour

Cautions; Contra-indications; Side-effects: see under Chlorpromazine Hydrochloride but is less sedating; should not be used in apathetic or withdrawn states

Dose: initially 20–30 mg daily in divided doses, increasing to a max. of 150 mg daily if necessary; usual maintenance dose 20–50 mg daily

▼ **PoM Clopixol**® (Lundbeck)

Tablets, pink, f/c, clopenthixol 2 mg (as dihydrochloride). Price 20 tabs = **C**. Label: 2

Tablets, light brown, f/c, clopenthixol 10 mg (as dihydrochloride). Price 20 tabs = **D**. Label: 2

Tablets, brown, f/c, clopenthixol 25 mg (as dihydrochloride). Price 20 tabs = **E**. Label: 2

Depot injection (clopenthixol decanoate): section 4.2.2

DROPERIDOL

Indications: tranquillisation and emergency control in psychoses, particularly mania, and in behavioural disturbances

Cautions; Contra-indications; Side-effects: see under Haloperidol

Dose: by mouth, 5–20 mg every 4–8 hours; CHILD, 300–600 micrograms/kg

By intramuscular injection, up to 10 mg every 4–6 hours; CHILD, 200–500 micrograms/kg

By intravenous injection, 5–15 mg every 4–6 hours; CHILD 200–300 micrograms/kg

PoM Droleptan® (Janssen)

Tablets, yellow, scored, droperidol 10 mg. Price 20 tabs = **F**. Label: 2

Oral liquid (= elixir), droperidol 1 mg/ml. Diluent purified water, freshly boiled and cooled, or syrup, life of diluted elixir 14 days. Price 100 ml (with graduated cap) = **E**. Label: 2

Injection, droperidol 5 mg/ml. Price 2-ml amp = **C**

FLUPENTHIXOL

Indications: schizophrenia and related psychoses, particularly with apathy and withdrawal but not mania or psychomotor hyperactivity; short-term adjunctive treatment of severe anxiety

Cautions; Contra-indications; Side-effects: see under Chlorpromazine Hydrochloride but less sedating; extrapyramidal symptoms are more frequent (25% of patients) and tardive dyskinesia also occurs. Oral administration may cause restlessness and insomnia. Avoid in children, senile confusional states, excitable and overactive patients

Dose: initially 3–9 mg twice daily adjusted according to the response; max. 18 mg daily

PoM Depixol® (Lundbeck)

Tablets, yellow, s/c, flupenthixol 3 mg (as dihydrochloride). Price 20 tabs = **E**. Label: 4

Depot injection (flupenthixol decanoate): section 4.2.2

FLUPHENAZINE HYDROCHLORIDE

Indications: schizophrenia and related psychoses, tranquillisation in behavioural dis-

C = 51-100p, D = 101-180p, E = 181-300p, F = 301-450p, G = 451-650p, H = 651-900p, I = 901-1200p, J = over 1200p.

turbances, short-term adjunctive treatment of severe anxiety

Cautions; Contra-indications; Side-effects: see under Chlorpromazine Hydrochloride, but less sedating and fewer anticholinergic or hypotensive symptoms. Extrapyramidal symptoms, particularly dystonic reactions and akathisia, are more frequent, especially with doses over 3 mg daily and in elderly patients. Occasionally tardive dyskinesia also occurs. Caution when used in depression

Dose: psychoses initially 2.5–10 mg daily in 2–3 divided doses, adjusted according to the response to a max. of 20 mg daily

Severe anxiety, initially 1 mg twice daily, increased as necessary to 4 mg daily

Behavioural disorders, CHILD 250–500 micrograms daily, increasing if necessary to 1 mg according to age and response

Geriatric confusion and agitation, initially 1 mg daily adjusted according to response

PoM **Moditen**® (Squibb)

Tablets, pink, s/c, fluphenazine hydrochloride 1 mg. Price 20 tabs = **D**. Label: 2

Tablets, yellow, s/c, fluphenazine hydrochloride 2.5 mg. Price 20 tabs = **D**. Label: 2

Tablets, s/c, fluphenazine hydrochloride 5 mg. Price 20 tabs = **E**. Label: 2

Depot injections (fluphenazine decanoate): section 4.2.2

HALOPERIDOL

Indications: schizophrenia and related psychoses, particularly mania; tranquillisation and emergency control in behavioural disturbances; short-term adjunctive treatment of severe anxiety

Cautions; Contra-indications; Side-effects: see under Chlorpromazine Hydrochloride but less sedating, and fewer anticholinergic or hypotensive symptoms. Extrapyramidal symptoms, particularly dystonic reactions and akathisia are more frequent especially in thyrotoxic patients. Occasionally tardive dyskinesia also occurs. Rarely, alterations in liver function, gastrointestinal disturbances, and weight loss. Caution in depression. Avoid in basal ganglia disease. Drug interactions: see Appendix 1 (sections 2.5, 4.2, *4.2*, *4.9*)

Dose: by mouth, psychoses, initially 0.5–5 mg 2–3 times daily adjusted according to the response; max. 200 mg daily; usual maintenance dose 5–10 mg daily; CHILD initially 25–150 micrograms/kg daily divided into 2 doses, adjusted according to response; usual maintenance dose 50 micrograms/kg daily divided into 2 doses

Severe anxiety, adults 500 micrograms twice daily

By intramuscular or intravenous injection, (acute symptoms) 2–10 mg (increasing to 30 mg for emergency control) every 6 hours or 5 mg every hour if necessary

PoM **Haloperidol Tablets**, haloperidol 1.5 mg, price 20 tabs = **B**; 5 mg, price 20 tabs = **C**; 10 mg, price 20 tabs = **F**; 20 mg, price 20 tabs = **G**. Label: 2

PoM **Haloperidol Elixir**, haloperidol 2 mg/ml. Diluent purified water, freshly boiled and cooled, life of diluted elixir 14 days. Price 100 ml = **G**. Label: 2

PoM **Dozic**® (RP Drugs)

Oral liquid (=elixir), haloperidol 1 mg/ml. Price 100 ml (with pipette) = **E**. Label: 2

Oral liquid (=elixir), haloperidol 2 mg/ml. Price 100 ml (with pipette) = **E**. Label: 2

PoM **Fortunan**® (Steinhard)

Tablets, haloperidol 500 micrograms. Price 20 tabs = **B**. Label: 2

Tablets, scored, haloperidol 1.5 mg. Price 20 tabs = **C**. Label: 2

Tablets, green, scored, haloperidol 5 mg. Price 20 tabs = **E**. Label: 2

Tablets, pink, scored, haloperidol 10 mg. Price 20 tabs = **F**. Label: 2

Tablets, scored, haloperidol 20 mg. Price 20 tabs = **H**. Label: 2

PoM **Haldol**® (Janssen)

Tablets, blue, scored, haloperidol 5 mg. Price 20 tabs = **D**. Label: 2

Tablets, yellow, scored, haloperidol 10 mg. Price 20 tabs = **F**. Label: 2

Oral liquid (=elixir), haloperidol 2 mg/ml. Diluent purified water, freshly boiled and cooled, life of diluted elixir 14 days. Price 100 ml (with pipette) = **G**. Label: 2

Oral liquid concentrate (= concentrated elixir), haloperidol 10 mg/ml. Diluent purified water, freshly boiled and cooled, life of diluted concentrate 14 days. Alternatively, purified water, freshly boiled and cooled, containing 0.05% of methyl hydroxybenzoate and 0.005% of propyl hydroxybenzoate, life of diluted concentrate 2 months. Price 10 ml = **E**. Label: 2

Injection, haloperidol 5 mg/ml. Price 1-ml amp = **B**; 2-ml amp = **C**

Depot injection (haloperidol decanoate): section 4.2.2

PoM **Serenace**® (Searle)

Capsules, green, haloperidol 500 micrograms. Price 20 caps = **C**. Label: 2

Tablets, scored, haloperidol 1.5 mg. Price 20 tabs = **D**. Label: 2

Tablets, pink, scored, haloperidol 5 mg. Price 20 tabs = **F**. Label: 2

Tablets, pale pink, scored, haloperidol 10 mg. Price 20 tabs = **G**. Label: 2

Tablets, dark pink, scored, haloperidol 20 mg. Price 20 tabs = **I**. Label: 2

Oral liquid (=elixir), haloperidol 2 mg/ml. Diluent syrup or purified water, freshly boiled and cooled, or syrup for dilutions containing 1% or less of the elixir, life of diluted elixir 2 months. Price 100 ml = **H**. Label: 2

Injection, haloperidol 5 mg/ml. Price 1-ml amp = **C**

Injection, haloperidol 10 mg/ml. Price 2-ml amp = **E**

For all abbreviations and symbols see inside cover.   Relative prices: **A** = up to 20p, **B** = 21-50p,

METHOTRIMEPRAZINE

Indications: schizophrenia and related psychoses, adjunctive treatment in terminal care

Cautions; Contra-indications; Side-effects: see under Chlorpromazine Hydrochloride but more sedating. Postural hypotension may occur; caution in patients over 50 years

Dose: by mouth, initially 25–50 mg daily in divided doses increased as necessary; bedpatients initially 100–200 mg daily in 3 divided doses, increased if necessary to 1 g daily

By intramuscular or intravenous injection, adjunct in terminal care, 12.5–25 mg (severe agitation up to 50 mg) every 6–8 hours if necessary

PoM **Nozinan®** (M&B)
Injection, methotrimeprazine hydrochloride 25 mg/ml. Price 1-ml amp = **C**
PoM **Veractil®** (M&B)
Tablets, varnished, scored, methotrimeprazine maleate 25 mg. Price 20 tabs = **D**. Label: 2

OXYPERTINE

Indications: schizophrenia and related psychoses, particularly with apathy and withdrawal, also suitable in mania and psychomotor hyperactivity; tranquillisation in behavioural disturbances; short-term adjunctive treatment of severe anxiety

Cautions; Side-effects: see under Chlorpromazine Hydrochloride, but extrapyramidal symptoms may occur less frequently. With low doses agitation and hyperactivity occur and with high doses sedation. Occasionally gastro-intestinal disturbances, photophobia, and rashes may occur. Drug interactions: see Appendix 1 (section *4.3*)

Dose: psychoses, initially 80–120 mg daily in divided doses adjusted according to the response; max. 300 mg daily

Severe anxiety, initially 10 mg 3–4 times daily preferably after food

PoM **Integrin®** (Sterling Research)
Capsules, oxypertine 10 mg. Price 20 caps = **D**. Label: 2
Tablets, scored, oxypertine 40 mg. Price 20 tabs = **F**. Label: 2

PERICYAZINE

Indications: tranquillisation in behavioural disturbances, schizophrenia and related psychoses, short-term adjunctive treatment of severe anxiety

Cautions; Contra-indications; Side-effects: see under Chlorpromazine Hydrochloride, but more sedating. Extrapyramidal symptoms occur only with high doses, but hypotension occurs occasionally when treatment is initiated

Dose: psychoses, initially 15–30 mg (elderly patients 10 mg) daily divided into 2 doses, taking the larger dose at bedtime, adjusted according to the response; CHILD, initially 500 micrograms per year of age, adjusted according to the response; max. in children over 15 years 30 mg daily

PoM **Neulactil®** (M&B)
Tablets, yellow, scored, pericyazine 2.5 mg. Price 20 tabs = **B**. Label: 2
Tablets, yellow, scored, pericyazine 10 mg. Price 20 tabs = **C**. Label: 2
Tablets, yellow, scored, pericyazine 25 mg. Price 20 tabs = **E**. Label: 2
Syrup forte (= strong elixir), brown, pericyazine 10 mg/5 ml. Diluent syrup, life of diluted elixir 14 days. Price 100 ml = **E**. Label: 2

PERPHENAZINE

Indications: schizophrenia and related psychoses, tranquillisation and emergency control in behavioural disturbances, short-term adjunctive treatment of severe anxiety, terminal disease, intractable hiccup

Cautions; Contra-indications; Side-effects: see under Chlorpromazine Hydrochloride, but it is less sedating; extrapyramidal symptoms, especially dystonia, are more frequent, particularly at high dosage, tardive dyskinesia also occurs. Avoid in children

Dose: by mouth, initially 4 mg 3 times daily adjusted according to the response; max. 24 mg daily

By intramuscular injection (for relief of acute symptoms), 5–10 mg, followed if necessary by 5 mg every 6 hours; max. 15 mg daily

PoM **Fentazin®** (A&H)
Tablets, s/c, perphenazine 2 mg. Price 20 tabs = **C**. Label: 2
Tablets, s/c, perphenazine 4 mg. Price 20 tabs = **C**. Label: 2
Tablets, s/c, perphenazine 8 mg. Price 20 tabs = **C**. Label: 2
Liquid concentrate (= elixir concentrate), perphenazine 2 mg/ml. Diluent syrup (without preservative), life of diluted concentrate 14 days. Price 100 ml = **C** (Hosp. only). Label: 2
Injection, perphenazine 5 mg/ml. Price 1-ml amp = **A**

PIMOZIDE

Indications: schizophrenia and related psychoses, particularly when thought disorders and inertia are prominent but not mania or psychomotor hyperactivity

Cautions; Side-effects: see under Chlorpromazine Hydrochloride, but less sedating and extrapyramidal symptoms are less frequent except with higher doses. May aggravate endogenous depression, parkinsonism, and epilepsy

Dose: initially 4–10 mg (acutely disturbed patients 20 mg) daily as a single dose, adjusted according to the response; usual dose 2–20 mg daily, max. 20 mg daily; CHILD over 12 years 1–3 mg daily

---

C = 51-100p, **D** = 101-180p, **E** = 181-300p, **F** = 301-450p, **G** = 451-650p, **H** = 651-900p, **I** = 901-1200p, **J** = over 1200p.

PoM **Orap**® (Janssen)

Tablets, scored, pimozide 2 mg. Price 20 tabs = E. Label: 2

Tablets, green, scored, pimozide 4 mg. Price 20 tabs = **F**. Label: 2

Tablets, scored, pimozide 10 mg. Price 20 tabs = I. Label: 2

PROCHLORPERAZINE

Indications: schizophrenia and related psychoses, short-term adjunctive treatment of severe anxiety; see also section 4.6

Cautions; Contra-indications; Side-effects: see under Chlorpromazine Hydrochloride, but it is less sedating although extrapyramidal symptoms, particularly dystonic reactions, are more frequent especially with doses above 40 mg daily; tardive dyskinesia also occurs. Avoid in children (but see section 4.6 for use as anti-emetic)

Dose: by mouth, prochlorperazine maleate or mesylate, psychoses, 12.5 mg twice daily for 7 days adjusted to 75–100 mg daily according to response

Severe anxiety, 15–20 mg daily; max. 40 mg daily

By deep intramuscular injection, psychoses, prochlorperazine mesylate 12.5–25 mg 2–3 times daily

By rectum in suppositories, psychoses, the equivalent of prochlorperazine maleate 25 mg 2–3 times daily

Preparations

Section 4.6

PROMAZINE HYDROCHLORIDE

Indications: agitation, particularly in the elderly, short-term adjunctive treatment of severe anxiety; terminal disease

Cautions; Contra-indications; Side-effects: see under Chlorpromazine Hydrochloride

Dose: by mouth, 25–200 mg 4 times daily, adjusted according to response

By intramuscular or intravenous injection, 50 mg (25 mg in elderly or debilitated patients), repeated if necessary after 6–8 hours. Intravenous injections should be no stronger than 25 mg/ml

PoM **Sparine**® (Wyeth)

Tablets, yellow, s/c, promazine hydrochloride 25 mg. Price 20 tabs = **A**. Label: 2

Tablets, orange, s/c, promazine hydrochloride 50 mg. Price 20 tabs = **B**. Label: 2

Tablets, red, s/c, promazine hydrochloride 100 mg. Price 20 tabs = **C**. Label: 2

Suspension (= mixture), yellow, promazine hydrochloride 50 mg (as embonate)/5 ml (contains aluminium hydroxide). Diluent syrup, life of diluted mixture 14 days. Price 150 ml = **C**. Label: 2

Injection, promazine hydrochloride 50 mg/ml. Price 1-ml amp = **A**; 2-ml amp = **B**

SULPIRIDE

Indications: schizophrenia

Cautions; Contra-indications; Side-effects: see under Chlorpromazine Hydrochloride; also contra-indicated in phaeochromocytoma; reduce dose in renal impairment

Dose: initially 200–400 mg twice daily, adjusted according to response; max. 800 mg daily in patients with predominantly negative symptoms, and 2.4 g daily in patients with mainly positive symptoms

▼ PoM **Dolmatil**® (Squibb)

Tablets, scored, sulpiride 200 mg. Price 20 tabs = **F**. Label: 2

THIORIDAZINE

Indications: schizophrenia and related psychoses, tranquillisation and emergency control in behavioural disturbances, agitation in elderly patients, short-term adjunctive treatment of severe anxiety

Cautions; Contra-indications; Side-effects: see under Chlorpromazine Hydrochloride, but less sedating and extrapyramidal symptoms and hypothermia rarely occur; more likely to induce hypotension. Caution in depression. Pigmentary retinopathy (with reduced visual acuity, brownish colouring of vision, and impaired night vision) occurs rarely with high doses. Sexual dysfunction, particularly retrograde ejaculation, may occur

Dose: psychoses, 150 mg (200 mg in acutely disturbed patients) daily in divided doses, adjusted according to the response; max. 800 mg daily for up to 4 weeks. Usual maintenance dose 100–200 mg daily

Severe anxiety, 30–200 mg daily in divided doses

Behavioural disorders, CHILD under 5 years 1 mg/kg, 6–12 years ½–½ adult dose

PoM **Melleril**® (Sandoz)

Tablets, s/c, thioridazine 10 mg (as hydrochloride). Price 20 tabs = **B**. Label: 2

Tablets, s/c, thioridazine 25 mg (as hydrochloride). Price 20 tabs = **B**. Label: 2

Tablets, s/c, thioridazine 50 mg (as hydrochloride). Price 20 tabs = **C**. Label: 2

Tablets, s/c, thioridazine 100 mg (as hydrochloride). Price 20 tabs = **D**. Label: 2

Suspension 25 mg/5 ml (= mixture), thioridazine 25 mg/5 ml. Price 100 ml = **C**. Label: 2

Suspension 100 mg/5 ml (= strong mixture), thioridazine 100 mg/5 ml. Price 100 ml = **E**. Label: 2.

These suspensions should not be diluted but the two preparations may be mixed with each other to provide intermediate doses

Syrup (= elixir), orange, thioridazine 25 mg/5 ml. Diluent syrup (without preservative), life of diluted elixir 14 days. Price 100 ml = **C**. Label: 2

TRIFLUOPERAZINE

Indications: schizophrenia and related psychoses, tranquillisation in behavioural disturbances, short-term adjunctive treatment of severe anxiety

Cautions; Contra-indications; Side-effects: see under Chlorpromazine Hydrochloride but less sedating, and hypotension, hypothermia, and anticholinergic side-effects occur less frequently. Extrapyramidal symptoms, particularly dystonic reactions and akathisia, are more frequent (particularly when the daily dose exceeds 6 mg). Caution in children

Dose: by mouth, psychoses, initially 5 mg twice daily, *or* 10 mg daily in slow-release form, adjusted after 1 week, then at intervals of 3 days, according to the response; CHILD up to 12 years, initially 5 mg daily in divided doses, adjusted according to response, age, and body-weight

Severe anxiety, 2–4 mg daily in divided doses *or* 2–4 mg daily in slow-release form; CHILD 3–5 years up to 1 mg, 6–12 years up to 4 mg daily in divided doses

By deep intramuscular injection (for acute symptoms), 1–3 mg daily in divided doses to a max. of 6 mg daily; CHILD 50 micrograms/kg daily in divided doses

PoM **Stelazine**® (SK&F)

Tablets, blue, s/c, trifluoperazine 1 mg (as hydrochloride). Price 20 tabs = **B**. Label: 2
Tablets, blue, s/c, trifluoperazine 5 mg (as hydrochloride). Price 20 tabs = **B**. Label: 2
Spansule® (= capsules s/r), clear/yellow, enclosing dark blue, light blue, and white pellets, trifluoperazine 2 mg (as hydrochloride). Price 20 caps = **C**. Label: 2, 25
Spansule® (= capsules s/r), clear/yellow, enclosing dark blue, light blue, and white pellets, trifluoperazine 10 mg (as hydrochloride). Price 20 caps = **D**. Label: 2, 25
Spansule® (= capsules s/r), clear/yellow, enclosing dark blue, light blue, and white pellets, trifluoperazine 15 mg (as hydrochloride). Price 20 caps = **D**. Label: 2, 25
Syrup (= elixir), yellow, trifluoperazine 1 mg (as hydrochloride)/5 ml. Diluent syrup, life of diluted elixir 14 days. Price 100 ml = **C**. Label: 2
Liquid concentrate (= elixir concentrate), yellow, trifluoperazine 10 mg (as hydrochloride)/ml for dilution before use. Diluent syrup or water for preparations, life of diluted elixir 12 weeks or 1 week respectively. (Hosp. only)
Injection, trifluoperazine 1 mg (as hydrochloride)/ml. Price 1-ml amp = **B**

TRIFLUPERIDOL

Indications: schizophrenia and related psychoses, particularly mania
Cautions; Contra-indications; Side-effects: see under Haloperidol
Dose: initially 500 micrograms daily, adjusted by

500 micrograms every 3–4 days according to the response; max. 6–8 mg daily; CHILD 6–12 years initially 250 micrograms, adjusted according to the response; max. 2 mg daily

PoM **Triperidol**® (Lagap)

Tablets, scored, trifluperidol 500 micrograms. Price 20 tabs = **C**. Label: 2
Tablets, scored, trifluperidol 1 mg. Price 20 tabs = **D**. Label: 2

4.2.2 Antipsychotic depot injections

For maintenance therapy, long-acting depot injections of antipsychotic drugs are used because they are more convenient than oral preparations and ensure better patient compliance. However, they may give rise to a higher incidence of extrapyramidal reactions than oral preparations.

ADMINISTRATION. Depot antipsychotics are administered by deep intramuscular injection at intervals of 1 to 4 weeks. Patients should first be given a small test-dose as undesirable side-effects are prolonged. *Not more than 2 ml of oily injection should be administered at any one site.*

When transferring patients from one depot injection to another the following approximate equivalents may be used:

Clopenthixol decanoate	200 mg
Flupenthixol decanoate	40 mg
Fluphenazine decanoate	25 mg
Fluphenazine enanthate	25 mg
Haloperidol decanoate	100 mg
Pipothiazine palmitate	50 mg

SELECTION. **Fluphenazine** or **clopenthixol** may be suitable for the treatment of excited or agitated patients. **Flupenthixol** can cause over-excitement in such patients but there is no clear-cut division in the usage of these drugs. In children fluphenazine is generally used as experience with the other depot preparations is limited. **Fluspirilene** (Redeptin®) has a shorter duration of action than the depot injections. The incidence of extrapyramidal reactions is similar for all these drugs.

CAUTIONS. Treatment requires careful monitoring for optimum effect; extrapyramidal symptoms occur frequently. When transferring from oral to depot therapy, dosage by mouth should be gradually phased out. Caution in arteriosclerosis.
CONTRA-INDICATIONS. Do not use in children, confusional states, coma caused by CNS depressants, parkinsonism, intolerance to antipsychotics.
SIDE-EFFECTS. Pain may occur at injection site and occasionally erythema, swelling, and nodules. For side-effects of specific antipsychotics see under the relevant monograph.

CLOPENTHIXOL DECANOATE

Indications: maintenance in schizophrenia and related psychoses, particularly with aggression and agitation
Cautions; Contra-indications; Side-effects: see under Chlorpromazine Hydrochloride (section 4.2.1) and notes above, but it is less sedating

C = 51-100p, D = 101-180p, E = 181-300p, F = 301-450p, G = 451-650p, H = 651-900p, I = 901-1200p, J = over 1200p.

Dose: by deep intramuscular injection into the gluteal muscle, test dose 100 mg, then after 7–28 days 100–200 mg or more, followed by 200–400 mg repeated at intervals of 2–4 weeks, adjusted according to the response; max. 600 mg weekly

PoM **Clopixol**® (Lundbeck)
Injection (oily), clopenthixol decanoate 200 mg/ml. Price 1-ml amp = **F**; 10-ml vial = **J**
▼ PoM **Clopixol Conc.**® (Lundbeck)
Injection (oily), clopenthixol decanoate 500 mg/ml. Price 1-ml amp with needle = **H**

FLUPENTHIXOL DECANOATE

Indications: maintenance in schizophrenia and related psychoses
Cautions; Contra-indications; Side-effects: see under Chlorpromazine Hydrochloride (section 4.2.1) and notes above, but it may have a mood elevating effect. Extrapyramidal symptoms usually appear 1–3 days after administration and continue for about 5 days but may be delayed. With high doses, periodic blood counts are advisable. An alternative antipsychotic drug may be necessary if symptoms such as aggression or agitation appear
Dose: by deep intramuscular injection into the gluteal muscle, test dose 20 mg, then after 5–10 days 20–40 mg repeated at intervals of 2–4 weeks, adjusted according to the response; max. 400 mg weekly

PoM **Depixol**® (Lundbeck)
Injection (oily), flupenthixol decanoate 20 mg/ml. Price 1-ml amp or syringe = **D**; 2-ml amp or syringe = **E**; 10-ml vial = **J**
PoM **Depixol Conc.**® (Lundbeck)
Injection (oily), flupenthixol decanoate 100 mg/ml. Price 1-ml amp = **G**; 5-ml vial = **J**

FLUPHENAZINE DECANOATE

Indications: maintenance in schizophrenia and related psychoses
Cautions; Contra-indications; Side-effects: see under Chlorpromazine Hydrochloride (section 4.2.1) and notes above. Extrapyramidal symptoms usually appear a few hours after the dose has been administered and continue for about 2 days but may be delayed
Dose: by deep intramuscular injection into the gluteal muscle, test dose 12.5 mg (6.25 mg in elderly patients), then after 4–7 days 12.5–100 mg repeated at intervals of 14–40 days, adjusted according to the response

PoM **Modecate**® (Squibb)
Injection (oily), fluphenazine decanoate 25 mg/ml. Price 0.5-ml amp = **D**; 1-ml amp or syringe = **E**; 2-ml amp or syringe = **G**; 10-ml vial = **J**
PoM **Modecate Concentrate**® (Squibb)
Injection (oily), fluphenazine decanoate 100 mg/ml. Price 0.5-ml amp = **G**; 1-ml amp = **I**

FLUPHENAZINE ENANTHATE

Indications; Cautions; Contra-indications; Side-effects: see under Fluphenazine Decanoate but it has less prolonged effect and higher incidence of extrapyramidal symptoms
Dose: by deep intramuscular injection into the gluteal muscle, test dose 12.5 mg (6.25 mg in elderly patients), then after 4–7 days 12.5–100 mg repeated at intervals of 10–21 days, adjusted according to the response

PoM **Moditen Enanthate**® (Squibb)
Injection (oily), fluphenazine enanthate 25 mg/ml. Price 1-ml amp = **E**

FLUSPIRILENE

Indications: maintenance in schizophrenia and related psychoses
Cautions; Contra-indications; Side-effects: see under Chlorpromazine Hydrochloride (section 4.2.1) and notes above, but less sedating. Extrapyramidal symptoms are less frequent than for the oily preparations (see above). They usually appear 6–12 hours after the dose and continue for about 48 hours but may be delayed. Common side-effects are restlessness, and sweating. With prolonged use, tissue damage (subcutaneous nodules) may occur at injection site
Dose: by deep intramuscular injection, 2 mg, increased by 2 mg at weekly intervals, according to the response; usual maintenance dose 2–8 mg weekly; max. 20 mg weekly

PoM **Redeptin**® (SK&F)
Injection (aqueous suspension), fluspirilene 2 mg/ml. Price 1-ml amp = **D**; 3-ml amp = **E**; 6-ml vial = **F**

HALOPERIDOL DECANOATE

Indications: maintenance in schizophrenia and related psychoses
Cautions; Contra-indications; Side-effects: see under Haloperidol (section 4.2.1) and notes above
Dose: by deep intramuscular injection into the gluteal muscle, every 4 weeks, mild cases and elderly patients up to 100 mg; moderate cases 100–200 mg; severe cases 200–300 mg or more

▼ PoM **Haldol Decanoate**® (Janssen)
Injection (oily), haloperidol 100 mg (as decanoate)/ml. Price 1-ml amp = **G**

PIPOTHIAZINE PALMITATE

Indications: maintenance in schizophrenia and related psychoses
Cautions; Contra-indications; Side-effects: see under Chlorpromazine Hydrochloride (section 4.2.1) and notes above
Dose: by deep intramuscular injection into the gluteal muscle, test dose 25 mg, then a further 25–50 mg after 4–7 days, then adjusted according to the response at intervals of 4 weeks; usual

---

maintenance range 50–100 mg (max. 200 mg) every 4 weeks

▼ PoM **Piportil Depot**® (M&B)
Injection (oily), pipothiazine palmitate 50 mg/ml. Price 1-ml amp = **G**; 2-ml amp = **H**

4.2.3 Lithium salts

Lithium salts are used for their mood-regulating action in the treatment of manic illness and in the prevention of manic and depressive illnesses. Lithium treatment quietens the overactive euphoric patient. The decision to give prophylactic treatment usually requires specialist advice, and must be based on careful consideration of the likelihood of recurrence in the individual patient, and the benefit weighed against the risks. Lithium treatment is unsuitable for children.

Treatment should be discontinued only if relief from affective illness is absent or insignificant.

In the initial stages supplementary treatment with **antipsychotic drugs** (section 4.2.1) is usually required because it may take a few days for lithium to exert its effect. High doses of haloperidol, fluphenazine, or flupenthixol may be hazardous when used with lithium; irreversible toxic encephalopathy has been reported.

Lithium salts have a narrow therapeutic/toxic ratio and should therefore not be prescribed unless facilities for monitoring plasma concentrations are available. Patients should be carefully selected. Doses are adjusted to achieve plasma concentrations of 0.6 to 1.2 mmol Li^+/litre (lower end of the range for maintenance therapy and elderly patients) on samples taken 12 hours after the preceding dose. Overdosage, usually with plasma concentrations over 1.5 mmol Li^+/litre, may be fatal and toxic effects include tremor, ataxia, dysarthria, nystagmus, renal impairment, and fits. If these potentially hazardous signs occur, treatment should be stopped, plasma-lithium concentrations redetermined, and steps taken to reverse lithium toxicity.

Lithium toxicity is made worse by sodium depletion. Concurrent use of diuretics that inhibit the uptake of sodium by the distal tubule (for example thiazides) should be avoided. In mild cases withdrawal of lithium and administration of generous amounts of sodium and fluid will reverse the toxicity. Plasma concentrations in excess of 2.5 mmol Li^+/litre are usually associated with serious toxicity requiring emergency treatment as indicated under Emergency Treatment of Poisoning. When toxic concentrations are reached there may be a delay of 1 or 2 days before maximum toxicity occurs.

In long-term use, therapeutic concentrations of lithium have been thought to cause histological and functional changes in the kidney. The significance of such changes is not clear but is of sufficient concern to discourage long-term use of lithium unless it is definitely indicated. Patients should be maintained on lithium treatment after 3–5 years only if, on assessment, benefit persists. Conventional and sustained-release tablets are available but it should be noted that **different preparations vary widely in bioavailability** and a change in the formulation used requires the same precautions as initiation of treatment. There seem few if any reasons for preferring one or other of the simple salts of lithium; the carbonate has been the more widely used but the citrate is also available.

LITHIUM CARBONATE

Indications: prophylaxis in manic-depressive illness, treatment of mania

Cautions: plasma concentrations must be measured regularly (every month on stabilised regimens), and thyroid function monitored; maintain adequate sodium and fluid intake. Avoid in impaired renal function, cardiac disease, and conditions with sodium imbalance such as Addison's disease (dose adjustment may be necessary in diarrhoea, vomiting, and heavy sweating). Caution in pregnancy (fetal intoxication), breast-feeding, elderly patients (reduce dose), diuretic treatment, myasthenia gravis. Drug interactions: see Appendix 1 (sections 4.2, *6.1, 15*)

Side-effects: gastro-intestinal disturbances, fine tremor, polyuria and polydipsia (may disappear with continued treatment); also weight gain and oedema (may respond to dose reduction). Signs of lithium intoxication are blurred vision, increasing gastro-intestinal disturbances (anorexia, vomiting, diarrhoea), increasing CNS disturbances (mild drowsiness and sluggishness increasing to giddiness with ataxia, coarse tremor, lack of co-ordination, dysarthria) require withdrawal of treatment. With severe overdosage (plasma concentrations above 2 mmol/litre) hyperreflexia and hyperextension of limbs, fits, toxic psychoses, syncope, oliguria, circulatory failure, coma, and occasionally, death. Goitre, raised antidiuretic hormone concentration, hypothyroidism, hypokalaemia, ECG changes, exacerbation of psoriasis, and kidney changes may also occur

Dose: initially 0.25–2 g daily, adjusted to achieve a plasma concentration of 0.6–1.2 mmol Li^+/litre by tests on samples taken 12 hours after the preceding dose on the fourth or seventh day of treatment, then weekly until dosage has remained constant for 4 weeks and monthly thereafter. Daily doses are usually divided, and sustained-release preparations are normally given twice daily

PoM **Camcolit 250**® (Norgine)
Tablets, f/c, scored, lithium carbonate 250 mg (6.8 mmol Li^+). Price 20 tabs = **B**. Label: 27
PoM **Camcolit 400**® (Norgine)
Tablets, f/c, scored, lithium carbonate 400 mg (10.8 mmol Li^+). Price 20 tabs = **C**. Label: 27
PoM **Liskonum**® (SK&F)
Tablets, s/r, f/c, scored, lithium carbonate 450 mg (12.2 mmol Li^+). Price 20 tabs = **C**. Label: 25, 27

C = 51-100p, **D** = 101-180p, **E** = 181-300p, **F** = 301-450p, **G** = 451-650p, **H** = 651-900p, **I** = 901-1200p, **J** = over 1200p.

PoM **Phasal**® (Lagap)
Tablets, s/r, lithium carbonate 300 mg (8.1 mmol Li⁺). Price 20 tabs = **C**. Label: 25, 27
PoM **Priadel**® (Delandale)
Tablets, s/r, scored, lithium carbonate 400 mg (10.8 mmol Li⁺). Price 20 tabs = **C**. Label: 25, 27, counselling advised, no hot drinks

LITHIUM CITRATE

Indications; Cautions; Side-effects: see under Lithium Carbonate and notes above
Dose: 564 mg twice daily adjusting dose to achieve plasma concentrations of 0.6–1.2 mmol Li⁺/litre as described under Lithium Carbonate

▼ PoM **Litarex**® (CP)
Tablets, s/r, lithium citrate 564 mg (6 mmol Li⁺). Price 20 tabs = **C**. Label: 25, 27

4.3   Antidepressant drugs

4.3.1 Tricyclic and related antidepressant drugs
4.3.2 Monoamine-oxidase inhibitors (MAOIs)
4.3.3 Combined antidepressant preparations
4.3.4 Other antidepressant drugs

Tricyclic and related antidepressants (antidepressives) are the drugs of choice in the treatment of depressive illness, unless it is so severe that electroconvulsive therapy is immediately indicated. They are preferred to MAOIs because they are more effective antidepressants and do not show the dangerous interactions with some foods and drugs that are characteristic of the MAOIs. **Lithium** (section 4.2.3) has a mood-regulating action and is used specifically in the treatment of manic depressive illnesses.

Prescribing more than one antidepressant of the tricyclic type is **not** recommended. It may constitute a hazard and there is no evidence that side-effects are minimised.

Mixtures of antidepressants with tranquillisers are included in section 4.3.3; their use is **not** recommended.

Other drugs used to treat depression (flupenthixol and tryptophan) are included in section 4.3.4.

It should be noted that although anxiety is often present in depressive illness and may be the presenting symptom, the use of antipsychotics or anxiolytics may mask the true diagnosis. They should therefore be used with caution though they are useful aids in the management of agitated depression.

DRUG INTERACTIONS. The effects of antidepressant drugs are modified by a number of other drugs. See Appendix 1 (sections *2.5, 4.1, 4.8, 4.9*) and under individual entries.

4.3.1   Tricyclic and related antidepressant drugs

The term 'tricyclic' is misleading as there are now 1-, 2-, and 4-ring structured drugs with broadly similar properties.

These drugs are most effective for treating moderate to severe endogenous depressive illness associated with psychomotor and physiological changes such as loss of appetite and eating and sleeping disturbances; improvement in sleep is usually the first benefit of therapy. Since there may be an interval of 2 to 4 weeks before the antidepressant action takes place electroconvulsive treatment may be required in severe depression when delay is hazardous or intolerable.

DOSAGE. About 10 to 20% of patients fail to respond to tricyclic and related antidepressant drugs and inadequate plasma concentrations may account for some of these failures. It is important to achieve plasma concentrations which are sufficiently high for effective treatment but not high enough to cause toxic effects.

MANAGEMENT. The patient's condition must be checked frequently, especially in the early weeks of treatment, to detect any suicidal tendencies. Limited quantities of antidepressant drugs should be prescribed at any one time as they are dangerous in overdosage. Some of the newer drugs, for example mianserin, nomifensine, and trazodone seem less dangerous in overdose than the older tricyclic compounds.

Treatment should be continued for 2 to 4 weeks before suppression of symptoms can be expected and thereafter should be maintained at the optimum level for at least another month before any attempt is made at dose reduction. Treatment should not be withdrawn prematurely, otherwise symptoms are likely to recur. The natural history of depressive illness suggests that remission usually occurs after 3 months to a year or more and some patients appear to benefit from maintenance therapy with about half the therapeutic dosage for several months to prevent relapse. It may be appropriate during the early stages of treatment to add a hypnotic (section 4.1.1) to correct the sleeping pattern and an anxiolytic (section 4.1.2) to allay anxiety or agitation.

SELECTION. Antidepressant drugs can be roughly divided into those with additional sedative properties, for example **amitriptyline**, and those with less, for example **imipramine**. Agitated and anxious patients tend to respond best to the sedative compounds whereas withdrawn and apathetic patients will often obtain most benefit from less sedating compounds.

Amitriptyline may be given in divided doses or the entire daily dose may be given at night to promote sleep and avoid daytime drowsiness. **Imipramine** can also be given once daily but as it has a much less sedative action there is less advantage in this.

Imipramine or the more sedating amitriptyline are well established and relatively safe and effective, but nevertheless have more marked anticholinergic or cardiac side-effects than some of the newer compounds (**doxepin, lofepramine, mianserin, nomifensine, trazodone**, and **viloxazine**); this may be important in individual patients.

Antidepressants with **sedative** properties include amitriptyline (Tryptizol®, Lentizol® etc.), dothiepin (Prothiaden®), doxepin (Sinequan®), maprotiline (Ludiomil®), mianserin (Bolvidon®, Norval®), trazodone (Molipaxin®), and trimipramine (Surmontil®).

Less sedative antidepressants include butriptyline (Evadyne®), clomipramine (Anafranil®), desipramine (Pertofran®), imipramine (Tofranil® etc.), iprindole (Prondol®), lofepramine (Gamanil®), nomifensine (Merital®), nortriptyline (Allegron®, Aventyl®), and viloxazine (Vivalan®). Protriptyline has a **stimulant** action.

SIDE-EFFECTS. Arrhythmias and heart block occasionally follow the use of tricyclic antidepressants, particularly amitriptyline, and may be a factor in the sudden death of patients with cardiac disease. Neutropenia and agranulocytosis are uncommon but well recognised adverse reactions of mianserin and aplastic anaemia has been rarely reported; patients being treated with this drug therefore require careful supervision. Other side-effects of tricyclic and related antidepressants are troublesome rather than serious and may include drowsiness, dry mouth, blurred vision, constipation, urinary retention, and sweating, attributed to anticholinergic activity. The patient should be encouraged to persist with treatment as some tolerance to these side-effects seems to develop. They are further reduced if, when initiating therapy, low doses are given and then gradually increased.

This gradual introduction of treatment is particularly important in the elderly, who, because of the hypotensive effects of these drugs, are prone to attacks of dizziness or even syncope. The tricyclic and related antidepressants should be prescribed with caution in epilepsy as they lower the convulsive threshold.

HYPERTENSIVE PATIENTS. Antidepressants may interfere with antihypertensive therapy. They diminish the action of bethanidine, clonidine, debrisoquine, and guanethidine. Beta-adrenoceptor blocking drugs may be used in conjunction with antidepressants as this combination does not interact. Alternatively, **mianserin** may be used with most antihypertensive agents as it does not interfere with re-uptake of amines into the neurone.

LACK OF RESPONSE. In patients who do not respond to antidepressants, the diagnosis, dosage, compliance, and possible continuation of psychosocial or physical aggravating causes should all be carefully reviewed; other drug treatment may be successful. The patient may respond to low-dose **flupenthixol** (Fluanxol®, section 4.3.4) or MAOIs (section 4.3.2). **Tryptophan** (section 4.3.4) appears to benefit some patients when given alone or as adjunctive therapy.

NOCTURNAL ENURESIS IN CHILDREN. Certain tricyclic antidepressants (**amitriptyline, imipramine,** and less often **nortriptyline**) are used to treat nocturnal enuresis in children. Their use should be reserved for when alternative methods have failed. Although they are effective, relapse occurs commonly after withdrawal of the drug. Also,

behavioural disturbances may occur and cases of poisoning have been reported. It is recommended that they should be avoided in children under 6 years of age, and that treatment should not exceed 3 months unless a full physical examination (including an electrocardiogram) is given (see section 7.4.2).

AMITRIPTYLINE HYDROCHLORIDE

Indications: depressive illness, particularly with anxiety, nocturnal enuresis in children

Cautions: initially, sedation may affect the ability to drive or operate machinery; effects of alcohol may be increased; diabetes, cardiac disease (particularly with arrhythmias, see contra-indications below), epilepsy, pregnancy, hepatic impairment, thyroid disease, psychoses (may aggravate mania), glaucoma, urinary retention. Avoid abrupt cessation of therapy. Also caution in anaesthesia (increased risk of arrhythmias). See notes above for nocturnal enuresis. Drug interactions: see Appendix 1 (sections 2.5, 2.7, 4.3, 4.3)

Contra-indications: recent myocardial infarction, heart block, mania

Side-effects: dry mouth, sedation, blurred vision, constipation, nausea, difficulty with micturition (due to anticholinergic action). Other common side-effects are cardiovascular (arrhythmias, postural hypotension, tachycardia, syncope, particularly with high doses), sweating, tremor, rashes, behavioural disturbances (particularly with children), confusion (particularly in the elderly), interference with sexual function, blood sugar changes, and weight changes. Less commonly, black tongue, paralytic ileus, convulsions, agranulocytosis, leucopenia, eosinophilia, purpura, thrombocytopenia, and jaundice

Dose: by mouth, initially 50–75 mg (elderly patients and adolescents 25–50 mg) daily in divided doses *or* as a single dose at bedtime increased gradually as necessary to a max. of 150 mg; usual maintenance dose 50–100 mg daily

Nocturnal enuresis, CHILD 6–10 years 10–20 mg, 11–16 years 25–50 mg at bedtime for up to 3 months and gradually withdrawn

By intramuscular or intravenous injection, 10–20 mg 4 times daily

PoM **Amitriptyline Tablets,** f/c or s/c, amitriptyline hydrochloride 10 and 25 mg, price 20 tabs (both) = **A**; 50 mg, price 20 tabs = **B**. Label: 2
PoM **Domical**® (Berk)
Tablets, blue, f/c, amitriptyline hydrochloride 10 mg. Price 20 tabs = **A**. Label: 2
Tablets, orange, f/c, amitriptyline hydrochloride 25 mg. Price 20 tabs = **A**. Label: 2
Tablets, red-brown, f/c, amitriptyline hydrochloride 50 mg. Price 20 tabs = **C**. Label: 2
PoM **Elavil**® (DDSA)
Tablets, blue, f/c, amitriptyline hydrochloride 10 mg. Price 20 tabs = **A**. Label: 2
Tablets, yellow, f/c, amitriptyline hydrochloride 25 mg. Price 20 tabs = **A**. Label: 2

PoM **Lentizol**® (Warner)
Capsules, s/r, pink, enclosing white pellets, amitriptyline hydrochloride 25 mg. Price 20 caps = **C**. Label: 2, 25
Capsules, s/r, pink/red, enclosing white pellets, amitriptyline hydrochloride 50 mg. Price 20 caps = **D**. Label: 2, 25

PoM **Tryptizol**® (Morson)
Capsules, s/r, orange, amitriptyline hydrochloride 75 mg. Price 20 caps = **D**. Label: 2, 25
Tablets, blue, f/c, amitriptyline hydrochloride 10 mg. Price 20 tabs = **B**. Label: 2
Tablets, yellow, f/c, amitriptyline hydrochloride 25 mg. Price 20 tabs = **B**. Label: 2
Tablets, brown, f/c, amitriptyline hydrochloride 50 mg. Price 20 tabs = **C**. Label: 2
Mixture, pink, amitriptyline 10 mg (as embonate)/5 ml. Diluent syrup, life of diluted mixture 14 days. Price 100 ml = **C**. Label: 2
Injection, amitriptyline hydrochloride 10 mg/ml. Price 10-ml vial = **B**

BUTRIPTYLINE
Indications: depressive illness, particularly with anxiety
Cautions; Contra-indications; Side-effects: see under Amitriptyline Hydrochloride, but less sedating
Dose: 25 mg 3 times daily, increased gradually as necessary to a max. of 150 mg; usual maintenance dose 25 mg 3 times daily

PoM **Evadyne**® (Ayerst)
Tablets, orange, f/c, butriptyline 25 mg (as hydrochloride). Price 20 tabs = **C**. Label: 2
Tablets, pink, f/c, butriptyline 50 mg (as hydrochloride). Price 20 tabs = **D**. Label: 2

CLOMIPRAMINE HYDROCHLORIDE
Indications: depressive illness, adjunctive treatment of phobic and obsessional states; cataplexy associated with narcolepsy
Cautions; Contra-indications; Side-effects: see under Amitriptyline Hydrochloride. Postural hypotension may occur on intravenous infusion
Dose: by mouth, initially 10 mg daily, increased gradually as necessary to 30–150 mg or more in severe depression and phobic and obsessional states, in divided doses or as a single dose at bedtime; elderly patients 10 mg daily, up to 30–75 mg
By intramuscular injection, up to 25 mg 6 times daily or more as necessary
By intravenous infusion, initially to assess tolerance, 25–50 mg over 45–120 minutes, adjusted as required, usually to about 100 mg daily, for 7–10 days

PoM **Anafranil**® (Geigy)
Capsules, yellow/caramel, clomipramine hydrochloride 10 mg. Price 20 caps = **C**. Label: 2
Capsules, orange/caramel, clomipramine hydrochloride 25 mg. Price 20 caps = **D**. Label: 2
Capsules, blue/caramel, clomipramine hydrochloride 50 mg. Price 20 caps = **E**. Label: 2
Syrup (= elixir), orange, clomipramine hydro-

chloride 25 mg/5 ml. Diluent purified water, freshly boiled and cooled; for dilutions below 15 mg/5 ml equal parts of syrup and tragacanth mucilage (freshly prepared), life of diluted elixir few days only. Price 150 ml = **G**. Label: 2
Injection, clomipramine hydrochloride 12.5 mg/ml. Price 2-ml amp = **B**

PoM **Anafranil SR**® (Geigy)
Tablets, s/r, pink, f/c, clomipramine hydrochloride 75 mg. Price 20 tabs = **G**. Label: 2, 25

DESIPRAMINE HYDROCHLORIDE
Indications: depressive illness
Cautions; Contra-indications; Side-effects: see under Amitriptyline Hydrochloride, but less sedating. Drug interactions: see Appendix 1 (section 4.3)
Dose: 75 mg (elderly patients 25 mg) daily in divided doses or as a single dose at bedtime, increased as necessary to a max. of 200 mg. Usual maintenance dose 100–150 mg daily in divided doses

PoM **Pertofran**® (Geigy)
Tablets, pink, s/c, desipramine hydrochloride 25 mg. Price 20 tabs = **C**. Label: 2

DOTHIEPIN HYDROCHLORIDE
Indications: depressive illness, particularly with anxiety
Cautions; Contra-indications; Side-effects: see under Amitriptyline Hydrochloride
Dose: initially 75 mg (elderly patients 50–75 mg) daily in divided doses or as a single dose at bedtime, increased gradually as necessary to 150 mg daily

PoM **Prothiaden**® (Boots)
Capsules, red/brown, dothiepin hydrochloride 25 mg. Price 20 caps = **C**. Label: 2
Tablets, red, s/c, dothiepin hydrochloride 75 mg. Price 20 tabs = **E**. Label: 2

DOXEPIN
Indications: depressive illness, particularly with anxiety
Cautions; Contra-indications; Side-effects: see under Amitriptyline Hydrochloride
Dose: initially 30–75 mg daily in 3 divided doses, increased gradually to a max. of 300 mg daily in divided doses; up to 100 mg may be given as a single dose at bedtime

PoM **Sinequan**® (Pfizer)
Capsules, orange, doxepin 10 mg (as hydrochloride). Price 20 caps = **C**. Label: 2
Capsules, orange/blue, doxepin 25 mg (as hydrochloride). Price 20 caps = **C**. Label: 2
Capsules, blue, doxepin 50 mg (as hydrochloride). Price 20 caps = **D**. Label: 2
Capsules, yellow/blue, doxepin 75 mg (as hydrochloride). Price 20 caps = **E**. Label: 2

IMIPRAMINE HYDROCHLORIDE

Indications: depressive illness, nocturnal enuresis in children

Cautions; Contra-indications; Side-effects: see under Amitriptyline Hydrochloride, but less sedating. Drug interactions: see Appendix 1 (section 4.3)

Dose: initially 75 mg daily in divided doses increased gradually to 200 mg; up to 150 mg may be given as a single dose at bedtime; elderly patients 10–25 mg 1–3 times daily

Nocturnal enuresis, CHILD 6–7 years 25 mg, 8–11 years 25–50 mg, over 11 years 50–75 mg at bedtime for up to 8 weeks, then gradually withdrawn

PoM **Imipramine Tablets,** s/c, imipramine hydrochloride 10 and 25 mg. Price 20 tabs (both) = **A.** Label: 2

PoM **Praminil**® (DDSA)
Tablets, brownish-pink, s/c, imipramine hydrochloride 10 mg. Price 20 tabs = **B.** Label: 2
Tablets, brown, s/c, imipramine hydrochloride 25 mg. Price 20 tabs = **C.** Label: 2

PoM **Tofranil**® (Geigy)
Tablets, red-brown, s/c, imipramine hydrochloride 10 mg. Price 20 tabs = **B.** Label: 2
Tablets, red-brown, s/c, imipramine hydrochloride 25 mg. Price 20 tabs = **C.** Label: 2
Syrup (= mixture), imipramine hydrochloride 25 mg/5 ml. Diluent purified water, freshly boiled and cooled; for dilutions below 15 mg/5 ml equal parts of syrup and tragacanth mucilage (freshly prepared), life of diluted mixture 14 days. Price 150 ml = **E.** Label: 2

IPRINDOLE

Indications: depressive illness

Cautions; Contra-indications; Side-effects: see under Amitriptyline Hydrochloride, but less sedating, and fewer and milder side-effects, particularly anticholinergic and cardiovascular effects. Caution in liver disease; jaundice, although rare, may develop, usually in the first 14 days of treatment

Dose: initially 15–30 mg 3 times daily, increased gradually as necessary to a max. of 60 mg 3 times daily; usual maintenance dose 30 mg 3 times daily

PoM **Prondol**® (Wyeth)
Tablets, yellow, iprindole 15 mg (as hydrochloride). Price 20 tabs = **B.** Label: 2
Tablets, yellow, iprindole 30 mg (as hydrochloride). Price 20 tabs = **C.** Label: 2

LOFEPRAMINE

Indications: depressive illness

Cautions; Contra-indications; Side-effects: see under Amitriptyline Hydrochloride, but less sedating and milder anticholinergic side-effects

Dose: 140–210 mg daily in divided doses

▼ PoM **Gamanil**® (Merck)
Tablets, lacquer-coated, brown-violet, lofep-

ramine 70 mg (as hydrochloride). Price 20 tabs = **F.** Label: 2

MAPROTILINE HYDROCHLORIDE

Indications: depressive illness, particularly with anxiety

Cautions; Contra-indications; Side-effects: see under Amitriptyline Hydrochloride, but less sedating and anticholinergic effects occur less frequently. Rashes commonly occur and there is an increased risk of convulsions at higher dosage

Dose: initially 25–75 mg (elderly patients 25–30 mg) daily in 3 divided doses *or* as a single dose at bedtime, increased gradually as necessary to a max. of 150 mg daily

PoM **Ludiomil**® (Ciba)
Tablets, pale orange, f/c, maprotiline hydrochloride 10 mg. Price 20 tabs = **C.** Label: 2
Tablets, greyish-red, f/c, maprotiline hydrochloride 25 mg. Price 20 tabs = **C.** Label: 2
Tablets, light orange, f/c, maprotiline hydrochloride 50 mg. Price 20 tabs = **E.** Label: 2
Tablets, brownish-orange, f/c, maprotiline hydrochloride 75 mg. Price 28 tabs = **F.** Label: 2

MIANSERIN HYDROCHLORIDE

Indications: depressive illness, particularly with anxiety

Cautions; Contra-indications; Side-effects: see under Amitriptyline Hydrochloride, but fewer and milder anticholinergic, cardiovascular and epileptiform effects, and many of the drug interactions of the tricyclic antidepressants are absent. See also notes above; arthritis, arthralgia, and agranulocytosis may occur

Dose: initially 30–40 mg daily in divided doses *or* as a single dose at bedtime, increased gradually as necessary; usual dose range 30–90 mg, max. 200 mg daily in divided doses

PoM **Mianserin Tablets,** mianserin hydrochloride 10 mg, price 20 tabs = **D**; 20 mg, price 20 tabs = **E**; 30 mg, price 20 tabs = **F.** Label: 2, 25
PoM **Bolvidon**® (Organon)
Tablets, f/c, mianserin hydrochloride 10 mg. Price 20 tabs = **D.** Label: 2, 25
Tablets, f/c, mianserin hydrochloride 20 mg. Price 20 tabs = **E.** Label: 2, 25
Tablets, f/c, mianserin hydrochloride 30 mg. Price 20 tabs = **F.** Label: 2, 25
PoM **Norval**® (Bencard)
Tablets, orange, f/c, mianserin hydrochloride 10 mg. Price 20 tabs = **D.** Label: 2, 25
Tablets, orange, f/c, mianserin hydrochloride 20 mg. Price 20 tabs = **E.** Label: 2, 25
Tablets, orange, f/c, mianserin hydrochloride 30 mg. Price 20 tabs = **F.** Label: 2, 25

NOMIFENSINE HYDROGEN MALEATE

Indications: depressive illness

Cautions; Contra-indications; Side-effects: see under Amitriptyline Hydrochloride, but less

---

C = 51-100p, **D** = 101-180p, **E** = 181-300p, **F** = 301-450p, **G** = 451-650p, **H** = 651-900p, **I** = 901-1200p, **J** = over 1200p.

sedating, and fewer and milder side-effects, particularly anticholinergic and cardiovascular effects; avoid in renal impairment
Dose: initially 25–50 mg 2–3 times daily, increased gradually as necessary after 7–10 days to a max. of 200 mg daily in divided doses. Up to 100 mg may be given as a single dose in the morning

▼ PoM **Merital**® (Hoechst)
Capsules, orange, nomifensine hydrogen maleate 25 mg. Price 20 caps = **E**. Label: 2
Capsules, orange/caramel, nomifensine hydrogen maleate 50 mg. Price 20 caps = **F**. Label: 2
▼ PoM **Merital AM**® (Hoechst)
Tablets, salmon, scored, nomifensine hydrogen maleate 100 mg. Price 30 tabs = **H**. Label: 2

NORTRIPTYLINE
Indications: depressive illness, nocturnal enuresis in children
Cautions; Contra-indications; Side-effects: see under Amitriptyline Hydrochloride but less sedating. Anticholinergic effects occur more frequently. Drug interactions: see Appendix 1 (section 4.3)
Dose: initially 10–25 mg (elderly patients 10 mg) 3–4 times daily, increased gradually as necessary to a max. of 100 mg daily in divided doses; usual maintenance dose 30–75 mg daily
Nocturnal enuresis, CHILD 6–7 years 10 mg, 8–11 years 10–20 mg, over 11 years 25–35 mg, at night

PoM **Allegron**® (Dista)
Tablets, yellow, nortriptyline 10 mg (as hydrochloride). Price 20 tabs = **B**. Label: 2
Tablets, orange, scored, nortriptyline 25 mg (as hydrochloride). Price 20 tabs = **C**. Label: 2
PoM **Aventyl**® (Lilly)
Capsules, yellow/white, nortriptyline 10 mg (as hydrochloride). Price 20 caps = **B**. Label: 2
Capsules, yellow/white, nortriptyline 25 mg (as hydrochloride). Price 20 caps = **C**. Label: 2
Liquid (= elixir), nortriptyline 10 mg (as hydrochloride)/5 ml. Diluent syrup, life of diluted elixir 14 days. Price 120 ml = **D**. Label: 2

PROTRIPTYLINE HYDROCHLORIDE
Indications: depressive illness, particularly with apathy and withdrawal
Cautions; Contra-indications; Side-effects: see under Amitriptyline Hydrochloride but less sedating. Cardiovascular side-effects are more common. May aggravate anxiety and tension and cause insomnia. Also rashes associated with photosensitisation may occur (avoid direct exposure to sunlight). Caution in the elderly, particularly when daily dose exceeds 20 mg
Dose: initially 5–10 mg 3–4 times daily (elderly patients 5 mg 3 times daily) taken not later than 4 p.m., increased gradually as necessary in severe depression to 60 mg daily

PoM **Concordin**® (MSD)
Tablets, pink, f/c, protriptyline hydrochloride 5 mg. Price 20 tabs = **B**. Label: 2, 11
Tablets, f/c, protriptyline hydrochloride 10 mg. Price 20 tabs = **C**. Label: 2, 11

TRAZODONE HYDROCHLORIDE
Indications: depressive illness, particularly with anxiety
Cautions; Contra-indications; Side-effects: see under Amitriptyline Hydrochloride but fewer and milder side-effects, particularly anticholinergic and cardiovascular effects. Marked sedative effects have been reported
Dose: initially 150 mg (elderly patients 100 mg) daily in divided doses after food *or* as a single dose at bedtime; usual maintenance dose 200–300 mg daily; max. 600 mg daily

PoM **Molipaxin**® (Roussel)
Capsules, violet/green, trazodone hydrochloride 50 mg. Price 20 caps = **F**. Label: 2, 21
Capsules, violet/fawn, trazodone hydrochloride 100 mg. Price 20 caps = **G**. Label: 2, 21
Liquid (= elixir), trazodone hydrochloride 50 mg/5 ml. Price 150 ml = **G**. Label: 2, 21

TRIMIPRAMINE
Indications: depressive illness, particularly with anxiety and insomnia
Cautions; Contra-indications; Side-effects: see under Amitriptyline Hydrochloride but more sedating. Anticholinergic and cardiovascular side-effects commonly occur and occasionally paraesthesia. Caution in hepatic impairment
Dose: initially 50–75 mg daily in divided doses *or* as a single dose 2 hours before bedtime (elderly patients 10–25 mg 3 times daily), increased as necessary to a max. of 300 mg daily; usual maintenance dose 75–150 mg daily

PoM **Surmontil**® (M&B)
Capsules, green/white, trimipramine 50 mg (as maleate). Price 20 caps = **D**. Label: 2
Tablets, compression coated, trimipramine 10 mg (as maleate). Price 20 tabs = **C**. Label: 2
Tablets, compression coated, trimipramine 25 mg (as maleate). Price 20 tabs = **C**. Label: 2

VILOXAZINE HYDROCHLORIDE
Indications: depressive illness, particularly when associated with apathy and withdrawal
Cautions; Contra-indications; Side-effects: see under Amitriptyline Hydrochloride, but less sedating and anticholinergic and cardiovascular side-effects are fewer and milder; nausea and headache may occur. Drug interactions: see Appendix 1 (section *4.8*)
Dose: initially 50–100 mg 3 times daily after food not later than 6 p.m. (elderly patients 100 mg daily), increased gradually as necessary; max. 400 mg daily

PoM **Vivalan®** (ICI)
Tablets, yellow, f/c, viloxazine 50 mg (as hydrochloride). Price 20 tabs = **D**. Label: 2, 21

4.3.2 Monoamine-oxidase inhibitors (MAOIs)

Monoamine-oxidase inhibitors are used much less frequently than tricyclic and related antidepressants because of the dangers of dietary and drug interactions and the fact that it is easier to prescribe MAOIs when tricyclic antidepressants have been unsuccessful than vice versa. **Tranylcypromine** (Parnate®) is the most **hazardous** of the MAOIs because of its stimulant action. The drugs of choice are **phenelzine** or **isocarboxazid** which are less stimulant and therefore safer.

Phobic patients and depressed patients with atypical, hypochondriacal, or hysterical features are said to respond best to MAOIs. However, MAOIs should be tried in any patients who are refractory to treatment with other antidepressants as there is occasionally a dramatic response. Response to treatment may be delayed for 3 weeks or more and may take an additional 1 or 2 weeks to become maximal.

MAOIs act by inhibiting monoamine oxidase, thereby causing an accumulation of amine neurotransmitters. The metabolism of some amine drugs such as sympathomimetics and tricyclic and related antidepressants is also inhibited and their pressor action may therefore be potentiated. The pressor effect of the tyramine present in some foods may also be dangerously potentiated.

Sympathomimetics are present in many proprietary cough mixtures and decongestant nasal drops. See Appendix 1 (section 4.3) and Treatment Card. These interactions may cause a dangerous rise in blood pressure. An early warning symptom may be a throbbing headache. The danger of interaction persists for up to 14 days after treatment with MAOIs is discontinued. Treatment cards which list the necessary precautions are distributed by the Pharmaceutical Society and given to patients at pharmacies etc.

Tricyclic and related antidepressants should **not** be given to patients for 14 days after treatment with MAOIs has been discontinued. Some psychiatrists use selected tricyclics in conjunction with MAOIs but this is hazardous, indeed potentially lethal, except in experienced hands and there is no evidence that the combination is more effective than when either constituent is used alone. The combination of tranylcypromine with clomipramine is particularly **dangerous**.

PHENELZINE
Indications: depressive illness
Cautions: may affect mental concentration and ability to drive or operate machinery. Avoid abrupt discontinuation of treatment, certain drugs and foods (see Treatment Card above). Drug interactions: see Appendix 1 (sections 4.3, 6.1)
Contra-indications: hepatic, cardiovascular, or cerebrovascular disease, phaeochromocytoma, epilepsy, children, elderly and debilitated patients
Side-effects: dizziness, postural hypotension, less commonly agitation, headache, tremor, constipation, dry mouth, blurred vision, difficulty in micturition, liver damage, rashes, psychotic episodes in susceptible patients; severe hypertensive reactions to certain drugs and foods
Dose: 15 mg 3 times daily, increased if necessary to 4 times daily after 2 weeks, then reduced gradually to lowest possible maintenance dose

PoM **Nardil®** (Warner)
Tablets, orange, s/c, phenelzine 15 mg (as sulphate). Price 20 tabs = **C**. Label: 3, 10 MAOI card, counselling advised, gluten

IPRONIAZID
Indications: depressive illness
Cautions; Contra-indications: see under Phenelzine
Side-effects: see under Phenelzine, but more toxic; rarely vasculitis and peripheral neuritis
Dose: 100–150 mg daily as a single dose, reducing gradually to a maintenance dose of 25–50 mg daily

PoM **Marsilid®** (Roche)
Tablets, orange, scored, iproniazid 25 mg (as phosphate). Price 20 tabs = **B**. Label: 3, 10 MAOI card

---

TREATMENT CARD
Carry this card with you at all times. Show it to any doctor who may treat you other than the doctor who prescribed this medicine, and to your dentist if you require dental treatment.

INSTRUCTIONS TO PATIENTS
Please read carefully
While taking this medicine and for 14 days after your treatment finishes you must observe the following simple instructions:-

1 Do not eat CHEESE, PICKLED HERRING OR BROAD BEAN PODS.

2 Do not eat or drink BOVRIL, OXO, MARMITE or ANY SIMILAR MEAT OR YEAST EXTRACT.

3 Eat only FRESH foods and avoid food that you suspect could be stale or 'going off'. This is especially important with meat, fish, poultry or offal. Avoid game.

4 Do not take any other MEDICINES (including tablets, capsules, nose drops, inhalations or suppositories) whether purchased by you or previously prescribed by your doctor, without first consulting your doctor or your pharmacist.

NB *Treatment for coughs and colds, pain relievers, tonics and laxatives are medicines.*

5 Avoid alcoholic drinks.

Keep a careful note of any food or drink that disagrees with you, avoid it and tell your doctor.

Report any unusual or severe symptoms to your doctor and follow any other advice given by him.

| M.A.O.I. | Prepared by The Pharmaceutical Society and the British Medical Association on behalf of the Health Departments of the United Kingdom. |

Printed in UK for HMSO D8919816 5/85 12773   33383

Tablets, yellow, scored, iproniazid 50 mg (as phosphate). Price 20 tabs = **C**. Label: 3, 10 MAOI card

ISOCARBOXAZID
Indications: depressive illness
Cautions; Contra-indications: see under Phenelzine
Side-effects: see under Phenelzine; rarely anaemia, hepatitis, peripheral oedema, and rashes
Dose: initially up to 30 mg daily in single or divided doses; usual maintenance dose 10–20 mg daily

PoM **Marplan**® (Roche)
Tablets, pink, scored, isocarboxazid 10 mg. Price 20 tabs = **B**. Label: 3, 10 MAOI card

TRANYLCYPROMINE
Indications: depressive illness
Cautions; Contra-indications: see under Phenelzine; also contra-indicated in hyperthyroidism
Side-effects: insomnia, dizziness, muscular weakness, dry mouth, hypotension; hypertensive crises with throbbing headache requiring discontinuation of treatment occur more frequently than with other MAOIs; liver damage occurs less frequently than with phenelzine
Dose: initially 10 mg twice daily not later than 3 p.m., increasing the second daily dose to 20 mg after 1 week if necessary; usual maintenance dose 10 mg daily

PoM **Parnate**® (SK&F)
Tablets, red, s/c, tranylcypromine 10 mg (as sulphate). Price 20 tabs = **C**. Label: 3, 10 MAOI card

4.3.3   Compound antidepressant preparations
Antipsychotic drugs such as the phenothiazine derivatives or anxiolytics such as the benzodiazepines can be usefully given with antidepressants but the use of preparations listed below is **not** recommended because the dosage of the individual components should be adjusted separately to be appropriate for the individual patient. Whereas antidepressants are given continuously over several months, the phenothiazines and benzodiazepines are usually prescribed intermittently in the lowest effective dosage.

NHS PoM **Limbitrol 5**® (Sauter)
Capsules, pink/green, amitriptyline 12.5 mg (as hydrochloride), chlordiazepoxide 5 mg. Price 20 caps = **C**. Label: 2
NHS PoM **Limbitrol 10**® (Sauter)
Capsules, pink/dark-green, amitriptyline 25 mg (as hydrochloride), chlordiazepoxide 10 mg. Price 20 caps = **D**. Label: 2
PoM **Motipress**® (Squibb)
Tablets, yellow, s/c, fluphenazine hydrochloride 1.5 mg, nortriptyline 30 mg (as hydrochloride). Price 28 tabs = **E**. Label: 2

PoM **Motival**® (Squibb)
Tablets, pink, s/c, fluphenazine hydrochloride 500 micrograms, nortriptyline 10 mg (as hydrochloride). Price 20 tabs = **C**. Label: 2
PoM **Parstelin**® (SK&F)
Tablets, green, s/c, tranylcypromine 10 mg (as sulphate), trifluoperazine 1 mg (as hydrochloride). Price 20 tabs = **C**. Label: 3, 10 MAOI card
Caution: contains MAOI
PoM **Triptafen**® (A&H)
Tablets, pink, s/c, amitriptyline hydrochloride 25 mg, perphenazine 2 mg. Price 20 tabs = **C**. Label: 2
PoM **Triptafen-M**® (A&H)
Tablets, pink, s/c, amitriptyline hydrochloride 10 mg, perphenazine 2 mg. Price 20 tabs = **B**. Label: 2

4.3.4   Other antidepressant drugs
Flupenthixol (Fluanxol®) has antidepressant properties, and low doses (1.5 to 3 mg daily) are given by mouth for this purpose. Its advantage over the tricyclic and related antidepressants is that, with the low doses employed, side-effects are fewer and overdosage less toxic. It should be withdrawn if there has been no response after 1 week at maximum dosage.

Tryptophan appears to benefit some patients when given alone or as adjunctive therapy. Its antidepressant effect may take up to 4 weeks to develop. Preparations containing pyridoxine are unsuitable for patients taking levodopa.

FLUPENTHIXOL
Indications: depressive illness. For use in psychoses, see section 4.2.1
Cautions: cardiovascular disease (including cardiac disorders and cerebral arteriosclerosis), senile confusional states, parkinsonism, renal and hepatic disease; avoid in excitable and overactive patients
Side-effects: restlessness, insomnia, rarely extrapyramidal symptoms
Dose: initially 1 mg (elderly patients 500 micrograms) in the morning, increased after 1 week to 2 mg (elderly patients 1 mg) if necessary. Max. 3 mg (elderly patients 2 mg) daily, doses above 2 mg (elderly patients 1 mg) being divided in 2 portions, the second given before 4 p.m.

PoM **Fluanxol**® (Lundbeck)
Tablets, red, s/c, flupenthixol 500 micrograms (as dihydrochloride). Price 20 tabs = **D**. Label: 4
Tablets, red, s/c, flupenthixol 1 mg (as dihydrochloride). Price 20 tabs = **E**. Label: 4

TRYPTOPHAN
Indications: adjunctive treatment of depressive illness, alone or in conjunction with other antidepressants
Cautions: active bladder disease, disorders of tryptophan metabolism. May initially affect ability to drive or operate machinery. Reduce dose when used in conjunction with MAOIs and discontinue if blurred vision or headache occur during tryptophan/MAOI therapy. Drug interactions: see Appendix 1 (section *4.3*)

For all abbreviations and symbols see inside cover.

Relative prices: **A** = up to 20p, **B** = 21-50p,

Side-effects: nausea, drowsiness, headache
Dose: 1–2 g 3 times daily, preferably after meals.
In conjunction with a monoamine-oxidase
inhibitor, 500 mg daily for 1 week, gradually
increased

PoM **Optimax®** (Merck)
Tablets, yellow, f/c, scored, L-tryptophan
500 mg, pyridoxine hydrochloride 5 mg, ascorbic acid 10 mg. Price 20 tabs = **E**. Label: 2
Powder, L-tryptophan 1 g, pyridoxine hydrochloride 10 mg, ascorbic acid 20 mg/6 g. Price
20 × 6-g sachets = **G**. Label: 2, 13
PoM **Optimax WV®** (Merck)
Tablets, yellow, f/c, scored, L-tryptophan
500 mg. Price 20 tabs = **E**. Label: 2
PoM **Pacitron®** (Berk)
Tablets, orange, f/c, L-tryptophan 500 mg. Price
20 tabs = **E**. Label: 2

4.4   Central nervous stimulants

4.4.1 Weak central nervous stimulants
4.4.2 Amphetamines and cocaine
See section 3.5 for respiratory stimulants.

4.4.1   Weak central nervous stimulants

Caffeine is a weak, widely used, stimulant present
in tea and coffee. It is included in many analgesic
preparations (section 4.7.1.3) but does not contribute to their analgesic or anti-inflammatory
effect. Over-indulgence may lead to a state of
arousal and anxiety.

Pemoline may be useful in the management of
hyperactive children. Other weak central nervous
stimulants are **fencamfamin** and **prolintane** which
are included in some vitamin preparations. Their
value is doubtful but they have been advocated
for the management of senility, debility, and relief
of fatigue. They should not be used to treat
depression.

PEMOLINE

Indications: debility and fatigue, hyperkinesia in
children
Cautions: cardiovascular disease, insomnia.
Drug interactions: see Appendix 1 (section *4.3*)
Contra-indications: glaucoma, extrapyramidal
disorders, hyperexcitable states (thyrotoxicosis)
Side-effects: insomnia, tachycardia, agitation
Dose: 20 mg in the morning and midday, gradually increased to a max. of 120 mg daily; CHILD
over 6 years (also elderly patients), 10–20 mg
morning and midday

PoM **Pemoline Tablets,** pemoline 20 mg. Price 20
tabs = **B**
PoM **Ronyl®** (Lipha)
Tablets, scored, pemoline 20 mg. Price 20 tabs =
B

PoM **Volital®** (LAB)
Tablets, scored, pemoline 20 mg. Price 20 tabs =
B

Preparations containing a stimulant and vitamins
NHS PoM **Reactivan®** (Merck)
Tablets, yellow, s/c, fencamfamin hydrochloride 10 mg,
ascorbic acid 100 mg, cyanocobalamin 10 micrograms,
pyridoxine phosphate 20 mg, thiamine phosphate
10 mg. Price 20 tabs = **C**
Dose: 2 tablets in the morning and 1 at midday if
necessary
NHS PoM **Villescon®** (Boehringer Ingelheim)
Tablets, orange, s/c, prolintane hydrochloride 10 mg,
ascorbic acid 50 mg, nicotinamide 15 mg, pyridoxine
hydrochloride 1.5 mg, riboflavine 3 mg, thiamine
mononitrate 5 mg. Price 20 tabs = **C**
Dose: 1 tablet twice daily before 4 p.m. for 1–2 weeks;
CHILD over 8 years 1 tablet after breakfast
Liquid (= elixir), red, prolintane hydrochloride 2.5 mg,
nicotinamide 5 mg, pyridoxine hydrochloride 500 micrograms, riboflavine sodium phosphate 1.36 mg, thiamine
hydrochloride 1.67 mg/5 ml. Diluent water for preparations, life of diluted elixir 14 days. Price 100 ml = **B**
Dose: 10 ml twice daily before 4 p.m. for 1–2 weeks;
CHILD 5–12 years 2.5–10 ml twice daily.

4.4.2   Amphetamines and cocaine

The amphetamines have a limited field of usefulness and their use should be **discouraged** as
they may cause dependence and psychotic states.

Patients with narcolepsy may derive benefit
from treatment with amphetamines. They have
also been advocated for the management of hyperactive children; beneficial effects have been
described. However, they must be used very selectively as they retard growth and the effect of long-
term therapy has not been evaluated.

Amphetamines have **no place** in the management of **depression** or **obesity**.

Cocaine is a drug of addiction which causes
central nervous stimulation. Its clinical use is
mainly as a topical local anaesthetic (see sections
11.7 and 15.2). It has been included in analgesic
elixirs for the relief of pain in terminal care (section 4.7.2) but this use is obsolescent.

DEXAMPHETAMINE SULPHATE

Indications: narcolepsy, hyperkinesia in children
Cautions: anorexia, insomnia, impaired renal
function, unstable personality. Drug
interactions: see Appendix 1 (sections *2.4*, *4.3*)
Contra-indications: cardiovascular disease,
hyperexcitable states (thyrotoxicosis),
glaucoma, extrapyramidal disorders
Side-effects: dependence and tolerance occur
readily, also agitation, restlessness, insomnia,
headache, dizziness, tremor, personality
change, anorexia, arrhythmias, dry mouth,
diarrhoea, or constipation. In children, anorexia, weight loss, growth inhibition, and tear-
fulness. Large doses cause disorientation and
aggression, leading to paranoid psychosis, convulsions, and coma
Dose: narcolepsy, 10 mg daily in divided doses
gradually increased to a max. of 60 mg daily
Hyperkinesia, CHILD 3–5 years 2.5 mg in the
morning gradually increased to a max. of 20 mg

C = 51-100p, D = 101-180p, E = 181-300p, F = 301-450p, G = 451-650p, H = 651-900p, I = 901-1200p, J = over 1200p.

daily; 6–12 years 5–10 mg in the morning, gradually increased to a max. of 40 mg daily in 2 divided doses

CD Dexedrine® (SK&F)
Tablets, yellow, scored, dexamphetamine sulphate 5 mg. Price 20 tabs = **A**

COMPOUND PREPARATIONS

CD Durophet ® (Riker)
Capsules (Durophet 7.5 mg), s/r, amphetamine 3.75 mg, dexamphetamine 3.75 mg (both resin complexes). Price 30 caps = **C**. Label: 25
Capsules (Durophet 12.5 mg), s/r, white/grey, amphetamine 6.25 mg, dexamphetamine 6.25 mg (both resin complexes). Price 30 caps = **C**. Label: 25
Capsules (Durophet 20 mg), s/r, grey, amphetamine 10 mg, dexamphetamine 10 mg (both resin complexes). Price 30 caps = **C**. Label: 25

4.5   Appetite suppressants

4.5.1 Bulk-forming drugs
4.5.2 Centrally-acting appetite suppressants

The development of obesity appears to be multi-factorial. Aggravating factors may be depression or other psychosocial problems or drug treatment.

The main treatment of the obese patient is an appropriate diet, carefully explained to the patient, with support and encouragement from the doctor. Attendance at groups (for example 'weight-watchers') helps some individuals. Drugs can play only a limited role and should never be used as the sole element of treatment as their effects tend to be disappointing.

Centrally-acting appetite suppressants (section 4.5.2) carry the risk of dependence and other adverse effects. They should **not** be given to patients with a past history of drug abuse or psychiatric illness. Also they are **not recommended** for periods of treatment beyond 3 to 6 months because of the risks of dependence and lack of efficacy in extended use.

4.5.1   Bulk-forming drugs

The most commonly used bulk-forming drug is **methylcellulose**. It is claimed to reduce intake by producing feelings of satiety but there is little evidence to support this claim.

METHYLCELLULOSE

Indications: obesity
Cautions: maintain adequate fluid intake
Contra-indications: gastro-intestinal obstruction
Side-effects: flatulence, abdominal distension, intestinal obstruction

Celevac® (WBP)
Tablets, pink, methylcellulose '450' 500 mg. Price 20 tabs = **A**. Label: 22, 24, 27
Dose: 3 tablets, chewed or crushed, with a tumblerful of liquid half an hour before food or when hungry

Cellucon® (Medo)
Tablets, buff, methylcellulose '2500' 500 mg. Price 20 tabs = **A**. Label: 22, 24, 27
Dose: 1–4 tablets, chewed or crushed, with a tumblerful of liquid half an hour before food or when hungry

Nilstim® (De Witt)
Tablets, green, cellulose (microcrystalline) 220 mg, methylcellulose '2500' 400 mg. Price 20 tabs = **A**. Label: 22, 24, 27
Dose: 2 tablets, chewed or crushed, with a tumblerful of liquid 15 minutes before the 2 main meals or when hungry

STERCULIA

Indications; Cautions; Side-effects: see under Methylcellulose

Prefil® (Norgine)
Granules, brown, coated, sterculia 55%. Price 200 g = **D**. Label: 22, 27
Dose: two 5-ml spoonfuls followed by a tumblerful of liquid ½–1 hour before food, reduced in patients accustomed to a low-residue diet

4.5.2   Centrally-acting appetite suppressants

The use of amphetamine-like drugs, including phenmetrazine, in the treatment of obesity is **not** justified as any possible benefits are outweighed by the risks involved.

The centrally-acting appetite suppressants below may be used as adjunctive treatment in some patients with moderate to severe obesity. Patients should be given close support and supervision and treatment limited to short periods. These drugs should be avoided in children because of the possibility of growth suppression, and should not be used for cosmetic purposes in mild obesity.

Diethylpropion (Apisate®, Tenuate Dospan®), **mazindol** (Teronac®), and **phentermine** (Duromine®, Ionamin®) are used as appetite suppressants. They have anorectic properties comparable with amphetamine but their stimulant action and risk of dependence is considerably less. Drug abuse, particularly with diethylpropion, is, however, an increasing problem. They are preferred for their stimulant action in lethargic, rather depressed patients.

Fenfluramine (Ponderax®) differs from most other appetite suppressants in not being stimulant; indeed it has some sedative properties. Dependence is rare but abrupt withdrawal may induce depression.

Thyroid hormones have no place in the treatment of obesity except in hypothyroid patients.

DIETHYLPROPION HYDROCHLORIDE

Indications: short-term adjunct in moderate to severe obesity
Cautions: cardiovascular disease, peptic ulceration, epilepsy, depression, diabetes, unstable personality

Contra-indications: glaucoma, hyperexcitable states (thyrotoxicosis)

Side-effects: agitation, insomnia, tachycardia, gastro-intestinal disturbances, dizziness, tremor, restlessness, dry mouth, headache, chills; tolerance and amphetamine-type dependence may occur. Also psychotic episodes in predisposed patients

CD Apisate® (Wyeth)
Tablets, s/r, yellow, diethylpropion hydrochloride 75 mg, thiamine hydrochloride 5 mg, pyridoxine hydrochloride 2 mg, riboflavine 4 mg, nicotinamide 30 mg. Price 20 tabs = **B**. Label: 25
Dose: 1 tablet, morning and/or mid-afternoon for not longer than 8 weeks

CD Tenuate Dospan® (Merrell)
Tablets, s/r, scored, diethylpropion hydrochloride 75 mg. Price 20 tabs = **C**. Label: 25
Dose: 1 tablet mid-morning for not longer than 8 weeks

FENFLURAMINE HYDROCHLORIDE

Indications: short-term adjunct in moderate to severe obesity

Cautions: depression; may affect mental concentration and ability to drive or operate machinery and increase the effects of alcohol. Drug interactions: see Appendix 1 (sections 2.5, 4.3)

Side-effects: sedation, headache, dizziness, and gastro-intestinal disturbances. Less commonly, dry mouth, sleep disturbances, tachycardia, fluid retention, urinary frequency, chills, alopecia, and haemolytic anaemia. Dosage should be discontinued gradually as rebound depression can occur rarely when therapy is discontinued abruptly. Tolerance may also occur

Dose: initially 20 mg morning and evening, increasing to a max. of 80 mg daily then gradually reduced; doses are preferably taken ½ hour before meals

PoM Ponderax® (Servier)
Tablets, pale blue, s/c, fenfluramine hydrochloride 20 mg. Price 20 tabs = **C**. Label: 2
Pacaps® (= capsules s/r), clear/blue, enclosing white pellets, fenfluramine hydrochloride 60 mg. Price 20 caps = **E**. Label: 2, 25
Dose: 1–2 capsules daily, preferably before breakfast

MAZINDOL

Indications: short-term adjunct in moderate to severe obesity

Cautions; Contra-indications; Side-effects: see under Diethylpropion Hydrochloride. Avoid in peptic ulceration. Drug interactions: see Appendix 1 (section 2.5)

Dose: 2 mg after breakfast for up to 12 weeks

PoM Teronac® (Sandoz)
Tablets, scored, mazindol 2 mg. Price 20 tabs = **D**. Label: 4

PHENTERMINE

Indications: short-term adjunct in moderate to severe obesity

Cautions; Contra-indications; Side-effects: see under Diethylpropion Hydrochloride

Dose: 15–30 mg before breakfast

PoM Duromine® (Riker)
Capsules, s/r, green/grey, phentermine 15 mg (as resin complex). Price 30 caps = **D**. Label: 25
Capsules, s/r, maroon/grey, phentermine 30 mg (as resin complex). Price 30 caps = **D**. Label: 25

PoM Ionamin® (Lipha)
Capsules, s/r, grey/yellow, phentermine 15 mg (as resin complex). Price 20 caps = **C**. Label: 25
Capsules, s/r, yellow, phentermine 30 mg (as resin complex). Price 20 caps = **D**. Label: 25

4.6 Drugs used in nausea and vertigo

Drug treatment of nausea and vertigo is discussed under the following headings:
Vestibular disorders
Nausea of pregnancy
Symptomatic relief of nausea from underlying disease

Anti-emetics should be prescribed only when the cause of vomiting is known, particularly in children, otherwise the symptomatic relief that they produce may delay identification and treatment of the underlying disease. When the cause can be treated (as in diabetic ketoacidosis and digitalis intoxication), anti-emetics are generally unnecessary. Patients may be taking medicines to treat other conditions; the prescriber should ascertain whether they could be the cause of nausea, in which case the problem may be resolved by dose reduction or by changing to a less nauseant preparation. If antinauseant drug treatment is indicated the choice of drug depends on the aetiology of vomiting.

VESTIBULAR DISORDERS

Anti-emetics may be required in motion sickness, Ménière's disease, positional vertigo, labyrinthitis, and operative manipulation of the otovestibular apparatus. **Hyoscine** and the **antihistamines** are the drugs of choice. If possible they should be administered prophylactically at least 30 minutes before the emetic stimulus. Patients should be **warned** that these compounds may cause drowsiness, impair driving performance, and enhance the effects of alcohol and central nervous depressants.

MOTION SICKNESS. The most effective drug for the prevention of motion sickness is **hyoscine**. Adverse effects (drowsiness, blurred vision, dry mouth, urinary retention) are more frequent than with the **antihistamines** but are not generally prominent at the doses employed.

Antihistamines such as **cinnarizine, cyclizine, dimenhydrinate, mepyramine,** and **promethazine**

C = 51-100p, D = 101-180p, E = 181-300p, F = 301-450p, G = 451-650p, H = 651-900p, I = 901-1200p, J = over 1200p.

are slightly less effective but generally better tolerated. There is no evidence that one antihistamine is superior to another but their duration of action and incidence of adverse effects (drowsiness and anticholinergic effects) differ. If a sedative effect is desired promethazine and dimenhydrinate are useful, but generally a less sedating antihistamine like cyclizine or cinnarizine is preferred. To prevent motion sickness the first dose is usually taken half an hour (2 hours for cinnarizine) before the start of the journey. Metoclopramide and the phenothiazine derivatives (except promethazine) are ineffective in motion sickness.

OTHER LABYRINTHINE DISORDERS. Vertigo and nausea associated with Ménière's disease and middle-ear surgery disorders may be difficult to treat. **Hyoscine, antihistamines**, and **phenothiazine derivatives** (such as chlorpromazine, prochlorperazine, and thiethylperazine) are effective in the prophylaxis and treatment of such conditions. **Betahistine** and **cinnarizine** have been promoted as specific treatment for Ménière's disease. In the acute attack **chlorpromazine, cyclizine, prochlorperazine**, or **thiethylperazine** may be given rectally or by intramuscular injection.

Treatment of vertigo in its chronic forms is seldom fully effective but antihistamines (such as dimenhydrinate) or phenothiazine derivatives (such as prochlorperazine) may help.

NAUSEA OF PREGNANCY

Nausea and vomiting in the first trimester of pregnancy does **not** generally require drug therapy, which should be avoided because of teratogenic risk. If vomiting is severe, an antihistamine or a phenothiazine derivative (promethazine or thiethylperazine) may be useful.

SYMPTOMATIC RELIEF OF NAUSEA FROM UNDERLYING DISEASE

A **phenothiazine derivative**, in low doses, is the drug of choice for the prophylaxis and treatment of nausea and vomiting associated with uraemia, diffuse neoplastic disease, radiation sickness, acute viral gastro-enteritis, and the emesis caused by drugs such as oestrogens, narcotics, general anaesthetics, and cytotoxic drugs. Rectal or parenteral administration is required if the vomiting has already started. **Chlorpromazine** is usually suitable and although a sedative effect is common, adverse extrapyramidal effects are not generally prominent at the doses required for full anti-emetic action.

Prochlorperazine, perphenazine, trifluoperazine, and **thiethylperazine** are less sedating than chlorpromazine but severe dystonic reactions sometimes occur, especially in children.

Metoclopramide is an effective anti-emetic with a spectrum of activity closely resembling that of the phenothiazine derivatives but it may be less potent. It has a peripheral action in addition to

its central effect and therefore may be superior to the phenothiazine derivatives in the emesis associated with gastroduodenal, hepatic, and biliary disease. The high-dose preparation is of value in the prevention of nausea and vomiting associated with cytotoxic drug therapy. Acute dystonic reactions may occur, particularly with children, but they are less frequent than with phenothiazine derivatives.

Domperidone (Motilium®) is used for the prevention and relief of nausea and vomiting, especially when associated with cytotoxic drug therapy. It has the advantage over metoclopramide and the phenothiazine derivatives of being less likely to cause central effects such as sedation and dystonic reactions. It may be given for the treatment of levodopa- and bromocriptine-induced vomiting in parkinsonism (section 4.9.1). In patients with cardiac disease or hypokalaemia and in those receiving cytotoxic therapy, intravenous injections are occasionally associated with arrhythmias; they are no longer generally available and can only be obtained by special request for a named patient. Domperidone acts at the chemoreceptor trigger zone and so is unlikely to be effective in motion sickness and other vestibular disorders.

Although antihistamines are active in most of these conditions, they are not usually drugs of choice.

Nabilone (Cesamet®) is a synthetic cannabinoid with anti-emetic properties, reported to be superior to prochlorperazine. It is beneficial in the relief of nausea and vomiting associated with cytotoxic drug therapy. Side-effects, which are more frequent than with prochlorperazine, include somnolence, dizziness, and dry mouth and will occur in about half of patients given standard doses. Repeated use should be avoided because of possible neurotoxic effects.

BETAHISTINE HYDROCHLORIDE

Indications: vertigo and hearing disturbances in labyrinthine disorders
Cautions: asthma, peptic ulcer. Drug interactions: see Appendix 1 (section 4.6)
Contra-indications: phaeochromocytoma
Side-effects: nausea; rarely headache, rashes
Dose: 8–16 mg 3 times daily, after food, increased as necessary to a max. of 48 mg daily

PoM **Serc®** (Duphar)
Tablets, scored, betahistine hydrochloride 8 mg. Price 20 tabs = D. Label: 21

BUCLIZINE HYDROCHLORIDE

Indications: nausea, vertigo, labyrinthine disorders
Cautions; Side-effects: see under Cyclizine. Avoid in children

PoM **Equivert®** (Pfizer)
Tablets, yellow, buclizine hydrochloride 25 mg, nicotinic acid 25 mg. Price 20 tabs = C. Label: 2, 22
Dose: 1 tablet 3 times daily before food

CHLORPROMAZINE HYDROCHLORIDE

Indications: severe nausea and vomiting (see notes above); vertigo
Cautions; Contra-indications; Side-effects: see section 4.2.1
Dose: by mouth, 25–50 mg 3 times daily
By subcutaneous or intramuscular injection, 12.5–50 mg 3 times daily
By rectum in suppositories, chlorpromazine 100 mg up to 3 times daily

Preparations
Section 4.2.1

CINNARIZINE

Indications: nausea, vertigo, labyrinthine disorders, motion sickness
Cautions; Side-effects: see under Cyclizine. Rarely allergic rashes
Dose: 15–30 mg 3 times daily; CHILD 6–12 years half adult dose

Stugeron® (Janssen)
Tablets, scored, cinnarizine 15 mg. Price 20 tabs = **C**. Label: 2
Stugeron Forte: see section 2.6.3

CYCLIZINE

Indications: nausea, vomiting, vertigo, motion sickness, labyrinthine disorders
Cautions: patient's ability to drive or operate machinery may be impaired; alcohol increases CNS depression; liver disease, epilepsy, prostatic hypertrophy, glaucoma. Drug interactions: see Appendix 1 (sections *4.1, 4.6, 4.9*)
Side-effects: drowsiness, headache, dry mouth, gastro-intestinal disturbances, blurred vision, rarely paradoxical excitation ·
Dose: by mouth, cyclizine hydrochloride 50 mg 3 times daily; CHILD 1–10 years 25 mg 3 times daily
By intramuscular or intravenous injection, adults and children over 10 years, cyclizine lactate 50 mg 3 times daily

Valoid® (Calmic)
Tablets, scored, cyclizine hydrochloride 50 mg. Price 20 tabs = **C**. Label: 2
PoM *Injection,* cyclizine lactate 50 mg/ml. Price 1-ml amp = **B**

DIMENHYDRINATE

Indications: nausea, vomiting, vertigo, motion sickness, labyrinthine disorders
Cautions; Side-effects: see under Cyclizine but more sedating
Dose: 50–100 mg 2–3 times daily; CHILD 1–5 years 12.5–25 mg, 6–12 years 25–50 mg 2–3 times daily

Dramamine® (Searle)
Tablets, yellow, scored, dimenhydrinate 50 mg. Price 20 tabs = **C**. Label: 2

DIPHENHYDRAMINE HYDROCHLORIDE

Indications: nausea, vertigo, labyrinthine disorders
Cautions; Side-effects: see under Cyclizine
Dose: 25–50 mg 3–4 times daily

Preparations
See section 3.4.1

DOMPERIDONE

Indications: nausea and vomiting, particularly in gastro-intestinal disorders or during treatment with cytotoxic drugs
Cautions: see notes above. Drug interactions: see Appendix 1 (section *6.7*)
Contra-indications: chronic administration; routine postoperative administration
Side-effects: raised prolactin concentrations (significance uncertain)
Dose: by mouth or by intramuscular injection or intravenous injection or infusion, 10–20 mg every 4–8 hours; CHILD, nausea and vomiting following cytotoxic therapy or radiotherapy, 200–400 micrograms/kg
By rectum in suppositories, 60 mg every 4–8 hours, adjusted as required; CHILD, half adult dose

▼ PoM **Motilium®** (Janssen)
Tablets, f/c, domperidone 10 mg (as maleate). Price 20 tabs = **E**
Suspension (= mixture), sugar-free, domperidone 5 mg/5 ml. Price 200 ml = **D**
Injection, domperidone 5 mg/ml (Named patient basis only)
Suppositories, domperidone 30 mg. Price 10 suppos = **E**

HYOSCINE HYDROBROMIDE
(Scopolamine)

Indications: nausea, vomiting, vertigo, labyrinthine disorders, motion sickness
Cautions: elderly patients, urinary retention, cardiovascular disease, paralytic ileus, pyloric stenosis
Contra-indications: glaucoma
Side-effects: drowsiness, dry mouth, dizziness, blurred vision, difficulty with micturition
Dose: by mouth or by subcutaneous injection, 300–600 micrograms 4 times daily; CHILD 3–5 years 75–100 micrograms, 6–12 years 100–300 micrograms

PoM **Hyoscine Tablets,** hyoscine hydrobromide 300 micrograms, price 20 tabs = **A**; 600 micrograms, price 20 tabs = **B**. Label: 3
PoM **Hyoscine Injection,** hyoscine hydrobromide 400 and 600 micrograms/ml. Price 1-ml amp (both) = **B**

MECLOZINE HYDROCHLORIDE

Indications: nausea
Cautions; Side-effects: see under Cyclizine

C = 51-100p, **D** = 101-180p, **E** = 181-300p, **F** = 301-450p, **G** = 451-650p, **H** = 651-900p, **I** = 901-1200p, **J** = over 1200p.

NHS PoM **Ancoloxin®** (DF)

Tablets, meclozine hydrochloride 25 mg, pyridoxine hydrochloride 50 mg. Price 20 tabs = **C**. Label: 2

Dose: 1–2 tablets 2–3 times daily; severe nausea and vomiting of pregnancy, 2 tablets at bedtime and if necessary 1 in the morning

MEPYRAMINE MALEATE

Indications: nausea, vomiting, vertigo, labyrinthine disorders, motion sickness
Cautions; Side-effects: see under Cyclizine
Dose: 100 mg 3 times daily, increased if necessary to 1 g daily; CHILD 7–14 years 50 mg 3–4 times daily

Preparations
See section 3.4.1

METOCLOPRAMIDE HYDROCHLORIDE

Indications: nausea and vomiting, particularly in gastro-intestinal disorders, during treatment with cytotoxic drugs or radiotherapy, and postoperative conditions; migraine—section 4.7.4.1
Cautions; Side-effects: see section 1.2
Dose: by mouth, or by intramuscular or intravenous injection, up to 10 mg (5 mg in young adults up to 20 years) 3 times daily; CHILD (see cautions) up to 1 year 1 mg twice daily, 1–2 years 1 mg 2–3 times daily, 3–5 years 2 mg 2–3 times daily, 6–14 years 2.5–5 mg 3 times daily
By intravenous infusion, nausea and vomiting associated with cytotoxic drugs, up to 2 mg/kg every 2 hours up to a max. of 10 mg/kg/24 hours. The initial dose should be given before starting cytotoxic treatment

▼ PoM **Maxolon High Dose®** (Beecham)

Injection, metoclopramide 5 mg (as hydrochloride)/ml. Price 20-ml amp = **E**. For intravenous infusion in nausea and vomiting associated with cytotoxic chemotherapy only
For other preparations see section 1.2

NABILONE

Indications: nausea and vomiting caused by cytotoxic drugs
Cautions: may affect patient's ability to drive or operate machinery and increase the effects of alcohol; severe hepatic impairment; history of psychosis
Side-effects: drowsiness, postural hypotension, tachycardia, dry mouth, decreased appetite, abdominal cramps; also confusion, disorientation, euphoria, hallucinations, psychosis, depression, headache, blurred vision, tremors, decreased concentration and co-ordination
Dose: 1–2 mg twice daily throughout each cycle of cytotoxic therapy and, if necessary, for 24 hours after the last dose of each cycle; max. 6 mg daily. The first dose should be taken the night before initiation of cytotoxic treatment, and the second dose 1–3 hours before the first dose of cytotoxic drug

▼ PoM **Cesamet®** (Lilly)

Capsules, blue/white, nabilone 1 mg. Price 5 caps = **H** (Hosp. only). Label: 2

PERPHENAZINE

Indications: severe nausea, vomiting (see notes above)
Cautions; Contra-indications; Side-effects: see section 4.2.1
Dose: by mouth, 4 mg 3 times daily, increased if necessary to a max. of 24 mg in 24 hours
By intramuscular injection, 5–10 mg initially, then 5 mg every 6 hours, max. 15 mg in 24 hours

Preparations
Section 4.2.1

PROCHLORPERAZINE

Indications: severe nausea, vomiting, vertigo, labyrinthine disorders, cytotoxic therapy (see notes above)
Cautions; Contra-indications: see under Chlorpromazine Hydrochloride (section 4.2.1). Avoid in children weighing less than 10 kg
Side-effects: dry mouth, drowsiness, which may affect the ability to drive or operate machinery or increase the CNS depressant effect of alcohol. Side-effects are rare with anti-emetic doses, but with high doses extrapyramidal symptoms may occur, particularly in children, elderly, and debilitated patients
Dose: by mouth, nausea and vomiting, prochlorperazine maleate or mesylate, acute attack, 20 mg initially then 10 mg after 2 hours; prevention 5–10 mg 2–3 times daily; CHILD 1–5 years 2.5 mg twice daily, 6–12 years 5 mg 2–3 times daily
Labyrinthine disorders, 5 mg 3 times daily, gradually increased if necessary to 30 mg daily in divided doses, then reduced after several weeks to 5–10 mg daily; CHILD as above
By deep intramuscular injection, 12.5 mg when required followed if necessary after 6 hours by an oral dose
By rectum in suppositories, 25 mg; CHILD daily in divided doses, 1–2 years up to 7.5 mg, 3–5 years up to 10 mg, 6–12 years up to 15 mg

PoM **Stemetil®** (M&B)

Tablets, prochlorperazine maleate 5 mg. Price 20 tabs = **C**. Label: 2
Tablets, scored, prochlorperazine maleate 25 mg. Price 20 tabs = **D**. Label: 2
Syrup (= elixir), green, prochlorperazine mesylate 5 mg/5 ml. Diluent syrup, life of diluted elixir 14 days. Price 125 ml = **D**. Label: 2
Injection, prochlorperazine mesylate 12.5 mg/ml. Price 1- and 2-ml amp (both) = **B**
Suppositories, prochlorperazine maleate 5 mg (as prochlorperazine). Price 10 suppos = **F**. Label: 2
Suppositories, prochlorperazine maleate 25 mg (as prochlorperazine). Price 10 suppos = **F**. Label: 2

PoM **Vertigon**® (SK&F)
Spansule® (= capsules s/r), clear/purple, enclosing yellowish-green and white pellets, prochlorperazine 10 mg (as maleate). Price 20 caps = **C**. Label: 2, 25
Spansule® (= capsules s/r), clear/purple, enclosing yellowish-green and white pellets, prochlorperazine 15 mg (as maleate). Price 20 caps = **D**. Label: 2, 25
Dose: initially 10–15 mg once or twice daily. Maintenance 10–15 mg daily

PROMETHAZINE HYDROCHLORIDE
Indications: nausea, vomiting, vertigo, labyrinthine disorders, motion sickness
Cautions; Side-effects: see under Cyclizine but more sedating; intramuscular injection may be painful
Dose: by mouth, 25–75 mg daily in single or divided doses; CHILD 6–12 months 5–10 mg, 1–5 years 5–15 mg, 6–12 years 10–25 mg daily in single or divided doses
By deep intramuscular injection, 25–50 mg when necessary; CHILD 6–12 years 6.25–12.5 mg
By slow intravenous injection, section 3.4.1

Preparations
See section 3.4.1

PROMETHAZINE THEOCLATE
Indications: nausea, vertigo, labyrinthine disorders, motion sickness (acts longer than the hydrochloride)
Cautions; Side-effects: see under Cyclizine but more sedating
Dose: 25–75 mg, max. 100 mg, daily; CHILD 5–10 years 12.5–37.5 mg daily
For severe vomiting in pregnancy, 25 mg at bedtime, increased if necessary to a max. of 100 mg daily

Avomine® (M&B)
Tablets, scored, promethazine theoclate 25 mg. Price 10 tabs = **B**. Label: 2

THIETHYLPERAZINE
Indications: severe nausea, vomiting, vertigo, labyrinthine disorders, cytotoxic therapy (see notes above)
Cautions; Contra-indications: see under Chlorpromazine Hydrochloride (section 4.2.1)
Side-effects: dry mouth, postural hypotension, drowsiness (which may affect the ability to drive or operate machinery and increase CNS effects of alcohol). Extrapyramidal effects are rare but females under 30 years are particularly susceptible
Dose: by mouth, thiethylperazine maleate 10 mg 2–3 times daily
By intramuscular injection, thiethylperazine 6.5 mg when necessary
By rectum in suppositories, thiethylperazine 6.5 mg night and morning

Note: thiethylperazine 6.5 mg ≡ thiethylperazine malate 10.86 mg ≡ thiethylperazine maleate 10.28 mg

PoM **Torecan**® (Sandoz)
Tablets, s/c, thiethylperazine *maleate* 10 mg. Price 20 tabs = **C**. Label: 2
Injection, thiethylperazine 6.5 mg (as *malate*)/ ml. Price 1-ml amp = **A**
Suppositories, thiethylperazine 6.5 mg (as *maleate*). Price 6 suppos = **C**. Label: 2

TRIFLUOPERAZINE
Indications: severe nausea and vomiting (see notes above)
Cautions; Contra-indications; Side-effects: see section 4.2.1. Side-effects occur infrequently with anti-emetic doses
Dose: by mouth, 2–4 mg daily in divided doses *or* as a single dose of a sustained-release preparation; CHILD 3–5 years up to 1 mg daily, 6–12 years up to 4 mg daily
By deep intramuscular injection, 1–3 mg daily in divided doses; CHILD 50 micrograms/kg daily in divided doses

Preparations
Section 4.2.1

4.7 Analgesics
4.7.1 Analgesics used for mild to moderate pain
4.7.1.1 Non-narcotic analgesics
4.7.1.2 Narcotic analgesics used for mild to moderate pain
4.7.1.3 Compound analgesic preparations
4.7.2 Narcotic and other analgesics used for severe pain
4.7.3 Trigeminal neuralgia
4.7.4 Antimigraine drugs
4.7.4.1 Treatment of the acute migraine attack
4.7.4.2 Prophylaxis of migraine

4.7.1 Analgesics used for mild to moderate pain
The non-narcotic drugs, aspirin and paracetamol, are particularly suited to the relief of pain in musculoskeletal conditions, whereas the narcotic analgesics are more suited for the relief of severe pain of visceral origin.

Analgesic requirements may be profoundly affected by the attitude of both the patient and the prescriber to the pain; in many cases where analgesics might normally have been given, a placebo has provided substantial relief. For advice on pain relief in terminal care see Prescribing in Terminal Care.

4.7.1.1 NON-NARCOTIC ANALGESICS

Aspirin and paracetamol are the main drugs in this group. They are usually sufficient to treat

---

C = 51-100p, **D** = 101-180p, **E** = 181-300p, **F** = 301-450p, **G** = 451-650p, **H** = 651-900p, **I** = 901-1200p, **J** = over 1200p.

most types of moderate pain and it is rarely necessary to use other analgesics.

Aspirin is the analgesic of choice for headache,
transient musculoskeletal pain, and dysmenorrhoea. It also has anti-inflammatory properties
which may sometimes be useful. Aspirin tablets
or dispersible aspirin tablets are adequate for most
purposes as they act rapidly and are inexpensive.

Gastric irritation may be a problem; it is minimised by taking the dose after food. Numerous
formulations are available which improve gastric
tolerance, for example the buffered aspirin preparations such as aloxiprin, micro-encapsulated
aspirin (Levius®) and enteric-coated aspirin (Nu-
Seals®). Some of these preparations have a slow
onset of action and are therefore unsuitable for
single-dose analgesic use though their prolonged
action may be useful for the relief of night pain.

Aspirin is **not** recommended for use in infants
under one year because of the danger of metabolic
acidosis and fatal poisoning which may occur after
repeated dosage, but single doses may be used for
minor infections in young children.

Aspirin Mixture BPC 1963 is an unstable mixture that should **not** be prescribed. The appropriate quantity of aspirin in the form of dispersible
tablets should be ordered to be taken in water.

Paracetamol is similar in efficacy to aspirin, but
has no demonstable anti-inflammatory activity; it
is less irritant to the stomach. Paediatric paracetamol elixir is preferable to aspirin in infants.
Overdosage with paracetamol is particularly
dangerous as it may cause hepatic damage which
is sometimes not apparent for 4 to 6 days. **Benorylate** is an aspirin–paracetamol ester which
releases paracetamol slowly and so hepatotoxicity
in overdosage may be reduced.

Anti-inflammatory analgesics (see section
10.1.1.2) are particularly useful for the treatment
of patients with chronic disease accompanied by
pain and inflammation. Some of them are also
used in the short-term treatment of mild to moderate pain including transient musculoskeletal
pain. They may be particularly suitable for the
relief of pain in *dysmenorrhoea* because of their
ability to inhibit prostaglandin synthetase. They
may often be usefully added to existing narcotic
analgesic regimens rather than increasing the dose
of narcotic when treating pain caused by some
secondary bone tumours many of which produce
lysis of bone and release prostaglandins. In this
case it is generally advisable to select one of the
longer-acting anti-inflammatory analgesics, for
example diflunisal (given as 500 mg every 12
hours). They have the advantage of lessening the
risk of gastro-intestinal complications and encouraging better patient compliance.

ASPIRIN

Indications: mild to moderate pain, pyrexia (see
notes above); see also section 10.1.1.1
Cautions: asthma, impaired renal or hepatic
function, dehydration, pregnancy; children (see

notes above). Drug interactions: see Appendix
1 (sections *2.2*, *2.8*, *2.8E*, *4.7*, *4.8*, *8*, *10*)
Contra-indications: gastro-intestinal ulceration
(see notes above), haemophilia, concurrent
anticoagulant therapy
Side-effects: generally mild and infrequent but
high incidence of gastro-intestinal irritation
with slight asymptomatic blood loss, increased
bleeding time, bronchospasm and skin reactions in hypersensitive patients. Prolonged
administration, see section 10.1.1.1
Dose: 300–900 mg every 4–6 hours when necessary; max. 4 g daily; CHILD 1–2 years 75–150 mg
every 6 hours, 3–5 years 225–300 mg every 8
hours, 6–12 years 300–400 mg every 6 hours

Aspirin Tablets, aspirin 300 mg. Price 20 tabs =
A. Label: 21
Aspirin Tablets, Dispersible, aspirin 300 mg.
Price 20 tabs = **A.** Label: 13, 21
Aspirin Tablets, Paediatric Dispersible, aspirin
75 mg. Price 20 tabs = **A.** Label: 13, 21
ℕℍ𝕊 **Aspergum®** (Plough)
Tablets, chewing gum, s/c, aspirin 227 mg. Price
20 tabs = **C.** Label: 21
Dose: 1–2 tablets chewed every 4–6 hours when
necessary; max. 8 tablets daily; CHILD 6–9 years
up to 3 tablets daily, 10–14 years up to 5 tablets
daily
ℕℍ𝕊 **Claradin®** (Nicholas)
Tablets, effervescent, scored, aspirin 300 mg.
Price 20 tabs = **B.** Label: 13, 21
ℕℍ𝕊 **Laboprin®** (LAB)
Tablets, mottled white/brown, aspirin 300 mg
with lysine 245 mg. Price 24 tabs = **C.** Label: 21
ℕℍ𝕊 **Paynocil®** (Beecham)
Tablets, scored, aspirin 600 mg, glycine 300 mg.
To be dissolved on the tongue. Price 30 tabs =
C. Label: 21, 24
ℕℍ𝕊 **Solprin®** (R&C)
Tablets, dispersible, aspirin 300 mg. Price 20
tabs = **A.** Label: 13, 21

Preparations for intestinal release
ℕℍ𝕊 **Breoprin®** (Sterling Research)
Tablets, s/r, scored, aspirin 648 mg (for intestinal
release). Price 20 tabs = **D.** Label: 25
Dose: 1–2 tablets every 8 hours; max. 6 tablets
daily
Caprin® (Sinclair)
Tablets, s/r, pink, aspirin 324 mg (for intestinal
release). Price 20 tabs = **B.** Label: 25
Dose: 1–4 tablets 3–4 times daily
ℕℍ𝕊 **Levius®** (Farmitalia Carlo Erba)
Tablets, s/r, aspirin 500 mg. Price 30 tabs = **B.**
Label: 25
Nu-Seals Aspirin® (Lilly)
Tablets, red, e/c, aspirin 300 mg. Price 20 tabs =
B. Label: 5, 25
Tablets, red, e/c, aspirin 600 mg. Price 20 tabs =
C. Label: 5, 25
Palaprin Forte® (Nicholas)
Tablets, orange, scored, aloxiprin 600 mg ≡
aspirin 500 mg. To be taken dispersed in water,
chewed, sucked, or swallowed whole. Price 20
tabs = **B.** Label: 12, 21

PARACETAMOL

Indications: mild to moderate pain, pyrexia
Cautions: hepatic impairment, alcoholism. Drug interactions: see Appendix 1 (sections *2.8C*, *4.7*, *5.1*)
Side-effects: liver damage in prolonged use or overdosage
Dose: 0.5–1 g every 4–6 hours to a max. of 4 g daily; CHILD up to 1 year 60–120 mg, 1–5 years 120–250 mg, 6–12 years 250–500 mg; these doses may be repeated every 4–6 hours when necessary

Paracetamol Tablets, paracetamol 500 mg. Price 20 tabs = **A**
Paracetamol Elixir, Paediatric, red, paracetamol 120 mg/5 ml. Do not dilute. Price 100 ml = **B**
Calpol® (Calmic)
Infant suspension (= mixture), pink, paracetamol 120 mg/5 ml. Price 100 ml = **C**
NHS *Six plus suspension* (= mixture), orange, paracetamol 250 mg/5 ml. Price 100 ml = **C**
Paldesic® (RP Drugs)
Syrup (= elixir), paracetamol 120 mg/5 ml. Price 60 ml = **A** (Hosp. only)
Panadol® (Winthrop)
NHS *Caplets®* (= tablets), paracetamol 500 mg. Price 20 tabs = **B**
NHS *Tablets*, scored, paracetamol 500 mg. Price 20 tabs = **A**
Elixir, yellow, paracetamol 120 mg/5 ml. Diluent syrup, life of diluted elixir 14 days. Price 60 ml = **C**
NHS **Panadol Soluble®** (Winthrop)
Tablets, effervescent, scored, paracetamol 500 mg. Price 12 tabs = **B**. Label: 13
NHS **Panasorb®** (Winthrop)
Tablets, paracetamol 500 mg in sorbitol basis. Price 20 tabs = **C**
Salzone® (Wallace Mfg)
Syrup (= elixir), paracetamol 120 mg/5 ml. Diluent syrup, life of diluted elixir 14 days. Price 75 ml = **C**

BENORYLATE
(Aspirin-paracetamol ester)
Indications: mild to moderate pain; pyrexia; see also section 10.1.1.1
Cautions; Contra-indications; Side-effects: see under Aspirin and under Paracetamol. Side-effects resemble aspirin rather than paracetamol but tolerance is better and hepatotoxicity may be less than with paracetamol
Dose: 1.5–2 g every 8 hours, preferably after food; CHILD, see section 10.1.1.1

Preparations
See section 10.1.1.1

DIFLUNISAL
Indications: mild to moderate pain; see also section 10.1.1.2

Cautions; Contra-indications; Side-effects: see section 10.1.1.2. Tablets should be swallowed whole
Dose: 250–500 mg twice daily preferably after food

Preparations
See section 10.1.1.2

FENOPROFEN
Indications: mild to moderate pain, pyrexia; see also section 10.1.1.2
Cautions; Contra-indications; Side-effects: See section 10.1.1.2
Dose: 200–400 mg 3–4 times daily, after food; max. 3 g daily

NHS PoM **Progesic®** (Lilly)
Tablets, yellow, fenoprofen 200 mg (as calcium salt). Price 20 tabs = **D**. Label: 21
Fenopron: see section 10.1.1.2

IBUPROFEN
Indications: mild to moderate pain; see also section 10.1.1.2
Cautions; Side-effects: see section 10.1.1.2
Dose: 1.2 g daily in divided doses, preferably after food, increased if necessary to a max. of 2.4 g daily; CHILD, see section 10.1.1.2

Preparations
See section 10.1.1.2

MEFENAMIC ACID
Indications: mild to moderate pain, pyrexia in children; menorrhagia; see also section 10.1.1.2
Cautions; Contra-indications; Side-effects: see section 10.1.1.2; exclude pathological conditions before treating menorrhagia
Dose: 500 mg 3 times daily after food; CHILD over 6 months 25 mg/kg daily in divided doses for not longer than 7 days, except in juvenile chronic arthritis

Preparations
See section 10.1.1.2

NAPROXEN SODIUM
Indications: mild to moderate pain; see also Naproxen, section 10.1.1.2
Cautions; Side-effects: see section 10.1.1.2
Dose: 550 mg initially, then 275 mg 6–8 hourly when necessary, preferably after food
Note: 275 mg naproxen sodium ≡ 250 mg naproxen but the sodium salt has a more rapid action

Naprosyn: see section 10.1.1.2
▼ PoM **Synflex®** (Syntex)
Tablets, orange, naproxen sodium 275 mg. Price 20 tabs = **E**

C = 51-100p, D = 101-180p, E = 181-300p, F = 301-450p, G = 451-650p, H = 651-900p, I = 901-1200p, J = over 1200p.

SODIUM SALICYLATE

Indications: mild to moderate pain, pyrexia; see also section 10.1.1.1

Cautions; Contra-indications; Side-effects: see under Aspirin. Avoid in children, except for rheumatic fever. Caution in patients on low-sodium diets and in congestive heart failure; avoid in acute renal disease

Dose: 0.5–1 g every 4 hours, when required, after food

Sodium Salicylate Mixture, sodium salicylate 250 mg/5 ml (see Formulary). Price 100 ml = **A**. Label: 21
Sodium Salicylate Mixture, Strong, sodium salicylate 500 mg/5 ml (see Formulary). Price 100 ml = **A**. Label: 21

SUPROFEN

Indications: mild to moderate pain; see also section 10.1.1.2
Cautions; Side-effects: see section 10.1.1.2
Dose: 200 mg 3–4 times daily

Preparations
See section 10.1.1.2

4.7.1.2   NARCOTIC ANALGESICS USED FOR MILD TO MODERATE PAIN

The risk of addiction, though possible, occurs rarely with drugs of this group. However they should be prescribed with caution in patients with a history of drug abuse; there is an increasing problem of drug abuse with the dextro-propoxyphene/paracetamol compound preparations (co-proxamol). Narcotic analgesics used in severe pain are listed in section 4.7.2, have an appreciable risk of addiction, and share many of the same side-effects as those listed below.

The temptation to prescribe these drugs freely should be **avoided**; the non-narcotic analgesics, though freely available to the public, are adequate for most purposes.

Codeine is used for the relief of mild to moderate pain but is too constipating for long-term use.

Dihydrocodeine (DF 118®) is similar in potency to codeine. It is suitable for use in ambulant patients with moderate pain but may cause dizziness and constipation. It may be given by mouth or by injection.

Pentazocine (Fortral®) given by *injection* is more potent than dihydrocodeine or codeine. Disadvantages are that hallucinations and thought disturbances may sometimes occur. It should be avoided after myocardial infarction as it may increase pulmonary and aortic blood pressure as well as cardiac work. Several formulations are available but it is usually given orally for mild pain and parenterally for severe pain.

Dextropropoxyphene given alone is a very mild analgesic and is somewhat less potent than codeine. Combinations of dextropropoxyphene and paracetamol (co-proxamol) or aspirin have a more

powerful effect. However the chief disadvantage of combinations with paracetamol is that overdosage, which may be deliberate and combined with alcohol, is complicated by respiratory depression and acute heart failure due to dextropropoxyphene and hepatotoxicity due to paracetamol. Rapid treatment, as described under Emergency Treatment of Poisoning, is essential.

CODEINE PHOSPHATE

Indications: mild to moderate pain
Cautions: liver disease, late pregnancy; avoid in renal impairment; avoid in children under 1 year. Drug interactions: see Appendix 1 (sections *1*, *2.3*, *4.1*, *4.3*)
Contra-indications: respiratory depression
Side-effects: tolerance and dependence, particularly on injection, sedation, dizziness, nausea, constipation; may enhance the effects of alcohol
Dose: by mouth, 10–60 mg every 4 hours when necessary, to a max. of 200 mg daily; CHILD 1–12 years, 3 mg/kg daily in divided doses
By intramuscular injection, up to 30 mg when necessary

PoM **Codeine Phosphate Tablets,** codeine phosphate 15 and 30 mg, price 20 tabs (both) = **B**; 60 mg, price 20 tabs = **D**
Codeine Phosphate Syrup, codeine phosphate 25 mg/5 ml. Price 100 ml = **C**
CD **Codeine Phosphate Injection,** (USP), codeine phosphate 60 mg/ml. Price 1-ml amp = **C**

DEXTROPROPOXYPHENE HYDROCHLORIDE

Indications: mild to moderate pain
Cautions: see under Codeine Phosphate; see also notes above. Drug interactions: see Appendix 1 (sections *2.8C*, *4.8*)
Side-effects: see under Codeine Phosphate; with daily doses above 720 mg toxic psychoses and convulsions may occur
Dose: 65 mg every 6–8 hours when necessary
Note: 65 mg dextropropoxyphene hydrochloride ≡ 100 mg dextropropoxyphene napsylate

PoM **Dextropropoxyphene Capsules,** the equivalent of dextropropoxyphene hydrochloride 65 mg (as napsylate). Price 20 caps = **C**. Label: 2
NHS PoM **Doloxene®** (Lilly)
Capsules, orange, the equivalent of dextropropoxyphene hydrochloride 65 mg (as napsylate). Price 20 caps = **C**. Label: 2

DIHYDROCODEINE TARTRATE

Indications: moderate to severe pain
Cautions; Side-effects: see under Codeine Phosphate. Caution in respiratory disease; reduce dose in elderly and debilitated patients, hypothyroidism.
Dose: by mouth, 30 mg every 4–6 hours when necessary, after food; CHILD over 4 years 0.5–1 mg/kg

By deep subcutaneous or intramuscular injection, 50 mg every 4–6 hours when necessary; CHILD over 4 years 0.5–1 mg/kg

PoM **Dihydrocodeine Tablets,** dihydrocodeine tartrate 30 mg. Price 20 tabs = **C**. Label: 21

PoM **Dihydrocodeine Elixir,** dihydrocodeine tartrate 10 mg/5 ml. Diluent syrup (without preservative), life of diluted elixir 14 days. Price 150 ml = **D**. Label: 21

CD **Dihydrocodeine Injection,** dihydrocodeine tartrate 50 mg/ml. Price 1-ml amp = **B**

NHS **DF 118®** (DF)

PoM *Tablets*, dihydrocodeine tartrate 30 mg. Price 20 tabs = **C**. Label: 21

PoM *Elixir*, brown, dihydrocodeine tartrate 10 mg/5 ml. Diluent syrup (without preservative), life of diluted elixir 14 days. Price 150 ml = **D**. Label: 21

CD *Injection*, dihydrocodeine tartrate 50 mg/ml. Price 1-ml amp = **B**

PENTAZOCINE

Indications: moderate to severe pain

Cautions; Side-effects: see under Codeine Phosphate. Occasionally hallucinations occur. Avoid in patients dependent on narcotics and in arterial or pulmonary hypertension and heart failure

Dose: by mouth, pentazocine hydrochloride 25–100 mg every 3–4 hours after food; CHILD 6–12 years 25 mg

By subcutaneous, intramuscular, or intravenous injection, moderate pain, pentazocine 30 mg, severe pain 45–60 mg every 3–4 hours when necessary; CHILD over 1 year, by subcutaneous or intramuscular injection, up to 1 mg/kg, by intravenous injection up to 500 micrograms/kg

By rectum in suppositories, pentazocine 50 mg up to 4 times daily

PoM **Pentazocine Tablets,** pentazocine hydrochloride 25 mg. Price 20 tabs = **D**. Label: 21

PoM **Pentazocine Lactate Injection,** pentazocine 30 mg (as lactate)/ml. Price 1-ml amp = **C**; 2-ml amp = **D**

PoM **Pentazocine Suppositories,** pentazocine 50 mg (as lactate). Price 20 suppos = **H**

NHS PoM **Fortral®** (Sterling Research)

Capsules, grey/yellow, pentazocine hydrochloride 50 mg. Price 20 caps = **F**. Label: 21

Tablets, f/c, pentazocine hydrochloride 25 mg. Price 20 tabs = **D**. Label: 21

Injection, pentazocine 30 mg (as lactate)/ml. Price 1-ml amp = **C**; 2-ml amp = **D**

Suppositories, pentazocine 50 mg (as lactate). Price 20 suppos = **H**

4.7.1.3 COMPOUND ANALGESIC PREPARATIONS

Compound analgesic preparations of, for example, aspirin, paracetamol, and codeine are **not** recommended. Single-ingredient preparations (sections 4.7.1.1 and 4.7.1.2) should be prescribed in preference because compound preparations

rarely have any advantage; they may increase the cost of treatment unnecessarily and complicate the treatment of overdosage. The dangers of co-proxamol (dextropropoxyphene-paracetamol) overdosage are described in section 4.7.1.2.

It is even more desirable to **avoid** mixtures of analgesics with laxatives, antihistamines, or hypnotics; the individual components should be prescribed separately so that the dose of each can be adjusted as appropriate.

Analgesic preparations containing muscle relaxants are discussed in section 10.2.2.

Caffeine is a weak stimulant that is often included, in small doses, in analgesic preparations. It does not contribute to the analgesic or anti-inflammatory effect of the preparation and may possibly aggravate the gastric irritation caused by aspirin. Moreover, in excessive dosage or on withdrawal caffeine may itself induce headache.

NEW NAMES FOR COMPOUND ANALGESICS. Following the exclusion of certain proprietary analgesics from NHS prescribing the following approved names have been adopted:

Co-codamol Compounded preparations of codeine phosphate and paracetamol in the proportions 2 parts to 125 parts

Co-codaprin Compounded preparations of codeine phosphate and aspirin in the proportions 1 part to 50 parts

Co-dydramol Compounded preparations of dihydrocodeine tartrate and paracetamol in the proportions 1 part to 50 parts

Co-proxamol Compounded preparations of dextropropoxyphene hydrochloride and paracetamol in the proportions 1 part to 10 parts

Aspirin, Paracetamol, and Codeine Tablets, aspirin 250 mg, paracetamol 250 mg, codeine phosphate 6.8 mg. Price 20 tabs = **C**. Label: 21
Dose: 1–2 tablets every 4–6 hours when necessary

Co-codamol Tablets and Dispersible Tablets (Codeine and Paracetamol Tablets and Dispersible Tablets). When co-codamol tablets or dispersible tablets are prescribed and no strength is stated tablets, or dispersible tablets, respectively, containing codeine phosphate 8 mg and paracetamol 500 mg should be dispensed. Price 20 tabs (both) = **B**. Label (dispersible tablets): 13
Dose: 1–2 tablets every 4–6 hours when necessary; max. 8 tablets daily

Co-codaprin Tablets (Aspirin and Codeine Tablets). When co-codaprin tablets are prescribed and no strength is stated tablets containing aspirin 400 mg and codeine phosphate 8 mg should be dispensed. Price 20 tabs = **A**. Label: 21
Dose: 1–2 tablets every 4–6 hours when necessary

Co-codaprin Tablets, Dispersible (Aspirin and Codeine Tablets, Dispersible). When co-codaprin tablets, dispersible are prescribed and no strength is stated tablets containing aspirin 400 mg and codeine phosphate 8 mg in an effervescent basis should be dispensed. Price 20 tabs = **B**. Label: 13, 21

PoM **Co-dydramol Tablets** (Dihydrocodeine and Paracetamol Tablets). When co-dydramol tablets are prescribed and no strength is stated tablets containing dihydrocodeine tartrate 10 mg and paracetamol 500 mg should be dispensed. Price 20 tabs = **B**. Label: 21
Dose: 1–2 tablets every 4–6 hours when necessary; max. 8 tablets daily

C = 51-100p, D = 101-180p, E = 181-300p, F = 301-450p, G = 451-650p, H = 651-900p, I = 901-1200p, J = over 1200p.

PoM **Co-proxamol Tablets** (Dextropropoxyphene and Paracetamol Tablets). When co-proxamol tablets are prescribed and no strength is stated tablets containing dextropropoxyphene hydrochloride 32.5 mg and paracetamol 325 mg should be dispensed. Price 20 tabs = **B**. Label: 2, 10 patient information leaflet
Dose: 2 tablets 3–4 times daily; max. 8 tablets daily

NHS **Antoin**® (Cox Pharmaceuticals)
Dispersible tablets, scored, aspirin 400 mg, codeine phosphate 5 mg, caffeine citrate 15 mg. Price 20 tabs = **B**. Label: 13, 21
Dose: 1–2 tablets in water 3–4 times daily; max. 10 tablets daily

PoM **Aspav**® (Cox Pharmaceuticals)
Dispersible tablets, aspirin 500 mg, papaveretum 10 mg. Price 20 tabs = **C**. Label: 13, 21
Dose: 1–2 tablets in water every 4–6 hours if necessary; max. 8 tablets daily

NHS **Cafadol**® (Typharm)
Tablets, yellow, scored, paracetamol 500 mg, caffeine 30 mg. Price 20 tabs = **B**
Dose: 2 tablets every 3–4 hours, max. 8 tablets daily; CHILD 5–12 years 1 tablet

NHS PoM **Carisoma Co**® (Pharmax)
Tablets, orange, carisoprodol 175 mg, paracetamol 350 mg. Price 20 tabs = **B**. Label: 2
Dose: 1–2 tablets 3 times daily

NHS **Codis**® (R&C)
Dispersible tablets, aspirin 500 mg, codeine phosphate 8 mg. Price 20 tabs = **C**. Label: 13, 21
Dose: 1–2 tablets in water every 4 hours, max. 8 tablets daily

NHS PoM **Delimon**® (Consolidated)
Tablets, scored, morazone hydrochloride 150 mg, paracetamol 400 mg. Price 10 tabs = **B**
Dose: ½–1 tablet when necessary

NHS PoM **Distalgesic**® (Dista)
Tablets, f/c, co-proxamol 357.5 mg (dextropropoxyphene hydrochloride 32.5 mg, paracetamol 325 mg). Price 20 tabs = **B**. Label: 2, 10 patient information leaflet
Dose: 2 tablets 3–4 times daily; max. 8 tablets daily

NHS PoM **Distalgesic Soluble**® (Dista)
Dispersible tablets, dextropropoxyphene napsylate 50 mg, paracetamol 325 mg. Price 20 tabs = **D**. Label: 2, 10 patient information leaflet, 13
Dose: 2 tablets in water 3–4 times daily; max. 8 tablets daily

NHS PoM **Dolasan**® (Lilly)
Tablets, orange, dextropropoxyphene napsylate 100 mg, aspirin 325 mg. Price 20 tabs = **D**. Label: 2, 21
Dose: 1 tablet 3–4 times daily; max. 4 tablets daily

NHS PoM **Doloxene Compound**® (Lilly)
Capsules, grey/red, dextropropoxyphene napsylate 100 mg, aspirin 375 mg, caffeine 30 mg. Price 20 caps = **C**. Label: 2, 21
Dose: 1 capsule 3–4 times daily; max. 4 capsules daily

NHS PoM **Equagesic**® (Wyeth)
Tablets, pink/white/yellow, ethoheptazine citrate 75 mg, meprobamate 150 mg, aspirin 250 mg. Price 20 tabs = **B**. Label: 2, 21
Dose: muscle pain, 1–2 tablets 3–4 times daily

NHS **Femerital**® (MCP)
Tablets, scored, ambucetamide 100 mg, paracetamol 250 mg. Price 20 tabs = **B**
Dose: dysmenorrhoea, 1–2 tablets 3 times daily starting 2 days before menstruation

NHS PoM **Fortagesic**® (Sterling Research)
Tablets, pentazocine 15 mg (as hydrochloride), paracetamol 500 mg. Price 20 tabs = **D**. Label: 2, 21
Dose: 2 tablets up to 4 times daily; CHILD 7–12 years 1 tablet every 4 hours, max. 4 tablets daily

NHS **Hypon**® (Calmic)
Tablets, yellow, aspirin 325 mg, caffeine 10 mg, codeine phosphate 5 mg. Price 20 tabs = **B**. Label: 21

Dose: 2 tablets every 4 hours, max. 12 tablets daily; CHILD 1 tablet

NHS PoM **Lobak**® (Sterling Research)
Tablets, scored, chlormezanone 100 mg, paracetamol 450 mg. Price 20 tabs = **E**. Label: 2
Dose: muscle pain, 1–2 tablets 3 times daily, max. 8 tablets daily

NHS **Medised**® (Martindale)
Tablets, scored, paracetamol 500 mg, promethazine hydrochloride 10 mg. Price 12 tabs = **C**. Label: 2
Dose: 2 tablets (usually at night), repeated if necessary every 4 hours; max. 8 tablets daily
Suspension (= mixture), paracetamol 120 mg, promethazine hydrochloride 2.5 mg/5 ml. Price 140 ml = **C**. Label: 1
Dose: CHILD 3–12 months 5 ml, 1–5 years 10 ml, 6–12 years 20 ml, up to 4 times daily

NHS **Medocodene**® (Medo)
Tablets, yellow, scored, co-codamol 508 mg (paracetamol 500 mg, codeine phosphate 8 mg). Price 20 tabs = **B**
Dose: 1–2 tablets every 4 hours, max. 8 tablets daily; CHILD 6–12 years ½–1 tablet

NHS **Myolgin**® (Cox Pharmaceuticals)
Dispersible tablets, scored, paracetamol 200 mg, aspirin 200 mg, codeine phosphate 5 mg, caffeine citrate 15 mg. Price 20 tabs = **B**. Label: 13, 21
Dose: 1–2 tablets in water 3–4 times daily; max. 16 tablets daily

NHS PoM **Napsalgesic**® (Dista)
Tablets, yellow, f/c, dextropropoxyphene napsylate 50 mg, aspirin 500 mg. Price 20 tabs = **C**. Label: 2, 21
Dose: 4–6 (max.) tablets daily in divided doses

NHS **Neurodyne**® (Rorer)
Capsules, co-codamol 508 mg (paracetamol 500 mg, codeine phosphate 8 mg). Price 20 caps = **C**
Dose: 1–2 capsules every 4 hours, max. 8 capsules daily

NHS PoM **Norgesic**® (Riker)
Tablets, scored, orphenadrine citrate 35 mg, paracetamol 450 mg. Price 20 tabs = **C**
Dose: muscle pain, 2 tablets 3 times daily

NHS PoM **Paedo-Sed**® (Pharmax)
Syrup (= elixir), yellow, dichloralphenazone 200 mg, paracetamol 100 mg/5 ml. Diluent syrup, life of diluted elixir 14 days. Price 100 ml = **C**
Dose: CHILD up to 6 months 2.5 ml, 6–12 months 5 ml, 1–4 years 10 ml, over 4 years 15–20 ml

NHS **Panadeine**® (Winthrop)
Tablets, scored, co-codamol 508 mg (codeine phosphate 8 mg, paracetamol 500 mg). Price 20 tabs = **B**
Dose: 2 tablets up to 4 times daily; CHILD 7–12 years ½–1 tablet

NHS PoM **Panadeine Forte**® (Winthrop)
Tablets, red, f/c, codeine phosphate 15 mg, paracetamol 500 mg. Price 20 tabs = **C**. Label: 2
Dose: 2 tablets 4 times daily

NHS **Panadeine Soluble**® (Winthrop)
Effervescent tablets, co-codamol 508 mg (codeine phosphate 8 mg, paracetamol 500 mg). Price 20 tabs = **C**. Label: 13
Dose: 2 tablets in water up to 4 times daily; CHILD ½–1 tablet

NHS **Paracodol**® (Fisons)
Effervescent tablets, co-codamol 508 mg (paracetamol 500 mg, codeine phosphate 8 mg). Price 20 tabs = **C**. Label: 13
Dose: 1–2 tablets in water every 4–6 hours, max. 8 tablets daily; CHILD 6–12 years ½–1 tablet, max. 4 tablets daily

NHS **Paradeine**® (Scotia)
Tablets, paracetamol 500 mg, codeine phosphate 10 mg, phenolphthalein 2.5 mg. Price 20 tabs = **B**
Dose: 1–2 tablets 4 times daily

NHS **Parahypon**® (Calmic)
Tablets, pink, scored, paracetamol 500 mg, codeine phosphate 5 mg, caffeine 10 mg. Price 20 tabs = **C**

Relative prices: **A** = up to 20p, **B** = 21-50p,

Dose: 2 tablets up to 4 times daily; CHILD 6–12 years 1 tablet up to 4 times daily

NHS **Parake**® (Galen)

Tablets, co-codamol 508 mg (paracetamol 500 mg, codeine phosphate 8 mg). Price 20 tabs = **C**
Dose: 2 tablets every 4 hours, max. 8 tablets daily

NHS **Paralgin**® (Norton)

Tablets, scored, paracetamol 450 mg, caffeine 20 mg, codeine phosphate 6 mg. Price 20 tabs = **B**
Dose: 2 tablets 3–4 times daily; CHILD 7–12 years ½–1 tablet

NHS PoM **Paramol**® (DF)

Tablets, scored, co-dydramol 510 mg (paracetamol 500 mg, dihydrocodeine tartrate 10 mg). Price 20 tabs = **B**. Label: 21
Dose: 1 tablet every 4 hours increased to a max. of 8 tablets daily

NHS **Pardale**® (Martindale)

Tablets, scored, paracetamol 400 mg, codeine phosphate 9 mg, caffeine hydrate 10 mg. Price 20 tabs = **C**
Dose: 1–2 tablets 3–4 times daily, max. 8 tablets daily

PoM **Paxidal**® (Wallace Mfg)

Tablets, paracetamol 325 mg, meprobamate 135 mg, caffeine 65 mg. Price 12 tabs = **B**. Label: 2
Dose: 2 tablets 3 times daily

NHS **Pharmidone**® (Farmitalia Carlo Erba)

Tablets, yellow, scored, codeine phosphate 10 mg, diphenhydramine hydrochloride 5 mg, paracetamol 400 mg, caffeine 50 mg. Price 12 tabs = **B**. Label: 2
Dose: 1–2 tablets every 4 hours, max. 10 tablets daily

NHS **Propain**® (Luitpold)

Tablets, yellow, scored, codeine phosphate 10 mg, diphenhydramine hydrochloride 5 mg, paracetamol 400 mg, caffeine 50 mg. Price 20 tabs = **C**. Label: 2
Dose: 1–2 tablets every 4 hours, max. 10 tablets daily

NHS PoM **Robaxisal Forte**® (Robins)

Tablets, pink/white, scored, methocarbamol 400 mg, aspirin 325 mg. Price 20 tabs = **C**. Label: 2, 21
Dose: muscle pain, 2 tablets 4 times daily

NHS **Safapryn**® (Pfizer)

Tablets, pink, s/c, paracetamol 250 mg, aspirin e/c 300 mg. Price 20 tabs = **B**. Label: 5, 25
Dose: 1–3 tablets 3–4 times daily, max. 10 tablets daily

NHS **Safapryn-Co**® (Pfizer)

Tablets, green, s/c, paracetamol 250 mg, codeine phosphate 8 mg, aspirin e/c 300 mg. Price 20 tabs = **B**. Label: 5, 25
Dose: 1–3 tablets 3–4 times daily, max. 10 tablets daily

NHS **Solpadeine**® (Sterling Research)

Effervescent tablets, paracetamol 500 mg, codeine phosphate 8 mg, caffeine 30 mg. Contains 18.5 mmol Na+/tablet; avoid in renal impairment. Price 20 tabs = **C**. Label: 13
Dose: 2 tablets in water 3–4 times daily; CHILD 7–12 years ½–1 tablet

NHS PoM **Solpadeine Forte**® (Sterling Research)

Effervescent tablets, paracetamol 500 mg, codeine phosphate 15 mg, caffeine 30 mg. Contains 18.5 mmol Na+/tablet; avoid in renal impairment. Price 20 tabs = **C**. Label: 2, 13
Dose: 2 tablets in water up to 4 times daily

NHS **Syndol**® (Merrell)

Tablets, yellow, scored, paracetamol 450 mg, codeine phosphate 10 mg, doxylamine succinate 5 mg, caffeine 30 mg. Price 20 tabs = **D**. Label: 2
Dose: 1–2 tablets every 4–6 hours, max. 8 tablets daily

NHS PoM **Trancoprin**® (Winthrop)

Tablets, scored, aspirin 300 mg, chlormezanone 100 mg. Price 20 tabs = **C**. Label: 2, 21
Dose: 1–2 tablets 3 times daily, max. 8 tablets daily

NHS **Unigesic**® (Unimed)

Capsules, grey/yellow, paracetamol 500 mg, caffeine 30 mg. Price 20 caps = **D**
Dose: 1–2 capsules every 4 hours, max. 8 capsules daily

NHS **Veganin**® (Warner)

Tablets, scored, aspirin 250 mg, paracetamol 250 mg, codeine phosphate 6.8 mg. Price 20 tabs = **B**. Label: 21
Dose: 1–2 tablets every 3–4 hours, max. 8 tablets daily; CHILD 6–12 years ½–1 tablet

NHS PoM **Zactirin**® (Wyeth)

Tablets, ethoheptazine citrate 75 mg, aspirin 325 mg. Price 20 tabs = **B**. Label: 2, 21
Dose: 2 tablets 2–3 times daily; max. 8 tablets daily

4.7.2   Narcotic and other analgesics used for severe pain

These analgesics are used to relieve moderate to severe pain, but with repeated administration they cause tolerance and dependence. This is no deterrent in the control of pain in terminal disease and the recommended practice is to adjust both the dose and frequency of administration so that the patient never suffers pain; both dose and frequency may need to be gradually increased as tolerance develops, to maintain adequate analgesia. Combining two or more narcotic analgesics is usually unnecessary and a higher dose of one will be as effective. However in certain conditions it is more satisfactory to choose one drug for background pain relief and another for exacerbations.

CAUTIONS. In general all narcotic analgesics should be used with caution, if at all, in patients taking monoamine-oxidase inhibitors, those with a history of drug abuse, and those with hypotension, asthma, decreased respiratory reserve, hepatic impairment, raised intracranial pressure, or head injury, and during pregnancy and breast-feeding. Drug interactions: see Appendix 1 (sections *1*, *2.3*, *4.1*, *4.3*).

SIDE-EFFECTS. The narcotic analgesics used for severe pain and those used in mild to moderate pain (section 4.7.1.2) share many side-effects though qualitative and quantitative differences exist. They all cause constipation (by reduction of intestinal motility), respiratory depression, cough suppression, urinary retention, nausea, and tolerance, and are liable to cause dependence.

CHOICE OF ANALGESIC. **Morphine** remains the most valuable narcotic analgesic for severe pain although it frequently causes nausea and vomiting, and it is the standard against which other narcotic analgesics are compared.

The initial dose depends largely on the patient's previous treatment. To replace a weak narcotic analgesic, 5–10 mg of morphine should be prescribed, for an intermediate narcotic, 10 mg, and for a strong narcotic, 20 mg or more. If the first dose of morphine is no more effective than the previous medicine it should be increased by 50%.

Morphine often confers a state of euphoria and mental detachment which may enhance the sense of well-being. Concurrent administration of small doses of chlorpromazine or other phenothiazine derivatives (section 4.6) reduces the tendency to nausea and vomiting. Preparations containing morphine with an anti-emetic such as cyclizine (Cyclimorph®) are available but should only be used intermittently to avoid the overdosage of

---

C = 51–100p, **D** = 101–180p, **E** = 181–300p, **F** = 301–450p, **G** = 451–650p, **H** = 651–900p, **I** = 901–1200p, **J** = over 1200p.

anti-emetic that may result when they are used in regular 4-hourly dosage regimens in terminal care. Mixed opium alkaloids such as **papaveretum** (Omnopon®) do not appear to have any advantage over morphine. Morphine is often formulated as an elixir for oral use (see below).

Diamorphine (heroin) is a powerful narcotic analgesic. It is more likely to produce euphoria and addiction than morphine but causes relatively less nausea, constipation, and hypotension. It is often formulated as an elixir for oral use (see below) but has little advantage over morphine in such preparations are chemically unstable, the diamorphine being gradually deacetylated to morphine. The greater solubility of diamorphine hydrochloride allows effective doses to be injected in smaller volumes and this is important in the emaciated patient.

Phenazocine (Narphen®) is also effective in severe pain. It is particularly useful in biliary colic as it has less tendency to increase biliary pressure than other narcotic analgesics. It may be administered sublingually if nausea and vomiting are a problem.

Pethidine produces a prompt but short-lasting analgesia and even in high doses it is a less potent analgesic than morphine. It is unsuitable for the relief of pain in terminal disease. It remains the drug of choice for the relief of pain when intracranial damage is known or suspected and for analgesia in labour. In the neonate it is associated with less respiratory depression than other narcotic analgesics but this is probably because its pharmacological actions are, in general, weaker. See also section 15.1.4.1 for its use in surgical anaesthesia.

Methadone (Physeptone®) and **levorphanol** (Dromoran®) are less sedating than morphine and act for more prolonged periods. They are suitable drugs for providing background pain relief in terminal disease. Methadone twice daily is commonly used for this purpose and supplemented by dextromoramide or dipipanone for severe exacerbations. Such combinations often control pain over long periods. In prolonged use, methadone should not be administered more often than twice daily to avoid the risk of accumulation and narcotic overdosage.

Dextromoramide (Palfium®) and **dipipanone** are less sedating than morphine but their actions are too short for providing background pain relief in severe chronic terminal pain; they are however effective in controlling severe exacerbations of pain.

The peri-operative use of **fentanyl** (Sublimaze®) and **phenoperidine** (Operidine®) is discussed in section 15.1.4.

Dihydrocodeine and **pentazocine** injections (section 4.7.1.2) are also used in severe pain.

NEWER ANALGESICS. **Buprenorphine** (Temgesic®) is suitable for sublingual or parenteral use. It has a much longer duration of action than morphine and is thought to have a low dependence potential. When administered sublingually it is very effective in relieving pain, but vomiting may be a problem and may last for 8–12 hours. Unlike most narcotic

analgesics its effects are only partially reversed by naloxone but doxapram (Dopram®) may be used to reverse profound respiratory depression. **Meptazinol** (Meptid®) is claimed to have a low incidence of respiratory depression. It has a reported length of action of 2 to 7 hours with onset within 15 minutes, but there is an incidence of nausea and vomiting.

Nefopam (Acupan®) is not related to the narcotic analgesics and its mode of action is unknown. It may have a place in the relief of persistent pain unresponsive to non-narcotic analgesics. It causes little or no respiratory depression, but anticholinergic side-effects may be troublesome.

Nalbuphine (Nubain®) is a new analgesic equipotent with morphine for pain relief, but which may have fewer side-effects and less abuse potential. Nausea and vomiting occur less than with other narcotics but respiratory depression is similar to that with morphine.

MORPHINE SALTS

Indications: severe pain, left ventricular failure, pulmonary oedema

Cautions; Contra-indications; Side-effects: see notes above. Avoid in renal impairment

Dose: by mouth or by subcutaneous, intramuscular or intravenous injection, morphine hydrochloride, sulphate, or tartrate 10–20 mg; CHILD up to 1 month 150 micrograms/kg, 1–12 months 200 micrograms/kg, 1–5 years 2.5–5 mg, 6–12 years 5–10 mg; these doses may be repeated every 4 hours, or more in terminal pain. See also notes above

Left ventricular failure and pulmonary oedema, *by intravenous injection,* morphine sulphate 5–10 mg as a single dose

By rectum, in suppositories, morphine hydrochloride or sulphate, 15–30 mg every 4 hours

CD Morphine Sulphate Injection, morphine sulphate 10, 15, 20, and 30 mg/ml, price 1- and 2-ml amp (all) = **B**

CD Morphine Suppositories, morphine hydrochloride or sulphate 15 mg, price 12 suppos = **E**; 30 mg, price 12 suppos = **F**. The strength of the suppositories and the morphine salt contained in them must be specified by the prescriber

CD Opium Tincture, morphine 1% (10 mg/ml). Price 10 ml = **B**

Dose: 1–2 ml; CHILD 1–5 years 0.25–0.5 ml, 6–12 years 0.5–1 ml

CD Cyclimorph-10® (Calmic)

Injection, morphine tartrate 10 mg, cyclizine tartrate 50 mg/ml. Price 1-ml amp = **C**

Dose: by subcutaneous, intramuscular, or intravenous injection, 1 ml, repeated not more often than 4-hourly, with not more than 3 doses in any 24-hour period; CHILD 1–5 years 0.25–0.5 ml as a single dose, 6–12 years 0.5–1 ml as a single dose

CD Cyclimorph-15® (Calmic)

Injection, morphine tartrate 15 mg, cyclizine tartrate 50 mg/ml. Price 1-ml amp = **C**

Dose: by subcutaneous, intramuscular, or intravenous injection, 1 ml, repeated not more often than 4-hourly, with not more than 3 doses in any 24-hour period

CD Duromorph® (LAB)
Injection, s/r, morphine 64 mg/ml (aqueous suspension). Price 1-ml amp = **C**
Dose: by subcutaneous or intramuscular injection, in terminal pain, 1–1.5 ml every 9 hours

CD MST Continus® (Napp)
Tablets, s/r, brown, f/c, morphine sulphate 10 mg. Price 20 tabs = **E**. Label: 25
Tablets, s/r, purple, f/c, morphine sulphate 30 mg. Price 20 tabs = **G**. Label: 25
Tablets, s/r, orange, f/c, morphine sulphate 60 mg. Price 10 tabs = **G**. Label: 25
Tablets, s/r, grey, f/c, morphine sulphate 100 mg. Price 10 tabs = **I**. Label: 25
Dose: initially 10–20 mg twice daily, adjusted according to response

CD Nepenthe (Evans)
Oral solution (= elixir), brown, anhydrous morphine 8.4 mg/ml (500 micrograms from opium tincture, 7.9 mg from morphine). Diluent syrup, life of diluted elixir 4 weeks. Price 100 ml = **F**
Dose: 1–2 ml, repeated not more often than 4-hourly when necessary; CHILD 6–12 years 0.5–1 ml, as a single dose
Injection, anhydrous morphine 8.4 mg/ml (500 micrograms from papaveretum, 7.9 mg from morphine hydrochloride). Price 0.5-ml amp = **B**
Dose: by subcutaneous or intramuscular injection, 1–2 ml, repeated not more often than 4-hourly when necessary; CHILD 6–12 years 0.5–1 ml as a single dose

Morphine Analgesic Elixirs
See below

BUPRENORPHINE

Indications: moderate to severe pain
Cautions; Contra-indications; Side-effects: see notes above, but side-effects are less marked than for morphine, the risk of dependence is lower, and it may give rise to mild withdrawal symptoms in cases of narcotic dependence. Commonest side-effects are drowsiness, nausea, vomiting, dizziness, and sweating; rarely respiratory depression. Effects only partially reversed by naloxone
Dose: by sublingual administration, initially 200 micrograms every 8 hours, increasing if necessary to 200–400 micrograms every 6–8 hours
By intramuscular or slow intravenous injection, 300–600 micrograms every 6–8 hours

PoM Temgesic® (R&C)
▼*Tablets* (sublingual), buprenorphine 200 micrograms (as hydrochloride). Price 20 tabs = **E**. Label: 2, 26
Injection, buprenorphine 300 micrograms (as hydrochloride)/ml. Price 1- and 2-ml amp (both) = **C**

DEXTROMORAMIDE

Indications: severe pain, particularly exacerbations in terminal disease
Cautions; Contra-indications; Side-effects: see notes above but less sedating than morphine

and development of tolerance and dependence is slower. Avoid in obstetric analgesia (increased risk of neonatal depression)
Dose: by mouth, 5 mg increasing to 20 mg, when required
By subcutaneous or intramuscular injection, 5 mg increasing to 15 mg, when required
By rectum in suppositories, 10 mg when required

CD Palfium® (MCP)
Tablets, scored, dextromoramide 5 mg (as tartrate). Price 20 tabs = **D**
Tablets, peach, scored, dextromoramide 10 mg (as tartrate). Price 20 tabs = **E**
Injection, dextromoramide 5 mg (as tartrate)/ml. Price 1-ml amp = **A**
Injection, dextromoramide 10 mg (as tartrate)/ml. Price 1-ml amp = **B**
Suppositories, dextromoramide 10 mg (as tartrate). Price 10 suppos = **E**

DIAMORPHINE HYDROCHLORIDE

Indications: severe pain
Cautions; Contra-indications; Side-effects: see notes above but more potent than morphine, causes greater respiratory depression, and is more liable to induce dependence
Dose: by mouth, or by subcutaneous, intramuscular, or intravenous injection, 5–10 mg every 4 hours

CD Diamorphine Tablets, diamorphine hydrochloride 10 mg (for oral administration). Price 20 tabs = **C**
CD Diamorphine Injection, powder for reconstitution, diamorphine hydrochloride. Price 5-, 10-, and 30-mg amp (all) = **C**; 100-mg amp = **E**
Diamorphine Analgesic Elixirs
See below

DIPIPANONE HYDROCHLORIDE

Indications: moderate to severe pain, particularly exacerbations in terminal disease
Cautions; Contra-indications; Side-effects: see notes above but less sedating than morphine

CD Diconal® (Calmic)
Tablets, pink, scored, dipipanone hydrochloride 10 mg, cyclizine hydrochloride 30 mg. Price 20 tabs = **D**
Dose: 1 tablet gradually increased to 3 tablets every 6 hours

---

LEVORPHANOL TARTRATE

Indications: severe pain, see notes above
Cautions; Contra-indications; Side-effects: see notes above
Dose: by mouth, 1.5–4.5 mg 1–2 times daily
By subcutaneous or intramuscular injection, 2–4 mg, repeated when necessary
By slow intravenous injection, 1–2 mg, repeated when necessary

---

C = 51-100p, D = 101-180p, E = 181-300p, F = 301-450p, G = 451-650p, H = 651-900p, I = 901-1200p, J = over 1200p.

CD Dromoran® (Roche)
Tablets, levorphanol tartrate 1.5 mg. Price 20 tabs = **C**
Injection, levorphanol tartrate 2 mg/ml. Price 1-ml amp = **B**

MEPTAZINOL
Indications: moderate to severe pain, including postoperative and obstetric pain and renal colic
Cautions; Contra-indications; Side-effects: see under Buprenorphine
Dose: by mouth, 200 mg every 3–6 hours as required
By intramuscular injection, 75–100 mg every 2–4 hours if necessary; obstetric analgesia, 100–150 mg according to patient's weight (2 mg/kg)
By slow intravenous injection, 50–100 mg every 2–4 hours if necessary

▼ PoM **Meptid®** (Wyeth)
Tablets, orange, f/c, meptazinol 200 mg. Price 20 tabs = **E**
Injection, meptazinol 100 mg (as hydro-chloride)/ml. Price 1-ml amp = **C**

METHADONE HYDROCHLORIDE
Indications: severe pain, see notes above
Cautions; Contra-indications; Side-effects: see notes above, but less sedating than morphine. Injections may cause local pain and tissue damage. Drug interactions: see Appendix 1 (section 4.7)
Dose: by mouth or by subcutaneous or intramuscular injection, 5–10 mg every 6–8 hours, adjusted according to response

CD Physeptone® (Calmic)
Tablets, scored, methadone hydrochloride 5 mg. Price 20 tabs = **C**
Injection, methadone hydrochloride 10 mg/ml. Price 1-ml amp = **B**

NALBUPHINE HYDROCHLORIDE
Indications: moderate to severe pain; peri-operative analgesia
Cautions; Contra-indications; Side-effects: see notes above. Sedation is the commonest side-effect; reduce dose in renal impairment
Dose: by subcutaneous, intramuscular, or intravenous injection, 10–20 mg every 3–6 hours, adjusted as required

▼ PoM **Nubain®** (Du Pont)
Injection, nalbuphine hydrochloride 10 mg/ml. Price 2-ml amp = **D**

NEFOPAM HYDROCHLORIDE
Indications: moderate pain
Cautions: hepatic disease, glaucoma, urinary retention
Contra-indications: convulsive disorders, myocardial infarction
Side-effects: nausea, nervousness, insomnia, dry mouth; less frequently blurred vision, drowsiness, sweating, tachycardia, headache

Dose: by mouth, initially 60 mg 3 times daily, adjusted according to response; usual range 30–90 mg 3 times daily
By intramuscular injection, 20 mg every 6 hours
Note: 20 mg by injection = 60 mg by mouth

▼ PoM **Acupan®** (Riker)
Tablets, f/c, nefopam hydrochloride 30 mg. Price 20 tabs = **E**
Injection, nefopam hydrochloride 20 mg/ml. Price 1-ml amp = **C**

PAPAVERETUM
Indications: moderate to severe pain
Cautions; Contra-indications; Side-effects: see notes above
Dose: by mouth or by subcutaneous, intramuscular, or intravenous injection, 10–20 mg every 4 hours if necessary; CHILD (by injection), 1–12 years 200–300 micrograms/kg max. as a single dose
Note: papaveretum contains anhydrous morphine 50% as hydrochloride with the hydrochlorides of other opium alkaloids. 10 mg papaveretum is equivalent in morphine content to 6.25 mg of morphine sulphate

CD Papaveretum Injection, papaveretum 10 and 20 mg/ml, price 1-ml amp (both) = **B**
CD Omnopon® (Roche)
Tablets, buff, papaveretum 10 mg. Price 20 tabs = **C**
Injection, papaveretum 20 mg/ml. Price 1-ml amp = **A**

PETHIDINE HYDROCHLORIDE
Indications: moderate to severe pain, obstetric analgesia
Cautions; Contra-indications; Side-effects: see notes above. Avoid in severe renal impairment. Drug interactions: see Appendix 1 (section 4.7)
Dose: by mouth, 50–150 mg every 4 hours; CHILD 0.5–2 mg/kg
By subcutaneous or intramuscular injection, 25–100 mg, repeated after 4 hours; CHILD, *by intramuscular injection,* 0.5–2 mg/kg
By slow intravenous injection, 25–50 mg, repeated after 4 hours
Obstetric analgesia, *by subcutaneous or intramuscular injection,* 50–100 mg, repeated 1–3 hours later if necessary; max. 400 mg in 24 hours

CD Pethidine Tablets, pethidine hydrochloride 25 and 50 mg. Price 20 tabs (both) = **B**
CD Pethidine Injection, pethidine hydrochloride 50 mg/ml. Price 1- and 2-ml amp (both) = **A**
CD Pamergan P100® (Martindale)
Injection, pethidine hydrochloride 50 mg, promethazine hydrochloride 25 mg/ml. Price 2-ml amp = **B**
Dose: by intramuscular injection, for obstetric analgesia, 1–2 ml every 4 hours if necessary; severe pain, 1–2 ml every 4–6 hours if necessary

CD Pethilorfan® (Roche)

Injection, pethidine hydrochloride 50 mg, levallorphan tartrate 625 micrograms/ml. Price 1- and 2-ml amp (both) = **A**

Dose: by subcutaneous, intramuscular, or intravenous injection, for obstetric analgesia, 1–3 ml; severe pain, 1–2 ml when necessary; CHILD 0.01–0.04 ml/kg (pethidine 0.5–2 mg/kg) as a single dose

PHENAZOCINE HYDROBROMIDE

Indications: severe pain, biliary or pancreatic pain

Cautions; Contra-indications; Side-effects: see notes above, but less sedating than morphine and dependence is slower to develop

Dose: by mouth or sublingually, 5 mg every 4– 6 hours when necessary; single doses may be increased to 20 mg

CD Narphen® (S&N Pharm.)

Tablets, scored, phenazocine hydrobromide 5 mg. Price 20 tabs = **E**

ANALGESIC ELIXIRS OF DIAMORPHINE AND MORPHINE

Both **morphine** and **diamorphine** are suitable for oral use in the relief of pain in terminal care. Many patients are adequately treated with morphine hydrochloride (or diamorphine hydrochloride). Routine administration of **cocaine** with the opiates is no longer recommended.

Prochlorperazine (Stemetil®) may be used for its anti-emetic and tranquillising action; **chlorpromazine** is an alternative but is more depressant. Such mixtures are usually preferable to the traditional 'Brompton Cocktail' elixirs (see below) which contain diamorphine or morphine with cocaine in a sweetened alcoholic basis. Many patients dislike the alcohol; the inclusion of chlorpromazine in such elixirs opposes the stimulant action of cocaine.

Simple Elixirs

Simple elixirs of **morphine** or **diamorphine** should be prescribed by writing the formula in full, for example:

Morphine hydrochloride 5 mg
Chloroform water to 5 ml

The total quantity to be supplied should be added in both words and figures, together with the other details required for controlled drug prescriptions (see Controlled Drugs and Drug Dependence). It is usual to adjust the strength so that the dose volume is 5 or 10 ml. These simple elixirs are now generally preferred to the traditional compound elixirs given below.

Traditional Compound Elixirs in a sweetened alcoholic basis

CD Diamorphine and Cocaine Elixir, diamorphine hydrochloride 5 mg, cocaine hydrochloride 5 mg/5 ml (see Formulary). Price 100 ml = **D**

CD Diamorphine, Cocaine, and Chlorpromazine Elixir, as above with chlorpromazine hydrochloride 6.25 mg/5 ml (see Formulary). Price 100 ml = **D**

* Morphine and Cocaine Elixir, morphine hydrochloride 5 mg, cocaine hydrochloride 5 mg/5 ml (see Formulary). Price 100 ml = **D**

* Morphine, Cocaine, and Chlorpromazine Elixir, as above with chlorpromazine hydrochloride 6.25 mg/5 ml (see Formulary). Price 100 ml = **D**

*CD if morphine content is increased, otherwise PoM When these preparations are ordered without qualification the proportion of diamorphine hydrochloride or of morphine hydrochloride is as stated above, but it may be varied when specified by the prescriber. For details see Formulary.

4.7.3 Trigeminal neuralgia

Carbamazepine (section 4.8.1), taken during the acute stages of trigeminal neuralgia, reduces the frequency and severity of attacks if given continuously. It has no effect on other forms of headache. A dose of 100 mg once or twice a day should be given initially and the dose slowly increased until the best response is obtained; most patients require 200 mg 3–4 times daily but a few may require an increased total daily dosage of up to 1.6 g. Plasma concentrations should be monitored when high doses are given. Occasionally extreme dizziness is encountered which is a further reason for starting treatment with a small dose and increasing it slowly.

Some cases of trigeminal neuralgia respond to **phenytoin** (section 4.8.1) and either carbamazepine or phenytoin may be of value for the pain of *diabetic neuropathy*.

4.7.4 Antimigraine drugs

These drugs are discussed under treatment of the acute migraine attack (section 4.7.4.1) and prophylaxis of migraine (section 4.7.4.2).

4.7.4.1 TREATMENT OF THE ACUTE MIGRAINE ATTACK

Most migraine headaches respond to analgesics such as **aspirin** or **paracetamol** (section 4.7.1.1) but as peristalsis is often reduced during migraine attacks the medication may not be sufficiently well absorbed to be effective; dispersible or effervescent preparations should therefore preferably be used.

Ergotamine is used in patients who do not respond to analgesics. It relieves migraine headache by constricting cranial arteries but visual and other prodromal symptoms are not affected and vomiting may be made worse. This can be relieved by the addition of an **anti-emetic** (see below).

The value of ergotamine is limited by difficulties in absorption and by its side-effects, particularly nausea, vomiting, abdominal pain, and muscular cramps. In some patients repeated administration may cause habituation. Rarely headache may be provoked, either by chronic overdosage or by rapid withdrawal of the drug. Doses of 6 to 8 mg per attack and 10 to 12 mg per week should **not** be exceeded. Ergotamine treatment should **not** be

---

C = 51-100p, **D** = 101-180p, **E** = 181-300p, **F** = 301-450p, **G** = 451-650p, **H** = 651-900p, **I** = 901-1200p, **J** = over 1200p.

repeated at intervals of less than 4 days and it should **never** be prescribed prophylactically.

There are various ergotamine preparations designed to improve absorption and best results are obtained when the dose is given early in an attack. An aerosol form (Medihaler-Ergotamine®) is acceptable to some patients. Sublingual ergotamine (Lingraine®) probably has no advantage over oral treatment.

Dihydroergotamine (Dihydergot®) is less effective than ergotamine and is of doubtful value.

Anti-emetics (section 4.6), such as **metoclopramide** by mouth or, if vomiting is likely, by intramuscular injection, or the phenothiazine and antihistamine anti-emetics, relieve the nausea associated with migraine attacks. Prochlorperazine may be given rectally if vomiting is a problem. Metoclopramide has the added advantage of promoting gastric emptying and normal peristalsis. A single dose should be given at the onset of symptoms. Oral analgesic preparations containing metoclopramide are available.

Diazepam and similar anxiolytics (section 4.1.2) may be useful adjuvant medication to counteract muscle spasm and anxiety often present in a migraine attack.

ANALGESICS

Aspirin Preparations
Paracetamol Preparations
Section 4.7.1.1

ANALGESICS WITH ANTI-EMETICS

Migraleve® (International Labs)
Tablets, all f/c, *pink tablets*, buclizine hydrochloride 6.25 mg, paracetamol 500 mg, codeine phosphate 8 mg, dioctyl sodium sulphosuccinate 10 mg; *yellow tablets*, paracetamol 500 mg, codeine phosphate 8 mg, dioctyl sodium sulphosuccinate 20 mg. Price 16 tabs (pink) + 8 tabs (yellow) = **E**; 24 pink = **E**; 24 yellow = **D**. Label: 17
Dose: 2 pink tablets at onset of attack, or at night during periods of impending attack then 2 yellow tablets every 3–4 hours if necessary; max. in 24 hours 2 pink and 6 yellow; CHILD 10–14 years, half adult dose

PoM **Migravess®** (Miles)
Tablets, effervescent, scored, metoclopramide hydrochloride 5 mg, aspirin 325 mg. Price 20 tabs = **E**. Label: 13, 17
Forte tablets, effervescent, scored, metoclopramide hydrochloride 5 mg, aspirin 450 mg. Price 20 tabs = **F**. Label: 13, 17
Dose: 2 tablets dissolved in water at onset of attack then every 4 hours when necessary; max. 6 tablets in 24 hours; CHILD 10–15 years, half adult dose

PoM **Paramax®** (Beecham)
Tablets, scored, paracetamol 500 mg, metoclopramide hydrochloride 5 mg. Price 20 tabs = **D**. Label: 17
Sachets, effervescent powder, the contents of 1 sachet = 1 tablet; to be dissolved in ¼ tumblerful of liquid before administration. Price 30 sachets = **F**. Label: 13, 17
Dose: 1–2 tablets at onset of attack then every

4 hours when necessary to a max. of 6 tablets in 24 hours; CHILD max. in 24 hours 12–14 years 3 tablets, 15–20 years 5 tablets

ERGOTAMINE TARTRATE
Indications: migraine attack, vascular headache
Cautions: renal, hepatic, and cardiovascular disease, hyperthyroidism; withdraw treatment if numbness or tingling of extremities develops; unsuitable for prophylaxis. Drug interactions: see Appendix 1 (sections *2.4*, 4.7)
Contra-indications: pregnancy, breast-feeding, peripheral vascular disease, sepsis
Side-effects: headache, nausea, and vomiting; repeated high dosage may cause ergotism with gangrene and confusion

PoM **Cafergot®** (Sandoz)
Tablets, pink, s/c, ergotamine tartrate 1 mg, caffeine 100 mg. Price 20 tabs = **C**. Label: 18
Dose: 2 tablets at onset, then 1 tablet every 30 minutes if necessary; max. 6 tablets per attack and 10 tablets weekly
Suppositories, ergotamine tartrate 2 mg, caffeine 100 mg. Price 6 suppos = **C**. Label: 18
Dose: 1 suppository, repeated if necessary; max. 3 suppositories per attack and 5 suppositories weekly

PoM **Lingraine®** (Winthrop)
Tablets (for sublingual use), green, ergotamine tartrate 2 mg. Price 12 tabs = **G**. Label: 18, 26
Dose: 1 tablet at onset repeated after 30 minutes if necessary; max. 3 tablets daily and 6 tablets weekly

PoM **Medihaler-Ergotamine®** (Riker)
Aerosol inhalation (oral), ergotamine tartrate 360 micrograms/metered inhalation. Price 75-dose unit = **F**. Label: 18
Dose: 360 micrograms repeated every 5 minutes if necessary; max. 6 inhalations daily and 15 inhalations weekly

PoM **Migril®** (Wellcome)
Tablets, scored, ergotamine tartrate 2 mg, cyclizine hydrochloride 50 mg, caffeine hydrate 100 mg. Price 20 tabs = **G**. Label: 2, 18
Dose: 1–2 tablets at onset, followed after 30 minutes by ½–1 tablet, repeated every 30 minutes if necessary; max. 4 tablets per attack and 6 tablets weekly

DIHYDROERGOTAMINE MESYLATE
Indications: migraine attack
Cautions; Contra-indications; Side-effects: see under Ergotamine Tartrate, but less effective and side-effects are milder. Avoid intra-arterial injection, and injection in coronary disease and uncontrolled hypertension
Dose: by mouth, mild attacks, 2–3 mg repeated every 30 minutes if necessary to a max. of 10 mg daily
Prophylaxis, 1–2 mg 3 times daily
By subcutaneous or intramuscular injection, 1–2 mg repeated once after 30 minutes if necessary

PoM **Dihydergot®** (Sandoz)
Tablets, scored, dihydroergotamine mesylate 1 mg. Price 20 tabs = **D**. Label: 17

Relative prices: **A** = up to 20p, **B** = 21-50p,

Oral solution, dihydroergotamine mesylate 2 mg/ml. 20 drops ≈ 1 ml. Do not dilute. Price 15-ml dropper bottle = **E**. Label: 17, counselling advised, use of dropper

Injection, dihydroergotamine mesylate 1 mg/ml. Price 1-ml amp = **B**

ISOMETHEPTENE MUCATE

Indications: migraine attack, headache
Cautions: cardiovascular disease
Contra-indications: glaucoma
Side-effects: dizziness, circulatory disturbances

PoM **Midrid**® (Carnrick)
Capsules, red, isometheptene mucate 65 mg, dichloral-phenazone 100 mg, paracetamol 325 mg. Price 20 caps = **E**. Label: 2, 17
Dose: migraine, 2 capsules at onset of attack, followed by 1 capsule every hour if necessary; max. 5 capsules in 12 hours; headache 1–2 capsules every 4 hours when necessary; max. 8 capsules daily

4.7.4.2 PROPHYLAXIS OF MIGRAINE

Prophylaxis is rarely indicated in patients who have one attack per month or less. A small dose of a benzodiazepine anxiolytic (section 4.1.2) is the first line of treatment in patients in whom nervous tension is playing a part. Depression is sometimes a factor and tricyclic antidepressants may help even when the patient is not obviously depressed. Combined oral contraceptives may precipitate migraine or worsen the pre-existing disease.

Clonidine (Dixarit®) is helpful in some patients but may aggravate depression and cause insomnia. It appears to diminish the responsiveness of the cranial vessels to either dilatation or constriction.

Pizotifen (Sanomigran®) is an antihistamine and antiserotonergic drug which is structurally related to the tricyclic antidepressants. Its efficacy is greater than that of clonidine but it causes anticholinergic side-effects and weight gain.

Methysergide (Deseril®) is also an antiserotonergic drug, but chronic use can cause retroperitoneal fibrosis and fibrosis of the heart valves and pleura; for this reason its use is no longer justified.

Some (but not all) beta-adrenoceptor blocking drugs are effective in about 60% of patients. These are atenolol, nadolol, propranolol, and timolol (see section 2.4). **Propranolol** is the most commonly used, in an initial dose of 40 mg two to three times daily by mouth. The value of these drugs is limited by their contra-indications (see section 2.4) and by interaction with ergotamine (see Appendix 1, section *2.4*).

There is recent evidence that the calcium-channel blockers, e.g. verapamil (Cordilox® etc.) and nifedipine (Adalat®) may be useful in migraine prophylaxis.

CLONIDINE HYDROCHLORIDE

Indications: prevention of recurrent migraine,

vascular headache, menopausal flushing
Cautions: depressive illness, concurrent antihypertensive therapy. Drug interactions: see Appendix 1 (section 2.5)
Side-effects: dry mouth, sedation, dizziness, nausea, nocturnal restlessness; occasionally rashes
Dose: 50 micrograms twice daily, increased after 2 weeks to 75 micrograms twice daily if necessary

PoM **Dixarit**® (WBP)
Tablets, blue, s/c, clonidine hydrochloride 25 micrograms. Price 20 tabs = **D**

METHYSERGIDE

Indications: prevention of severe recurrent migraine and migrainous neuralgia (see notes above)
Cautions: peptic ulceration; avoid abrupt withdrawal of treatment; withdraw treatment for reassessment after 6 months (see also notes above)
Contra-indications: renal, hepatic, pulmonary, and cardiovascular disease, collagen disorders, pregnancy, breast-feeding
Side-effects: nausea, drowsiness, and dizziness occur frequently in initial treatment; psychic reactions, oedema, arterial spasm, paraesthesias of extremities, postural hypotension, and tachycardia also occur. Retroperitoneal and other abnormal fibrotic reactions may occur on prolonged administration, requiring immediate withdrawal of treatment
Dose: 1 mg at bedtime, gradually increased to 1–2 mg 2–3 times daily with food (see notes above)

PoM **Deseril**® (Sandoz)
Tablets, yellow, s/c, methysergide 1 mg (as hydrogen maleate). Price 20 tabs = **D**. Label: 2, 21

PIZOTIFEN

Indications: prevention of recurrent migraine, vascular headache
Cautions: may affect the ability to drive or operate machinery and increase effects of alcohol. Drug interactions: see Appendix 1 (section *2.5*)
Contra-indications: urinary retention; closed-angle glaucoma
Side-effects: anticholinergic effects, drowsiness, weight gain; occasionally nausea, dizziness, muscle pain
Dose: 1.5 mg at night *or* 500 micrograms 3 times daily, adjusted according to response within the range 0.5–6 mg daily; max. single dose 3 mg; CHILD up to 1.5 mg daily; max. single dose at night 1 mg

PoM **Sanomigran**® (Sandoz)
Tablets, ivory-yellow, s/c, pizotifen 500 micrograms (as hydrogen malate). Price 20 tabs = **D**. Label: 2
Tablets, ivory-yellow, s/c, pizotifen 1.5 mg (as hydrogen malate). Price 28 tabs = **H**. Label: 2
Elixir, sugar-free, pizotifen 250 micrograms (as

hydrogen malate)/5 ml. Price 100 ml = **D**. Label: 2

PROCHLORPERAZINE

Indications: prevention of severe recurrent migraine

Cautions; Contra-indications; Side-effects: see section 4.6

Dose: by mouth, 5 mg 3–4 times daily *or* 5–10 mg as a single dose before anticipated migraine-precipitating event. To abort an attack 20 mg *by mouth* followed after 2 hours by 10 mg if necessary *or by rectum* 25 mg *or by deep intramuscular injection* 12.5 mg

Preparations
Section 4.6

4.8   Antiepileptics

In this section drugs are discussed under the following subsections:

4.8.1 Control of epilepsy
4.8.2 Drugs used in status epilepticus

4.8.1   Control of epilepsy

The object of treatment is to prevent the occurrence of fits by maintaining an effective plasma concentration of the drug. Dose and frequency are determined by the plasma half-life. Careful adjustment of doses is necessary, starting with low doses and increasing gradually until fits are controlled or there are overdose effects.

Frequency of administration should be kept as low as possible to encourage better patient compliance. Most antiepileptics, when used in average dosage, may be given twice daily. Phenobarbitone, which has a long half-life, may often be given as a daily dose at bedtime. However, with large doses, antiepileptics may need to be administered 3 or 4 times daily to avoid adverse effects associated with high peak plasma concentrations. Young children metabolise antiepileptics more rapidly than adults and therefore require more frequent dose and a higher dose per kilogram body-weight.

Therapy with several drugs concurrently should be avoided. Patients are best controlled with one antiepileptic. Combinations of drugs have been used on the grounds that their therapeutic effects were additive while their individual toxicity was reduced but there is no evidence for this. A second drug should only be added to the regimen if fits continue despite high plasma concentrations or toxic effects. The use of more than two antiepileptics is rarely justified.

Another disadvantage of multiple therapy is that drug interactions occur between the various antiepileptics (see Appendix 1, section 4.8). By inducing liver microsomal enzymes, phenobarbitone, phenytoin, and primidone increase each other's metabolism and can reduce plasma concentrations of carbamazepine. Also, primidone is partially metabolised to phenobarbitone. Compound preparations should be avoided because

the dose of each antiepileptic should be adjusted separately.

Once a successful regimen is established it should be maintained until there is freedom from fits for at least two years. Treatment should not be withdrawn abruptly as this may precipitate convulsions. Change-over from one antiepileptic to another should be made cautiously over several weeks.

DRIVING. Patients suffering from epilepsy may drive a motor vehicle (but not a heavy goods or public service vehicle) provided that they have had a fit-free period of two years or, if subject to attacks only while asleep, have established a three-year period of asleep attacks without awake attacks. Patients affected by drowsiness should not drive or operate machinery.

PREGNANCY. Although several antiepileptics are teratogenic in *animals*, the increased risk of congenital malformations is in practice slight. Abrupt withdrawal of antiepileptics also carries risk of increased seizure frequency or status epilepticus. See under Prescribing in Pregnancy.

Drug treatment of epilepsy is discussed under the headings tonic-clonic (grand mal) seizures; partial (focal) seizures; absence seizures (petit mal); myoclonic-atonic seizures (myoclonic jerks) (all in section 4.8.1) and status epilepticus (section 4.8.2).

Neonatal fits, infantile spasms (West's syndrome), and febrile convulsions are outside the scope of this book.

TONIC-CLONIC (GRAND MAL) AND PARTIAL (FOCAL) SEIZURES

The same range of drugs is used to treat both tonic-clonic seizures and partial fits. Phenytoin and carbamazepine are the drugs of choice as they usually give adequate control and the use of the more sedating compounds such as phenobarbitone or primidone is usually unnecessary. Carbamazepine may be preferred to phenytoin in patients with partial seizures, particularly complex partial (temporal lobe or psychomotor) seizures because side-effects are less of a problem.

Phenytoin (Epanutin®) is as effective as carbamazepine in tonic-clonic seizures but is ineffective in absence seizures. Disadvantages are that it has a narrow therapeutic index and readily produces nystagmus, slurred speech, and ataxia in overdose. Monitoring of plasma concentration greatly assists dosage adjustment. A few missed doses or a small change in drug absorption will result in a marked change in plasma concentration.

Phenytoin may cause coarse facies, acne, hirsutism, and gingival hyperplasia and for these reasons may be particularly undesirable in adolescent patients. Carbamazepine is often used as an alternative for this reason.

Carbamazepine (Tegretol®) is the drug of choice in controlling both simple and complex partial seizures. It is effective in controlling tonic-clonic fits regardless of whether they are primary (idiopathic) or secondary to a focal discharge. It is less sedating than phenobarbitone, but side-effects such as diplopia and dizziness may be dose-limiting. Monitoring plasma carbamazepine concentrations is helpful in determining the optimum dosage.

Phenobarbitone is an effective drug but it is sedative in adults and may cause behavioural disturbances and hyperkinesia in children. Rebound fits may be a problem on withdrawal. Monitoring plasma concentrations is less useful than with other drugs because tolerance occurs. **Methylphenobarbitone** is largely converted to phenobarbitone in the liver and has no advantages. **Primidone** (Mysoline®) is partially converted to phenobarbitone, but the unchanged drug and a second metabolite (both with short half-lives) may also be active. A small starting dose is essential.

Sodium valproate (Epilim®) is active in controlling tonic-clonic fits, particularly if they are primary (idiopathic). Routine monitoring is unjustified at present because the activity of the drug may not be accurately reflected by its plasma concentration.

Sulthiame (Ospolot®) is a weak antiepileptic but readily causes drug interactions by inhibition of metabolism, particularly with phenytoin, and it is rarely used. Hyperventilation is common.

Clonazepam (Rivotril®) and other **benzodiazepines** are, in general, too sedating for chronic use in doses which control tonic-clonic or partial fits. **Clobazam** may be used as intermittent adjunctive therapy in the treatment of epilepsy (section 4.1.2). The effectiveness of benzodiazepines may appear to wane after a period of weeks or months.

ABSENCE SEIZURES (PETIT MAL)

Ethosuximide (Emeside®, Zarontin®) and **sodium valproate** (Epilim®) are the drugs of choice in children who have simple absence seizures. In complex absences with co-existing tonic-clonic fits, against which ethosuximide is not active, additional treatment with another suitable drug (see above) may be necessary. Monitoring plasma ethosuximide concentrations is helpful in determining the optimum dosage.

Since sodium valproate, unlike ethosuximide, will also treat tonic-clonic seizures, it may be preferred for absences associated with tonic-clonic seizures.

MYOCLONIC-ATONIC SEIZURES (MYOCLONIC JERKS)

There are a variety of syndromes occurring in childhood in which myoclonic jerks and atonic seizures occur. They have responded poorly to the traditional drugs.

Sodium valproate (Epilim®) and **clonazepam** (Rivotril®) are the drugs of first choice. Sodium

valproate should be tried before clonazepam, which is more sedating.

BECLAMIDE

Indications: behavioural disorders, tonic-clonic and partial seizures

Cautions: previous antiepileptic medication should be continued for 4 weeks then gradually reduced

Side-effects: dizziness, weight loss, rashes, renal and gastro-intestinal disturbances, and leucopenia are uncommon

Dose: initially 3–4 g daily in divided doses, reduced as necessary; maintenance dose usually 1.5–3 g daily in divided doses; CHILD up to 5 years 0.75–1 g daily in divided doses, 6–12 years 1.5 g daily in divided doses

PoM **Nydrane**® (Lipha)
Tablets, scored, beclamide 500 mg. Price 20 tabs = **C**

CARBAMAZEPINE

Indications: all forms of epilepsy except absence seizures; trigeminal neuralgia (section 4.7.3)

Cautions: see notes above; hepatic impairment; breast-feeding. Drug interactions: see Appendix 1 (sections *2.8A*, *3*, *4.2*, *4.8*, *4.8*, *5.1*, *6.2*, *6.3*, *7*)

Contra-indications: previous sensitivity to carbamazepine, atrioventricular conduction abnormalities; porphyrias; patients on monamine-oxidase inhibitors or within 2 weeks of MAOI therapy

Side-effects: dizziness, drowsiness, visual, and gastro-intestinal disturbances (often associated with peak plasma concentrations); a generalised erythematous rash may occur in about 3% of patients; leucopenia and other blood disorders have occurred rarely

Dose: initially, 100–200 mg 1–2 times daily, increased slowly to a usual dose of 0.8–1.2 g daily according to the patient's needs; in some cases 1.6 g (or even 1.8 g) daily may be needed; CHILD daily in divided doses, up to one year 100–200 mg, 1–5 years 200–400 mg, 5–10 years 400–600 mg, 10–15 years 0.6–1 g

Note: plasma concentration for optimum response 3–10 micrograms/ml

PoM **Tegretol**® (Geigy)
Tablets, scored, carbamazepine 100 mg. Price 20 tabs = **C**. Label: 2
Tablets, scored, carbamazepine 200 mg. Price 20 tabs = **D**. Label: 2
Tablets, scored, carbamazepine 400 mg. Price 20 tabs = **E**. Label: 2
Syrup (= mixture), carbamazepine 100 mg/5 ml. Diluent tragacanth mucilage for 1 + 1 dilution, life of diluted mixture 14 days. Price 100 ml = **D**. Label: 2

CLONAZEPAM

Indications: all forms of epilepsy. For status epilepticus see section 4.8.2

Cautions: may affect the ability to drive or operate machinery and increase the effects of alcohol; breast-feeding; see notes above. Drug interactions: see Appendix 1 (section 4.8)

Side-effects: drowsiness, fatigue, dizziness, muscle hypotonia, hypersalivation in infants, paradoxical aggression, irritability and mental changes

Dose: 1 mg, initially at night for 4 nights, increased over 2–4 weeks to a usual daily maintenance dose of 4–8 mg; CHILD up to 1 year 250 micrograms increased as above to 0.5–1 mg, 1–5 years 250 micrograms increased to 1–3 mg, 6–12 years 500 micrograms increased to 3–6 mg

PoM **Rivotril**® (Sauter)
Tablets, beige, scored, clonazepam 500 micrograms. Price 20 tabs = **C**. Label: 2
Tablets, scored, clonazepam 2 mg. Price 20 tabs = **D**. Label: 2

ETHOSUXIMIDE

Indications: absence seizures
Cautions: see notes above. Drug interactions: see Appendix 1 (section 4.8)
Contra-indications: porphyrias
Side-effects: gastro-intestinal disturbances, drowsiness, dizziness, ataxia, headache, depression, and mild euphoria. Psychotic states, rashes, liver changes, and haematological disorders such as leucopenia and agranulocytosis occur rarely
Dose: initially, 500 mg daily, increased according to patient's needs by 250 mg at intervals of 4–7 days to a max. of 2 g daily; CHILD up to 6 years 250 mg daily, over 6 years 500 mg, increased gradually to a max. of 1 g daily
Note: plasma concentration for optimum response 50–100 micrograms/ml

PoM **Ethosuximide Capsules,** ethosuximide 250 mg. Price 20 caps = **C**. Label: 1
PoM **Ethosuximide Elixir,** ethosuximide 250 mg/5 ml. Diluent as below. Price 100 ml = **D**. Label: 1
PoM **Emeside**® (LAB)
Capsules, orange, ethosuximide 250 mg. Price 20 caps = **C**. Label: 1
Syrup (= elixir), black currant or orange, ethosuximide 250 mg/5 ml. Diluent syrup, life of diluted elixir 14 days. Price 100 ml = **D**. Label: 1
PoM **Zarontin**® (P-D)
Capsules, orange, ethosuximide 250 mg. Price 20 caps = **D**. Label: 1
Syrup (= elixir), red, ethosuximide 250 mg/5 ml. Diluent syrup, life of diluted elixir 14 days. Price 100 ml = **D**. Label: 1

METHYLPHENOBARBITONE

Indications: tonic-clonic and partial seizures
Cautions; Contra-indications; Side-effects: see under Phenobarbitone
Dose: 100–600 mg daily, according to the patient's needs

CD **Prominal**® (Winthrop)
Tablets, methylphenobarbitone 30 mg. Price 20 tabs = **C**. Label: 2
Tablets, methylphenobarbitone 60 mg. Price 20 tabs = **C**. Label: 2
Tablets, methylphenobarbitone 200 mg. Price 20 tabs = **D**. Label: 2

PHENOBARBITONE

Indications: all forms of epilepsy except absence seizures. For status epilepticus see section 4.8.2
Cautions: elderly, children, impaired renal or hepatic function, severe respiratory depression, breast-feeding; avoid sudden withdrawal, or use with other CNS sedatives, particularly alcohol; prolonged dosage may produce dependence; see also notes above. Drug interactions: see Appendix 1 (sections *2.1, 2.8A, 4.8, 4.8, 5.1, 5.2, 6.3, 7, 8*)
Contra-indications: porphyrias
Side-effects: drowsiness, lethargy, mental depression, ataxia and allergic skin reactions; paradoxical excitement, restlessness and confusion in the elderly and hyperkinesia in children; megaloblastic anaemia (may be treated with folic acid)
Dose: by mouth, 60–300 mg at night; CHILD 5–10 mg/kg daily
By intramuscular or intravenous injection, 50–200 mg, repeated after 6 hours if necessary; max. 600 mg daily
Note: for therapeutic purposes phenobarbitone and phenobarbitone sodium may be considered equivalent in effect

CD **Phenobarbitone Tablets,** phenobarbitone 15, 30, 60, and 100 mg. Price 20 tabs (all) = **A**. Label: 2
CD **Phenobarbitone Sodium Tablets,** phenobarbitone sodium 30 and 60 mg. Price 20 tabs (both) = **A**. Label: 2
CD **Phenobarbitone Elixir,** yellow, phenobarbitone 30 mg/10 ml (see Formulary). Price 100 ml = **B**. Label: 2
CD **Phenobarbitone Injection,** phenobarbitone sodium 200 mg/ml in propylene glycol 90% and water for injections 10%. Price 1-ml amp = **B**
CD **Gardenal Sodium**® (M&B)
Injection, phenobarbitone sodium 200 mg/ml. Price 1-ml amp = **B**
CD **Luminal**® (Winthrop)
Tablets, phenobarbitone 15 mg. Price 20 tabs = **A**. Label: 2
Tablets, phenobarbitone 30 mg. Price 20 tabs = **B**. Label: 2
Tablets, phenobarbitone 60 mg. Price 20 tabs = **B**. Label: 2
CD **Phenobarbitone Spansule**® (SK&F)
Spansule® (= capsules s/r), clear/blue enclosing blue and white pellets, phenobarbitone 60 mg. Price 20 caps = **B**. Label: 2, 25
Spansule® (= capsules s/r), clear/blue enclosing blue and white pellets, phenobarbitone 100 mg. Price 20 caps = **B**. Label: 2, 25

PHENYTOIN

Indications: tonic-clonic and partial seizures
Cautions; Side-effects; Dose: see under Phenytoin Sodium
Note: phenytoin 100 mg ≡ phenytoin sodium 108 mg

PoM **Epanutin**® (P-D)
Suspension (= mixture), red, phenytoin 30 mg/5 ml. Diluent syrup, life of diluted mixture 14 days. Price 100 ml = **C**. Label: 27
Infatabs® (= tablets, chewable), yellow, scored, phenytoin 50 mg. Price 20 tabs = **C**. Label: 24

PHENYTOIN SODIUM

Indications: all forms of epilepsy except absence seizures
Cautions: hepatic impairment (reduce dose), change-over from other drugs should be made cautiously; avoid sudden withdrawal; see also notes above. Drug interactions: see Appendix 1 (sections *2.8D*, *3*, *4.2*, *4.8*, *4.8*, *5.1*, *6.2*, *6.3*, *7*, *8*)
Contra-indications: porphyrias
Side-effects: nausea, vomiting, mental confusion, dizziness, headache, tremor, insomnia occur commonly. Ataxia, slurred speech, nystagmus and blurred vision are signs of overdosage. Skin eruptions (sometimes severe), coarse facies, acne and hirsutism, fever and hepatitis; lupus erythematosus, erythema multiforme; lymphadenopathy; gingival hypertrophy and tenderness; haematological effects, including megaloblastic anaemia due to folate deficiency, leucopenia, thrombocytopenia, agranulocytosis, and aplastic anaemia are rare. Plasma calcium may be lowered, causing rickets and osteomalacia
Dose: by mouth, daily as a single dose or 2 divided doses, with water, 150–300 mg increased gradually to 600 mg according to the patient's needs; CHILD 5–8 mg/kg daily in 1 or 2 doses
By intravenous injection—section 4.8.2
Note: plasma concentration for optimum response 10–20 micrograms/ml

PoM **Phenytoin Tablets,** s/c, phenytoin sodium 50 and 100 mg. Price 20 tabs (both) = **A**. Label: 27
PoM **Epanutin**® (P-D)
Capsules, white/purple, phenytoin sodium 25 mg. Price 20 caps = **B**. Label: 27
Capsules, white/pink, phenytoin sodium 50 mg. Price 20 caps = **B**. Label: 27
Capsules, white/orange, phenytoin sodium 100 mg. Price 20 caps = **B**. Label: 27

PRIMIDONE

Indications: all forms of epilepsy except absence seizures. For use in benign essential tremor see section 4.9.3
Cautions; Contra-indications; Side-effects: see under Phenobarbitone. Drowsiness, ataxia, nausea, visual disturbances, and rashes, particularly at first, but usually reversible on continued administration. Drug interactions: see Appendix 1 (sections *2.8A*, 4.8, *4.8*, *6.3*, 7)
Dose: initially, 125 mg daily at bedtime, increased by 125 mg every 3 days to 500 mg daily in 2 divided doses then increased by 250 mg every 3 days to a max. of 1.5 g daily in divided doses; CHILD 20–30 mg/kg daily in 2 divided doses

PoM **Mysoline**® (ICI)
Tablets, scored, primidone 250 mg. Price 20 tabs = **B**. Label: 2
Oral suspension (= mixture), primidone 250 mg/5 ml. Diluent propyl hydroxybenzoate 0.015%, methyl hydroxybenzoate 0.15%, carmellose sodium '50' 1%, sucrose 20%, in freshly boiled and cooled purified water. Price 100 ml = **B**. Label: 2

SODIUM VALPROATE

Indications: all forms of epilepsy
Cautions: avoid when possible in hepatic impairment; monitor liver function before and at 2-month intervals during first 6 months of therapy; monitor platelet function before major surgery; may give false-positive urine tests for ketones in diabetes mellitus; see also notes above. Drug interactions: see Appendix 1 (sections 4.8, *4.8*)
Side-effects: gastric irritation, nausea; hyperammonaemia, increased appetite and weight gain; transient hair loss (regrowth may be curly), oedema, thrombocytopenia, and inhibition of platelet aggregation; impaired hepatic function leading rarely to fatal hepatic failure (see Cautions—withdraw treatment immediately if vomiting, anorexia, jaundice, drowsiness, or loss of seizure control occurs); rarely pancreatitis (estimate plasma amylase in acute abdominal pain)
Dose: initially, 600 mg daily in divided doses, preferably after food, increasing by 200 mg/day at 3-day intervals to a max. of 2.5 g daily in divided doses, according to the patient's needs; CHILD up to 20 kg (about 4 years), initially 20 mg/kg daily in divided doses increased gradually to a max. of 40 mg/kg daily; over 20 kg, initially 400 mg daily in divided doses increased gradually to 30 mg/kg daily, according to the patient's needs

PoM **Epilim**® (Labaz)
Tablets (crushable), scored, sodium valproate 100 mg. Price 20 tabs = **C**
Tablets, e/c, lilac, sodium valproate 200 mg. Price 20 tabs = **D**. Label: 5, 25
Tablets, e/c, lilac, sodium valproate 500 mg. Price 20 tabs = **F**. Label: 5, 25
Liquid (= elixir), red, sugar-free, sodium valproate 200 mg/5 ml. Do not dilute. Price 100 ml = **E**
Syrup (= elixir), red, sodium valproate 200 mg/5 ml. Diluent syrup (without preservative), life of diluted elixir 14 days. Price 100 ml = **E**

SULTHIAME

Indications: myoclonic seizures, partial seizures, hyperkinesia, and possibly tonic-clonic seizures

Cautions: impaired renal function; change-over from other drugs should be made cautiously over several weeks; see also notes above. Drug interactions: see Appendix 1 (section *4.8*)

Side-effects: paraesthesias of face and extremities, gastric disturbances, headache, vertigo, ataxia, hyperventilation, anorexia, and loss of weight

Dose: initially 100 mg twice daily increased to 200 mg 3 times daily according to the patient's needs; CHILD, daily in divided doses, 3–5 mg/kg increasing to 10–15 mg/kg

PoM **Ospolot**® (Bayer)
Tablets, lacquer coated, scored, sulthiame 50 mg. Price 20 tabs = **D**
Tablets, lacquer coated, scored, sulthiame 200 mg. Price 20 tabs = **D**
Suspension (= mixture), yellow, sulthiame 50 mg/5 ml. Diluent tragacanth mucilage, life of diluted mixture 14 days; *or* carmellose sodium 1% with methyl hydroxybenzoate 0.07% in recently boiled and cooled purified water, life of diluted mixture 2 months. Price 100 ml = **C**

COMPOUND PREPARATIONS

Compound preparations in fixed proportions should be **avoided** because the dose of each antiepileptic should be adjusted separately according to the patient's response.

CD **Epanutin with Phenobarbitone** ® (P-D)
Capsules, yellow/white, phenytoin sodium 100 mg, phenobarbitone 50 mg. Price 20 caps = **B**. Label: 2, 27

4.8.2   Drugs used in status epilepticus

Major status epilepticus should be treated first with intravenous **diazepam** or **clonazepam** (Rivotril®) but they should be used with caution because of the risk of respiratory depression; there may be a high incidence of venous thrombophlebitis. Intramuscular injection is unsatisfactory as the drugs are too slowly absorbed. When diazepam is given intravenously the risk of thrombophlebitis is minimised by using an emulsion (Diazemuls®). If intravenous administration is not possible, diazepam may be given as a rectal solution (Stesolid®). Absorption from suppositories is too slow for treatment of status epilepticus. If status epilepticus continues or returns, an intravenous infusion of **chlormethiazole** (Heminevrin®) should be used.

Paraldehyde also remains a valuable drug. It may be given diluted with sodium chloride 0.9% by intravenous injection or may be given by intramuscular or rectal administration.

Phenobarbitone sodium (section 4.8.1) is occasionally used but it is less satisfactory for urgent treatment because it enters the brain too slowly and is metabolised and excreted too slowly. Slow intravenous injections of **phenytoin sodium** may be tried in patients who have not been taking it by mouth; a loading dose of 13 to 15 mg/kg

may be successful in controlling the condition and preventing subsequent recurrence of seizures.

DIAZEPAM

Indications: status epilepticus; convulsions due to poisoning (see Emergency Treatment of Poisoning)

Cautions; Side-effects: see section 4.1.2. When given intravenously facilities for reversing respiratory depression with mechanical ventilation should be at hand

Dose: by intramuscular injection or slow intravenous injection, as a 0.5% solution or emulsion, 10–20 mg at a rate of 0.5 ml (2.5 mg) per 30 seconds, repeated if necessary after 30–60 minutes; may be followed by *slow intravenous infusion* to a max. of 3 mg/kg over 24 hours; CHILD 200–300 micrograms/kg

By rectum in solution, adults and children over 3 years 10 mg; CHILD 1–3 years and elderly patients 5 mg; repeat after 5 minutes if necessary

PoM **Diazemuls**® (KabiVitrum)
Injection (emulsion), diazepam 5 mg/ml (0.5%). See Appendix 2. Price 2-ml amp = **B**
PoM **Stesolid**® (CP)
Injection, diazepam 5 mg/ml (0.5%). See Appendix 2. Price 2- and 4-ml amp (both) = **B**
Rectal tubes (= rectal solution), diazepam 2 mg/ml. Price 5 × 2.5-ml tubes = **F**
Rectal tubes (= rectal solution), diazepam 4 mg/ml. Price 5 × 2.5-ml tubes = **G**
PoM **Valium**® (Roche)
Injection, diazepam 5 mg/ml (0.5%) in solvent. See Appendix 2. Price 2- and 4-ml amp (both) = **B**

CLONAZEPAM

Indications: status epilepticus

Cautions; Side-effects: see section 4.8.1. Hypotension and apnoea may occur and resuscitation facilities must be available

Dose: by slow intravenous injection or infusion, 1 mg over 30 seconds; CHILD all ages, 500 micrograms

PoM **Rivotril**® (Sauter)
Injection, clonazepam 1 mg/ml in solvent, for dilution with 1 ml water for injections immediately before injection or as described in Appendix 2. Price 1-ml amp (with 1 ml water for injections) = **C**

CHLORMETHIAZOLE EDISYLATE

Indications: status epilepticus

Cautions: obstructive pulmonary disease; sedative effects may be enhanced by other central depressants, phenothiazines or butyrophenones; during continuous infusion deep sleep may quickly lapse into unconsciousness and patients must be constantly observed

Side-effects: tingling in the nose, sneezing, conjunctival irritation, headache, slight hypotension, respiratory depression, local thrombophlebitis at site of continuous infusion

---

Dose: by intravenous infusion, as a 0.8% solution, 40–100 ml (320–800 mg) at a rate of 60–150 drops per minute

PoM Heminevrin® (Astra)
Intravenous infusion 0.8%, chlormethiazole edisylate 8 mg/ml. Price 500-ml bottle = **G**

PARALDEHYDE

Indications: status epilepticus
Cautions: bronchopulmonary disease, hepatic impairment
Side-effects: rashes; injections are painful
Dose: by deep intramuscular injection, as a single dose, 5–10 ml; not more than 5 ml at any one site; CHILD up to 3 months 0.5 ml, 3–6 months 1 ml, 6–12 months 1.5 ml, 1–2 years 2 ml, 3–5 years 3–4 ml, 6–12 years 5–6 ml
By slow intravenous injection, diluted with several times its volume of sodium chloride intravenous infusion 0.9%, up to 4–5 ml
By rectum, 4–5 ml, administered as a 10% enema in isotonic sodium chloride solution; CHILD as for intramuscular dose
Note: do not use paraldehyde if it has a brownish colour or an odour of acetic acid. Avoid contact with rubber and plastics.

PoM Paraldehyde Injection, sterile paraldehyde. Price 5- and 10-ml amp (both) = **C**

PHENYTOIN SODIUM

Indications: status epilepticus; prophylaxis of seizures in neurosurgery
Cautions; Side-effects: see under Phenytoin Sodium, section 4.8.1. Do not give with lignocaine hydrochloride. Injection solutions are alkaline and may be irritant. May cause hypotension, asystole, bradycardia, and confusion. Resuscitation facilities must be available
Contra-indications: should not be given intravenously in patients with bradycardia, supraventricular tachycardias, or heart block
Dose: by slow intravenous injection, status epilepticus, 13–15 mg/kg at a rate not exceeding 50 mg per minute; CHILD up to 5 mg/kg
By intramuscular injection, prophylaxis in neurosurgery, 100–200 mg 3–4 times daily during surgery and postoperatively

PoM Epanutin Ready Mixed Parenteral® (P-D)
Injection, phenytoin sodium 50 mg/ml with propylene glycol 40% and alcohol 10% in water for injections. Price 5-ml amp = **F**

4.9 Drugs used in parkinsonism and related disorders

4.9.1 Dopaminergic drugs used in parkinsonism
4.9.2 Anticholinergic drugs used in parkinsonism
4.9.3 Drugs used in choreas, tics, and related disorders

In idiopathic Parkinson's disease, progressive degeneration of pigment-containing cells of the substantia nigra leads to deficiency of the inhibitory neurotransmitter dopamine. This, in turn, results in a neurohumoral imbalance in the basal ganglia, causing the characteristic signs and symptoms of the illness to appear. The pathogenesis of this process is still obscure and current therapy aims simply to correct the imbalance. Although this approach fails to prevent the progression of the disease, it greatly improves the quality and expectancy of life of most patients.

Levodopa, used in conjunction with **dopa-decarboxylase inhibitors** (section 4.9.1), is the treatment of choice for patients disabled by idiopathic Parkinson's disease. It is less effective in patients with post-encephalitic parkinsonism and should be avoided in neuroleptic-induced parkinsonism.

Parkinsonism caused by generalised degenerative brain disease does not respond to levodopa.

Anticholinergic drugs (section 4.9.2) are the other main class of drugs used in Parkinson's disease. They are less effective than levodopa in idiopathic Parkinson's disease although they often usefully supplement its action. Patients with mild symptoms may be treated with anticholinergic drugs before they are eventually transferred to levodopa therapy as symptoms progress. Anticholinergic drugs are particularly valuable in treating drug-induced parkinsonism or in patients with post-encephalitic parkinsonism.

Other antiparkinsonian drugs include amantadine and bromocriptine (section 4.9.1).

The patient should be advised at the outset of the limitations of treatment and possible side-effects. About 10 to 20% of patients are unresponsive to treatment.

For drug interactions of antiparkinsonian drugs, see Appendix 1 (section 4.9).

4.9.1 Dopaminergic drugs used in parkinsonism

Levodopa is the treatment of choice for disabled patients. It is least valuable in elderly patients and in those with long-standing disease who rarely tolerate a dose large enough to overcome their deficit. It is also less valuable in patients with post-encephalitic disease who are particularly susceptible to the side-effects.

Levodopa, the amino-acid precursor of dopamine, acts mainly by replenishing depleted striatal dopamine. It improves bradykinesia and rigidity more rapidly than tremor. It is generally administered in conjunction with an extra-cerebral dopa-decarboxylase inhibitor (**carbidopa**, as in Sinemet® or **benserazide**, as in Madopar®) which prevents the peripheral degradation of levodopa to dopamine.

The presence of the inhibitor enables the effective dose of levodopa to be greatly reduced, while peripheral side-effects such as nausea and vomiting and cardiovascular effects are minimised. There is less delay in onset of therapeutic effect and a smoother clinical response is obtained. A disadvantage is that there is an increased inci-

---

C = 51-100p, D = 101-180p, E = 181-300p, F = 301-450p, G = 451-650p, H = 651-900p, I = 901-1200p, J = over 1200p.

dence of abnormal involuntary movements. When Sinemet® is used in low dosage the dose of carbidopa may be insufficient to achieve full inhibition of extracerebral dopa-decarboxylase; Sinemet-Plus® (containing 25 mg of carbidopa for each 100 mg of levodopa) should then be used so that the daily dose of carbidopa is at least 75 mg. This will ensure maximum effectiveness of the levodopa with a minimum of adverse peripheral effects.

Treatment with levodopa should be initiated with low doses and gradually increased, by small increments, at intervals of 2 to 3 days. (It is rarely necessary to exceed a daily dose of 1 gram when levodopa is used in conjunction with a dopa-decarboxylase inhibitor.) When titrated in this way the final dose is usually a compromise between increased mobility and dose-limiting side-effects. Intervals between doses may be critical and should be chosen to suit the needs of the individual patient. Nausea and vomiting are rarely dose-limiting if levodopa is given in this way but doses should be taken after meals. Domperidone may be useful in controlling vomiting (section 4.6). The most frequent dose-limiting side-effects of levodopa are involuntary movements and psychiatric complications.

Treatment with levodopa should not be discontinued abruptly. As the patient ages, the maintenance dose may need to be reduced. When substituting the combined levodopa-decarboxylase inhibitor preparations for levodopa alone, treatment should be discontinued for 12 hours before starting therapy with the combined preparation.

During the first 6 to 18 months of levodopa therapy there may be a slow improvement in the response of the patient which is maintained for 1½ to 2 years; thereafter a slow decline may occur. Particularly troublesome is the 'on-off' effect the incidence of which increases as the treatment progresses. This is characterised by fluctuations in performance with normal performance during the 'on' period and weakness and akinesia lasting for 2 to 4 hours during the 'off' period.

Monoamine-oxidase inhibitors must be withdrawn at least 14 days before treatment. Close observation is especially necessary in patients with a past history of psychiatric illness, dementia, open-angle glaucoma, or skin melanoma. Antipsychotic drugs should not be administered concurrently.

Selegiline (Eldepryl®) is a recently-introduced monoamine-oxidase-B inhibitor used in severe parkinsonism in conjunction with levodopa to reduce 'end-of-dose' akinesia. Unlike other monoamine-oxidase inhibitors, it does not cause episodes of hypertension.

Bromocriptine (Parlodel®) acts by direct stimulation of surviving dopamine receptors. Although effective, it has no advantages over levodopa. Its use should be restricted to the treatment of previously untreated disabled patients and those who despite careful titration cannot tolerate levodopa. When used with levodopa, abnormal involuntary movements and confusional states are common, and the doses of the two drugs should be balanced for optimum effect.

Amantadine (Symmetrel®) has modest antiparkinsonian effects. It improves mild bradykinetic disabilities as well as tremor and rigidity. Unfortunately only a small proportion of patients derive much benefit from this drug and tolerance to its effects occurs. However it has the advantage of being relatively free from side-effects.

LEVODOPA

Indications: parkinsonism (but not drug-induced extrapyramidal symptoms), see notes above

Cautions: pulmonary disease, peptic ulceration, cardiovascular disease, diabetes, open-angle glaucoma, skin melanoma, psychiatric illness. In prolonged therapy, psychiatric, hepatic, haematological, renal, and cardiovascular surveillance is advisable. Discontinue treatment 8 hours before surgery (increased risk of arrhythmias). Warn patients who benefit from therapy to resume normal activities gradually. Drug interactions: see Appendix 1 (sections *2.5*, *4.3*, *4.9*, *15*)

Contra-indications: closed-angle glaucoma

Side-effects: anorexia, nausea, insomnia, agitation, postural hypotension, dizziness, tachycardia, arrhythmias, discoloration of urine and other body fluids, rarely hypersensitivity; abnormal involuntary movements and psychiatric symptoms may be dose-limiting

Dose: initially 125–500 mg daily in divided doses after meals, increased according to response (see notes above)

PoM **Levodopa Capsules,** levodopa 125 and 250 mg, price 20 caps (both) = **B**; 500 mg, price 20 caps = **C**. Label: 14, 21

PoM **Levodopa Tablets,** levodopa 500 mg. Price 20 tabs = **C**. Label: 14, 21

PoM **Brocadopa®** (Brocades)
Capsules, levodopa 125 mg. Price 20 caps = **B**. Label: 14, 21
Capsules, levodopa 250 mg. Price 20 caps = **B**. Label: 14, 21
Capsules, levodopa 500 mg. Price 20 caps = **C**. Label: 14, 21

PoM **Larodopa®** (Roche)
Tablets, scored, levodopa 500 mg. Price 20 tabs = **D**. Label: 14, 21

LEVODOPA WITH BENSERAZIDE

Indications; Cautions; Contra-indications; Side-effects: see under Levodopa and notes above

Dose: expressed as levodopa, initially 50–100 mg twice daily, adjusted according to response; usual maintenance dose 400–800 mg daily in divided doses after meals

Note: when transferring patients from levodopa 3 capsules Madopar 125® should be substituted for 2 g levodopa

PoM **Madopar®** (Roche)
Capsules (Madopar 62.5), blue/grey, levodopa

50 mg, benserazide 12.5 mg (as hydrochloride). Price 20 caps = **D**. Label: 14, 21

Capsules (Madopar 125), blue/pink, levodopa 100 mg, benserazide 25 mg (as hydrochloride). Price 20 caps = **E**. Label: 14, 21

Capsules (Madopar 250), blue/caramel, levodopa 200 mg, benserazide 50 mg (as hydrochloride). Price 20 caps = **F**. Label: 14, 21

LEVODOPA WITH CARBIDOPA

Indications; Cautions; Contra-indications; Side-effects: see under Levodopa and notes above
Dose: expressed as levodopa, initially 100–125 mg 3–4 times daily adjusted according to response; usual maintenance dose 0.75–1.5 g daily in divided doses after food. See also under Sinemet-Plus®
Note: when transferring patients from levodopa, 3 tablets Sinemet-275 should be substituted for 4 g levodopa

PoM **Sinemet®** (MSD)
Tablets (Sinemet-110), blue, scored, levodopa 100 mg, carbidopa 10 mg (as monohydrate). Price 20 tabs = **D**. Label: 14, 21
Tablets (Sinemet-275), blue, scored, levodopa 250 mg, carbidopa 25 mg (as monohydrate). Price 20 tabs = **F**. Label: 14, 21
PoM **Sinemet-Plus®** (MSD)
Tablets, yellow, scored, levodopa 100 mg, carbidopa 25 mg (as monohydrate). Price 20 tabs = **E**. Label: 14, 21
Dose: initially 1 tablet 3 times daily, adjusted according to response to 8 daily in divided doses; larger doses by gradual substitution of Sinemet for Sinemet-Plus

AMANTADINE HYDROCHLORIDE

Indications: parkinsonism (but not drug-induced extrapyramidal symptoms)
Cautions: cardiovascular, hepatic, or renal disease, recurrent eczema, psychosis, elderly patients, breast-feeding. Avoid abrupt discontinuation of treatment. Drug interactions: see Appendix 1 (section *4.9*)
Contra-indications: epilepsy, gastric ulceration
Side-effects: nervousness, inability to concentrate, insomnia, dizziness, gastro-intestinal disturbances, skin discoloration, dry mouth, peripheral oedema; rarely leucopenia
Dose: 100 mg daily increased if necessary to 100 mg twice daily (not later than 4 p.m.), usually in conjunction with other treatment

PoM **Symmetrel®** (Geigy)
Capsules, brownish-red, amantadine hydrochloride 100 mg. Price 20 caps = **F**
Syrup (=elixir), amantadine hydrochloride 50 mg/5 ml. Diluent syrup, life of diluted elixir 4 weeks. Price 150 ml = **F**

BROMOCRIPTINE

Indications: parkinsonism (but not drug-induced extrapyramidal symptoms)
Cautions; Side-effects: see section 6.7.1

Dose: first week 1–1.25 mg at night, second week 2–2.5 mg at night, third week 2.5 mg twice daily, then 3 times daily increasing by 2.5 mg every 3–14 days according to response to a usual range of 10–80 mg daily given in 3 divided doses, with food

PoM **Parlodel®** (Sandoz)
Tablets, scored, bromocriptine 1 mg (as mesylate). Price 20 tabs = **E**. Label: 21
Tablets, scored, bromocriptine 2.5 mg (as mesylate). Price 20 tabs = **G**. Label: 21
Capsules, blue/white, bromocriptine 5 mg (as mesylate). Price 20 caps = **I**. Label: 21
Capsules, bromocriptine 10 mg (as mesylate). Price 10 caps = **I**. Label: 21

SELEGILINE

Indications: adjunct in Parkinson's disease treated with levodopa, particularly in patients who have developed 'end-of-dose' akinesia
Cautions: side-effects of levodopa may be increased, concurrent levodopa dosage may need to be reduced by 20–50%
Side-effects: hypotension, nausea and vomiting, confusion, agitation
Dose: initially 5 mg in the morning, increasing to 10 mg if necessary

▼ PoM **Eldepryl®** (Britannia)
Tablets, scored, selegiline hydrochloride 5 mg. Price 20 tabs = **H**

4.9.2 Anticholinergic drugs used in parkinsonism

These drugs exert their antiparkinsonian effect by correcting the relative cholinergic excess which is thought to occur in parkinsonism as a result of dopamine deficiency. They produce at most only a 20% reduction in disability from tremor and rigidity, and do not significantly help bradykinesia. Anticholinergic drugs exert a synergistic effect when used with levodopa and are useful in reducing sialorrhoea.

The anticholinergic drugs also reduce drug-induced symptoms of parkinsonism as for example with antipsychotic drugs (section 4.2.1). There is no justification for giving anticholinergic drugs simultaneously with antipsychotics unless parkinsonian adverse effects occur. Tardive dyskinesia is not improved by the anticholinergic drugs and may be made worse.

No important differences exist between the many synthetic drugs available but certain patients appear to tolerate one preparation better than another. Doses may be taken before food if dry mouth is troublesome, or after food if gastrointestinal symptoms predominate.

The most commonly used drugs are **orphenadrine hydrochloride** (Disipal®) and **benzhexol** (Artane®). Benzhexol may have a mood-elevating effect which is useful in the management of phenothiazine-induced parkinsonism. **Benztropine** (Cogentin®) and **procyclidine** (Kemadrin®) are also used. Benztropine is similar to benzhexol

---

C = 51-100p, **D** = 101-180p, **E** = 181-300p, **F** = 301-450p, **G** = 451-650p, **H** = 651-900p, **I** = 901-1200p, **J** = over 1200p.

but is excreted more slowly; changes in dose therefore need to be carried out very gradually. Procyclidine may be given parenterally and is an effective treatment for drug-induced acute dystonic reactions.

BENZHEXOL HYDROCHLORIDE

Indications: parkinsonism, particularly with apathy and depression; drug-induced extrapyramidal symptoms.

Cautions: urinary retention, glaucoma, cardiovascular disease, hepatic or renal impairment; avoid abrupt discontinuation of treatment. Drug interactions of anticholinergic drugs: see Appendix 1 (sections *1*, 4.9, 5.2)

Contra-indications: tardive dyskinesia

Side-effects: dry mouth, gastro-intestinal disturbances, dizziness, blurred vision; less commonly tachycardia, hypersensitivity, nervousness, and with high doses in susceptible patients, mental confusion, excitement, and psychiatric disturbances which may necessitate discontinuation of treatment

Dose: 1 mg daily, gradually increased; usual maintenance dose 5–15 mg daily in 3–4 divided doses

PoM **Benzhexol Tablets,** benzhexol hydrochloride 2 mg, price 20 tabs = **B**; 5 mg, price 20 tabs = **C**. Counselling advised, before or after food (see notes above)

PoM **Artane®** (Lederle)
Tablets, scored, benzhexol hydrochloride 2 mg. Price 20 tabs = **B**. Counselling advised, before or after food (see notes above)
Tablets, scored, benzhexol hydrochloride 5 mg. Price 20 tabs = **C**. Counselling advised, before or after food (see notes above)
Sustets® (=capsules s/r), turquoise, benzhexol hydrochloride 5 mg. Price 20 caps = **D**. Label: 25, counselling advised, before or after food (see notes above)
Dose: 1–3 capsules daily in divided doses or as a single dose in the morning
Powder (for oral use), benzhexol hydrochloride. Price 25 g = **J**

PoM **Bentex®** (Steinhard)
Tablets, scored, benzhexol hydrochloride 2 mg. Price 20 tabs = **B**. Counselling advised, before or after food (see notes above)
Tablets, scored, benzhexol hydrochloride 5 mg. Price 20 tabs = **C**. Counselling advised, before or after food (see notes above)

PoM **Broflex®** (Bio-Medical)
Syrup (=elixir), pink, benzhexol hydrochloride 5 mg/5 ml. Diluent syrup, life of diluted elixir 14 days. Price 100 ml = **C**. Counselling advised, before or after food (see notes above)

ORPHENADRINE HYDROCHLORIDE

Indications: parkinsonism, particularly with apathy and depression; drug-induced extrapyramidal symptoms

Cautions; Contra-indications; Side-effects: see under Benzhexol Hydrochloride, but more euphoric; may cause insomnia; less effective in controlling tremor

Dose: by mouth, adults and children, daily in divided doses, 150 mg gradually increased; max. 400 mg daily
By intramuscular injection, adults and children, 20–40 mg when necessary

PoM **Biorphen®** (Bio-Medical)
Elixir, sugar-free, orphenadrine hydrochloride 25 mg/5 ml. Price 100 ml = **C**

PoM **Disipal®** (Brocades)
Tablets, yellow, s/c, orphenadrine hydrochloride 50 mg. Price 20 tabs = **B**
Injection, orphenadrine hydrochloride 20 mg/ml. Price 2-ml amp = **B**

BENZTROPINE MESYLATE

Indications: parkinsonism, drug-induced extrapyramidal symptoms

Cautions; Contra-indications; Side-effects: see under Benzhexol Hydrochloride, but causes sedation rather than stimulation; persons affected should not drive or operate machinery; avoid alcohol (CNS depression); avoid in children under 3 years

Dose: by mouth, 0.5–1 mg daily usually at bedtime, gradually increased; max. 6 mg daily; usual maintenance dose 1–4 mg daily in single or divided doses
By intramuscular or intravenous injection, 1–2 mg, repeated if symptoms reappear

PoM **Cogentin®** (MSD)
Tablets, scored, benztropine mesylate 2 mg. Price 20 tabs = **B**. Label: 2
Injection, benztropine mesylate 1 mg/ml. Price 2-ml amp = **C**

METHIXENE HYDROCHLORIDE

Indications: parkinsonism, drug-induced extrapyramidal symptoms, senile tremor, more effective in controlling tremor than rigidity

Cautions; Contra-indications; Side-effects: see under Benzhexol Hydrochloride

Dose: 2.5 mg 3 times daily gradually increased; usual maintenance dose 15–60 mg (elderly patients 15–30 mg) daily in divided doses

PoM **Tremonil®** (Sandoz)
Tablets, scored, methixene hydrochloride 5 mg. Price 20 tabs = **C**. Label: 2

PROCYCLIDINE HYDROCHLORIDE

Indications: parkinsonism, drug-induced extrapyramidal symptoms

Cautions; Contra-indications; Side-effects: see under Benzhexol Hydrochloride; may cause drowsiness

Dose: by mouth, 2.5 mg 3 times daily, gradually increased if necessary; usual max. 30 mg daily
By intramuscular or intravenous injection, 5–10 mg, repeated if necessary after 20 minutes; max. 20 mg daily

PoM **Arpicolin**® (RP Drugs)
Syrup (= elixir), red, procyclidine hydrochloride 2.5 mg/5 ml. Price 100 ml = **C**
Syrup (= elixir), procyclidine hydrochloride 5 mg/5 ml. Price 100 ml = **D**

PoM **Kemadrin**® (Wellcome)
Tablets, scored, procyclidine hydrochloride 5 mg. Price 20 tabs = **C**
Injection, procyclidine hydrochloride 5 mg/ml. Price 2-ml amp = **C**

4.9.3 Drugs used in choreas, tics, and related disorders

Tetrabenazine (Nitoman®) is mainly used to control movement disorders in Huntington's chorea and related disorders. It may act by depleting nerve endings of dopamine. It was formerly used as an antipsychotic drug.

Haloperidol may be useful in improving motor tics, stuttering, hiccup, and symptoms of Gilles de la Tourette syndrome and related choreas. Other antipsychotic drugs such as **chlorpromazine** and **perphenazine** are used to relieve intractable hiccup (section 4.2.1).

Propranolol or another beta-adrenoceptor blocking drug (see section 2.4) may be useful in treating essential tremor or tremors associated with anxiety or thyrotoxicosis. Propranolol is given in a dosage of 40 mg 2 or 3 times daily, increased if necessary; 80 to 160 mg daily is usually required for maintenance.

Primidone (section 4.8.1) in some cases provides relief from benign essential tremor. A small dose such as 125 mg 3 times daily may be effective.

HALOPERIDOL

Indications: motor tics, stuttering, adjunctive treatment in choreas and Gilles de la Tourette syndrome
Cautions; Contra-indications; Side-effects: see section 4.2.1
Dose: by mouth, 0.5–1.5 mg 3 times daily adjusted according to the response; 10 mg daily or more may occasionally be necessary in Gilles de la Tourette syndrome; CHILD, stuttering 50 micrograms/kg daily, Gilles de la Tourette syndrome up to 10 mg daily

Preparations
Section 4.2.1

TETRABENAZINE

Indications: movement disorders due to Huntington's chorea, senile chorea, and related neurological conditions
Cautions: drug interactions: see Appendix 1 (sections 4.2, *4.3, 4.9*)
Side-effects: drowsiness, gastro-intestinal disturbances, rarely depression, extrapyramidal dysfunction
Dose: initially 25 mg 3 times daily, gradually increased (elderly patients 12.5 mg daily, increasing to 3 times daily if necessary); max. 200 mg daily

PoM **Nitoman**® (Roche)
Tablets, pale orange-brown, scored, tetrabenazine 25 mg. Price 20 tabs = **C**. Label: 1

5: Drugs used in the treatment of
INFECTIONS

In this chapter, drug treatment is discussed under the following headings:

5.1 Antibacterial drugs
5.2 Antifungal drugs
5.3 Antiviral drugs
5.4 Antiprotozoal drugs
5.5 Anthelmintics

5.1 Antibacterial drugs

5.1.1   Penicillins
5.1.2   Cephalosporins and cephamycins
5.1.3   Tetracyclines
5.1.4   Aminoglycosides
5.1.5   Macrolides
5.1.6   Clindamycin and lincomycin
5.1.7   Other antibiotics
5.1.8   Sulphonamides and trimethoprim
5.1.9   Antituberculous drugs
5.1.10 Antileprotic drugs
5.1.11 Other antimicrobial drugs

CHOICE OF A SUITABLE DRUG. Before selecting an antibiotic for the treatment of an infection the clinician must first consider two factors—the patient and the known or likely causative organism. Factors related to the patient which must be considered include history of allergy to antibiotics, renal and hepatic function, resistance to infection (i.e. whether a compromised host), ability to tolerate oral drugs, severity of illness, race, age and, if female, whether pregnant or taking an oral contraceptive.

The known or likely organism and its antibiotic sensitivity, considered in association with the above factors, should guide the prescriber towards one or more antibiotics, the final choice depending on the microbiological, pharmacological, and toxicological properties of the various possible drugs for any particular infection.

An example of a rational approach to the selection of an antibiotic is the treatment of a urinary-tract infection in a patient complaining of nausea in early pregnancy. The causative organism is reported as being resistant to ampicillin but sensitive to nitrofurantoin (which can cause nausea), gentamicin (which can only be given by injection and is best avoided in pregnancy), tetracycline and co-trimoxazole (which are both contra-indicated in pregnancy), and cephalexin. The safest antibiotics in pregnancy are the penicillins and cephalosporins and, therefore, cephalexin would be indicated for this patient.

The principles involved in the selection of an antibiotic must allow for a number of variables including changing renal and hepatic function, increasing bacterial resistance, and new information on side-effects of drugs. Duration of therapy, dosage, and route of administration of the drug depend on site and type of infection and its severity.

ANTIBIOTIC POLICIES. Many health authorities now place limits on the antibiotics that may be used in their hospitals, to achieve reasonable economy consistent with adequate cover, and to reduce the development of resistant organisms. An authority may indicate a range of drugs for general use, and permit treatment with other drugs only on the advice of the microbiologist or physician responsible for the control of infectious diseases.

BEFORE STARTING THERAPY. The following precepts should be considered before starting antibiotic therapy:

Viral infections should not be treated with antibiotics.

The 'blind' prescribing of an antibiotic for a patient ill with unexplained pyrexia usually leads to further difficulty in establishing the diagnosis.

An up-to-date knowledge of prevalent organisms and their current sensitivity is of great help in choosing an antibiotic before bacteriological confirmation is available.

The dose of an antibiotic will vary according to a number of factors including age, weight, renal function, and severity of infection. The prescribing of the so-called 'standard' dose in serious infections may result in failure of treatment or even death of the patient. Most antibiotics are rapidly excreted from the body and should be administered every 6 hours for the treatment of serious infections. Less severe infections as seen in general practice usually respond to administration every 8 hours. Agents with prolonged plasma half-lives such as trimethoprim need only be given every 12 hours. The aminoglycoside antibiotics should not be given more frequently than every 8 hours and the interval between doses must be increased in patients with renal failure.

The route of administration of an antibiotic will often depend on the severity of the infection. Life-threatening infections require intravenous therapy.

Duration of therapy depends on the nature of the infection and the response to treatment. Courses should not be unduly prolonged as they are wasteful and may lead to side-effects. However, in certain infections such as endocarditis or tuberculosis it is necessary to continue treatment for relatively long periods. Conversely a single dose of an antibiotic may cure uncomplicated urinary-tract infections.

Suggested initial antibacterial therapy for various infections is shown in Table 1. Sites of infection are arranged in the same order as the chapters of this book. When a pathogenic organism has been isolated treatment may, if indicated, be changed to a more appropriate agent. If no bacterium is cultured a decision whether the antibiotic treatment should be continued or stopped has to be made on clinical grounds. The possible infections for which antibacterial prophylaxis is useful are listed in Table 2.

Table 1. Summary of antibacterial therapy[1]

Infection	Suggested antibacterial	Comment
1: Gastro-intestinal system		
Gastro-enteritis	Antibiotic not usually indicated	Frequently nonbacterial aetiology
Bacillary dysentery	Antibiotic usually not indicated	Co-trimoxazole in severe illness
Campylobacter enteritis	Erythromycin	
Invasive salmonellosis	Co-trimoxazole *or* ampicillin	
Typhoid fever	Chloramphenicol *or* co-trimoxazole *or* amoxycillin	
Biliary-tract infection	Gentamicin *or* a cephalosporin	
Peritonitis	Gentamicin + metronidazole (*or* clindamycin)	
2: Cardiovascular system		
Endocarditis caused by:		
Staph. aureus	Flucloxacillin + fusidic acid (*or* gentamicin)	Treat for at least 4 weeks
Strep. faecalis	Benzylpenicillin (*or* ampicillin) + gentamicin	Treat for at least 4 weeks
Strep. viridans	Benzylpenicillin (+ gentamicin)	Treat for at least 4 weeks; gentamicin may be stopped after 10–14 days
3: Respiratory system		
Exacerbations of chronic bronchitis	Tetracycline *or* ampicillin *or* ampicillin derivative *or* co-trimoxazole (*or* trimethoprim)	Note that 20% of pneumococci and some *H. influenzae* strains are tetracycline-resistant
Pneumonia:		
Previously healthy chest	Penicillin *or* ampicillin *or* ampicillin derivative	Add flucloxacillin if *Staphylococcus* suspected e.g. in influenza or measles; use erythromycin if *Legionella* infection is suspected
Previously unhealthy chest	Flucloxacillin + ampicillin (*or* cotrimoxazole *or* erythromycin)	
4: Central nervous system		
Meningitis caused by:		
Meningococcus	Benzylpenicillin	Intrathecal therapy not necessary
Pneumococcus	Benzylpenicillin	
Haemophilus influenzae	Chloramphenicol	
7: Genital system		
Syphilis	Procaine penicillin (*or* tetracycline *or* erythromycin if penicillin-allergic)	Treat for 10–21 days
Gonorrhoea	Procaine penicillin with probenecid *or* ampicillin with probenecid (*or* co-trimoxazole, spectinomycin, *or* cefuroxime if penicillin-allergic)	Single-dose treatment
Non-gonococcal urethritis	Tetracycline	Treat for 10–21 days
7: Urinary tract		
Acute pyelonephritis or prostatitis	Co-trimoxazole (*or* trimethoprim) *or* gentamicin *or* cephalosporin	Do not give co-trimoxazole (*or* trimethoprim) in pregnancy. Treat prostatitis with co-trimoxazole (*or* trimethoprim) for 4 weeks

C = 51-100p, D = 101-180p, E = 181-300p, F = 301-450p, G = 451-650p, H = 651-900p, I = 901-1200p, J = over 1200p.

Table 1. Summary of antibacterial therapy (*continued*)

Infection	Suggested antibacterial	Comment
'Lower' UTI	1 Sulphonamide *or* 2 Ampicillin *or* 3 Trimethoprim *or* oral cephalosporin	Select in order. A single 3-g dose of amoxycillin may cure uncomplicated infections
9: Blood Septicaemia Initial 'blind' therapy	Aminoglycoside + a penicillin *or* a cephalosporin	Choice of agents depends on local bacterial resistance patterns and clinical presentation
10: Musculoskeletal system Osteomyelitis and septic arthritis	Clindamycin *or* flucloxacillin *or* fusidic acid. If *H. influenzae* give ampicillin *or* co-trimoxazole	Under 5 years of age may be *H. influenzae* Treat acute disease for at least 6 weeks and chronic infection for at least 12 weeks
11: Eye Purulent conjunctivitis	Chloramphenicol *or* gentamicin eye-drops	
12: Ear, nose, and oropharynx Dental infections	Amoxycillin (*or* ampicillin ester)	Metronidazole for anaerobic infections or those not responding to amoxycillin
Sinusitis	Erythromycin *or* co-trimoxazole	
Otitis media	Benzylpenicillin Phenoxymethylpenicillin Amoxycillin (*or* ampicillin ester) if under 5 years (*or* erythromycin if penicillin-allergic)	Initial i/m therapy (if possible) with benzylpenicillin, then oral therapy with phenoxymethylpenicillin Under 5 years of age may be *H. influenzae*
Tonsillitis	Benzylpenicillin Phenoxymethylpenicillin	Initial i/m therapy (in severe infection) with benzylpenicillin, then oral therapy with phenoxymethylpenicillin. Most infections are caused by viruses
13: Skin Impetigo	Topical chlortetracycline *or* oral flucloxacillin if systemic toxicity	
Erysipelas	Benzylpenicillin Phenoxymethylpenicillin	Initial i/m therapy (if possible) with benzylpenicillin, then oral therapy with phenoxymethylpenicillin
Cellulitis	Flucloxacillin (*or* erythromycin if penicillin-allergic)	
Acne	Tetracycline	Treat for at least 3–4 months

[1]Where ampicillin is suggested in the table amoxycillin or an ester of ampicillin may be used, and where flucloxacillin is suggested cloxacillin may be used.

Table 2. Summary of antibacterial prophylaxis[1]

Infection	Antibacterial and adult dose
Prevention of recurrence of rheumatic fever	Phenoxymethylpenicillin 500 mg daily *or* sulphadimidine (avail. hosp. only) 500 mg daily (250 mg for children)

Table 2. Summary of antibacterial prophylaxis (*continued*)

Infection	Antibacterial and adult dose
Prevention of secondary case of meningococcal meningitis	Rifampicin 600 mg every 12 hours for 2 days; *or* minocycline 100 mg every 12 hours for 5 days; *or* sulphadimidine (avail. hosp. only) 2 g/day for 5 days (if strain known to be sensitive). Reduce dose for children
Prevention of secondary case of diphtheria in non-immune patient	Erythromycin 500 mg every 6 hours for 5 days
Prevention of endocarditis in patients with heart-valve lesion, septal defect, patent ductus, or prosthetic valve	*Dental procedures*—under local anaesthesia, oral amoxycillin 3 g 1 hour before procedure *or*, if already taking a penicillin *or* if penicillin-allergic, oral erythromycin 1.5 g (as stearate) 1 hour before procedure, then 500 mg 6 hours later; general anaesthesia (no special risk), i/m amoxycillin 1 g before induction, then oral amoxycillin 500 mg 6 hours later; special risk (patients with a prosthetic heart valve or who have had endocarditis), i/m amoxycillin 1 g + i/m gentamicin 120 mg before induction, then oral amoxycillin 500 mg 6 hours later; special risk patients who are penicillin-allergic *or* already taking a penicillin, i/v vancomycin 1 g over 20–30 minutes then i/v gentamicin 1.5 mg/kg before induction *Genito-urinary and colonic procedures*-i/v gentamicin 1.5 mg/kg (reduce dose in renal impairment) + i/v ampicillin 1 g 30 minutes before procedure and repeated twice at 8-hourly intervals, *or* if penicillin-allergic replace ampicillin with i/v erythromycin 500 mg (as lactobionate); metronidazole may also be added
Prevention of gas-gangrene in high lower-limb amputations or following major trauma	Benzylpenicillin 300–600 mg every 6 hours for 5 days; *or* procaine penicillin 2.4 g every 12 hours for 5 days; *or* if penicillin-allergic give metronidazole 500 mg every 6 hours
Prevention of tuberculosis in susceptible close contacts	Isoniazid alone for 12 months *or* isoniazid + ethambutol for 6–9 months
Prevention of infection in abdominal surgery Operations on stomach or oesophagus for carcinoma, or cholecystectomy in patients with possibly infected bile	Single immediate pre-operative dose of gentamicin *or* a cephalosporin
Resections of colon and rectum for carcinoma, and resections in inflammatory bowel disease	Single immediate pre-operative dose of gentamicin + metronidazole
Hysterectomy	Metronidazole as suppository *or* single i/v dose

[1]Where ampicillin is suggested in the table amoxycillin or an ester of ampicillin may be used, and where flucloxacillin is suggested cloxacillin may be used.

5.1.1 Penicillins

5.1.1.1 Penicillinase-sensitive penicillins
5.1.1.2 Penicillinase-resistant penicillins
5.1.1.3 Broad-spectrum penicillins
5.1.1.4 Antipseudomonal penicillins
5.1.1.5 Other penicillins

The penicillins are bactericidal and act by interfering with bacterial cell wall synthesis. They dif-

fuse well into body tissues and fluids, but penetration into the cerebrospinal fluid is poor except when the meninges are inflamed. They are excreted in the urine in therapeutic concentrations. Probenecid blocks the renal tubular excretion of the penicillins, producing higher and more prolonged plasma concentrations. (For suggested doses see section 10.1.4)

The most important side-effect of the penicillins

C = 51-100p, D = 101-180p, E = 181-300p, F = 301-450p, G = 451-650p, H = 651-900p, I = 901-1200p, J = over 1200p.

is hypersensitivity, which causes rashes and, occasionally, anaphylaxis, which can be fatal. Patients who are allergic to one penicillin will be allergic to all as the hypersensitivity is related to the basic penicillin structure. A rare but serious toxic effect of the penicillins is encephalopathy due to cerebral irritation. This may result from excessively high doses but can also develop with normal doses given to patients with renal failure. Encephalopathy may follow intrathecal injection of the penicillins and this route of administration is best **avoided**, unless absolutely necessary, as chemical irritation of the brain can produce convulsions and sometimes death.

A second problem relating to high doses of penicillin, or normal doses given to patients with renal failure, is the accumulation of electrolyte since most injectable penicillins contain either sodium or potassium.

Diarrhoea frequently occurs during oral penicillin therapy. It is commonest with ampicillin and its derivatives, which can also cause pseudomembranous colitis.

UNITS. International units are no longer used for penicillins and all doses are stated in milligrams.

5.1.1.1 PENICILLINASE-SENSITIVE PENICILLINS

Benzylpenicillin (Penicillin G, Crystapen®), the first of the penicillins, remains an important and useful antibiotic; it is inactivated by bacterial penicillinases (beta-lactamases). It is the drug of choice for streptococcal, pneumococcal, gonococcal, and meningococcal infections and also for actinomycosis, anthrax, diphtheria, gas-gangrene, syphilis, tetanus, and yaws. Pneumococci and gonococci have recently been isolated which have decreased sensitivity to penicillin. Benzylpenicillin is inactivated by gastric acid and absorption from the gut is low; therefore it is best given by injection. Benzylpenicillin may cause convulsions after high doses by intravenous or intrathecal injection or in renal failure.

Procaine penicillin (Depocillin®) is a sparingly soluble salt of benzylpenicillin. It is used in intramuscular depot preparations which provide therapeutic tissue concentrations for up to 24 hours. It is commonly used for the treatment of syphilis and gonorrhoea.

Benethamine penicillin and **benzathine penicillin** are benzylpenicillin salts with a very low solubility which gives a prolonged action after intramuscular injection, though producing low plasma concentrations, and so can be used for prophylaxis, combined with soluble and procaine penicillin.

Phenoxymethylpenicillin (Penicillin V) has a similar antibacterial spectrum to benzylpenicillin, but is less active. It is gastric acid-stable, so is suitable for oral administration. It should not be used for serious infections because absorption can be unpredictable and plasma concentrations variable. It is indicated principally for respiratory-tract infections in children, for streptococcal tonsillitis, and for continuing treatment after one or more injections of benzylpenicillin when clinical response has begun. It should not be used for meningococcal or gonococcal infections. Phenoxymethylpenicillin is used for prophylaxis against streptococcal infections following rheumatic fever.

Penamecillin and **phenethicillin** have similar antibacterial activity, but they are no more effective than phenoxymethylpenicillin.

BENZYLPENICILLIN
(Penicillin G)

Indications: tonsillitis, otitis media, erysipelas, streptococcal endocarditis, meningococcal and pneumococcal meningitis, prophylaxis in limb amputation

Cautions: history of allergy; renal impairment

Contra-indications: penicillin hypersensitivity

Side-effects: sensitivity reactions including urticaria, fever, joint pains; angioedema; anaphylactic shock in hypersensitive patients; diarrhoea after administration by mouth

Dose: by intramuscular injection, 300–600 mg 2–4 times daily; CHILD up to 12 years, 10–20 mg/kg daily; NEONATE, 30 mg/kg daily

By intravenous infusion, up to 24 g daily

By intrathecal injection, 6–12 mg daily
Prophylaxis in dental procedures and limb amputation, section 5.1, Table 2

PoM **Crystapen**® (Glaxo)
Injection, powder for reconstitution, benzylpenicillin sodium (unbuffered). Price 300- and 600-mg vial (both) = **A**
Injection, powder for reconstitution, benzylpenicillin sodium (buffered). Price 3-g vial = **B**; 6-g vial = **C**
Intrathecal injection, powder for reconstitution, benzylpenicillin sodium (unbuffered). Price 12-mg amp = **D**
PoM **Crystapen G**® (Glaxo)
Tablets, yellow, f/c, benzylpenicillin potassium 250 mg. Price 20 tabs = **B**. Label: 9, 23
Syrup (= elixir), yellow, benzylpenicillin potassium 125 mg/5 ml when reconstituted with water for preparations. Diluent syrup, life of diluted elixir 7 days. Price 100 ml = **C**. Label: 9, 23
Syrup (= elixir), yellow, benzylpenicillin potassium 250 mg/5 ml when reconstituted with water for preparations. Diluent as above. Price 100 ml = **C**. Label: 9, 23

BENETHAMINE PENICILLIN

Indications: penicillin-sensitive   infections; prophylaxis

Cautions; Contra-indications; Side-effects: see under Benzylpenicillin

PoM **Triplopen**® (Glaxo)
Injection, powder for reconstitution, benethamine penicillin 475 mg, procaine penicillin

Relative prices: **A** = up to 20p, **B** = 21-50p,

250 mg, benzylpenicillin sodium 300 mg. Price per vial = **B**
Dose: by deep intramuscular injection, 1 vial every 2–3 days

BENZATHINE PENICILLIN

Indications: penicillin-sensitive infections
Cautions; Contra-indications; Side-effects: see under Benzylpenicillin
Dose: by mouth, 458 mg every 6–8 hours
By intramuscular injection, treatment of infections, 229–916 mg every 5–7 days; rheumatic fever prophylaxis 916 mg every 3 weeks

PoM **Penidural®** (Wyeth)
Suspension (= mixture), pink, benzathine penicillin 229 mg/5 ml. Diluent syrup, life of diluted mixture 14 days. Price 100 ml = **D**. Label: 9
Paediatric drops, pink, benzathine penicillin 115 mg/ml. Price 10 ml = **D**. Label: 9, counselling advised, use of pipette
PoM **Penidural-LA®** (Wyeth)
Injection, benzathine penicillin 229 mg/ml. Price 10-ml vial = **E**

PENAMECILLIN

Indications: penicillin-sensitive infections
Cautions; Contra-indications; Side-effects: see under Benzylpenicillin
Dose: 350 mg every 8 hours

PoM **Havapen®** (Wyeth)
Tablets, penamecillin 350 mg. Price 20 tabs = **D**. Label: 9, 23

PHENETHICILLIN

Indications: penicillin-sensitive infections
Cautions; Contra-indications; Side-effects: see under Benzylpenicillin
Dose: 250 mg every 6 hours, at least 30 minutes before food; CHILD, under 2 years ¼ adult dose, 2–10 years ½ adult dose

PoM **Broxil®** (Beecham)
Capsules, black/ivory, phenethicillin 250 mg (as potassium salt). Price 20 caps = **E**. Label: 9, 23
Tablets, yellow, scored, phenethicillin 250 mg (as potassium salt). Price 20 tabs = **E**. Label: 9, 23
Syrup (= elixir), phenethicillin 125 mg (as potassium salt)/5 ml when reconstituted with water for preparations. Diluent syrup, life of diluted elixir 7 days. Price 100 ml = **D**. Label: 9, 23

PHENOXYMETHYLPENICILLIN
(Penicillin V)

Indications: tonsillitis, otitis media, erysipelas, rheumatic fever prophylaxis, endocarditis prophylaxis
Cautions; Contra-indications; Side-effects: see under Benzylpenicillin. Drug interactions: see Appendix 1 (section 5.1)
Dose: 250–500 mg every 6 hours, at least 30 min-

utes before food; CHILD, every 6 hours, up to 1 year 62.5 mg, 1–5 years 125 mg, 6–12 years 250 mg

PoM **Phenoxymethylpenicillin Potassium Capsules**, phenoxymethylpenicillin 250 mg (as potassium salt). Price 20 caps = **B**. Label: 9, 23
PoM **Phenoxymethylpenicillin Potassium Tablets**, phenoxymethylpenicillin 125 mg (as potassium salt), price 20 tabs = **A**; 250 and 300 mg, price 20 tabs (both) = **B**. Label: 9, 23
PoM **Phenoxymethylpenicillin Elixir**, phenoxymethylpenicillin 62.5 mg (as potassium salt)/5 ml when reconstituted with water for preparations. Diluent syrup, life of diluted elixir 7 days. Price 100 ml = **B**. Label: 9, 23
Phenoxymethylpenicillin 125 mg (as potassium salt)/5 ml when reconstituted with water for preparations. Diluent as above. Price 100 ml = **C**. Label: 9, 23
Phenoxymethylpenicillin 125 mg (as potassium salt)/single-dose sachet (granules). Price 12 sachets = **C**. Label: 9, 13, 23
Phenoxymethylpenicillin 250 mg (as potassium salt)/5 ml when reconstituted with water for preparations. Diluent as above. Price 100 ml = **C**. Label: 9, 23
PoM **Phenoxymethylpenicillin Mixture**, phenoxymethylpenicillin 125 mg (as calcium or potassium salt)/5 ml. Diluent fractionated coconut oil, life of diluted mixture 14 days. Price 100 ml = **C**. Label: 9, 23
PoM **Apsin VK®** (APS)
Tablets, f/c, scored, phenoxymethylpenicillin 250 mg (as potassium salt). Price 20 tabs = **B**. Label: 9, 23
Syrup (= elixir), orange, phenoxymethylpenicillin 125 mg (as potassium salt)/5 ml when reconstituted with water for preparations. Diluent syrup, life of diluted elixir 7 days. Price 100 ml = **B**. Label: 9, 23
Syrup (= elixir), orange, phenoxymethylpenicillin 250 mg (as potassium salt)/5 ml when reconstituted with water for preparations. Diluent as above. Price 100 ml = **C**. Label: 9, 23
PoM **Crystapen V®** (Glaxo)
Tablets, orange, f/c, phenoxymethylpenicillin 250 mg (as potassium salt). Price 20 tabs = **B**. Label: 9, 23
Syrup (= elixir), red, phenoxymethylpenicillin 125 mg (as potassium salt)/5 ml when reconstituted with water for preparations. Diluent syrup, life of diluted elixir 7 days. Price 100 ml = **C**. Label: 9, 23
Syrup (= elixir), red, phenoxymethylpenicillin 250 mg (as potassium salt)/5 ml when reconstituted with water for preparations. Diluent as above. Price 100 ml = **C**. Label: 9, 23
PoM **Distaquaine V-K®** (Dista)
Tablets, scored, phenoxymethylpenicillin 125 mg (as potassium salt). Price 20 tabs = **B**. Label: 9, 23
Tablets, scored, phenoxymethylpenicillin 250 mg (as potassium salt). Price 20 tabs = **B**. Label: 9, 23

C = 51-100p, **D** = 101-180p, **E** = 181-300p, **F** = 301-450p, **G** = 451-650p, **H** = 651-900p, **I** = 901-1200p, **J** = over 1200p.

Elixir, orange, phenoxymethylpenicillin 62.5 mg (as potassium salt)/5 ml when reconstituted with water for preparations. Diluent syrup, life of diluted elixir 7 days. Price 100 ml = **B**. Label: 9, 23

Syrup (= elixir), orange, phenoxymethylpenicillin 125 mg (as potassium salt)/5 ml when reconstituted with water for preparations. Diluent as above. Price 100 ml = **C**. Label: 9, 23

Syrup (= elixir), orange, phenoxymethylpenicillin 250 mg (as potassium salt)/5 ml when reconstituted with water for preparations. Diluent as above. Price 100 ml = **D**. Label: 9, 23

PoM **Econocil VK**® (DDSA)
Capsules, pink, phenoxymethylpenicillin 250 mg (as potassium salt). Price 20 caps = **B**. Label: 9, 23
Tablets, phenoxymethylpenicillin 125 mg (as potassium salt). Price 20 tabs = **A**. Label: 9, 23
Tablets, phenoxymethylpenicillin 250 mg (as potassium salt). Price 20 tabs = **B**. Label: 9, 23

PoM **Stabillin V-K**® (Boots)
Tablets, phenoxymethylpenicillin 250 mg (as potassium salt). Price 20 tabs = **B**. Label: 9, 23
Elixir, phenoxymethylpenicillin 62.5 mg (as potassium salt)/5 ml when reconstituted with water for preparations. Diluent syrup, life of diluted elixir 7 days. Price 100 ml = **B**. Label: 9, 23
Elixir, phenoxymethylpenicillin 125 mg (as potassium salt)/5 ml when reconstituted with water for preparations. Diluent as above. Price 100 ml = **B**. Label: 9, 23
Elixir, phenoxymethylpenicillin 250 mg (as potassium salt)/5 ml when reconstituted with water for preparations. Diluent as above. Price 100 ml = **C**. Label: 9, 23

PoM **V-Cil-K**® (Lilly)
Capsules, pink, phenoxymethylpenicillin 250 mg (as potassium salt). Price 20 caps = **B**. Label: 9, 23
Tablets, phenoxymethylpenicillin 125 mg (as potassium salt). Price 20 tabs = **A**. Label: 9, 23
Tablets, phenoxymethylpenicillin 250 mg (as potassium salt). Price 20 tabs = **B**. Label: 9, 23
Pedipacs®, granules, phenoxymethylpenicillin 125 mg (as potassium salt)/single-dose sachet. Price 12 sachets = **C**. Label: 9, 13, 23
Paediatric syrup (= elixir), phenoxymethylpenicillin 62.5 mg (as potassium salt)/5 ml when reconstituted with water for preparations. Diluent syrup, life of diluted elixir 7 days. Price 100 ml = **B**. Label: 9, 23
Paediatric syrup (= elixir), phenoxymethylpenicillin 125 mg (as potassium salt)/5 ml when reconstituted with water for preparations. Diluent as above. Price 100 ml = **C**. Label: 9, 23
Syrup (= elixir), phenoxymethylpenicillin 250 mg (as potassium salt)/5 ml when reconstituted with water for preparations. Diluent as above. Price 100 ml = **C**. Label: 9, 23

PROCAINE PENICILLIN

Indications: prevention of endocarditis during dental procedures, gas-gangrene following amputation; syphilis, gonorrhoea
Cautions; Contra-indications; Side-effects: see under Benzylpenicillin; **not** for intravenous administration
Dose: by intramuscular injection, 300 mg 1–2 times daily
Gonorrhoea, men, 2.4 g; women, 4.8 g as a single dose
Syphilis, 1.2 g daily for at least 10 days
See also section 5.1, Table 1

PoM **Bicillin**® (Brocades)
Injection, powder for reconstitution, procaine penicillin 3 g, benzylpenicillin sodium 600 mg. Price per vial = **B**
Dose: when reconstituted with 7.5 ml water for injections, 1 ml 1–2 times daily
PoM **Depocillin**® (Brocades)
Injection, powder for reconstitution, procaine penicillin. Price 3-g vial = **B**

5.1.1.2   PENICILLINASE-RESISTANT PENICILLINS

Most staphylococci are now resistant to benzylpenicillin because they produce penicillinases. **Cloxacillin** (Orbenin®) and **flucloxacillin** (Floxapen®), however, are not inactivated by these enzymes and are thus effective in infections caused by penicillin-resistant *Staphylococci*, which is the sole indication for their use. They are acid-stable and can, therefore, be given by mouth as well as by injection.

Flucloxacillin is better absorbed from the gut than cloxacillin and is, therefore, to be preferred for oral therapy.

Methicillin (Celbenin®) is also effective against penicillin-resistant *Staph. aureus*, but can only be given by injection because it is not acid-stable and is now seldom used.

Staph. aureus strains resistant to methicillin and cloxacillin have emerged in some hospitals; some of these organisms are only sensitive to vancomycin (section 5.1.7).

CLOXACILLIN

Indications: infections due to penicillinase-producing staphylococci
Cautions; Contra-indications; Side-effects: see under Benzylpenicillin (section 5.1.1.1)
Dose: by mouth, 500 mg every 6 hours, at least 30 minutes before food
By intramuscular injection, 250 mg every 4–6 hours
By intravenous injection or infusion, 500 mg every 4–6 hours
Doses may be doubled in severe infections
CHILD, any route, under 2 years ¼ adult dose; 2–10 years ½ adult dose

PoM **Orbenin**® (Beecham)
Capsules, orange/black, cloxacillin 250 mg (as

sodium salt). Price 20 caps = **F**. Label: 9, 23

Capsules, orange/black, cloxacillin 500 mg (as sodium salt). Price 20 caps = **H**. Label: 9, 23

Syrup (= elixir), cloxacillin 125 mg (as sodium salt)/5 ml when reconstituted with water for preparations. Diluent syrup, life of diluted elixir 7 days. Price 100 ml = **F**. Label: 9, 23

Injection, powder for reconstitution, cloxacillin (as sodium salt). Price 250-mg vial = **C**; 500-mg vial = **E**; 1-g vial = **F**

FLUCLOXACILLIN

Indications: infections due to penicillinase-producing staphylococci

Cautions; Contra-indications; Side-effects: see under Benzylpenicillin (section 5.1.1.1)

Dose: by mouth, 250 mg every 6 hours, at least 30 minutes before food

By intramuscular injection, 250 mg every 6 hours

By slow intravenous injection or infusion, 0.25–1 g every 6 hours

Doses may be doubled in severe infections

CHILD, any route, under 2 years ¼ adult dose; 2–10 years ½ adult dose

PoM **Flucloxacillin Capsules,** flucloxacillin 250 mg (as sodium salt), price 20 caps = **F**; 500 mg, price 20 caps = **H**. Label: 9, 23

PoM **Floxapen®** (Beecham)

Capsules, black/caramel, flucloxacillin 250 mg (as sodium salt). Price 20 caps = **F**. Label: 9, 23

Capsules, black/caramel, flucloxacillin 500 mg (as sodium salt). Price 20 caps = **H**. Label: 9, 23

Syrup (= mixture), flucloxacillin 125 mg (as magnesium salt)/5 ml when reconstituted with water for preparations. Diluent syrup, life of diluted mixture 14 days. Price 100 ml = **F**. Label: 9, 23

Syrup forte (= mixture), flucloxacillin 250 mg (as magnesium salt)/5 ml when reconstituted with water for preparations. Diluent as above. Price 100 ml = **H**. Label: 9, 23

Injection, powder for reconstitution, flucloxacillin (as sodium salt). Price 250-mg vial = **C**; 500-mg vial = **E**; 1-g vial = **F**

PoM **Ladropen®** (Berk)

Capsules, brown/orange, flucloxacillin 250 mg (as sodium salt). Price 20 caps = **F**. Label: 9, 23

Capsules, brown/orange, flucloxacillin 500 mg (as sodium salt). Price 20 caps = **H**. Label: 9, 23

PoM **Stafoxil®** (Brocades)

Capsules, cream/brown, flucloxacillin 250 mg (as sodium salt). Price 28 caps = **G**. Label: 9, 23

Capsules, cream/brown, flucloxacillin 500 mg (as sodium salt). Price 28 caps = **I**. Label: 9, 23

METHICILLIN SODIUM

Indications: infections due to penicillinase-producing staphylococci

Cautions; Contra-indications; Side-effects: see under Benzylpenicillin (section 5.1.1.1)

Dose: by intramuscular injection or slow intravenous injection or infusion, 1 g every 4–6 hours

PoM **Celbenin®** (Beecham)

Injection, powder for reconstitution, methicillin sodium. Price 1-g vial = **E**

5.1.1.3 BROAD-SPECTRUM PENICILLINS

Ampicillin (Penbritin®) is active against certain Gram-positive and Gram-negative organisms but is inactivated by penicillinases including those produced by *Staph. aureus* and by common Gram-negative bacilli such as *Escherichia coli*. Almost all staphylococci, one-third of *E. coli* strains and up to one-tenth of *Haemophilus influenzae* strains are now resistant. Ampicillin should therefore not be used for the 'blind' treatment of infections, especially in hospital patients.

It can be given by mouth before food, and by injection, and is well excreted in the bile and urine. It is principally indicated for the treatment of exacerbations of chronic bronchitis and middle ear infections, both of which are usually due to *Streptococcus pneumoniae* and *H. influenzae*, and for urinary-tract infections.

Less than half the dose of ampicillin is absorbed after oral administration, and absorption is further decreased by the presence of food in the gut. Higher plasma concentrations are obtained with the ampicillin esters **bacampicillin** (Ambaxin®), **pivampicillin** (Pondocillin®), and **talampicillin** (Talpen®); their absorption is little affected by the presence of food, and the incidence of diarrhoea is less than with ampicillin. These antibiotics should be given every 8 hours for moderate or severe infections, especially outside the renal tract.

Maculopapular rashes commonly occur with the ampicillins but are not usually related to true penicillin allergy. They are almost invariable in patients with glandular fever or chronic lymphatic leukaemia who are given these antibiotics.

Amoxycillin (Amoxil®) is a derivative of ampicillin which differs by only one hydroxyl group and has a similar antibacterial spectrum. It is, however, better absorbed when given by mouth, producing higher plasma and tissue concentrations; unlike ampicillin, absorption is not affected by the presence of food in the stomach.

Augmentin® consists of amoxycillin with the beta-lactamase inhibitor **clavulanic acid**, which itself has no significant antibacterial activity but which, by inactivating penicillinases, makes the product active against penicillinase-producing bacteria that are resistant to amoxycillin. These include most *Staph. aureus*, one-third of *E. coli* strains, and up to 10% of *H. influenzae* strains, as well as many *Bacteroides* and *Klebsiella* spp.

Ciclacillin (Calthor®) is another derivative of ampicillin. It is less active than ampicillin but, like amoxycillin, is better absorbed from the gastro-intestinal tract.

Mezlocillin (Baypen®) is a derivative of ampicillin which is active against certain ampicillin-

---

C = 51-100p, D = 101-180p, E = 181-300p, F = 301-450p, G = 451-650p, H = 651-900p, I = 901-1200p, J = over 1200p.

resistant bacteria. However, like ampicillin, it is inactivated by beta-lactamases.

Piperacillin (Pipril®) is a related antibiotic which is more active than mezlocillin against *Pseudomonas aeruginosa*.

AMOXYCILLIN

Indications: see under Ampicillin; also typhoid fever and dental prophylaxis

Cautions; Contra-indications; Side-effects: see under Benzylpenicillin (section 5.1.1.1); also erythematous rashes in glandular fever and chronic lymphatic leukaemia; reduce dose in renal impairment

Dose: by mouth, 250 mg every 8 hours, doubled in severe infections; CHILD up to 10 years, 125 mg every 8 hours

Dental prophylaxis, section 5.1, Table 2

By intramuscular injection, 500 mg every 8 hours; CHILD, 50–100 mg/kg daily in divided doses

By intravenous injection or infusion (in severe infections), 1 g every 6 hours; CHILD, 50–100 mg/kg daily in divided doses

PoM **Amoxil**® (Bencard)

Capsules, maroon/gold, amoxycillin 250 mg (as trihydrate). Price 20 caps = **F**. Label: 9

Capsules, maroon/gold, amoxycillin 500 mg (as trihydrate). Price 20 caps = **H**. Label: 9

Dispersible tablets, amoxycillin 500 mg (as trihydrate). Price 20 tabs = **H**. Label: 9, 13

Syrup (= mixture), amoxycillin 125 mg (as trihydrate)/5 ml when reconstituted with water for preparations. Diluent syrup, life of diluted mixture 14 days. Price 100 ml = **E**. Label: 9

Syrup forte (= strong mixture), amoxycillin 250 mg (as trihydrate)/5 ml when reconstituted with water for preparations. Diluent as above. Price 100 ml = **F**. Label: 9

Paediatric suspension, amoxycillin 125 mg (as trihydrate)/1.25 ml when reconstituted with water for preparations. Price 20 ml = **F**. Label: 9, counselling advised, use of pipette

Sachets, powder, amoxycillin (as trihydrate). Price per 3-g sachet = **E**. Label: 9, 13

Dose: urinary-tract infections, 3 g in water, repeated after 12 hours; gonorrhoea, single 3-g dose in water

Injection, powder for reconstitution, amoxycillin (as sodium salt). Price 250-mg vial = **B**; 500-mg vial = **C**; 1-g vial = **D**

▼ PoM **Augmentin**® (Beecham)

Tablets, f/c, amoxycillin 250 mg (as trihydrate), clavulanic acid 125 mg (as potassium salt). Price 20 tabs = **G**. Label: 9

Dose: 1 tablet every 8 hours, increased to 2 tablets in severe infections

Dispersible tablets, amoxycillin 250 mg (as trihydrate), clavulanic acid 125 mg (as potassium salt). Price 20 tabs = **H**. Label: 9, 13

Dose: see under tablets above

Junior suspension (= mixture), amoxycillin 125 mg (as trihydrate), clavulanic acid 62 mg (as potassium salt)/5 ml (sugar-free) when reconstituted with water for preparations. Price 100 ml = **F**. Label: 9

Dose: CHILD 6–12 years, 5 ml every 8 hours, increased to 10 ml in severe infections

Paediatric suspension (= mixture), amoxycillin 125 mg (as trihydrate), clavulanic acid 31 mg (as potassium salt)/5 ml (sugar-free) when reconstituted with water for preparations. Diluent not more than an equal volume of water for preparations, life of diluted mixture 7 days. Price 100 ml = **E**. Label: 9

Dose: CHILD 3–8 months, 1.25 ml every 8 hours; 9 months–2 years, 2.5 ml every 8 hours; 3–6 years, 5 ml every 8 hours, increased to 10 ml in severe infections

AMPICILLIN

Indications: urinary-tract infections, otitis media, chronic bronchitis, invasive salmonellosis, gonorrhoea

Cautions; Contra-indications; Side-effects: see under Benzylpenicillin (section 5.1.1.1); also erythematous rashes in glandular fever and chronic lymphatic leukaemia; reduce dose in renal impairment. Drug interactions: see Appendix 1 (section 7)

Dose: by mouth, 0.25–1 g every 6 hours, at least 30 minutes before food

Gonorrhoea, 2 g as a single dose with probenecid 1 g; repeated for women

Urinary-tract infections, 500 mg every 8 hours

By intramuscular injection or intravenous injection or infusion, 500 mg every 4–6 hours; higher doses in meningitis

CHILD, any route, ½ adult dose

PoM **Ampicillin Capsules,** ampicillin 250 mg, price 20 caps = **C**; 500 mg, price 20 caps = **D**. Label: 9, 23

PoM **Ampicillin Mixture,** ampicillin 125 mg/5 ml when reconstituted with water for preparations. Diluent syrup, life of diluted mixture 7 days, price 100 ml = **C**; 250 mg/5 ml, price 100 ml= **D**. Label: 9, 23

PoM **Amfipen**® (Brocades)

Capsules, red/grey, ampicillin 250 mg. Price 20 caps = **C**. Label: 9, 23

Capsules, red/grey, ampicillin 500 mg. Price 20 caps = **D**. Label: 9, 23

Syrup (= mixture), pink, ampicillin 125 mg/5 ml when reconstituted with water for preparations. Diluent syrup, life of diluted mixture 7 days. Price 100 ml = **C**. Label: 9, 23

Syrup forte (= strong mixture), pink, ampicillin 250 mg/5 ml when reconstituted with water for preparations. Diluent as above. Price 100 ml = **D**. Label: 9, 23

Injection, powder for reconstitution, ampicillin (as sodium salt). Price 250-mg vial = **B**; 500-mg vial = **C**

PoM **Britcin**® (DDSA)

Capsules, red/grey, ampicillin 250 mg (as trihydrate). Price 20 caps = **C**. Label: 9, 23

Capsules, red/grey, ampicillin 500 mg (as trihydrate). Price 20 caps = **D**. Label: 9, 23

PoM **Penbritin**® (Beecham)

Capsules, black/red, ampicillin 250 mg (as trihydrate). Price 20 caps = **D**. Label: 9, 23

Capsules, black/red, ampicillin 500 mg (as trihydrate). Price 20 caps = **F**. Label: 9, 23
Paediatric tablets, scored, ampicillin 125 mg (as trihydrate). Price 20 tabs = **C**. Label: 9, 23
Syrup (= mixture), ampicillin 125 mg (as trihydrate)/5 ml when reconstituted with water for preparations. Diluent syrup, life of diluted mixture 7 days. Price 100 ml = **D**. Label: 9, 23
Syrup forte (= strong mixture), ampicillin 250 mg (as trihydrate)/5 ml when reconstituted with water for preparations. Diluent as above. Price 100 ml = **E**. Label: 9, 23
Paediatric suspension, pink, ampicillin 125 mg (as trihydrate)/1.25 ml. Price 25 ml = **E**. Label: 9, 23, counselling advised, use of pipette
Injection, powder for reconstitution, ampicillin (as sodium salt). Price 250-mg vial = **B**; 500-mg vial = **C**

PoM Vidopen® (Berk)
Capsules, pink/red, ampicillin 250 mg (as trihydrate). Price 20 caps = **C**. Label: 9, 23
Capsules, pink/red, ampicillin 500 mg (as trihydrate). Price 20 caps = **D**. Label: 9, 23
Syrup (= mixture), pink, ampicillin 125 mg (as trihydrate)/5 ml when reconstituted with water for preparations. Diluent syrup, life of diluted mixture 7 days. Price 100 ml = **C**. Label: 9, 23
Syrup forte (= strong mixture), pink, ampicillin 250 mg (as trihydrate)/5 ml when reconstituted with water for preparations. Diluent as above. Price 100 ml = **C**. Label: 9, 23

Preparations containing ampicillin and a penicillinase-resistant penicillin
PoM Ampiclox® (Beecham)
Injection, ampicillin 250 mg (as sodium salt), cloxacillin 250 mg (as sodium salt). Price per vial = **D**
Dose: by intramuscular injection or intravenous injection or infusion, 1–2 vials every 4–6 hours; CHILD up to 2 years ¼ adult dose, 2–10 years ½ adult dose
PoM Ampiclox Neonatal® (Beecham)
Suspension, ampicillin 60 mg (as trihydrate), cloxacillin 30 mg (as sodium salt)/0.6 ml when reconstituted with water for preparations. Price 10 ml = **E**. Label: 9, counselling advised, use of pipette
Dose: 0.6 ml every 4 hours.
Injection, powder for reconstitution, ampicillin 50 mg (as sodium salt), cloxacillin 25 mg (as sodium salt). Price per vial = **B**
Dose: by intramuscular injection or intravenous injection or infusion, 1 vial every 8 hours
PoM Magnapen® (Beecham)
Capsules, black/turquoise, ampicillin 250 mg (as trihydrate), flucloxacillin 250 mg (as sodium salt). Price 20 caps = **F**. Label: 9, 23
Dose: 1 capsule every 6 hours
Syrup (= mixture), ampicillin 125 mg (as trihydrate), flucloxacillin 125 mg (as sodium salt)/5 ml when reconstituted with water for preparations. Diluent syrup, life of diluted mixture 7 days. Price 100 ml = **F**. Label: 9, 23
Dose: 10 ml every 6 hours; CHILD up to 2 years ¼ adult dose, 2–10 years ½ adult dose

Injection 500 mg, powder for reconstitution, ampicillin 250 mg (as sodium salt), flucloxacillin 250 mg (as sodium salt). Price per vial = **D**
Dose: by intramuscular injection or intravenous injection or infusion, 1 vial every 6 hours; CHILD up to 2 years ¼ adult dose, 2–10 years ½ adult dose; doses may be doubled in severe infections
Injection 1 g, powder for reconstitution, ampicillin 500 mg (as sodium salt), flucloxacillin 500 mg (as sodium salt). Price per vial = **E**

BACAMPICILLIN HYDROCHLORIDE
Indications: see under Ampicillin
Cautions; Contra-indications; Side-effects: see under Benzylpenicillin (section 5.1.1.1); also erythematous rashes in glandular fever and chronic lymphatic leukaemia; avoid in severe liver disease and renal impairment
Dose: 400 mg 2–3 times daily, doubled in severe infections

▼ **PoM Ambaxin®** (Upjohn)
Tablets, scored, bacampicillin hydrochloride 400 mg. Price 20 tabs = **F**. Label: 9

CICLACILLIN
Indications: bronchitis, urinary-tract infections, soft-tissue infections
Cautions; Contra-indications; Side-effects: see under Benzylpenicillin (section 5.1.1.1); also erythematous rashes in glandular fever and chronic lymphatic leukaemia
Dose: 250–500 mg every 6 hours; longer interval between doses in renal impairment

PoM Calthor (Ayerst)
Tablets, scored, ciclacillin 250 mg. Price 20 tabs = **E**. Label: 9
Tablets, scored, ciclacillin 500 mg. Price 20 tabs = **G**. Label: 9
Suspension (= mixture), pink, ciclacillin 125 mg/5 ml when reconstituted with water for preparations. Diluent syrup, life of diluted mixture 7 days. Price 120 ml = **E**. Label: 9
Suspension (= mixture), ciclacillin 250 mg/5 ml when reconstituted with water for preparations. Diluent as above. Price 120 ml = **F**. Label: 9

MEZLOCILLIN
Indications: infections due to *E. coli, Pseudomonas*, and *Proteus* spp.
Cautions; Contra-indications; Side-effects: see under Benzylpenicillin (section 5.1.1.1); increase interval between doses in renal impairment
Dose: by intravenous injection, 2 g every 6–8 hours
By intravenous infusion, in serious infections, 5 g every 6–8 hours
By intramuscular injection, 0.5–2 g

▼ **PoM Baypen®** (Bayer)
Injection, powder for reconstitution, mezlocillin (as sodium salt). Price 500-mg vial = **D**; 1-g vial = **E**; 2-g vial = **F**

C = 51-100p, D = 101-180p, E = 181-300p, F = 301-450p, G = 451-650p, H = 651-900p, I = 901-1200p, J = over 1200p.

Infusion, powder for reconstitution, mezlocillin (as sodium salt). Price 5-g vial = **H** (also available with 50 ml water for injections and transfer needle)

PIPERACILLIN

Indications: severe infections due to sensitive Gram-positive, Gram-negative, and anaerobic bacteria; peri-operative prophylaxis

Cautions; Contra-indications; Side-effects: see under Benzylpenicillin (section 5.1.1.1); increase interval between doses in moderate or severe renal impairment

Dose: by intramuscular injection or slow intravenous injection or infusion, 100–150 mg/kg daily (in divided doses), increased to 200–300 mg/kg daily in severe infections, and to at least 16 g/day in life-threatening infections; max. intramuscular dose 2 g

▼ PoM **Pipril**® (Lederle)
Injection, powder for reconstitution, piperacillin (as sodium salt). Price 1-g vial = **E**; 2-g vial = **G**; 4-g vial = **I**
Infusion, powder for reconstitution, piperacillin 4 g (as sodium salt), with 50-ml bottle water for injections and transfer needle. Price complete unit = **J**

PIVAMPICILLIN

Indications: see under Ampicillin

Cautions; Contra-indications; Side-effects: see under Benzylpenicillin (section 5.1.1.1); also erythematous rashes in chronic lymphatic leukaemia; liver- and kidney-function tests required in long-term use; avoid in severe liver disease and renal impairment. Drug interactions: see Appendix 1 (section 5.1)

Dose: 500 mg every 12 hours, doubled in severe infections

▼ PoM **Pondocillin**® (Burgess)
Tablets, f/c, pivampicillin 500 mg. Price 20 tabs = **F**. Label: 5, 9
Suspension (= mixture), pivampicillin 162 mg/5 ml when reconstituted with water for preparations. Price 50 ml = **D**; 100 ml = **E**. Label: 5, 9

Compound preparation
▼ PoM **Miraxid**® (Leo)
Tablets, f/c, pivampicillin 125 mg, pivmecillinam hydrochloride 100 mg. Price 20 tabs = **E**. Label: 9, 21
  Dose: 2 tablets twice daily, increased to 3 tablets twice daily for severe infections; CHILD 6–10 years 1 tablet twice daily
Paediatric suspension (= mixture), pivampicillin 62.5 mg, pivmecillinam   46.2 mg/unit-dose sachet. Price 10 sachets = **E**. Label: 5, 9, 13, 21
  Dose: under 6 years 1 sachet twice daily increased to 2 sachets twice daily for severe infections, 6–10 years 2 sachets twice daily increased to 3 sachets twice daily for severe infections

TALAMPICILLIN HYDROCHLORIDE

Indications: see under Ampicillin

Cautions; Contra-indications; Side-effects: see under Benzylpenicillin (section 5.1.1.1); avoid in severe hepatic or renal impairment; also erythematous rashes in glandular fever and chronic lymphatic leukaemia

Dose: 250–500 mg every 8 hours

PoM **Talpen**® (Beecham)
Tablets, red, f/c, talampicillin hydrochloride 250 mg. Price 20 tabs = **F**. Label: 9
Syrup (= mixture), talampicillin hydrochloride 125 mg (as napsylate)/5 ml when reconstituted with water for preparations. Diluent syrup, life of diluted mixture 7 days. Price 100 ml = **E**. Label: 9

5.1.1.4   ANTIPSEUDOMONAL PENICILLINS

The carboxypenicillins, **carbenicillin** (Pyopen®) and **ticarcillin** (Ticar®), are principally indicated for the treatment of serious infections caused by *Ps. aeruginosa* although they also have activity against certain other Gram-negative bacilli including *Proteus* spp. and *Bacteroides fragilis*. Carbenicillin has been replaced by ticarcillin which is more active against these organisms.

Carbenicillin and ticarcillin are not absorbed when given by mouth but the phenyl ester of carbenicillin, **carfecillin** (Uticillin®) is absorbed, carbenicillin being released into the blood in only low concentrations although urinary excretion is adequate for the treatment of *Pseudomonas* and *Proteus* infections of the lower urinary tract. For *Pseudomonas* septicaemias, especially in the neutropenic patient or in those with endocarditis, ticarcillin should be given in combination with an aminoglycoside antibiotic such as gentamicin or tobramycin as there is a synergistic effect (but not mixed together in the same syringe or infusion).

The ureidopenicillins, **azlocillin** (Securopen®) and piperacillin (section 5.1.1.3) both have greater activity than ticarcillin against *Ps. aeruginosa*.

AZLOCILLIN

Indications: infections due to *Pseudomonas aeruginosa*

Cautions; Contra-indications; Side-effects: see under Benzylpenicillin (section 5.1.1.1); also longer dose interval in renal impairment

Dose: by intravenous injection, 2 g every 8 hours
By intravenous infusion, in serious infections, 5 g every 8 hours

▼ PoM **Securopen**® (Bayer)
Injection, powder for reconstitution, azlocillin (as sodium salt). Price 500-mg vial = **D**; 1-g vial = **F**; 2-g vial = **G**
Infusion, powder for reconstitution, azlocillin (as sodium salt). Price 5-g vial = **J** (also available

with 50 ml water for injections and transfer needle)

CARBENICILLIN

Indications: infections due to *Pseudomonas aeruginosa* and *Proteus* spp.

Cautions; Contra-indications: see under Benzylpenicillin (section 5.1.1.1); reduce dose in renal impairment

Side-effects: see under Benzylpenicillin (section 5.1.1.1); also hypokalaemia, alteration in platelet function

Dose: by slow intravenous injection or rapid infusion, severe systemic infections, 5 g every 4–6 hours; CHILD 250–400 mg/kg daily in divided doses

By intramuscular injection, urinary-tract infections, 2 g every 6 hours; CHILD 50–100 mg/kg daily in divided doses

PoM **Pyopen**® (Beecham)
Injection, powder for reconstitution, carbenicillin (as sodium salt). Price 1-g vial = **D**; 5-g vial = **H**

Infusion set, powder for reconstitution, carbenicillin 5 g (as sodium salt) in infusion bottle, with transfer needle and diluent. Price complete unit = **H**

CARFECILLIN SODIUM

Indications: urinary-tract infections due to *Pseudomonas* and *Proteus* spp.

Cautions; Contra-indications; Side-effects: see under Benzylpenicillin (section 5.1.1.1)

Dose: 0.5–1 g 3 times daily

PoM **Uticillin**® (Beecham)
Tablets, carfecillin sodium 500 mg. Price 20 tabs = **H**. Label: 9

TICARCILLIN

Indications: infections due to *Pseudomonas* and *Proteus* spp.

Cautions; Contra-indications; Side-effects: see under Benzylpenicillin (section 5.1.1.1)

Dose: by intramuscular or slow intravenous injection, or rapid intravenous infusion, 15–20 g daily in divided doses; CHILD 200–300 mg/kg daily in divided doses

PoM **Ticar**® (Beecham)
Injection, powder for reconstitution, ticarcillin (as sodium salt). Price 1-g vial = **E**; 3-g vial = **G**; 5-g vial = **I**

Infusion, powder for reconstitution, ticarcillin 5 g (as sodium salt) in infusion bottle, with transfer needle and diluent. Price complete unit = **I**

5.1.1.5   OTHER PENICILLINS

Mecillinam (Selexidin®) and **pivmecillinam** (Selexid®) have significant activity against many Gram-negative bacilli including salmonellae, but excluding *Ps. aeruginosa*. Pivmecillinam is given by mouth and subsequently hydrolysed to mecillinam, which is the active agent and must itself be given by injection.

MECILLINAM

Indications: severe infections due to Gramnegative enteric bacteria

Cautions; Contra-indications; Side-effects: see under Benzylpenicillin (section 5.1.1.1); also liver- and kidney-function tests required in long-term use

Dose: by intramuscular injection or slow intravenous injection or infusion, 5–15 mg/kg every 6–8 hours

PoM **Selexidin**® (Leo)
Injection, powder for reconstitution, mecillinam. Price 200-mg vial = **C**; 400-mg vial = **D**

PIVMECILLINAM HYDROCHLORIDE

Indications: urinary-tract infections due to enterobacteria, salmonellosis

Cautions; Contra-indications; Side-effects: see under Benzylpenicillin (section 5.1.1.1); also liver- and kidney-function tests required in long-term use

Dose: salmonellosis, 1.2–2.4 g daily for 14 days
Urinary-tract infections, 200–400 mg every 6–8 hours

PoM **Selexid**® (Leo)
Tablets, f/c, pivmecillinam hydrochloride 200 mg. Price 20 tabs = **F**. Label: 9, 21

Suspension, granules, pivmecillinam hydrochloride 100 mg/single-dose sachet. Price 20 sachets = **F**. Label: 9, 13, 21

Compound Preparation
see under Pivampicillin (section 5.1.1.3)

5.1.2   Cephalosporins and cephamycins

The cephalosporins are broad-spectrum antibiotics but in spite of the number of cephalosporins currently available there are few absolute indications for their use. All have a similar antibacterial spectrum although individual agents have differing activity against certain organisms. The pharmacology of the cephalosporins is similar to that of the penicillins, excretion being principally renal. Cephalexin, cephradine, cefaclor, and cefadroxil are all active when given by mouth but parenteral administration may be required in severe infections.

The principal side-effect of the cephalosporins is hypersensitivity and about 10% of penicillinsensitive patients will also be allergic to the cephalosporins. Haemorrhage due to interference with blood clotting factors has been associated with several cephalosporins and there have been recent reports of severe bleeding in patients receiving latamoxef, particularly in elderly or debilitated patients. For drug interactions of the cephalosporins see Appendix 1 (section 5.1).

C = 51-100p, **D** = 101-180p, **E** = 181-300p, **F** = 301-450p, **G** = 451-650p, **H** = 651-900p, **I** = 901-1200p, **J** = over 1200p.

The first cephalosporins were **cephaloridine** (Ceporin®) and **cephalothin** (Keflin®). Cephalothin is less active and less stable than the newer cephalosporins. Cephaloridine can be nephrotoxic and is potentiated by potent tubular diuretics such as frusemide and ethacrynic acid. These two have been replaced by the newer cephalosporins, **cephradine** (Velosef®), **cephazolin** (Kefzol®), **cefuroxime** (Zinacef®), and **cephamandole** (Kefadol®).

Cefuroxime and **cephamandole** are 'second generation' cephalosporins and are slightly less susceptible than the other cephalosporins to inactivation by penicillinases. They are, therefore, active against certain bacteria which are resistant to the other drugs and have greater activity against *H. influenzae* and *Neisseria gonorrhoeae*.

Cefotaxime (Claforan®), **ceftazidime** (Fortum®), **ceftizoxime** (Cefizox®) and **latamoxef** (Moxalactam®) are 'third generation' cephalosporins with greater activity than the 'second generation' cephalosporins against certain Gram-negative bacilli. However, they are less active than cefuroxime and cephamandole against Gram-positive bacilli, most notably *Staph. aureus*. Their broad antibacterial spectrum may encourage superinfection with resistant bacteria or fungi.

Cefsulodin (Monaspor®) has good activity against *Ps. aeruginosa* and infections caused by this organism are the only indication for its use.

Cefadroxil (Baxan®) is a new oral cephalosporin with a slightly longer plasma half-life than the other cephalosporins, but is less active against *H. influenzae*. As the half-life is still only about one and a half hours, the dosage interval should be 8 hours for infections of moderate severity.

Cefoxitin (Mefoxin®), a cephamycin antibiotic, is active against bowel flora including *Bacteroides fragilis* and because of this it has been recommended for the treatment of abdominal sepsis such as peritonitis.

CEFACLOR

Indications: infections due to sensitive Gram-positive and Gram-negative bacteria, but see notes above
Cautions: penicillin sensitivity
Contra-indications: cephalosporin hypersensitivity
Side-effects: allergic reactions including urticaria and rashes; hypersensitivity reactions including anaphylaxis; nausea, vomiting, diarrhoea
Dose: 250 mg every 8 hours; max. 4 g daily; CHILD, 20–40 mg/kg daily in divided doses; max. 1 g daily

PoM **Distaclor**® (Dista)
Capsules, violet/white, cefaclor 250 mg. Price 20 caps = **G**. Label: 9
Suspension (= mixture), pink, cefaclor 125 mg/5 ml when reconstituted with water for preparations. Diluent water for preparations or syrup, life of diluted mixture 14 days. Price 100 ml = **F**. Label: 9

Suspension (= mixture), pink, cefaclor 250 mg/5 ml when reconstituted with water for preparations. Diluent as above. Price 100 ml = **G**. Label: 9

CEFADROXIL

Indications: see under Cefaclor; see also notes above
Cautions; Contra-indications; Side-effects: see under Cefaclor; also reduce dose in renal impairment, false-positive Coombs' test may develop, false-positive results for glucose in urine with reducing substances
Dose: patients over 40 kg, 0.5–1 g twice daily (but see also notes above); skin, soft tissue, and simple urinary-tract infections, 1 g daily; CHILD under 1 year, 25 mg/kg daily in divided doses; 1–6 years, 250 mg twice daily; over 6 years, 500 mg twice daily

▼ PoM **Baxan**® (Bristol-Myers)
Capsules, cefadroxil 500 mg (as monohydrate). Price 20 caps = **G**. Label: 9
Suspension (= mixture), cefadroxil 125 mg (as monohydrate)/5 ml when reconstituted with water for preparations. Price 60 ml = **D**. Label: 9
Suspension (= mixture), cefadroxil 250 mg (as monohydrate)/5 ml when reconstituted with water for preparations. Price 60 ml = **F**. Label: 9
Suspension (= mixture), cefradroxil 500 mg (as monohydrate)/5 ml when reconstituted with water for preparations. Price 100 ml = **H**. Label: 9

CEFOTAXIME

Indications: see under Cefaclor; see also notes above
Cautions; Contra-indications; Side-effects: see under Cefaclor; also reduce dose in severe renal impairment, false-positive results for glucose in urine with reducing substances
Dose: by intramuscular or intravenous injection, 1 g every 12 hours; in moderate to serious infection 1 g every 8 hours; life-threatening infection 2 g every 8 hours; exceptionally, for life-threatening infections due to organisms less sensitive to cefotaxime, up to 12 g daily
Gonorrhoea 1 g as a single dose
In severe renal impairment, doses to be halved after initial dose of 1 g. NEONATE, 50 mg/kg daily in 2–4 divided doses; in severe infections 150–200 mg/kg daily. CHILD, 100–150 mg/kg daily in 2–4 divided doses; in severe infections, up to 200 mg/kg daily
By intravenous infusion, 1–2 g over 20–60 minutes

▼ PoM **Claforan**® (Roussel)
Injection, powder for reconstitution, cefotaxime (as sodium salt). Price 500-mg vial = **E**; 1-g vial = **G**; 2-g vial = **I**

CEFOXITIN

Indications: see under Cefaclor; more active against Gram-negative bacteria

Cautions; Contra-indications; Side-effects: see under Cefaclor; also reduce dose in renal impairment, false-positive results for glucose in urine with reducing substances

Dose: by intramuscular injection or slow intravenous injection or infusion, 1–2 g every 6–8 hours, increased in severe infections; max. 12 g daily; CHILD over 3 months, 80–160 mg/kg daily in divided doses

PoM **Mefoxin**® (MSD)
Injection, powder for reconstitution, cefoxitin (as sodium salt). Price 1-g vial = **G**; 2-g vial = **I**

CEFSULODIN SODIUM

Indications: infections due to sensitive strains of *Ps. aeruginosa*

Cautions; Contra-indications; Side-effects: see under Cefaclor; also reduce dose in renal impairment

Dose: by intramuscular or intravenous injection, 1–4 g daily in 2–4 divided doses; CHILD 20–50 mg/kg daily

▼ PoM **Monaspor**® (Ciba)
Injection, powder for reconstitution, cefsulodin sodium. Price 50-mg vial = **G**; 1-g vial = **I**

CEFTAZIDIME

Indications: see under Cefaclor; see also notes above

Cautions; Contra-indications; Side-effects: see under Cefaclor; also reduce dose in renal impairment, false-positive Coombs' test may develop, false-positive results for glucose in urine with reducing substances

Dose: by intramuscular injection or intravenous injection or infusion, 1–6 g daily in divided doses; CHILD, up to 2 months 25–60 mg/kg daily in 2 divided doses, over 2 months 30–100 mg/kg daily in 2–3 divided doses
Pseudomonal lung infection in cystic fibrosis, ADULT with normal renal function 100–150 mg/kg daily in 3 divided doses

▼ PoM **Fortum**® (Glaxo)
Injection, powder for reconstitution, ceftazidime (as pentahydrate), with sodium carbonate. Price 500-mg vial = **G**; 1-g vial = **I**; 2-g vial (for injection and for infusion) = **J**

CEFTIZOXIME

Indications: see under Cefaclor; see also notes above

Cautions; Contra-indications; Side-effects: see under Cefaclor; also reduce dose in renal impairment; false-positive Coombs' test may develop, false-positive results for glucose in urine with reducing substances

Dose: by intramuscular injection or slow intravenous injection or infusion, up to 8 g daily, in divided doses; CHILD over 3 months 30–60 mg/

kg daily in divided doses, increased to 100–150 mg/kg daily for severe infections
Gonorrhoea, *by intramuscular injection*, 1 g as a single dose
Urinary-tract infections, *by intramuscular or slow intravenous injection or infusion*, 0.5–1 g every 12 hours

▼ PoM **Cefizox**® (Wellcome)
Injection, powder for reconstitution, ceftizoxime (as sodium salt). Price 500-mg vial = **E**; 1-g vial = **G**; 2-g vial = **I**

CEFUROXIME

Indications: see under Cefaclor; more active against *H. influenzae* and *N. gonorrhoeae*

Cautions; Contra-indications; Side-effects: see under Cefaclor; also positive Coombs' test may develop; reduce dose in renal impairment

Dose: by intramuscular or intravenous injection, 750 mg every 8 hours
Gonorrhoea, 1.5 g as a single dose by intramuscular injection
Surgical prophylaxis, 1.5 g by intravenous injection at induction
By intravenous injection or infusion, in severe infections, 1.5 g every 6–8 hours
CHILD, 30–100 mg/kg daily in divided doses

PoM **Zinacef**® (Glaxo)
Injection, powder for reconstitution, cefuroxime (as sodium salt). Price 250-mg vial = **C**; 750-mg vial = **E**; 1.5-g vial = **G**

CEPHALEXIN

Indications: see under Cefaclor

Cautions; Contra-indications; Side-effects: see under Cefaclor; also reduce dose in renal impairment, false-positive results for glucose in urine with reducing substances

Dose: 250 mg every 6 hours *or* 500 mg every 8–12 hours; CHILD, 25–50 mg/kg daily in divided doses

PoM **Cephalexin Capsules,** cephalexin 250 mg, price 20 caps = **E**; 500 mg, price 20 caps = **F**. Label: 9
PoM **Cephalexin Tablets,** cephalexin 250 mg, price 20 tabs = **E**; 500 mg, price 20 tabs = **F**. Label: 9
PoM **Cephalexin Mixture,** cephalexin 125 mg/5 ml when reconstituted with water for preparations. Diluent, see below under Ceporex or Keflex. Price 100 ml = **D**. Label: 9
Cephalexin 250 mg/5 ml when reconstituted with water for preparations. Diluent as above. Price 100 ml = **E**. Label: 9
Cephalexin 500 mg/5 ml when reconstituted with water for preparations. Diluent as above. Price 100 ml = **G**. Label: 9
PoM **Ceporex**® (Glaxo)
Capsules, caramel/grey, cephalexin 250 mg. Price 20 caps = **E**. Label: 9
Capsules, caramel/grey, cephalexin 500 mg. Price 20 caps = **G**. Label: 9

C = 51-100p, D = 101-180p, E = 181-300p, F = 301-450p, G = 451-650p, H = 651-900p, I = 901-1200p, J = over 1200p.

Tablets, pink, f/c, cephalexin 250 mg. Price 20 tabs = **E**. Label: 9

Tablets, pink, f/c, cephalexin 500 mg. Price 20 tabs = **G**. Label: 9

Paediatric drops, orange, cephalexin 125 mg/1.25 ml when reconstituted with water for preparations. Price 10 ml = **D**. Label: 9, counselling advised, use of pipette

Suspension, yellow, cephalexin 125 mg/5 ml. Do not dilute. Price 100 ml = **D**. Label: 9

Suspension, yellow, cephalexin 250 mg/5 ml. Do not dilute. Price 100 ml = **E**. Label: 9

Syrup (= mixture), orange, cephalexin 125 mg/5 ml when reconstituted with water for preparations. Diluent water for preparations, life of diluted mixture 7 days. Price 100 ml = **D**. Label: 9

Syrup (= mixture), orange, cephalexin 250 mg/5 ml when reconstituted with water for preparations. Diluent as above. Price 100 ml = **E**. Label: 9

Syrup (= mixture), orange, cephalexin 500 mg/5 ml when reconstituted with water for preparations. Diluent as above. Price 100 ml = **G**. Label: 9

PoM **Keflex**® (Lilly)

Capsules, green/white, cephalexin 250 mg. Price 20 caps = **F**. Label: 9

Capsules, green, cephalexin 500 mg. Price 20 caps = **H**. Label: 9

Tablets, peach, cephalexin 250 mg. Price 20 tabs = **F**. Label: 9

Tablets, peach, cephalexin 500 mg. Price 20 tabs = **H**. Label: 9

Suspension (= mixture), pink, cephalexin 125 mg/5 ml after reconstitution with water for preparations. Diluent syrup, life of diluted mixture 10 days. Price 100 ml = **E**. Label: 9

Suspension (= mixture), orange, cephalexin 250 mg/5 ml after reconstitution with water for preparations. Diluent as above. Price 100 ml = **F**. Label: 9

CEPHALORIDINE

Indications: see under Cefaclor

Cautions; Contra-indications; Side-effects: see under Cefaclor; also avoid in renal impairment; positive Coombs' test may develop. Drug interactions: see Appendix 1 (section 5.1)

Dose: by intramuscular injection or intravenous injection or infusion, 0.5–1 g every 8–12 hours; max. 6 g daily (4 g in patients over 50 years or within 2 days of surgery); CHILD, 20–40 mg/kg daily in divided doses, max. 4 g daily

PoM **Ceporin**® (Glaxo)

Injection, powder for reconstitution, cephaloridine. Price 250- and 500-mg vial (both) = **B**; 1-g vial = **C**

CEPHALOTHIN

Indications: see under Cefaclor

Cautions; Contra-indications; Side-effects: see under Cefaclor; also avoid in renal impairment,

intramuscular injections painful. Drug interactions: see Appendix 1 (section 5.1)

Dose: by intravenous injection or infusion, 1 g every 4–6 hours; max. 12 g daily; CHILD, 80–160 mg/kg daily in divided doses

PoM **Keflin**® (Lilly)

Injection, powder for reconstitution, cephalothin (as sodium salt). Price 1-g vial = **E**

CEPHAMANDOLE

Indications: see under Cefaclor

Cautions; Contra-indications; Side-effects: see under Cefaclor; also reduce doses in renal impairment, false-positive results for glucose in urine with reducing substances. Drug interactions: see Appendix 1 (section 5.1)

Dose: by deep intramuscular injection or intravenous injection or infusion, 0.5–2 g every 4–8 hours; CHILD, 50–100 mg/kg daily in divided doses

PoM **Kefadol**® (Dista)

Injection, powder for reconstitution, cephamandole (as nafate) with sodium carbonate. Price 500-mg vial = **D**; 1-g vial = **F**; 2-g vial = **G** (Hosp. only)

CEPHAZOLIN

Indications: see under Cefaclor

Cautions; Contra-indications; Side-effects: see under Cefaclor; also reduce doses in renal impairment, false-positive results for glucose in urine with reducing substances

Dose: by intramuscular injection or intravenous injection or infusion, 0.5–1 g every 6–12 hours; CHILD, 25–50 mg/kg daily (in divided doses), increased to 100 mg/kg daily in severe infections

PoM **Kefzol**® (Lilly)

Injection, powder for reconstitution, cephazolin (as sodium salt). Price 500-mg vial = **E**; 1-g vial = **F**

CEPHRADINE

Indications: see under Cefaclor

Cautions; Contra-indications; Side-effects: see under Cefaclor; also reduce doses in renal impairment, false-positive results for glucose in urine with reducing substances

Dose: by mouth, 250–500 mg every 6 hours *or* 0.5–1 g every 12 hours; CHILD, 25–50 mg/kg daily in divided doses

By intramuscular injection or intravenous injection or infusion, 0.5–1 g every 6 hours, increased to 8 g daily in severe infections; CHILD, 50–100 mg/kg daily in 4 divided doses

PoM **Velosef**® (Squibb)

Capsules, orange/blue, cephradine 250 mg. Price 20 caps = **F**. Label: 9

Capsules, blue, cephradine 500 mg. Price 20 caps = **H**. Label: 9

Syrup (= elixir), cephradine 125 mg/5 ml when

---

reconstituted with water for preparations. Diluent syrup, life of diluted elixir 7 days. Price 100 ml = **E**. Label: 9

Syrup (= elixir), cephradine 250 mg/5 ml when reconstituted with water for preparations. Diluent as above. Price 100 ml = **F**. Label: 9

Injection, powder for reconstitution, cephradine. Price 500-mg vial = **C**; 1-g vial = **E**

LATAMOXEF SODIUM

Indications: see notes above

Cautions: penicillin sensitivity; reduce dose in renal impairment; possibly disulfiram reaction with alcohol. Drug interactions: see Appendix 1 (sections *2.8B*, 5.1)

Side-effects: hypersensitivity reactions; haematological effects including eosinophilia, reversible leucopenia, thrombocytopenia, and decreased prothrombin; rarely diarrhoea

Dose: by deep intramuscular injection or intravenous injection or infusion, 0.25–3 g every 12 hours, increased up to 4 g every 8 hours in severe infections; INFANT up to 1 week, 25 mg/kg every 12 hours; 1–4 weeks, 25 mg/kg every 8 hours; CHILD, 50 mg/kg every 12 hours. Doses may be doubled in severe infections

▼ PoM **Moxalactam®** (Lilly)
Injection, powder for reconstitution, latamoxef sodium. Price 500-mg vial = **F**; 1-g vial = **G**; 2-g vial = **J**

5.1.3 Tetracyclines

The tetracyclines are broad-spectrum antibiotics whose usefulness has decreased as a result of increasing bacterial resistance. They remain, however, the treatment of choice for infections caused by chlamydia (causing trachoma, psittacosis, urethritis, and lymphogranuloma venereum), rickettsia (including Q-fever), mycoplasma (respiratory and genital tract infections), and brucella. They are also used for the treatment of exacerbations of chronic bronchitis because of their activity against *H.influenzae*. For use of demeclocycline in inappropriate secretion of antidiuretic hormone see section 6.5.3.

Microbiologically, there is little to choose between the various tetracyclines, the only exception being **minocycline** (Minocin®) which has a broader spectrum, is active against *Neisseria meningitidis* and is used for meningococcal prophylaxis; however it may cause dizziness and vertigo.

The tetracyclines are deposited in growing bone and teeth (being bound to calcium) causing staining and occasionally dental hypoplasia, and should **not** be given to children under 12 years or to pregnant women. With the exception of **doxycycline** (Vibramycin®) and **minocycline** the tetracyclines may exacerbate renal failure and should **not** be given to patients with kidney disease. Absorption of tetracyclines is decreased by milk (except minocycline), antacids, and calcium, iron, and magnesium salts.

TETRACYCLINE

Indications: exacerbations of chronic bronchitis; infections due to brucella, chlamydia, mycoplasma, and rickettsia; severe acne vulgaris

Cautions: breast-feeding; rarely causes photosensitivity. Avoid intravenous administration in hepatic impairment. Drug interactions: see Appendix 1 (sections *2.8C*, 5.1, *7*, *9*)

Contra-indications: renal failure, pregnancy, children under 12 years of age

Side-effects: nausea, vomiting, diarrhoea; superinfection with resistant organisms; rarely allergic reactions

Dose: by mouth, 250–500 mg every 6 hours
Acne, see section 13.6
Syphilis, 30–40 g in divided doses over 10–15 days
Non-gonococcal urethritis, 500 mg 4 times daily for 10–21 days
By intramuscular injection, 100 mg every 8–12 hours, or every 4–6 hours in severe infections
By intravenous infusion, 500 mg every 12 hours; max. 2 g daily

PoM **Tetracycline Capsules,** tetracycline hydrochloride 250 mg. Price 20 caps = **B**. Label: 7, 9, 23

PoM **Tetracycline Tablets,** f/c or s/c, tetracycline hydrochloride 250 mg. Price 20 tabs = **B**. Label: 7, 9, 23

PoM **Tetracycline Mixture,** tetracycline hydrochloride 125 mg (as tetracycline)/5 ml. Diluent syrup, life of diluted mixture 14 days. Price 100 ml = **D**. Label: 7, 9, 23

PoM **Achromycin®** (Lederle)
Capsules, orange, tetracycline hydrochloride 250 mg. Price 20 caps = **C**. Label: 7, 9, 23
Tablets, orange, f/c, tetracycline hydrochloride 250 mg. Price 20 tabs = **C**. Label: 7, 9, 23
Powder, tetracycline hydrochloride. Price 25-g bottle = **I**. Label: 7, 9, 23
Syrup (= mixture), red, tetracycline hydrochloride 125 mg (as tetracycline)/5 ml. Diluent syrup, life of diluted mixture 14 days. Price 100 ml = **D**. Label: 7, 9, 23
Intramuscular injection, powder for reconstitution, tetracycline hydrochloride 100 mg, procaine hydrochloride 40 mg. Price per vial = **D**
Intravenous injection, powder for reconstitution, tetracycline hydrochloride. Price 250-mg vial = **D**; 500-mg vial = **E**

PoM **Achromycin V®** (Lederle)
Capsules, pink, tetracycline hydrochloride 250 mg (as tetracycline) with buffer. Price 20 caps = **E**. Label: 7, 9, 23
Syrup (= mixture), red, tetracycline hydrochloride 125 mg (as tetracycline)/5 ml with buffer. Do not dilute. Price 100 ml = **E**. Label: 7, 9, 23

PoM **Deteclo®** (Lederle)
Tablets, blue, f/c, tetracycline hydrochloride 115.4 mg, chlortetracycline hydrochloride 115.4 mg, demeclocycline hydrochloride 69.2 mg. Price 20 tabs = **E**. Label: 7, 9, 11, 23
Syrup (= mixture), red, tetracycline hydrochloride 28.85 mg (as tetracycline),

chlortetracycline hydrochloride 28.85 mg (as chlortetracycline), and demeclocycline hydrochloride 17.3 mg (as demeclocycline)/5 ml when reconstituted with water for preparations. Do not dilute. Price 100 ml = **E**. Label: 7, 9, 11, 23
Dose: 1 tablet or 20 ml mixture every 12 hours

PoM **Economycin**® (DDSA)
Capsules, orange, tetracycline hydrochloride 250 mg. Price 20 caps = **B**. Label: 7, 9, 23
Tablets, orange, f/c, tetracycline hydrochloride 250 mg. Price 20 tabs = **B**. Label: 7, 9, 23

PoM **Sustamycin**® (MCP)
Capsules, s/r, blue, tetracycline hydrochloride 250 mg. Price 20 caps = **E**. Label: 7, 9, 23, 25
Dose: 2 capsules initially, then 1 every 12 hours

PoM **Tetrabid**® (Organon)
Capsules, s/r, purple/yellow, tetracycline hydrochloride 250 mg. Price 20 caps = **E**. Label: 7, 9, 23, 25
Dose: 2 capsules initially, then 1 every 12 hours

PoM **Tetrachel**® (Berk)
Capsules, orange, tetracycline hydrochloride 250 mg. Price 20 caps = **B**. Label: 7, 9, 23
Tablets, orange, f/c, tetracycline hydrochloride 250 mg. Price 20 tabs = **B**. Label: 7, 9, 23

PoM **Tetrex**® (Bristol-Myers)
Capsules, yellow/orange, tetracycline 250 mg (as phosphate complex). Price 20 caps = **E**. Label: 7, 9, 23

CHLORTETRACYCLINE HYDROCHLORIDE

Indications: see under Tetracycline
Cautions; Contra-indications; Side-effects: see under Tetracycline
Dose: 250–500 mg every 6 hours

PoM **Aureomycin**® (Lederle)
Capsules, yellow, chlortetracycline hydrochloride 250 mg. Price 20 caps = **F**. Label: 7, 9, 23
Powder, chlortetracycline hydrochloride. Price 25-g bottle = **I**. Label: 7, 9, 23

CLOMOCYCLINE SODIUM

Indications: see under Tetracycline
Cautions; Contra-indications; Side-effects: see under Tetracycline
Dose: 170–340 mg every 6–8 hours

PoM **Megaclor**® (Pharmax)
Capsules, red, clomocycline sodium 170 mg. Price 20 caps = **E**. Label: 7, 9, 23

DEMECLOCYCLINE HYDROCHLORIDE

Indications: see under Tetracycline
Cautions; Contra-indications; Side-effects: see under Tetracycline, but photosensitivity is more common
Dose: 150 mg every 6 hours *or* 300 mg every 12 hours

PoM **Ledermycin**® (Lederle)
Capsules, red, demeclocycline hydrochloride 150 mg. Price 20 caps = **F**. Label: 7, 9, 11, 23
Tablets, red, f/c, demeclocycline hydrochloride 300 mg. Price 20 tabs = **H**. Label: 7, 9, 11, 23
Drops, yellow, demeclocycline hydrochloride 60 mg (as demeclocycline)/ml. Price 10 ml = **F**. Label: 7, 9, 11, 23, counselling advised, use of pipette
Syrup (= mixture), red, demeclocycline hydrochloride 75 mg (as demeclocycline)/5 ml. Do not dilute. Price 100 ml = **F**. Label: 7, 9, 11, 23

DOXYCYCLINE

Indications: see under Tetracycline; also chronic prostatitis
Cautions; Contra-indications; Side-effects: see under Tetracycline, but may be used in renal impairment
Dose: 200 mg on first day, then 100 mg daily

PoM **Doxatet**® (Cox Pharmaceuticals)
Tablets, green, f/c, doxycycline 100 mg (as hydrochloride). Price 20 tabs = **H**. Label: 6, 9, 27

PoM **Doxylar**® (Lagap)
Capsules, doxycycline 100 mg (as hydrochloride). Price 20 caps = **H**. Label: 6, 9, 27

PoM **Nordox**® (Norton)
Capsules, green, doxycycline 100 mg. Price 20 caps = **H**. Label: 6, 9, 27

PoM **Vibramycin**® (Pfizer)
Capsules, green, doxycycline 100 mg (as hydrochloride). Price 20 caps = **I**. Label: 6, 9, 27
Syrup (= mixture), red, doxycycline 50 mg (as calcium chelate)/5 ml. Diluent syrup, life of diluted mixture 14 days. Price 30 ml = **D**. Label: 6, 9, 27

PoM **Vibramycin-D**® (Pfizer)
Dispersible tablets, off-white, doxycycline 100 mg. Price 10 tabs = **G**. Label: 6, 9, 13

LYMECYCLINE

Indications: see under Tetracycline
Cautions; Contra-indications; Side-effects: see under Tetracycline
Dose: 408 mg every 12 hours

PoM **Tetralysal**® (Farmitalia Carlo Erba)
Capsules, lymecycline 204 mg. Price 20 caps = **D**. Label: 7, 9, 23

MINOCYCLINE

Indications: see under Tetracycline; also meningococcal carrier state
Cautions; Contra-indications: see under Tetracycline, but may be used in renal impairment
Side-effects: see under Tetracycline; also dizziness and vertigo (more common in women)
Dose: 200 mg initially, then 100 mg every 12 hours
Acne, initially 100–200 mg daily, then 50 mg twice daily

PoM **Minocin**® (Lederle)
Tablets, beige, f/c, minocycline 50 mg (as hydrochloride). Price 20 tabs = **G**. Label: 6, 9
Tablets, orange, f/c, minocycline 100 mg (as hydrochloride). Price 20 tabs = **I**. Label: 6, 9

OXYTETRACYCLINE

Indications: see under Tetracycline
Cautions; Contra-indications; Side-effects: see under Tetracycline
Dose: 250–500 mg every 6 hours

PoM **Oxytetracycline Capsules,** oxytetracycline hydrochloride 250 mg, price 20 caps = **B**; oxytetracycline 250 mg (as hydrochloride), price 20 caps = **D**. Label: 7, 9, 23

PoM **Oxytetracycline Tablets,** f/c or s/c, oxytetracycline dihydrate 250 mg, price 20 tabs = **A**; oxytetracycline 250 mg (as dihydrate), price 20 tabs = **A**. Label: 7, 9, 23

PoM **Oxytetracycline Mixture,** oxytetracycline 125 mg (as calcium salt)/5 ml. Diluent syrup, life of diluted mixture 14 days. Price 100 ml = **C**. Label: 7, 9, 23

PoM **Berkmycin**® (Berk)
Tablets, yellow, f/c, oxytetracycline dihydrate 250 mg. Price 20 tabs = **B**. Label: 7, 9, 23

PoM **Chemocycline**® (Consolidated)
Tablets, yellow, s/c, oxytetracycline dihydrate 250 mg. Price 20 tabs = **B**. Label: 7, 9, 23
Syrup (= mixture), oxytetracycline 125 mg (as calcium salt)/5 ml. Diluent syrup, life of diluted mixture 14 days. Price 100 ml = **C**. Label: 7, 9, 23

PoM **Galenomycin**® (Galen)
Tablets, brown, s/c, oxytetracycline dihydrate 250 mg. Price 20 tabs = **B**. Label: 7, 9, 23

PoM **Imperacin**® (ICI)
Tablets, yellow, f/c, oxytetracycline dihydrate 250 mg. Price 20 tabs = **B**. Label: 7, 9, 23

PoM **Oxymycin**® (DDSA)
Tablets, oxytetracycline dihydrate 250 mg. Price 20 tabs = **B**. Label: 7, 9, 23

PoM **Terramycin**® (Pfizer)
Capsules, yellow, oxytetracycline 250 mg (as hydrochloride). Price 20 caps = **C**. Label: 7, 9, 23
Tablets, yellow, s/c, oxytetracycline 250 mg (as dihydrate). Price 20 tabs = **C**. Label: 7, 9, 23

PoM **Unimycin**® (Unigreg)
Capsules, yellow/red, oxytetracycline hydrochloride 250 mg. Price 20 caps = **B**. Label: 7, 9, 23

COMPOUND PREPARATIONS

NHS PoM **Bisolvomycin**® (Boehringer Ingelheim)
Capsules, turquoise/grey, oxytetracycline hydrochloride 250 mg, bromhexine hydrochloride 8 mg. Price 20 caps = **D**. Label: 7, 9, 23

PoM **Chymocyclar**® (Armour)
Capsules, pink, tetracycline hydrochloride 250 mg, pancreatic enzymes (trypsin and chymotrypsin) 50 000 Armour units. Price 20 caps = **E**. Label: 7, 9, 23, 25

PoM **Mysteclin**® (Squibb)
Capsules, pink/brown, tetracycline hydrochloride 250 mg, nystatin 250 000 units. Price 20 caps = **D**. Label: 7, 9, 23
Tablets, orange, s/c, tetracycline hydrochloride 250 mg, nystatin 250 000 units. Price 20 tabs = **D**. Label: 7, 9, 23
Syrup, yellow, tetracycline 125 mg (as hydrochloride), amphotericin 25 mg/5 ml. Price 100 ml = **D**. Label: 7, 9, 23

5.1.4 Aminoglycosides

This group includes amikacin, gentamicin, kanamycin, neomycin, netilmicin, streptomycin, and tobramycin. All are bactericidal and active against some Gram-positive and many Gram-negative organisms. Streptomycin and kanamycin are also active against *Mycobacterium tuberculosis* while amikacin, gentamicin, and tobramycin have activity against *Strep. faecalis* (in conjunction with a penicillin) and *Ps. aeruginosa.*

The aminoglycosides are not absorbed from the gut unless there is inflammatory bowel disease or liver failure and must, therefore, be given by injection to treat systemic infections. Excretion is principally via the kidney and if there is renal impairment accumulation occurs in the blood with increased risk of side-effects which are dose-related.

The important side-effects are ototoxicity, and to a lesser degree nephrotoxicity, and occur most commonly in the elderly and in patients with renal failure. Where possible, the aminoglycosides should be avoided in pregnancy as they cross the placenta and can cause fetal eighth nerve damage. Care must therefore be taken with the dose of this group of antibiotics and, if possible, plasma concentrations should be monitored to prevent toxicity and, at the same time, ensure efficacy.

Plasma concentrations are measured approximately one hour after an intramuscular injection or 20 minutes after an intravenous injection, and also just before the next dose. One-hour concentrations of **gentamicin** should not exceed 10 micrograms/ml while the pre-dose (trough) concentrations should be less than 2 micrograms/ml.

Simultaneous administration of the aminoglycosides with the potentially ototoxic diuretics, frusemide, ethacrynic acid, and related compounds should be avoided. If it is necessary to administer an aminoglycoside and one of these diuretics to a patient the doses should be separated by as long a period as practicable.

Aminoglycosides may impair neuromuscular transmission and should not be given to patients with myasthenia gravis. Large doses given prophylactically during surgery have also been responsible for a transient myasthenic syndrome in patients with otherwise normal neuromuscular function.

Gentamicin is the most important of the aminoglycosides and is widely used for the treatment of serious infections. It is the aminoglycoside of choice in the United Kingdom. It has a broad spectrum but is inactive against anaerobes and has poor activity against haemolytic streptococci and pneumococci. When used for the 'blind' therapy of undiagnosed serious infections it is usually given in conjunction with a penicillin and/or metronidazole.

The daily dose is up to 5 mg/kg. Higher doses are occasionally indicated for serious infections, especially in the neonate or compromised host. When high doses are being given if there is renal failure, or if treatment lasts longer than 7 days, plasma concentrations **must** be measured. If renal

---

function is normal gentamicin is given in divided doses every 8 hours.

If there is impairment of renal function the time between doses must be increased and if renal impairment is severe the individual dose should also be reduced. Nomograms are available for the calculation of the dose, which depends on the patient's age, weight, and renal function.

Kanamycin (Kannasyn®, Kantrex®) has been replaced by gentamicin as the drug of first choice for serious infections caused by Gram-negative bacilli.

Amikacin (Amikin®) is a derivative of kanamycin and has one important advantage over gentamicin in that it is stable to 8 of the 9 classified aminoglycoside-inactivating enzymes whereas gentamicin is inactivated by 5. It is principally indicated for the treatment of serious infections caused by Gram-negative bacilli which are resistant to gentamicin, and is given by intramuscular or intravenous injection.

Tobramycin (Nebcin®) is similar to gentamicin. It is slightly more active against *Ps. aeruginosa* but shows less activity against certain other Gram-negative bacteria. Tobramycin is claimed to be less toxic than gentamicin.

Netilmicin (Netillin®) also has similar activity to gentamicin, but is claimed to cause less ototoxicity and nephrotoxicity. It is active against a number of gentamicin-resistant Gram-negative bacilli but is less active against *Ps. aeruginosa* than gentamicin or tobramycin.

Neomycin is too toxic for parenteral administration and can only be used for infections of the skin or mucous membranes or to reduce the bacterial population of the colon prior to bowel surgery or in hepatic failure. Topical application may lead to hypersensitivity, and oral administration to malabsorption. Small amounts of neomycin may be absorbed from the gut in patients with hepatic failure and, as these patients may also be uraemic, cumulation may occur with resultant ototoxicity. Similarly, ototoxicity may result from topical application to large areas, for example burns. **Framycetin** is almost identical with neomycin in its actions and uses.

Streptomycin is today almost entirely reserved for the treatment of tuberculosis (section 5.1.9).

GENTAMICIN

Indications: septicaemia and neonatal sepsis; meningitis and other CNS infections; biliary tract infection, acute pyelonephritis or prostatitis, endocarditis caused by *Strep. viridans* or *faecalis* (with a penicillin)

Cautions: increase dose interval in renal impairment (see below). Drug interactions: see Appendix 1 (sections 5.1, *5.1*, 8, *15*)

Contra-indications: pregnancy, myasthenia gravis

Side-effects: vestibular damage, reversible nephrotoxicity

Dose: by intramuscular injection or slow intravenous injection or infusion, 2–5 mg/kg daily, in divided doses every 8 hours. In renal impair-

ment the interval between successive doses should be increased to 12 hours when the creatinine clearance is 30–70 ml/minute, 24 hours for 10–30 ml/minute, 48 hours for 5–10 ml/minute, and 3–4 days after dialysis for less than 5 ml/minute

CHILD, up to 2 weeks, 3 mg/kg every 12 hours; 2 weeks–12 years, 2 mg/kg every 8 hours

By intrathecal injection, 1 mg daily, with 2–4 mg/kg daily *by intramuscular injection* in divided doses every 8 hours

PoM **Gentamicin Injection,** gentamicin 40 mg (as sulphate)/ml, price 1-ml amp = C; 2-ml amp or vial = D, 2-ml syringe = E; 60 mg (as sulphate)/ml, price 1-ml amp = D; 2-ml amp = E; 80 mg (as sulphate)/ml, price 1.5-ml syringe = F

PoM **Gentamicin Injection, Intrathecal,** gentamicin 1 mg (as sulphate)/ml, price 2-ml amp = C; gentamicin 5 mg (as sulphate)/ml, price 1-ml amp = C

PoM **Gentamicin Injection, Paediatric,** gentamicin 5 mg (as sulphate)/ml, price 2-ml amp = B; 10 mg (as sulphate)/ml, price 2-ml vial = C

PoM **Gentamicin Powder,** (for preparing injections), gentamicin (as sulphate), price 1-g vial = J

PoM **Cidomycin®** (Roussel)
Injection, gentamicin 40 mg (as sulphate)/ml. Price 2-ml amp or vial = D
Paediatric injection, gentamicin 10 mg (as sulphate)/ml. Price 2-ml vial = C
Intrathecal injection, gentamicin 5 mg (as sulphate)/ml. Price 1-ml amp = C
Powder (for preparing injections), gentamicin (as sulphate). Price 1-g bottle = J

PoM **Garamycin®** (Kirby-Warrick)
Injection, gentamicin 40 mg (as sulphate)/ml. Price 2-ml amp or vial = D (Hosp. only)
Paediatric injection, gentamicin 10 mg (as sulphate)/ml. Price 2-ml vial = C (Hosp. only)

PoM **Genticin®** (Nicholas)
Injection, gentamicin 40 mg (as sulphate)/ml. Price 2-ml amp or vial = D
Paediatric injection, gentamicin 10 mg (as sulphate)/ml. Price 2-ml vial = C
Intrathecal injection, gentamicin 1 mg (as sulphate)/ml. Price 2-ml amp = C
Powder (for preparing injections), gentamicin (as sulphate). Price 1-g vial = J

PoM **Lugacin®** (Lagap)
Injection, gentamicin 40 mg (as sulphate)/ml. Price 2-ml amp = D

AMIKACIN

Indications: serious Gram-negative infections resistant to gentamicin

Cautions; Contra-indications; Side-effects: see under Gentamicin

Dose: by intramuscular injection or slow intravenous injection or infusion, 15 mg/kg daily in 2 divided doses

PoM **Amikin®** (Bristol-Myers)
Injection, amikacin 250 mg (as sulphate)/ml. Price 2-ml vial = I

Paediatric injection, amikacin 50 mg (as sulphate)/ml. Price 2-ml amp = **E**

FRAMYCETIN SULPHATE

Indications: see under Neomycin Sulphate
Cautions; Contra-indications; Side-effects: see under Gentamicin
Dose: by mouth, 2–4 g daily

PoM **Soframycin**® (Roussel)
Tablets, scored, framycetin sulphate 250 mg. Price 20 tabs = **G**
Powder (for preparing intrathecal or subconjunctival injections and topical solutions), framycetin sulphate. Price 500-mg vial = **F**

KANAMYCIN

Indications: serious Gram-negative infections resistant to gentamicin
Cautions; Contra-indications; Side-effects: see under Gentamicin
Dose: by intramuscular injection, 250 mg every 6 hours *or* 500 mg every 12 hours
By slow intravenous infusion, 15–30 mg/kg daily in divided doses every 8–12 hours

PoM **Kannasyn**® (Winthrop)
Solution (= injection), kanamycin 250 mg (as sulphate)/ml. Price 4-ml vial = **J**
Powder (for preparing injections), kanamycin (as acid sulphate). Price 1-g vial = **J**
PoM **Kantrex**® (Bristol-Myers)
Injection, kanamycin 333 mg (as sulphate)/ml. Price 3-ml single-dose vial (1 g) = **F**

NEOMYCIN SULPHATE

Indications: bowel sterilisation prior to surgery
Cautions; Contra-indications; Side-effects: see under Gentamicin; avoid in renal impairment. Drug interactions: see Appendix 1 (sections *2.8, 2.8B, 5.1, 15*)
Dose: by mouth, 1 g every 4 hours

PoM **Neomycin Elixir,** neomycin sulphate 100 mg/ 5 ml (see Formulary). Price 100 ml = **C**
PoM **Mycifradin**® (Upjohn)
Powder (for preparing irrigations and topical solutions), neomycin sulphate. Price 500-mg vial = **D**
PoM **Nivemycin**® (Boots)
Tablets, neomycin sulphate 500 mg. Price 20 tabs = **E**
Elixir, neomycin sulphate 100 mg/5 ml. Price 100 ml = **C**

NETILMICIN

Indications: serious Gram-negative infections resistant to gentamicin
Cautions; Contra-indications; Side-effects: see under Gentamicin
Dose: by intramuscular injection or intravenous injection or infusion, 4–6 mg/kg daily, in divided doses every 8 or 12 hours; in severe infections, up to 7.5 mg/kg daily in divided doses every 8 hours (usually for 48 hours)

INFANT age up to 1 week, 3 mg/kg every 12 hours; age over 1 week, 2.5–3 mg/kg every 8 hours; CHILD 2–2.5 mg/kg every 8 hours

▼ PoM **Netillin**® (Kirby-Warrick)
Injection, netilmicin 10 mg (as sulphate)/ml. Price 1.5-ml amp = **D**
Injection, netilmicin 50 mg (as sulphate)/ml. Price 1-ml amp = **E**
Injection, netilmicin 100 mg (as sulphate)/ml. Price 1-ml amp = **F**; 1.5-ml amp or vial = **F**

TOBRAMYCIN

Indications: see under Gentamicin and notes above
Cautions; Contra-indications; Side-effects: see under Gentamicin
Dose: by intramuscular injection or intravenous injection or infusion, 3–5 mg/kg daily in divided doses every 8 hours; INFANT age up to 1 week 2 mg/kg twice daily; age over 1 week 2–2.5 mg/ kg every 8 hours

PoM **Nebcin**® (Lilly)
Injection, tobramycin 10 mg (as sulphate)/ml. Price 2-ml vial = **C**
Injection, tobramycin 40 mg (as sulphate)/ml. Price 1-ml vial = **D**; 2-ml vial = **E**

5.1.5 Macrolides

Erythromycin has a similar, although not identical, antibacterial spectrum to that of penicillin and is thus an alternative in penicillin-allergic patients. Indications include respiratory infections in children, whooping-cough, legionnaire's disease, and campylobacter enteritis. It has activity against gut anaerobes and has been used with neomycin for prophylaxis prior to bowel surgery. It is active against many penicillin-resistant staphylococci, and also chlamydia and mycoplasmas.

Erythromycin estolate, if given for more than 14 days, may cause cholestatic jaundice. This may rarely occur with other erythromycin preparations.

ERYTHROMYCIN

Indications: alternative to penicillin in hypersensitive patients; sinusitis, diphtheria and whooping cough prophylaxis; legionnaire's disease; chronic prostatitis
Cautions: hepatic impairment. Drug interactions: see Appendix 1 (sections *2.8B, 3, 4.7, 4.8*)
Contra-indications: estolate contra-indicated in liver disease
Side-effects: nausea, vomiting, diarrhoea after large doses
Dose: by mouth, 250–500 mg every 6 hours; CHILD, 125–250 mg every 6 hours
Syphilis, 20 g in divided doses over 10 days
By slow intravenous injection or infusion, 2 g daily in divided doses, increased to 4 g in severe infections; CHILD, 30–50 mg/kg daily in divided doses

---

PoM **Erythromycin Tablets,** e/c, s/c or f/c, erythromycin 250 mg, price 20 tabs = **C**; 500 mg, price 20 tabs = **F**. Label: 5, 9, 25

PoM **Erythromycin Stearate Tablets,** erythromycin 250 mg (as stearate), price 20 tabs = **E**; 500 mg, price 20 tabs = **F**. Label: 9, 21

PoM **Arpimycin®** (RP Drugs)

Mixture, pink, erythromycin 125 mg (as ethylsuccinate)/5 ml when reconstituted with water for preparations. Diluent syrup, life of diluted mixture 7 days. Price 100 ml = **D**. Label: 9

Mixture, pink, erythromycin 250 mg (as ethylsuccinate)/5 ml when reconstituted with water for preparations. Diluent as above. Price 100 ml = **D**. Label: 9

Mixture, pink, erythromycin 500 mg (as ethylsuccinate)/5 ml when reconstituted with water for preparations. Diluent as above. Price 100 ml = **F**. Label: 9

PoM **Erycen®** (Berk)

Tablets, orange, e/c, f/c, erythromycin 250 mg. Price 20 tabs = **C**. Label: 5, 9, 25

PoM **Erythrocin®** (Abbott)

Tablets, f/c, erythromycin 250 mg (as stearate). Price 20 tabs = **E**. Label: 9, 21

Tablets, f/c, erythromycin 500 mg (as stearate). Price 20 tabs = **F**. Label: 9, 21

Intravenous injection, powder for reconstitution, erythromycin (as lactobionate). Price 1-g vial = **G**

PoM **Erythrolar®** (Lagap)

Suspension (= mixture), erythromycin 250 mg (as ethylsuccinate)/5 ml when reconstituted with water for preparations. Diluent syrup, life of diluted mixture 5 days. Price 100 ml = **D**. Label: 9

PoM **Erythromid®** (Abbott)

Tablets, orange, e/c, f/c, erythromycin 250 mg. Price 20 tabs = **C**. Label: 5, 9, 25

PoM **Erythromid DS®** (Abbott)

Tablets, e/c, f/c, erythromycin 500 mg. Price 20 tabs = **E**. Label: 5, 9, 25

PoM **Erythroped®** (Abbott)

Suspension PI (= paediatric mixture), erythromycin 125 mg (as ethylsuccinate)/5 ml when reconstituted with water for preparations. Diluent syrup, life of diluted mixture 5 days. Price 100 ml = **D**. Label: 9

Suspension (= mixture), erythromycin 250 mg (as ethylsuccinate)/5 ml when reconstituted with water for preparations. Diluent as above. Price 100 ml = **E**. Label: 9

Suspension forte (= strong mixture), erythromycin 500 mg (as ethylsuccinate)/5 ml when reconstituted with water for preparations. Diluent as above. Price 100 ml = **F**. Label: 9

▼ PoM **Erythroped A®** (Abbott)

Tablets, yellow, f/c, erythromycin 500 mg (as ethylsuccinate). Price 20 tabs = **F**. Label: 9

PoM **Ilosone®** (Dista)

Capsules, ivory/red, erythromycin 250 mg (as estolate). Price 20 caps = **E**. Label: 9

Tablets, pink, erythromycin 500 mg (as estolate). Price 20 tabs = **G**. Label: 9

Suspension (= mixture), orange, erythromycin 125 mg (as estolate)/5 ml. Diluent syrup, life of diluted mixture 14 days. Price 100 ml = **E**. Label: 9

Suspension forte (= strong mixture), orange, erythromycin 250 mg (as estolate)/5 ml. Diluent as above. Price 100 ml = **G**. Label: 9

PoM **Ilotycin®** (Lilly)

Tablets, red, e/c, erythromycin 250 mg. Price 20 tabs = **D**. Label: 5, 9, 25

PoM **Retcin®** (DDSA)

Tablets, red, e/c, erythromycin 250 mg. Price 20 tabs = **C**. Label: 5, 9, 25

5.1.6   Clindamycin and lincomycin

These antibiotics have only a limited use because of their serious side-effects.

Clindamycin (Dalacin C®), which is more active and better absorbed from the gut, has generally replaced **lincomycin** (Lincocin®).

They are active against Gram-positive cocci, including penicillin-resistant staphylococci and also against many anaerobes, especially *Bacteroides fragilis*. They are well concentrated in bone and excreted in bile and urine.

Clindamycin is recommended for staphylococcal bone and joint infections, and intra-abdominal sepsis.

The most serious toxic effect of clindamycin and lincomycin is pseudomembranous colitis which may be fatal and is commonest in middle-aged and elderly females, especially following operation. This complication may occur with most antibiotics but is more frequently seen with clindamycin and is due to a toxin produced by *Clostridium difficile*, an anaerobic organism resistant to many antibiotics including clindamycin. It is sensitive to vancomycin (section 5.1.7) and metronidazole (section 5.1.11.1) administered by mouth.

CLINDAMYCIN

Indications: staphylococcal bone and joint infections, peritonitis

Cautions: discontinue immediately if diarrhoea or colitis develops; impaired hepatic or renal function. Drug interactions: see Appendix 1 (section *15*)

Contra-indications: diarrhoeal states

Side-effects: diarrhoea (discontinue treatment), nausea, vomiting, pseudomembranous colitis

Dose: by mouth, 150–300 mg every 6 hours with water; CHILD, 3–6 mg/kg every 6 hours with water

By intramuscular injection or slow intravenous infusion, 0.6–2.7 g daily in 2–4 divided doses; CHILD, 15–40 mg/kg daily in 3–4 divided doses

PoM **Dalacin C®** (Upjohn)

Capsules, lavender, clindamycin 75 mg (as hydrochloride). Price 20 caps = **F**. Label: 9, 27, counselling advised, see above (diarrhoea)

Capsules, lavender/maroon, clindamycin 150 mg (as hydrochloride). Price 20 caps = **G**. Label: 9, 27, counselling advised, see above (diarrhoea)

Paediatric suspension (= mixture), pink, clin-

---

damycin 75 mg (as palmitate hydrochloride)/ 5 ml when reconstituted with water for preparations. Diluent water for preparations, life of diluted mixture 14 days. Price 100 ml = **F**. Label: 9, 27, counselling advised, see above (diarrhoea)

Injection, clindamycin 150 mg (as phosphate)/ ml. Price 2-ml amp = **E**; 4-ml amp = **G**

LINCOMYCIN

Indications: see under Clindamycin, also notes above

Cautions; Contra-indications; Side-effects: see under Clindamycin. Drug interactions: see Appendix 1 (sections 5.1, *15*)

Dose: by mouth, 500 mg every 6–8 hours

By intramuscular injection, 600 mg every 12–24 hours

By slow intravenous infusion, 600 mg every 8–12 hours

PoM **Lincocin**® (Upjohn)
Capsules, blue, lincomycin 500 mg (as hydrochloride). Price 20 caps = **H**. Label: 9, 23, counselling advised, see above (diarrhoea)
Syrup (= elixir), red, lincomycin 250 mg (as hydrochloride)/5 ml. Diluent syrup, life of diluted elixir 14 days. Price 100 ml = **G**. Label: 9, 23, counselling advised, see above (diarrhoea)
Injection, lincomycin 300 mg (as hydrochloride)/ ml. Price 2-ml amp = **D**

5.1.7 Other antibiotics

Antibacterials discussed in this section include acrosoxacin, chloramphenicol, colistin, fusidic acid, polymyxin B, spectinomycin, and vancomycin.

Acrosoxacin (Eradacin®) is used only in the treatment of gonorrhoea in patients allergic to penicillins or who have strains resistant to penicillins and other antibiotics.

ACROSOXACIN

(Rosoxacin)
Indications: gonorrhoea
Cautions: impaired renal or hepatic function; patient's ability to drive or operate machinery may be impaired; avoid repeated doses in patients under 18 years
Side-effects: dizziness, drowsiness, headache, gastro-intestinal disturbances
Dose: 300 mg as a single dose on an empty stomach

▼ PoM **Eradacin**® (Sterling Research)
Capsules, red/yellow, acrosoxacin 150 mg. Price 2 caps = **E**. Label: 2, 23

Chloramphenicol is a potent, potentially toxic, broad-spectrum antibiotic which should be reserved for the treatment of life-threatening infections, particularly those caused by *Haemophilus influenzae*, and also for typhoid fever.

Chloramphenicol is widely over prescribed. Its toxicity renders it unsuitable for systemic use except in the circumstances indicated above.

Eye-drops of chloramphenicol (see section 11.3.1) are useful for the treatment of bacterial conjunctivitis.

CHLORAMPHENICOL

Indications: see notes above
Cautions: avoid repeated courses and prolonged treatment; reduce doses in hepatic or renal impairment; periodic blood counts required; interferes with development of immunity; may cause 'grey syndrome' in neonates (monitor plasma concentrations). Drug interactions: see Appendix 1 (sections *2.8B*, *4.8*, 5.1, *6.1*)
Contra-indications: pregnancy, breast-feeding
Side-effects: leucopenia, thrombocytopenia, irreversible aplastic anaemia, peripheral neuritis, optic neuritis, erythema multiforme, nausea, vomiting, diarrhoea
Dose: by mouth, 500 mg every 6 hours
By intramuscular injection or intravenous injection or infusion, 50 mg/kg daily in divided doses every 6 hours; CHILD, pyogenic meningitis, 50–100 mg/kg daily in divided doses every 6 hours; INFANTS under 2 weeks 25 mg/kg daily in divided doses every 6 hours

PoM **Chloromycetin**® (P-D)
Capsules, white/grey, chloramphenicol 250 mg. Price 20 caps = **D**
Suspension (= mixture), chloramphenicol 125 mg (as palmitate)/5 ml. Diluent syrup, life of diluted mixture 14 days. Price 100 ml = **D**
Injection, powder for reconstitution, chloramphenicol (as sodium succinate). Price 300 mg vial = **D**; 1.2-g vial = **D**
Powder, chloramphenicol. Price 5-g vial = **D**
PoM **Kemicetine**® (Farmitalia Carlo Erba)
Injection, powder for reconstitution, chloramphenicol (as sodium succinate). Price 1-g vial = **C**

Colistin is a polymyxin antibiotic active against Gram-negative organisms including *Ps. aeruginosa*.

It is **not** absorbed when given by mouth but is sometimes prescribed in infantile gastro-enteritis (but see section 1.4) and used topically for skin infection and as ear drops. It is also used in bowel sterilisation regimens in neutropenic patients. For use in bladder irrigation see section 7.4.4.

COLISTIN

Indications: see notes above
Cautions: reduce dose in renal impairment. Drug interactions: see Appendix 1 (section *15*)
Contra-indications: myasthenia gravis
Side-effects: perioral paraesthesia, vertigo, muscle weakness, apnoea
Dose: by mouth, 1.5–3 million units every 8 hours
By intramuscular injection or intravenous injection or infusion, 2 million units every 8 hours

PoM Colomycin® (Pharmax)
Tablets, scored, colistin sulphate 1.5 million units. Price 20 tabs = **J**
Syrup (= elixir), pink, colistin sulphate 250 000 units/5 ml when reconstituted with water for preparations. Diluent syrup, life of diluted elixir 14 days. Price 80 ml = **F**
Injection, powder for reconstitution, colistin sulphomethate sodium. Price 500 000-unit and 1 million-unit vial (both) = **D**

Fusidic acid and its salts are narrow-spectrum antibiotics. The only indication for their use is in infections caused by penicillin-resistant staphylococci, especially osteomyelitis, as they are well concentrated in bone; a second antistaphylococcal antibiotic is usually required.

SODIUM FUSIDATE
Indications: see notes above
Cautions: liver-function tests required
Side-effects: nausea, vomiting, rashes, jaundice, reversible change in liver function
Dose: by mouth, 500 mg every 8 hours
By slow intravenous infusion, 500 mg over 6 hours, 3 times daily

PoM Fucidin® (Leo)
Tablets, e/c, sodium fusidate 250 mg. Price 10 tabs = **G**. Label: 5, 9, 25
Suspension (= mixture), orange, fusidic acid 250 mg (≡sodium fusidate 175 mg)/5 ml. Do not dilute. Price 25 ml = **H**. Label: 9, 21
Intravenous infusion, powder for reconstitution, diethanolamine fusidate 580 mg (≡sodium fusidate 500 mg), with buffer. Price per vial (with diluent) = **F**

Polymyxin B sulphate is effective against Gram-negative organisms, particularly *Ps. aeruginosa*. It is a toxic antibiotic and there are very few indications for its use. For use in bladder irrigation see section 7.4.4.

POLYMYXIN B SULPHATE
Indications: see notes above
Cautions: impaired renal function. Drug interactions: see Appendix 1 (section 15)
Contra-indications: myasthenia gravis
Side-effects: circumoral and peripheral paraesthesia; haematuria, proteinuria, tubular necrosis; vertigo, muscle weakness, apnoea
Dose: by slow intravenous infusion, 15 000–25 000 units/kg daily in divided doses

PoM Aerosporin® (Calmic)
Injection, powder for reconstitution, polymyxin B sulphate. Price 500 000-unit vial = **H**
PoM Polybactrin® (Calmic)
Soluble GU, powder for reconstitution, polymyxin B sulphate 75 000 units, neomycin sulphate 20 000 units, bacitracin 1000 units. For bladder irrigation. Price per vial = **F**

Spectinomycin is active against Gram-negative organisms, including *N. gonorrhoeae*. Its only indication is the treatment of gonorrhoea caused by penicillin-resistant organisms or in a penicillin-allergic patient.

SPECTINOMYCIN
Indications: see notes above
Side-effects: nausea, vomiting, headache, dizziness, urticaria, fever
Dose: by deep intramuscular injection, 2 g in men and 4 g in women

PoM Trobicin® (Upjohn)
Injection, powder for reconstitution, spectinomycin (as hydrochloride). Price 2-g vial (with diluent) = **F**

Vancomycin is a bactericidal antibiotic. It is the drug of choice for antibiotic-associated pseudomembranous colitis, for which it is given by mouth, and the oral dose indicated below is considered to be adequate. It also has a limited use by the intravenous route in the prophylaxis and treatment of endocarditis and other serious infections caused by Gram-positive cocci including multiply-resistant staphylococci. It has a relatively long plasma half-life of approximately 6 hours therefore administration every 12 hours is usually adequate; plasma concentrations should be monitored (especially in patients with renal impairment).

VANCOMYCIN
Indications: see notes above
Cautions: extravasation at injection site may cause necrosis and thrombophlebitis, blood counts and liver- and kidney-function tests required. Drug interactions: see Appendix 1 (section 5.1)
Contra-indications: if possible avoid parenteral administration in patients with renal impairment or a history of deafness
Side-effects: after parenteral administration nausea, chills, fever, urticaria, rashes, eosinophilia, tinnitus (discontinue use), renal impairment
Dose: by mouth, 125 mg every 6 hours
By intravenous infusion, 500 mg over 20–30 minutes every 6 hours *or* 1 g every 12 hours

PoM Vancocin® (Lilly)
Powder (for oral use), vancomycin (as hydrochloride). Price 10-g bottle = **J**
Injection, powder for reconstitution, vancomycin (as hydrochloride). Price 500-mg vial = **I**

5.1.8 Sulphonamides and trimethoprim
The importance of the sulphonamides as chemotherapeutic agents has decreased as a result of increasing bacterial resistance and their replacement by antibiotics which are generally more active and less toxic.

The principal indication for sulphonamides used alone is urinary-tract infections caused by

---

sensitive organisms and for this purpose **sulphamethizole** is effective.

The addition of the folic acid antagonist trimethoprim to sulphamethoxazole (co-trimoxazole) increases the activity of the sulphonamide against Gram-negative bacteria except *Pseudomonas*.

Indications for **co-trimoxazole** (Bactrim®, Septrin® etc.) include urinary-tract infections, prostatitis, exacerbations of chronic bronchitis, invasive salmonella infections, brucellosis, and *Pneumocystis carinii* infections. Pentamidine has also been used for *Pneumocystis* pneumonia but is not generally available.

Trimethoprim is increasingly being used alone for the treatment of urinary- and respiratory-tract infections. Side-effects are less than with co-trimoxazole especially in older patients.

Side-effects of the sulphonamides include rashes, which are common, the Stevens-Johnson syndrome (erythema multiforme), renal failure (especially with the less soluble preparations), and blood dyscrasias, notably marrow depression and agranulocytosis.

Side-effects of co-trimoxazole are similar to those of the sulphonamides but a particular watch should be kept for haematological effects and special care should be taken in patients who may be folate deficient such as the elderly and chronic sick. The effect on the fetus is unknown and the drugs should not be used in pregnancy.

The **longer-acting sulphonamides** (sulfametopyrazine, sulphadimethoxine, and sulphamethoxypyridazine) which are usually highly bound to plasma proteins, have the advantage of less frequent administration, but toxic effects due to accumulation are more likely to occur.

The **poorly-absorbed sulphonamides** (calcium sulphaloxate, phthalylsulphathiazole, and sulphaguanidine) have been widely used for the treatment of intestinal infections and pre-operative bowel preparation but can no longer be recommended for these indications (for use in acute and chronic diarrhoeas see sections 1.4.3 and 1.5).

For *topical preparations* of sulphonamides used in the treatment of burns see section 13.10.1.1.

CO-TRIMOXAZOLE

A mixture of sulphamethoxazole 5 parts, trimethoprim 1 part

Indications: invasive salmonellosis, typhoid fever, bone and joint infections due to *H. influenzae*, urinary-tract infections, sinusitis, exacerbations of chronic bronchitis, gonorrhoea in penicillin-allergic patients

Cautions: blood counts in prolonged treatment, maintain adequate fluid intake, renal impairment, breast-feeding; photosensitivity. Drug interactions: see Appendix 1 (sections *2.8B*, *4.8*, *6.1*, *8*, *15*)

Contra-indications: pregnancy, infants under 6 weeks, renal or hepatic failure, jaundice, blood disorders

Side-effects: nausea, vomiting, rashes, erythema multiforme, epidermal necrolysis, eosinophilia, agranulocytosis, granulocytopenia, purpura, leucopenia; megaloblastic anaemia due to trimethoprim

Dose: by mouth, 960 mg every 12 hours, increased to 1.44 g in severe infections; 480 mg every 12 hours if treated for more than 14 days; CHILD, every 12 hours, 6 weeks to 5 months, 120 mg; 6 months to 5 years, 240 mg; 6–12 years, 480 mg

Gonorrhoea, 1.92 g every 12 hours for 2 days, or 2.4 g followed by a further dose of 2.4 g after 8 hours

By intramuscular injection or intravenous infusion, 960 mg every 12 hours

Note: 480 mg of co-trimoxazole consists of sulphamethoxazole 400 mg and trimethoprim 80 mg

PoM **Co-trimoxazole Tablets,** co-trimoxazole 480 mg. Price 20 tabs = **C**. Label: 9

PoM **Co-trimoxazole Tablets, Dispersible,** co-trimoxazole 480 mg. Price 20 tabs = **C**. Label: 9, 13

PoM **Co-trimoxazole Tablets, Double-strength,** co-trimoxazole 960 mg. Price 20 tabs = **E**. Label: 9

PoM **Co-trimoxazole Tablets, Double-strength, Dispersible,** co-trimoxazole 960 mg. Price 20 tabs = **E**. Label: 9, 13

PoM **Co-trimoxazole Tablets, Paediatric,** co-trimoxazole 120 mg. Price 20 tabs = **B**. Label: 9

PoM **Co-trimoxazole Mixture,** co-trimoxazole 480 mg/5 ml. Diluent syrup, life of diluted mixture 14 days. Price 100 ml = **E**. Label: 9

PoM **Co-trimoxazole Mixture, Paediatric,** co-trimoxazole 240 mg/5 ml. Diluent as above. Price 100 ml = **D**. Label: 9

PoM **Co-trimoxazole Intramuscular Injection,** co-trimoxazole 320 mg/ml in solvent. Price 3-ml amp = **D**

PoM **Co-trimoxazole Solution, Strong Sterile,** co-trimoxazole 96 mg/ml. **Co-trimoxazole Intravenous Infusion** is prepared by diluting this solution with 25 to 35 times its volume of glucose intravenous infusion 5% or sodium chloride intravenous infusion 0.9% before use. Price 5-ml amp = **C**

PoM **Bactrim®** (Roche)

Drapsules® (= tablets), orange, f/c, co-trimoxazole 480 mg. Price 20 tabs = **D**. Label: 9

Tablets (dispersible), greenish-yellow, scored, co-trimoxazole 480 mg. Price 20 tabs = **D**. Label: 9, 13

Double-strength tablets, scored, co-trimoxazole 960 mg. Price 20 tabs = **E**. Label: 9

Paediatric tablets, scored, co-trimoxazole 120 mg. Price 20 tabs = **B**. Label: 9

Adult suspension (= mixture), yellow, co-trimoxazole 480 mg/5 ml. Diluent syrup, life of diluted mixture 14 days. Price 100 ml = **E**. Label: 9

Paediatric syrup (= paediatric mixture), pink, co-trimoxazole 240 mg/5 ml. Diluent as above. Price 100 ml = **D**. Label: 9

Intramuscular injection, co-trimoxazole 320 mg/ml. Price 3-ml amp = **D**

C = 51-100p, D = 101-180p, E = 181-300p, F = 301-450p, G = 451-650p, H = 651-900p, I = 901-1200p, J = over 1200p.

Intravenous infusion, co-trimoxazole 96 mg/ml. To be diluted before use. Price 5-ml amp = **C** (Hosp. only)

PoM **Chemotrim**® (RP Drugs)
Paediatric suspension (= paediatric mixture), pale pink, co-trimoxazole 240 mg/5 ml. Diluent syrup, life of diluted mixture 14 days. Price 125 ml = **E**. Label: 9

PoM **Comox**® (Norton)
Tablets, scored, co-trimoxazole 480 mg. Price 20 tabs = **E**. Label: 9
Dispersible tablets, orange, co-trimoxazole 480 mg. Price 20 tabs = **E**. Label: 9, 13
Forte tablets, scored, co-trimoxazole 960 mg. Price 20 tabs = **E**. Label: 9
Paediatric suspension (= paediatric mixture), pink, co-trimoxazole 240 mg/5 ml. Price 100 ml = **D**. Label: 9

PoM **Cotrimox**® (Unimed)
Tablets, co-trimoxazole 480 mg. Price 20 tabs = **E**. Label: 9

PoM **Fectrim**® (DDSA)
Tablets (dispersible), co-trimoxazole 480 mg. Price 20 tabs = **D**. Label: 9, 13
Forte tablets (dispersible), co-trimoxazole 960 mg. Price 20 tabs = **E**. Label: 9, 13
Paediatric tablets, co-trimoxazole 120 mg. Price 20 tabs = **B**. Label: 9

PoM **Laratrim**® (Lagap)
Tablets, co-trimoxazole 480 mg. Price 20 tabs = **D**. Label: 9
Forte tablets, co-trimoxazole 960 mg. Price 20 tabs = **E**. Label: 9
Paediatric suspension (= paediatric mixture), co-trimoxazole 240 mg/5 ml. Price 100 ml = **D**. Label: 9

PoM **Septrin**® (Wellcome)
Tablets, co-trimoxazole 480 mg. Price 20 tabs = **E**. Label: 9
Dispersible tablets, orange, co-trimoxazole 480 mg. Price 20 tabs = **E**. Label: 9, 13
Forte tablets, co-trimoxazole 960 mg. Price 20 tabs = **F**. Label: 9
Paediatric tablets, co-trimoxazole 120 mg. Price 20 tabs = **C**. Label: 9
Adult suspension (= mixture), co-trimoxazole 480 mg/5 ml. Diluent syrup, life of diluted mixture 14 days. Price 100 ml = **F**. Label: 9
Paediatric suspension (= paediatric mixture), pink, co-trimoxazole 240 mg/5 ml. Diluent as above. Price 100 ml = **E**. Label: 9
Intramuscular injection, co-trimoxazole 320 mg/ml. Price 3-ml amp = **E**
Intravenous infusion, co-trimoxazole 96 mg/ml. To be diluted before use. Price 5-ml amp = **D**

CALCIUM SULPHALOXATE

Indications: see notes on poorly-absorbed sulphonamides
Cautions; Contra-indications; Side-effects: see under Co-trimoxazole; side-effects less common because of limited absorption
Dose: 1 g every 8 hours

PoM **Enteromide**® (Consolidated)
Tablets, calcium sulphaloxate 500 mg. Price 20 tabs = **C**

PHTHALYLSULPHATHIAZOLE

Indications: see notes on poorly-absorbed sulphonamides
Cautions; Contra-indications; Side-effects: see under Co-trimoxazole; side-effects less common because of limited absorption
Dose: 2–12 g daily in divided doses

PoM **Thalazole**® (M&B)
Tablets, scored, phthalylsulphathiazole 500 mg. Price 20 tabs = **B**. Label: 9

SULFAMETOPYRAZINE

Indications: urinary-tract infections, chronic bronchitis
Cautions; Contra-indications; Side-effects: see under Co-trimoxazole
Dose: 2 g once weekly

PoM **Kelfizine W**® (Farmitalia Carlo Erba)
Tablets, sulfametopyrazine 2 g. Tablets to be taken in water. Price 1 tab = **C**. Label: 9, 13

SULPHADIAZINE

Indications: meningococcal meningitis
Cautions; Contra-indications; Side-effects: see under Co-trimoxazole; avoid in severe renal impairment
Dose: by intramuscular injection or intravenous infusion, 1–1.5 g every 4 hours for 2 days, followed by oral treatment

PoM **Sulphadiazine Injection**, sulphadiazine 250 mg (as sodium salt)/ml. Price 4-ml amp = **C**
PoM **Streptotriad**® (M&B)
Tablets, pink, scored, sulphadiazine 100 mg, streptomycin 65 mg (as sulphate), sulphadimidine 100 mg, sulphathiazole 100 mg. Price 20 tabs = **D**. Label: 9, 27
PoM **Sulphatriad**® (M&B)
Tablets, scored, sulphadiazine 185 mg, sulphamerazine 130 mg, sulphathiazole 185 mg. Price 20 tabs = **B**. Label: 9, 27

SULPHADIMETHOXINE

Indications: urinary-tract infections, bronchitis
Cautions; Contra-indications; Side-effects: see under Co-trimoxazole
Dose: 1–2 g initially, then 0.5–1 g daily

PoM **Madribon**® (Roche)
Tablets, scored, sulphadimethoxine 500 mg. Price 20 tabs = **C**. Label: 9, 27

SULPHADIMIDINE

Indications: urinary-tract infections
Cautions; Contra-indications; Side-effects: see under Co-trimoxazole
Dose: by mouth or by intravenous or intramuscular injection, 2 g initially, then 0.5–1 g every 6–8 hours

PoM **Sulphamezathine**® (ICI)
Injection, sulphadimidine sodium 333 mg/ml. Price 3-ml (1-g) amp = **B**

SULPHAFURAZOLE

Indications: urinary-tract infections
Cautions; Contra-indications; Side-effects: see under Co-trimoxazole
Dose: 2 g initially, then 1 g every 4–6 hours

PoM **Gantrisin**® (Roche)
Tablets, sulphafurazole 500 mg. Price 20 tabs = **B**. Label: 9, 27
Syrup (= mixture), sulphafurazole 500 mg (as acetyl derivative)/5 ml. Diluent syrup, life of diluted mixture 14 days. Price 100 ml = **C**. Label: 9, 27

SULPHAGUANIDINE

Indications: see notes on poorly-absorbed sulphonamides
Cautions; Contra-indications; Side-effects: see under Co-trimoxazole; rashes frequent
Dose: 3 g every 6–8 hours for 3 days

PoM **Sulphaguanidine Tablets**, sulphaguanidine 500 mg. Price 20 tabs = **C**. Label: 9

SULPHAMETHIZOLE

Indications: urinary-tract infections
Cautions; Contra-indications; Side-effects: see under Co-trimoxazole
Dose: 200 mg 5 times daily; CHILD up to 5 years 50 mg; 6–12 years 100 mg

PoM **Sulphamethizole Tablets**, sulphamethizole 100 mg. Price 20 tabs = **A**. Label: 9
PoM **Urolucosil**® (Warner)
Tablets, scored, sulphamethizole 100 mg. Price 20 tabs = **A**. Label: 9
Suspension (= mixture), sulphamethizole 100 mg/5 ml. Diluent syrup, life of diluted mixture 28 days. Price 200 ml = **D**. Label: 9

SULPHAMETHOXYPYRIDAZINE

Indications: urinary-tract infections
Cautions; Contra-indications; Side-effects: see under Co-trimoxazole
Dose: 1–2 g initially, then 500 mg daily

PoM **Lederkyn**® (Lederle)
Tablets, peach, sulphamethoxypyridazine 500 mg. Price 20 tabs = **E**. Label: 9, 27

SULPHAUREA

Indications: urinary-tract infections
Cautions; Contra-indications; Side-effects: see under Co-trimoxazole

PoM **Uromide**® (Consolidated)
Tablets, yellow, sulphaurea 500 mg, phenazopyridine hydrochloride 50 mg. Price 20 tabs = **C**. Label: 9, 14, 22

TRIMETHOPRIM

Indications: urinary-tract infections, acute and chronic bronchitis
Cautions: reduce dose in moderate renal impairment, predisposition to folate deficiency, blood counts required on long-term therapy

Contra-indications: severe renal impairment, pregnancy, neonates
Side-effects: gastro-intestinal disturbances including nausea and vomiting, pruritus, rashes, depression of haemopoiesis
Dose: by mouth, acute infections, 200 mg every 12 hours; urinary-tract infections, 300 mg daily *or* 200 mg twice daily; chronic infections and prophylaxis, 100 mg at night; CHILD, twice daily, 2–5 months 25 mg, 6 months–5 years 50 mg, 6–12 years 100 mg
By slow intravenous injection or infusion, 150–250 mg every 12 hours; CHILD under 12 years, 6–9 mg/kg daily in 2–3 divided doses

PoM **Trimethoprim Tablets**, trimethoprim 100 mg, price 20 tabs = **C**; 200 mg, price 20 tabs = **D**; 300 mg, price 20 tabs = **H**. Label: 9
PoM **Trimethoprim Mixture**, sugar-free, trimethoprim 50 mg/5 ml. Diluents, see below. Price 100 ml = **D**. Label: 9
PoM **Trimethoprim Injection**, trimethoprim 20 mg (as lactate)/ml. Price 5-ml amp = **C**
PoM **Ipral**® (Squibb)
Tablets, trimethoprim 100 mg. Price 20 tabs = **C**. Label: 9
Tablets, trimethoprim 200 mg. Price 20 tabs = **D**. Label: 9
Paediatric suspension (= mixture), sugar-free, trimethoprim 50 mg/5 ml. Diluents sorbitol solution, syrup, or water for preparations, life of diluted mixture 14 days. Price 100 ml = **D**. Label: 9
PoM **Monotrim**® (Duphar)
Tablets, scored, trimethoprim 100 mg. Price 20 tabs = **C**. Label: 9
Tablets, scored, trimethoprim 200 mg. Price 20 tabs = **D**. Label: 9
Suspension (= mixture), sugar-free, trimethoprim 50 mg/5 ml. Diluents sorbitol solution or water for preparations, life of diluted mixture 14 days. Price 100 ml = **D**. Label: 9
Injection, trimethoprim 20 mg (as lactate)/ml. Price 5-ml amp = **C**
PoM **Syraprim**® (Wellcome)
Tablets, scored, trimethoprim 100 mg. Price 20 tabs = **E**. Label: 9
Tablets, scored, trimethoprim 300 mg. Price 20 tabs = **H**. Label: 9
Injection, trimethoprim 20 mg (as lactate)/ml. Price 5-ml amp = **D**
PoM **Tiempe**® (DDSA)
Tablets, trimethoprim 100 mg. Price 20 tabs = **C**. Label: 9
Tablets, trimethoprim 200 mg. Price 20 tabs = **D**. Label: 9
PoM **Trimogal**® (Lagap)
Tablets, trimethoprim 100 mg. Price 20 tabs = **C**. Label: 9
Tablets, trimethoprim 200 mg. Price 20 tabs = **D**. Label: 9
PoM **Trimopan**® (Berk)
Tablets, scored, trimethoprim 100 mg. Price 20 tabs = **C**. Label: 9
Tablets, scored, trimethoprim 200 mg. Price 20 tabs = **D**. Label: 9

C = 51-100p, **D** = 101-180p, **E** = 181-300p, **F** = 301-450p, **G** = 451-650p, **H** = 651-900p, **I** = 901-1200p, **J** = over 1200p.

Suspension (= mixture), sugar-free, trimetho-
prim 50 mg/5 ml. Diluent syrup, life of diluted
mixture 14 days. Price 100 ml = **D**. Label: 9
PoM **Unitrim®** (Unimed)
Tablets, trimethoprim 100 mg. Price 20 tabs =
E. Label: 9

5.1.9   Antituberculous drugs

The treatment of tuberculosis has two phases—
an *initial phase* using at least three drugs and a
continuation phase with two drugs.

Treatment requires specialised knowledge,
particularly where the organisms are resistant to
the first-line drugs isoniazid, rifampicin, streptomycin, and ethambutol, or where the disease
involves non-respiratory organs.

INITIAL PHASE. The concurrent use of at least three
drugs during the initial phase is designed to reduce
the population of viable bacteria as rapidly as
possible and to minimise the risk of ineffective
treatment in those patients infected by drug-resist-
ant bacteria. Treatment of choice for the initial
phase is the daily use of isoniazid and rifampicin
supplemented by ethambutol or streptomycin.
The further addition of pyrazinamide in the initial
phase produces the most intensive bactericidal
effect and permits the duration of the continuation
phase to be reduced to a minimum. These drugs
should be continued for at least 8 weeks and
preferably until the result of drug-sensitivity testing is known.

CONTINUATION PHASE. After the initial phase,
treatment is continued with only two drugs, one
of which, in the absence of contra-indications,
should always be isoniazid. The second drug may
be rifampicin, ethambutol, or streptomycin
(which can be given twice weekly with a high
dose of isoniazid to allow treatment to be fully
supervised).

DURATION OF TREATMENT. The duration of treatment depends on the combination of drugs used.
Where isoniazid and rifampicin are given daily
throughout treatment a *9-month course* is sufficient for patients with respiratory disease regardless of its extent. If in the initial phase pyrazinamide and either ethambutol or streptomycin
are included with isoniazid and rifampicin, which
are then used in the continuation phase, a total
of *6 months treatment* gives equally good results.
Where twice weekly streptomycin and isoniazid
are used in the continuation phase to allow supervision, a total treatment period of *18 months*
should be given.

The major causes of treatment failure are incor-
rect prescribing by the physician and inadequate
compliance by the patient.

Isoniazid (Rimifon®) is cheap and highly effective. Its only common side-effect is peripheral
neuropathy which is more likely to occur when
high dosage is used (as in meningitis) or where
there are pre-existing risk factors. In these circumstances pyridoxine 10 mg daily should be
given prophylactically from the start of treatment.
Other side-effects such as hepatitis and psychosis
are rare.

Streptomycin is given intramuscularly in a
standard dose of 1 g daily, reduced to 500 to
750 mg in small patients or those over the age of
40 years. Measurement of plasma drug concentrations should be performed, particularly in
patients with impaired renal function in whom
streptomycin must be used with great care.

Rifampicin (Rifadin®, Rimactane®) is an essential component of any short course regimen. It
should be given in a single daily dose of 450 mg
in adults of less than 50 kg and 600 mg in those
above that weight.

During the first two months of rifampicin
administration transient disturbance of liver function with elevated serum transaminases is common but generally does not require interruption
of treatment. Occasionally more serious liver toxicity requires a change of treatment particularly
in those with pre-existing liver disease.

On intermittent treatment six toxicity syndromes have been recognised—influenzal,
abdominal, and respiratory symptoms, shock,
renal failure, and thrombocytopenic purpura—
and can occur in 20 to 30% of patients.

Rifampicin induces hepatic enzymes which
accelerate the metabolism of several drugs including oestrogens, corticosteroids, sulphonylureas,
and anticoagulants. The effectiveness of oral contraceptives is reduced and, where appropriate,
alternative family planning advice should be
offered. The drug should be avoided in pregnancy
as the effect on the fetus is unknown.

Ethambutol (Myambutol®) is a valuable drug
for use in conjunction with isoniazid or rifampicin.
Side-effects are rare, and largely confined to visual
disturbances in the form of loss of acuity, colour
blindness, and restriction of visual fields. These
toxic effects are more common where excessive
dosage is used or the patient's renal function is
impaired, in which case the drug should be
avoided. The earliest features of ocular toxicity
are subjective and patients should be advised to
report any visual disturbance immediately. Early
discontinuation of the drug is almost always followed by recovery of eyesight. Patients who cannot understand warnings about visual side-effects
should, if possible, be given an alternative drug.

Ophthalmic examination should be performed
prior to treatment and, in children, at intervals
during treatment.

Pyrazinamide (Zinamide®) is a bactericidal
drug active against *Mycobacterium tuberculosis*
but not *M. bovis*. It is particularly useful in
tuberculous meningitis because of good meningeal
penetration.

Second-line drugs available for infections
caused by resistant organisms, or when first-line
drugs cause unacceptable side-effects, include
capreomycin (Capastat®), cycloserine, and prothionamide (Trevintix®).

Relative prices: **A** = up to 20p, **B** = 21-50p,

CAPREOMYCIN

Indications: tuberculosis resistant to first-line drugs

Cautions: renal, hepatic, or auditory impairment; breast-feeding; do not give with streptomycin or other ototoxic drugs

Contra-indications: pregnancy

Side-effects: hypersensitivity reactions including urticaria and rashes, changes in liver function, renal damage, hearing loss with tinnitus and vertigo, pain and induration at injection site

Dose: by intramuscular injection, 1 g daily (not more than 20 mg/kg)

PoM **Capastat**® (Dista)
Injection, powder for reconstitution, capreomycin sulphate 1 million units (capreomycin approx. 1 g). Price per vial = **D**

CYCLOSERINE

Indications: tuberculosis resistant to first-line drugs

Cautions: reduce dose in renal impairment

Contra-indications: epilepsy, depression, severe anxiety, psychotic states, alcoholism

Side-effects: mainly neurological, including headache, dizziness, vertigo, drowsiness, convulsions; allergic rashes

Dose: usually 250 mg every 12 hours; max. 1 g daily

PoM **Cycloserine Capsules,** cycloserine 125 mg, price 20 caps = **F**; 250 mg, price 20 caps = **H**. Label: 2, 8

ETHAMBUTOL HYDROCHLORIDE

Indications: tuberculosis, in combination with other drugs, usually rifampicin and/or isoniazid; prophylaxis—section 5.1, Table 2

Cautions: reduce dose in renal impairment, warn patients to report visual changes—see notes above

Contra-indications: young children, elderly patients, optic neuritis

Side-effects: optic neuritis, red/green colour blindness, peripheral neuritis

Dose: 15 mg/kg daily; CHILD 25 mg/kg daily for 60 days, followed by 15 mg/kg daily

PoM **Myambutol**® (Lederle)
Tablets, yellow, ethambutol hydrochloride 100 mg. Price 20 tabs = **D**. Label: 8
Tablets, grey, ethambutol hydrochloride 400 mg. Price 20 tabs = **G**. Label: 8
Powder (for oral use), ethambutol hydrochloride. Price 50-g bottle = **J**. Label: 8
PoM **Mynah 200**® (Lederle)
Tablets, ethambutol hydrochloride 200 mg, isoniazid 100 mg. Price 20 tabs = **F**. Label: 8, 22
PoM **Mynah 250**® (Lederle)
Tablets, yellow, ethambutol hydrochloride 250 mg, isoniazid 100 mg. Price 20 tabs = **F**. Label: 8, 22

PoM **Mynah 300**® (Lederle)
Tablets, orange, ethambutol hydrochloride 300 mg, isoniazid 100 mg. Price 20 tabs = **G**. Label: 8, 22
PoM **Mynah 365**® (Lederle)
Tablets, pink, ethambutol hydrochloride 365 mg, isoniazid 100 mg. Price 20 tabs = **G**. Label: 8, 22

ISONIAZID

Indications: tuberculosis, in combination with other drugs; prophylaxis—section 5.1, Table 2

Cautions: impaired liver and kidney function, epilepsy, alcoholism, breast-feeding. Drug interactions: see Appendix 1 (section *4.8*)

Contra-indications: drug-induced liver disease

Side-effects: nausea, vomiting, hypersensitivity reactions including rashes, peripheral neuritis with high doses (pyridoxine prophylaxis, see notes above), convulsions, psychotic episodes, agranulocytosis

Dose: by mouth or intramuscular injection, pulmonary tuberculosis, 300 mg daily *or* up to 1 g (14 mg/kg) twice weekly; CHILD 6 mg/kg daily
Tuberculous meningitis, 10 mg/kg daily

PoM **Isoniazid Tablets,** isoniazid 50 mg, price 20 tabs = **A**; 100 mg, price 20 tabs = **B**. Label: 8, 22
PoM **Isoniazid Elixir,** isoniazid 50 mg/5 ml (see Formulary). Price 100 ml = **B**. Label: 8, 22
PoM **Rimifon**® (Roche)
Injection, isoniazid 25 mg/ml. Price 2-ml amp = **A**

PROTHIONAMIDE

Indications: tuberculosis resistant to first-line drugs

Cautions: diabetes, liver-function tests

Contra-indications: see under Cycloserine; also history of liver disease

Side-effects: gastro-intestinal disturbances including anorexia, nausea, vomiting, and upper abdominal pain in a minority of patients; rarely mental disturbances (including depression), convulsions, headache, vertigo, peripheral neuritis, photophobia, acne, exacerbation of existing seborrhoea, urticaria, hypoglycaemia, and jaundice

Dose: ADULT and child over 10 years 0.5–1 g daily, in divided doses *or* as a single dose at night; CHILD up to 10 years, initially 10 mg/kg daily, increased over 15 days to 20 mg/kg if tolerated

PoM **Trevintix**® (M&B)
Tablets, prothionamide 125 mg. Price 20 tabs = **D**. Label: 8, 21

PYRAZINAMIDE

Indications: tuberculosis, especially tuberculous meningitis

Cautions: impaired renal function, diabetes, gout, liver-function tests required. Drug interactions: see Appendix 1 (section *10*)

Contra-indications: liver damage

C = 51-100p, **D** = 101-180p, **E** = 181-300p, **F** = 301-450p, **G** = 451-650p, **H** = 651-900p, **I** = 901-1200p, **J** = over 1200p.

Side-effects: hepatotoxicity including fever, anorexia, hepatomegaly, jaundice, fulminating liver failure; nausea, vomiting, arthralgia, sideroblastic anaemia, urticaria
Dose: 20–30 mg/kg daily; max. 3 g daily

PoM **Zinamide®** (MSD)
Tablets, scored, pyrazinamide 500 mg. Price 20 tabs = **D**

RIFAMPICIN

Indications: tuberculosis, in combination with other drugs, usually isoniazid and ethambutol; leprosy (section 5.1.10)
Cautions: reduce dose in hepatic impairment; alcoholism, pregnancy. Discolours soft contact lenses. See also notes above. Drug interactions: see Appendix 1 (sections *2.1*, *2.3*, *2.4*, *2.8A*, *3*, *4.7*, *5.1*, *5.1*, *6.1*, *6.3*, *7*, *8*)
Contra-indications: jaundice
Side-effects: gastro-intestinal symptoms including anorexia, nausea, vomiting, diarrhoea; influenzal syndrome including chills, fever, dizziness, bone pain; respiratory symptoms including shortness of breath, wheezing; collapse and shock; acute renal failure; thrombocytopenic purpura; hepatic reactions with alterations of liver function, jaundice; urticaria and rashes; urine, saliva, and other body secretions coloured orange-red
Dose: 450–600 mg (about 10 mg/kg) daily preferably before breakfast; CHILD up to 20 mg/kg daily to a max. of 600 mg
Dose in hepatic impairment should not exceed 8 mg/kg daily

PoM **Rifampicin Capsules**, rifampicin 150 mg. Price 20 caps = **F**; 300 mg, price 20 caps = **H**. Label: 8, 14, 22, counselling advised, see lenses above

PoM **Rifampicin Mixture**, rifampicin 100 mg/5 ml. Price 100 ml = **F**. Label: 8, 14, 22, counselling advised, see lenses above

PoM **Rifampicin and Isoniazid 150 + 100 Tablets**, rifampicin 150 mg, isoniazid 100 mg. Price 20 tabs = **G**. Label: 8, 14, 22, counselling advised, see lenses above

PoM **Rifampicin and Isoniazid 300 + 150 Tablets**, rifampicin 300 mg, isoniazid 150 mg. Price 20 tabs = **I**. Label: 8, 14, 22, counselling advised, see lenses above

PoM **Rifadin®** (Merrell)
Capsules, blue/red, rifampicin 150 mg. Price 20 caps = **F**. Label: 8, 14, 22, counselling advised, see lenses above
Capsules, red, rifampicin 300 mg. Price 20 caps = **H**. Label: 8, 14, 22, counselling advised, see lenses above
Syrup (= mixture), red, rifampicin 100 mg/5 ml. Do not dilute. Price 120 ml = **F**. Label: 8, 14, 22, counselling advised, see lenses above
PoM **Rifinah 150®** (Merrell)
Tablets, pink, rifampicin 150 mg, isoniazid 100 mg. Price 20 tabs = **G**. Label: 8, 14, 22, counselling advised, see lenses above

Dose: patients under 50 kg, 3 tablets daily, preferably before breakfast
PoM **Rifinah 300®** (Merrell)
Tablets, orange, rifampicin 300 mg, isoniazid 150 mg. Price 20 tabs = **I**. Label: 8, 14, 22, counselling advised, see lenses above
Dose: patients over 50 kg, 2 tablets daily, preferably before breakfast
PoM **Rimactane®** (Ciba)
Capsules, red, rifampicin 150 mg. Price 20 caps = **F**. Label: 8, 14, 22, counselling advised, see lenses above
Capsules, red/brown, rifampicin 300 mg. Price 20 caps = **H**. Label: 8, 14, 22, counselling advised, see lenses above
Syrup (= mixture), red, rifampicin 100 mg/5 ml. Do not dilute. Price 100 ml = **F**. Label: 8, 14, 22, counselling advised, see lenses above
Intravenous infusion, powder for reconstitution, rifampicin. Price 300-mg vial (with diluent) = **H**
PoM **Rimactazid 150®** (Ciba)
Tablets, pink, s/c, rifampicin 150 mg, isoniazid 100 mg. Price 20 tabs = **G**. Label: 8, 14, 22, counselling advised, see lenses above
Dose: patients under 50 kg, 3 tablets daily, preferably before breakfast
PoM **Rimactazid 300®** (Ciba)
Tablets, orange, s/c, rifampicin 300 mg, isoniazid 150 mg. Price 20 tabs = **I**. Label: 8, 14, 22, counselling advised, see lenses above
Dose: patients over 50 kg, 2 tablets daily, preferably before breakfast

STREPTOMYCIN

Indications: tuberculosis, especially in patients with impaired liver function
Cautions; Contra-indications; Side-effects: see under Aminoglycosides, section 5.1.4; also hypersensitivity reactions, paraesthesia of mouth
Dose: by *intramuscular injection*, 1 g daily; in patients over 40 years, 750 mg; in small patients, 500 mg

PoM **Streptomycin Sulphate** (Evans)
Injection, powder for reconstitution, streptomycin (as sulphate). Price 1-g vial = **B**

5.1.10   Antileprotic drugs

Treatment of leprosy varies with the type of disease, and advice from a member of the Panel of Leprosy Opinion is essential. Details of the Panel can be found in *Memorandum on Leprosy*, DHSS, London, H. M. Stationery Office, 1977 [in Scotland, NHS Circular 1978(GEN)44].

Dapsone, a sulphone, is the most widely used drug for the treatment of leprosy. However, dapsone resistance has recently become an increasing problem, and if the patient has severe (multibacillary) infection dapsone should be given initially in combination with **rifampicin** (section 5.1.9) and **clofazimine** (Lamprene®). Rifampicin should be continued for at least 4 weeks, clofazimine for one year, and dapsone for life.

Patients with few organisms (paucibacillary) are treated with dapsone for from 3 to 10 years depending on precise classification of the disease and response to therapy.

Lepra reactions, fever, erythema nodosum, painful polyneuritis, and iritis may complicate treatment, especially with dapsone, and are treated with clofazimine (which has an anti-inflammatory action), or prednisolone. Neurological involvement commonly occurs in leprosy and therefore neuropathy resulting from treatment with dapsone may be overlooked.

DAPSONE

Indications: leprosy, dermatitis herpetiformis
Cautions: cardiac or pulmonary disease; breast-feeding. Drug interactions: see Appendix 1 (section 5.1)
Contra-indications: pregnancy
Side-effects: neuropathy, allergic dermatitis, anorexia, nausea, vomiting, headache, insomnia, tachycardia, anaemia, hepatitis, agranulocytosis, lepra reactions (discontinue if eye or nerve trunks affected)
Dose: leprosy, 25–50 mg twice weekly, gradually increased to 400 mg twice weekly or 100 mg daily

PoM **Dapsone Tablets,** dapsone 50 and 100 mg. Price 20 tabs (both) = **B.** Label: 8

CLOFAZIMINE

Indications: leprosy
Cautions: hepatic and renal impairment—function tests required
Side-effects: nausea, giddiness, headache, and diarrhoea with high doses, red coloration of skin and urine, blue-black discoloration of lesions
Dose: previously untreated patients, 100 mg 3 times weekly; sulphone-resistant patients, 100 mg daily (initially with rifampicin)
Lepra reactions, 300 mg daily for 3 months

PoM **Lamprene**® (Geigy)
Capsules, brown, clofazimine 100 mg. Price 20 caps = **D.** Label: 8, 14, 21

5.1.11   Other antimicrobial drugs

5.1.11.1 Metronidazole and tinidazole
5.1.11.2 Urinary antimicrobial drugs

5.1.11.1   METRONIDAZOLE AND TINIDAZOLE

Metronidazole (Flagyl® etc.) is an antimicrobial drug with high activity against anaerobic bacteria and protozoa. Indications include surgical and gynaecological sepsis in which its activity against colonic anaerobes, especially *Bacteroides fragilis*, is important, trichomonal vaginitis (section 5.4.3), non-specific vaginitis, and *Entamoeba histolytica* and *Giardia lamblia* infections (section 5.4.2). Side-effects are uncommon but neuropathy can occur during prolonged therapy. Gastro-intestinal

disturbances may be minimised by taking tablets with or after food, but the mixture (which contains benzoyl metronidazole) should be taken at least 1 hour before food.

Tinidazole (Fasigyn®) is similar to metronidazole but has a longer plasma half-life, thus allowing less frequent administration.

METRONIDAZOLE

Indications: see notes above
Cautions: active CNS disease, disulfiram-like reaction with alcohol, hepatic impairment. Drug interactions: see Appendix 1 (section 2.8B, 5.1)
Side-effects: nausea, vomiting and gastro-intestinal disturbances, drowsiness, headache, rashes, leucopenia, darkening of urine, peripheral neuropathy in prolonged treatment, dizziness, ataxia, transient epileptiform seizures with high doses
Dose: anaerobic infections, *by mouth*, 400 mg every 8 hours; *by rectum*, 1 g every 8 hours for 3 days, then 1 g every 12 hours; *by intravenous infusion*, 500 mg every 8 hours for up to 7 days; CHILD, any route, 7.5 mg/kg every 8 hours
Non-specific vaginitis, *by mouth*, 400 mg twice daily for 7 days *or* 2 g as a single dose
Trichomoniasis, *by mouth*, 200 mg every 8 hours for 7 days *or* 800 mg in the morning and 1.2 g at night for 2 days *or* 2 g as a single dose
Amoebiasis, *by mouth*, 800 mg every 8 hours for 5 days
Giardiasis, *by mouth*, 2 g daily for 3 days
Acute ulcerative gingivitis, see section 12.3.2

PoM **Metronidazole Tablets,** metronidazole 200 mg, price 20 tabs = **D**; 400 mg, price 20 tabs = **F.** Label: 4, 9, 21, 25
PoM **Metronidazole Intravenous Infusion,** metronidazole 5 mg/ml. Price 20-ml amp = **E**; 100-ml vial = **F**; 100-ml bottle = **G**; 100-ml plastic bag = **G**
PoM **Metronidazole Suppositories,** metronidazole 500 mg, price 10 suppos = **F**; 1 g, price 10 suppos = **H.** Label: 4
PoM **Flagyl**® (M&B)
Tablets, scored, metronidazole 200 mg. Price 20 tabs = **E.** Label: 4, 9, 21, 25
Tablets, yellow, scored, metronidazole 400 mg. Price 20 tabs = **F.** Label: 4, 9, 21, 25
Intravenous infusion, metronidazole 5 mg/ml. Price 20-ml amp = **E**; 100-ml bottle = **F**; 100-ml Viaflex bag = **G**
▼ *Suppositories,* metronidazole 500 mg, price 10 suppos = **H**; 1 g, price 10 suppos = **I.** Label: 4
▼ PoM **Flagyl S**® (M&B)
Suspension (= mixture), metronidazole 200 mg (as benzoyl metronidazole)/5 ml. Diluent syrup, life of diluted mixture 14 days. Price 100 ml = **F.** Label: 4, 9, 23
PoM **Metrolyl**® (Lagap)
Tablets, scored, metronidazole 200 mg. Price 20 tabs = **D.** Label: 4, 9, 21, 25
Tablets, scored, metronidazole 400 mg. Price 20 tabs = **E.** Label: 4, 9, 21, 25

C = 51-100p, **D** = 101-180p, **E** = 181-300p, **F** = 301-450p, **G** = 451-650p, **H** = 651-900p, **I** = 901-1200p, **J** = over 1200p.

Intravenous infusion, metronidazole 5 mg/ml. Price 100-ml vial, Steriflex® bag (both) = **F**

▼ *Suppositories*, metronidazole 500 mg. Price 10 suppos = **G**. Label: 4

▼ *Suppositories*, metronidazole 1 g. Price 10 suppos = **H**. Label: 4

PoM **Nidazol**® (Steinhard)
Tablets, scored, metronidazole 200 mg. Price 20 tabs = **D**. Label: 4, 9, 21, 25

PoM **Vaginyl**® (DDSA)
Tablets, scored, metronidazole 200 mg. Price 20 tabs = **D**. Label: 4, 9, 21, 25
Tablets, scored, metronidazole 400 mg. Price 20 tabs = **E**. Label: 4, 9, 21, 25

▼ PoM **Zadstat**® (Lederle)
Tablets, scored, metronidazole 200 mg. Price 20 tabs = **D**. Label: 4, 9, 21, 25
Intravenous infusion, metronidazole 5 mg/ml. Price 100-ml Steriflex minipack = **G**
Suppositories, metronidazole 500 mg. Price 10 suppos = **F**. Label: 4

TINIDAZOLE

Indications: anaerobic bacterial and protozoal infections
Cautions; Side-effects: see under Metronidazole
Dose: by mouth, 2 g initially, followed by 1 g daily *or* 500 mg twice daily, usually for 5–6 days
Abdominal surgery prophylaxis and acute ulcerative gingivitis, a single 2-g dose
By intraveneous infusion, 800 mg daily until treatment by mouth can be given

▼ PoM **Fasigyn**® (Pfizer)
Tablets, f/c, tinidazole 500 mg. Price 20 tabs = **I**. Label: 4, 9, 21, 25
Intravenous infusion, tinidazole 2 mg/ml. Price 400- and 800-ml bottle (both) = **J**

5.1.11.2   URINARY ANTIMICROBIAL DRUGS

Urinary-tract infection commonly implies a functional or anatomical disorder of the urinary tract. Most of the organisms involved are bowel commensals, the commonest being *Escherichia coli*. Proteus, micrococci, coliforms, and faecal streptococci are also prevalent. *Pseudomonas* and *Klebsiella* spp. may be derived from hospital bacterial flora and *Staphylococcus epidermidis* may occur following catheterisation or instrumentation. Chlamydia are intracellular bacteria which may cause urethritis in males or cervicitis in females.

Urinary infection in pregnancy is often asymptomatic yet requires prompt treatment in order to prevent progression to pyelonephritis. Infection is associated with anaemia, prematurity, and stillbirth. Penicillins, cephalosporins, and nitrofurantoin are safe but co-trimoxazole and the sulphonamides, nalidixic acid, and tetracyclines are to be avoided in pregnant patients.

In uncomplicated infections ampicillin (section 5.1.1.3), co-trimoxazole and trimethoprim (section 5.1.8), nitrofurantoin, and nalidixic acid are all effective. Hexamine should **not** be used any longer as it is only bacteriostatic, requires acidification of the urine, and frequently causes side-effects. Chronic prostatitis is very difficult to eradicate and requires a lipid-soluble antibiotic which will penetrate prostatic tissue. Long-term treatment may be needed using various antibiotics in rotation; these include co-trimoxazole, erythromycin (section 5.1.5), and doxycycline (section 5.1.3).

Where infection is localised and associated with the presence of a urinary catheter, the use of a simple bladder instillation is often effective (see section 7.4.4).

Although aseptic instrumentation of the urinary tract does not require antibiotic cover (except in patients with heart-valve lesions) a parenteral bactericidal agent such as gentamicin (section 5.1.4) or a cephalosporin (section 5.1.2) is necessary should bacteraemia or septicaemia occur.

Noxythiolin (Noxyflex®) is a topical antimicrobial agent with antibacterial and antifungal properties. Indications include treatment of bladder infections by instillation (see section 7.4.4) and intraperitoneal use during colonic surgery.

In renal failure, impaired renal function will cause accumulation of many antibiotics or their metabolites with resultant toxicity. Drugs to be avoided include tetracyclines, hexamine mandelate, and nitrofurantoin. Peritoneal or haemodialysis is often able to remove the drug and supplementary doses can be given later. Aminoglycosides are more successfully cleared by haemodialysis; they should be used with great caution in renal failure. Adequacy of dosage of any drug should be accurately checked by plasma concentrations.

NITROFURANTOIN

Indications: urinary-tract infections
Cautions: ineffective in alkaline urine. Drug interactions: see Appendix 1 (section 5.1)
Contra-indications: impaired renal function, infants less than 1 month old, glucose-6-phosphate dehydrogenase deficiency
Side-effects: nausea, vomiting, rashes, peripheral neuropathy, pulmonary infiltration, allergic liver damage
Dose: 100 mg every 6 hours with food

PoM **Nitrofurantoin   Tablets,** nitrofurantoin 50 mg, price 20 tabs = **C**; 100 mg, price 20 tabs = **D**. Label: 9, 14, 21

PoM **Berkfurin**® (Berk)
Tablets, yellow, scored, nitrofurantoin 50 mg. Price 20 tabs = **C**. Label: 9, 14, 21

PoM **Ceduran**® (Tillotts)
Tablets, brown, scored, nitrofurantoin 100 mg, deglycyrrhizinised liquorice 250 mg. Price 20 tabs = **E**. Label: 9, 14, 21

PoM **Furadantin**® (Norwich-Eaton)
Tablets, yellow, scored, nitrofurantoin 50 mg. Price 20 tabs = **D**. Label: 9, 14, 21
Tablets, yellow, scored, nitrofurantoin 100 mg. Price 20 tabs = **E**. Label: 9, 14, 21

Suspension (= mixture), yellow, nitrofurantoin
25 mg/5 ml. Do not dilute. Price 300 ml = **F**.
Label: 9, 14, 21
PoM **Furan**® (Chelsea)
Tablets, yellow, scored, nitrofurantoin 50 mg.
Price 20 tabs = **A**. Label: 9, 14, 21
Tablets, yellow, scored, nitrofurantoin 100 mg.
Price 20 tabs = **B**. Label: 9, 14, 21
PoM **Macrodantin**® (Norwich-Eaton)
Capsules, yellow/white, nitrofurantoin 50 mg.
Price 20 caps = **D**. Label: 9, 14, 21
Capsules, yellow, nitrofurantoin 100 mg. Price
20 caps = **F**. Label: 9, 14, 21
PoM **Urantoin**® (DDSA)
Tablets, yellow, scored, nitrofurantoin 50 mg.
Price 20 tabs = **B**. Label: 9, 14, 21
Tablets, yellow, scored, nitrofurantoin 100 mg.
Price 20 tabs = **D**. Label: 9, 14, 21

CINOXACIN

Indications: urinary-tract infections
Cautions: moderately impaired renal function
Contra-indications: severe renal impairment
Side-effects: gastro-intestinal symptoms including anorexia, nausea, vomiting, cramps,
diarrhoea; hypersensitivity reactions including
urticaria, rashes, peripheral and oral oedema;
dizziness, headache, photophobia, tinnitus,
perineal burning, changes in liver-function tests
Dose: 500 mg every 12 hours; prophylaxis,
500 mg at night

PoM **Cinobac**® (Lilly)
Capsules, green/orange, cinoxacin 500 mg. Price
20 caps = **I**. Label: 9

HEXAMINE

Indications: see notes above
Cautions: urine must be acidic
Contra-indications: impaired renal and hepatic
function, dehydration, metabolic acidosis
Side-effects: gastro-intestinal disturbances,
frequent and painful micturition, bladder irritation, haematuria, proteinuria, rashes
Dose: hexamine hippurate, 1 g every 12 hours;
hexamine mandelate, 1 g every 6 hours

Hiprex® (Riker)
Tablets, hexamine hippurate 1 g. Price 20 tabs = **D**.
Label: 9
Mandelamine® (Warner)
Tablets, brown, e/c, hexamine mandelate 250 mg. Price
20 tabs = **B**. Label: 5, 9, 25
Tablets, brown, e/c, hexamine mandelate 500 mg. Price
20 tabs = **B**. Label: 5, 9, 25

NALIDIXIC ACID

Indications: urinary-tract infections
Cautions: impaired renal or hepatic function,
breast-feeding, avoid strong sunlight, interference with tests using copper salts (e.g.
Benedict's test). Drug interactions: see Appendix 1 (sections *2.8C*, 5.1)
Contra-indications: infants under 3 months,
epilepsy, CNS lesions

Side-effects: gastro-intestinal disturbances
including nausea, vomiting, diarrhoea; haemolysis in G6PD deficiency; allergic reactions
including urticaria, rashes, fever, arthralgia,
eosinophilia; also myalgia, muscle weakness,
phototoxicity, jaundice, visual disturbances,
convulsions
Dose: 1 g every 6 hours for 7 days, reducing to
500 mg every 6 hours

PoM **Nalidixic Acid Tablets,** nalidixic acid 500 mg.
Price 20 tabs = **D**. Label: 9, 11
PoM **Nalidixic Acid Mixture,** nalidixic acid
300 mg/5 ml. Diluent see below. Price 100 ml =
F. Label: 9, 11
PoM **Mictral**® (Winthrop)
Granules, effervescent, nalidixic acid 660 mg,
sodium citrate 3.75 g/sachet (Na+ 41 mmol/
sachet). Price 9 sachets = **F**. Label: 9, 11, 13
Dose: 1 sachet in water 3 times daily for 3 days
PoM **Negram**® (Sterling Research)
Tablets, beige, nalidixic acid 500 mg. Price 20
tabs = **F**. Label: 9, 11
Suspension (= mixture), pink, nalidixic acid
300 mg/5 ml. Diluent syrup, life of diluted mix-
ture 14 days. Price 100 ml = **G**. Label: 9, 11
PoM **Uriben**® (RP Drugs)
Tablets, nalidixic acid 500 mg. Price 20 tabs = **D**.
Label: 9, 11
Suspension (= mixture), pink, nalidixic acid
300 mg/5 ml. Diluent syrup, life of diluted mix-
ture 14 days. Price 100 ml = **F**. Label: 9, 11

NITROFURAZONE

Indications: bladder infections (see section 7.4.4)
Cautions: sensitisation may develop; impaired
renal function
Dose: as an irrigation or by instillation, 1 in 6
solution in sterile water

PoM **Furacin**® (Norwich-Eaton)
Solution (sterile), yellow, nitrofurazone 0.2%.
Price 50 ml = **G**

NOXYTHIOLIN

Indications: see notes above
Side-effects: burning sensation on application to
bladder (relieved by addition of amethocaine)
Dose: bladder instillation, 100 ml of a 2.5% solution instilled 1–2 times daily
Intraperitoneal use, 100 ml of a 2.5% solution
instilled prior to closure

PoM **Noxyflex**® (Geistlich)
Solution, powder for reconstitution, noxythiolin
2.5 g, amethocaine hydrochloride 10 mg. Price
per vial = **G**
PoM **Noxyflex S**® (Geistlich)
Solution, powder for reconstitution, noxythiolin.
Price 2.5-g vial = **G**

5.2 Antifungal drugs

It is important to remember that fungal infections
are frequently associated with a defect in host

C = 51-100p, **D** = 101-180p, **E** = 181-300p, **F** = 301-450p, **G** = 451-650p, **H** = 651-900p, **I** = 901-1200p, **J** = over 1200p.

resistance which should, if possible, be corrected otherwise drug therapy may fail. Similarly, treatment of dermatophyte infection may be unsuccessful until the animal source has been removed or controlled.

Amphotericin (Fungilin®) is not absorbed from the gut and is the only polyene antibiotic which can be given parenterally. It is the most important drug for the treatment of systemic fungal infections and is active against most fungi and yeasts. It is highly protein bound and penetrates poorly into body fluids and tissues. Amphotericin is a toxic drug and side-effects are common.

Flucytosine (Alcobon®) is a synthetic antifungal drug which is only active against yeasts and has been used for the treatment of systemic candidiasis, cryptococcosis, and torulopsosis. It is well absorbed from the gut and distributed widely in the body. Side-effects are uncommon but bone-marrow depression can occur and weekly blood counts are necessary during prolonged therapy. It can be given with amphotericin and synergy has been demonstrated. Resistance to flucytosine is not uncommon and can develop during therapy; sensitivity testing is, therefore, essential before treatment.

Griseofulvin is selectively concentrated in keratin and is the drug of choice for widespread or intractable dermatophyte infections—a topical imidazole or **Whitfield's ointment** (see section 13.10.2) is used for localised lesions. The drug is well absorbed from the gut but is inactive when applied topically. It is more effective in skin than in nail infections and treatment must be continued for several weeks or even months. Side-effects are uncommon.

The imidazole group of antifungal drugs includes clotrimazole, econazole, ketoconazole, and miconazole. The imidazoles are active against a wide range of fungi and yeasts. The main indications for their use at present are vaginal candidiasis and dermatophyte infections. **Miconazole** is also available for oral and parenteral administration, but the injection contains Cremophor EL®, which may give rise to hypersensitivity reactions. **Ketoconazole** (Nizoral®) is significantly better absorbed after oral administration than the other imidazoles, but has been associated with fatal hepatotoxicity. The CSM has advised that prescribers should weigh the potential benefits of ketoconazole treatment against the liver damage risk and should carefully monitor patients both clinically and biochemically. It should not be given for superficial fungal infections unless topically applied antifungal agents (or griseofulvin) have failed or are contra-indicated because of local hypersensitivity reactions. The imidazoles are not effective in aspergillus infections.

Nystatin (Nystan®) is a polyene antibiotic which is not absorbed when given by mouth and is too toxic for parenteral use. It is active against a number of yeasts and fungi but is principally used for *Candida albicans* infections of skin and mucous membranes. It is also used in the treatment of intestinal candidiasis.

For antifungal preparations used in genital infections see section 7.2.2 and in skin infections, see section 13.10.2. For use in bladder irrigation see section 7.4.4.

AMPHOTERICIN

Indications: candidiasis, systemic fungal infections

Cautions: when given parenterally, renal-function tests required, frequent change of injection site, avoid use with other nephrotoxic drugs

Side-effects: when given parenterally, fever, anorexia, nausea, vomiting, hypokalaemia, nephrotoxicity (reduced by intravenous infusion of mannitol), tinnitus

Dose: by mouth, up to 200 mg every 6 hours

By intravenous infusion, 250 micrograms/kg daily, gradually increased if tolerated to 1 mg/ kg daily; max. in severely ill patients 1.5 mg/kg daily or on alternate days

PoM **Fungilin®** (Squibb)
Tablets, yellow, scored, amphotericin 100 mg. Price 20 tabs = E. Label: 9
Lozenges—see section 12.3.2
Suspension (= mixture), yellow, amphotericin 100 mg/ml. Do not dilute. Price 12 ml = E. Label: 9, counselling advised, use of pipette
PoM **Fungizone®** (Squibb)
Intravenous infusion, powder for reconstitution, amphotericin (as sodium deoxycholate complex). Price 50-mg vial = E

FLUCYTOSINE

Indications: systemic yeast infections

Cautions: renal and hepatic impairment, blood disorders, liver-function tests and blood counts required, plasma concentrations monitored in renal impairment; pregnancy, breast-feeding

Side-effects: nausea, vomiting, diarrhoea, rashes, thrombocytopenia, leucopenia

Dose: by mouth or intravenous infusion, 100–200 mg/kg daily in 4 divided doses; reduce dose in renal impairment

PoM **Alcobon®** (Roche)
Tablets, scored, flucytosine 500 mg. Price 20 tabs = H (Hosp. only)
Intravenous infusion, flucytosine 10 mg/ml. Price 250-ml infusion bottle and giving set = I (Hosp. only)

GRISEOFULVIN

Indications: dermatophyte infections

Cautions: rarely aggravation or precipitation of systemic lupus erythematosus. Drug interactions: see Appendix 1 (sections *2.8A*, 5.2, 7)

Contra-indications: liver failure, porphyria

Side-effects: headache, nausea, vomiting, rashes, photosensitivity

Dose: 0.5–1 g daily, in divided doses or as a single dose; CHILD, 10 mg/kg daily in divided doses or as a single dose

PoM **Griseofulvin Tablets,** griseofulvin 125 mg,

price 20 tabs = **B**; 500 mg, price 20 tabs = **E**. Label: 9, 21

PoM **Fulcin**® (ICI)
Tablets, scored, griseofulvin 125 mg. Price 20 tabs = **B**. Label: 9, 21
Tablets, f/c, griseofulvin 500 mg. Price 20 tabs = **E**. Label: 9, 21
Suspension (= mixture), brown, griseofulvin 125 mg/5 ml. Diluent syrup, life of diluted mixture 14 days. Price 100 ml = **C**. Label: 9, 21

PoM **Grisovin**® (Glaxo)
Tablets, f/c, griseofulvin 125 mg. Price 20 tabs = **B**. Label: 9, 21
Tablets, f/c, griseofulvin 500 mg. Price 20 tabs = **E**. Label: 9, 21

KETOCONAZOLE

Indications: dermatophyte infections; systemic fungal infections, candidiasis; prophylaxis in immunosuppressed patients
Cautions: avoid in hepatic impairment; pregnancy (toxicity in *animal* studies). Drug interactions: see Appendix 1 (sections *2.8C*, 5.2, *8*)
Side-effects: rarely nausea, rashes, pruritus; fatal liver damage—for CSM advice see notes above
Dose: 200 mg once daily with food, until at least 1 week after symptoms have cleared and cultures become negative; max. 400 mg daily. CHILD, 3 mg/kg daily
Vaginal candidiasis, 400 mg daily with food for 5 days

▼ PoM **Nizoral**® (Janssen)
Tablets, scored, ketoconazole 200 mg. Price 20 tabs = **H**. Label: 5, 9, 21
Suspension (= mixture), pink, ketoconazole 100 mg/5 ml. Price 100 ml = **H**. Label: 5, 9, 21

MICONAZOLE

Indications: systemic fungal infections, candidiasis, dermatophyte infections
Cautions: change infusion site to avoid phlebitis; pregnancy. Drug interactions: see Appendix 1 (sections *2.8B*, *4.8*, *6.1*)
Side-effects: nausea and vomiting, pruritus, rashes
Dose: by mouth, 250 mg every 6 hours
By intravenous infusion, initially, 600 mg every 8 hours; CHILD, max. 15 mg/kg every 8 hours up to 40 mg/kg/day
For use as a bladder washout, see section 7.4.4

Daktarin® (Janssen)
PoM *Tablets*, scored, miconazole 250 mg. Price 20 tabs = **J**. Label: 9, 21
Oral gel, sugar-free, miconazole 25 mg/ml. Price 40 g = **E**. Label: 9, 21, counselling advised, hold in mouth
PoM *Intravenous solution*, miconazole 10 mg/ml with Cremophor EL. For dilution and use as an infusion. Price 20-ml amp = **D** (Hosp. only)

NATAMYCIN

Indications: candidiasis
Dose: by inhalation, 2.5 mg every 8 hours

PoM **Pimafucin**® (Brocades)
Oral suspension—see section 12.3.2
Suspension for inhalation, natamycin 25 mg/ml. Price 20 ml = **F**

NYSTATIN

Indications: candidiasis
Side-effects: nausea, vomiting, diarrhoea
Dose: by mouth, intestinal candidiasis 500 000 units every 6 hours, doubled in severe infections; CHILD 100 000 units 4 times daily
For use as a mouth-wash in oral candidiases, see section 12.3.2

PoM **Nystatin Mixture**, nystatin 100 000 units/ml. Do not dilute. Price 30 ml = **E**. Label: 9, counselling advised, measure with pipette

PoM **Nystan**® (Squibb)
Tablets, brown, s/c, nystatin 500 000 units. Price 20 tabs = **D**. Label: 9
Pastilles—see section 12.3.2
Suspension (= mixture), yellow, nystatin 100 000 units/ml. Do not dilute. Measure with pipette. Price 30 ml with pipette = **E**. Label: 9, counselling advised, measure with pipette

PoM **Nystatin-Dome**® (Bayer)
Suspension (= mixture), yellow, nystatin 100 000 units/ml. Price 30 ml with 1-ml spoon = **E**. Label: 9, counselling advised, measure with 1-ml spoon

5.3 Antiviral drugs

The specific therapy of virus infections is generally unsatisfactory and treatment is, therefore, primarily symptomatic. Fortunately, the majority of infections resolve spontaneously.

Acyclovir is active against *Herpes simplex* and varicella/zoster viruses. Uses include the treatment of *H. simplex* virus infections of the skin and mucous membranes, including initial and recurrent infections. To be effective the drug should be given as early as possible in the illness. Unfortunately, acyclovir will not eradicate herpes viruses from root ganglia and will not therefore produce a lasting cure in recurrent infections. Topical and oral preparations are used in the treatment of *H. simplex* infections of the skin and mucous membranes. Intravenous injection is used to treat severe *H. simplex* infections and to treat varicella/zoster infections in the immunocompromised patient. Care should be taken with the dose of acyclovir in patients with renal impairment. See also section 13.10.3; for use in herpetic conjunctivitis see section 11.3.1.

Idoxuridine is active against herpes viruses; it is too toxic for systemic administration, a problem with many antiviral drugs, but has been used in the treatment of *Herpes simplex* lesions of the skin, eye, and external genitalia with variable results. Idoxuridine is also used for the topical treatment of shingles, in which it is claimed to reduce the duration of pain and lessen the incidence of post-herpetic neuralgia. However, to be effective, it must be applied early in the illness as soon as the first skin lesions appear. For use in herpetic skin diseases, see section 13.10.3; for use in herpetic conjunctivitis, see section 11.3.1; for use in oral lesions, see section 12.3.2.

Amantadine (Symmetrel®), given by mouth, has been used for the prophylaxis of influenza A infections and for the treatment of shingles.

Vidarabine (Vira-A®) is used in immuno-suppressed patients for the treatment of serious infections caused by herpes viruses; these include varicella, zoster, and *Herpes simplex* infections. For use in herpetic conjunctivitis, see section 11.3.1.

Inosine pronobex (Imunovir®) is a newly introduced drug for the management of *H. simplex* infections.

ACYCLOVIR

Indications: Herpes simplex infections (see notes above)

Cautions: maintain adequate hydration; reduce dose in renal impairment; pregnancy. Drug interactions: see Appendix 1 (section 5.3)

Side-effects: reversible increases in plasma urea and creatinine and liver-related enzymes, decreases in haematological indices, neurological reactions, rashes

Dose: by mouth, 200 mg 5 times daily, usually for 5 days

By slow intravenous infusion, 5 mg/kg over 1 hour, repeated every 8 hours

▼ PoM **Zovirax**® (Wellcome)

Tablets, blue, acyclovir 200 mg. Price 10 tabs = I. Label: 9

Suspension (= mixture), off-white, acyclovir 200 mg/5 ml. Diluent syrup or sorbitol solution for 1 + 1 dilution, life of diluted mixture 28 days. Price 125 ml = J. Label: 9

Intravenous infusion, powder for reconstitution, acyclovir (as sodium salt). Price 250-mg vial = I

AMANTADINE HYDROCHLORIDE

Indications: influenza A prophylaxis, herpes zoster

Cautions; Contra-indications; Side-effects: see section 4.9.1

Dose: 100 mg every 12 hours

PoM **Symmetrel**® (Geigy)

Capsules, brown, amantadine hydrochloride 100 mg. Price 20 caps = F

Syrup (= elixir), amantadine hydrochloride 50 mg/5 ml. Diluent syrup, life of diluted elixir 28 days. Price 150 ml = F

INOSINE PRANOBEX

Indications: mucocutaneous *Herpes simplex* infections

Cautions: avoid in renal impairment; history of gout or hyperuricaemia

Side-effects: reversible increases in serum and urinary uric acid

Dose: 4 g daily in divided doses for 7–14 days

▼ PoM **Imunovir**® (Burgess)

Tablets, inosine pranobex 500 mg. Price 20 tabs = H. Label: 9

VIDARABINE

Indications: chicken-pox and herpes zoster infections in immunosuppressed patients

Cautions: reduce dose in renal impairment; blood counts required

Contra-indications: pregnancy, breast-feeding

Side-effects: anorexia, nausea, vomiting, diarrhoea; tremor, ataxia, dizziness, confusion; decreased haematocrit, white cell count, and platelet count

Dose: by slow intravenous infusion, 10 mg/kg daily for at least 5 days

PoM **Vira-A**® (P-D)

Injection, vidarabine 200 mg/ml. For dilution and use as an infusion. Price 5-ml vial = J

5.4   Antiprotozoal drugs

Prophylaxis and treatment of protozoal infections frequently require expert management and advice is available from the Liverpool School of Tropical Medicine (051-708 9393), the Hospital for Tropical Diseases (01-387 4411), or the East Birmingham Hospital (021-772 4311).

Many of the drugs and proprietary preparations mentioned in the notes in section 5.4 are not generally available in the U.K. Details are given only for those which are available.

5.4.1   Antimalarials
5.4.2   Amoebicides
5.4.3   Trichomonacides
5.4.4   Antigiardial drugs
5.4.5   Leishmaniacides
5.4.6   Trypanocides
5.4.7   Drugs for toxoplasmosis

5.4.1   Antimalarials

TREATMENT OF BENIGN TERTIAN MALARIA. **Chloroquine** is the drug of choice for the treatment of benign tertian malaria, which is usually caused by *Plasmodium vivax* and less commonly by *P. ovale* and *P. malariae*. Dosage by mouth is summarised in Table 3.

If the patient is vomiting or seriously ill, chloroquine sulphate can be given by intramuscular or slow intravenous injection in a dose equivalent to 200–300 mg of chloroquine in 250 ml of sodium chloride intravenous infusion. If after 6 hours the patient still cannot take tablets a second injection should be given. The drug should not be given intravenously to infants as it can have cardiovascular side-effects. Chloroquine causes cerebral and ocular changes if given in excessive dosage.

Table 3. Chloroquine therapeutic dosage

Age (years)	Day	Dose (tablets)
Up to 1	1	½ initially
		½ after 6–8 hours
	2–5	½ daily
1–2	1	1 initially
		¾ after 6–8 hours
	2–5	½ daily
3–5	1	2 initially
		1 after 6–8 hours
	2–5	½ daily
6–12	1	2 initially
		1 after 6–8 hours
	2–5	1 daily
13–15	1	3–4 initially
		1–2 after 6–8 hours
	2–4	1–2 daily
Adult	1	4 initially
		2 after 6–8 hours
	2–3	1 twice daily

Note: Tablets contain equivalent of 150 mg chloroquine (base)

ERADICATION OF BENIGN TERTIAN MALARIA. **Primaquine** in a dose of 15 mg daily (7.5 mg for children) should be given for 14 to 21 days following the treatment of benign tertian malaria with chloroquine, to destroy parasites in the liver and prevent relapses. Before starting primaquine the blood should be tested for glucose-6-phosphate dehydrogenase (G-6-PD) activity as the drug can cause haemolysis in patients who are deficient in the enzyme.

TREATMENT OF MALIGNANT TERTIAN MALARIA. **Chloroquine** in the dosage schedule outlined above is also effective in malignant tertian malaria. However, strains of *P. falciparum* resistant to chloroquine are becoming increasingly common particularly in South-east Asia including the Indian subcontinent, Central and South America, and Central and East Africa.

If the patient has come from one of these areas, or is seriously ill, **quinine** should be given by intravenous infusion over 2–4 hours in a dose of 10 mg/kg of base. For Thai strains of *P. falciparum* a loading dose of 20 mg/kg of base is advocated. The total dose should not normally exceed 2 g over 24 hours and 3 doses should be given at intervals of 8 hours depending on the size of the patient, severity of infection, and evidence of renal or liver disease (when the intervals should be increased). Following a course of quinine the patient should be given Fansidar® (3 tablets). Some strains of *P. falciparum* are now resistant to both chloroquine and Fansidar®. In these cases quinine with tetracycline seems to be effective; however, expert advice should be sought since other drugs may become available. If quin-

ine is not available the same dose of quinidine may be used as an alternative.

For patients who are not seriously ill quinine can be given by mouth in a dose of 600 mg every 8 hours for at least 3 days, followed by a single dose of 3 tablets of Fansidar®. Quinine is well tolerated by children, although the salts are bitter; infants from birth to 1 year are given one-tenth the adult dose, and for older children the dose is calculated from the formula:

$$\text{Approximate dose} = \frac{\text{age}}{20} \times \text{adult dose}$$

Quinine should not be given intravenously to infants but may be given by intramuscular injection in a dose not exceeding 5 mg/kg.

CHEMOPROPHYLAXIS. The chemoprophylaxis of malaria is becoming more complex as a result of drug resistance, and varies for different areas of the world. Up-to-the-minute advice may be obtained from the centres listed at the beginning of section 5.4. The most important point to remember is that **prophylaxis is relative and not absolute**, and that breakthrough can occur with any of the drugs recommended anywhere in the world.

Prophylactic drugs should be taken from the day before travel into an endemic area until at least 4 weeks after leaving it. For the **Indian subcontinent** give chloroquine 300 mg once weekly and proguanil 200 mg daily. For **Southeast Asia**, **Central** and **South America**, and **Oceania** give Fansidar® or Maloprim® 1 tablet once weekly together with chloroquine 300 mg once weekly. [**Important: see p. 453**].

For the **Middle East** and **Africa**, give chloroquine 300 mg once weekly, except **Angola**, the **Comoros Islands**, **Kenya**, **Madagascar** (Republic of Malagasy), **Malawi**, **Namibia**, **Sudan**, **Tanzania**, **Uganda**, and **Zambia**, where Fansidar® or Maloprim® should be used as above in conjunction with chloroquine. For these countries some authorities consider the use of chloroquine 300 mg *or* amodiaquine 400 mg once weekly together with proguanil 200 mg daily a less toxic alternative, even though the risk of breakthrough may be greater than with Fansidar® or Maloprim®. Fansidar® is contra-indicated in sulphonamide sensitivity. [**Important: see p. 453**].

PROPHYLAXIS IN CHILDREN. Except where indicated in the appropriate entry, drugs are given following the same regimens as in adults, but with doses reduced as follows, using body-weight if available: under 5 kg (under 1 year), one-quarter adult dose; 5 to 20 kg (1 to 5 years) one-half adult dose; 20 to 40 kg (6 to 12 years), three-quarters adult dose; and over 40 kg (over 12 years), adult dose. Prophylaxis is required in breast-fed infants; although antimalarials are excreted in milk, the amounts are too variable to give reliable protection.

PROPHYLAXIS IN PREGNANCY. Chloroquine may be given in usual doses in areas where *P. falciparum*

C = 51-100p, D = 101-180p, E = 181-300p, F = 301-450p, G = 451-650p, H = 651-900p, I = 901-1200p, J = over 1200p.

is sensitive. The centres listed in section 5.4 should be consulted for advice on prophylaxis in chloroquine-resistant areas.

AMODIAQUINE

Indications: chemoprophylaxis of malaria
Cautions: see under Chloroquine
Side-effects: nausea, vomiting, diarrhoea, lethargy; rarely agranulocytosis and other blood disorders, hepatitis, peripheral neuropathy; on prolonged treatment corneal deposits, blue-grey pigmentation of skin, finger nails, hard palate
Dose: see notes above

Camoquin® (P-D)
Tablets, yellow, f/c, scored, amodiaquine 200 mg (as hydrochloride). Price 20 tabs = **D**

CHLOROQUINE

Indications: benign and malignant tertian malaria, amoebiasis.
Cautions: impaired renal or hepatic function, psoriasis, porphyria, ocular examinations in long-term treatment
Side-effects: headache, nausea, vomiting, diarrhoea, rashes; pruritus; rarely psychotic episodes, convulsions; corneal and retinal changes with prolonged high dosage (may be irreversible)
Dose: see Table 3 and notes above
Note: chloroquine base 150 mg ≡ chloroquine sulphate 200 mg ≡ chloroquine phosphate 250 mg (approx.)

Avloclor® (ICI)
Tablets, scored, chloroquine phosphate 250 mg. Price 20 tabs = **B**
Malarivon® (Wallace Mfg)
Syrup (= elixir), chloroquine phosphate 80 mg/5 ml. Price 75 ml = **C**
Nivaquine® (M&B)
Tablets, scored, chloroquine sulphate 200 mg. Price 20 tabs = **C**
Syrup (= elixir), red, chloroquine sulphate 68 mg/5 ml. Diluent syrup, life of diluted elixir 14 days. Price 60 ml = **C**
PoM *Injection,* chloroquine 40 mg (as sulphate)/ml. Price 5-ml amp = **B**

HYDROXYCHLOROQUINE SULPHATE

Indications: malaria
Cautions; Side-effects: see under Chloroquine
Dose: malaria, treatment, 800 mg initially, 400 mg after 6–8 hours, then 400 mg daily for 2 days
Prophylaxis, 400 mg weekly

Plaquenil® (Sterling Research)
Tablets, orange, s/c, hydroxychloroquine sulphate 200 mg. Price 20 tabs = **G**

PRIMAQUINE

Indications: eradication of benign tertian malaria
Cautions: see notes above; pregnancy

Side-effects: anorexia, nausea, vomiting, jaundice; less commonly bone-marrow depression, methaemoglobinaemia, haemolytic anaemia
Dose: see notes above

Primaquine Tablets, s/c, primaquine 7.5 mg (as phosphate). Price 20 tabs = **A**

PROGUANIL HYDROCHLORIDE

Indications: chemoprophylaxis of malaria
Side-effects: mild gastric intolerance
Dose: see notes above

Paludrine® (ICI)
Tablets, scored, proguanil hydrochloride 100 mg. Price 20 tabs = **A**. Label: 21

PYRIMETHAMINE

Indications: chemoprophylaxis of malaria
Cautions: hepatic or renal impairment, folate supplements in pregnancy, blood counts required with high doses. Drug interactions: see Appendix 1 (section *8*)
Side-effects: depression of haemopoiesis with prolonged treatment, rashes
Dose: see notes above

Daraprim® (Wellcome)
Tablets, scored, pyrimethamine 25 mg. Price 20 tabs = **C**
PoM **Fansidar**® (Roche)
Tablets, scored, pyrimethamine 25 mg, sulfadoxine 500 mg. Price 20 tabs = **F**
Dose: see notes above
PoM **Maloprim**® (Wellcome)
Tablets, scored, pyrimethamine 12.5 mg, dapsone 100 mg. Price 20 tabs = **C**
Dose: 1 tablet weekly; CHILD 5–9 years ½ tablet weekly

QUININE

Indications: malignant tertian malaria
Cautions: atrial fibrillation, conduction defects, heart block, pregnancy. Drug interactions: see Appendix 1 (section *2.1*)
Contra-indications: haemoglobinuria, optic neuritis
Side-effects: cinchonism, including tinnitus, headache, nausea, abdominal pain, rashes, visual disturbances, blindness; hypersensitivity reactions including angioedema
Dose: see notes above
Note: quinine (anhydrous base) 100 mg ≡ quinine bisulphate 169 mg ≡ quinine dihydrochloride 122 mg ≡ quinine hydrochloride 122 mg ≡ quinine sulphate 121 mg

PoM **Quinine Bisulphate Tablets,** s/c, or f/c, quinine bisulphate 300 mg. Price 20 tabs = **C**
PoM **Quinine Dihydrochloride Tablets,** quinine dihydrochloride 300 mg. Price 20 tabs = **D**
PoM **Quinine Hydrochloride Tablets,** quinine hydrochloride 300 mg. Price 20 tabs = **D**
PoM **Quinine Sulphate Tablets,** s/c or f/c, quinine sulphate 125 mg. Price 20 tabs = **B**

PoM **Quinine Sulphate Tablets,** s/c or f/c, quinine sulphate 200, and 300 mg. Price 20 tabs (both) = C

5.4.2 Amoebicides

Metronidazole (section 5.1.11.1) is the drug of choice for acute invasive amoebic dysentery for it is very effective against vegetative amoebae in ulcers at a dosage of 800 mg three times a day for 5 days. It is also effective against amoebae which may have migrated to the liver. Much of it is absorbed and excreted in the urine, which becomes dark in colour. Side-effects include anorexia, giddiness, and lassitude. It is given either for 10 days, or for 5 days followed by a 10-day course of diloxanide furoate.

Metronidazole is relatively ineffective in chronic intestinal amoebiasis in which only cysts are present in the stool.

Diloxanide furoate (Furamide®) is the drug of choice in chronic infections in which only cysts and not vegetative forms of *E. histolytica* are present in the faeces. It is relatively free from toxic effects in therapeutic doses and the usual course is of 10 days, given alone for chronic infections or following 5 days of metronidazole in acute dysenteric infections.

Emetine hydrochloride and **emetine and bismuth iodide** have now been largely replaced by metronidazole and are rarely used for they are associated with more nausea and have a smaller margin of safety between the therapeutic and the cardiotoxic dose.

For the treatment of amoebic abscesses of the liver **metronidazole** is effective in doses of 400 mg 3 times daily for 5–10 days and the course may be repeated after 2 weeks if necessary.

If metronidazole is not available emetine may be used but its side-effects are more marked. Diloxanide is not effective against hepatic amoebiasis, but a 10-day course should be given at the completion of metronidazole or emetine treatment to destroy the cysts in the gut.

Chloroquine (section 5.4.1) is concentrated in the liver and for adults a dosage of 600 mg (base) daily for 5 days followed by 300 mg (base) daily for 14 to 21 days is effective but is slower and less certain in its action than metronidazole. For abscesses containing more than 100 ml of pus (i.e. approximately 60 to 100 mm in diameter) aspiration carried out in conjunction with drug therapy will greatly reduce the period of disability.

DILOXANIDE FUROATE

Indications: chronic amoebiasis—see notes above
Side-effects: flatulence, vomiting, urticaria, pruritus
Dose: 500 mg every 8 hours for 10 days—see notes above

PoM **Entamizole®** (Boots)
Tablets, off-white, diloxanide furoate 250 mg, metronidazole 200 mg. Label: 4, 9, 21, 25

Dose: amoebiasis 2 tablets 3 times daily for 5 days; CHILD 5–12 years ½–1 tablet, according to age, for 5 days
Treatment may be extended to 10 days in refractory cases; not suitable for prophylactic use
PoM **Furamide®** (Boots)
Tablets, scored, diloxanide furoate 500 mg. Label: 9

5.4.3 Trichomonacides

Metronidazole (section 5.1.11.1) is the treatment of choice for *Trichomonas vaginalis* infection. It is given by mouth after meals; 200 mg 3 times daily for 7 days, 800 mg in the morning and 1.2 g at night for 2 days, or a single 2-g dose have given satisfactory results.

If metronidazole is ineffective, **nimorazole** (Naxogin®) may be tried; it is usually given as a single 2-g dose, with food.

Alcohol should be avoided during treatment with both metronidazole and nimorazole.

NIMORAZOLE

Indications: trichomoniasis (acute ulcerative gingivitis, see section 12.3.2)
Contra-indications: active CNS disease, severe renal failure
Side-effects: nausea, vomiting, rashes, vertigo, drowsiness, ataxia (discontinue treatment), intolerance to alcohol
Dose: see notes above

Naxogin 500® (Farmitalia Carlo Erba)
Tablets, scored, nimorazole 500 mg. Price 4 tabs = B. Label: 4, 21

5.4.4 Antigiardial drugs

Metronidazole (section 5.1.11.1) is the treatment of choice for *Giardia lamblia* infections, given by mouth in a dosage of 2 g daily for 3 days, or 400 mg every 8 hours for 7 days.

Alternative treatments are **tinidazole** (section 5.1.11.1) 1.5–2 g as a single dose or **mepacrine hydrochloride** 100 mg every 8 hours for 5–8 days.

5.4.5 Leishmaniacides

Cutaneous leishmaniasis frequently heals spontaneously without specific treatment. If the skin lesions are extensive or unsightly, treatment is indicated, as it is in visceral leishmaniasis (kala-azar).

Sodium stibogluconate (Pentostam®), an organic pentavalent antimony compound, is the treatment of choice. The dose is 10 mg/kg daily for 30 days by intramuscular or intravenous injection. Skin lesions are treated for 10 days.

SODIUM STIBOGLUCONATE

Indications: leishmaniasis
Cautions: intravenous injections must be given slowly and stopped if coughing or substernal pain develops
Contra-indications: pneumonia, myocarditis, nephritis, hepatitis

---

C = 51-100p, D = 101-180p, E = 181-300p, F = 301-450p, G = 451-650p, H = 651-900p, I = 901-1200p, J = over 1200p.

Side-effects: anorexia, vomiting, coughing, substernal pain
Dose: see notes above

PoM **Pentostam**® (Wellcome)
Injection, sodium stibogluconate equivalent to pentavalent antimony 100 mg/ml. Price 100-ml bottle = **J**

5.4.6 Trypanocides

The prophylaxis and treatment of trypanosomiasis is difficult and differs according to the strain of organism. Expert advice should therefore be obtained.

5.4.7 Drugs for toxoplasmosis

Most infections caused by *Toxoplasma gondii* are self-limiting, and treatment is not necessary. Exceptions are patients with eye involvement, and those who are immunosuppressed. The treatment of choice is a combination of pyrimethamine and a sulphonamide, given for several weeks. Pyrimethamine is a folate antagonist, and adverse reactions to this combination are relatively common.

5.5 Anthelmintics

Prophylaxis and treatment of helminth infections frequently requires expert management and advice is available from the Liverpool School of Tropical Medicine (051-708 9393), the Hospital for Tropical Diseases (01-387 4411), or the East Birmingham Hospital (021-772 4311).

Many of the drugs and proprietary preparations mentioned in the notes in section 5.5 are not generally available in the U.K. Details are given only for those which are available.

5.5.1 Drugs for threadworms
5.5.2 Ascaricides
5.5.3 Taenicides
5.5.4 Drugs for hookworms
5.5.5 Schistosomicides
5.5.6 Filaricides
5.5.7 Drugs for guinea worms
5.5.8 Drugs for strongyloidiasis

5.5.1 Drugs for threadworms

(pinworms, *Enterobius vermicularis*)

Anthelmintics are relatively ineffective in threadworm infections, and their use should be combined with hygienic measures to break the cycle of auto-infection. All members of the family require treatment.

Adult threadworms do not live for longer than 6 weeks and for development of fresh worms, ova must be swallowed and exposed to the action of digestive juices in the upper intestinal tract. Direct multiplication of worms does not take place in the large bowel. Adult female worms lay ova on the peri-anal skin and cause pruritus by so doing; scratching the area then leads to ova being transmitted on fingers to the mouth, often via food

eaten with unwashed hands. Washing the hands and fingers with the aid of a nail brush before each meal and after each visit to the toilet is essential. A bath taken immediately after rising will remove ova laid during the night and limit their dissemination.

Mebendazole (Vermox®) in a single dose of 100 mg is the drug of choice for patients of all ages over 2 years.

Piperazine salts including the citrate and phosphate are used. Piperazine may be given in doses equivalent to the following quantities of piperazine hydrate: up to 2 years 50–75 mg/kg, 2–4 years 750 mg, 5–12 years 1.5 g, adults and children over 12 years 2 g. These doses are given daily for 7 days.

Pyrantel (Combantrin®) given as a single dose of 10 mg/kg (max. 1 g) is equally effective.

MEBENDAZOLE

Indications: threadworm,   roundworm, whipworm, and hookworm infections
Cautions: pregnancy (toxicity in *animal* studies)
Contra-indications: children under 2 years
Side-effects: rarely abdominal pain, diarrhoea
Dose: see notes above and sections 5.5.2 and 5.5.4

PoM **Vermox**® (Janssen)
Tablets, pink, scored, chewable, mebendazole 100 mg. Price 6 tabs = **E**
Suspension (= mixture), mebendazole 100 mg/5 ml. Price 30 ml = **E**

PIPERAZINE

Indications: threadworm infections
Cautions: impaired renal function, psychiatric states, neurological disease
Contra-indications: epilepsy, renal failure, liver disease
Side-effects: nausea, vomiting, diarrhoea, urticaria; rarely dizziness, paraesthesia, muscular incoordination
Dose: see notes above
Note: 100 mg piperazine hydrate ≡ 125 mg piperazine citrate ≡ 104 mg piperazine phosphate

Piperazine Citrate Elixir, green, piperazine citrate equivalent to piperazine hydrate 750 mg/5 ml (see Formulary). Price 100 ml = **B**
Antepar® (Wellcome)
Tablets, yellow, scored, piperazine hydrate 500 mg (as phosphate). Price 28 tabs = **E**. Label: 24
Elixir, orange, piperazine hydrate 750 mg/5 ml (as hydrate and citrate). Diluent syrup, life of diluted elixir 14 days. Price 100 ml = **D**
Ascalix® (Wallace Mfg)
Syrup (= elixir), piperazine hydrate 750 mg (as citrate)/5 ml. Price 75 ml = **D**. Also 4 g in 20-ml sachet, price each = **A**; 4 g in 30-ml bottle, price each = **B**
Pripsen® (R&C)
Oral powder, cream, piperazine phosphate 4 g

Relative prices: **A** = up to 20p, **B** = 21-50p,

and sennosides 15.3 mg/sachet. Price 2 sachets = **C**. Label: 13

Dose: stirred into a small glass of milk or water, adults and children over 6 years, 1 sachet; INFANTS 3 months–1 year, 5 ml granules; CHILDREN 1–6 years, 10 ml granules. Repeat after 14 days

5.5.2 Ascaricides
(common roundworm infections)

Levamisole is very effective against ascaris and is generally considered to be the drug of choice. It is very well tolerated; mild nausea or vomiting has been reported in about 1% of treated patients; it is given as a single dose of 150 mg in adults.

Mebendazole (section 5.5.1) is also active against *Ascaris lumbricoides*; the usual dose is 100 mg twice daily for 1 day (3 days for whipworm).

Pyrantel (Combantrin®) is also an effective broad-spectrum anthelmintic and a single dose of 10 mg/kg (max. 1 g) is usually sufficient to eradicate ascaris; it may occasionally produce mild nausea but experience shows it to be a very safe drug.

PYRANTEL
Indications: roundworm, hookworm, and whip-worm infections
Cautions: liver disease
Side-effects: see notes above
Dose: ADULT and CHILD over 6 months, see notes above and section 5.5.4

PoM **Combantrin**® (Pfizer)
Tablets, orange, pyrantel 125 mg (as embonate). Price 6 tabs = **C**; 25 tabs = **E**

5.5.3 Taenicides
(tapeworms)

Niclosamide (Yomesan®) is the most widely used drug for tapeworm infections and side-effects is limited to occasional gastro-intestinal upset, light-headedness, and pruritus. Fears of developing cysticercosis in *T. solium* infections have proved unfounded. All the same, it is wise to anticipate this possibility by using an anti-emetic on wakening.

Praziquantel is as effective as niclosamide and is given as a single dose of 5–10 mg/kg after a light breakfast.

NICLOSAMIDE
Indications: tapeworm infections—see notes above
Side-effects: gastro-intestinal discomfort
Dose: 2 g on an empty stomach taken as two 1-g doses separated by a 1-hour interval, followed by a purgative after 2 hours; CHILD up to 2 years, 500 mg, 2–6 years, 1 g

Yomesan® (Bayer)
Tablets, yellow, chewable, niclosamide 500 mg. Price 4 tabs = **D**. Label: 24, 27

5.5.4 Drugs for hookworms
(ancylostomiasis, necatoriasis)

Hookworms live in the upper small intestine and draw blood from the point of their attachment to their host. An iron-deficiency anaemia may thereby be produced and, if present, effective treatment of the infection requires not only expulsion of the worms but treatment of the anaemia.

Tetrachloroethylene is still the most widely used drug for hookworm infection. It is best administered in a suspension rather than in capsules so that effective action of the drug on the worms in the upper intestine can be assured. Alcohol and fatty foods should be avoided following treatment with tetrachloroethylene as they increase its absorption and therefore hepatotoxicity. Toxic effects are rare but occasionally nausea and headache or drowsiness may be experienced. It should be avoided in debilitated patients or young children.

Bephenium is widely used and its side-effects are limited to occasional nausea and vomiting. A single dose of 2.5 g is given and repeated after 1–2 days. It is thought to be more effective against *Ancylostoma duodenale* than against *Necator americanus*. **Pyrantel** (section 5.5.2) is very effective against hookworms and, like bephenium, has side-effects limited to occasional nausea and vomiting. A single dose of 10 mg/kg to a maximum of 1 g is given for 3 days.

Bitoscanate and **thiabendazole** (section 5.5.8) are also used, as is levamisole. **Mebendazole** (section 5.5.1) has a useful broad-spectrum activity, and is effective against hookworms; the usual dose is 100 mg twice daily for 3 days.

BEPHENIUM
Indications: roundworm and hookworm infections
Side-effects: nausea, vomiting, diarrhoea, headache, vertigo
Dose: see notes above

Alcopar® (Wellcome)
Granules, yellow/green, bephenium 2.5 g (as hydroxynaphthoate)/sachet. Price per sachet = **B**. Label: 13

5.5.5 Schistosomicides
(bilharziasis)

Adult *Schistosoma haematobium* worms live in the genito-urinary veins and adult *S. mansoni* in those of the colon and mesentery. *S. japonicum* is more widely distributed in veins of the alimentary tract and portal system.

Praziquantel (Biltricide®) is effective against all human schistosomes. The dose is 40 mg/kg as a single oral dose. No serious toxic effects have been reported. Of all the available schistosomicides, it has the most attractive combination of effectiveness, broad-spectrum activity, and low toxicity.

Oxamniquine (Mansil®, Vansil®) is effective against *S. mansoni* infections only. It is a quinoline

---

C = 51-100p, D = 101-180p, E = 181-300p, F = 301-450p, G = 451-650p, H = 651-900p, I = 901-1200p, J = over 1200p.

compound given by mouth in doses of 15–60 mg/ kg daily for 1 to 3 days. Toxicity is insignificant.

Metriphonate (Bilarcil®) is an organophosphorus compound which is only effective against *S. haematobium* infections. It is given by mouth in 3 doses of 7.5 mg/kg at intervals of 2 to 4 weeks. Toxicity is negligible, but as it reduces plasmacholinesterase concentrations it should be used with caution in patients likely to be frequently exposed to organophosphorus insecticides.

Hycanthone, lucanthone, niridazole, and stibocaptate have now been superseded.

5.5.6   Filaricides

Diethylcarbamazine (Banocide®) is highly effective against microfilariae and adults of *Loa loa* and of *Wuchereria bancrofti* and against the microfilariae of *Onchocerca volvulus*. It is less effective against adult *O. volvulus*. The destruction of the microfilariae is associated with release of antigens and a resulting allergic response. Headache, nausea, and sometimes vomiting are complained of and in onchocerciasis the filarial dermatitis may be temporarily aggravated and conjunctivitis and punctate keratitis temporarily increased. Antihistamines may be helpful in controlling these reactions but topical corticosteroids may be required for the skin irritation in severely affected patients.

With the object of limiting allergic responses in onchocerciasis, treatment is commenced with a dose of 1 mg/kg bodyweight, gradually increased over 3 days to 6 mg/kg daily in divided doses; this dosage is maintained for 21 days. Close medical supervision is necessary particularly in the early phase of treatment. **Diethylcarbamazine** is the treatment of choice for all patients with filarial infection; onchocerciasis is the most resistant of these but even heavily infected patients usually respond to 3–4 courses given at intervals of several months as required.

In very persistent cases **suramin** may be used for it is active against adult worms although it has little action on microfilariae. It is nephrotoxic and it is for this reason that its use is usually withheld except in chronically relapsing cases. When used, a preliminary test dose of 200 mg is administered intravenously and if well tolerated is followed by an increasing weekly dose of 0.4, 0.6, 0.8, and 1 g dissolved in 10 ml of water for injections given intravenously. The whole course of treatment

lasts 5 weeks. It is important to ensure that the urine is free from albumin and casts which if present contra-indicate further suramin treatment.

DIETHYLCARBAMAZINE CITRATE

Indications: filariasis

Cautions; Side-effects: see notes above

Dose: see notes above

Banocide® (Wellcome)

Tablets, scored, diethylcarbamazine citrate 50 mg. Price 20 tabs = C. Label: 9

5.5.7   Drugs for guinea worms
(dracontiasis)

Guinea worms, *Dracunculus medinensis*, may be killed and their removal from the tissues facilitated by a course of **niridazole** (Ambilhar®). Use of niridazole does not obviate the concomitant need for sterile dressing of the ulcer caused by a guinea worm and for its extraction, wherever possible, under sterile conditions. In India, mebendazole has been reported as effective at a dosage of 200 mg twice daily for 7 days.

5.5.8   Drugs for strongyloidiasis

Adult *Strongyloides stercoralis* live in the gut and produce larvae which penetrate the gut wall and invade the tissues, setting up a cycle of autoinfection. **Thiabendazole** is the drug of choice, at a dosage of 25 mg/kg every 12 hours for 3 days.

THIABENDAZOLE

Indications: strongyloid, threadworm, guinea worm, roundworm, and hookworm infections

Cautions: hepatic or renal impairment, if drowsiness occurs warn patients not to drive, discontinue if hypersensitivity reactions occur

Side-effects: anorexia, nausea, vomiting, dizziness, diarrhoea, headache, pruritus, drowsiness; hypersensitivity reactions including fever, chills, angioedema, rashes, erythema multiforme; rarely tinnitus, collapse, parenchymal liver damage

Dose: see notes above

Mintezol® (MSD)

Tablets, orange, chewable, thiabendazole 500 mg. Price 6 tabs = C. Label: 3, 21, 24

6: Drugs used in the treatment of disorders of the
ENDOCRINE SYSTEM

In this chapter, drug treatment is discussed under the following headings:

6.1 Drugs used in diabetes
6.2 Thyroid and antithyroid drugs
6.3 Corticosteroids
6.4 Sex hormones
6.5 Hypothalamic and pituitary hormones
6.6 Drugs affecting bone metabolism
6.7 Other endocrine drugs

6.1 Drugs used in diabetes

Two groups of drugs are used in the treatment of diabetes, insulin preparations (section 6.1.1) and oral hypoglycaemic drugs (section 6.1.2).

The treatment of diabetic ketoacidosis or hyperosmolar non-ketotic 'coma' (section 6.1.3) and hypoglycaemia (section 6.1.4) is also discussed.

6.1.1 Insulin

6.1.1.1 Short-acting insulin preparations
6.1.1.2 Intermediate- and long-acting insulin preparations

Insulin plays a key role in the body's regulation of carbohydrate, fat, and protein metabolism. Diabetes mellitus is due to a deficiency in insulin synthesis and secretion, and the severity of the metabolic disturbance is directly related to the extent of the insulin deficiency. Patients with extreme deficiency require long-term replacement therapy with insulin, while those with a less marked deficiency may be able to maintain apparently normal health by dietary restriction of carbohydrate alone.

Insulin is a polypeptide hormone of complex structure; it is extracted from beef or pork pancreas and purified by crystallisation, or it can be made biosynthetically by recombinant DNA technology using *Escherichia coli*. All insulin preparations are to a greater or lesser extent immunogenic in man but immunological resistance to insulin action is uncommon. When it does occur, it may be overcome by changing to a pure pork or biosynthetic preparation.

Insulin is inactivated by gastro-intestinal enzymes if given by mouth, and it must therefore be given by injection; the subcutaneous route is ideal for most circumstances. Insulin is usually injected into the upper arms, thighs, buttocks, or abdomen. There may be increased absorption from a limb site if that limb is used in strenuous exercise. Insulin can also be given by continuous subcutaneous infusion using soluble insulin in an infusion pump. This technique now has an established place in the treatment of diabetes, and provides continuous basal insulin infusion with preprandial boosts. Its chief benefit is the considerable improvement in quality of life enjoyed by some patients, and, at times, the elimination of troublesome hypoglycaemia. There is, at present, only slender evidence of a beneficial effect on diabetic complications, and no proof of harmful effects. It is unsuitable for emotionally or psychiatrically disturbed patients, and thus does not provide a general solution for 'brittle' diabetics. There are many disadvantages to this technique, especially the tendency to rapid development of ketoacidosis, together with the bulkiness of the apparatus, risk of mechanical failure, difficulties with vigorous physical activities, some tendency to gain weight, and sometimes problems from skin sepsis. Patients using it must be well-motivated, reliable, and able to monitor their own blood glucose, and must have access to expert advice both day and night.

When treating diabetic ketoacidosis (section 6.1.3), insulin should be given by intravenous and/or intramuscular injection, since absorption from subcutaneous depots may be slow and erratic.

Minor allergic reactions at the sites of injections are still common during the first few weeks of treatment; they are usually transient and require no treatment. Lipo-atrophy is uncommon with highly-purified insulin preparations: if it does develop, it can sometimes be reversed by the use of injections of neutral pork insulin.

CHOICE OF TREATMENT. About 25% of diabetics require insulin treatment; apart from those presenting in ketoacidosis, insulin is needed by most of those with a rapid onset of symptoms, weight loss, weakness, and sometimes vomiting, often associated with ketonuria. The majority of those who are obese can be managed by restriction of carbohydrate or energy intake alone or with the subsequent administration of oral hypoglycaemic drugs. Most children require insulin from the outset.

MANAGEMENT OF DIABETIC PATIENTS. Since insulin secretion fluctuates from minute to minute in normal subjects, it is impossible to maintain normoglycaemia in the majority of diabetics by insulin injections once, twice, or even thrice daily. Symptoms are relieved rapidly as glycosuria is controlled. The aim of treatment is to achieve the best possible control of plasma glucose without disabling hypoglycaemia, and close co-operation is needed between the patient and the medical team. To achieve control, mixtures of available insulin preparations may be required (such as Insulin Injection and Isophane Insulin Injection) and these combinations have to be worked out for the individual patient. Insulin requirements may be affected by variations in lifestyle, infection, and steroids, and sometimes by a very small amount when the oral contraceptive pill is taken. In pregnancy insulin requirements should be

---

C = 51-100p, D = 101-180p, E = 181-300p, F = 301-450p, G = 451-650p, H = 651-900p, I = 901-1200p, J = over 1200p.

assessed frequently by an experienced diabetic physician.

The energy and carbohydrate intake must be adequate to allow normal growth and development but obesity must be avoided. The carbohydrate intake must be regulated in non-obese patients on insulin and should be distributed throughout the day. Fine control of plasma glucose can be achieved by moving portions of carbohydrate from one meal to another without altering the total intake.

Insulin doses are determined on an individual basis, by gradually increasing the dose but avoiding troublesome hypoglycaemic reactions. Care should be taken to avoid inducing obesity by the administration of too much insulin.

There are three main types of insulin preparations:
1. those of **short** duration which have a relatively rapid onset of action, for example Insulin Injection (Soluble);
2. those with an **intermediate** action, for example Isophane Insulin Injection and Insulin Zinc Suspension, Amorphous (Insulin Semilente); and
3. those whose action is slower in onset and lasts for **long** periods, for example Insulin Zinc Suspension (Insulin Lente and Ultralente) and Protamine Zinc Insulin.

The duration of action of different insulin preparations varies considerably from one patient to another, and needs to be assessed for every individual. The durations of action indicated below are only approximations. The type of insulin used and its dose and frequency of administration depend on the particular needs of the patient. Most patients are best started on insulins of intermediate action twice daily and a short-acting insulin can later be added to cover any hyperglycaemia which may follow breakfast or evening meal.

HUMAN INSULINS. There are differences in the amino-acid sequence in animal and human insulins, and until recently all available insulins reflected the sequence in the animal (ox or pig) from which they had been prepared. Recently insulin of human sequence prepared by modification of porcine material (emp) or biosynthetically (crb) has become available. Preparations of human sequence insulin should theoretically be less immunogenic, but in trials no real advantage has been shown. Human sequence insulins are as effective as the highly-purified animal insulins and should be used in approximately the same dosage.

CONVERSION TO 100 UNITS PER ML. Insulin preparations of 100 units/ml strength were introduced into the United Kingdom in March 1983 to replace the existing 20, 40, and 80 unit strengths. All patients using insulin were to be transferred to the 100 unit/ml strength within 2 years. At the same time patients were issued with U-100 syringes, graduated in units rather than marks, for use with the 100 unit/ml strength insulin. Three syringes are available under the National Health Service: 0.5-ml syringes for injections up to 50 units, 1-ml syringes for injections up to 100 units, and a preset syringe for partially-sighted patients. The introduction of a single insulin strength is intended to reduce the potential for error that exists with the other strengths and to reduce injection volume.

6.1.1.1   SHORT-ACTING INSULIN PREPARATIONS

Insulin Injection (soluble or regular insulin) is a clear solution of insulin with an acid pH (about 3.2). When injected subcutaneously, its effect is maximal in 2–4 hours and lasts for up to 12 hours, although the duration of action is affected by the amount given. It is the only appropriate insulin for use in diabetic emergencies of all kinds, and at the time of operation. In maintenance regimens it is usual to give the first dose 15 to 30 minutes before breakfast. See section 6.1.3 for use in ketoacidosis.

Neutral Insulin Injection has the advantage of being neutral in reaction and very similar in action to soluble insulin. The neutral solution allows more rapid absorption and reduces the incidence of discomfort at the site of injection. See section 6.1.3 for use in ketoacidosis.

INSULIN INJECTION
(Soluble Insulin)
  Indications: diabetes mellitus; diabetic keto-acidosis (section 6.1.3)
  Cautions: see notes above; reduce dose in renal impairment. Drug interactions: see Appendix 1 (section 6.1)
  Side-effects: see notes above; local reactions and lipo-atrophy at injection site; overdose causes hypoglycaemia
  Dose: by subcutaneous, intramuscular, or intravenous injection or intravenous infusion, according to patient's requirements

Insulin Injection, 20 units/ml, price 10-ml vial = **D**; 40 units/ml, price 10-ml vial = **E**; 80 units/ml, price 10-ml vial = **F**; 320 units/ml, price 5-ml vial = **G**

Highly purified insulins
Insulin Injection (bovine, highly purified), 100 units/ml, price 10-ml vial = **G**

NEUTRAL INSULIN INJECTION
(Neutral Insulin)
  Indications: diabetes mellitus; diabetic keto-acidosis (section 6.1.3)
  Cautions; Side-effects; Dose: see under Insulin Injection

Highly purified insulins
Neutral Insulin Injection (bovine, highly purified), 100 units/ml. Price 10-ml vial = **G**
Actrapid MC® (Novo)
  Injection, neutral insulin (porcine, highly purified) 100 units/ml, price 10-ml vial = **H**

For all abbreviations and symbols see inside cover.   Relative prices: **A** = up to 20p, **B** = 21-50p,

Hypurin Neutral® (CP)
Injection, neutral insulin (bovine, highly purified) 40 units/ml, price 10-ml vial = **E**; 100 units/ml, price 10-ml vial = **G**

Neusulin® (Wellcome)
Injection, neutral insulin (bovine, highly purified) 40 units/ml, price 10-ml vial = **E**; 100 units/ml, price 10-ml vial = **G**

Quicksol® (Boots)
Injection, neutral insulin (bovine, highly purified) 100 units/ml, price 10-ml vial = **G**

Velosulin® (Nordisk Wellcome)
Injection, neutral insulin (porcine, highly purified) 100 units/ml, price 10-ml vial = **G**

Human insulins

▼ **Human Actrapid®** (Novo)
Injection, neutral insulin (human, emp) 100 units/ml, price 10-ml vial = **H**

▼ **Human Velosulin®** (Nordisk Wellcome)
Injection, neutral insulin (human, emp) 100 units/ml, price 10-ml vial = **G**

▼ **Humulin S®** (Lilly)
Injection, neutral insulin (human, crb) 100 units/ml, price 10-ml vial = **G**

6.1.1.2 INTERMEDIATE- AND LONG-ACTING INSULIN PREPARATIONS

When given by subcutaneous injection these preparations have an onset of action in approximately 1–2 hours, a maximal effect at 4–12 hours, and a duration of 16–35 hours. They are used to provide background levels in insulin regimens. Some are given twice daily in conjunction with the short-acting insulins, and others are given once daily, particularly in elderly patients. They are unsuitable for intramuscular or intravenous administration.

Isophane Insulin Injection is a suspension of insulin with protamine which is of particular value for initiation of twice-daily insulin regimens. It can readily be combined with neutral insulin to produce a stable mixture retaining the properties of its two components. Patients usually mix isophane with neutral insulin but ready-mixed preparations (Initard 50/50® and Mixtard 30/70®) may be appropriate; Initard 50/50® has a more intense initial effect than Mixtard 30/70®.

Biphasic Insulin Injection (Rapitard MC®) is another ready-mixed insulin suitable for twice-daily injection.

Insulin Zinc Suspension (Amorphous) has an intermediate duration and **Insulin Zinc Suspension (crystalline)** a more prolonged duration of action. These preparations may be used independently or in **Insulin Zinc Suspension** (30% amorphous, 70% crystalline). The duration of action of these insulins may be modified for use in once-daily regimens, although insulin zinc suspension and insulin zinc suspension (amorphous) are usually given twice daily. Porcine and human insulin zinc suspensions have a shorter duration of action than bovine insulins of similar formulation.

Protamine Zinc Insulin is usually given once daily in conjunction with a short-acting insulin. It has the drawback of binding with the short-acting insulins when mixed in the same syringe, and is now rarely used.

BIPHASIC INSULIN INJECTION
A suspension of crystalline bovine insulin (3 parts) in a neutral solution of porcine insulin (1 part)
Indications: diabetes mellitus (intermediate acting)
Cautions; Side-effects: see under Insulin Injection (section 6.1.1.1)
Dose: by subcutaneous injection, according to patient's requirements

Rapitard MC® (Novo)
Injection, biphasic insulin injection (highly purified) 100 units/ml, price 10-ml vial = **G**

INSULIN ZINC SUSPENSION
(Insulin Zinc Suspension, Mixed; I.Z.S.)
Indications: diabetes mellitus (long acting)
Cautions; Side-effects: see under Insulin Injection (section 6.1.1.1)
Dose: by subcutaneous injection, according to patient's requirements

Insulin Zinc Suspension, Lente, 40 units/ml, price 10-ml vial = **E**; 80 units/ml, price 10-ml vial = **F**
Highly purified insulins
Insulin Zinc Suspension Lente (bovine, highly purified) 100 units/ml. Price 10-ml vial = **G**

Hypurin Lente® (CP)
Injection, insulin zinc suspension (bovine, highly purified) 40 units/ml, price 10-ml vial = **E**; 80 units/ml, price 10-ml vial = **F**; 100 units/ml, price 10-ml vial = **H**

Lentard MC® (Novo)
Injection, insulin zinc suspension (bovine and porcine, highly purified) 100 units/ml, price 10-ml vial = **G**

Monotard MC® (Novo)
Injection, insulin zinc suspension (porcine, highly purified) 100 units/ml, price 10-ml vial = **H**

Neulente® (Wellcome)
Injection, insulin zinc suspension (bovine, highly purified) 40 units/ml, price 10-ml vial = **E**; 80 units/ml, price 10-ml vial = **G**; 100 units/ml, price 10-ml vial = **G**

Tempulin® (Boots)
Injection, insulin zinc suspension (bovine, highly purified) 100 units/ml, price 10-ml vial = **G**

Human insulins

▼ **Human Monotard®** (Novo)
Injection, insulin zinc suspension (human, emp) 100 units/ml, price 10-ml vial = **H**

C = 51-100p, **D** = 101-180p, **E** = 181-300p, **F** = 301-450p, **G** = 451-650p, **H** = 651-900p, **I** = 901-1200p, **J** = over 1200p.

INSULIN ZINC SUSPENSION (AMORPHOUS)

(Amorph. I.Z.S.)

Indications: diabetes mellitus (intermediate acting)

Cautions; Side-effects: see under Insulin Injection (section 6.1.1.1)

Dose: by subcutaneous injection, according to patient's requirements

Insulin Zinc Suspension (Amorphous), Semi-lente, 40 units/ml, price 10-ml vial = **E**
Semitard MC® (Novo)
Injection, insulin zinc suspension (amorphous) (porcine, highly purified) 100 units/ml, price 10-ml vial = **H**

INSULIN ZINC SUSPENSION (CRYSTALLINE)

(Cryst. I.Z.S.)

Indications: diabetes mellitus

Cautions; Side-effects: see under Insulin Injection (section 6.1.1.1)

Dose: by subcutaneous injection, according to patient's requirements
Note: preparations of animal insulin are long acting; preparations of human insulin are intermediate acting

Insulin Zinc Suspension (Crystalline), Ultra-lente, 40 units/ml, price 10-ml vial = **E**; 80 units/ml, price 10-ml vial = **F**
Ultratard MC® (Novo)
Injection, insulin zinc suspension, crystalline (bovine, highly purified) 100 units/ml, price 10-ml vial = **G**

Human insulins
Human Ultratard® (Novo)
Injection, insulin zinc suspension, crystalline (human, emp) 100 units/ml, price 10-ml vial = **H**
▼ **Humulin Zn®** (Lilly)
Injection, insulin zinc suspension, crystalline (human crb) 100 units/ml, price 10-ml vial = **G**

ISOPHANE INSULIN INJECTION

(Isophane Insulin (NPH); Isophane Protamine Insulin Injection)

Indications: diabetes mellitus (intermediate acting)

Cautions; Side-effects: see under Insulin Injection (section 6.1.1.1); protamine may cause allergic reactions

Dose: by subcutaneous injection, according to patient's requirements

Isophane Insulin Injection, 40 units/ml, price 10-ml vial = **E**; 80 units/ml, price 10-ml vial = **F**

Highly purified insulins
Isophane Insulin Injection, bovine, highly purified, 100 units/ml. Price 10-ml vial = **G**

Hypurin Isophane® (CP)
Injection, isophane insulin (bovine, highly purified) 100 units/ml, price 10-ml vial = **H**
Insulatard® (Nordisk Wellcome)
Injection, isophane insulin (porcine, highly purified) 100 units/ml, price 10-ml vial = **G**
Monophane® (Boots)
Injection, isophane insulin (bovine, highly purified) 100 units/ml, price 10-ml vial = **G**
Neuphane® (Wellcome)
Injection, isophane insulin (bovine, highly purified) 40 units/ml, price 10-ml vial = **E**; 80 units/ml, price 10-ml vial = **G**; 100 units/ml, price 10-ml vial = **G**

Mixed highly purified insulins
Initard 50/50® (Nordisk Wellcome)
Injection, isophane insulin (porcine, highly purified) 50%, neutral insulin (porcine, highly purified) 50%. 100 units/ml, price 10-ml vial = **G**
Mixtard 30/70® (Nordisk Wellcome)
Injection, isophane insulin (porcine, highly purified) 70%, neutral insulin (porcine, highly purified) 30%. 100 units/ml, price 10-ml vial = **G**

Human insulins
▼ **Human Actraphane®** (Novo)
Injection, isophane insulin (human, emp) 70%, neutral insulin (human, emp) 30%. 100 units/ml, price 10-ml vial = **H**
▼ **Human Initard 50/50®** (Nordisk Wellcome)
Injection, isophane insulin (human, emp) 50%, neutral insulin (human, emp) 50%. 100 units/ml, price 10-ml vial = **G**
▼ **Human Insulatard®** (Nordisk Wellcome)
Injection, isophane insulin (human, emp) 100 units/ml, price 10-ml vial = **G**
▼ **Human Mixtard 30/70®** (Nordisk Wellcome)
Injection, isophane insulin (human, emp) 70%, neutral insulin (human, emp) 30%. 100 units/ml, price 10-ml vial = **G**
▼ **Human Protaphane®** (Novo)
Injection, isophane insulin (human, emp) 100 units/ml, price 10-ml vial = **H**
▼ **Humulin I®** (Lilly)
Injection, isophane insulin (human, crb) 100 units/ml, price 10-ml vial = **G**

PROTAMINE ZINC INSULIN INJECTION

Indications: diabetes mellitus (long acting)

Cautions; Side-effects: see under Insulin Injection (section 6.1.1.1); protamine may cause allergic reactions; see also notes above

Dose: by subcutaneous injection, according to patient's requirements

Protamine Zinc Insulin Injection, 40 units/ml, price 10-ml vial = **E**; 80 units/ml, price 10-ml vial = **F**

Hypurin Protamine Zinc® (CP)
Injection, protamine zinc insulin (bovine, highly purified) 80 units/ml, price 10-ml vial = **G**; 100 units/ml, price 10-ml vial = **H**

6.1.2 Oral hypoglycaemic drugs

6.1.2.1 Sulphonylureas
6.1.2.2 Biguanides
6.1.2.3 Guar gum

Oral hypoglycaemic drugs should not be used until patients have been shown not to respond adequately to a period of at least one month's restriction of energy and carbohydrate intake. They should be used to augment the effect of diet, and not to replace it. Selection of suitable patients is described in section 6.1.1, choice of treatment.

6.1.2.1 SULPHONYLUREAS AND RELATED DRUGS

The sulphonylureas act mainly by augmenting insulin secretion and consequently are effective only when some residual pancreatic beta-cell activity is present. All may lead to hypoglycaemia 4 hours or more after food but this is usually an indication of overdose. Hypoglycaemia occurs most commonly when long-acting sulphonylureas are given to elderly patients or if a meal is missed.
Tolbutamide (Pramidex®, Rastinon®) has a short duration of action and is usually given twice daily. **Chlorpropamide** (Diabinese®, Melitase®) has a more prolonged action, and need only be given once daily, usually with breakfast or the first main meal. It may cause prolonged hypoglycaemia, particularly in the elderly and in those with renal disease; a short-acting drug such as tolbutamide is preferable in the elderly.
Glibenclamide (Daonil®, Euglucon®) has a duration of action intermediate between tolbutamide and chlorpropamide, but is usually given once daily.
Other sulphonylureas include acetohexamide (Dimelor®), glibornuride (Glutril®), gliclazide (Diamicron®), glipizide (Glibenese®, Minodiab®), gliquidone (Glurenorm®), and tolazamide (Tolanase®).
Glymidine (Gondafon®) is a related compound which shows most of the properties of the sulphonylureas. It may be tried cautiously in sulphonylurea hypersensitivity.

CAUTIONS AND CONTRA-INDICATIONS. These drugs tend to encourage weight gain and should only be prescribed if poor control and symptoms persist despite adequate attempts at dieting. They should not be used during breast-feeding, and caution is needed in the elderly and those with renal failure because of the hazard of hypoglycaemia. The short-acting tolbutamide may be used in renal impairment, as may gliquidone and gliclazide as the latter are principally metabolised and inactivated in the liver; they should be used with caution in patients with impaired hepatic function.
Insulin therapy should be instituted temporarily during intercurrent illness (such as myocardial infarction, coma, infection, and trauma) and during surgery since control of diabetes with the sulphonylureas is usually inadequate in such circumstances. Insulin therapy is also usually substituted during pregnancy. Sulphonylureas are contra-indicated in the presence of ketosis. Drug interactions: see Appendix 1 (section 6.1).

SIDE-EFFECTS. These are generally mild and infrequent.
Chlorpropamide may cause facial flushing after drinking alcohol; this effect is not normally witnessed with other sulphonylureas.
Sensitivity reactions (usually in first 6–8 weeks of therapy) include transient rashes which rarely progress to erythema multiforme and exfoliative dermatitis, fever, and jaundice; photosensitivity has also rarely been reported with chlorpropamide. Blood dyscrasias are rare but include thrombocytopenia, agranulocytosis, and aplastic anaemia.

ACETOHEXAMIDE

Indications: diabetes mellitus
Cautions; Contra-indications; Side-effects: see notes above
Dose: initially 0.25–1.5 g daily, adjusted according to response; up to 500 mg given as a single daily dose, higher doses divided

PoM **Dimelor®** (Lilly)
Tablets, yellow, scored, acetohexamide 500 mg. Price 20 tabs = **C**

CHLORPROPAMIDE

Indications: diabetes mellitus (for use in diabetes insipidus, see section 6.5.2)
Cautions; Contra-indications; Side-effects: see notes above
Dose: initially 250 mg daily (elderly patients 100–125 mg), adjusted according to response; max. 500 mg daily; taken with breakfast

PoM **Chlorpropamide Tablets,** chlorpropamide 100 mg, price 20 tabs = **B**; 250 mg, price 20 tabs = **C**. Label: 4
PoM **Diabinese®** (Pfizer)
Tablets, scored, chlorpropamide 100 mg. Price 20 tabs = **C**. Label: 4
Tablets, scored, chlorpropamide 250 mg. Price 20 tabs = **D**. Label: 4
PoM **Glymese®** (DDSA)
Tablets, scored, chlorpropamide 250 mg. Price 20 tabs = **B**. Label: 4
PoM **Melitase®** (Berk)
Tablets, scored, chlorpropamide 100 mg. Price 20 tabs = **B**. Label: 4
Tablets, scored, chlorpropamide 250 mg. Price 20 tabs = **C**. Label: 4

GLIBENCLAMIDE

Indications: diabetes mellitus
Cautions; Contra-indications; Side-effects: see notes above

C = 51-100p, D = 101-180p, E = 181-300p, F = 301-450p, G = 451-650p, H = 651-900p, I = 901-1200p, J = over 1200p.

Dose: initially 5 mg daily (elderly patients 2.5 mg), adjusted according to response; max. 15 mg daily; taken with breakfast

PoM **Glibenclamide Tablets,** glibenclamide 2.5 mg, price 20 tabs = **D**; 5 mg, price 20 tabs = **E**

PoM **Daonil**® (Hoechst)
Tablets, scored, glibenclamide 5 mg. Price 20 tabs = **E**

PoM **Semi-Daonil**® (Hoechst)
Tablets, scored, glibenclamide 2.5 mg. Price 20 tabs = **D**

PoM **Euglucon**® (Roussel)
Tablets, glibenclamide 2.5 mg. Price 20 tabs = **D**
Tablets, scored, glibenclamide 5 mg. Price 20 tabs = **E**

PoM **Libanil**® (APS)
Tablets, glibenclamide 2.5 mg. Price 20 tabs = **D**
Tablets, scored, glibenclamide 5 mg. Price 20 tabs = **D**

PoM **Malix**® (Lagap)
Tablets, glibenclamide 2.5 mg. Price 20 tabs = **C**
Tablets, glibenclamide 5 mg. Price 20 tabs = **D**

GLIBORNURIDE
Indications: diabetes mellitus
Cautions; Contra-indications; Side-effects: see notes above
Dose: initially 12.5 mg daily, adjusted according to response; max. 75 mg daily; up to 50 mg may be given as a single dose with breakfast; higher doses, the remainder in the evening

PoM **Glutril**® (Roche)
Tablets, scored, glibornuride 25 mg. Price 20 tabs = **D**

GLICLAZIDE
Indications: diabetes mellitus
Cautions; Contra-indications: see notes above
Side-effects: gastro-intestinal disturbances, nausea, headache, rashes
Dose: initially, 40–80 mg daily, adjusted according to response; max. 320 mg daily; up to 80 mg as a single dose, with breakfast; higher doses divided with the main meals

PoM **Diamicron**® (Servier)
Tablets, scored, gliclazide 80 mg. Price 20 tabs = **E**

GLIPIZIDE
Indications: diabetes mellitus
Cautions; Contra-indications; Side-effects: see notes above
Dose: initially 2.5–5 mg daily, adjusted according to response; max. 40 mg daily; up to 15 mg may be given as a single dose before breakfast; higher doses divided before main meals

PoM **Glipizide Tablets,** glipizide 5 mg. Price 20 tabs = **C**

PoM **Glibenese**® (Pfizer)
Tablets, scored, glipizide 5 mg. Price 20 tabs = **D**

PoM **Minodiab**® (Farmitalia Carlo Erba)
Tablets, scored, glipizide 5 mg. Price 20 tabs = **C**

GLIQUIDONE
Indications: diabetes mellitus
Cautions; Contra-indications; Side-effects: see notes above
Dose: initially 15 mg daily, adjusted according to response; max. 180 mg daily; up to 60 mg as a single dose with breakfast, higher doses divided with meals

PoM **Glurenorm**® (Winthrop)
Tablets, scored, gliquidone 30 mg. Price 20 tabs = **E**

GLYMIDINE
Indications: diabetes mellitus
Cautions; Contra-indications; Side-effects: see notes above
Dose: initially 1.5 g daily, with breakfast, adjusted according to response; max. 2 g daily (1.5 g at breakfast and 500 mg in late afternoon)

PoM **Gondafon**® (Schering)
Tablets, scored, glymidine 500 mg. Price 20 tabs = **E**

TOLAZAMIDE
Indications: diabetes mellitus
Cautions; Contra-indications; Side-effects: see notes above
Dose: initially 100–250 mg daily with breakfast adjusted according to response; max. 1 g daily

PoM **Tolanase**® (Upjohn)
Tablets, scored, tolazamide 100 mg. Price 20 tabs = **B**
Tablets, scored, tolazamide 250 mg. Price 20 tabs = **D**

TOLBUTAMIDE
Indications: diabetes mellitus
Cautions; Contra-indications; Side-effects: see notes above
Dose: 0.5–1.5 g (max. 2 g) daily in divided doses

PoM **Tolbutamide Tablets,** tolbutamide 500 mg. Price 20 tabs = **B**

PoM **Glyconon**® (DDSA)
Tablets, scored, tolbutamide 500 mg. Price 20 tabs = **B**

PoM **Pramidex**® (Berk)
Tablets, scored, tolbutamide 500 mg. Price 20 tabs = **B**

PoM **Rastinon**® (Hoechst)
Tablets, scored, tolbutamide 500 mg. Price 20 tabs = **C**

6.1.2.2 BIGUANIDES

Metformin (Glucophage®), the only available biguanide, acts in a different way from the sulphonylureas, and should not be regarded as interchangeable with them. It is thought to exert its hypoglycaemic effect mainly by increasing peripheral utilisation of glucose and is only effective in diabetics with functioning pancreatic islet cells. Metformin is most frequently used in overweight diabetics who will not, or cannot, lose weight. It does not exert a hypoglycaemic action in non-diabetic subjects unless given in overdose.

Metformin is not free from the hazard of lactic acidosis which, however, occurs almost exclusively in renal failure patients, in whom it should not be used.

METFORMIN HYDROCHLORIDE
Indications: diabetes mellitus (see notes above)
Cautions: see notes above; breast-feeding. Drug interactions: see Appendix 1 (section 6.1)
Contra-indications: renal or hepatic failure, predisposition to lactic acidosis, heart failure, severe infection or trauma, dehydration, alcoholism
Side-effects: anorexia, nausea, vomiting, diarrhoea (usually transient), lactic acidosis (withdraw treatment), decreased vitamin-B_{12} absorption
Dose: 500 mg every 8 hours *or* 850 mg every 12 hours after food; max. 3 g daily in divided doses

PoM **Glucophage**® (Lipha)
Tablets, f/c, metformin hydrochloride 500 mg. Price 20 tabs = **B**. Label: 21
Tablets, f/c, metformin hydrochloride 850 mg. Price 20 tabs = **C**. Label: 21

6.1.2.3 GUAR GUM

Guar gum, if taken in adequate quantities, results in some reduction of postprandial plasma-glucose concentrations, probably by retarding carbohydrate absorption.

GUAR GUM
Indications: control of postprandial plasma-glucose concentrations in diabetes mellitus
Cautions: maintain adequate fluid intake
Contra-indications: gastro-intestinal obstruction
Side-effects: flatulence, abdominal distension, intestinal obstruction

Glucotard® (MCP)
Sachets (containing mini-tablets), guar gum 5 g/sachet. Price 20 sachets = **E**. Label: 27, counselling advised, food
Dose: 5 g 3 times daily immediately before meals with fluids
Guarem® (Rybar)
Granules, cream, guar gum 5 g/sachet. Price 20 sachets = **E**. Label: 13, counselling advised, food

Dose: 5 g stirred into 200 ml liquid 3 times daily before meals
Lejguar® (Britannia)
Granules, white/yellow, guar gum 90%. Price 250 g (with 3.5-g scoop) = **G**. Label: 13, counselling advised, food
Dose: 7 g 3 times daily for 6 weeks, reducing to 7 g twice daily; 3.5 g in 100 ml liquid, followed by a further 100 ml, before food and 3.5 g with liquid during the meal

6.1.3 Treatment of diabetic ketoacidosis

A clear solution (**insulin injection** or **neutral insulin injection**) is the only form of insulin that may be given intravenously and it should be used in the management of diabetic ketoacidotic and hyperosmolar nonketotic coma. It is preferable to use the type of insulin (standard, highly purified, or human sequence) that the patient has been using previously. It is necessary to achieve and to maintain an adequate plasma-insulin concentration until the metabolic disturbance is brought under control.

If a slow infusion pump is available, insulin is probably best given by the intravenous route; a single bolus (however large) will only achieve an adequate concentration for a short period of time. Adequate plasma concentrations are usually maintained with infusion rates of 5 units/hour for adults and 0.1 units/kg/hour for children. Insulin is diluted in sodium chloride 0.9% infusion to a concentration of 1 unit/ml.

If the response is judged inadequate the infusion rate may be doubled or quadrupled. When plasma glucose has fallen to 10 mmol/litre the rate of infusion can be dropped to about 0.02 units/kg/hour (1 to 2 units/hour for adults) and continued until the patient is ready to take food by mouth. The insulin infusion should not be stopped before subcutaneous insulin is started.

If facilities for administering insulin by continuous infusion are inadequate it may be given by intramuscular injection. Absorption of insulin after intramuscular administration is usually rapid but may be impaired in patients who are hypotensive or who have poor peripheral circulation. An initial loading dose of 20 units is followed by 6 units given every hour until the plasma glucose concentration is less than 10 mmol/litre. Doses are then given by intramuscular injection every 2 hours.

In the presence of hypotension and poor tissue perfusion the intravenous route of insulin administration is preferable. Depots of insulin may build up during treatment and late hypoglycaemia should be watched for and treated appropriately.

6.1.4 Treatment of hypoglycaemia

Initially, glucose or 3 or 4 lumps of sugar should be taken with a little water. If necessary, this may be repeated in 10 to 15 minutes.

If hypoglycaemia causes unconsciousness, up to 50 ml of **50% glucose intravenous infusion** should be given intravenously (see section 9.2.2), or glucose or sucrose may be given by stomach tube.

Glucagon can be given as an alternative to parenteral glucose in hypoglycaemia. It is a polypeptide hormone produced by the alpha cells of the islets of Langerhans. Its action is to increase plasma glucose concentration by mobilising glycogen stored in the liver.

Glucagon is used to treat acute hypoglycaemic reactions and it has the advantage that it can be injected by any route (intramuscular, subcutaneous, or intravenous) in a dose of 1 mg (1 unit) in circumstances when an intravenous injection of glucose would be difficult or impossible to administer.

It may be issued to close relatives of insulin-treated patients for emergency use in hypoglycaemic attacks. It is often advisable to prescribe on an 'if necessary' basis to all hospitalised insulin-treated patients, so that it may be given rapidly by the nurses during an hypoglycaemic emergency. If not effective in 20 minutes intravenous glucose should be given.

Diazoxide (Eudemine®), administered by mouth, is useful in the management of patients with chronic hypoglycaemia from excess endogenous insulin secretion, either from an islet cell tumour or islet cell hyperplasia. It has no place in the management of acute hypoglycaemia.

___

DIAZOXIDE

Indications: chronic intractable hypoglycaemia (for use in hypertensive crisis see section 2.5.1)
Cautions: ischaemic heart disease, pregnancy, labour, impaired renal function; haematological examinations and blood pressure monitoring required during prolonged treatment. Drug interactions: see Appendix 1 (section *6.1*)
Side-effects: anorexia, nausea, vomiting, hypertrichosis, hyperuricaemia, hypotension, oedema, tachycardia, arrhythmias, extrapyramidal effects; hypertrichosis on prolonged treatment
Dose: by mouth, adults and children, initially 5 mg/kg daily in 2–3 divided doses

PoM **Eudemine**® (A&H)
Tablets, s/c, diazoxide 50 mg. Price 20 tabs = **D**

GLUCAGON

Indications: acute hypoglycaemia
Cautions: see notes above. Ineffective in chronic hypoglycaemia, starvation, and adrenal insufficiency
Contra-indications: insulinoma, phaeochromocytoma, glucagonoma
Side-effects: nausea, vomiting, rarely hypersensitivity reactions
Dose: by subcutaneous, intramuscular, or intravenous injection, adults and children 0.5–1 unit repeated after 20 minutes if necessary
Note: 1 unit of glucagon = 1 mg of glucagon or glucagon hydrochloride

PoM **Glucagon Injection,** powder for reconstitution, glucagon (as hydrochloride, with lactose). Price 1-unit vial = **F**; 10-unit vial = **J** (both with diluent)

6.2   Thyroid and antithyroid drugs

6.2.1 Thyroid hormones
6.2.2 Antithyroid drugs

6.2.1   Thyroid hormones

Thyroid hormones are used in hypothyroidism (myxoedema), and also in diffuse non-toxic goitre, lymphadenoid goitre, and thyroid carcinoma. Neonatal hypothyroidism requires prompt treatment for normal development.

Thyroxine sodium (Eltroxin®) is the treatment of choice for maintenance therapy. The initial dose should not exceed 50 to 100 micrograms daily, preferably before breakfast, or 25 micrograms in elderly patients or those with cardiac disease, increased by 25 to 50 micrograms at intervals of 2 to 4 weeks. The usual maintenance dose to relieve hypothyroidism is 100 to 200 micrograms daily. If side-effects develop, dosage should be reduced or withheld for 1 to 2 days before re-introduction at a lower dosage.

In infants a daily dose of 50 micrograms and in children over 1 year of age 2.5 to 5 micrograms/kg should be given initially; subsequent therapy can be judged from clinical response, skeletal maturation, and plasma-thyroxine (T_4) and thyroid-stimulating hormone measurements.

Liothyronine sodium (Tertroxin®) has a similar action to thyroxine but is more rapidly metabolised; 20 micrograms is equivalent to 100 micrograms of thyroxine. Its effects develop after a few hours and disappear within 24 to 48 hours of discontinuing treatment. It may be used in severe hypothyroid states when a rapid response is desired. Liothyronine or thyroxine may be used in conjunction with carbimazole as part of the blocking-replacement regimen in the treatment of hyperthyroidism.

Liothyronine by intravenous injection is the treatment of choice in hypothyroid coma. Adjunctive therapy includes intravenous fluids, hydrocortisone, and antibiotics; assisted ventilation is often required.

Dried **thyroid** should **not** be used as its effects are unpredictable.

LIOTHYRONINE SODIUM

(L-Tri-iodothyronine sodium)
Indications: see notes above
Cautions: adrenal insufficiency. Drug interactions: see Appendix 1 (sections *2.8, 2.8B,* 6.2)
Contra-indications: angina, cardiovascular disorders
Side-effects: arrhythmias, anginal pain, tachycardia, cramps in skeletal muscles, headache, restlessness, excitability, flushing, sweating, diarrhoea, excessive weight loss

___

Dose: by mouth, initially 10–20 micrograms daily in 2–3 divided doses gradually increased to 20 micrograms 3 times daily; elderly patients should receive smaller initial doses, gradually increased; CHILD, adult dose reduced in proportion to body-weight

By slow intravenous injection, hypothyroid coma, 5-20 micrograms repeated 12-hourly or more frequently (4-hourly if necessary); alternatively 50 micrograms initially then 25 micrograms 8-hourly, reducing to 25 micrograms twice daily

PoM **Tertroxin**® (Glaxo)
Tablets, scored, liothyronine sodium 20 micrograms. Price 20 tabs = **A**
PoM **Triiodothyronine** (Glaxo)
Injection, powder for reconstitution, liothyronine sodium (with dextran). Price 20-microgram amp = **F**

THYROXINE SODIUM
Indications: hypothyroidism
Cautions; Contra-indications; Side-effects: see under Liothyronine Sodium; has a delayed effect and cumulative action
Dose: see notes above

PoM **Thyroxine Tablets**, thyroxine sodium 25, 50, and 100 micrograms. Price 20 tabs (all) = **A**
PoM **Eltroxin**® (Glaxo)
Tablets, scored, thyroxine sodium 50 micrograms. Price 20 tabs = **A**
Tablets, thyroxine sodium 100 micrograms. Price 20 tabs = **A**

6.2.2 Antithyroid drugs

Antithyroid drugs are used to prepare patients for thyroidectomy. They are also used for prolonged periods in the hope of inducing life-long remission. In the United Kingdom carbimazole is the most commonly used drug. Propylthiouracil may be used in patients who suffer sensitivity reactions to carbimazole as sensitivity is rarely displayed to both drugs. Both drugs act primarily by interfering with the synthesis of thyroid hormones.

Carbimazole (Neo-Mercazole®) inhibits thyroxine synthesis. It should be given in an initial daily dose of 30 to 60 mg and maintained at this dose until the patient becomes euthyroid, usually 4 to 8 weeks; the dose may then be progressively reduced to a maintenance dose of between 5 and 15 mg daily. Children may be given 15 mg daily, adjusted according to response. Rashes are common, and **propylthiouracil** may then be substituted.

It is no longer considered necessary to space doses of antithyroid drugs evenly throughout the 24 hours and the dose may be given once daily although divided doses are still commonly used. Over-treatment with the rapid development of hypothyroidism is not uncommon and should be avoided particularly during pregnancy since it can cause fetal goitre.

Unless operation or use of radioactive iodine is planned, treatment should be for at least a year, and preferably two.

Potassium perchlorate (Peroidin®) blocks iodine uptake by the thyroid; it is used occasionally when toxic reactions appear with other antithyroid drugs, but may cause hypoplastic or aplastic anaemia and is now used infrequently.

Before partial thyroidectomy **iodine** should be given for about 2 weeks as well as carbimazole or propylthiouracil. Iodine should not be given to patients treated with potassium perchlorate since it leads to an exacerbation of thyrotoxicosis. Iodine can be prescribed as Aqueous Iodine Solution in a dose of 0.1–0.3 ml 3 times daily. Iodine should **not** be used for long-term treatment since its antithyroid action tends to diminish. It may be used as emergency treatment for thyrotoxic crisis since it reduces thyroid hormone release. It may also be used as pre-operative treatment for 10–14 days since there is some evidence that it reduces the vascularity of the thyroid. It may be used in conjunction with propranolol to prepare mildly thyrotoxic patients for operation but it is preferable to render the patient euthyroid with carbimazole prior to surgery.

Radioactive sodium iodide (^{131}I) solution is used for the treatment of thyrotoxicosis, principally in patients over 45 years of age. It may be used in younger patients when compliance is a problem, in the care of patients in whom control with antithyroid drugs is difficult, and in patients who relapse after thyroidectomy.

Propranolol is useful in patients being prepared for thyroidectomy. It is also used in doses of up to 5 mg intravenously in the treatment of thyrotoxic crises ('thyroid storm') in combination with sedation with chlorpromazine.

Propranolol has also been used as an adjunct to radioactive iodine treatment instead of conventional antithyroid drugs. One of its advantages is that it permits laboratory assessment of radio-iodine therapy since laboratory tests of thyroid function are not altered by beta-blockers. In addition beta-blockers are useful in neonatal thyrotoxicosis and in supraventricular arrhythmias due to hyperthyroidism. Presumably all beta-blockers will manifest an antithyroid action, but those without intrinsic sympathomimetic activity, for example **propranolol**, **nadolol**, and **sotalol**, appear preferable. Most experience has been gained with propranolol. For doses and preparations see section 2.4.

For the use of **protirelin** in the diagnosis of hyperthyroidism see section 6.7.2.

CARBIMAZOLE
Indications: thyrotoxicosis
Cautions: pregnancy
Contra-indications: tracheal obstruction, breast-feeding
Side-effects: nausea, headache, rashes, arthralgia; rarely alopecia, agranulocytosis, jaundice
Dose: see notes above

C = 51-100p, **D** = 101-180p, **E** = 181-300p, **F** = 301-450p, **G** = 451-650p, **H** = 651-900p, **I** = 901-1200p, **J** = over 1200p.

PoM **Neo-Mercazole**® (Nicholas)
Tablets, pink, scored, carbimazole 5 mg. Price
20 tabs = **B**

IODINE
Indications: pre-operative treatment of
thyrotoxicosis
Cautions: pregnancy, children
Contra-indications: breast-feeding
Side-effects: hypersensitivity reactions including
coryza-like symptoms, headache, lachrymation, conjunctivitis, pain in salivary glands,
laryngitis, bronchitis, rashes;` on prolonged
treatment depression, insomnia, impotence;
goitre in infants of mothers taking iodides

Aqueous Iodine Solution (Lugol's Solution),
iodine 5%, potassium iodide 10% in purified
water, freshly boiled and cooled, total iodine
130 mg/ml. Price 100 ml = **D**
Dose: 0.1–0.3 ml 3 times daily

POTASSIUM PERCHLORATE
Indications: thyrotoxicosis, but see notes
Cautions: pregnancy
Contra-indications: large or retrosternal goitres
Side-effects: nausea, vomiting, rashes, fever,
fatal aplastic anaemia, agranulocytosis, leucopenia, thrombocytopenia, pancytopenia,
nephrotic syndrome
Dose: initially 200 mg every 6–8 hours; max. 1 g
daily; reduce to 100 mg every 6–8 hours after
2–4 weeks

PoM **Peroidin**® (Larkhall)
Tablets, potassium perchlorate 200 mg. Price 20
tabs = **D**

PROPYLTHIOURACIL
Indications: thyrotoxicosis
Cautions; Contra-indications; Side-effects: see
under Carbimazole; also rarely tendency to
haemorrhage; reduce dose in renal impairment;
caution in breast-feeding
Dose: 300–450 mg daily in divided doses

PoM **Propylthiouracil Tablets,** propylthiouracil
50 mg. Price 20 tabs = **C**

6.3   Corticosteroids

6.3.1 Replacement therapy
6.3.2 Suppression of disease processes
6.3.3 Disadvantages of corticosteroids
6.3.4 Clinical management

6.3.1   Replacement therapy

The adrenal cortex normally secretes hydrocortisone (cortisol) which has predominantly glucocorticoid activity as well as weak mineralocorticoid actions. It also secretes the
mineralocorticoid aldosterone.

In deficiency states, physiological replacement
is best achieved with a combination of oral
hydrocortisone (section 6.3.4) and the mineralocorticoid **fludrocortisone** (Florinef®); hydrocortisone alone does not usually provide sufficient
mineralocorticoid activity for complete replacement. Cortisone is no longer used in replacement
therapy.

Management with the more potent synthetic
glucocorticoids such as prednisolone (with fludrocortisone) though practicable, offers no advantage. They tend to have less mineralocorticoid
activity than hydrocortisone and their greater
potency is only of advantage in the treatment of
inflammatory and neoplastic disease.

In *Addison's disease* or following adrenalectomy, **hydrocortisone** 20 to 30 mg daily by mouth
is usually required. This should be given in 2
doses, the larger in the morning and the smaller
in the evening, mimicking the normal diurnal
rhythm of cortisol secretion. The optimum daily
dose should be determined for each individual on
the basis of clinical response and also, if possible,
by monitoring the plasma-cortisol concentration.
Glucocorticoid therapy should be supplemented
by fludrocortisone 50 to 300 micrograms daily.

In *acute adrenocortical insufficiency*, **hydrocortisone** is given intravenously (as sodium phosphate or succinate) in doses of 100 mg every 6 to
8 hours in sodium chloride intravenous infusion
0.9%. **Prednisolone sodium phosphate** injection
(Codelsol®) is an alternative preparation.

In *hypopituitarism* glucocorticoids should be
given as in adrenocortical insufficiency, but since
the production of aldosterone is also regulated by
the renin-angiotensin system a mineralocorticoid
is not required. Additional replacement therapy
with thyroxine (section 6.2.1) and sex hormones
(section 6.4) should be given as indicated by the
pattern of hormone deficiency that is present.

Corticosteroid cover for *adrenalectomy, hypo-
physectomy* or operations on patients on long-
term treatment with corticosteroids is determined
logically from the knowledge that in a normal
person major stress will not lead to the secretion
of more than 300 mg of cortisol in 24 hours. Once
the stress is over, cortisol production rapidly
returns to the usual 20 to 30 mg per 24 hours. A
simple way of mimicking this is to administer
hydrocortisone, initially parenterally but changing
to oral therapy once this is possible.

On the day of operation hydrocortisone 100 mg
is given intramuscularly (as sodium phosphate or
succinate) with the premedication, and repeated
8-hourly. In the absence of any complications, the
dose can be halved every 24 hours until a normal
maintenance dose of 25 mg per 24 hours is reached
on the 5th postoperative day. In the case of
adrenalectomy it is not necessary to start mineralocorticoid therapy immediately and this can
be withheld until the patient can take tablets. If
there are postoperative complications, hydrocortisone may have to be continued at a slightly
higher dose (50 to 75 mg per 24 hours) and min-

eralocorticoid given parenterally as **deoxycortone pivalate** (Percorten M®).

Dexamethasone and **betamethasone** have little if any mineralocorticoid action and because of their longer action are favoured for suppressing corticotrophin secretion in *congenital adrenal hyperplasia*. In common with all glucocorticoids their suppressive action on the hypothalamic-pituitary-adrenal axis is greatest and most prolonged when they are given at night. In normal subjects a single dose of 1 mg of dexamethasone at night is sufficient to inhibit corticotrophin secretion for 24 hours. This is the basis of the 'overnight dexamethasone suppression test' for diagnosing Cushing's syndrome.

Although most types of *Cushing's syndrome* are treated surgically, that which occasionally accompanies carcinoma of the bronchus is not usually amenable to surgery. **Metyrapone** (section 6.7.2), which interferes directly with steroid synthesis in the adrenal glands, has been found helpful in controlling the symptoms of the disease. Variable dose schedules of metyrapone are in use, but if high doses are given they should be combined with corticosteroid replacement and used under specialist advice.

See also trilostane (section 6.7.4) and aminoglutethimide (see section 8.3.4).

FLUDROCORTISONE ACETATE

Indications: mineralocorticoid replacement in adrenocortical insufficiency

Cautions; Contra-indications; Side-effects: section 6.3.3

Dose: adrenocortical insufficiency, 50–300 micrograms daily; CHILD 5 micrograms/kg daily

PoM **Florinef**® (Squibb)
Tablets, pink, scored, fludrocortisone acetate 100 micrograms. Price 20 tabs = C. Label: 10 steroid card

---

DEOXYCORTONE PIVALATE

Indications: mineralocorticoid replacement in adrenocortical insufficiency

Cautions; Contra-indications; Side-effects: section 6.3.3

Dose: by *intramuscular injection*, 50-100 mg every 2–4 weeks

PoM **Percorten M Crystules**® (Ciba)
Injection (aqueous suspension), deoxycortone pivalate 25 mg/ml. Price 1-ml amp = C. Label: 10 steroid card

For monographs on systemic glucocorticoids, see section 6.3.4

6.3.2 Suppression of disease processes

Betamethasone, dexamethasone, hydrocortisone, prednisolone, and prednisone are used for their anti-inflammatory effect; the Table shows equivalent anti-inflammatory doses.

Table: Equivalent Doses of Glucocorticoids

Drug	Equivalent anti-inflammatory dose (mg)
Betamethasone	0.75
Cortisone acetate	25
Dexamethasone	0.75
Hydrocortisone	20
Methylprednisolone	4
Prednisolone	5
Prednisone	5
Triamcinolone	4

High potency is of no advantage, though the effect on water and electrolyte retention is important. **Prednisolone** is the glucocorticoid most commonly used by mouth for continued treatment. **Prednisone** is only active after conversion in the body to prednisolone. **Betamethasone** and **dexamethasone** are as satisfactory. All must be given in divided doses for a continuous effect. Cortisone acetate and hydrocortisone are not used for inflammatory disease suppression, as they cause fluid retention owing to their higher mineralocorticoid content (section 6.3.1).

Hydrocortisone sodium succinate or **hydrocortisone sodium phosphate** can be given by intravenous injection in *shock* (see also sections 6.3.4 and 3.4.3), although critical evidence of the value of such treatment is lacking. It begins to act within one hour, and since this use is temporary the dangers of high dosage do not apply. Injections of prednisolone can be used in the same way. Betamethasone and dexamethasone are used when water retention would be a disadvantage, as for example in treating traumatic *cerebral oedema* with doses of 16 to 20 mg daily.

The action of corticosteroids in suppressing inflammatory reactions may be useful in conditions such as *rheumatoid arthritis, rheumatic fever, chronic active hepatitis, ulcerative colitis,* and *Crohn's disease*. The prognosis of serious conditions such as *systemic lupus erythematosus* and *polyarteritis nodosa* can be improved. The effects of the disease process may be suppressed and symptoms relieved, but the underlying condition is not cured, although it may ultimately burn itself out. It is usual to commence therapy in these conditions at fairly high dose, such as 40 to 60 mg prednisolone daily, and then to reduce the dose to the lowest commensurate with disease control. If serious side-effects occur in response to the large doses of corticosteroids required to suppress the disease process, it is sometimes possible to reduce the dose of corticosteroid by giving a small dose of an immunosuppressive drug (see section 8.2.1).

Because corticosteroids reduce antibody formation, they may be used to suppress or modify *allergic reactions*. This may benefit some types of *asthma* and *skin diseases*. It may also lead to remissions of acquired *haemolytic anaemia*, the

---

C = 51-100p, D = 101-180p, E = 181-300p, F = 301-450p, G = 451-650p, H = 651-900p, I = 901-1200p, J = over 1200p.

nephrotic syndrome, and some cases of *thrombocytopenic purpura*.

For the use of the corticosteroids in the treatment of *reticuloses* and some types of *leukaemia*, see section 8.2.2.

Corticosteroids are extensively used on the skin, and also as aerosols, eye-drops, enemas, and intra-articular injections. The formulation here is of the greatest importance and partly determines the choice of drug. A potent drug such as betamethasone valerate may be more effective than any strength of a weaker one such as hydrocortisone.

The use of corticosteroids in the treatment of many other disease processes is described elsewhere in the following sections:

colon and rectum, sections 1.5, 1.7.2 and 1.7.3
asthma, section 3.2
rheumatic diseases, section 10.1.2
eye, section 11.4
otitis externa, section 12.1.1
allergic rhinitis, section 12.2.1
aphthous ulcers, section 12.3.1
skin, section 13.4

6.3.3 Disadvantages of corticosteroids

Overdosage or prolonged use may exaggerate some of the normal physiological actions of corticosteroids. Mineralocorticoid effects include hypertension, sodium and water retention, potassium loss, and muscle weakness. Glucocorticoid effects include diabetes and osteoporosis which is a danger, particularly in the elderly, as it may result in vertebral collapse. Mental disturbances may occur; a serious paranoid state or depression with risk of suicide may be induced, particularly in patients with a history of mental disorder. Euphoria is frequently observed. Peptic ulceration is a recognised complication which may result in haemorrhage or perforation. Mineralocorticoid effects are most marked with fludrocortisone and deoxycortone, but are significant with cortisone, hydrocortisone, corticotrophin, and tetracosactrin. Mineralocorticoid effects are negligible with the high potency glucocorticoids betamethasone, dexamethasone, methylprednisolone, and triamcinolone and occur only slightly with prednisolone and prednisone.

In children, administration of corticosteroids may result in suppression of growth. Corticosteroids given in high dosage during pregnancy may affect adrenal development in the child.

Modification of tissue reactions may result in spread of infection. Suppression of clinical signs may allow septicaemia or tuberculosis to reach an advanced stage before being recognised. Systemic corticosteroid therapy should be avoided in patients with psoriasis, as subsequent reduction in dose is commonly followed by a severe and persistent exacerbation.

ADRENAL SUPPRESSION. The administration of exogenous corticosteroids suppresses the secretion of corticotrophin and may lead to adrenal atrophy which can persist for years after stopping prolonged corticosteroid therapy; any illness or surgical emergency may then require further corticosteroid therapy to compensate for lack of sufficient adrenocortical response.

High doses of corticosteroids may cause Cushing's syndrome, with moon face, striae, and acne; it is usually reversible on withdrawal of treatment, but this must always be gradually tapered to avoid symptoms of acute adrenal insufficiency (see 'steroid card', section 6.3.4).

Drug interactions: see Appendix 1 (sections *2.2*, *2.5*, *6.1*, 6.3).

6.3.4 Clinical management

Corticosteroids should not be used unless the benefits justify the hazards and the lowest dose that will produce an acceptable response should be used. Dosage varies widely in different diseases and in different patients. Whenever possible local treatment with intra-articular injections, inhalations, eye-drops, or enemas should be used in preference to systemic treatment.

In status asthmaticus, acute hypersensitivity reactions such as *angioedema* of the upper respiratory tract and anaphylactic *shock*, and other serious acute conditions, an immediate systemic corticosteroid effect is required. In such cases **hydrocortisone** (as the sodium succinate or sodium phosphate) given by intravenous injection in a dose of 100 to 300 mg may be required. Doses of up to 500 mg of hydrocortisone intravenously have been used in severe shock, particularly when due to Gram-negative septicaemia. High doses should be given because the risk of complications is negligible with short-term therapy. Emergency treatment with adrenaline (see section 3.4.3) should also be given.

If the use of corticosteroids can save or prolong life, as in exfoliative dermatitis, pemphigus, or acute leukaemia, high doses must be given, as the complications of therapy are likely to be less serious than the effects of the disease itself.

When long-term corticosteroid therapy is used to relieve discomfort and disability in relatively benign chronic diseases such as rheumatoid arthritis the danger of treatment may become greater than the disabilities produced by the disease. To minimise side-effects the maintenance dose should be kept as low as possible, seldom exceeding the equivalent of 10 mg of prednisolone daily or ideally 5–6 mg daily (see also section 10.1.2.1).

When treatment is to be discontinued, the dose should be reduced gradually over a period of several weeks or months depending on the dosage and duration of the therapy.

In an attempt to reduce pituitary-adrenal suppression in patients requiring long-term corticosteroid therapy, intermittent treatment has been used, either in short courses, or by giving the corticosteroid as a single (higher) dose on alternate days instead of daily. This is satisfactory in some cases and should be considered when prolonged treatment is necessary, for example in asthma and some of the rheumatic diseases.

STEROID CARDS. Patients should carry cards giving details of their dosage and possible complications. These 'steroid cards' can be obtained from local Family Practitioner Committees or

DHSS Printing and Stationery Unit
Room 110
North Fylde Central Office
Norcross
Blackpool FY5 3TA

In Scotland 'steroid cards' are available from Health Boards.
Pharmacists may obtain these cards from the Pharmaceutical Society of Great Britain.

ANAESTHESIA. Anaesthetists must know whether a patient is taking or has been taking corticosteroids as adrenal suppression may cause a precipitous fall in blood pressure during anaesthesia.

CHILDREN. In children the indications for corticosteroids are the same as for adults but risks are greater. The implications of starting these drugs are serious, and they should be used only when specifically indicated, in a minimal dosage, and for the shortest possible time. Prolonged or continuous treatment is rarely justified. Stunting of growth may be mitigated by giving corticotrophin, or by giving prednisolone as single doses on alternate days.

Stimulation of the adrenal cortex by **corticotrophin** or **tetracosactrin** has been used as an alternative to corticosteroids to control certain diseases but there is no close relationship between the dose producing satisfactory clinical improvement and the equivalent dose of oral corticosteroid producing the same degree of improvement.

BETAMETHASONE

Indications: suppression of inflammatory and allergic disorders; adrenal hyperplasia (section 6.3.1); cerebral oedema (section 6.3.2)
Cautions; Contra-indications; Side-effects: section 6.3.3
Dose: by mouth, 0.5–5 mg daily in divided doses
By intramuscular injection or slow intravenous injection or infusion, 4–20 mg, repeated up to 4 times in 24 hours; CHILD, *by slow intravenous injection*, up to 1 year 1 mg, 1–5 years 2 mg, 6–12 years 4 mg

PoM **Betnelan**® (Glaxo)
Tablets, scored, betamethasone 500 micrograms. Price 20 tabs = **C**. Label: 10 steroid card
PoM **Betnesol**® (Glaxo)
Tablets, pink, scored, soluble, betamethasone 500 micrograms (as sodium phosphate). Price 20 tabs = **C**. Label: 10 steroid card, 13

I am a patient on—

STEROID
TREATMENT

which must not be stopped abruptly

and in the case of intercurrrent illness may have to be increased

full details are available
from the hospital or general ⟶
practitioners shown overleaf
STC1

INSTRUCTIONS

1 *DO NOT STOP taking the steroid drug except on medical advice. Always have a supply in reserve.*

2 *In case of feverish illness, accident, operation (emergency or otherwise), diarrhoea or vomiting the steroid treatment MUST be continued. Your doctor may wish you to have a LARGER DOSE or an INJECTION at such times.*

3 *If the tablets cause indigestion consult your doctor AT ONCE.*

4 *Always carry this card while receiving steroid treatment and show it to any doctor, dentist, nurse or midwife or anyone else who is giving you treatment.*

5 *After your treatment has finished you must still tell any doctor, dentist, nurse or midwife or anyone else who is giving you treatment that you have had steroid treatment.*

C = 51-100p, D = 101-180p, E = 181-300p, F = 301-450p, G = 451-650p, H = 651-900p, I = 901-1200p, J = over 1200p.

Injection, betamethasone 4 mg (as sodium phosphate)/ml. Price 1-ml amp = **C**. Label: 10 steroid card

CORTISONE ACETATE
Indications: section 6.3.1
Cautions; Contra-indications; Side-effects: section 6.3.3
Dose: by mouth, replacement therapy, 25–37.5 mg daily in divided doses but see also section 6.3.1

PoM **Cortisone Tablets,** cortisone acetate 5 mg, price 20 tabs = **A**; 25 mg, price 20 tabs = **B**. Label: 10 steroid card
PoM **Cortelan**® (Glaxo)
Tablets, scored, cortisone acetate 25 mg. Price 20 tabs = **C**. Label: 10 steroid card
PoM **Cortistab**® (Boots)
Tablets, scored, cortisone acetate 5 mg. Price 20 tabs = **A**. Label: 10 steroid card
Tablets, scored, cortisone acetate 25 mg. Price 20 tabs = **C**. Label: 10 steroid card
Injection (aqueous suspension), cortisone acetate 25 mg/ml. Price 10-ml vial = **C**. Label: 10 steroid card
PoM **Cortisyl**® (Roussel)
Tablets, scored, cortisone acetate 25 mg. Price 20 tabs = **D**. Label: 10 steroid card

DEXAMETHASONE
Indications: suppression of inflammatory and allergic disorders; shock; diagnosis of Cushing's disease; adrenal hyperplasia (section 6.3.1); cerebral oedema (section 6.3.2)
Cautions; Contra-indications; Side-effects: section 6.3.3
Dose: by mouth, 0.5–2 mg daily in divided doses; up to 15 mg daily in severe disease
Adrenal hyperplasia, 0.5–1.5 mg daily in divided doses
By intramuscular injection or slow intravenous injection or infusion, initially 0.5–20 mg; CHILD 200–500 micrograms/kg daily
Shock, *by intravenous injection or infusion*, 2–6 mg/kg, repeated if necessary after 2–6 hours
Cerebral oedema, *by intravenous injection*, 10 mg initially, then 4 mg *by intramuscular injection* every 6 hours as required for 2–10 days
Note: 1.3 mg dexamethasone sodium phosphate ≡ 1.2 mg dexamethasone phosphate ≡ 1 mg dexamethasone

PoM **Dexamethasone Tablets,** dexamethasone 500 micrograms, price 20 tabs = **C**; 2 mg, price 20 tabs = **D**. Label: 10 steroid card
PoM **Decadron**® (MSD)
Tablets, scored, dexamethasone 500 micrograms. Price 20 tabs = **C**. Label: 10 steroid card
Injection, dexamethasone phosphate 4 mg/ml (as sodium salt) (= 3.33 mg dexamethasone/ml). Price 2-ml vial = **D**. Label: 10 steroid card
PoM **Decadron Shock-Pak**® (MSD)
Injection, dexamethasone 20 mg (as sodium phosphate)/ml. Price 5-ml vial = **J**. Label: 10 steroid card

PoM **Oradexon**® (Organon)
Tablets, dexamethasone 500 micrograms. Price 20 tabs = **C**. Label: 10 steroid card
Tablets, dexamethasone 2 mg. Price 20 tabs = **D**. Label: 10 steroid card
Injection, dexamethasone 4 mg (as sodium phosphate)/ml. Price 1-ml amp = **C**. Label: 10 steroid card
Injection, dexamethasone 4 mg (as sodium phosphate)/ml. Price 2-ml vial = **D**. Label: 10 steroid card

HYDROCORTISONE
Indications: adrenocortical insufficiency (section 6.3.1); suppression of inflammatory and allergic disorders; shock (section 6.3.2)
Cautions; Contra-indications; Side-effects: section 6.3.3
Dose: by mouth, replacement therapy, 20–30 mg daily in divided doses—see section 6.3.1
By intramuscular injection or slow intravenous injection or infusion, 100–500 mg, 3–4 times in 24 hours or as required; CHILD *by slow intravenous injection* up to 1 year 25 mg, 1–5 years 50 mg, 6–12 years 100 mg
Shock—see notes above

Oral preparations
PoM **Hydrocortisone Tablets,** hydrocortisone 10 and 20 mg, price 20 tabs (both) = **B**. Label: 10 steroid card
PoM **Hydrocortistab**® (Boots)
Tablets, scored, hydrocortisone 20 mg. Price 20 tabs = **B**. Label: 10 steroid card
PoM **Hydrocortone**® (MSD)
Tablets, scored, hydrocortisone 10 mg. Price 20 tabs = **B**. Label: 10 steroid card
Tablets, scored, hydrocortisone 20 mg. Price 20 tabs = **C**. Label: 10 steroid card

Parenteral preparations
PoM **Hydrocortisone Sodium Succinate Injection,** powder for reconstitution, hydrocortisone (as sodium succinate). Price 100-mg vial (with 2-ml amp water for injections) = **B**; 500-mg vial = **E**. Label: 10 steroid card
PoM **Efcortelan Soluble**® (Glaxo)
Injection, powder for reconstitution, hydrocortisone (as sodium succinate). Price 100-mg vial (with 2-ml amp water for injections) = **C**. Label: 10 steroid card
PoM **Efcortesol**® (Glaxo)
Injection, hydrocortisone 100 mg (as sodium phosphate)/ml. Price 1-ml amp = **C**; 5-ml amp = **F**. Label: 10 steroid card
PoM **Solu-Cortef**® (Upjohn)
Injection, powder for reconstitution, hydrocortisone (as sodium succinate). Price 100-mg vial (with 2-ml amp water for injections) = **C**. Label: 10 steroid card

METHYLPREDNISOLONE
Indications: suppression of inflammatory and allergic disorders; shock; cerebral oedema

Cautions; Contra-indications; Side-effects: section 6.3.3

Dose: by mouth, in inflammatory disorders up to 16 mg daily in 4 divided doses preferably with food; in allergic disorders initially, up to 40 mg daily, in divided doses

By intramuscular injection or slow intravenous injection or infusion, up to 120 mg daily for up to 3 days

Shock, *by intravenous infusion,* up to 30 mg/kg

PoM **Depo-Medrone**® (Upjohn)
Injection (aqueous suspension), methylprednisolone acetate 40 mg/ml. Price 1-ml vial = **E**; 2-ml vial or syringe = **F**; 5-ml vial = **H**. Label: 10 steroid card
Dose: by deep intramuscular injection, 40–120 mg, repeated every 2–3 weeks if required

PoM **Medrone**® (Upjohn)
Tablets, pink, scored, methylprednisolone 2 mg. Price 20 tabs = **D**. Label: 10 steroid card
Tablets, scored, methylprednisolone 4 mg. Price 20 tabs = **E**. Label: 10 steroid card
Tablets, scored, methylprednisolone 16 mg. Price 20 tabs = **H**. Label: 10 steroid card

PoM **Min-I-Mix Methylprednisolone**® (IMS)
Injection, powder for reconstitution, methylprednisolone sodium succinate. Price 0.5-g vial = **I**; 1-g vial = **J**. Label: 10 steroid card

PoM **Solu-Medrone**® (Upjohn)
Injection, powder for reconstitution, methylprednisolone (as sodium succinate). Price 40-mg mix-o-vial = **D**; 125-mg mix-o-vial = **F**; 500-mg vial (with solvent) = **I**; 1-, and 2-g vial (both with solvent) = **J**. Label: 10 steroid card

PREDNISOLONE

Indications: suppression of inflammatory and allergic disorders

Cautions; Contra-indications; Side-effects: section 6.3.3

Dose: by mouth, initially up to 30 mg daily in divided doses

By intravenous injection or infusion or intramuscular injection, initially 4–60 mg daily in divided doses (as sodium phosphate)

By intramuscular injection, prednisolone acetate 25–100 mg once or twice weekly

PoM **Prednisolone Tablets,** prednisolone 1 and 5 mg. Price 20 tabs (both) = **A**. Label: 10 steroid card

PoM **Codelsol**® (MSD)
Injection, prednisolone 16 mg (as sodium phosphate)/ml. Price 2-ml vial = **D**. Label: 10 steroid card

PoM **Delta-Phoricol**® (Wallace Mfg)
Tablets, prednisolone 5 mg. Price 20 tabs = **C**. Label: 10 steroid card

PoM **Deltacortril Enteric**® (Pfizer)
Tablets, brown, e/c, prednisolone 2.5 mg. Price 20 tabs = **B**. Label: 5, 10 steroid card, 25
Tablets, red, e/c, prednisolone 5 mg. Price 20 tabs = **B**. Label: 5, 10 steroid card, 25

PoM **Deltalone**® (DDSA)
Tablets, prednisolone 1 mg. Price 20 tabs = **A**. Label: 10 steroid card
Tablets, scored, prednisolone 5 mg. Price 20 tabs = **A**. Label: 10 steroid card

PoM **Deltastab**® (Boots)
Tablets, scored, prednisolone 1 mg. Price 20 tabs = **A**. Label: 10 steroid card
Tablets, scored, prednisolone 5 mg. Price 20 tabs = **A**. Label: 10 steroid card
Injection (aqueous suspension), prednisolone acetate 25 mg/ml. Price 5-ml vial = **C**. Label: 10 steroid card

PoM **Precortisyl**® (Roussel)
Tablets, prednisolone 1 mg. Price 20 tabs = **A**. Label: 10 steroid card
Tablets, scored, prednisolone 5 mg. Price 20 tabs = **A**. Label: 10 steroid card
Tablets, prednisolone 25 mg. Price 20 tabs = **D**. Label: 10 steroid card

PoM **Prednesol**® (Glaxo)
Tablets, pink, scored, soluble, prednisolone 5 mg (as sodium phosphate). Price 20 tabs = **D**. Label: 10 steroid card, 13

PoM **Sintisone**® (Farmitalia Carlo Erba)
Tablets, scored, prednisolone steaglate 6.65 mg (≡ prednisolone 5 mg). Price 20 tabs = **D**. Label: 10 steroid card

PREDNISONE

Indications: suppression of inflammatory and allergic disorders

Cautions; Contra-indications; Side-effects: section 6.3.3. Avoid in liver disease

Dose: initially up to 30 mg daily

PoM **Prednisone Tablets,** prednisone 1 and 5 mg. Price 20 tabs (both) = **A**. Label: 10 steroid card

PoM **Decortisyl**® (Roussel)
Tablets, scored, prednisone 5 mg. Price 20 tabs = **A**. Label: 10 steroid card

PoM **Econosone**® (DDSA)
Tablets, prednisone 1 mg. Price 20 tabs = **A**. Label: 10 steroid card
Tablets, prednisone 5 mg. Price 20 tabs = **A**. Label: 10 steroid card

TRIAMCINOLONE

Indications: suppression of inflammatory and allergic disorders

Cautions; Contra-indications; Side-effects: section 6.3.3. Triamcinolone has a particular tendency to cause a proximal myopathy and should be avoided in chronic therapy

Dose: by mouth, up to 24 mg daily in divided doses

By deep intramuscular injection, 40 mg of acetonide for depot effect, repeated at intervals according to the patient's response; max. single dose 100 mg

PoM **Triamcinolone Tablets,** triamcinolone 2 mg, price 20 tabs = **D**; 4 mg, price 20 tabs = **E**. Label: 10 steroid card

---

C = 51-100p, D = 101-180p, E = 181-300p, F = 301-450p, G = 451-650p, H = 651-900p, I = 901-1200p, J = over 1200p.

PoM **Kenalog**® (Squibb)

Injection (aqueous suspension), triamcinolone acetonide 40 mg/ml. Price 1-ml vial = **D**; 1-ml syringe = **E**; 2-ml syringe = **F**. Label: 10 steroid card

PoM **Ledercort**® (Lederle)

Tablets, blue, triamcinolone 2 mg. Price 20 tabs = **D**. Label: 10 steroid card

Tablets, triamcinolone 4 mg. Price 20 tabs = **F**. Label: 10 steroid card

6.4 Sex hormones

Sex hormones are described under the following section headings:

6.4.1 Female sex hormones
6.4.2 Male sex hormones and antagonists
6.4.3 Anabolic steroids

6.4.1 Female sex hormones

There are two groups of female sex hormones, the oestrogens (section 6.4.1.1) and progestogens (section 6.4.1.2). Combined hormone preparations for menopausal symptoms are listed in section 6.4.1.3 and for menstrual disorders in section 6.4.1.4. Combined and other preparations for use as contraceptives are in sections 7.3.1 and 7.3.2.

6.4.1.1 OESTROGENS

Oestrogens are necessary for the development of female secondary sexual characteristics; they stimulate myometrial hypertrophy, with endometrial hyperplasia which may lead to withdrawal bleeding when treatment is stopped, and they promote cornification of the vagina. They are used as oral contraceptives (see section 7.3.1) with **progestogens** since oestrogens suppress ovulation and inhibit production of follicle-stimulating hormone (FSH) from the anterior pituitary gland. They may also be used with benefit in some neoplastic conditions (section 8.3.1), particularly cancer of the prostate and some cases of breast cancer. Several gynaecological conditions also benefit from treatment with oestrogens but systemic administration is associated with an increased risk of thrombo-embolism and this should be borne in mind when they are prescribed.

Ethinyloestradiol is the oestrogen of choice for most conditions. The natural (as opposed to synthetic) oestrogens have not been shown to have any advantages. Stilboestrol is used mainly in neoplastic conditions (see section 8.3.1).

MENOPAUSAL SYMPTOMS. Hormone replacement therapy with oestrogens is **not** routinely indicated in postmenopausal women but small doses given for long periods will diminish postmenopausal osteoporosis. Menopausal vasomotor symptoms and senile vaginitis and vulvitis can, if severe, justify treatment for a few months. Topical preparations (see section 7.2.1) are used to treat senile vaginitis and vulvitis; patients who do not respond require systemic treatment, for example 10–20

micrograms of ethinyloestradiol daily. Unless the patient has been hysterectomised, the oestrogen should be given cyclically and a dose of a **progestogen** (section 6.4.1.2), such as norethisterone added. The addition of progestogen has been shown to prevent cystic hyperplasia of the endometrium and possible transformation to atypical hyperplasia and carcinoma. Recently, lower doses of progestogen have been shown to be as effective as the earlier higher doses. The use of oestrogens alone, except for short periods, is no longer recommended. See section 6.4.1.3 for suitable compound preparations.

MENSTRUAL DISORDERS. Oestrogens are used with progestogens in a number of menstrual disorders, such as spasmodic dysmenorrhoea (see also section 6.4.1.2), when they are given on a cyclical basis. They are more effective than treatment with progestogens alone in relieving pain of spasmodic dysmenorrhoea but also inhibit ovulation. For suitable oestrogen/progestogen preparations see section 6.4.1.4. Alternatively, the combined oral contraceptives (see section 7.3.1) may be used.

Oestrogens are also used in primary amenorrhoea or hypogonadism to induce an artificial menstruation. They are usually given on a cyclical basis with a progestogen as indicated above. High doses of ethinyloestradiol such as 1 mg daily, given for a few days and then withdrawn, are used to induce withdrawal bleeding.

SUPPRESSION OF LACTATION. Oestrogens are no longer used to suppress lactation because of their association with thrombo-embolism, and **bromocriptine** (section 6.7.1) is used where necessary.

ETHINYLOESTRADIOL

Indications: menopausal symptoms, primary amenorrhoea

Cautions: pregnancy, breast-feeding, diabetes, epilepsy, hypertension, migraine, cardiac or renal disease, history of jaundice, wearing of contact lenses; may interfere with results of thyroid-function tests and cortisol estimations by increasing concentrations of hormone-binding protein. Drug interactions: see Appendix 1 (sections 2.2, 2.5)

Contra-indications: oestrogen-dependent carcinoma, history of thrombo-embolism, hepatic impairment, endometriosis, porphyria, undiagnosed vaginal bleeding, history of herpes gestationis

Side-effects: nausea and vomiting, weight gain, breast enlargement and tenderness, withdrawal bleeding, sodium retention with oedema, changes in liver function, jaundice, rashes and chloasma, depression, headache, endometrial carcinoma in postmenopausal women

Dose: menopausal symptoms 10–20 micrograms daily continuously *or* for 21 days, repeated after 7 days, with progestogen from day 17 to day 26 of cycle

Primary amenorrhoea, up to 50 micrograms 3 times daily continuously with a progestogen for the last 5 days of month; to induce withdrawal bleeding 1 mg daily for a few days

PoM **Ethinyloestradiol Tablets,** ethinyloestradiol 10 micrograms, price 20 tabs = **A**; 50 micrograms, price 20 tabs = **B**; 1 mg, price 20 tabs = **C**

OESTRADIOL

Indications: menopausal symptoms, primary amenorrhoea

Cautions; Contra-indications; Side-effects: see under Ethinyloestradiol

Dose: by mouth, menopausal symptoms, oestradiol valerate 1–2 mg daily for 21 days, with 7-day interval before next course

By intramuscular injection, primary amenorrhoea, oestradiol benzoate 1–5 mg at 1–14 day intervals

By implantation, oestradiol, amenorrhoea, 25–50 mg, menopausal symptoms 25 mg

PoM **Oestradiol Implants** (Organon)
Implant, oestradiol 25 mg (duration 36 weeks). Price each = **F**
Implant, oestradiol 50 mg (duration 44 weeks). Price each = **G**
Implant, oestradiol 100 mg (duration 57 weeks). Price each = **J**

PoM **Benztrone**® (Paines & Byrne)
Injection (oily), oestradiol benzoate 1 mg/ml. Price 1-ml amp = **B**
Injection (oily), oestradiol benzoate 5 mg/ml. Price 1- and 2-ml amp (both) = **B**

PoM **Hormonin**® (Carnrick)
Tablets, pink, scored, oestradiol 600 micrograms, oestriol 270 micrograms, oestrone 1.4 mg. Price 20 tabs = **D**
Dose: menopausal symptoms, 2 tablets daily or on alternate days

PoM **Progynova**® (Schering)
Tablets, beige, s/c, oestradiol valerate 1 mg. Price 21-tab calendar pack = **E**
Tablets, blue, s/c, oestradiol valerate 2 mg. Price 21-tab calendar pack = **E**

OESTRIOL

Indications: post-menopausal vaginal and vulval conditions

Cautions; Contra-indications; Side-effects: see under Ethinyloestradiol

Dose: 250–500 micrograms daily, reducing as symptoms are controlled

PoM **Ovestin**® (Organon)
Tablets, oestriol 250 micrograms. Price 20 tabs = **B**

OESTROGENS, CONJUGATED

Indications: menopausal symptoms, primary amenorrhoea

Cautions; Contra-indications; Side-effects: see under Ethinyloestradiol

Dose: menopausal symptoms, postmenopausal osteoporosis, 0.625–1.25 mg daily for 21 days

from 5th day of cycle, repeated after 7 days if necessary, reduced to maintenance dose, and if necessary continued on a cyclical basis with a progestogen from day 17 to day 26 of cycle

Primary amenorrhoea, 1.25–3.75 mg daily in divided doses for 21 days, with a progestogen from 15th to 21st day

PoM **Premarin**® (Ayerst)
Tablets, maroon, s/c, conjugated oestrogens 625 micrograms. Price 20 tabs or 21-tab calendar pack = **C**
Tablets, yellow, s/c, conjugated oestrogens 1.25 mg. Price 20 tabs or 21-tab calendar pack = **D**
Tablets, purple, s/c, conjugated oestrogens 2.5 mg. Price 20 tabs = **E**

PIPERAZINE OESTRONE SULPHATE

Indications: menopausal symptoms

Cautions; Contra-indications; Side-effects: see under Ethinyloestradiol

Dose: initially 1.5–4.5 mg daily in single or divided doses for 21–28 days, repeated after 5–7 days if necessary, reduced to maintenance dose, and if necessary continued on a cyclical basis

Note: piperazine oestrone sulphate 1.5 mg = oestrone 930 micrograms

PoM **Harmogen**® (Abbott)
Tablets, peach, scored, piperazine oestrone sulphate 1.5 mg. Price 20 tabs = **D**

QUINESTRADOL

Indications: post-menopausal vaginal and vulval conditions

Cautions; Contra-indications; Side-effects: see under Ethinyloestradiol

Dose: 500 micrograms twice daily for 2–3 weeks

PoM **Pentovis**® (Warner)
Capsules, green, quinestradol 250 micrograms. Price 20 caps = **D**

QUINESTROL

Indications: inhibition and suppression of lactation

Cautions; Contra-indications; Side-effects: see under Ethinyloestradiol and notes above

Dose: inhibition, 4 mg within 6 hours of delivery and a further 4 mg if symptoms persist

Suppression, 4 mg immediately and a further 4 mg after 48 hours if necessary

PoM **Estrovis**® (Warner)
Tablets, pink, quinestrol 4 mg. Price 2 tabs = **E**

6.4.1.2 PROGESTOGENS

Progestogens modify some of the effects of oestrogens and act mainly on tissues sensitised by them; their effects are inhibited by excess of oestrogens. There are two main groups of progestogen, the

---

C = 51-100p, **D** = 101-180p, **E** = 181-300p, **F** = 301-450p, **G** = 451-650p, **H** = 651-900p, **I** = 901-1200p, **J** = over 1200p.

naturally occurring hormone *progesterone* and its analogues (allyloestrenol, dydrogesterone, hydroxyprogesterone, and medroxyprogesterone) and the *testosterone* analogues which include ethisterone and norethisterone. Progesterone and its analogues are less androgenic than the testosterone derivatives and neither **progesterone** nor **dydrogesterone** causes virilisation. Other synthetic derivatives are variably metabolised into testosterone and oestrogen; thus side-effects vary with the preparation and the dose.

Progestogens are useful in many menstrual disorders. They are used in the premenstrual syndrome, severe dysmenorrhoea, and dysfunctional uterine bleeding to relieve pain and prevent or arrest bleeding. **Norethisterone** and dydrogesterone (Duphaston®) are suitable and may be given alone on a cyclical basis during part of the menstrual cycle or in conjunction with the **oestrogens** (section 6.4.1.1). Suitable preparations are listed in section 6.4.1.4. Alternatively the combined oral contraceptives (see section 7.3.1) may be used. See also **bromocriptine** (section 6.7.1).

Where endometriosis requires drug treatment, it usually responds to a progestogen, for example norethisterone, which should be administered on a continuous basis. Alternatively, cyclical or continuous treatment with the oral contraceptives (see section 7.3.1) or **danazol** (section 6.7.3) may be given.

The progestogens desogestrel, ethynodiol diacetate, levonorgestrel, lynoestrenol, and norethisterone acetate are used in combined oral contraceptives and progestogen-only contraceptives (see sections 7.3.1 and 7.3.2). Levonorgestrel is the active isomer and has twice the potency of racemic norgestrel.

Progestogens are also used in conjunction with oestrogens (section 6.4.1.1) in hormone replacement therapy in menopausal women. Combined oestrogen/progestogen preparations are listed in section 6.4.1.3. See section 8.3.2 for use in neoplastic disease.

Progestogens have been used in habitual abortion but their efficacy is in doubt. If they are used for this purpose they should be of the true progesterone-derivative type, e.g. **hydroxyprogesterone hexanoate** (Proluton Depot®) to avoid any masculinisation of a female fetus.

ALLYLOESTRENOL

Indications: habitual abortion, failure of nidation
Cautions; Contra-indications; Side-effects: see under Progesterone and notes above
Dose: habitual abortion, 5–10 mg daily for at least 16 weeks
Failure of nidation, 10–20 mg daily from 16th to 26th day of each cycle until conception is achieved, then 10 mg daily for at least 16 weeks

PoM **Gestanin**® (Organon)
Tablets, allyloestrenol 5 mg. Price 20 tabs = **E**

DYDROGESTERONE

Indications: endometriosis, habitual abortion,

failure of nidation, menstrual disorders, amenorrhoea, dysfunctional uterine bleeding
Cautions; Contra-indications; Side-effects: see under Progesterone and notes above. Breakthrough bleeding may rarely occur (increase dose). Liver function disturbances and jaundice have not been reported
Dose: endometriosis, 10 mg 2–3 times daily from 5th to 25th day of cycle or continuously
Failure of nidation, irregular cycles, 10 mg twice daily from 11th to 25th day for at least 6 cycles
Habitual abortion, 10 mg twice daily from day 11 to day 25 of cycle until conception, then continuously until 20th week of pregnancy and gradually reduced
Dysfunctional uterine bleeding, 10 mg twice daily for 5–7 days to arrest bleeding; 10 mg twice daily from 11th to 25th day of cycle to prevent bleeding
Dysmenorrhoea, 10 mg twice daily from 5th to 25th day of cycle
Amenorrhoea, 10 mg twice daily from 11th to 25th day of cycle following oestrogen therapy from 1st to 25th day of cycle
Premenstrual syndrome, 10 mg twice daily from 12th to 26th day of cycle

PoM **Duphaston**® (Duphar)
Tablets, scored, dydrogesterone 10 mg. Price 20 tabs = **F**

ETHISTERONE

Indications: menstrual disorders
Cautions; Contra-indications; Side-effects: see under Norethisterone but more virilising
Dose: menorrhagia, 10–15 mg 3 times daily for 8 days prior to menstruation
Premenstrual syndrome, 5–10 mg daily for last 2 weeks of cycle

PoM **Gestone-oral**® (Paines & Byrne)
Tablets, ethisterone 10 mg. Price 20 tabs = **B**
Tablets, ethisterone 25 mg. Price 20 tabs = **C**

HYDROXYPROGESTERONE HEXANOATE

Indications: habitual abortion
Cautions; Contra-indications; Side-effects: see under Progesterone and notes above
Dose: by intramuscular injection, 250–500 mg weekly during first half of pregnancy

PoM **Proluton Depot**® (Schering)
Injection (oily), hydroxyprogesterone hexanoate 250 mg/ml. Price 1- and 2-ml amp (both) = **E**

MEDROXYPROGESTERONE ACETATE

Indications: endometriosis, dysfunctional uterine bleeding, secondary amenorrhoea
Cautions; Contra-indications; Side-effects: see under Progesterone and notes above; disturbances of normal menstrual cycle and irregular bleeding may occur
Dose: by mouth, 2.5–10 mg daily for 5–10 days beginning on 16th–21st day of cycle, repeated

for 2 cycles in dysfunctional uterine bleeding and 3 cycles in amenorrhoea
By deep intramuscular injection, endometriosis, 50 mg weekly or 100 mg every 2 weeks

PoM **Depo-Provera**® (Upjohn)
Injection (aqueous suspension), medroxyprogesterone acetate 50 mg/ml. Price 1-ml vial = **D**; 3-ml vial = **F**; 5-ml vial = **G**
PoM **Provera**® (Upjohn)
Tablets, scored, medroxyprogesterone acetate 5 mg. Price 20 tabs = **E**

NORETHISTERONE

Indications: dysfunctional uterine bleeding, menstrual disorders, endometriosis, postponement of menstruation
Cautions; Contra-indications; Side-effects: see under Progesterone but more virilising and greater incidence of liver disturbances and jaundice. Caution in asthma and epilepsy. Avoid in pregnancy. Side-effects rare below 15 mg daily. Headache and depression occur occasionally
Dose: endometriosis 10 mg daily starting on 5th day of cycle (increased if spotting occurs to 25 mg daily in divided doses to prevent breakthrough bleeding) for at least 6 months
Dysfunctional uterine bleeding, menorrhagia, 5 mg 3 times daily for 10 days to arrest bleeding; to prevent bleeding 5 mg twice daily from 19th to 26th day
Dysmenorrhoea, 5 mg 3 times daily from 5th to 25th day for 3–4 cycles
Premenstrual syndrome, 10–15 mg daily from 19th to 26th day for several cycles
Postponement of menstruation, 5 mg 3 times daily starting 3 days before anticipated onset

PoM **Norethisterone Tablets**, norethisterone 5 mg. Price 20 tabs = **D**
PoM **Primolut N**® (Schering)
Tablets, norethisterone 5 mg. Price 20 tabs = **E**
PoM **Utovlan**® (Syntex)
Tablets, scored, norethisterone 5 mg. Price 20 tabs = **D**

PROGESTERONE

Indications: dysfunctional uterine bleeding, habitual abortion, premenstrual syndrome
Cautions: diabetes, breast-feeding, hypertension; liver, cardiac, or renal disease
Contra-indications: undiagnosed vaginal bleeding, missed or incomplete abortion, history of thrombo-embolism, mammary carcinoma
Side-effects: acne, urticaria, oedema, weight gain, gastro-intestinal disturbances, changes in libido, breast discomfort, irregular menstrual cycles; rarely jaundice. Injection may be painful
Dose: by vagina or rectum, dysfunctional uterine bleeding, premenstrual syndrome, 200–400 mg twice daily (starting for premenstrual syndrome on 14th day, or 12th day if symptoms of ovulation are present) and continued until onset of menstruation
By intramuscular injection, habitual abortion, 5–

10 mg daily or up to 20 mg 2–3 times weekly; dysfunctional uterine bleeding, 5–10 mg daily 5–10 days before anticipated onset of menstruation

PoM **Cyclogest**® (Collins)
Suppositories, progesterone 200 mg. Price 20 suppos = **H**
Suppositories, progesterone 400 mg. Price 20 suppos = **I**
PoM **Gestone**® (Paines & Byrne)
Injection, progesterone 10 mg/ml. Price 1-ml amp = **B**
Injection, progesterone 25 mg/ml. Price 1-ml amp = **B**
Injection, progesterone 50 mg/ml. Price 1- and 2-ml amp (both) = **B**

6.4.1.3 COMBINED PREPARATIONS FOR MENOPAUSAL SYMPTOMS

Note: the preparations in this section are unsuitable for use as oral contraceptives (see section 7.3.1)
For *Cautions; Contra-indications; Side-effects:* see under Combined Oral Contraceptives, section 7.3.1. Hirsuitism may result from preparations with a testosterone component

PoM **Cyclo-Progynova 1 mg**® (Schering)
Calendar pack, all s/c, 11 beige tablets, oestradiol valerate 1 mg; 10 brown tablets, oestradiol valerate 1 mg and levonorgestrel 250 micrograms. Price per pack = **F**
Dose: 1 beige tablet daily for 11 days, starting on 5th day of menstrual cycle or at any time if cycles have ceased or are infrequent, then 1 brown tablet daily for 10 days, followed by a 7-day interval
PoM **Cyclo-Progynova 2 mg**® (Schering)
Calendar pack, all s/c, 11 white tablets, oestradiol valerate 2 mg; 10 brown tablets, oestradiol valerate 2 mg and levonorgestrel 250 micrograms. Price per pack = **F**
Dose: see above, but starting with 1 white tablet daily
PoM **Menophase**® (Syntex)
Calendar pack, 5 pink tablets, mestranol 12.5 micrograms; 8 orange tablets, mestranol 25 micrograms; 2 yellow tablets, mestranol 50 micrograms; 3 green tablets, mestranol 25 micrograms and norethisterone 1 mg; 6 blue tablets, mestranol 30 micrograms and norethisterone 1.5 mg; 4 lavender tablets, mestranol 20 micrograms and norethisterone 750 micrograms. Price per pack = **E**
Dose: 1 tablet daily, starting with a pink tablet on Sunday, then in sequence (without interruption)
PoM **Mixogen**® (Organon)
Tablets, ethinyloestradiol 4.4 micrograms, methyltestosterone 3.6 mg. Price 20 tabs = **B**
Dose: 1–2 tablets daily for 3 weeks, followed by a 7-day interval
Injection (oily), oestradiol benzoate 1 mg,

C = 51-100p, D = 101-180p, E = 181-300p, F = 301-450p, G = 451-650p, H = 651-900p, I = 901-1200p, J = over 1200p.

oestradiol phenylpropionate 4 mg, testosterone propionate 20 mg, testosterone phenylpropionate 40 mg, and testosterone isohexanoate 40 mg/ml. Price 1-ml amp = C
Dose: by deep intramuscular injection, 1 ml every 3–4 weeks

PoM **Prempak 0.625®** (Ayerst)
Calendar pack, all s/c, 21 maroon tablets, conjugated oestrogens 625 micrograms; 7 white tablets, norgestrel 500 micrograms. Price per pack = D
Dose: 1 maroon tablet daily for 14 days starting on 5th day of cycle or at any time if cycles have ceased or are infrequent, then 1 white and 1 maroon tablet daily for 7 days, followed by a 7-day interval

PoM **Prempak 1.25®** (Ayerst)
Calendar pack, all s/c, 21 yellow tablets, conjugated oestrogens 1.25 mg; 7 white tablets, norgestrel 500 micrograms. Price per pack = E
Dose: see above, but starting with 1 yellow tablet daily

PoM **Prempak-C 0.625®** (Ayerst)
Calendar pack, all s/c, 28 maroon tablets, conjugated oestrogens 625 micrograms; 12 light brown tablets, norgestrel 150 micrograms. Price per pack = F
Dose: 1 maroon tablet daily for 16 days, starting on 1st day of cycle or at any time if cycles have ceased or are infrequent, then 1 maroon and 1 brown tablet daily for 12 days. Subsequent courses should be repeated without interval

PoM **Prempak-C 1.25®** (Ayerst)
Calendar pack, all s/c, 28 yellow tablets, conjugated oestrogens 1.25 mg; 12 light brown tablets, norgestrel 150 micrograms. Price per pack = F
Dose: see above, but starting with 1 yellow tablet daily

6.4.1.4 COMBINED PREPARATIONS FOR MENSTRUAL DISORDERS

Cautions; Contra-indications; Side-effects: see under Combined Oral Contraceptives, section 7.3.1

PoM **Controvlar®** (Schering)
Tablets, pink, s/c, norethisterone acetate 3 mg, ethinyloestradiol 50 micrograms. Price 21 tabs = C
Dose: dysmenorrhoea, menstrual irregularities, menorrhagia, endometriosis, 1 tablet daily for 21 days, starting on 5th day of menstrual cycle, followed by a 7-day interval

PoM **Norlestrin®** (P-D)
Tablets, pink, f/c, norethisterone acetate 2.5 mg, ethinyloestradiol 50 micrograms. Price 21-tab calendar pack = C
Dose: dysmenorrhoea, menstrual irregularities, prevention of dysfunctional uterine bleeding, premenstrual tension, 1–2 tablets daily from 5th to 25th day of cycle; dysfunctional uterine bleeding 1–2 tablets daily until 5 days after bleeding stops

Ovran and **Ovranette: see section 7.3.1**

6.4.2   Male sex hormones and antagonists

Androgens cause masculinisation; they may be used as replacement therapy in castrated adults and in those who are hypogonadal due to either pituitary or testicular disease. In the normal male they depress spermatogenesis and inhibit pituitary gonadotrophin secretion. Androgens also have an anabolic action which has lead to the development of anabolic steroids (section 6.4.3).

Androgens are useless as a treatment of impotence unless it accompanies hypogonadism and should not be given until the hypogonadism has been properly investigated. Treatment should be under expert supervision.

When given to patients with hypopituitarism they can lead to normal sexual development and potency but not fertility. If fertility is desired, the correct treatment is with chorionic gonadotrophin injection (HCG) and with menotrophin (FSH) (section 6.5.1) which will stimulate spermatogenesis as well as androgen production.

Caution should be used when androgens or chorionic gonadotrophin are used in treating boys with delayed puberty since the fusion of epiphyses is hastened and may result in short stature.

Androgens are now rarely used in the treatment of disseminated carcinoma of the breast because of their masculinising effects in the female. The synthetic anabolic steroids (such as nandrolone) which cause less masculinisation are usually preferred (see section 8.3.3).

Intramuscular depot preparations of testosterone are preferred for replacement therapy. **Testosterone propionate** (Virormone®) or alternatively **Sustanon®**, which consists of a mixture of **testosterone esters** and has a longer duration of action, may be used. Satisfactory replacement therapy can sometimes be obtained with 1 ml of Sustanon 250®, given by intramuscular injection once a month, although more frequent dose intervals are often necessary. Implants of testosterone have been superseded.

Of the orally active preparations, methyltestosterone is not generally used and other preparations are preferred because like the other 17α-alkyl derivatives of testosterone it can sometimes cause dose-related but reversible cholestatic jaundice. **Mesterolone** (Pro-Viron®) is not a 17α-alkyl derivative and is less toxic to the liver.

ANTI-ANDROGENS. **Cyproterone acetate** (Androcur®) is used in the treatment of severe hypersexuality and sexual deviation in the male; it inhibits spermatogenesis and produces reversible infertility. Abnormal sperm forms are produced. Cyproterone acetate is also used in the treatment of hirsutism in women (see section 13.6). As hepatic tumours have been produced in *animal* studies, careful consideration should be given to the risk/benefit ratio before commencing treatment.

CYPROTERONE ACETATE
Indications: see notes above

Cautions: impaired ability to drive and operate machinery; ineffective in chronic alcoholism; monitor hepatic function, adrenocortical function and blood glucose every 4–6 weeks; diabetes mellitus, chronic hepatic disease, adrenocortical insufficiency, breast-feeding

Contra-indications: acute hepatic disease, malignant or wasting disease, severe depression, history of thrombo-embolic disorders, in immature youths may arrest bone maturation and testicular development

Side-effects: sedation and depression, weight gain, changes in hair pattern, gynaecomastia (rarely leading to galactorrhoea and benign breast nodules)

Dose: male hypersexuality, 50 mg twice daily after food

PoM **Androcur**® (Schering)
Tablets, scored, cyproterone acetate 50 mg. Price 10 tabs = **G**. Label: 2, 21
Cyprostat: see section 8.3.4
Diane: see section 13.6

MESTEROLONE
Indications: hypogonadism
Cautions; Contra-indications; Side-effects: see under Testosterone
Dose: 25 mg 3–4 times daily for several months, reduced to 50–75 mg daily in divided doses for maintenance

PoM **Pro-Viron**® (Schering)
Tablets, scored, mesterolone 25 mg. Price 20 tabs = **F**

METHYLTESTOSTERONE
Indications: hypogonadism
Cautions; Contra-indications; Side-effects: see under Testosterone; also dose-related cholestatic jaundice
Dose: initially 30–50 mg daily, in divided doses

PoM **Methyltestosterone Tablets,** methyltestosterone 5 and 10 mg, price 20 tabs (both) = **C**; 25 mg, price 20 tabs = **D**; 50 mg, price 20 tabs = **E**
PoM **Plex-Hormone**® (Consolidated)
Tablets, red, methyltestosterone 5 mg, deoxycortone acetate 500 micrograms, ethinyloestradiol 2 micrograms, tocopheryl acetate 5 mg. Price 20 tabs = **E**
Dose: 4–5 tablets daily for 10–14 days, followed if necessary after 10 days by a reduced dose for maintenance
PoM **Virormone-Oral**® (Paines & Byrne)
Tablets, methyltestosterone 5 mg. Price 20 tabs = **B**
Tablets, methyltestosterone 10 mg. Price 20 tabs = **C**
Tablets, methyltestosterone 25 mg. Price 20 tabs = **C**
Tablets, methyltestosterone 50 mg. Price 20 tabs = **E**

TESTOSTERONE
Indications: hypogonadism
Cautions: cardiac, renal, or hepatic impairment, circulatory failure, hypertension, epilepsy, migraine, thyroid disease, diabetes mellitus
Contra-indications: breast cancer in men, prostatic carcinoma, pregnancy, breast-feeding, nephrosis
Side-effects: oedema, increase in weight, hypercalcaemia, increased bone growth, priapism, premature closure of epiphyses in early puberty, prostatism in elderly patients, high doses cause virilism in women, and suppress spermatogenesis in men

Dose: by sublingual administration, initially 10–30 mg daily reducing to 10 mg daily for maintenance
By implantation, 200–600 mg; duration of effect 7–8 months

PoM **Testosterone Implants** (Organon)
Implant, testosterone 100 mg (duration 30 weeks). Price each = **E**
Implant, testosterone 200 mg (duration 34 weeks). Price each = **G**
PoM **Testoral Sublings**® (Organon)
Sublingual tablets, testosterone 10 mg. Price 20 tabs = **C**. Label: 26

TESTOSTERONE ESTERS
Indications; Cautions; Contra-indications; Side-effects: see under Testosterone

PoM **Primoteston Depot**® (Schering)
Injection (oily), testosterone enanthate 250 mg/ml. Price 1-ml amp = **F**
Dose: by intramuscular injection, initially 250 mg every 2–3 weeks; maintenance 250 mg every 3–6 weeks
PoM **Restandol**® (Organon)
Capsules, red-brown, testosterone undecanoate 40 mg in oily solution. Price 20 caps = **G**
Dose: 120–160 mg daily for 2–3 weeks; maintenance 40–120 mg daily
PoM **Sustanon 100**® (Organon)
Injection (oily), testosterone propionate 20 mg, testosterone phenylpropionate 40 mg, and testosterone isohexanoate 40 mg/ml. Price 1-ml amp = **D**
Dose: by deep intramuscular injection, 1 ml every 2 weeks
PoM **Sustanon 250**® (Organon)
Injection (oily), testosterone propionate 30 mg, testosterone phenylpropionate 60 mg, testosterone isohexanoate 60 mg, and testosterone decanoate 100 mg/ml. Price 1-ml amp = **E**
Dose: by deep intramuscular injection, 1 ml every 2–4 weeks
PoM **Virormone**® (Paines & Byrne)
Injection, testosterone propionate 10 mg/ml. Price 1-ml amp = **B**
Injection, testosterone propionate 25 mg/ml. Price 1-ml amp = **B**
Injection, testosterone propionate 50 mg/ml. Price 1- and 2-ml amp (both) = **B**
Dose: by intramuscular injection, 10–50 mg 2–3 times weekly

6.4.3 Anabolic steroids
All the anabolic steroids have some androgenic activity but they cause less virilisation than androgens in women. Their protein-building property led to the hope that they might be widely useful in medicine but this hope has not been realised. They have, for example, been given for osteo-

---

porosis in women and in cases of wasting. Their use as body builders or tonics is quite unjustified.

It is doubtful whether anabolic steroids should be used to increase height in children; apart from virilising properties, they may lead to premature closing of the epiphyses so that the eventual height is the same as or less than without treatment. Side-effects such as cholestatic jaundice may occur, particularly with the 17-α alkyl derivatives of testosterone (ethyloestrenol and stanozolol) which should be **avoided** in hepatic impairment. They reduce the itching of chronic biliary obstruction but usually make the jaundice worse. Some anabolic steroids produce hepatic tumours in long-term use.

Anabolic steroids are also used in the treatment of some aplastic anaemias (see section 9.1.3), in the palliative treatment of breast cancer (see section 8.3.3), and to stimulate fibrinolysis (see section 2.10). They are abused by some athletes although they have not been shown to have a beneficial effect.

ETHYLOESTRENOL

Indications: protein synthesis after major surgery or chronic debilitating disease

Cautions: cardiac and renal impairment, circulatory failure, hypertension, diabetes mellitus, epilepsy, migraine; monitor skeletal maturation in young patients. Drug interactions: see Appendix 1 (sections *2.8*, *2.8B*)

Contra-indications: hepatic impairment, prostatic carcinoma, pregnancy, breast-feeding

Side-effects: acne, oedema, jaundice on prolonged treatment, virilism with high doses, hypercalcaemia, menstrual irregularities

Dose: 2–4 mg daily for max. of 3 months

PoM **Orabolin**® (Organon)
Tablets, ethyloestrenol 2 mg. Price 20 tabs = **C**

NANDROLONE

Indications: protein synthesis after major surgery or chronic debilitating disease

Cautions; Contra-indications; Side-effects: see under Ethyloestrenol; does not cause cholestatic jaundice or liver function disturbance

Dose: by deep intramuscular injection, nandrolone decanoate 25–50 mg every 3 weeks; CHILD up to 400 micrograms/kg every 3 weeks; nandrolone phenylpropionate 25–50 mg weekly; CHILD up to 1 mg/kg/month

PoM **Deca-Durabolin**® (Organon)
Injection (oily), nandrolone decanoate 25 mg/ml. Price 1-ml amp or syringe = **E**
Injection (oily), nandrolone decanoate 50 mg/ml. Price 1-ml amp or syringe = **F**
Injection (oily), nandrolone decanoate 100 mg/ml. Price 1-ml amp = **H**

PoM **Durabolin**® (Organon)
Injection (oily), nandrolone phenylpropionate 25 mg/ml. Price 1-ml amp or syringe = **C**
Injection (oily), nandrolone phenylpropionate 50 mg/ml. Price 1-ml syringe = **E**

STANOZOLOL

Indications: protein synthesis after major surgery or chronic debilitating disease; hereditary angioedema (for use in aplastic anaemia, see section 9.1.3; for use as a fibrinolytic, see section 2.10)

Cautions; Contra-indications; Side-effects: see under Ethyloestrenol. Headache, euphoria, depression and cramp occur occasionally

Dose: by mouth, anabolic effect, 5 mg daily
Hereditary angioedema, 2.5–10 mg to control attacks, reduced for maintenance
By deep intramuscular injection, 50 mg every 2–3 weeks

PoM **Stromba**® (Sterling Research)
Tablets, scored, stanozolol 5 mg. Price 20 tabs = **G**
Injection (aqueous suspension), stanozolol 50 mg/ml. Price 1-ml amp = **F**

6.5   Hypothalamic and pituitary hormones

Hypothalamic and pituitary hormones are described under the following section headings:

6.5.1 Hypothalamic and anterior pituitary hormones

6.5.2 Posterior pituitary hormones

6.5.3 Antidiuretic hormone antagonists

6.5.1   Hypothalamic and anterior pituitary hormones

FEMALE INFERTILITY. **Clomiphene** is an antioestrogen which is capable of stimulating gonadotrophin release by inhibiting the negative feedback of gonadal steroids on the hypothalamus. It should only be administered under specialist supervision in carefully selected patients. Its main use is in inducing ovulation in patients with secondary amenorrhoea due to the Stein-Leventhal syndrome. In patients who produce a good oestrogen response to clomiphene but who show no biochemical evidence of corpus luteum formation, a single injection of **chorionic gonadotrophin** (HCG) 7 days after the clomiphene is sometimes of help.

Cyclofenil (Rehibin®) is used similarly to clomiphene in the treatment of anovulatory infertility or oligomenorrhoea associated with infertility. **Tamoxifen** (see section 8.3.4) which acts as an oestrogen antagonist is a further alternative in the treatment of anovulatory infertility, but again it should only be used under specialist supervision.

In women with proven hypopituitarism, ovulation and corpus luteum formation can be achieved with injections of **menotrophin** (Pergonal®, human follicle-stimulating hormone, FSH). This is followed by injection of **chorionic gonadotrophin**. Such treatment can only be undertaken in specialist centres and biochemical monitoring is essential to avoid ovarian hyperstimulation with possible rupture and to avoid the risk of multiple pregnancy. When this occurs dose reduction or temporary discontinuation of treatment is necessary. **Serum gonadotrophin** (Gonadotraphon FSH®) is similar to menotrophin but is rarely used.

MALE INFERTILITY. Oligospermia due to a failure of gonadotrophin production can sometimes be successfully treated with injections of chorionic gonadotrophin and menotrophin. This stimulates the production of testosterone in the testis. The treatment is useless in patients with either primary gonadal failure or mechanical blockage in the epididymis or vas deferens.

Gonadorelin (section 6.7.2) and **chorionic gonadotrophin** have both been used in the treatment of cryptorchidism and delayed puberty. Indiscriminate use should be **discouraged** since in the former condition it is of doubtful value and in the latter, detailed endocrinological investigation is required.

CORTICOTROPHINS. **Corticotrophin** and **tetracosactrin** have little therapeutic use in endocrinology and are used mainly as diagnostic agents (section 6.7.2). **Tetracosactrin** is preferred as adrenal stimulation may last for up to 48 hours after each injection; allergic reactions may occur. They have been used to stimulate an adrenal cortex suppressed by chronic corticosteroid administration or following the removal of a unilateral adrenal cortical tumour but even in this role they are of limited use since suppression is often at the hypothalamic or pituitary level.

Corticotrophin and tetracosactrin have been used as an alternative to corticosteroids to control certain conditions, especially Crohn's disease (see section 1.5) and rheumatic disease (see section 10.1.2.1), the alleged advantages being that there is no adrenocortical suppression and that linear growth may be inhibited to a lesser extent. Once a response has occurred, alternate-day therapy should be used if possible. The dose administered has to be judged by monitoring urinary 17-oxogenic steroid excretion since adrenal response is variable.

OTHER HORMONES. **Growth hormone** (somatotrophin, HGH) is effective in the treatment of short stature due to HGH deficiency. Only human growth hormone is active in man, and at present HGH preparations are only available at special centres. Treatment should be confined to patients with open epiphyses. Doses are usually given 2 to 3 times weekly. See section 6.7.1 for bromocriptine in acromegaly.

The clinical uses of **protirelin**, the hypothalamic releasing hormone for thyrotrophin (thyrotrophin-releasing hormone, TRH) and **gonadorelin**, the releasing hormone for the gonadotrophins (gonadotrophin-releasing hormone, LH-RH) are not established and their main uses are as diagnostic agents (section 6.7.2). Gonadorelin has been used in the treatment of functional hypothalamic amenorrhoea and hypogonadotrophic hypogonadism. It requires administration in a pulsatile fashion and its use is only appropriate to specialist endocrine units.

CHORIONIC GONADOTROPHIN
(HCG)

Indications: see notes above
Cautions: see notes above; cardiac or renal impairment, asthma, epilepsy, migraine, skin tests required if predisposed to allergies
Side-effects: oedema (particularly in males—reduce dose), headache, tiredness, mood changes, sensitivity reactions; sexual precocity with high doses; may aggravate ovarian hyperstimulation after menotrophin
Dose: by intramuscular injection, according to patient's requirements

PoM **Chorionic Gonadotrophin Injection,** powder for reconstitution, chorionic gonadotrophin. Price 500- and 1000-unit (both) = **C**; 5000-unit amp = **E** (all with solvent)
PoM **Gonadotraphon LH**® (Paines & Byrne)
Injection, powder for reconstitution, chorionic gonadotrophin. Price 500- and 1000-unit amp (both) = **C**; 5000-unit amp = **E** (all with solvent)
PoM **Pregnyl**® (Organon)
Injection, powder for reconstitution, chorionic gonadotrophin. Price 500-unit amp = **C**; 1500-unit amp = **D**; 5000-unit amp = **E** (all with solvent)
PoM **Profasi**® (Serono)
Injection, powder for reconstitution, chorionic gonadotrophin. Price 500- and 1000-unit amp (both) = **C**; 2000-unit amp = **D**; 5000-unit amp = **E** (all with solvent)

CLOMIPHENE CITRATE

Indications: anovulatory infertility—see notes above
Cautions: see notes above; polycystic ovary syndrome (cysts may enlarge during treatment), incidence of multiple births increased
Contra-indications: hepatic disease, ovarian cysts, endometrial carcinoma, pregnancy, abnormal uterine bleeding
Side-effects: visual disturbances, ovarian hyperstimulation (withdraw treatment), hot flushes, abdominal discomfort, occasionally nausea, vomiting, depression, insomnia, breast tenderness, weight gain, rashes, dizziness, hair loss
Dose: 50 mg daily for 5 days starting on 5th day of menstrual cycle or at any time if cycles have ceased; max. 6 courses. In absence of ovulation dose may be increased by 50-mg amounts each month to max. 200 mg daily for 5 days

PoM **Clomiphene Tablets,** clomiphene citrate 50 mg. Price 20 tabs = **H**
PoM **Clomid**® (Merrell)
Tablets, yellow, scored, clomiphene citrate 50 mg. Price 20 tabs = **H**
PoM **Serophene**® (Serono)
Tablets, scored, clomiphene citrate 50 mg. Price 20 tabs = **H**

C = 51-100p, D = 101-180p, E = 181-300p, F = 301-450p, G = 451-650p, H = 651-900p, I = 901-1200p, J = over 1200p.

CORTICOTROPHIN
(ACTH)

Indications: see notes above
Cautions; Contra-indications; Side-effects: see section 6.3.3; also caution in hypertension. Drug interactions: see Appendix 1 (sections *2.2*, *2.5*, *6.1*, 6.3)
Dose: by subcutaneous or intramuscular injection, depot preparations, initially 40–80 units daily, reduced according to response

PoM **Acthar Gel**® (Armour)
Injection, corticotrophin (with gelatin) 20 units/ml. Price 5-ml vial = **G**
Injection, corticotrophin (with gelatin) 40 units/ml. Price 2-ml vial = **F**; 5-ml vial = **H**
Injection, corticotrophin (with gelatin) 80 units/ml. Price 5-ml vial = **J**
PoM **ACTH/CMC** (Ferring)
Injection, corticotrophin (with carmellose) 60 units/ml. Price 5-ml vial = **G**

CYCLOFENIL

Indications: anovulatory infertility—see notes above
Contra-indications: see under Clomiphene Citrate
Side-effects: hot flushes, abdominal discomfort, nausea; rarely cholestatic jaundice
Dose: 200 mg twice daily for 10 days starting on 3rd day of natural or progesterone-induced bleeding, followed by 20 treatment-free days, repeated for at least 3 months

▼ PoM **Rehibin**® (Thames)
Tablets, scored, cyclofenil 100 mg. Price 20 tabs = **F**

GROWTH HORMONE
(HGH)

Indications: short stature
Contra-indications: diabetes mellitus
Side-effects: antibody formation
Dose: by intramuscular injection, according to patient's requirements

PoM **Crescormon**® (KabiVitrum)
Injection, powder for reconstitution, human growth hormone (from pituitary glands). Price 4-unit vial (with diluent) = **J**

MENOTROPHIN

Indications: see notes above
Cautions: ovarian cysts, adrenal or thyroid disorders, intracranial lesions, exclude endocrine disorders, skin tests required if predisposed to allergies
Side-effects: sensitivity reactions, ovarian hyperstimulation, enlargement, and possible rupture, multiple pregnancy
Dose: by deep intramuscular injection, according to patient's response

PoM **Gonadotraphon FSH**® (Paines & Byrne)
Injection, powder for reconstitution, serum gonadotrophin (from pregnant mares' serum). Price 1000-unit amp (with solvent) = **F**
PoM **Pergonal**® (Serono)
Injection, powder for reconstitution, menotrophin (from postmenopausal urine) as human follicle-stimulating hormone 75 units, human luteinising hormone 75 units, lactose 10 mg. Price per amp (with solvent) = **H**

TETRACOSACTRIN

Indications: see notes above
Cautions; Contra-indications; Side-effects: see section 6.3.3; hypersensitivity reactions may occur less frequently than with corticotrophin

PoM **Synacthen**® (Ciba)
Injection, tetracosactrin 250 micrograms (as acetate)/ml. Price 1-ml amp = **C**
Dose: therapeutic, by intravenous infusion, 250 micrograms (approx. 25 units) in 500 ml over 6 hours, adjusted according to response, by intramuscular injection, 250 micrograms every 3–4 hours
Diagnostic, by intramuscular injection, 250 micrograms as a single dose
PoM **Synacthen Depot**® (Ciba)
Injection (aqueous suspension), tetracosactrin 1 mg (as acetate)/ml, with zinc phosphate complex. Price 1-ml amp = **D**; 2-ml vial = **E**
Dose: by intramuscular injection, initially 0.5–1 mg twice weekly, or, in acute conditions, daily for 3 days, adjusted according to response; CHILD up to 1 year 250 micrograms daily, 1–5 years 250–500 micrograms daily, 6–12 years 0.25–1 mg daily, adjusted according to response

6.5.2   Posterior pituitary hormones

Vasopressin (antidiuretic hormone, ADH) is used in the treatment of diabetes insipidus of pituitary origin; it is of no value in the nephrogenic type. Vasopressin may cause sensitivity reactions. It is given as **lypressin** (8-lysine vasopressin, Syntopressin®) or as the vasopressin analogue **desmopressin** (DDAVP®) which has a longer duration of action due to slower clearance from the circulation and unlike lypressin and vasopressin does not have any vasoconstrictor effects.

In diabetes insipidus following pituitary surgery or trauma, treatment may be required only for a limited period and it is particularly important to take precautions to avoid overdosage and unnecessary prolongation of therapy.

The dose of desmopressin should be adjusted according to individual response and should produce a slight diuresis at least once every 24 hours to avoid water intoxication. Desmopressin is given intranasally for maintenance in doses of 10 to 20 micrograms once or twice daily for adults and 5 to 10 micrograms once or twice daily for children; a single dose usually suppresses diuresis for 12 hours. Desmopressin injection is used mainly for initial diagnosis of diabetes insipidus and postoperatively. The usual dose by intravenous or intramuscular injection is 1 to 4 micrograms daily for adults and 400 nanograms daily for children;

a single dose usually suppresses diuresis for 24 hours. Desmopressin injection is also used in other investigatory procedures and, in specialist centres, for boosting Factor VIII concentrations in mild to moderate haemophiliacs. Vasopressin infusion is used to control variceal bleeding in patients with portal hypertension but with variable results.

Terlipressin (Glypressin®) is a new derivative of vasopressin which is used in the treatment of bleeding oesophageal varices.

In diabetes insipidus of renal as well as of pituitary origin, some benefit may be obtained from the paradoxical antidiuretic effect of the **thiazide** and related **diuretics** such as chlorthalidone and hydrochlorothiazide. The usual initial dose of **chlorthalidone** is 100 mg twice daily, reduced to a maintenance dose of 50 mg daily (see section 2.2.1).

In diabetes insipidus of pituitary or hypothalamic origin **chlorpropamide** (section 6.1.2.1), but not other sulphonylureas, may reduce polyuria. It acts by sensitising the renal tubules to the action of endogenous vasopressin and is useful only in mild cases. The dose of chlorpropamide should not exceed 350 mg daily in adults or 200 mg daily in children and great care should be taken to avoid hypoglycaemic reactions which can be particularly dangerous in patients with hypopituitarism and in children.

Carbamazepine (see section 4.8.1) has been shown to have an antidiuretic action. Although its exact mode of action is not yet known, it is probably similar to that of chlorpropamide. It is used in a dose of 200 mg once or twice daily.

Oxytocin (see section 7.1.1) is also released from the posterior pituitary.

DESMOPRESSIN

Indications: diabetes insipidus; diagnostic procedures (section 6.7.2)
Cautions: see notes above; heart failure, asthma, epilepsy, migraine
Contra-indications: vascular disease, chronic nephritis
Dose: see notes above

PoM **DDAVP**® (Ferring)
Intranasal solution, desmopressin 100 micrograms/ml. Price 2.5-ml dropper bottle and catheter = **I**
Injection, desmopressin 4 micrograms/ml. Price 1-ml amp = **D**

LYPRESSIN

Indications: diabetes insipidus
Cautions; Contra-indications: see under Desmopressin; also vasconstriction—caution in hypertension
Side-effects: nausea, abdominal pain, urge to defaecate, nasal congestion with ulceration of mucosa
Dose: intranasally, 2.5–5 units 3–7 times daily

PoM **Syntopressin**® (Sandoz)
Nasal spray, lypressin 50 units/ml, providing 2.5 units/squeeze. Price 5-ml spray bottle = **F**

PITUITARY (POSTERIOR LOBE)

Indications: diabetes insipidus
Cautions; Contra-indications: see under Desmopressin; also vasoconstriction—contra-indicated in hypertension
Side-effects: see under Vasopressin; also allergic rhinitis, asthma, alveolitis
Dose: by insufflation, 60–90 antidiuretic units daily in divided doses

PoM **Di-Sipidin**® (Paines & Byrne)
Insufflation capsules, pituitary (posterior lobe) 30 antidiuretic units. Price 25 caps and with insufflator (both) = **F**

TERLIPRESSIN

Indications: bleeding from oesophageal varices
Cautions; Contra-indications; Side-effects: see under Vasopressin, but effects are reduced
Dose: by intravenous injection, 2 mg repeated every 4 to 6 hours until bleeding is controlled, to a max. of 24 hours

▼ PoM **Glypressin**® (Ferring)
Injection, terlipressin, powder for reconstitution. Price 1-mg vial with 5 ml diluent = **J** (Hosp. only)

VASOPRESSIN

Indications: diabetes insipidus; bleeding from oesophageal varices
Cautions; Contra-indications: see under Desmopressin
Side-effects: nausea, cramp, desire to defaecate, uterine cramps, hypersensitivity reactions, constriction of coronary arteries (may cause anginal attacks and myocardial ischaemia)
Dose: by subcutaneous or intramuscular injection, diabetes insipidus, 5–20 units at least twice daily
By intravenous infusion, variceal bleeding, 5–20 units over 15 minutes

PoM **Pitressin**® (P-D)
Injection, argipressin (synthetic vasopressin) 20 units/ml. Price 1-ml amp = **C** (Hosp. only)

6.5.3 Antidiuretic hormone antagonists

Demeclocycline (see section 5.1.3) may be used in the treatment of hyponatraemia resulting from inappropriate secretion of antidiuretic hormone. It is thought to act by directly blocking the renal tubular effect of antidiuretic hormone. Initially 0.9 to 1.2 g is given daily in divided doses, reduced to 600–900 mg daily in divided doses for maintenance.

C = 51-100p, **D** = 101-180p, **E** = 181-300p, **F** = 301-450p, **G** = 451-650p, **H** = 651-900p, **I** = 901-1200p, **J** = over 1200p.

6.6   Drugs affecting bone metabolism

This section includes calcitonin and salcatonin (section 6.6.1) and disodium etidronate (section 6.6.2).

See also mithramycin (section 8.1.2), calcium and phosphorus compounds (sections 9.5.1.1 and 9.5.2), vitamin D preparations (section 9.6.4), and oestrogens in postmenopausal osteoporosis (section 6.4.1.1).

6.6.1   Calcitonin and salcatonin

Calcitonin (Calcitare®) is involved with parathyroid hormone in the regulation of bone turnover and hence in the maintenance of calcium balance and homoeostasis. It is used to lower the plasma-calcium concentration in some patients with hypercalcaemia (notably when associated with malignant disease). In the treatment of severe Paget's disease of bone it is used mainly for relief of pain but it is also effective in relieving some of the neurological complications, for example deafness. The prolonged use of porcine calcitonin can lead to the production of neutralising antibodies. **Salcatonin** (Calsynar®, synthetic salmon calcitonin) is less immunogenic and thus more suitable for long-term therapy. When changing treatment in Paget's disease, calcitonin 80 units is equivalent to salcatonin 50 units.

CALCITONIN

Indications: Paget's disease of bone; hypercalcaemia

Cautions: see notes above; porcine calcitonin may contain trace amounts of thyroid. Skin test advisable in patients with history of allergy

Side-effects: nausea, vomiting, flushing, tingling of hands, unpleasant taste, inflammatory reactions at injection site

Dose: hypercalcaemia, *by subcutaneous or intramuscular injection*, initially 4–8 units/kg daily adjusted according to clinical and biochemical response

Paget's disease of bone, *by subcutaneous or intramuscular injection*, 80–160 units 3 times weekly increased to daily in patients with bone pain or nerve compression syndromes

PoM **Calcitare**® (Armour)
Injection, powder for reconstitution, porcine calcitonin. Price 160-unit vial (with gelatin diluent) = **I**

SALCATONIN

Indications: Paget's disease of bone; hypercalcaemia; bone pain in neoplastic disease; postmenopausal osteoporosis

Cautions; Side-effects: see under Calcitonin and notes above

Dose: hypercalcaemia, *by subcutaneous or intramuscular injection*, initially up to 8 units/kg every 6–8 hours adjusted according to clinical and biochemical response

Paget's disease of bone, *by subcutaneous or intramuscular injection*, 50–100 units 3 times weekly increased to daily, in single or divided doses, in patients with bone pain or nerve compression syndromes, usually for 3–6 months

Bone pain in neoplastic disease, *by subcutaneous or intramuscular injection*, 200 units every 6 hours for 48 hours

Postmenopausal osteoporosis, *by subcutaneous or intramuscular injection*, 100 units daily with calcium and vitamin D

PoM **Calsynar**® (Armour)
Injection, salcatonin 100 units/ml in saline/acetate. Price 1-ml amp = **H**
Injection, salcatonin 200 units/ml in saline/acetate. Price 2-ml vial = **J**

6.6.2   Disodium etidronate

Disodium etidronate (Didronel®) is used mainly in the treatment of Paget's disease of bone for the relief of pain. It is adsorbed onto hydroxyapatite crystals, so slowing both their rate of growth and dissolution, and reduces the increased rate of bone turnover associated with Paget's disease of bone. The initial dose is usually 5 mg/kg daily for up to 6 months, but 10 mg/kg daily may be used for up to 3 months if more rapid suppression of bone turnover is necessary; however doses higher than this may make symptoms worse. At least three months should elapse before retreatment.

DISODIUM ETIDRONATE

Indications: Paget's disease of bone

Cautions: enterocolitis; discontinue use if fractures occur; reduce dose in renal impairment (avoid if severe)

Side-effects: nausea, diarrhoea, increase in bone pain, increased risk of fractures with high doses

Dose: Paget's disease of bone, 5 mg/kg as a single daily dose for up to 6 months *or* 10 mg/kg for up to 3 months, avoiding food for 2 hours before and after treatment, particularly calcium and mineral containing products; see also notes above

Heterotropic ossification (complicating hip replacement) 20 mg/kg daily for 1 month before and 3 months after operation; heterotropic ossification (spinal cord injury) 20 mg/kg daily for 2 weeks, reducing to 10 mg/kg daily for 10 weeks

▼ PoM **Didronel**® (Brocades)
Tablets, disodium etidronate 200 mg. Price 20 tabs = **I**. Counselling advised, food and calcium (see dose above)

6.7   Other endocrine drugs

This section includes:
6.7.1 Bromocriptine
6.7.2 Diagnostic agents
6.7.3 Danazol
6.7.4 Trilostane

6.7.1 Bromocriptine

Bromocriptine (Parlodel®) is a stimulant of dopaminergic receptors in the brain. It inhibits release of prolactin by the pituitary and is used to prevent or suppress lactation when simpler measures have proved unsuccessful. It is also used in the treatment of hypogonadism, galactorrhoea, cyclical benign breast disease, and cyclical menstrual disorders. Bromocriptine is used in specialised units in the treatment of prolactinomas. It also inhibits the release of growth hormone and is used in acromegaly. For its use in the treatment of parkinsonism, see section 4.9.1.

BROMOCRIPTINE

Indications: see notes above

Cautions: monitor for pituitary enlargement, particularly during pregnancy, gynaecological examinations, monitor for peptic ulceration in acromegalic patients; non-hormonal contraceptive advice if appropriate; at high dosage caution in patients with psychotic disorders or severe cardiovascular disease. Drug interactions: see Appendix 1 (section 6.7)

Side-effects: nausea, vomiting, constipation, headache, dizziness, postural hypotension, drowsiness; with high doses, confusion, hallucinations, dyskinesia, dry mouth, leg cramps, pleural effusions with high doses (may necessitate withdrawal of treatment); digital vasospasm

Dose: prevention/suppression of lactation, 2.5 mg on 1st day (prevention) or daily for 2–3 days (suppression); then 2.5 mg twice daily for 14 days

Hypogonadism/galactorrhoea, infertility, initially 1–1.25 mg at bedtime, increased gradually; usual dose 7.5 mg daily in divided doses, increased if necessary to a max. of 30 mg daily. Usual dose in infertility without hyperprolactinaemia, 2.5 mg twice daily

Cyclical benign breast disease and cyclical menstrual disorders (particularly breast pain), 1–1.25 mg at bedtime, increased gradually; usual dose 2.5 mg twice daily

Acromegaly, initially 1–1.25 mg daily, gradually increased; usual dose 20 mg daily (occasional patients may require up to 60 mg daily)

Prolactinoma, initially 1.25 mg at bedtime; increased gradually to an average dose of 2.5 mg 3 times daily (occasional patients may require up to 30 mg daily)

Doses should be taken with food

PoM **Parlodel**® (Sandoz)

Tablets, scored, bromocriptine 1 mg (as mesylate). Price 20 tabs = **E**. Label: 21

Tablets, scored, bromocriptine 2.5 mg (as mesylate). Price 20 tabs = **G**. Label: 21

Capsules, blue/white, bromocriptine 5 mg (as mesylate). Price 20 caps = **I**. Label: 21

Capsules, bromocriptine 10 mg (as mesylate). Price 10 caps = **I**. Label: 21

6.7.2 Diagnostic agents for endocrine disorders

Tetracosactrin injection (section 6.5.1) is used to test adrenocortical function. The normal rise in plasma cortisol concentration which follows this administration does not occur in adrenocortical insufficiency.

Metyrapone (Metopirone®) by acting as a competitive inhibitor for 11β-hydroxylation, is capable of inhibiting cortisol production. In the presence of a normal functioning pituitary gland this results in an increase in ACTH production which in turn leads to increased synthesis and release of cortisol precursors from the adrenal cortex. These are measured in the urine as 17-oxogenic steroids. A normal response indicates adequate function of both pituitary and adrenal cortex; failure of response indicates malfunction of either or both endocrine glands. The function of the adrenal glands can be assessed independently with corticotrophin. See also section 6.3.1 for **dexamethasone** suppression test for diagnosis of Cushing's disease. In Cushing's syndrome a significant rise in 17-oxogenic steroids in response to metyrapone favours a diagnosis of a pituitary origin rather than the ectopic ACTH syndrome. For therapeutic purposes see section 6.3.1.

Protirelin (thyrotrophin-releasing hormone, TRH) is a useful diagnostic agent in difficult cases of hyperthyroidism; when injected intravenously into normal subjects it leads to a rapid rise in plasma thyrotrophin (TSH). Plasma thyrotrophin does not rise in patients with thyrotoxicosis because of feed-back inhibition of the pituitary by excess circulating thyroid hormone. Plasma thyrotrophin may not rise in patients with endocrine exophthalmos even when plasma thyroxine and triiodothyronine are within the normal range. Many patients with hypopituitarism show a reduced or delayed rise in thyrotrophin after protirelin. Protirelin also causes release of prolactin.

Impaired or absent responses are also seen in some euthyroid patients with subclinical toxic adenomas, multinodular goitres, acromegaly, and Cushing's syndrome. A normal TSH response to protirelin 200 micrograms rules out hyperthyroidism.

Gonadorelin (gonadotrophin-releasing hormone, LH-RH) when injected intravenously into normal subjects leads to a rapid rise in plasma-luteinising hormone (LH) and follicle-stimulating hormone (FSH) concentrations. It has not so far proved to be very helpful in differentiating hypothalamic from pituitary lesions.

Bovine **thyrotrophin** (thyroid stimulating hormone, TSH) is sometimes used to stimulate thyroidal activity. Its use is declining since alternative diagnostic tests are available and allergic side-effects from its use are common.

Desmopressin (section 6.5.2) is used to diagnose diabetes insipidus. Diabetes insipidus due to lack of antidiuretic hormone (cranial) is diagnosed where the ability to concentrate urine after water deprivation is restored following administration of desmopressin given either intramuscularly in

---

C = 51-100p, D = 101-180p, E = 181-300p, F = 301-450p, G = 451-650p, H = 651-900p, I = 901-1200p, J = over 1200p.

doses of 2 micrograms or intranasally in doses of 20 micrograms. Where the patient fails to concentrate urine following administration of desmopressin, the condition may be due to insensitivity of renal tubules to the hormone (nephrogenic).

The **glucose** tolerance test is used in the diagnosis of diabetes mellitus. Glucose 75 g is usually given orally whilst the patient is in the fasting state, and plasma glucose concentrations measured at intervals.

GONADORELIN
(LH–RH)
Indications: pituitary function assessment
Side-effects: rarely, nausea, headache, abdominal pain, increased menstrual bleeding
Dose: by intravenous injection, adults and childen 100 micrograms

▼ PoM **HRF**® (Ayerst)
Injection, powder for reconstitution, gonadorelin. Price 100-microgram vial = **H**; 500-microgram vial = **J** (both with diluent)
▼ PoM **Relecaf LH-RH**® (Hoechst)
Injection, gonadorelin 100 micrograms/ml. Price 1-ml amp = **H**
▼ PoM **Relecaf LH-RH/TRH**® (Hoechst)
Injection, gonadorelin 100 micrograms, protirelin 200 micrograms/ml. Price 1-ml amp = **I**. For assessment of anterior pituitary reserve in patients with suspected pituitary impairment, by intravenous injection, adults and children 1 ml

METYRAPONE
Indications: Cushing's syndrome (see section 6.3.1), anterior pituitary function assessment in hypopituitarism and after prolonged treatment with corticosteroids. See notes above
Cautions: gross hypopituitarism; many drugs interfere with estimation of steroids
Side-effects: nausea, vomiting, precipitation of hypo-adrenalism
Dose: in the assessment of pituitary function 750 mg every 4 hours for 6 doses; CHILD 15 mg/kg (minimum 250 mg)

PoM **Metopirone**® (Ciba)
Capsules, metyrapone 250 mg. Price 20 caps = **F**

PROTIRELIN
Indications: assessment of thyroid function and thyroid stimulating hormone reserve in hypopituitarism
Cautions: severe hypopituitarism, cardiac insufficiency, oral administration preferable in bronchial asthma and obstructive airways disease, early pregnancy
Side-effects: nausea; also after rapid intravenous administration desire to micturate, flushing, dizziness, syncope, strange taste
Dose: by mouth, adults and children 40 mg, after overnight fasting

By intravenous injection, adults and children 200 micrograms

PoM **TRH** (Roche)
Tablets, scored, protirelin 40 mg. Price 10 tabs = **H**
Injection, protirelin 100 micrograms/ml. Price 2-ml amp = **D**

THYROTROPHIN
Indications: see notes above
Cautions: angina, cardiac failure, hypopituitarism, patients receiving corticosteroids
Contra-indications: coronary thrombosis, adrenal insufficiency
Side-effects: nausea, vomiting, urticaria, transitory hypotension, thyroid swelling, allergy
Dose: by subcutaneous or intramuscular injection, 10 units

PoM **Thytropar**® (Armour)
Injection, powder for reconstitution, thyrotrophin. Price 10-unit vial = **J**

6.7.3   Danazol

Danazol (Danol®) inhibits pituitary gonadotrophin secretion, and is used in the treatment of endometriosis. It has also been used for menorrhagia, mammary dysplasia, and gynaecomastia. It is the drug of choice in the long-term management of hereditary angioedema.

DANAZOL
Indications: see notes above
Cautions: cardiac, hepatic, or renal impairment, epilepsy, diabetes mellitus, migraine; non-hormonal contraceptive methods should be used, if appropriate. Drug interactions: see Appendix 1 (section *2.8B*)
Contra-indications: pregnancy, ensure that patients with amenorrhoea are not pregnant
Side-effects: nausea, dizziness, rashes, backache, flushing, skeletal muscle spasm, hair loss; mild androgenic effects including acne, oily skin, oedema, mild hirsutism, voice changes
Dose: endometriosis, initially 400 mg daily in 2–4 divided doses, adjusted according to response, usually for 6 months; menorrhagia 100–400 mg daily in 2–4 divided doses adjusted according to response, starting on 1st day of menstrual cycle; benign breast disorders, initially 300 mg daily in divided doses, adjusted according to response
CHILD, precocious puberty, 100–400 mg daily according to age and response

PoM **Danol**® (Winthrop)
Capsules, pink/white, danazol 200 mg. Price 10 caps = **H**; 56-cap calendar pack = **J**
PoM **Danol-½**® (Winthrop)
Capsules, grey/white, danazol 100 mg. Price 20 caps = **H**

6.7.4   Trilostane
Trilostane (Modrenal®) inhibits the synthesis of

mineralocorticoids and glucocorticoids by the adrenal cortex, and its use is being evaluated for Cushing's syndrome and primary hyperaldosteronism. It appears to be less effective than metyrapone for the treatment of Cushing's syndrome.

TRILOSTANE

Indications: see notes above

Cautions: impaired liver and kidney function, monitor circulating corticosteroids and blood-electrolyte concentrations; non-hormonal con-

traceptive methods should be used, if appropriate. Drug interactions: see Appendix 1 (section 2.2)

Contra-indications: pregnancy

Side-effects: rarely flushing, nausea, rhinorrhoea with high doses

Dose: 60 mg 4 times daily for at least 3 days, then adjusted according to patient's response; usual dose range 120–480 mg daily in divided doses

▼ PoM **Modrenal**® (Sterling Research)
Capsules, pink/black, trilostane 60 mg. Price 20 caps = **H**

7: Drugs used in

OBSTETRICS, GYNAECOLOGY, and URINARY-TRACT DISORDERS

In this chapter, drugs are discussed under the following headings:

7.1 Drugs acting on smooth muscle
7.2 Treatment of vaginal and vulval conditions
7.3 Contraceptives
7.4 Drugs used in urinary-tract disorders

For hormonal therapy of gynaecological disorders see sections 6.4.1 and 6.5.1.

7.1 Drugs acting on smooth muscle

This section includes prostaglandins and oxytocics (section 7.1.1) and myometrial relaxants (section 7.1.2).

7.1.1 Prostaglandins and oxytocics

Myometrial stimulants are used to induce abortion or induce or augment labour and to minimise blood loss from the placental site. They include oxytocin, ergometrine, and the prostaglandins.

Alprostadil (prostaglandin E_1) is used to maintain patency of the ductus arteriosus in neonates with congenital heart defects, prior to corrective surgery in centres where intensive care is immediately available.

INDUCTION OF ABORTION. The prostaglandins **dinoprost** (Prostin F2 alpha®) and **dinoprostone** (Prostin E2®) can be used for the induction of abortion, including missed abortion and hydatidiform mole. They are contra-indicated in conditions where prolonged uterine contractions would be inappropriate, for example pelvic inflammatory disease and history of difficult labour.

The *intravenous route* is associated with a high incidence of side-effects, including phlebitis and intestinal colic, and its use is confined to cases of missed abortion and hydatidiform mole.

Extra- or intra-amniotic injection is preferable for the induction of late therapeutic abortion. *Extra-amniotic* administration of dinoprostone through a transcervical catheter can be by either intermittent or continuous instillation. Extra-amniotic dinoprostone is also of value as an adjunct in 'priming' the cervix prior to suction termination of pregnancy. The *intra-amniotic* route can only be used after about 14–16 weeks gestation. Dinoprost is given by a single injection of 40 mg which can be repeated if necessary. Prostaglandin administration can be combined with an oxytocin infusion but the risk of uterine rupture is increased.

INDUCTION AND AUGMENTATION OF LABOUR. **Oxytocin** (Syntocinon®) is administered by slow intravenous infusion, preferably using an infusion pump, to induce or augment labour, often in conjunction with amniotomy. Uterine activity must be monitored and hyperstimulation avoided. Large doses of oxytocin may result in excessive fluid retention.

Prostaglandins are not the drugs of choice for induction of labour at term because of the side-effects associated with intravenous administration and the risks to the fetus if hyperstimulation occurs after extra- or intra-amniotic administration. In the induction of preterm labour, if for example there is intrauterine fetal death or gross fetal malformation, prostaglandins may be more effective than oxytocin alone, and can also be combined with oxytocin infusion. Dinoprostone pessaries may be used in selected cases to ripen the cervix.

PREVENTION AND TREATMENT OF HAEMORRHAGE. Bleeding due to incomplete abortion can be controlled with **ergometrine** and **oxytocin** (Syntometrine®) given intravenously or intramuscularly, the dose being adjusted according to the patient's condition and blood loss. This is commonly used prior to surgical evacuation of the uterus, particularly when surgery is delayed. Oxytocin or ergometrine may be used alone but is usually less effective on the early pregnant uterus.

For prophylaxis of postpartum haemorrhage, **ergometrine** with or without oxytocin is commonly used; either 5 units **oxytocin** and 500 micrograms ergometrine maleate (1 ml Syntometrine®) by intramuscular injection at or after delivery of the anterior shoulder, or ergometrine maleate 125 to 250 micrograms by intravenous injection at or after delivery of the anterior shoulder.

Atonic postpartum haemorrhage can be controlled by ergometrine maleate 125 to 250 micrograms by intravenous injection, or by oxytocin intravenous infusion when the patient does not respond to ergometrine.

ALPROSTADIL

Indications: congenital heart defects in neonates prior to corrective surgery

Cautions: see notes above; avoid use in hyaline membrane disease, history of haemorrhage, monitor arterial pressure

Side-effects: apnoea (particularly in infants under 2 kg), flushing, bradycardia, hypotension, tachycardia, cardiac arrest, oedema, diarrhoea, fever, convulsions, disseminated intravascular coagulation, hypokalaemia; cortical proliferation of long bones, weakening of the wall of the ductus arteriosus and pulmonary artery may follow prolonged use

Dose: by intravenous infusion, initially 100

nanograms/kg/minute, then decreased to lowest effective dose

▼ PoM **Prostin VR**® (Upjohn)
Injection, alprostadil 500 micrograms/ml in alcohol. To be diluted before use. Price 1-ml amp = **J** (Hosp. only)

DINOPROST

Indications: see notes above
Cautions: asthma, glaucoma, multiple pregnancy; raised intra-ocular pressure; excessive dosage may cause uterine rupture; see also notes above
Contra-indications: hypertonic uterine inertia, mechanical obstruction of delivery, placenta praevia, predisposition to uterine rupture, severe toxaemia, untreated pelvic infection, fetal distress
Side-effects: nausea, vomiting, diarrhoea, flushing, shivering, headache, dizziness, temporary pyrexia and raised white blood cell count; all dose-related and more common after intravenous administration; also local tissue reaction and erythema
Dose: by intravenous infusion, induction of labour, fetal intra-uterine death, as a solution containing 15 micrograms/ml, 2.5 micrograms/minute (increased in fetal intra-uterine death to 5 micrograms if necessary) for at least 30 minutes
Therapeutic abortion, missed abortion, and hydatidiform mole, as a solution containing 50 micrograms/ml, 25 micrograms/minute for at least 30 minutes, then continued or increased to 50 micrograms/minute
By slow intra-amniotic injection, therapeutic termination of pregnancy in second trimester, 40 mg, repeated if necessary

PoM **Prostin F2 alpha**® (Upjohn)
Intravenous injection, dinoprost 5 mg (as trometamol salt)/ml. Dilute before use. Price 1.5-ml amp = **G**; 5-ml amp = **J** (Hosp. only)
Intra-amniotic injection, dinoprost 5 mg (as trometamol salt)/ml. Price 4-ml amp = **J**; 8-ml amp = **J** (Hosp. only)

DINOPROSTONE

Indications; Cautions; Contra-indications; Side-effects: see under Dinoprost and notes above; also avoid extra-amniotic route in cervicitis or vaginitis
Dose: by mouth, induction of labour, 500 micrograms, followed by 0.5–1 mg (max. 1.5 mg) at hourly intervals
By intravenous infusion, induction of labour, fetal intra-uterine death, as a solution containing 1.5 micrograms/ml, 250 nanograms/minute for at least 30 minutes (increased if necessary to 500 nanograms/minute in fetal intra-uterine death)
Therapeutic abortion, missed abortion, and hydatidiform mole, as a solution containing 5 micrograms/ml, 2.5 micrograms/minute for at

least 30 minutes then increased if necessary to 5 micrograms/minute; may be increased again after 4 hours
By extra-amniotic instillation, therapeutic abortion, as a solution containing 100 micrograms/ml, 100 micrograms, followed by 100–200 micrograms every 2 hours
By vagina in vaginal tablets, inserted high into the posterior fornix, induction of labour, 3 mg, followed after 6–8 hours by 3 mg if labour is not established

PoM **Prostin E2**® (Upjohn)
Tablets, dinoprostone 500 micrograms. Price 20 tabs = **J** (Hosp. only)
Intravenous injection, dinoprostone 1 mg/ml. Dilute before use. Price 0.75-ml amp = **G** (Hosp. only)
Intravenous injection, dinoprostone 10 mg/ml. Dilute before use. Price 0.5-ml amp = **J** (Hosp. only)
Extra-amniotic injection, dinoprostone 10 mg/ml. Price 0.5-ml amp (with diluent) = **J** (Hosp. only)
Vaginal tablets, dinoprostone 3 mg. Price per tab = **H**

ERGOMETRINE MALEATE

Indications: active management of third stage of labour, postpartum haemorrhage
Cautions: toxaemia, cardiac disease, hypertension, sepsis
Contra-indications: 1st and 2nd stages of labour, vascular disease, impaired hepatic and renal function, multiple pregnancy
Side-effects: nausea, vomiting, transient hypertension, vasoconstriction
Dose: by mouth, 0.5–1 mg (onset about 8 minutes, duration about 1 hour)
By intramuscular injection, 200–500 micrograms (onset about 2–7 minutes)
By intravenous injection for emergency control of haemorrhage, 100–500 micrograms (onset about 1 minute)
See also notes above

PoM **Ergometrine Tablets,** ergometrine maleate 250 micrograms, price 20 tabs = **C**; 500 micrograms, price 20 tabs = **D**
PoM **Ergometrine Injection,** ergometrine maleate 500 micrograms/ml. Price 1-ml amp = **B**
PoM **Syntometrine**® (Sandoz)
Injection, ergometrine maleate 500 micrograms, oxytocin 5 units/ml. Price 1-ml amp = **A**
Dose: by intramuscular injection, 1 ml; by intravenous injection, 0.5–1 ml

OXYTOCIN

Indications: induction and augmentation of labour; management of missed or incomplete abortion; postpartum haemorrhage; also facilitation of lactation (as nasal spray)
Cautions: hypertension, pressor drugs (may precipitate severe hypertension), multiple pregnancy, high parity, previous Caesarean section

---

C = 51-100p, **D** = 101-180p, **E** = 181-300p, **F** = 301-450p, **G** = 451-650p, **H** = 651-900p, **I** = 901-1200p, **J** = over 1200p.

Contra-indications: hypertonic uterine inertia, mechanical obstruction to delivery, failed trial labour, severe toxaemia, predisposition to amniotic fluid embolism, fetal distress, and placenta praevia

Side-effects: high doses cause violent uterine contractions leading to rupture and fetal asphyxiation, arrhythmias, maternal hypertension and subarachnoid haemorrhage, water intoxication

Dose: by slow intravenous infusion, induction and augmentation of labour, as a solution containing 1 unit per litre, 1–3 milliunits per minute, adjusted according to response

Missed abortion, as a solution containing 10–20 units/500 ml given at a rate of 10–30 drops/minute, increased in strength by 10–20 units/500 ml every hour to a max. strength of 100 units/500 ml.

Postpartum haemorrhage, 5–10 units/500 ml given at a rate of 15 drops/minute, adjusted according to response

By nasal instillation, facilitation of lactation, 1 squeeze (about 2 units) into one or both nostrils 2–5 minutes before feeding infant

PoM **Syntocinon**® (Sandoz)
Injection, oxytocin 1 unit/ml. Price 2-ml amp = **A**
Injection, oxytocin 5 units/ml. Price 1-ml amp = **A**
Injection, oxytocin 10 units/ml. Price 1-ml amp = **B**; 5-ml amp = **C**
Nasal spray, oxytocin 40 units/ml. Price 5-ml bottle = **D**

7.1.2   Myometrial relaxants

Beta$_2$-adrenoceptor stimulants (sympathomimetics) relax uterine muscle and may be used in selected cases in an attempt to inhibit premature labour. They may also be of value in reducing uterine tone in cases of acute fetal distress associated with excessive uterine activity in hypertonus induced by myometrial stimulants. They are given initially by intravenous infusion to stop contractions and continued by intramuscular injection or by mouth to prevent relapse, but are unlikely to be effective if labour is well advanced. Maternal pulse and blood pressure must be monitored throughout.

Beta$_2$-adrenoceptor stimulants should not be used unless a clear benefit is likely to result from attempting to reduce uterine activity. Tachycardia is the commonest side-effect and may be extreme if atropine is also administered.

Drugs used in the treatment of spasmodic dysmenorrhoea include prostaglandin-synthetase inhibitors such as **aspirin**, **mefenamic acid** and **naproxen sodium** (see section 4.7.1.1) and antispasmodics such as **hyoscine butylbromide** (Buscopan®). See sections 6.4.1.2 and 6.4.1.4 for hormone treatment.

DYSMENORRHOEA

ALVERINE CITRATE
Indications: spasmodic dysmenorrhoea
Cautions; Side-effects: see section 1.2
Dose: 60-120 mg 1–3 times daily

Spasmonal® (Norgine)
Capsules, blue/grey, alverine citrate 60 mg. Price 20 caps = **D**

HYOSCINE BUTYLBROMIDE
Indications: spasmodic dysmenorrhoea
Cautions; Contra-indications; Side-effects: see section 1.2
Dose: by mouth, 20 mg 4 times daily, starting 2 days before expected date of menstruation and continuing for 3 days after commencement
By intramuscular or intravenous injection, 20 mg every 30–60 minutes when necessary

PoM **Buscopan**® (Boehringer Ingelheim)
Tablets, s/c, hyoscine butylbromide 10 mg. Price 20 tabs = **C**
Injection, see section 1.2

PREMATURE LABOUR

ISOXSUPRINE HYDROCHLORIDE
Indications: premature labour
Cautions: may cause hypotension in the newborn; see notes above
Contra-indications: recent arterial haemorrhage, heart disease, premature detachment of placenta, severe anaemia, ruptured membranes, infection
Side-effects: hypotension, transient tachycardia, flushing, nausea, vomiting
Dose: by intravenous infusion, initially 200-300 micrograms/minute gradually increased to 500 micrograms/minute until labour is arrested; subsequently *by intramuscular injection,* 10 mg every 3 hours for 24 hours, then every 4–6 hours for 48 hours; then *by mouth,* 20 mg 4 times daily

PoM **Duvadilan**® (Duphar)
Tablets, pink, scored, isoxsuprine hydrochloride 20 mg. Price 20 tabs = **C**
Injection, isoxsuprine hydrochloride 5 mg/ml. Price 2-ml amp = **B**

ORCIPRENALINE SULPHATE
Indications: premature labour
Cautions; Contra-indications; Side-effects: see under Ritodrine Hydrochloride
Dose: by intravenous infusion, 2.5 micrograms/minute for 5 minutes, increased until contractions are suppressed; max. 2.5 mg in 24 hours

PoM **Alupent Obstetric**® (Boehringer Ingelheim)
Injection, orciprenaline sulphate 500 micro-

grams/ml. To be diluted before use. Price
10-ml amp = **C**

RITODRINE HYDROCHLORIDE

Indications: premature labour; fetal asphyxia due
to hypertonic uterine action

Cautions: diabetes mellitus (monitor blood sugar
during intravenous treatment), treatment with
corticosteroids, anaesthetics, potassium-deplet-
ing diuretics; monitor blood pressure and pulse

Contra-indications: cardiac disorders, haemorrhage, hypertension, pre-eclampsia, cord compression, thyrotoxicosis, ruptured membranes,
infection, treatment with monoamine-oxidase
inhibitors, tricyclic antidepressants, beta-
adrenoceptor blocking drugs, antihypertensives

Side-effects: nausea, vomiting, flushing, sweating, tremor; tachycardia and hypotension with
high doses

Dose: by intravenous infusion, premature labour,
initially 50 micrograms/minute, gradually
increased to 150–350 micrograms/minute and
continued for 12–48 hours after contractions
have ceased; or *by intramuscular injection,*
10 mg every 3–8 hours continued for 12–48
hours after contractions have ceased; then *by
mouth,* 10 mg 30 minutes before termination of
intravenous infusion, repeated every 2 hours
for 24 hours, followed by 10–20 mg every 4–6
hours, max. 120 mg daily
Fetal asphyxia due to hypertonic uterine action,
by intravenous infusion, 50 micrograms/minute
increased as necessary to a max. of 350
micrograms/minute

PoM **Yutopar**® (Duphar)
Tablets, buff, scored, ritodrine hydrochloride
10 mg. Price 20 tabs = **F**
Injection, ritodrine hydrochloride 10 mg/ml.
Price 5-ml amp = **E**

SALBUTAMOL

Indications: premature labour

Cautions; Contra-indications; Side-effects: see
under Ritodrine Hydrochloride

Dose: by intravenous infusion, 10 micrograms/
minute gradually increased to 45 micrograms/
minute until contractions have ceased, then
gradually reduced; or *by intravenous or intramuscular injection,* 100–250 micrograms
repeated according to patient's response; subsequently *by mouth* 4 mg every 6–8 hours

PoM **Ventolin**® (A&H)
Solution for intravenous infusion, salbutamol
1 mg (as sulphate)/ml. Price 5-ml amp = **F**
Tablets, see section 3.1.1.1
Injection, see section 3.1.1.1

TERBUTALINE SULPHATE

Indications: premature labour

Cautions; Contra-indications; Side-effects: see
under Ritodrine Hydrochloride

Dose: by intravenous infusion, 10 micro-
grams/minute (as a 0.0005% solution) for 1
hour, gradually increased to a max. of 25
micrograms/minute until contractions have
ceased, then reduced; subsequently *by subcutaneous injection,* 250 micrograms every 6
hours for 3 days, and *by mouth,* 5 mg every 8
hours until 37th week of pregnancy

PoM **Bricanyl**® (Astra)
Injection, terbutaline sulphate 500 micrograms/
ml. Price 1-ml amp = **B**
Tablets, see section 3.1.1.1

7.2 Treatment of vaginal and vulval conditions

Topical applications to the vulva and vagina
include pessaries, dusting-powders, creams, and
medicated tampons. Symptoms are likely to be
primarily referable to the vulva, but infections
almost invariably involve the vagina also, so that
external applications to the vulva at best are likely
to give only symptomatic relief and will not cure
infections.

Creams are usually preferable to ointments,
which are not water permeable and adversely
affect evaporation and dispersal of natural
secretions. Aqueous medicated douches may
disturb normal vaginal acidity and bacterial flora.

Topical anaesthetic agents (see section 13.3)
give only symptomatic relief and may cause sensitivity reactions. They are indicated only in cases
of pruritus where specific local causes have been
excluded.

Systemic drugs are required in the treatment
of infections, especially those which are sexually
transmitted, which, whilst manifest primarily by
genital tract symptoms, may also affect other tissues (see section 5.1).

7.2.1 Topical hormones
7.2.2 Anti-infective drugs

7.2.1 Topical hormones

When there is a lack of endogenous oestrogens
(as in postmenopausal women) **dienoestrol cream**
0.01% may be used as an adjunct to other treatment in order to improve the quality of the vaginal
epithelium in conditions such as atrophic vaginitis
and kraurosis vulvae and increase natural resistance to infection. Topical oestrogens are also used
prior to vaginal surgery for prolapse when there
is epithelial atrophy. They should be used in the
minimum effective amount and treatment discontinued as soon as possible to minimise absorption
of the oestrogen.

OESTROGENS, TOPICAL

Indications: see notes above

Cautions: examine patients periodically during
prolonged treatment; porphyria

Contra-indications: undiagnosed vaginal
bleeding, pregnancy, endometriosis, mammary
or genital carcinoma, thrombosis, severe cardiac disease

Side-effects: see section 6.4.1.1

C = 51-100p, **D** = 101-180p, **E** = 181-300p, **F** = 301-450p, **G** = 451-650p, **H** = 651-900p, **I** = 901-1200p, **J** = over 1200p.

PoM **Stilboestrol Pessaries,** stilboestrol 500 micrograms. Price 12 pessaries = **D**
Insert 2 pessaries at night for 1–2 weeks then reduced

PoM **Hormofemin**® (Medo)
Cream, dienoestrol 0.025%. Price 40 g with 4-g applicator = **E**
Insert ½–1 applicatorful daily for 1–2 weeks then reduced

PoM **Ortho Dienoestrol** (Ortho-Cilag)
Cream, dienoestrol 0.01%. Price 78 g with applicator = **E**
Insert 1–2 applicatorfuls daily for 1–2 weeks, then gradually reduced to 1 applicatorful 1–3 times weekly if necessary

▼ PoM **Ovestin**® (Organon)
Intravaginal cream, oestriol 0.1%. Price 15 g with applicator = **F**
Insert 1 applicatorful daily for 3 weeks, then reduced; postmenopausal surgery, 1 applicatorful daily for 2 weeks, resuming 2 weeks after surgery

PoM **Premarin**® (Ayerst)
Vaginal cream, conjugated oestrogens 625 micrograms/g. Price 42.5 g with calibrated applicator = **E**
Insert 1–2 g daily starting on the 5th day of the cycle, gradually increased if necessary to max. 4 g, daily for 3 weeks, followed by a 1-week interval; postmenopausal surgery, 1–2 g daily for 10 days before and after surgery

PoM **Tampovagan Stilboestrol and Lactic Acid**® (Norgine)
Pessaries, stilboestrol 500 micrograms, lactic acid 5%. Price 10 pessaries = **E**
Insert 2 pessaries at night for 1–2 weeks then reduce

7.2.2 Anti-infective drugs

Effective specific treatments are available for the common vaginal infections and the causal organism should be identified before instituting treatment.

Vaginal candidiasis is treated primarily by pessaries or cream which should be inserted high into the vagina, including the time of menstruation, using a special applicator for the cream. Candidal vulvitis is treated with cream but there is almost invariably associated vaginal infection which should also be treated.

Nystatin is a well established treatment. One pessary is inserted nightly for 14 to 28 nights. It may be supplemented with cream for vulvitis and other superficial sites of infection. Imidazole drugs appear to be equally effective in shorter courses, for example **clotrimazole** and **econazole** for 3 days or **miconazole** for 5, 7, or 14 days according to the preparation used; **isoconazole** is given as a single dose and clotrimazole (as Canesten 1®) may also be used in this way, which is an advantage when patient compliance is a problem. Tampons coated with miconazole are also available. Vaginal applications may be supplemented with cream for vulvitis and other superficial sites of infection.

Recurrence is common if the full course of treatment has not been completed and is also particularly likely if there are predisposing factors such as antibiotic therapy, steroid contraceptive use, pregnancy, or diabetes mellitus. Possible reservoirs of infection may also lead to recontamination and should be treated. These include other skin sites such as the digits, nail beds, and umbilicus as well as the gut and the bladder. Also, the partner may be the source of reinfection and should be treated with the cream at the same time. Concurrent oral treatment may be necessary in resistant or recurrent infection, using **nystatin** or **miconazole** tablets (see section 5.2). Vaginal preparations intended to restore the normal acidity (Aci-jel®) may also prevent re-infection and permit the re-establishment of the normal vaginal flora.

Trichomonal infections commonly involve the lower urinary tract as well as the genital system and require systemic treatment with either metronidazole or nimorazole. **Metronidazole** (see section 5.1.11.1) is given as a 200-mg tablet 3 times daily for 7 days or 800 mg in the morning and 1.2 g at night for 2 days. To achieve a high cure rate the course should be repeated after an interval of 7 days. The partner should be given the same course of treatment. Side-effects are more common with the short course of metronidazole and following the ingestion of alcohol.

Nimorazole (see section 5.4.3) is administered as a single oral dose of 2 g to each partner when metronidazole is ineffective.

Bacterial infections of the lower genital tract may be caused by a wide range of organisms. The treatment of gonorrhoea and syphilis is described in section 5.1, Table 1. Infections with Gram-negative organisms are particularly common in association with gynaecological operations and trauma. Metronidazole is effective against certain Gram-negative organisms, especially *Bacteroides* spp. and may be used as a prophylactic measure in gynaecological surgery.

Antibacterial creams such as Sultrin® may be used in the treatment of mixed bacterial infections, for example, in infants. They are ineffective against *Candida* spp. and *Trichomonas vaginalis*.

Acyclovir preparations (see section 5.3 for tablets and infusion and section 13.10.3 for cream) may be used in the treatment of genital infection due to *Herpes simplex* virus, the HSV type 2 being a major cause of genital ulceration. These preparations all have a beneficial effect on virus shedding and healing, generally giving relief from pain and other symptoms.

GENITAL ANTIFUNGAL PREPARATIONS

Indications: vaginal and vulval candidiasis
Side-effects: local irritation, possibly including burning, oedema, erythema
Administration: insert pessaries or cream high into the vagina and complete the course regardless of intervening menstruation

---

Canesten® (Bayer)
Cream (topical), clotrimazole 1%. Price 20 g = **E**; 50 g = **F**
Apply to anogenital area 2–3 times daily
PoM *Vaginal cream*, clotrimazole 2%. Price 35 g (with 5-g applicators) = **G**
Insert 5 g twice daily for 3 days or once nightly for 6 nights
PoM *Vaginal tablets*, clotrimazole 100 mg. Price 6 tabs with applicator = **E**
PoM *Vaginal tablets*, clotrimazole 200 mg. Price 3 tabs with applicator = **E**
Insert 200 mg for 3 nights *or* 100 mg for 6 nights
PoM *Duopak*, clotrimazole 100-mg vaginal tablets and cream (topical) 1%. Price 6 tabs and 20 g cream = **F**

PoM **Canesten 1®** (Bayer)
Vaginal tablets, clotrimazole 500 mg. Price 1 tab with applicator = **E**
Insert 1 at night as a single dose

Ecostatin® (Squibb)
Cream (topical), econazole nitrate 1%. Price 15 g = **D**; 30 g = **E**
Apply to anogenital area twice daily
PoM *Pessaries*, econazole nitrate 150 mg. Price 3 pessaries with applicator = **F**
Insert 1 pessary for 3 nights
PoM *Twinpack*, econazole nitrate pessaries and cream as above. Price 3 pessaries and 15 g cream = **G**

PoM **Flagyl®** (M&B)
Compak, tablets, scored, metronidazole 200 mg, with pessaries, yellow, nystatin 100000 units. Price 21 tablets and 14 pessaries (with applicator) = **F**
Dose: for mixed trichomonal and candidal infections, 1 tablet 3 times daily with water after food for 7 days and 1 pessary inserted twice daily for 7 days or 1 at night for 14 nights

PoM **Fungilin®** (Squibb)
Cream, amphotericin 3%. Price 15 g = **D**
Apply to anogenital area 2–4 times daily

PoM **Gyno-Daktarin®** (Janssen)
Intravaginal cream, miconazole nitrate 2%. Price 78 g with applicators = **G**
Insert 1 applicatorful at night for 7 nights
Pessaries, miconazole nitrate 100 mg. Price 14 pessaries = **F**
Insert 2 pessaries for 7 nights
Tampons, coated with miconazole nitrate 100 mg. Price 10 tampons = **F**
Insert 1 tampon night and morning for 5 days
Combipack, miconazole nitrate pessaries and cream (topical) 2%. Price 14 pessaries and 15 g cream = **G**

PoM **Gyno-Pevaryl®** (Ortho-Cilag)
Pessaries, econazole nitrate 150 mg. Price 3 pessaries = **F**
Insert 1 pessary for 3 nights
Combipack, econazole nitrate pessaries as above, econazole nitrate 1% cream (to be applied to anogenital area). Price 3 pessaries and 15 g cream = **G**

PoM **Monistat®** (Ortho-Cilag)
Vaginal cream, miconazole nitrate 2%. Price 78 g with applicator = **F**

Insert 1 applicatorful (approx. 5 g) at night for 14 nights; also apply to anogenital area
Pessaries, miconazole nitrate 100 mg. Price 14 pessaries = **F**
Insert 100 mg at night for 14 days

▼ PoM **Nizoral®** (Janssen)
Cream (topical), ketoconazole 2%. Price 15 g = **D**
Apply to anogenital area once or twice daily

PoM **Nyspes®** (DDSA)
Pessaries, buff, nystatin 100000 units. Price 15 pessaries = **D**
Insert 1–2 pessaries for at least 14 nights

PoM **Nystan®** (Squibb)
Cream and *Ointment*, see section 13.10.2
Gel (topical), nystatin 100000 units/g. Price 30 g = **E**
Apply to anogenital area 2–4 times daily
Vaginal cream, nystatin 100000 units/4-g application. Price 60 g with applicator = **F**
Pessaries, yellow, nystatin 100000 units. Price 15 pessaries with applicator = **D**
Insert 1–2 applicatorfuls of cream or 1–2 pessaries at night for at least 14 nights
Triple pack, nystatin tablets 500000 units, nystatin gel 100000 units/g. Nystavescent® pessaries as below. Price 42 tablets+28 pessaries +30 g gel = **H**
Dose: 1 tablet 3 times daily for 14 days, with gel and pessaries as above

PoM **Nystavescent®** (Squibb)
Pessaries, yellow, effervescent, nystatin 100000 units. Price 15 pessaries with applicator = **D**
Insert as for Nystan® (above)

Pevaryl® (Ortho-Cilag)
Cream, econazole nitrate 1%. Price 30 g = **E**
Apply to anogenital area 2–3 times daily
Lotion and *Dusting-powder*, see section 13.10.2

PoM **Pimafucin®** (Brocades)
Cream, natamycin 2%. Price 30 g = **D**
Apply to anogenital area 2–3 times daily
Vaginal tablets (=pessaries), natamycin 25 mg. Price 20 tabs = **D**
Insert 1 pessary for 20 nights *or*, in candidal infections, 1 pessary twice daily for 10 days *or* 1 pessary for 20 nights

▼ PoM **Travogyn®** (Schering)
Cream (topical), isoconazole nitrate 1%. Price 20 g = **E**
Apply to anogenital area twice daily
Vaginal tablets (=pessaries), isoconazole nitrate 300 mg. Price 2 tabs = **F**
Insert 2 pessaries as a single dose preferably at night

VAGINAL ANTIBACTERIAL PREPARATIONS

Indications: bacterial vaginitis and cervicitis
Side-effects: sensitivity

PoM **Sultrin®** (Ortho-Cilag)
Cream, sulphathiazole 3.42%, sulphacetamide 2.86%, sulphabenzamide 3.7%. Price 78 g with applicator = **E**
Vaginal tablets, sulphathiazole 172.5 mg, sul-

phacetamide   143.75 mg,   sulphabenzamide 184 mg. Price 20 tabs with applicator = **E**

Insert 1 pessary or applicatorful of cream twice daily for 10 days, then once daily if necessary

VAGINAL ANTISEPTIC PREPARATIONS

Aci-Jel® (Ortho-Cilag)

Vaginal jelly, acetic acid 0.92% in a buffered (pH 4) basis. Price 85 g with applicator = **E**

Non-specific infections, insert 1 applicatorful twice daily to restore vaginal acidity

Betadine® (Napp)

Caution: avoid in pregnancy and in breast-feeding

Pessaries, brown, povidone-iodine 200 mg. Price 28 pessaries with applicator = **G**

Vaginal gel, brown, povidone-iodine 10%. Price 80 g with applicator = **E**

In vaginal infections insert 1 moistened pessary or 1 applicatorful (5 g) of gel twice daily for 2–4 weeks

Antiseptic Vaginal Cleansing Kit, solution, povidone-iodine 10%. For dilution before use. Price 250 ml with measuring bottle and applicator = **E**

Vaginal cleansing in vaginal infections or pre-operatively, douche daily for 14 days

PoM **Penotrane**® (WBP)

Pessaries, hydrargaphen 1.5 mg. Price 15 pessaries = **D**

In vaginal infections insert 2 pessaries of 1.5 mg for 15 nights, repeated if necessary at the start of the next menstrual cycle. Do not use with copper-containing intra-uterine devices

7.3   Contraceptives

The criteria by which contraceptive methods should be judged are effectiveness, acceptability, and freedom from side-effects.

Hormonal contraception is the most effective method of fertility control, short of sterilisation, but has unwanted major and minor side-effects, especially for certain groups of women.

Intra-uterine devices, usually made of inert plastic, have a high use-effectiveness but may produce undesirable side-effects, especially menorrhagia, or be otherwise unsuitable in a significant proportion of women. The use of intra-uterine devices is generally inadvisable in nulliparous women because of the risk of inducing pelvic sepsis and infertility. In order to minimise side-effects smaller devices with a copper coating have been introduced. Their contraceptive efficacy is as good as with the inert devices.

Barrier methods alone (condoms, diaphragms, and caps) are less effective but can be very reliable for well motivated couples if used in conjunction with a **spermicide**. Occasionally sensitivity reactions occur.

7.3.1 Combined oral contraceptives
7.3.2 Progestogen-only contraceptives
7.3.3 Spermicidal contraceptives

7.3.1   Combined oral contraceptives

Oral contraceptives containing an oestrogen and a progestogen are the most effective preparations for general use. The oestrogen content ranges from 20 to 50 micrograms (see Table) and generally a preparation with the lowest oestrogen and progestogen content which gives good cycle control and minimal side-effects in the individual patient is chosen. With low-oestrogen preparations (30 or 35 micrograms of oestrogen) the margin of safety is reduced and regularity of pill taking becomes more critical. Below 30 micrograms the preparations may be less effective.

The chemical nature and biological activity of the 6 progestogens in use varies. In general, higher doses of progestogen reduce menstrual loss (even to the point of amenorrhoea in susceptible individuals) and induce greater weight gain.

The dosage regimen for *combined oral contraceptives* is usually 1 tablet daily for 21 days, followed by a 7-day interval during which menstrual bleeding occurs. It is usually recommended that the first course is started on the 5th day of the cycle; ovulation may then not be inhibited during the cycle and additional contraceptive precautions should therefore be taken during the first 14 days of that cycle or when changing from a high to a low oestrogen preparation. Additional contraceptive precautions are unnecessary in the first cycle if the tablets are started on the first day of the cycle.

The course of tablets should be taken at approximately the same time each day. If it is delayed by longer than 12 hours, contraceptive protection may be lost. The patient should then be advised to complete the course but to use an additional method of contraception for the next 14 days. It is important that if more than 2 consecutive tablets have been missed, oral contraceptives should be discontinued immediately and a method of non-hormonal contraception used until menstruation occurs.

Phased formulations more closely mimic normal endogenous cyclical hormonal activity. The total dose of oestrogen is slightly increased and the total dose of progestogen decreased over the cycle, compared with low-oestrogen (30-microgram) preparations. They are generally recommended for a day 1 start.

Critical factors which limit effectiveness are vomiting and diarrhoea and some antibiotics, for example ampicillin, which interfere with absorption. Drugs which induce hepatic mono-oxidase activity (for example barbiturates, phenytoin, rifampicin) also increase the risk of failure.

Following childbirth oral contraception can be started at any time, but preferably not earlier than 2 weeks postpartum because of the increased risk of thrombosis. Lactation may be affected by combined oral contraceptives as described under Prescribing during Breast-feeding.

Combined oral contraceptives carry a small risk of thrombo-embolic and cardiovascular complications. This increases with oestrogen content, age, obesity, and cigarette smoking, and with

Table. Hormone content of combined oral contraceptives

Preparation	Progestogen
Oestrogen: Ethinyloestradiol 20 micrograms	
Loestrin 20	Norethisterone acetate 1 mg
Oestrogen: Ethinyloestradiol 30 micrograms	
Conova 30	Ethynodiol diacetate 2 mg
Eugynon 30	Levonorgestrel 250 micrograms
Loestrin 30	Norethisterone acetate 1.5 mg
Marvelon	Desogestrel 150 micrograms
Microgynon 30	Levonorgestrel 150 micrograms
Ovran 30	Levonorgestrel 250 micrograms
Ovranette	Levonorgestrel 150 micrograms
Oestrogen: Ethinyloestradiol 35 micrograms	
BiNovum	Norethisterone 0.5 and 1mg
Brevinor	Norethisterone 500 micrograms
Neocon 1/35	Norethisterone 1 mg
Norimin	Norethisterone 1 mg
Ovysmen	Norethisterone 500 micrograms
Synphase	Norethisterone 0.5 and 1 mg
TriNovum	Norethisterone 0.5/0.75/1 mg
Oestrogen: Ethinyloestradiol 30/40 micrograms	
Logynon	Levonorgestrel 50/75/125 micrograms
Logynon ED	Levonorgestrel 50/75/125 micrograms
Trinordiol	Levonorgestrel 50/75/125 micrograms
Oestrogen: Ethinyloestradiol 50 micrograms	
Anovlar 21	Norethisterone acetate 4 mg
Eugynon 50	Levonorgestrel 250 micrograms
Gynovlar 21	Norethisterone acetate 3 mg
Minilyn	Lynoestrenol 2.5 mg
Minovlar and ED	Norethisterone acetate 1 mg
Norlestrin	Norethisterone acetate 2.5 mg
Orlest 21	Norethisterone acetate 1 mg
Ovran	Levonorgestrel 250 micrograms
Oestrogen: Mestranol 50 micrograms	
Norinyl-1	Norethisterone 1 mg
Ortho-Novin 1/50	Norethisterone 1 mg

predisposing conditions such as diabetes, hypertension, and familial hyperlipidaemia.

Hypertension may develop as the result of therapy but when it is due to contraceptive usage reversion to normotension occurs on cessation of treatment.

Oestrogen-containing oral contraceptives should be discontinued (and adequate alternative contraceptive arrangements made) 4 weeks before major elective surgery; they should normally be recommenced at the first menses occurring at least 2 weeks after the procedure. When discontinuation is not possible, e.g. after trauma or if, by oversight, a patient admitted for an elective procedure is still on an oestrogen-containing oral contraceptive, some consideration should be given to subcutaneous heparin prophylaxis. These recommendations do not apply to minor surgery with short duration of anaesthesia, e.g. laparoscopic sterilisation or tooth extraction, or to women taking oestrogen-free contraceptives.

POSTCOITAL CONTRACEPTION. Combined oral contraceptives may also be given for occasional emergency use after unprotected intercourse. Two tablets of a preparation containing levonorgestrel 250 micrograms and ethinyloestradiol 50 micrograms (Eugynon 50®, Ovran®, Schering PC4®) are taken within 72 hours, and a further 2 tablets 12 hours later. The patient should be advised to consult her doctor if menstruation does not occur within 3 weeks.

ORAL CONTRACEPTIVES (Combined)

Indications: contraception; menstrual symptoms, see section 6.4.1.4

Cautions: see notes above; diabetes, hypertension, cardiac or renal disease, migraine, epilepsy, depression, asthma, multiple sclerosis, wearing of contact lenses, varicose veins; cigarette-smokers, patients over 35 years, obesity, breast-feeding. Drug interactions: see Appendix 1 (sections *2.5, 2.8, 2.8A, 3, 4.3, 6.1, 7*)

Contra-indications: pregnancy; thrombosis and history of thrombo-embolic disease, recurrent jaundice, acute and chronic liver disease, Dubin-Johnson and Roter syndromes, sickle-cell anaemia, hyperlipidaemia, mammary or endometrial carcinoma, oestrogen-dependent tumours, severe migraine, undiagnosed vaginal bleeding, history of pruritus of pregnancy or herpes gestationis, deterioration of otosclerosis

Side-effects: nausea, vomiting, headache, breast tenderness, changes in body weight, thrombosis (more common in blood groups A, B, and AB than O), changes in libido, depression, chloasma, hypertension, impairment of liver function, benign hepatic tumours, reduced menstrual loss, 'spotting' in early cycles, amenorrhoea; rarely photosensitivity

Dose: 1 tablet at the same time each day for 21 days starting on 5th day of cycle, and repeated after a 7-day interval (unless other instructions are given) irrespective of menstrual pattern

PoM **Anovlar 21**® (Schering)
Tablets, green, s/c, norethisterone acetate 4 mg, ethinyloestradiol 50 micrograms. Price 21-tab calendar pack = **C**

PoM **Brevinor**® (Syntex)
Tablets, norethisterone 500 micrograms, ethinyloestradiol 35 micrograms. Price 21-tab calendar pack = **B**

PoM **Conova 30**® (Gold Cross)
Tablets, f/c, ethynodiol diacetate 2 mg, ethinyloestradiol 30 micrograms. Price 21-tab calendar pack = **C**

PoM **Eugynon 30**® (Schering)
Tablets, s/c, levonorgestrel 250 micrograms, ethinyloestradiol 30 micrograms. Price 21-tab calendar pack = **C**

PoM **Eugynon 50**® (Schering)
Tablets, s/c, levonorgestrel 250 micrograms, ethinyloestradiol 50 micrograms. Price 21-tab calendar pack = **C**

PoM **Gynovlar 21**® (Schering)
Tablets, pink, s/c, norethisterone acetate 3 mg, ethinyloestradiol 50 micrograms. Price 21-tab calendar pack = **C**

PoM **Loestrin 20**® (P-D)
Tablets, blue-grey, f/c, norethisterone acetate 1 mg, ethinyloestradiol 20 micrograms. Price 21-tab calendar pack = **C**

PoM **Loestrin 30**® (P-D)
Tablets, green, f/c, norethisterone acetate 1.5 mg, ethinyloestradiol 30 micrograms. Price 21-tab calendar pack = **D**

▼ PoM **Marvelon**® (Organon)
Tablets, desogestrel 150 micrograms, ethinyloestradiol 30 micrograms. Price 21-tab calender pack = **C**
Dose: 1 tablet daily for 21 days, starting on 1st day of cycle, and repeated after a 7-day interval

PoM **Microgynon 30**® (Schering)
Tablets, beige, s/c, levonorgestrel 150 micrograms, ethinyloestradiol 30 micrograms. Price 21-tab calendar pack = **B**

PoM **Minilyn**® (Organon)
Tablets, lynoestrenol 2.5 mg, ethinyloestradiol 50 micrograms. Price 22-tab calendar pack = **C**
Dose: 1 tablet daily for 22 days starting on 1st day of cycle, and repeated after a 6-day interval

PoM **Minovlar**® (Schering)
Tablets, ochre, s/c, norethisterone acetate 1 mg, ethinyloestradiol 50 micrograms. Price 21-tab calendar pack = **C**

PoM **Minovlar ED**® (Schering)
As for Minovlar and in addition 7 ochre lactose tablets. Price 28-tab calendar pack = **C**
Dose: 1 tablet daily starting in red sector on 1st day of cycle continuing in sequence without interruption

PoM **Neocon 1/35**® (Ortho-Cilag)
Tablets, peach, norethisterone 1 mg, ethinyl-oestradiol 35 micrograms. Price 21-tab calendar pack = **C**

PoM **Norimin**® (Syntex)
Tablets, yellow, norethisterone 1 mg, ethinyl-oestradiol 35 micrograms. Price 21-tab calendar pack = **B**

PoM **Norinyl-1**® (Syntex)
Tablets, norethisterone 1 mg, mestranol 50 micrograms. Price 21-tab calendar pack = **B**

PoM **Norlestrin**® (P-D)
Tablets, pink, f/c, norethisterone acetate 2.5 mg, ethinyloestradiol 50 micrograms. Price 21-tab calendar pack = **C**

PoM **Orlest 21**® (P-D)
Tablets, yellow, f/c, norethisterone acetate 1 mg, ethinyloestradiol 50 micrograms. Price 21-tab calendar pack = **B**

PoM **Ortho-Novin 1/50**® (Ortho-Cilag)
Tablets, norethisterone 1 mg, mestranol 50 micrograms. Price 21-tab calendar pack = **C**

PoM **Ovran**® (Wyeth)
Tablets, levonorgestrel 250 micrograms, ethinyloestradiol 50 micrograms. Price 21-tab calendar pack = **B**
Dose: contraception, spasmodic dysmenorrhoea, see above; endometriosis 1-2 tablets daily without interruption; postponement of menstruation 1 tablet daily, preferably beginning before last 5 days of cycle, increased if spotting occurs to 2 tablets daily

PoM **Ovran 30**® (Wyeth)
Tablets, levonorgestrel 250 micrograms, ethinyloestradiol 30 micrograms. Price 21-tab calendar pack = **B**

PoM **Ovranette**® (Wyeth)
Tablets, levonorgestrel 150 micrograms, ethinyloestradiol 30 micrograms. Price 21-tab calendar pack = **B**
Dose: see above and under Ovran

PoM **Ovysmen**® (Ortho-Cilag)
Tablets, norethisterone 500 micrograms, ethinyloestradiol 35 micrograms. Price 21-tab calendar pack = **C**

Phased formulations
PoM **BiNovum**® (Ortho-Cilag)
Calendar pack, 7 white tablets, norethisterone 500 micrograms, ethinyloestradiol 35 micrograms; 14 peach tablets, norethisterone 1 mg, ethinyloestradiol 35 micrograms. Price 21 tabs = **C**
Dose: 1 tablet daily for 21 days, starting with a white tablet on 1st day of cycle, and repeated after a 7-day interval

PoM **Logynon**® (Schering)
Calendar pack, all s/c, 6 light brown tablets, levonorgestrel 50 micrograms, ethinyloestradiol 30 micrograms; 5 white tablets, levonorgestrel 75 micrograms, ethinyloestradiol 40 micrograms; 10 ochre tablets, levonorgestrel 125 micrograms, ethinyloestradiol 30 micrograms. Price 21 tabs = **C**
Dose: 1 tablet daily for 21 days, starting with tablet marked 1 on 1st day of cycle, and repeated after a 7-day interval

PoM **Logynon ED**® (Schering)
As for Logynon and in addition 7 white placebo tablets. Price 28-tab calendar pack = C
Dose: 1 tablet daily starting in red sector on 1st day of cycle continuing in sequence without interruption

▼ PoM **Synphase**® (Syntex)
Calendar pack, 7 white tablets, norethisterone 500 micrograms, ethinyloestradiol 35 micrograms; 9 yellow tablets, norethisterone 1 mg, ethinyloestradiol 35 micrograms; 5 white tablets, norethisterone 500 micrograms, ethinyloestradiol 35 micrograms. Price 21 tabs = C
Dose: 1 tablet daily for 21 days, starting with tablet marked 1 on the 5th day of the cycle, and repeated after a 7-day interval

PoM **Trinordiol**® (Wyeth)
Calendar pack, all s/c, 6 light brown tablets, levonorgestrel 50 micrograms, ethinyloestradiol 30 micrograms; 5 white tablets, levonorgestrel 75 micrograms, ethinyloestradiol 40 micrograms; 10 ochre tablets, levonorgestrel 125 micrograms, ethinyloestradiol 30 micrograms. Price 21 tabs = C
Dose: 1 tablet daily for 21 days, starting with tablet marked 1 on 1st day of cycle, and repeated after a 7-day interval

PoM **TriNovum**® (Ortho-Cilag)
Calendar pack, 7 white tablets, norethisterone 500 micrograms, ethinyloestradiol 35 micrograms; 7 light peach tablets, norethisterone 750 micrograms, ethinyloestradiol 35 micrograms; 7 peach tablets, norethisterone 1 mg, ethinyloestradiol 35 micrograms. Price 21 tabs = C
Dose: 1 tablet daily for 21 days, starting with a white tablet on 1st day of cycle, and repeated after a 7-day interval

Postcoital contraceptive

▼ PoM **Schering PC4**® (Schering)
Tablets, s/c, levonorgestrel 250 micrograms, ethinyloestradiol 50 micrograms. Price 4 tabs = **D**. For postcoital contraception
Dose: 2 tablets as soon as possible after coitus (up to 72 hours) then 2 tablets after 12 hours

7.3.2 Progestogen-only contraceptives

When oestrogens are contra-indicated, progestogen-only preparations may offer a suitable alternative but have a higher failure rate than combined preparations. They are suitable for older patients who may be at risk from oestrogen, heavy smokers, and those in whom oestrogens cause severe side-effects. Menstrual irregularities (oligomenorrhoea, menorrhagia) are more common but patients tend to revert to a more regular cyclical menstrual pattern on long treatment. Oral preparations are started on the 1st day of the cycle and taken every day at the same time without a break. Contraceptive efficacy may be impaired if the dose is delayed by more than 3 hours. The patient should be advised to complete the course as usual but to use an additional form of contraception for the next 14 days. It is important

that if more than 2 consecutive tablets have been missed, oral contraceptives should be discontinued immediately and a method of non-hormonal contraception used until menstruation occurs. Additional contraceptive precautions are also necessary for the first 14 days when initiating treatment with progestogen-only contraceptives and when changing from a combined oral contraceptive to a progestogen-only preparation. In the latter case, treatment should start on the day following completion of the combined oral contraceptive course so that there is no break in tablet taking.

For other critical factors affecting contraceptive efficacy such as vomiting, diarrhoea, and antibiotic intake and for comment on progestogen-only contraceptives and surgical operations, see under Combined Oral Contraceptives, section 7.3.1.

Medroxyprogesterone acetate (Depo-Provera®) is a long-acting progestogen given by intramuscular injection. It is useful for short-term interim contraception, for example, before vasectomy becomes effective or after rubella vaccination. It may also be used as a long-term contraceptive for women who are unable to use any other method, after counselling on the long and short-term effects. Transient infertility and irregular cycles may occur after discontinuation of treatment. Heavy bleeding has been reported in patients given medroxyprogesterone acetate in the immediate puerperium. **Norethisterone enanthate** (Noristerat®) is a long-acting progestogen given as an oily injection which provides contraception for 8 weeks.

Progestogen-only preparations can be administered in the early puerperium without adverse effects; established lactation is not affected.

Progesterone has been incorporated into an intra-uterine contraceptive device.

PROGESTOGEN-ONLY CONTRACEPTIVES

Indications: contraception
Cautions: see notes above; diabetes, hypertension, cardiac or renal disease, migraine, epilepsy, depression, asthma, multiple sclerosis, wearing of contact lenses, varicose veins, obesity. Drug interactions: see under Combined Oral Contraceptives, section 7.3.1
Contra-indications: pregnancy, undiagnosed vaginal bleeding, past ectopic pregnancy, hypertriglyceridaemia; active liver disease, recurrent cholestatic jaundice, and history of jaundice in pregnancy; after evacuation of hydatidiform mole (until return to normal of urine and plasma gonadotrophin values); carcinoma of breast
Side-effects: menstrual irregularities (see also notes above); nausea and vomiting, headache, migraine, breast discomfort, weight changes, depression, skin disorders
Dose: by mouth, 1 tablet daily at the same time, preferably early in the evening, starting on 1st day of cycle then continuously

---

Oral preparations

PoM **Femulen**® (Gold Cross)
Tablets, ethynodiol diacetate 500 micrograms.
Price 28-tab calendar pack = **C**

PoM **Micronor**® (Ortho-Cilag)
Tablets, norethisterone 350 micrograms. Price
28-tab calendar pack = **C**

PoM **Microval**® (Wyeth)
Tablets, levonorgestrel 30 micrograms. Price
35-tab calendar pack = **C**

PoM **Neogest**® (Schering)
Tablets, brown, s/c, levonorgestrel 37.5 micrograms. Price 35-tab calendar pack = **C**

PoM **Norgeston**® (Schering)
Tablets, s/c, levonorgestrel 30 micrograms. Price
35-tab calendar pack = **C**

PoM **Noriday**® (Syntex)
Tablets, yellow, norethisterone 350 micrograms.
Price 28-tab calendar pack = **C**

Parenteral preparations

PoM **Depo-Provera**® (Upjohn)
Injection (aqueous suspension), medroxyprogesterone acetate 50 mg/ml. Price 3-ml vial = **F**
Dose: by deep intramuscular injection, 150 mg
in first 3–5 days of cycle or first 6 weeks after
parturition (duration 3 months); for long-term
contraception repeated 3 monthly

▼ PoM **Noristerat**® (Schering)
Injection (oily), norethisterone enanthate 200
mg/ml. Price 1-ml amp = **E**
Dose: by deep intramuscular injection, short-
term contraception, 200 mg in first 5 days of
cycle or immediately after parturition (duration
8 weeks); may be repeated once again after 8
weeks

7.3.3 Spermicidal contraceptives

Spermicidal contraceptives are useful additional
safeguards but do **not** give adequate protection if
used alone; they are suitable for use in conjunction with barrier methods. They have two
components: a spermicide and a vehicle which
itself may have some inhibiting effect on sperm
migration. They are formulated as pessaries,
creams, pastes, gels, aerosol foams, and soluble
films. The commonly used spermicides are all
phenoxypolyethoxyethanol derivatives.

DIRECTIONS. *Creams, Gels* (diaphragms, caps),
apply over surface and rim of diaphragm or cap
within one hour of intercourse then subsequently
one applicatorful; (condoms) insert 1 applicatorful before intercourse. *Pessaries*, insert 1
pessary before intercourse. *Foams*, insert 1 applicatorful before intercourse. A fresh application
or an additional pessary must be inserted if intercourse is repeated or delayed by more than one
hour.

Delfen® (Ortho-Cilag)
Cream, nonoxinol '9' 5%. Price 70 g = **D**
Foam, nonoxinol '9' 12.5%, pressurised aerosol
unit. Price 20 g (with applicator) = **F**; 20 g
refill = **E**

Double Check® (FP)
Pessaries, nonoxinol '9' 6%. Price 10
pessaries = **C**

Duracreme® (LRC)
Cream, nonoxinol '9' 2%. Price 100-g tube = **D**;
applicator = **B**

Duragel® (LRC)
Gel, nonoxinol '9' 2%. Price 100-g tube = **D**;
applicator = **B**

Emko® (Syntex)
Foam, nonoxinol '9' 8%, benzethonium chloride
0.2%, pressurised aerosol unit. Price 40 g (with
applicator) = **G**; 40-g refill = **F**; 90-g refill = **G**

Genexol® (Rendell)
Pessaries, nonoxinols '10' and '11' 5%, in a palm
kernel oil basis. Price 12 pessaries = **C**. For use
with condoms only

Ortho-Creme® (Ortho-Cilag)
Cream, nonoxinol '9' 2%. Price 70 g = **D**; applicator = **C**

Orthoforms® (Ortho-Cilag)
Pessaries, nonoxinol '9' 5%. Price 15
pessaries = **D**

Ortho-Gynol® (Ortho-Cilag)
Jelly, *p*-di-isobutylphenoxypolyethoxyethanol
1%. Price 81 g = **D**; applicator = **C**

Rendells® (Rendell)
Pessaries, nonoxinols '10' & '11' 5%, in a basis
containing fractionated palm kernel oil. Price
12 pessaries = **C**. For use with condoms only

Staycept® (Syntex)
Jelly, octoxinol 1%. Price 80 g = **D**
Pessaries, nonoxinol '9' 6%. Price 10
pessaries = **C**
When used with diaphragm or cap, one pessary
inside device before it is placed in position and
insert a second pessary before intercourse

7.4 Drugs used in urinary-tract disorders

7.4.1 Drugs used in urinary retention
7.4.2 Drugs used in urinary frequency, nocturnal enuresis, and incontinence
7.4.3 Drugs used as urinary analgesics or to
alter urinary pH
7.4.4 Bladder instillations

For drugs used in the treatment of urinary infections see chapter 5.

7.4.1 Drugs used in urinary retention

In the absence of obstruction to the bladder outlet,
the parasympathomimetics have a limited role in
the relief of urinary retention, for example in
neurological disease or post-operatively.

Acute retention is painful and is initially treated
by catheterisation. Thereafter, provided an
obstructive cause is excluded, further episodes
may be treated medically.

Chronic retention is painless and often long-
standing. Catheterisation is unnecessary unless
there is deterioration of renal function. After the
cause has initially been established and treated,
drugs may be required to increase detrusor muscle

---

tone. Drugs with anticholinergic or sympathomimetic properties should be avoided in such patients as they may precipitate urinary retention by a secondary effect on the bladder.

Carbachol, orally or by subcutaneous injection, may relieve acute or chronic urinary retention. It improves voiding efficiency by increasing detrusor muscle contraction. Generalised parasympathomimetic side-effects such as sweating, bradycardia, and intestinal colic may occur, particularly in the elderly. **Bethanechol** (Myotonine Chloride®) has a similar action. **Distigmine** (Ubretid®) inhibits the action of cholinesterase and prolongs the effect of acetylcholine at neuromuscular junctions. It may help patients with an upper motor neurone neurogenic bladder. **Phenoxybenzamine** (Dibenyline®) is an alpha-adrenoceptor blocking drug which reduces the muscle tone in the bladder neck, proximal urethra, and prostate and may help in some cases of neurogenic bladder. It may also be useful in some patients with benign prostatic hypertrophy who are awaiting prostatectomy. Its use should not be continued if there is no response after 2 to 3 weeks.

BETHANECHOL CHLORIDE
Indications: urinary retention (see section 1.6.2 for use in gastro-intestinal disease)
Cautions: asthma, cardiovascular disease, epilepsy, parkinsonism, vagotonia, hyperthyoidism, elderly patients
Contra-indications: intestinal or urinary obstruction, recent myocardial infarction, recent intestinal anastomosis
Side-effects: parasympathomimetic effects such as nausea, vomiting, sweating, blurred vision, bradycardia, and intestinal colic
Dose: 10–30 mg 3–4 times daily half an hour before food

PoM **Myotonine Chloride®** (Glenwood)
Tablets, pale blue, scored, bethanechol chloride 10 mg. Price 20 tabs = **C**. Label: 22
Tablets, pale blue, scored, bethanechol chloride 25 mg. Price 20 tabs = **C**. Label: 22

CARBACHOL
Indications: urinary retention
Cautions; Contra-indications; Side-effects: see under Bethanechol Chloride but side-effects are more frequent
Dose: by mouth, 2 mg 3 times daily half an hour before food
By subcutaneous injection (acute symptoms, postoperative urinary retention) 250 micrograms, repeated twice if necessary at 30-minute intervals

PoM **Carbachol Tablets**, carbachol 2 mg. Price 20 tabs = **B**. Label: 22
PoM **Carbachol Injection**, carbachol 250 micrograms/ml. Price 1-ml amp = **B**

DISTIGMINE BROMIDE
Indications: urinary retention due to upper motor lesions (see section 1.6.2 for use in gastro-intestinal disease)
Cautions; Contra-indications; Side-effects: see under Bethanechol Chloride; side-effects are mild but more prolonged
Dose: by mouth, 5 mg daily or on alternate days, half an hour before breakfast
By intramuscular injection, 500 micrograms daily or 12 hours after surgery to prevent urinary retention

PoM **Ubretid®** (Berk)
Tablets, scored, distigmine bromide 5 mg. Price 20 tabs = **I**. Label: 22
Injection, distigmine bromide 500 micrograms/ml. Price 1-ml amp = **C**

PHENOXYBENZAMINE HYDROCHLORIDE
Indications: urinary retention due to neurogenic bladder or benign prostatic hypertrophy
Cautions; Contra-indications; Side-effects: see section 2.5.4
Dose: by mouth, 10 mg twice daily; CHILD 300–500 micrograms/kg daily

PoM **Dibenyline®** (SK&F)
Capsules, red/white, phenoxybenzamine hydrochloride 10 mg. Price 20 caps = **E**

7.4.2 Drugs used in urinary frequency, nocturnal enuresis, and incontinence
Emepronium (Cetiprin®), **flavoxate** (Urispas®), and **propantheline** (Pro-Banthine®) are anticholinergic drugs used to treat *urinary frequency*. They increase bladder capacity by diminishing unstable detrusor contractions. Emepronium and propantheline are anticholinergic drugs and flavoxate is an antispasmodic with anticholinergic properties. All these drugs may cause dry mouth and blurred vision and may precipitate glaucoma. **Emepronium** is poorly and irregularly absorbed from the gastro-intestinal tract and must be given with fluid or it may cause ulceration of the mouth, gums, or oesophagus. The **tricyclic antidepressants** imipramine, amitriptyline, and nortriptyline (see section 4.3.1) are sometimes effective in the management of the unstable bladder because of their anticholinergic properties.

Nocturnal enuresis is a normal occurrence in young children but persists in as many as 5% by 10 years of age. In the absence of urinary-tract infection simple measures such as bladder training or the use of an alarm system may be successful. The most widely used drug treatment is with tricyclic antidepressants such as **imipramine** (see section 4.3.1). The sympathomimetic drugs **ephedrine** and **pseudoephedrine** may also be useful. Drug therapy is not appropriate for children under 7 years of age. The possible side-effects and potential toxicity of these agents if taken in overdose should be borne in mind when they are prescribed.

C = 51-100p, **D** = 101-180p, **E** = 181-300p, **F** = 301-450p, **G** = 451-650p, **H** = 651-900p, **I** = 901-1200p, **J** = over 1200p.

EMEPRONIUM BROMIDE

Indications: urinary frequency and incontinence
Cautions: gastric retention, prostatic hypertrophy; see also notes above
Contra-indications: achalasia, obstructive oeso-phageal lesions, oesophagitis, glaucoma
Side-effects: mild peripheral anticholinergic side-effects (see under Atropine Sulphate, section 1.2), also see notes above
Dose: 200 mg 3 times daily or, for nocturnal symptoms, 400 mg at night, with at least 100 ml of fluid. The tablets should be taken while sitting or standing

PoM **Cetiprin**® (KabiVitrum)
Tablets, f/c, emepronium bromide 100 mg. Price 20 tabs = **D**. Label: 27, counselling advised, posture (see dose above)

EPHEDRINE HYDROCHLORIDE

Indications: nocturnal enuresis
Cautions; Contra-indications; Side-effects: see under Ephedrine Hydrochloride (section 3.1.1.2) and notes in section 3.10
Dose: CHILD 6–8 years 30 mg, 9–12 years 45 mg, 13–15 years 60 mg at bedtime

PoM **Ephedrine Hydrochloride Tablets,** ephedrine hydrochloride 15, 30, and 60 mg. Price 20 tabs (all) = **A**
PoM **Ephedrine Elixir,** ephedrine hydrochloride 15 mg/5 ml. Dilution only to be in accordance with the manufacturer's instructions. Price 100 ml = **B**

FLAVOXATE HYDROCHLORIDE

Indications: urinary frequency and incontinence, dysuria
Cautions: gastric retention, glaucoma
Contra-indications: obstructive lesions, achalasia
Side-effects: headache, nausea, fatigue, blurred vision, dry mouth, diarrhoea
Dose: 200 mg 3 times daily

PoM **Urispas**® (Syntex)
Tablets, s/c, flavoxate hydrochloride 100 mg. Price 20 tabs = **B**

PHENYLPROPANOLAMINE HYDROCHLORIDE

Indications: diurnal enuresis with bladder neck weakness (under specialist supervision).
Cautions; Contra-indications; Side-effects: see under Ephedrine Hydrochloride (section 3.1.1.2) and notes in section 3.10; also can induce arrhythmias, hypertension and thyroid dysfunction

NHS **Eskornade**® (SK&F)
Spansule® (=capsules s/r), grey/clear, enclosing red, grey, and white pellets, phenylpropanolamine hydrochloride 50 mg, diphenylpyraline hydrochloride 5 mg, isopropamide 2.5 mg (as iodide). Price 20 caps = **D**. Label: 2, 25

Syrup (=elixir), green, phenylpropanolamine hydrochloride 15 mg, diphenylpyraline hydrochloride 1.5 mg, isopropamide 750 micrograms (as iodide)/5 ml. Diluent syrup, life of diluted elixir 14 days. Price 150 ml = **D**. Label: 2
Dose: CHILD over 7 years 5 ml of elixir every 12 hours, gradually increased if necessary to 10 ml every 12 hours; older child 1 capsule every 12 hours

POLDINE METHYLSULPHATE

Indications: nocturnal enuresis (see notes above)
Cautions; Contra-indications; Side-effects: see under Atropine Sulphate (section 1.2) but peripheral side-effects occur less frequently
Dose: CHILD 6–12 years 2 mg at night

PoM **Nacton**® (Bencard)
Tablets, scored, poldine methylsulphate 2 mg. Price 20 tabs = **B**

PROPANTHELINE BROMIDE

Indications: urinary frequency and incontinence
Cautions; Contra-indications; Side-effects: see under Atropine Sulphate (section 1.2) but peripheral side-effects occur less frequently
Dose: 15–30 mg 2–3 times daily one hour before meals; CHILD, nocturnal enuresis, 6–12 years 15–45 mg at night, max. 2 mg/kg daily in divided doses

Preparations
See section 1.2

PSEUDOEPHEDRINE HYDROCHLORIDE

Indications: nocturnal enuresis
Cautions; Contra-indications; Side-effects: see under Ephedrine Hydrochloride (section 3.1.1.2) but has been stated to have fewer cardiovascular and CNS effects. See also notes in section 3.10
Dose: 60 mg at night; CHILD 6–12 years 30–45 mg at night

Sudafed® (Calmic)
Tablets, pseudoephedrine hydrochloride 60 mg. Price 20 tabs = **C**
Elixir, pink, pseudoephedrine hydrochloride 30 mg/5 ml. Diluent syrup, life of diluted elixir 14 days. Price 100 ml = **C**

7.4.3   Drugs used as urinary analgesics or to alter urinary pH

Potassium citrate mixture by its alkalinising action may relieve the discomfort of cystitis caused by lower urinary tract infections. **Phenazopyridine** (Pyridium®) also gives palliative relief but colours the urine orange-red and, if renal function is impaired, may cause haemolysis. A **terpene** mixture (Rowatinex®) is claimed to be of benefit in urolithiasis for the expulsion of calculi. **Lignocaine**

Relative prices: **A** = up to 20p, **B** = 21-50p,

gel is a useful topical application in urethral pain or to relieve the discomfort of catheterisation.

Alkalinisation of urine may be undertaken with **sodium bicarbonate**, or alternatively sodium or potassium citrate. *Acidification* of urine may be undertaken with **ascorbic acid** or occasionally with ammonium chloride.

ASCORBIC ACID
Indications: acidification of urine
Dose: by mouth, 4 g daily in divided doses

Preparations
See section 9.6.3

LIGNOCAINE HYDROCHLORIDE
Indications: urethral analgesia
Side-effects: sensitivity with repeated use
Dose: (1 and 2% preparations) into urethra; men initially 5–10 ml then 3–5 ml; women 3–5 ml

Lignocaine Gel, lignocaine 1 or 2% with chlorhexidine gluconate solution 0.25% or hydroxybenzoates, in a sterile lubricant water-miscible basis. Price 15 ml (both) = **C**
PoM**Instillagel**® (Rimmer)
Gel, lignocaine hydrochloride 2%, chlorhexidine gluconate solution 0.25%, in a sterile lubricant basis in disposable syringe. Price 6- and 11-ml syringe (both) = **B**
Dose: 6–11 ml into urethra
Xylocaine® (Astra)
Gel, anhydrous lignocaine hydrochloride 2%, in a sterile lubricant water-miscible basis. Price 20 g = **C**
Antiseptic gel, lignocaine hydrochloride 2%, chlorhexidine gluconate solution 0.25%, in a sterile lubricant water-miscible basis. Price 15 ml = **C**

PHENAZOPYRIDINE HYDROCHLORIDE
Indications: urinary-tract pain
Contra-indications: renal and hepatic impairment
Side-effects: gastro-intestinal disturbances, headache, vertigo; in high dosage methaemoglobinaemia; rarely haemolytic anaemia. Colours the urine orange-red. Stones reported after long-term use
Dose: 200 mg 3 times daily after meals; CHILD over 8 years 100 mg

Pyridium® (Warner)
Tablets, brown, s/c, phenazopyridine hydrochloride 100 mg. Price 20 tabs = **B**. Label: 14, 21, counselling advised, gluten, staining

POTASSIUM CITRATE
Indications: relief of discomfort in mild urinary-tract infections; alkalinisation of urine
Cautions: renal impairment, cardiac disease. Drug interactions: see Appendix 1 (sections 2.2, 2.5)
Side-effects: hyperkalaemia on prolonged high dosage, mild diuresis

Dose: cystitis, adults and children over 6 years, 3 g, well diluted with water, 3 times daily; CHILD 1–6 years 1.5 g
Alkalinisation of urine, 3–6 g with water every 6 hours

Potassium Citrate Mixture, potassium citrate 1.5 g/5 ml (see Formulary). Price 100 ml = **A**. Label: 27
Effercitrate® (Typharm)
Tablets, effervescent, the equivalent of potassium citrate 1.5 g (13.9 mmolK+), citric acid 250 mg (1 tablet ≡ 5 ml potassium citrate mixture). Price 12 tabs = **D**. Label: 13

SODIUM BICARBONATE
Indications: alkalinisation of urine
Cautions; Side-effects: see section 1.1.1
Dose: 3 g in water every 2 hours until urinary pH exceeds 7; maintenance of alkaline urine 5-10 g daily

Sodium Bicarbonate Powder. Price 50 g = **A**. Label: 13

OTHER PREPARATIONS FOR URINARY DISORDERS

Ammonium Chloride Mixture (see Formulary). Price 100 ml = **A**.
Dose: 10–20 ml up to 3 times daily for the acidification of urine. To be taken well diluted with water
Rowatinex® (Tillotts)
Capsules, yellow, e/c, 0.1 ml of solution of composition below. Price 20 caps = **E**. Label: 25
Dose: 1 capsule 3–4 times daily
Solution, yellow, anethole 400 mg, borneol 1 g, camphene 1.5 g, cineole 300 mg, fenchone 400 mg, pinene 3.1 g, olive oil to 10 g. Price 10 ml = **G**. Label: 22, counselling advised, use of dropper
Dose: 3–5 drops 4–5 times daily before food

7.4.4 Bladder instillations
INFECTED BLADDERS. Various solutions are available as irrigations or washouts for the infected bladder. The simplest is **sterile sodium chloride solution** (normal saline). Aqueous **chlorhexidine** (Hibitane®), described in section 13.11, is effective against a wide range of common urinary-tract pathogens but not against most *Pseudomonas* spp. Solutions containing 1 in 10000 (0.01%) are usually preferred as stronger solutions irritate the mucosa and cause haematuria. **Polymyxin B sulphate with neomycin** (Polybactrin®, see section 5.1.7), **noxythiolin** (see section 5.1.11.2), and **colistin** (see section 5.1.7) are bactericidal to most pathogens and emergence of resistance is slow. **Nitrofurazone** (Furacin®), see section 5.1.11.2, has limited application as many urinary pathogens are resistant to it. Bladder irrigations of **amphotericin** 100 micrograms/ml (Fungizone Intravenous Infusion®) or **miconazole** (Daktarin Intravenous Solution®) (100 mg twice daily as undiluted solution or as a 12-hourly continuous

irrigation in 500 ml of sterile sodium chloride solution) may be of value in mycotic infections (see section 5.2).

DISSOLUTION OF BLOOD CLOTS. Clot retention is usually treated by irrigation with **sterile sodium chloride solution** but **sterile sodium citrate solution for bladder irrigation (3%)** may also be helpful. **Streptokinase-streptodornase** (Varidase Topical®) is an alternative. **Deoxyribonuclease** (Deanase®) is effective but may cause bladder irritation and hypersensitivity (see section 10.3.1).

LOCALLY-ACTING CYTOTOXIC DRUGS. **Ethoglucid** (Epodyl®, see section 8.1.1) is used in the control of rapidly recurring non-invasive bladder tumours of low grade malignancy. 100 ml of a 1–2% solution is left in the bladder for as long as possible (usually 1 hour). Treatment may be given weekly for 12 weeks and then monthly for a year. It may cause dysuria and frequency.

Thiotepa (see section 8.1.1) is used for bladder tumours of low to medium grade malignancy. A solution containing 30–60 mg in 50 ml of sterile water is retained in the bladder for 2 hours. It is given weekly for 4 weeks. The concentration should be reduced if there is evidence of bone-marrow suppression.

Doxorubicin (see section 8.1.2) is used to treat recurrent superficial bladder tumours, carcinoma-in-situ, and some papillary tumours. An instillation (50 mg in 50 ml of sterile sodium chloride solution) is retained in the bladder for one hour and treatment repeated monthly. Although systemic side-effects are few, it may cause frequency, urgency, dysuria, and occasionally reduction in bladder capacity.

INTERSTITIAL CYSTITIS. Dimethyl sulphoxide may be used for symptomatic relief in patients with interstitial cystitis (Hunner's ulcer). 50 ml of a 50% solution (Rimso-50®) is instilled into the bladder, retained for 15 minutes, and voided by the patient. Treatment is repeated at intervals of 2 weeks. Bladder spasm and hypersensitivity reactions may occur and long term use requires ophthalmic, renal, and hepatic assessment at 6-monthly intervals. Toxic complications include erythema, itching, and dermatitis.

Sterile Sodium Citrate Solution for Bladder Irrigation, sodium citrate 3%, dilute hydrochloric acid 0.2%, in purified water, freshly boiled and cooled, and sterilised. Price 100 ml = **A**

PoM **Rimso-50**® (Britannia)
Bladder instillation, sterile, dimethyl sulphoxide 50%, in aqueous solution. Price 50 ml = **J**

8: Drugs used in the treatment of
MALIGNANT DISEASE and for IMMUNOSUPPRESSION

Dosage in malignant disease. Because of the complexity of dosage regimens in the treatment of malignant disease, dose statements have been omitted from some of the drug entries in this chapter. *In all cases detailed specialist literature should be consulted.*

In this chapter, drug treatment is discussed under the following headings:

8.1 Cytotoxic drugs
8.2 Drugs affecting the immune response
8.3 Sex hormones and antagonists used in malignant disease

Malignant disease may be treated by surgery, radiotherapy, and/or chemotherapy. Certain tumours are highly sensitive to chemotherapy but many are not, and inappropriate drug administration in these circumstances can only increase morbidity or mortality. Cytotoxic drugs and corticosteroids are also used as immunosuppressants. The sex hormones are used to treat certain responsive tumours.

8.1   Cytotoxic drugs

8.1.1 Alkylating drugs
8.1.2 Cytotoxic antibiotics
8.1.3 Antimetabolites
8.1.4 Vinca alkaloids and etoposide
8.1.5 Other cytotoxic drugs
8.1.6 Antagonists used with cytotoxic drugs

Many drugs are now available which are active in malignant disease or as immunosuppressants for use in organ transplant recipients or patients with a range of medical conditions.

Great care is needed when prescribing these drugs as damage to normal tissue, which may be irreversible, is an almost invariable consequence of their use. These drugs should rarely, if ever, be used empirically in a patient with cancer, and administration should always be regarded as a clinical trial with clear objectives in mind.

In a minority of cancers, chemotherapy may be given with cure, or marked prolongation of survival, a realistic end-point. Here short-term drug-related toxicity, which may be severe, is acceptable. However, for the majority of patients, modest survival prolongation or palliation of symptoms will be the aim, and an attempt should be made to use relatively non-toxic treatments, or to consider the use of other effective modalities, e.g. radiotherapy.

Cytotoxic drugs may be used either singly, or in combination therapy. In the latter case, the initial letters of the drug names, or proprietary names, identify the regimen used and those referred to in this chapter are:

MOPP—mustine, vincristine (Oncovin®), procarbazine, and prednisolone
MVPP—mustine, vinblastine, procarbazine, and prednisolone
ABVD—doxorubicin (Adriamycin®), bleomycin, vinblastine, and dacarbazine.

Many other such combinations have been used. Drug combinations are frequently more toxic than single drugs but may have the advantage in certain tumours of enhanced response and increased survival, e.g. in Hodgkin's disease. However for some tumour types, single-agent chemotherapy remains the treatment of choice.

These drugs fall naturally into a number of classes, each with characteristic antitumour activity, sites of action, and toxicity. A knowledge of sites of metabolism and excretion is important, as impaired drug handling as a result of disease is not uncommon and may result in enhanced toxic effects. A number of side-effects are characteristic of particular agents or groups of drugs, e.g. neurotoxicity of vinca alkaloids, and details will be provided in the appropriate sections. Most toxic effects are, however, common to many of these drugs and will be briefly outlined here.

EXTRAVASATION OF INTRAVENOUS DRUGS. A number of drugs will cause severe local tissue necrosis if leakage into the extravascular compartment occurs. Recommended modes of administration must be adhered to. Infusion of vesicant drugs should be stopped immediately if local pain is experienced. Where doubt exists as to whether significant leakage has occurred, the infusion should be discontinued and the cannula resited in another vein.

NAUSEA AND VOMITING. Certain drugs, e.g. cisplatin and dacarbazine, will cause nausea and vomiting in almost all patients, while others cause this problem less commonly. Where vomiting is anticipated, or has occurred previously, a phenothiazine derivative or metoclopramide (see section 4.6) should be given prophylactically as well as during and after chemotherapy. Severe vomiting may necessitate the use of suppositories or parenteral anti-emetics. Vomiting refractory to these drugs may respond to one of the new preparations, e.g. high dose metoclopramide or nabilone. Experience with these is relatively limited.

BONE-MARROW SUPPRESSION. All cytotoxic drugs except vincristine and bleomycin cause marrow depression. This commonly occurs 7 to 10 days after administration, but is delayed for certain

---

C = 51-100p, D = 101-180p, E = 181-300p, F = 301-450p, G = 451-650p, H = 651-900p, I = 901-1200p, J = over 1200p.

drugs, such as carmustine, lomustine, and melphalan. Peripheral blood counts must be checked prior to each treatment, and doses should be reduced or therapy delayed if marrow recovery has not occurred. Fever occurring in a neutropenic patient (neutrophil count less than 800×10^9/litre) is an indication for immediate parenteral broadspectrum antibiotic therapy, once appropriate bacteriological investigations have taken place.

ALOPECIA. Reversible hair loss is a common complication of these drugs, although it varies in degree between drug preparations and individual patients. No pharmacological methods of preventing this are available.

Many cytotoxic drugs are very expensive, most are teratogenic, and all may cause life-threatening toxicity. Administration of these drugs should, where possible, be confined to those experienced in their use.

8.1.1   Alkylating drugs

Extensive experience is available with these drugs, which are among the most widely used in cancer chemotherapy. They act by damaging DNA, thus interfering with cell replication. In addition to the side-effects common to many cytotoxic drugs (section 8.1), there are two problems associated with prolonged usage. Firstly, gametogenesis is often severely affected. Almost all males will be rendered permanently sterile early in a treatment course. Females are less severely affected, though the span of reproductive life may be shortened by the onset of a premature menopause. Potency is not affected. Secondly, prolonged use of these drugs, particularly when combined with extensive irradiation, is associated with a marked increase in the incidence of acute non-lymphocytic leukaemia.

Cyclophosphamide (Endoxana®) is widely used in the treatment of chronic lymphocytic leukaemia, the lymphomas, and solid tumours. It may be given orally or intravenously and is inactive until metabolised by the liver. Acrolein, a urinary metabolite of cyclophosphamide, may cause haemorrhagic cystitis; this is a serious complication and an absolute contra-indication to further therapy. An increased fluid intake, for example 3 to 4 litres per day after intravenous injection, will help avoid this complication. When high dose therapy is used mesna (Uromitexan®, section 8.1.6) will also help prevent this complication.

Ifosfamide (Mitoxana®) is related to cyclophosphamide and is given with mesna to reduce endothelial toxicity. There is relatively little experience with this drug.

Chlorambucil (Leukeran®) is a useful agent commonly used to treat chronic lymphocytic leukaemia, the indolent non-Hodgkin's lymphomas, Hodgkin's disease, and ovarian carcinoma. Side-effects, apart from marrow suppression, are uncommon, although rashes may occur.

Melphalan (Alkeran®) is used to treat myeloma

and occasionally solid tumours and lymphomas. Marrow toxicity is delayed and it is usually given at intervals of 4–6 weeks.

Busulphan (Myleran®) is used almost exclusively to treat chronic myeloid leukaemia. Frequent blood counts are necessary as excessive myelosuppression may result in irreversible bone-marrow aplasia. Hyperpigmentation of the skin is a common side-effect and, rarely, progressive pulmonary fibrosis may occur.

Lomustine (CCNU®) is a lipid-soluble nitrosourea and may be given orally. It is mainly used to treat Hodgkin's disease and certain solid tumours. Marrow toxicity is delayed, and the drug is therefore given at intervals of 4 to 6 weeks. Permanent marrow damage may occur with prolonged use. Nausea and vomiting are common and moderately severe.

Carmustine (BiCNU®) is given intravenously. It has similar activity and toxicities.

Mustine is now much less commonly used. It is a very toxic drug which causes severe vomiting. The freshly prepared injection must be given into a fast-running intravenous infusion. Local extravasation causes severe tissue necrosis.

Estramustine (Estracyt®) is a stable combination of an oestrogen and mustine, designed to deliver mustine to the oestrogen receptor site of a tumour, for example prostate cancer. It is not extensively used in this country.

Treosulphan is used to treat ovarian carcinoma.

Thiotepa is usually used as an intracavitary drug for the treatment of malignant effusions or bladder cancer. It is also occasionally used to treat breast cancer, but requires parenteral administration.

Ethoglucid (Epodyl®) is used by the intracavitary route for bladder cancer.

Mitobronitol (Myelobromol®) is occasionally used to treat chronic myeloid leukaemia.

BUSULPHAN

Indications: chronic myeloid leukaemia
Cautions; Side-effects: see section 8.1 and notes above
Dose: induction of remission, 2–4 mg daily; maintenance, 0.5–2 mg daily

PoM **Myleran**® (Wellcome)
Tablets, busulphan 500 micrograms. Price 20 tabs = **D**
Tablets, busulphan 2 mg. Price 20 tabs = **E**

CARMUSTINE

Indications: see notes above
Cautions; Side-effects: see section 8.1 and notes above; irritant to tissues

PoM **BiCNU**® (Bristol-Myers)
Injection, powder for reconstitution, carmustine. Price 100-mg vial (with diluent) = **J**

CHLORAMBUCIL

Indications: see notes above (for use as an immunosuppressant see section 8.2.1)

Cautions; Side-effects: see section 8.1 and notes above

Dose: used alone, 5–10 mg daily for 3–6 weeks; maintenance, 2–4 mg daily

PoM **Leukeran**® (Wellcome)
Tablets, yellow, chlorambucil 2 mg. Price 20 tabs = **F**
Tablets, yellow, chlorambucil 5 mg. Price 20 tabs = **G**

CYCLOPHOSPHAMIDE
Indications: see notes above
Cautions; Side-effects: see section 8.1 and notes above; reduce dose in renal impairment. Drug interactions: see Appendix 1 (section *15*)

PoM **Cyclophosphamide Tablets,** compression-coated or s/c, cyclophosphamide 10 mg, price 20 tabs = **C**; 50 mg, price 20 tabs = **D**. Label: 27
PoM **Cyclophosphamide Injection,** powder for reconstitution, cyclophosphamide, price 100-mg vial = **C**; 200-mg vial = **D**; 500-mg vial = **E**; 1-g vial = **F**
PoM **Endoxana**® (Boehringer Ingelheim)
Tablets, compression-coated, cyclophosphamide 10 mg. Price 20 tabs = **C**. Label: 27
Tablets, compression-coated, cyclophosphamide 50 mg. Price 20 tabs = **D**. Label: 27
Injection, powder for reconstitution, cyclophosphamide. Price 107-mg vial = **C**; 214-mg vial = **D**; 535-mg vial = **E**; 1.069-g vial = **F**

ESTRAMUSTINE PHOSPHATE
Indications: prostatic carcinoma
Cautions; Contra-indications; Side-effects: see section 8.1 and under Ethinyloestradiol (section 6.4.1.1)
Dose: initially, 560 mg daily

▼ PoM **Estracyt**® (Lundbeck)
Capsules, estramustine phosphate 140 mg (as disodium salt). Price 10 caps = **I**. Label: 21

ETHOGLUCID
Indications: non-invasive bladder carcinoma, see section 7.4.4
Side-effects: frequency of micturition, dysuria, fall in leucocyte count
Dose: by *instillation*, 1% solution

PoM **Epodyl**® (ICI)
Liquid, sterile ethoglucid. Plastic syringes should not be used. Price 1-ml amp = **E**

IFOSFAMIDE
Indications: see notes above
Cautions; Side-effects: see section 8.1 and notes under Cyclophosphamide

PoM **Mitoxana**® (Boehringer Ingelheim)
Injection, powder for reconstitution, ifosfamide. Price 500-mg vial = **G**; 1-g vial = **I**; 2-g vial = **J** (Hosp. only)

LOMUSTINE
Indications: see notes above
Cautions; Side-effects: see section 8.1 and notes above
Dose: used alone, 120–130 mg/m² body-surface every 6–8 weeks

▼ PoM **CCNU**® (Lundbeck)
Capsules, blue/white, lomustine 10 mg. Price 20 caps = **I**
Capsules, blue, lomustine 40 mg. Price 10 caps = **I**

MELPHALAN
Indications: myelomatosis
Cautions; Side-effects: see section 8.1 and notes above; reduce dose in renal failure
Dose: by *mouth*, up to 10 mg daily for 7 days, repeated after 4–6 weeks

PoM **Alkeran**® (Wellcome)
Tablets, pink, melphalan 2 mg. Price 20 tabs = **G**
Tablets, pink, melphalan 5 mg. Price 20 tabs = **H**
Injection, powder for reconstitution, melphalan. Price 100-mg vial (with solvent and diluent) = **J**

MITOBRONITOL
Indications: chronic myeloid leukaemia
Cautions; Side-effects: see section 8.1
Dose: initially 250 mg daily

PoM **Myelobromol**® (Sinclair)
Tablets, mitobronitol 125 mg. Price 20 tabs = **H**

MUSTINE HYDROCHLORIDE
Indications: Hodgkin's disease—see notes above
Cautions; Side-effects: see section 8.1 and notes above; also caution in handling—vesicant and a nasal irritant

PoM **Mustine Hydrochloride Injection,** powder for reconstitution, mustine hydrochloride. Price 10-mg vial = **D**

THIOTEPA
Indications: see notes above and section 7.4.4
Cautions; Side-effects: see section 8.1. Drug interactions: see Appendix 1 (section *15*)

PoM **Thiotepa Injection,** powder for reconstitution, thiotepa (with sodium chloride and bicarbonate). Price 15-mg vial = **G**

TREOSULFAN
Indications: see notes above
Cautions; Side-effects: see section 8.1

PoM **Treosulfan** (Leo)
Capsules, treosulfan 250 mg. Price 20 caps = **G**. Label: 25

C = 51-100p, **D** = 101-180p, **E** = 181-300p, **F** = 301-450p, **G** = 451-650p, **H** = 651-900p, **I** = 901-1200p, **J** = over 1200p.

Injection, powder for reconstitution, treosulfan. Price 5 g in infusion bottle with transfer needle = **J**

8.1.2 Cytotoxic antibiotics

Drugs within this group are widely used as anti-cancer agents. Many act as radiomimetics and simultaneous use of radiotherapy with these drugs should be avoided as it may result in markedly enhanced normal tissue toxicity.

Doxorubicin (Adriamycin®) is one of the most successful and widely used antitumour drugs, and is used to treat the acute leukaemias, lymphomas, and a variety of solid tumours. It is given by fast running infusion, commonly at 21-day intervals. Local extravasation will cause severe tissue necrosis. Common toxic effects include nausea and vomiting, myelosuppression, alopecia, and mucositis. This drug is largely excreted by the biliary tract, and an elevated bilirubin concentration is an indication for reducing the dose. Supraventricular tachycardia related to drug administration is an uncommon complication. Higher cumulative doses are associated with development of a cardiomyopathy. It is customary to arbitrarily limit total doses to be administered to 450–550 mg/m^2 body-surface area as symptomatic and potentially fatal heart failure occurs increasingly commonly above this level. Patients with pre-existing cardiac disease, the elderly, and those who have received myocardial irradiation should be treated cautiously. Cardiac monitoring, for example by sequential radionuclide ejection fraction measurement, may assist in safely limiting total dosage. Evidence is available to suggest that weekly low dose administration may be associated with less cardiac damage.

Epirubicin (Pharmorubicin®) is new and is likely to have similar actions to doxorubicin.

Bleomycin is used to treat the lymphomas, certain solid tumours and, by the intracavitary route, malignant effusions. It is unusual in that it causes no marrow suppression. Dermatological toxicity is common; increased pigmentation particularly affecting the flexures and subcutaneous sclerotic plaques may occur. Mucositis is also relatively common and an association with Raynaud's phenomenon is reported. Hypersensitivity reactions manifest by chills and fevers commonly occur a few hours after drug administration and may be prevented by simultaneous administration of a corticosteroid, for example hydrocortisone intravenously. The principal problem associated with the use of bleomycin is progressive pulmonary fibrosis. This is dose related, occurring more commonly at cumulative doses greater than 300 mg and in the elderly. Basal lung crepitations or suspicious chest X-ray changes are an indication to stop therapy with this drug.

Actinomycin D (Cosmegen Lyovac®) is principally used to treat paediatric cancers. Its side-effects are similar to those of doxorubicin, except that cardiac toxicity is not a problem.

Mithramycin (Mithracin®) is no longer used as a cytotoxic, but has found a useful role in low dose in the emergency therapy of hypercalcaemia due to malignant disease.

Mitomycin (Mitomycin C Kyowa®) is used to treat upper gastro-intestinal and breast cancers. It causes delayed marrow toxicity and is usually administered at 6-weekly intervals. Prolonged use may result in permanent marrow damage. It is a relatively toxic drug and may cause lung fibrosis and renal damage.

ACTINOMYCIN D

(Dactinomycin)

Indications: see notes above

Cautions; Side-effects: see section 8.1 and notes above; irritant to tissues

PoM**Cosmegen Lyovac**® (MSD)

Injection, powder for reconstitution, actinomycin D (with mannitol). Price 500-microgram vial = **D**

BLEOMYCIN

Indications: squamous cell carcinoma—see notes above

Cautions; Side-effects: see section 8.1 and notes above; reduce dose in renal failure. Also caution in handling—irritant to skin

PoM**Bleomycin Injection**, powder for reconstitution, bleomycin (as sulphate). Price 15 mg = **J**

DOXORUBICIN HYDROCHLORIDE

Indications: see notes above and section 7.4.4

Cautions; Side-effects: see section 8.1 and notes above; also caution in handling—irritant to skin and tissues

PoM**Adriamycin**® (Farmitalia Carlo Erba)

Injection, powder for reconstitution, doxorubicin hydrochloride (with lactose). Price 10-mg vial = **I**; 50-mg vial = **J**

EPIRUBICIN HYDROCHLORIDE

Indications: see notes above

Cautions; Side-effects: see section 8.1 and notes above; also irritant to tissues

▼ PoM**Pharmorubicin**® (Farmitalia Carlo Erba)

Injection, powder for reconstitution, epirubicin hydrochloride. Price 10- and 50-mg vials (both) = **J**

MITHRAMYCIN

Indications: see notes above

Cautions; Side-effects: see section 8.1 and notes above; irritant to tissues

PoM**Mithracin**® (Pfizer)

Injection, powder for reconstitution, mithramycin (with mannitol and sodium phosphate). Price 2.5-mg vial = **I**

MITOMYCIN

Indications: see notes above

Cautions; Side-effects: see section 8.1 and notes above; also irritant to tissues

PoM **Mitomycin C Kyowa**® (Martindale)
Injection, powder for reconstitution, mitomycin. Price 2-mg vial = F; 10-mg vial = I; 20-mg vial = J (Hosp. only)

8.1.3 Antimetabolites

Antimetabolites are incorporated into new nuclear material or combine irreversibly with vital cellular enzymes, preventing normal cellular division.

Methotrexate inhibits the enzyme dihydrofolate reductase, essential for the synthesis of purines and pyrimidines. It may be given orally, intravenously, intramuscularly, or intrathecally. The use of high dose intravenous methotrexate (with folinic acid rescue) has largely failed to fulfill its earlier promise but clinical trials are still continuing. Its use in this procedure should be confined to such trials.

Methotrexate is used as maintenance therapy for childhood acute lymphoblastic leukaemia. Other uses include choriocarcinoma, non-Hodgkin lymphomas, and a number of solid tumours. Intrathecal methotrexate is used in the CNS prophylaxis of childhood acute lymphoblastic leukaemia, and as a therapy for established meningeal carcinoma or lymphoma.

Methotrexate causes myelosuppression and mucositis. It should be used with extreme caution in renal impairment, as the kidney is its main route of excretion. It should also be avoided when serous effusions exist, as it will accumulate in them and subsequently leak out causing myelosuppression.

Cytarabine (Cytosar® etc.) acts by interfering with pyrimidine synthesis. It may be given subcutaneously, intravenously, or intrathecally. Its predominant use is in the induction and maintenance therapy of acute myeloblastic leukaemia. It is a potent myelosuppressant and requires careful haematological monitoring.

Fluorouracil may be given orally or intravenously. It remains the treatment of choice for metastatic colon cancer, and is also used to treat other solid tumours, particularly breast cancer. It may also be used topically for certain malignant skin lesions. Toxicity is unusual, but may include myelosuppression, mucositis, and rarely a cerebellar syndrome.

Mercaptopurine (Puri-Nethol®) is used almost exclusively as maintenance therapy for the acute leukaemias. Drug doses should be reduced if the patient is receiving concurrent allopurinol as this drug interferes with the metabolism of mercaptopurine, resulting in higher drug concentrations and marrow toxicity.

Thioguanine (Lanvis®) is used orally to induce remission and for maintenance in acute myeloid leukaemia.

Azathioprine is an antimetabolite, but is commonly used as an immunosuppressant (section 8.2.1).

CYTARABINE
Indications: acute leukaemias
Cautions; Side-effects: see section 8.1 and notes above

▼ PoM **Alexan**® (Pfizer)
Injection, cytarabine 20 mg/ml. Price 2-ml amp = D; 5-ml amp = F
PoM **Cytosar**® (Upjohn)
Injection, powder for reconstitution, cytarabine. Price 100-mg vial (with diluent) = F

FLUOROURACIL
Indications: see notes above
Cautions; Side-effects: see section 8.1

PoM **Fluorouracil Capsules,** fluorouracil 250 mg. Price 10 caps = I. Label: 21
PoM **Fluorouracil Injection,** fluorouracil 25 mg (as sodium salt)/ml. Price 10-ml amp = D
▼ PoM **Efudix**® (Roche)
Cream, fluorouracil 5%. Price 20 g = F

MERCAPTOPURINE
Indications: acute leukaemias
Cautions; Side-effects: see section 8.1 and notes above; reduce dose in renal failure. Drug interactions: see Appendix 1 (section 8)
Dose: initially 2.5 mg/kg daily

PoM **Puri-Nethol**® (Wellcome)
Tablets, fawn, scored, mercaptopurine 50 mg. Price 20 tabs = H

METHOTREXATE
Indications: see notes above
Cautions; Side-effects: see section 8.1 and notes above; reduce dose in renal failure; dose-related toxicity in hepatic impairment. Drug interactions: see Appendix 1 (section 8)
Dose: by mouth, 10–25 mg weekly

PoM **Methotrexate Tablets,** methotrexate 2.5 mg, price 20 tabs = E; 10 mg, price 20 tabs = I
PoM **Methotrexate Injection,** methotrexate 2.5 mg (as sodium salt)/ml, price 1-ml amp = C, 2-ml vial = D; 25 mg/ml, price 1-ml vial = E, 2-ml vial = G, 4-ml vial = I, 8-, 10-, 20-, 40-, and 200-ml vial (all) = J; powder for reconstitution, price 500-mg, 1-, and 5-g vial (all) = J
PoM **Emtexate**® (Nordic)
Tablets, methotrexate 10 mg. Price 10 tabs = G
Injection, methotrexate 2.5 mg (as sodium salt)/ ml. Price 2-ml amp = D
Injection, methotrexate 25 mg (as sodium salt)/ ml. Price 2-ml vial = F; 10-, 20-, 40-, and 200-ml vial (all) = J
Injection, methotrexate 100 mg (as sodium salt)/ ml. Price 10- and 50-ml vial (both) = J
Injection, powder for reconstitution, methotrexate (as sodium salt). Price 0.5-, 1-, and 5-g vial (all) = J

THIOGUANINE
Indications: acute leukaemias

C = 51-100p, D = 101-180p, E = 181-300p, F = 301-450p, G = 451-650p, H = 651-900p, I = 901-1200p, J = over 1200p.

Cautions; Side-effects: see section 8.1 and notes above; reduce dose in renal failure
Dose: initially 2–2.5 mg/kg daily

PoM **Lanvis**® (Wellcome)
Tablets, yellow, scored, thioguanine 40 mg. Price 10 tabs = **I**

8.1.4   Vinca alkaloids and etoposide

These interfere with microtubule assembly, causing metaphase arrest. All vinca alkaloids have similar activity but vary in the predominant site of toxicity.

Vincristine (Oncovin®) is used to treat the acute leukaemias, particularly lymphoblastic leukaemia, lymphomas, and certain solid tumours. It is given intravenously with a maximum recommended dose of 2 mg.

Vincristine causes remarkably little myelosuppression. Its predominant toxicity affects the peripheral nerves and the autonomic nervous system. Deep tendon reflexes are usually lost and peripheral paraesthesia and numbness commonly occur. Abdominal bloating and constipation after treatment are also common as are manifestations of bowel atony. If these symptoms are severe or motor weakness is found, doses should be reduced. Vincristine should be stopped if these symptoms continue to progress; recovery in these instances is usually slow but complete. In addition alopecia may occur and, rarely, hyponatraemia as a result of inappropriate antidiuretic hormone secretion.

Vinblastine (Velbe®) is used intravenously to treat the lymphomas and certain solid tumours, for example, testicular teratoma. It causes more myelosuppression than vincristine, but less neurotoxicity, and is therefore commonly substituted for that drug.

Vindesine (Eldisine®) is the most recent addition to the vinca alkaloid group. It has a similar range of clinical activity, and side-effects intermediate between those of the above two drugs.

Etoposide (Vepesid®) may be given orally or intravenously, the dose when used orally being double that when given intravenously. There is limited clinical evidence to suggest that administration in divided doses over 3–5 days may be beneficial. It has useful activity in small cell carcinoma of the bronchus, the lymphomas, and testicular teratoma. Common toxic effects include alopecia, myelosuppression, nausea, and vomiting.

ETOPOSIDE
Indications: see notes above
Cautions; Contra-indications; Side-effects: see section 8.1 and notes above; irritant to tissues

▼ PoM **Vepesid**® (Bristol-Myers)
Capsules, etoposide 50 mg. Price 2 caps = **I**
Capsules, etoposide 100 mg. Price 1 cap = **I**

Injection, etoposide 20 mg/ml. To be diluted. Price 5-ml amp = **J**
Caution: may dissolve certain types of filter

VINBLASTINE SULPHATE
Indications: see notes above
Cautions; Side-effects: see section 8.1 and notes above; caution in handling—avoid contact with eyes; irritant to tissues

PoM **Vinblastine Injection,** powder for reconstitution, vinblastine sulphate. Price 10-mg vial (with diluent) = **H**
PoM **Velbe**® (Lilly)
Injection, powder for reconstitution, vinblastine sulphate. Price 10-mg amp (with diluent) = **I**

VINCRISTINE SULPHATE
Indications: see notes above
Cautions; Side-effects: see section 8.1 and notes above; caution in handling—avoid contact with eyes; irritant to tissues

PoM **Vincristine Injection,** powder for reconstitution, vincristine sulphate (with lactose). Price 1-mg vial = **H**; 2- and 5-mg vial (both) = **J** (all with diluent)
PoM **Oncovin**® (Lilly)
Injection, powder for reconstitution, vincristine sulphate (with lactose). Price 1-mg vial = **I**; 2- and 5-mg vial = **J** (all with diluent)
Injection, vincristine sulphate 1 mg, mannitol 100 mg/ml. Price 1-ml vial = **I**; 2-ml vial = **J**

VINDESINE SULPHATE
Indications: see notes above
Cautions; Side-effects: see section 8.1 and notes above; caution in handling—avoid contact with eyes; irritant to tissues

PoM **Eldisine**® (Lilly)
Injection, powder for reconstitution, vindesine sulphate (with mannitol). Price 5-mg vial (with diluent) = **J** (Hosp. only)

8.1.5   Other cytotoxic drugs

Amsacrine (Amsidine®) is a newly introduced drug with an action and toxic effects similar to those of doxorubicin. It is used as second-line treatment in refractory acute myeloid leukaemia. Side-effects include myelosuppression and mucositis; monitor electrolytes as fatal arrhythmias have occurred in hypokalaemia.

AMSACRINE
Indications: see notes above
Cautions; Side-effects: see section 8.1 and notes above; reduce dose in renal or hepatic impairment. Also caution in handling—irritant to skin and tissues

▼ PoM **Amsidine**® (P-D)
Concentrate for intravenous infusion, amsacrine 5 mg (as lactate)/ml, when reconstituted by mix-

Relative prices: **A** = up to 20p, **B** = 21-50p,

ing two solutions. Price 1.5-ml amp with 13.5-ml vial = **J** (Hosp. only)
Use glass infusion apparatus

Cisplatin has an alkylating action. It has useful antitumour activity in certain solid tumours including ovarian carcinoma and testicular teratoma. It is, however, a toxic drug. Common problems include severe nausea and vomiting, nephrotoxicity (the creatinine clearance should be closely monitored), myelotoxicity, ototoxicity (high tone hearing loss and tinnitus), peripheral neuropathy, and hypomagnesaemia. These toxic effects commonly necessitate dose reduction and/or drug withdrawal. It is preferable that treatment with this drug be supervised by specialists familiar with its use.

CISPLATIN
Indications: see notes above
Cautions; Side-effects: see section 8.1 and notes above; reduce dose in renal impairment. Drug interactions: see Appendix 1 (section 8)

PoM **Neoplatin**® (Bristol-Myers)
Injection, powder for reconstitution, cisplatin. Price 10-mg vial = **H**; 50-mg vial = **J**
▼ PoM **Platinex**® (Bristol-Myers)
Injection, cisplatin 500 micrograms/ml. Price 20-ml vial = **I**; 50- and 100-ml vial (both) = **J**
PoM **Platosin**® (Nordic)
Injection, powder for reconstitution, cisplatin. Price 10-mg vial = **E**; 25-mg vial = **H**; 50-mg vial = **J**

Dacarbazine is not commonly used on account of its toxicity. It has been used to treat melanoma and, in combination therapy, the soft tissue sarcomas. It is also a component of a commonly used second-line combination for Hodgkin's disease (ABVD). The predominant side-effects are myelosuppression and intense nausea and vomiting.

DACARBAZINE
Indications: see notes above
Cautions; Side-effects: see section 8.1; also caution in handling—irritant to skin and tissues

PoM **DTIC-Dome** (Bayer)
Injection, powder for reconstitution, dacarbazine. Price 100-mg vial = **G**; 200-mg vial = **H**

Hydroxyurea (Hydrea®) is an orally active drug used mainly in the treatment of chronic myeloid leukaemia. Myelosuppression, nausea, and skin reactions are the commonest toxic effects.

HYDROXYUREA
Indications: see notes above
Cautions; Side-effects: see section 8.1 and notes above
Dose: 20–30 mg/kg daily *or* 80 mg/kg every 3rd day

PoM **Hydrea**® (Squibb)
Capsules, pink/green, hydroxyurea 500 mg. Price 20 caps = **E**

Mitozantrone (Novantrone®) is structurally related to doxorubicin and preliminary work suggests that it has equal activity in breast cancer; it is well tolerated apart from myelosuppression and probable dose-related cardiotoxicity.

MITOZANTRONE
Indications: see notes above
Cautions; Side-effects: see section 8.1 and notes above

▼ PoM **Novantrone**® (Lederle)
Intravenous infusion, mitozantrone 2 mg (as hydrochloride)/ml, with sodium chloride and acetate buffer. Price 20-, 25-, and 30-mg vial (all) = **J**

Procarbazine (Natulan®) is a first-line drug in Hodgkin's disease, for example in MOPP chemotherapy. It is also used to treat non-Hodgkin lymphomas and small cell carcinoma of the bronchus. It is given orally. Toxic effects include nausea, myelosuppression, and a hypersensitivity rash preventing further use of this drug. It is a mild monoamine-oxidase inhibitor and appropriate dietary advice is recommended (see section 4.3.2). Alcohol ingestion may cause a disulfiram-like reaction.

PROCARBAZINE
Indications: see notes above
Cautions; Side-effects: see section 8.1 and notes above; reduce dose in renal failure. Drug interactions: see Appendix 1 (section 8)
Dose: initially 50 mg daily, gradually increased to 250–300 mg daily in divided doses

PoM **Natulan**® (Roche)
Capsules, yellow, procarbazine 50 mg (as hydrochloride). Price 20 caps = **D**. Label: 4

Razoxane (Razoxin®) has limited activity in the leukaemias, and is little used.

RAZOXANE
Indications: see notes above
Cautions; Side-effects: see section 8.1
Dose: 125 mg twice daily, with radiotherapy

▼ PoM **Razoxin**® (ICI)
Tablets, razoxane 125 mg. Price 10 tabs = **H**

8.1.6 Antagonists used with cytotoxic drugs

Urothelial toxicity, commonly manifest by haemorrhagic cystitis, is a problem peculiar to the use of cyclophosphamide or ifosfamide and is caused by a metabolite (acrolein). **Mesna** (Uromitexan®) reacts specifically with this metabolite in the urinary tract, preventing toxicity. There is no interaction with the parent drug. Mesna is given intra-

---

C = 51-100p, **D** = 101-180p, **E** = 181-300p, **F** = 301-450p, **G** = 451-650p, **H** = 651-900p, **I** = 901-1200p, **J** = over 1200p.

venously simultaneously from the beginning and also continued for an appropriate time after completing administration of cyclophosphamide and ifosfamide and is particularly indicated where these drugs are used in high dosage.

MESNA

Indications: see notes above
Side-effects: above max. therapeutic doses, gastro-intestinal disturbances, fatigue, headache

▼ PoM **Uromitexan**® (Boehringer Ingelheim)
Injection, mesna 100 mg/ml. Price 4-ml amp = D; 10-ml amp = E

8.2   Drugs affecting the immune response

8.2.1 Cytotoxic immunosuppressants
8.2.2 Corticosteroids and other immuno-suppressants
8.2.3 Immunostimulants

8.2.1   Cytotoxic immunosuppressants

These drugs are used to suppress rejection in organ transplant recipients and are also used to treat a variety of auto-immune and collagen diseases (see section 10.1.3). They are non-specific in their action and careful monitoring of peripheral blood counts is required, with dose adjustments for marrow toxicity. Patients receiving these drugs will be prone to atypical, for example fungal, infections.

Azathioprine (Imuran® etc.) is the most widely used drug for transplant recipients and is also used to treat a number of conditions, usually when corticosteroid therapy alone has provided inadequate control. This drug is metabolised to mercaptopurine, and doses should be reduced when concurrent therapy with allopurinol is given. The predominant toxic effect is myelosuppression, although hepatic toxicity is also well recognised.

Cyclophosphamide and chlorambucil (section 8.1.1) are less commonly prescribed as immuno-suppressants.

AZATHIOPRINE

Indications: see notes above
Cautions; Side-effects: see section 8.1 and notes above; also rashes. Reduce dose in severe renal failure. Drug interactions: see Appendix 1 (section 8)
Dose: by mouth, 1–5 mg/kg daily

PoM **Azamune**® (Penn)
Tablets, yellow, scored, azathioprine 50 mg. Price 20 tabs = H
PoM **Imuran**® (Wellcome)
Tablets, yellow, scored, azathioprine 50 mg. Price 20 tabs = H
Injection, powder for reconstitution, azathioprine (as sodium salt). Price 50-mg vial = I

8.2.2   Corticosteroids and other immunosuppressants

Prednisone and prednisolone are widely used in oncology. They have marked antitumour effect in acute lymphoblastic leukaemia, Hodgkin's disease, and the non-Hodgkin lymphomas. They are also active in hormone-sensitive breast cancer and may cause useful disease regression. Finally, they have a role in the palliation of symptomatic end-stage malignant disease when they may produce a sense of well-being.

The corticosteroids are also powerful immuno-suppressants. They are used to prevent organ transplant rejection, and in high dose to treat rejection episodes. For notes on corticosteroids see section 6.3.

Antilymphocyte immunoglobulin (Pressimmune®) is obtained from immunised horses. It has mainly been used to prevent transplant rejection.

Cyclosporin (Sandimmun®) is a fungal metabolite and potent immunosuppressant which is virtually non-myelotoxic. It has found particular use in the field of organ and tissue transplantation, for prevention of graft rejection following bone marrow, kidney, liver, pancreas, heart, and heart-lung transplantation, and for prophylaxis of graft-versus-host disease.

ANTILYMPHOCYTE IMMUNOGLOBULIN

Indications: see notes above
Cautions: test for hypersensitivity; acute infections
Side-effects: fever, shivering, nausea, hypotension, tachycardia; also anaphylactic reactions, urticaria, pruritus

PoM **Pressimmune**® (Hoechst)
Injection, antilymphocyte immunoglobulin (horse) 50 mg/ml. Price 5- and 10-ml amp (both) = J (Hosp. only)

CYCLOSPORIN

Indications: see notes above
Cautions: increased susceptibility to infections, especially when administered with other immunosuppressive agents; breast-feeding. Drug interactions: see Appendix 1 (section 8)
Side-effects: impairment of liver and renal function; tremor, gastro-intestinal disturbances, hirsutism

▼ PoM **Sandimmun**® (Sandoz)
Oral solution, oily, yellow, cyclosporin 100 mg/ml. Price 50 ml = J
Concentrate for intravenous infusion (oily), cyclosporin 50 mg/ml (formulation contains Cremophor EL®). To be diluted before use. Price 1-ml amp = D; 5-ml amp = H

8.2.3   Immunostimulants

A suspension of inactivated *Corynebacterium parvum* organisms may be used by the intracavitary route to treat malignant effusions. Pyrexia is a common side-effect. Treatment should be avoided within 10 days of thoracotomy.

CORYNEBACTERIUM PARVUM VACCINE

Indications: see notes above
Side-effects: pyrexia, abdominal pain, nausea and vomiting

PoM **Coparvax**® (Calmic)
Injection, powder for reconstitution, *Corynebacterium parvum* (inactivated). Price 7-mg vial = **J**

8.3 Sex hormones and antagonists in malignant disease

8.3.1 Oestrogens
8.3.2 Progestogens
8.3.3 Androgens and anabolic steroids
8.3.4 Hormone antagonists

These drugs are predominantly used in the treatment of breast and prostate cancers. Certain other tumours, however, are variably hormone responsive including endometrial and ovarian carcinoma and hypernephroma. In recent years hormone antagonists have assumed increasing importance in the management of the postmenopausal patient with breast cancer. Tamoxifen has replaced oestrogens as the drug of choice in this setting, and aminoglutethimide has replaced adrenalectomy as secondary therapy. The role of hormones in the adjuvant therapy of breast cancer is at present being re-evaluated.

8.3.1 Oestrogens

Stilboestrol is widely used in postmenopausal breast cancer and prostate cancer and will cause temporary disease regression in, respectively, approximately 30% and 80% of cases. Toxicity is relatively common, and dose-related side-effects include nausea, fluid retention, venous and, particularly in elderly males, arterial thrombosis. Hypercalcaemia may occur in breast cancer where widespread bone metastases are present. Impotence and gynaecomastia will always occur in the male, and withdrawal bleeding may be a problem in the female.

Fosfestrol (Honvan®) is activated by the enzyme acid phosphatase to produce stilboestrol. Side-effects are as for stilboestrol and, in addition, perineal pain may complicate intravenous use in prostate cancer.

Ethinyloestradiol is the most potent oestrogen available. Unlike other oestrogens it is not metabolised in the liver. It is used in breast cancer and may be better tolerated than stilboestrol in patients suffering from nausea.

Polyestradiol (Estradurin®) is a long-acting oestrogen preparation.

ETHINYLOESTRADIOL

Indications: see notes above

Cautions; Contra-indications; Side-effects: see section 6.4.1.1 and notes above
Dose: 1–3 mg daily

Preparations
See section 6.4.1.1

FOSFESTROL TETRASODIUM

Indications: see notes above
Cautions; Contra-indications; Side-effects: see under Ethinyloestradiol (section 6.4.1.1) and notes above
Dose: by mouth, 100–200 mg 3 times daily, reducing to 100–300 mg daily
By intravenous injection, 552–1104 mg daily for at least 5 days; maintenance 276 mg 1–4 times weekly

PoM **Honvan**® (Boehringer Ingelheim)
Tablets, fosfestrol tetrasodium 100 mg. Price 20 tabs = **E**
Injection, fosfestrol tetrasodium 55.2 mg/ml. Price 5-ml amp = **C**

POLYESTRADIOL PHOSPHATE

Indications: prostatic carcinoma
Cautions; Contra-indications; Side-effects: see under Ethinyloestradiol (section 6.4.1.1) and notes above
Dose: by deep intramuscular injection, 80–160 mg every 4 weeks; maintenance 40–80 mg

PoM **Estradurin**® (Lundbeck)
Injection, powder for reconstitution, polyestradiol phosphate (with mepivacaine and nicotinamide). Price 40-mg vial = **E**; 80-mg vial = **F** (both with diluent)

STILBOESTROL

Indications: see notes above
Cautions; Contra-indications; Side-effects: see under Ethinyloestradiol (section 6.4.1.1) and notes above
Dose: breast cancer, 10–20 mg daily
Prostatic cancer, 1–3 mg daily

PoM **Stilboestrol Tablets,** stilboestrol 1 and 5 mg, price 20 tabs (both) = **B**

8.3.2 Progestogens

These drugs are used largely as second- or third-line therapy in breast cancer. They are also used to treat endometrial carcinoma and hypernephroma. Side-effects occur less commonly than with oestrogens. **Norethisterone** (Utovlan®) and esters of **gestronol** (Depostat®), **hydroxyprogesterone** (Proluton Depot®), **medroxyprogesterone** (Farlutal®, Provera®), **megestrol** (Megace®) and **norethisterone** (SH 420®) may be used. Progestogens given parenterally in high dose are under evaluation in breast cancer. Although increased response rates have been reported, duration of survival has not been influenced. Side-effects include nausea and fluid retention.

C = 51-100p, **D** = 101-180p, **E** = 181-300p, **F** = 301-450p, **G** = 451-650p, **H** = 651-900p, **I** = 901-1200p, **J** = over 1200p.

GESTRONOL HEXANOATE

Indications: see notes above

Cautions; Contra-indications; Side-effects: see under Progesterone (section 6.4.1.2) and notes above

Dose: by intramuscular injection, 200–400 mg every 5–7 days

PoM **Depostat**® (Schering)
Injection (oily), gestronol hexanoate 100 mg/ml. Price 2-ml amp = **F**

HYDROXYPROGESTERONE HEXANOATE

Indications: see notes above

Cautions; Contra-indications; Side-effects: see under Progesterone (section 6.4.1.2) and notes above

Dose: by intramuscular injection, 1 g one or more times weekly

Preparations
See section 6.4.1.2

MEDROXYPROGESTERONE ACETATE

Indications: see notes above

Cautions; Contra-indications; Side-effects: see under Progesterone (section 6.4.1.2) and notes above

Dose: by mouth, 200–400 mg daily for up to 3 months to assess response

By intramuscular injection, 0.4–1 g one or more times weekly

PoM **Depo-Provera**® (Upjohn)
Injection, medroxyprogesterone acetate 150 mg/ml. Price 3-ml vial = **I**
PoM **Farlutal**® (Farmitalia Carlo Erba)
Tablets, scored, medroxyprogesterone acetate 100 mg. Price 20 tabs = **H**
Tablets, scored, medroxyprogesterone acetate 250 mg. Price 10 tabs = **H**
Tablets, scored, medroxyprogesterone acetate 500 mg. Price 5 tabs = **H**. Label: 27
Injection, medroxyprogesterone acetate 200 mg/ml. Price 2.5-ml vial = **I**; 5-ml vial = **J**
PoM **Provera 100 mg**® (Upjohn)
Tablets, scored, medroxyprogesterone acetate 100 mg. Price 20 tabs = **H**
PoM **Provera 200 mg**® (Upjohn)
Tablets, scored, medroxyprogesterone acetate 200 mg. Price 10 tabs = **H**

MEGESTROL ACETATE

Indications: see notes above

Cautions; Contra-indications; Side-effects: see under Progesterone (section 6.4.1.2) and notes above

Dose: breast cancer, 160 mg daily, endometrial cancer, 40–320 mg daily

PoM **Megace**® (Bristol-Myers)
Tablets, scored, megestrol acetate 40 mg. Price 20 tabs = **G**

NORETHISTERONE

Indications: see notes above

Cautions; Contra-indications; Side-effects: see section 6.4.1.2 and notes above

Dose: 40 mg daily, increased to 60 mg daily if required

Preparations
See section 6.4.1.2

NORETHISTERONE ACETATE

Indications: see notes above

Cautions; Contra-indications; Side-effects: see section 6.4.1.2 and notes above

Dose: 10 mg 3 times daily, increased to 60 mg daily if required

PoM **SH 420**® (Schering)
Tablets, norethisterone acetate 10 mg. Price 20 tabs = **G**

8.3.3   Androgens and anabolic steroids

The androgens are given parenterally and are predominantly used as second- or third-line therapy for metastatic breast cancer.

DROSTANOLONE PROPIONATE

Indications: see notes above

Cautions; Contra-indications; Side-effects: see under Ethyloestrenol (section 6.4.3) and notes above

Dose: by intramuscular injection, 300 mg weekly

PoM **Masteril**® (Syntex)
Injection, drostanolone propionate 100 mg/ml. Price 1-ml amp = **E**

NANDROLONE

Indications: see notes above

Cautions; Contra-indications; Side-effects: see under Ethyloestrenol (section 6.4.3) and notes above

Dose: by intramuscular injection, nandrolone decanoate 25–50 mg every 3 weeks; nandrolone phenylpropionate 25–50 mg weekly

Preparations
See section 6.4.3

8.3.4   Hormone antagonists

Aminoglutethimide (Orimeten®) is used in postmenopausal patients with breast cancer. It acts by inhibiting the conversion of androgens to oestrogens in peripheral tissues. In addition it acts as an inhibitor of adrenal steroid production and corticosteroid replacement must therefore be prescribed for the duration of therapy. Early toxicity is common and may include drowsiness, a transitory drug eruption, and drug fever. The dose is usually increased gradually. Hepatic enzyme induction occurs, and may require dose modification of other drugs, for example oral anticoagulants and oral hypoglycaemics.

Tamoxifen acts as an oestrogen antagonist and blocks receptor sites in target organs. This drug has replaced oestrogens as the treatment of choice for postmenopausal metastatic breast cancer. Side-effects are uncommon. However, patients with widespread bone metastases may experience exacerbation of bone pain and, occasionally, hypercalcaemia.

The anti-androgen **cyproterone** (Cyprostat®) is under evaluation as primary therapy for metastatic prostate cancer, but is not at present widely used in the United Kingdom.

AMINOGLUTETHIMIDE

Indications: metastatic mammary carcinoma in postmenopausal or oophorectomised women; Cushing's syndrome due to malignant disease
Cautions; Side-effects: see notes above. Drug interactions: see Appendix 1 (sections *2.8A*, *6.3*)
Dose: 250 mg twice daily for 2 weeks, increased to 250 mg 4 times daily

▼ PoM **Orimeten**® (Ciba)
Tablets, scored, aminoglutethimide 250 mg. Price 20 tabs = **H**

CYPROTERONE ACETATE

Indications: see notes above
Cautions; Side-effects: see section 6.4.2
Dose: 300 mg daily in 2–3 divided doses after food

▼ PoM **Cyprostat**® (Schering)
Tablets, scored, cyproterone acetate 50 mg. Price 20 tabs = **J**. Label: 2, 21

TAMOXIFEN
Indications: see notes above
Contra-indications: pregnancy
Side-effects: hot flushes, vaginal bleeding, gastro-intestinal disturbances dizziness; rarely fluid retention, visual disturbances; see also notes above
Dose: breast cancer, initially 20–40 mg daily

PoM **Tamoxifen Citrate Tablets,** tamoxifen (as citrate) 10 mg, price 20 tabs = **G**; 20 mg, price 20 tabs = **I**
PoM **Kessar**® (Farmitalia Carla Erba)
Tablets, tamoxifen 10 mg (as citrate). Price 20 tabs = **G**
Tablets, tamoxifen 20 mg (as citrate). Price 20 tabs = **H**
PoM **Noltam**® (Lederle)
Tablets, f/c, tamoxifen 10 mg (as citrate). Price 20 tabs = **G**
Tablets, f/c, scored, tamoxifen 20 mg (as citrate). Price 20 tabs = **H**
PoM **Nolvadex**® (ICI)
Tablets, tamoxifen 10 mg (as citrate). Price 20 tabs = **G**
PoM **Nolvadex-D**® (ICI)
Tablets, tamoxifen 20 mg (as citrate). Price 20 tabs = **I**
PoM **Nolvadex-Forte**® (ICI)
Tablets, scored, tamoxifen 40 mg (as citrate). Price 10 tabs = **I**
PoM **Tamofen**® (Tillotts)
Tablets, off-white, scored, tamoxifen 10 mg (as citrate). Price 20 tabs = **G**
PoM **Tamofen-20**® (Tillotts)
Tablets, off-white, tamoxifen 20 mg (as citrate). Price 20 tabs = **H**
PoM **Tamofen-40**® (Tillotts)
Tablets, off-white, tamoxifen 40 mg (as citrate). Price 10 tabs = **H**

C = 51-100p, **D** = 101-180p, **E** = 181-300p, **F** = 301-450p, **G** = 451-650p, **H** = 651-900p, **I** = 901-1200p, **J** = over 1200p.

9: Drugs affecting
NUTRITION and BLOOD

This section includes drugs for the treatment of anaemias, and foods, food supplements, vitamins, and electrolytes used in nutritional disorders. It does not include information on preparations of human blood or blood products which, in the United Kingdom, are supplied through the Department of Health and Social Security (England and Wales), the Scottish National Blood Transfusion Association (Scotland), and the Regional Transfusion Centre (Northern Ireland). Immunoglobulin injections are discussed in Chapter 14.

This chapter is arranged in the following sections:

9.1 Drugs used in anaemias
9.2 Electrolyte and water replacement
9.3 Intravenous feeding
9.4 Foods for special diets and nutritional support
9.5 Minerals
9.6 Vitamins
9.7 Bitters and tonics

9.1   Drugs used in anaemias

9.1.1   Iron-deficiency anaemias
9.1.1.1   Oral iron therapy
9.1.1.2   Parenteral iron therapy
9.1.2   Megaloblastic anaemias
9.1.3   Hypoplastic and haemolytic anaemias

Before initiating treatment it is essential to determine which type of anaemia is present. Iron salts may be harmful and result in iron overload if given alone to patients with anaemias other than those due to iron deficiency.

9.1.1   Iron-deficiency anaemias

Other than in the special cases indicated below, the only justification for iron treatment is the presence of a demonstrable iron-deficiency state. However, prophylaxis is justifiable in pregnancy, menorrhagia, after subtotal or total gastrectomy (where iron deficiency anaemia may be expected in up to 60% of patients), and in the management of low birth-weight infants such as premature babies, twins, and infants after Caesarean section. The National Blood Transfusion Service provides iron prophylaxis for female blood donors in some centres.

9.1.1.1   ORAL IRON THERAPY

Iron salts should be given by mouth unless there are good reasons for using another route. The commonly used ferrous salts show only marginal differences in efficiency of absorption of iron. Ferric salts are much less well absorbed than ferrous salts. Haemoglobin regeneration rate is little affected by the salt used provided sufficient iron is given, and in most patients the time factor is not critical. Choice of preparation is thus usually decided by incidence of side-effects and cost.

The oral dose of elemental iron should be 100 to 200 mg daily. It is customary to start treatment with dried **ferrous sulphate**, 200 mg being given three times daily initially. Iron is best absorbed in the fasting state but ferrous sulphate may be given after food to minimise gastric intolerance. If side-effects arise, dosage can be reduced or a change made to an alternative iron salt. It should be remembered, however, that an apparent improvement in tolerance on changing to another salt may be due to its lower content of elemental iron.

Table 1: Iron Salts

Iron salt	Amount	Content of ferrous iron
Ferrous fumarate	200 mg	65 mg
Ferrous gluconate	300 mg	35 mg
Ferrous glycine sulphate	225 mg	40 mg
Ferrous succinate	100 mg	35 mg
Ferrous sulphate	300 mg	60 mg
Ferrous sulphate, dried	200 mg	60 mg

THERAPEUTIC RESPONSE. The haemoglobin concentration should rise by about 100 to 200 mg per 100 ml per day. When the haemoglobin figure has risen to a normal level, treatment should be continued for a further three months in an attempt to replenish the iron stores. Epithelial tissue changes such as atrophic glossitis and koilonychia are usually improved although the response is often slow.

ADJUVANTS. Some oral preparations contain adjuvants such as ascorbic acid, or the iron is in the form of a chelate, which can be shown experimentally to produce a modest increase in absorption of iron. However, the therapeutic advantage is minimal and cost may be increased. There can be neither theoretical nor clinical justification for the inclusion of other therapeutically active ingredients, especially the B group of vitamins, in orally administered preparations, except for folic acid in conjunction with an iron salt as prophylactic therapy for pregnant women (iron and folic acid preparations—see below).

SLOW-RELEASE CAPSULES AND TABLETS. These are designed to release iron gradually as the capsule or tablet passes along the gut so that a smaller amount of ionic iron is present in the lumen at any one time. It is claimed that each dose unit contains enough iron for 24 hours, thus giving simple once daily dosage.

These preparations are likely to carry the iron

past the first part of the duodenum into an area of the gut where conditions for iron absorption are poor. The low incidence of side-effects may well be because of the small amounts of iron available under these conditions and so the preparations have no therapeutic advantage and should not be used.

SIDE-EFFECTS. Because iron salts are astringent, gastro-intestinal irritation may occur, necessitating care in administration as described above. Nausea and epigastric pain may occur and are dose-related but the relationship between dose and altered bowel habit, giving rise to constipation or diarrhoea, is less clear. The incidence of side-effects due to ferrous sulphate is no greater than with other iron salts when compared on the basis of equivalent amounts of elemental iron.

FERROUS FUMARATE
Indications: iron-deficiency anaemia
Cautions; Side-effects; Dose: see under Ferrous Sulphate

Fersaday® (DF)
Tablets, orange, f/c, ferrous fumarate 304 mg (100 mg iron). Price 28 tabs = **B**
Fersamal® (DF)
Tablets, brown, ferrous fumarate 200 mg (65 mg iron). Price 20 tabs = **A**
Syrup (= mixture), brown, ferrous fumarate 140 mg (45 mg iron)/5 ml. Diluent syrup, life of diluted mixture 14 days. Price 200 ml = **D**
Galfer® (Galen)
Capsules, red/green, ferrous fumarate 290 mg (100 mg iron). Price 20 caps = **B**
Meterfer® (Sinclair)
Tablets, blue, f/c, ferrous fumarate equivalent to 100 mg iron. Price 20 tabs = **B**
Plancaps® (Unimed)
Capsules, ferrous fumarate 290 mg (100 mg iron). Price 20 caps = **D**

FERROUS GLUCONATE
Indications: iron-deficiency anaemia
Cautions; Side-effects; Dose: see under Ferrous Sulphate

Ferrous Gluconate Tablets, red, s/c, ferrous gluconate 300 mg (35 mg iron). Price 20 tabs = **A**
Fergon® (Winthrop)
Tablets, red, s/c, ferrous gluconate 300 mg (35 mg iron). Price 20 tabs = **B**

FERROUS GLYCINE SULPHATE
Indications: iron-deficiency anaemia
Cautions; Side-effects; Dose: see under Ferrous Sulphate

Fe-Cap® (MCP)
Capsules, yellow/white, ferrous glycine sulphate 565 mg (100 mg iron). Price 30 caps = **C**
Ferrocontin Continus® (Napp)
Tablets, s/r, red, f/c, ferrous glycine sulphate 562.5 mg (100 mg iron). Price 20 tabs = **B**. Label: 25

Kelferon® (MCP)
Tablets, pink, s/c, ferrous glycine sulphate 225 mg (40 mg iron). Price 20 tabs = **A**
Plesmet® (Napp)
Syrup (= elixir), ferrous glycine sulphate 141 mg (25 mg iron)/5 ml. Diluent syrup, life of diluted elixir 14 days. Price 100 ml = **C**

FERROUS SUCCINATE
Indications: iron-deficiency anaemia
Cautions; Side-effects; Dose: see under Ferrous Sulphate

Ferrous Succinate Tablets, orange, s/c, ferrous succinate 100 mg (35 mg iron). Price 20 tabs = **B**
Ferromyn® (Calmic)
Tablets, orange, s/c, ferrous succinate 100 mg (35 mg iron). Price 20 tabs = **C**
Elixir, brown, ferrous succinate 106 mg (37 mg iron)/5 ml. Diluent syrup, life of diluted elixir 14 days. Price 100 ml = **E**

FERROUS SULPHATE
Indications: iron-deficiency anaemia
Cautions: drug interactions: see Appendix 1 (sections *5.1*, 9, *9*, *10*)
Side-effects: large doses may produce gastro-intestinal irritation, vomiting, diarrhoea; continued administration may result in constipation
Dose: ferrous iron, therapeutic, 120–180 mg daily in divided doses; prophylactic, 60 mg daily; CHILD, therapeutic, daily in divided doses, up to 1 year 36 mg, 1–5 years 72 mg, 6–12 years 120 mg

Ferrous Sulphate Tablets, f/c or s/c, dried ferrous sulphate 200 mg (60 mg iron) and 300 mg (90 mg iron). Price 20 tabs (both) = **A**
Ferrous Sulphate Mixture, Paediatric, ferrous sulphate 60 mg (12 mg iron)/5 ml (see Formulary). Price 100 ml = **A**. Label: 27
To be taken well diluted with water
Feospan® (SK&F)
Spansule® (= capsules s/r), clear/red, enclosing green and red pellets, dried ferrous sulphate 150 mg (45 mg iron). Price 20 caps = **C**. Label: 25
Ferro-Gradumet® (Abbott)
Filmtabs® (= tablets f/c), s/r, red, dried ferrous sulphate 325 mg (105 mg iron). Price 20 tabs = **B**. Label: 25
Ironorm® (Wallace Mfg)
Drops (= elixir), ferrous sulphate 116 mg (25 mg iron)/ml. Price 15 ml = **C**. Label: 27
Slow-Fe® (Ciba)
Tablets, s/r, dried ferrous sulphate 160 mg (48 mg iron). Price 20 tabs = **B**. Label: 25

IRON AND FOLIC ACID
Indications: prevention of iron and folic acid deficiencies in pregnancy
Cautions: the small doses of folic acid recommended for prophylaxis are inadequate for the treatment of megaloblastic anaemias. Drug interactions: see under Ferrous Sulphate
Side-effects: see under Ferrous Sulphate
Dose: prophylactic, the equivalent of approximately 100 mg of iron with 200–500 micrograms of folic acid, daily

---

PoM **Iron and Folic Acid Tablets,** ferrous fumarate 304 mg (100 mg iron), folic acid 350 micrograms. Price 20 tabs = **B**

PoM **Co-Ferol**® (Cox Pharmaceuticals)
Tablets, red, s/c, ferrous fumarate 120 mg (40 mg iron), folic acid 200 micrograms. Price 20 tabs = **A**

PoM **Fe-Cap Folic**® (MCP)
Capsules, yellow/red, ferrous glycine sulphate 450 mg (80 mg iron), folic acid 350 micrograms. Price 30 caps = **C**

PoM **Fefol**® (SK&F)
Spansule® (= capsules s/r), clear/green, enclosing red, yellow, and white pellets, dried ferrous sulphate 150 mg (47 mg iron), folic acid 500 micrograms. Price 20 caps = **C**. Label: 25

PoM **Ferrocap-F 350**® (Consolidated)
Capsules, s/r, pink, enclosing brown, white, and yellow granules, ferrous fumarate 330 mg (110 mg iron), folic acid 350 micrograms. Price 20 caps = **C**. Label: 25

PoM **Ferrocontin Folic Continus**® (Napp)
Tablets, orange, f/c, ferrous glycine sulphate 562.5 mg (100 mg iron) for sustained release, folic acid 500 micrograms. Price 20 tabs = **B**. Label: 25

PoM **Ferrograd Folic**® (Abbott)
Filmtabs® (= tablets f/c), red/yellow, dried ferrous sulphate 325 mg (105 mg iron) for sustained release, folic acid 350 micrograms. Price 20 tabs = **B**. Label: 25

PoM **Folex-350**® (Rybar)
Tablets, pink, s/c, ferrous fumarate 308 mg (100 mg iron), folic acid 350 micrograms. Price 20 tabs = **B**

PoM **Galfer FA**® (Galen)
Capsules, red/yellow, ferrous fumarate 290 mg (100 mg iron), folic acid 350 micrograms. Price 20 caps = **C**

PoM **Kelfolate**® (MCP)
Tablets, yellow, s/c, ferrous glycine sulphate 225 mg (40 mg iron), folic acid 150 micrograms. Price 20 tabs = **A**

PoM **Meterfolic**® (Sinclair)
Tablets, grey, f/c, ferrous fumarate equivalent to 100 mg iron, folic acid 350 micrograms. Price 20 tabs = **B**

PoM **Pregaday**® (DF)
Tablets, brown, f/c, ferrous fumarate 304 mg (100 mg iron), folic acid 350 micrograms. Price 28 tabs = **B**

PoM **Pregfol**® (Wyeth)
Capsules, dark claret, dried ferrous sulphate 270 mg (81 mg iron), folic acid 500 micrograms. Price 20 caps = **B**

PoM **Slow-Fe Folic**® (Ciba)
Tablets, s/r, cream, f/c, dried ferrous sulphate 160 mg (50 mg iron), folic acid 400 micrograms. Price 20 tabs = **B**. Label: 25

POLYSACCHARIDE-IRON COMPLEX

Indications: iron-deficiency anaemia
Cautions; Side-effects: see under Ferrous Sulphate
Dose: the equivalent of iron, therapeutic, 100 mg once or twice daily; prophylactic, 50 mg daily; CHILD, 1–5 years 50 mg daily, 6–12 years 100 mg daily

Niferex® (Tillotts)
Tablets, brown, polysaccharide-iron complex equivalent to 50 mg of iron. Price 20 tabs = **C**

Elixir, brown, polysaccharide-iron complex equivalent to 100 mg of iron/5 ml. Diluent water for preparations or sorbitol solution, life of diluted elixir 14 days. Price 100 ml = **E**; 30-ml dropper bottle for paediatric use = **D**. Counselling advised, use of dropper
Dose: infant, 1 drop (approx. 0.04 ml) per pound body-weight 3 times daily

Niferex-150® (Tillotts)
Capsules, brown/orange, polysaccharide-iron complex equivalent to 150 mg of iron. Price 20 caps = **D**

SODIUM IRONEDETATE

Indications: iron-deficiency anaemia
Cautions; Side-effects: see under Ferrous Sulphate
Dose: the equivalent of iron, up to 55 mg 3 times daily; CHILD ¼–½ adult dose

Sytron® (P-D)
Elixir, sodium ironedetate equivalent to 27.5 mg of iron/5 ml. Diluent water for preparations, life of diluted elixir 14 days. Price 100 ml = **B**

COMPOUND IRON PREPARATIONS

These preparations contain an iron salt and, usually, one or more vitamins or small amounts of substances intended to provide a 'mineral supplement'. There is no justification for prescribing such preparations, except for preparations of iron and folic acid for prophylactic use in pregnancy (see above).

Ferrous Sulphate Tablets, Compound, green, s/c, dried ferrous sulphate equivalent to 170 mg of FeSO₄, copper sulphate 2.5 mg, manganese sulphate 2.5 mg. Price 20 tabs = **A**

NHS **BC 500 with Iron**® (Ayerst)
Tablets, red, f/c, ferrous fumarate 200 mg (65 mg iron), thiamine mononitrate 25 mg, riboflavine 12.5 mg, nicotinamide 100 mg, pyridoxine hydrochloride 10 mg, ascorbic acid 500 mg (as sodium salt), calcium pantothenate 20 mg. Price 20 tabs = **C**

NHS **FEAC**® (Robins)
Tablets, s/r, red, f/c, dried ferrous sulphate 150 mg (45 mg iron), thiamine mononitrate 7.5 mg, riboflavine 5 mg, nicotinamide 25 mg, pyridoxine hydrochloride 2.5 mg, ascorbic acid 150 mg. Price 20 tabs = **C**. Label: 25

NHS **Fe-Cap C**® (MCP)
Capsules, yellow/orange, ferrous glycine sulphate 565 mg (100 mg iron), ascorbic acid 300 mg. Price 20 caps = **B**

NHS PoM **Fefol-Vit**® (SK&F)
Spansule® (= capsules s/r), clear/white, enclosing red, orange, yellow, and white pellets, dried ferrous sulphate 150 mg (47 mg iron), folic acid 500 micrograms, thiamine mononitrate 2 mg, riboflavine 2 mg, nicotinamide 10 mg, pyridoxine hydrochloride 1 mg, ascorbic acid 50 mg. Price 20 caps = **C**. Label: 25

PoM **Fefol Z**® (SK&F)

Spansule® (= capsules s/r), blue/clear, enclosing red, yellow, and white pellets, dried ferrous sulphate 150 mg (47 mg iron), folic acid 500 micrograms, zinc sulphate monohydrate 61.8 mg (22.5 mg zinc). Price 20 caps = **D**. Label: 25

Feospan Z® (SK&F)

Spansule® (= capsules s/r), pink/clear, enclosing green, red, and white pellets, dried ferrous sulphate 150 mg (47 mg iron), zinc sulphate monohydrate 61.8 mg (22.5 mg zinc). Price 20 caps = **D**. Label: 25

NHS PoM **Ferfolic**® (Sinclair)

Tablets, orange, s/c, ferrous gluconate 250 mg (30 mg iron), folic acid 5 mg, thiamine hydrochloride 3 mg, riboflavine 1 mg, nicotinamide 10 mg, ascorbic acid 10 mg. Price 20 tabs = **B**

NHS PoM **Ferfolic SV**® (Sinclair)

Tablets, pink, s/c, ferrous gluconate 250 mg (30 mg iron), folic acid 5 mg. Price 20 tabs = **B**

NHS **Fergluvite**® (Sinclair)

Tablets, yellow, s/c, ferrous gluconate 250 mg (30 mg iron), thiamine hydrochloride 3 mg, riboflavine 1 mg, nicotinamide 10 mg, ascorbic acid 10 mg. Price 20 tabs = **B**

NHS **Ferrocap**® (Consolidated)

Capsules, s/r, green/orange, enclosing brown and white granules, ferrous fumarate 330 mg (110 mg iron), thiamine hydrochloride 5 mg. Price 20 caps = **B**. Label: 25

NHS **Ferrograd C**® (Abbott)

Filmtabs® (= tablets f/c), red, dried ferrous sulphate 325 mg (105 mg iron) for sustained release, ascorbic acid 500 mg (as sodium salt). Price 20 tabs = **C**. Label: 25

NHS **Ferromyn B**® (Calmic)

Tablets, brown, ferrous succinate 106 mg (37 mg iron), thiamine hydrochloride 1 mg, riboflavine 1 mg, nicotinamide 10 mg. Price 20 tabs = **C**

Elixir, brown, ferrous succinate 106 mg (37 mg iron), thiamine hydrochloride 1 mg, riboflavine 1 mg, nicotinamide 10 mg/5 ml. Diluent syrup, life of diluted elixir 14 days. Price 100 ml = **E**

Ferromyn S® (Calmic)

Tablets, orange, ferrous succinate 106 mg (37 mg iron), succinic acid 110 mg. Price 20 tabs = **C**

PoM **Ferromyn S Folic**® (Calmic)

Tablets, red, ferrous succinate 106 mg (37 mg iron), folic acid 100 micrograms, succinic acid 110 mg. Price 20 tabs = **C**

NHS **Fesovit**® (SK&F)

Spansule® (= capsules s/r), colourless/yellow, enclosing red, orange, and white pellets, dried ferrous sulphate 150 mg (47 mg iron), thiamine mononitrate 2 mg, riboflavine 2 mg, nicotinamide 10 mg, pyridoxine hydrochloride 1 mg, ascorbic acid 50 mg. Price 20 caps = **C**. Label: 25

NHS **Fesovit Z**® (SK&F)

Spansule® (= capsules s/r), orange/clear, enclosing red, orange, and white pellets, dried ferrous sulphate 150 mg (47 mg iron), thiamine mononitrate 2 mg, riboflavine 2 mg, nicotinamide 10 mg, pyridoxine hydrochloride 1 mg, ascorbic acid 50 mg, zinc sulphate monohydrate 61.8 mg (22.5 mg zinc). Price 20 caps = **D**. Label: 25

PoM **Folicin**® (Paines & Byrne)

Tablets, s/c, dried ferrous sulphate 200 mg (60 mg iron), folic acid 2.5 mg, copper sulphate 2.5 mg, manganese sulphate 2.5 mg. Price 20 tabs = **A**

NHS **Forceval**® (Unigreg)

Capsules, ferrous fumarate 30.8 mg (10 mg iron), vitamin A 5000 units, thiamine mononitrate 10 mg, riboflavine 5 mg, nicotinamide 20 mg, pyridoxine hydrochloride 500 micrograms, cyanocobalamin 2 micrograms, ascorbic acid 50 mg, vitamin D 600 units, vitamin E 10 mg, calcium pantothenate 2 mg, choline bitartrate 40 mg, calcium 70 mg, copper 500 micrograms, inositol 60 mg, iodine 100 micrograms, lysine hydrochloride 60 mg, magnesium 2 mg, manganese 500 micrograms, phos-

phorus 55 mg, potassium 3 mg, zinc 500 micrograms. Price 20 caps = **D**

Junior capsules, red, ferrous fumarate 15.4 mg (5 mg iron), vitamin A 1650 units, thiamine hydrochloride 1.5 mg, riboflavine 1 mg, nicotinamide 7.5 mg, pyridoxine hydrochloride 1 mg, cyanocobalamin 2 micrograms, ascorbic acid 25 mg, vitamin D_3 200 units, vitamin E 5 mg, calcium pantothenate 1 mg, copper 250 micrograms, iodine 50 micrograms, lysine hydrochloride 10 mg, magnesium 1 mg, manganese 250 micrograms, potassium 1.5 mg, zinc 250 micrograms. Price 20 caps = **D**

NHS **Galfer-Vit**® (Galen)

Capsules, maroon/orange, ferrous fumarate 305 mg (100 mg iron), thiamine mononitrate 2 mg, riboflavine 2 mg, nicotinamide 10 mg, pyridoxine hydrochloride 4 mg, sodium ascorbate 56 mg. Price 20 caps = **C**

NHS **Gastrovite**® (MCP)

Tablets, pink, s/c, ferrous glycine sulphate 225 mg (40 mg iron), ascorbic acid 15 mg, ergocalciferol 200 units, calcium gluconate 100 mg. Price 20 tabs = **B**

NHS **Gevral**® (Lederle)

Capsules, brown, ferrous fumarate 30.8 mg (10 mg iron), vitamin A 5000 units, thiamine mononitrate 5 mg, riboflavine 5 mg, nicotinamide 15 mg, pyridoxine hydrochloride 500 micrograms, cyanocobalamin 1 microgram, ascorbic acid 50 mg, vitamin D 500 units, d-α-tocopheryl acetate 10 units, calcium pantothenate 5 mg, choline bitartrate 50 mg, copper 1 mg (as oxide), iodine 100 micrograms (as potassium iodide), inositol 50 mg, lysine hydrochloride 25 mg, magnesium 1 mg (as oxide), manganese 1 mg (as dioxide), calcium 145 mg and phosphorus 110 mg (as dibasic calcium phosphate), potassium 5 mg (as sulphate), zinc 500 micrograms (as oxide). Price 30 caps = **D**

NHS PoM **Givitol**® (Galen)

Capsules, red/maroon, ferrous fumarate 305 mg (100 mg iron), folic acid 500 micrograms, thiamine mononitrate 2 mg, riboflavine 2 mg, nicotinamide 10 mg, pyridoxine hydrochloride 4 mg, sodium ascorbate 56 mg. Price 20 caps = **C**

NHS **Glykola**® (Sinclair)

Elixir, red, ferric chloride solution 0.01 ml (500 micrograms iron), caffeine 20 mg, calcium glycerophosphate 30 mg, kola liquid extract 0.12 ml/5 ml. Diluent water for preparations, life of diluted elixir 14 days. Price 100 ml = **C**

NHS **Glykola Infans**® (Sinclair)

Elixir paediatric, reddish-brown, ferric chloride solution 0.016 ml (800 micrograms iron), citric acid 40 mg, compound gentian infusion 1 ml, kola liquid extract 0.066 ml, manganese glycerophosphate 10 mg/5 ml. Price 100 ml = **C**

NHS PoM **Irofol C**® (Abbott)

Filmtabs® (= tablets, f/c), red, dried ferrous sulphate 325 mg (105 mg iron) for sustained release, folic acid 350 micrograms, ascorbic acid 500 mg (as sodium salt). Price 20 tabs = **C**. Label: 25

NHS **Ironorm**® (Wallace Mfg)

PoM *Capsules*, dried ferrous sulphate 195 mg (59 mg iron), folic acid 1.7 mg, thiamine hydrochloride 1 mg, riboflavine 2 mg, nicotinamide 10 mg, cyanocobalamin 5 micrograms, ascorbic acid 15 mg, intrinsic factor concentrate 10 mg, liver fraction II 130 mg. Price 20 caps = **C**

Tonic with iron (= elixir), ferric ammonium citrate 250 mg (50 mg iron), thiamine hydrochloride 500 micrograms, riboflavine 250 micrograms, nicotinamide 3.75 mg, pyridoxine hydrochloride 125 micrograms, cyanocobalamin 2.5 micrograms, calcium glycerophosphate 10.75 mg, calcium pantothenate 125 micrograms, proteolysed liver extract ≡ 2 g fresh liver, manganese glycerophosphate 1 mg, potassium glycerophosphate 1.75 mg, sodium glycerophosphate 21.25 mg/5 ml. Price 150 ml = **C**

C = 51-100p, **D** = 101-180p, **E** = 181-300p, **F** = 301-450p, **G** = 451-650p, **H** = 651-900p, **I** = 901-1200p, **J** = over 1200p.

NHS PoM **Pregnavite Forte F**® (Bencard)

Tablets, lilac, s/c, dried ferrous sulphate 84 mg (25.2 mg iron), folic acid 120 micrograms, vitamin A 1333 units, thiamine hydrochloride 500 micrograms, riboflavine 500 micrograms, nicotinamide 5 mg, pyridoxine hydrochloride 330 micrograms, ascorbic acid 13.3 mg, vitamin D 133 units, calcium phosphate 160 mg. Price 20 tabs = **B**

NHS **Sidros**® (Arun)

Tablets, red, s/c, ferrous gluconate 300 mg (35 mg iron), ascorbic acid 30 mg. Price 20 tabs = **B**

NHS **Tonivitan A & D**® (Medo)

Syrup (= elixir), green, ferric ammonium citrate 150 mg (22 mg iron), vitamin A 700 units, ergocalciferol 70 units, calcium glycerophosphate 25 mg, copper sulphate 400 micrograms, manganese glycerophosphate 400 micrograms/5 ml. Price 125 ml = **C**

9.1.1.2   PARENTERAL IRON THERAPY

The only valid reason for administering iron preparations parenterally is failure of oral therapy. Such failure may be due to lack of patient co-operation with oral treatment, gastro-intestinal side-effects, continuing severe blood loss, and resistant malabsorption. Provided that the oral iron preparation is taken reliably and is absorbed, then with equivalent doses of iron the rate of haemoglobin response is not significantly faster when the intramuscular or intravenous instead of the oral route is used. The need for a rapid cure of the anaemia is therefore not met by intramuscular administration of iron.

For parenteral administration, it is customary to give a course of deep *intramuscular* injections lasting about 10 days. The manufacturer's dosage schedules should be consulted; these usually include a supplement for the reconstitution of the iron stores.

Iron dextran (Imferon®) may also be administered as a single dose by slow intravenous infusion over 6 to 8 hours at a rate not exceeding 1 ml/minute provided that there is no reaction within 30 minutes of administration of a 0.5-ml test dose. Although the incidence of side-effects is low, disquieting adverse reactions may occur, especially in allergic subjects, and intravenous infusion is contra-indicated in asthmatic patients. Iron dextran should only be administered *intravenously* in selected cases where proper indications exist for its use, that is, when continuing blood loss is likely to be permanent and oral prophylaxis cannot keep pace, when a patient requiring parenteral iron has a small muscle mass or a haemostatic defect contra-indicating intramuscular injection or when reasons of psychological or social pressure make iron treatment by other means impracticable.

Preparations suitable for parenteral use contain iron either in the form of **Iron Dextran Injection**, containing a complex of ferric hydroxide with dextrans of high molecular weight, or as **Iron Sorbitol Injection** (Jectofer®), containing a complex of iron, sorbitol and citric acid. The latter preparation is **not** suitable for intravenous injection and, although the low mean molecular weight

allows rapid absorption from the injection site, excretion in the saliva and substantial urinary losses from each dose also occur.

To prevent leakage along the needle track with subsequent staining of the skin, intramuscular injections should be deep for both preparations.

IRON DEXTRAN INJECTION
Contains 5% (50 mg/ml) of iron

Indications: iron deficiency anaemia (see notes above)

Cautions: when given by slow intravenous infusion patient should be under observation the whole time and for an hour afterwards. Antihistamines should be available. Caution in patients with a history of allergic conditions

Contra-indications: severe liver disease, acute renal failure and renal infections; intravenous infusion in asthmatic patients

Side-effects: staining of the skin if leakage along needle track occurs, transient nausea, vomiting, flushing; occasionally severe dyspnoea; rarely severe anaphylaxis

Dose: by deep intramuscular injection or intravenous infusion, see notes above and manufacturer's literature

PoM **Imferon**® (Fisons)

Injection, iron dextran injection. Price 2-ml amp = **C**; 5-ml amp = **D**

Intravenous infusion, iron dextran injection. Price 20-ml amp = **F** (Hosp. only)

IRON SORBITOL INJECTION
Contains 5% (50 mg/ml) of iron

Indications: iron-deficiency anaemia

Cautions: 24 hours should elapse between iron administered orally and start of therapy with iron sorbitol injection. When another injectable iron preparation has been used, a week should elapse between the last injection and the start of therapy with iron sorbitol

Contra-indications: liver disease, kidney disease (particularly pyelonephritis), untreated urinary-tract infections

Dose: by intramuscular injection, see notes above and manufacturer's literature

PoM **Jectofer**® (Astra)

Injection, iron sorbitol injection. Price 2-ml amp = **B**

9.1.2   Drugs used in megaloblastic anaemias

Most megaloblastic anaemias are due to lack of either **vitamin B$_{12}$** or **folic acid** and it is essential to establish in every case which deficiency is present and the underlying cause. In emergencies, where delay might be dangerous, it is sometimes necessary to administer both substances after the bone marrow test while plasma assay results are awaited. Normally, however, appropriate treat-

---

ment should be instituted only when the results of tests are available. Vitamin B_{12} is also needed in the treatment of megaloblastosis due to prolonged nitrous oxide anaesthesia, which inactivates the vitamin, and in the rare syndrome of congenital transcobalamin II deficiency

Vitamin B_{12} should be given prophylactically to patients who have undergone total gastrectomy or total ileal resection.

Hydroxocobalamin has completely replaced cyanocobalamin and is now the form of vitamin B_{12} of choice for therapy; when vitamin B_{12} is prescribed hydroxocobalamin should be given. It is retained in the body longer than cyanocobalamin and thus for maintenance therapy need only be given at intervals of 3 months. Although a haematological response in vitamin-B_{12} deficiency may be obtained by small doses, it is customary to start treatment with 1 mg by intramuscular injection repeated 5 times at intervals of 2 to 3 days to replenish the depleted body stores. Thereafter, maintenance treatment, which is usually for life, can be instituted. There is no evidence that larger doses provide any additional benefit in vitamin-B_{12} neuropathy.

Apart from the rare dietary deficiency, all other causes of vitamin-B_{12} deficiency are attributable to malabsorption and there is little place for the use of vitamin B_{12} orally and none for vitamin B_{12} intrinsic factor complexes given by the same route.

Many causes of **folic acid** deficiency are self-limiting, or may yield to treatment, and there are thus few indications for long-term therapy. Even when untreated malabsorption is present, an oral dose of 5 to 10 mg daily of folic acid is usually sufficient to bring about a haematological response. However, treatment should continue for 3 to 4 months to replenish the body stores. Folic acid therapy should not be used indiscriminately in undiagnosed megaloblastic anaemia unless vitamin B_{12} is administered concurrently otherwise neuropathy may be precipitated. Caution should be exercised when administering folic acid to epileptic subjects and to patients who may have folate-dependent tumours.

Folic acid is widely used during pregnancy in the prevention of megaloblastic anaemia (for preparations with iron salts see section 9.1.1.1) and can also be used prophylactically in chronic haemolytic states such as thalassaemia major or sickle-cell anaemia.

There is **no** justification for prescribing multiple-ingredient vitamin preparations containing these substances.

HYDROXOCOBALAMIN

Indications: Addisonian pernicious anaemia, subacute combined degeneration of the spinal cord, other causes of vitamin-B_{12} deficiency, nitrous oxide-induced megaloblastosis
Cautions: should not be given before diagnosis has been fully established
Dose: by intramuscular injection, initially 1 mg repeated 5 times at intervals of 2–3 days; main-

tenance dose 1 mg every 3 months; CHILD, dosage as for adult

PoM **Hydroxocobalamin Injection,** hydroxocobalamin 250 micrograms/ml and 1 mg/ml. Price 1-ml amp (both) = **A**
NHS PoM **Cobalin-H®** (Paines & Byrne)
Injection, hydroxocobalamin 1 mg/ml. Price 1-ml amp = **A**
NHS PoM **Neo-Cytamen®** (DF)
Injection, hydroxocobalamin 250 micrograms/ml. Price 1-ml amp = **A**
Injection, hydroxocobalamin 1 mg/ml. Price 1-ml amp = **A**

CYANOCOBALAMIN

Indications: see notes above
Dose: by intramuscular injection, initially 1 mg repeated 10 times at intervals of 2–3 days, maintenance 1 mg every month, but see notes above

NHS PoM **Cyanocobalamin Injection,** cyanocobalamin 1 mg/ml. Price 1-ml amp = **A**
NHS **Cytacon®** (DF)
Tablets, f/c, cyanocobalamin 50 micrograms. Price 20 tabs = **B**
Liquid (= elixir), red, cyanocobalamin 35 micrograms/5 ml. Price 100 ml = **B**
NHS PoM **Cytamen®** (DF)
Injection, cyanocobalamin 250 micrograms/ml. Price 1-ml amp = **A**
Injection, cyanocobalamin 1 mg/ml. Price 1-ml amp = **A**
NHS PoM **Hepacon B_{12}®** (Consolidated)
Injection, cyanocobalamin 1 mg/ml. Price 1-ml amp = **A**
NHS PoM **Hepacon-B Forte®** (Consolidated)
Injection, folic acid 2.5 mg, liver extract equivalent to vitamin B_{12} 15 micrograms, cocarboxylase 50 mg. Price 2-ml amp = **B**
NHS PoM **Hepacon Liver Extract®** (Consolidated)
Injection, liver extract equivalent to vitamin B_{12} 50 micrograms/ml. Price 2-ml amp = **B**
Injection, liver extract equivalent to vitamin B_{12} 500 micrograms/ml. Price 2-ml amp = **B**

FOLIC ACID

Indications: megaloblastic anaemia due to folic acid deficiency
Cautions: should never be given alone in the treatment of Addisonian pernicious anaemia and other vitamin B_{12}-deficiency states because it may precipitate the onset of subacute combined degeneration of the spinal cord. Do not use in malignant disease unless megaloblastic anaemia due to folate deficiency is an important complication
Dose: initially, 15 mg daily for 14 days or until a haematopoietic response has been obtained; maintenance, 5 mg every 1–7 days; CHILD, initially daily for 2 days, up to 1 year 500 micrograms/kg, 1–5 years 5 mg, 6–12 years 10 mg; maintenance, half the initial dose

PoM **Folic Acid Tablets,** folic acid 100 micrograms and 5 mg. Price 20 tabs (both) = **A**
PoM **Lexpec®** (RP Drugs)
Syrup (= elixir), sugar-free, folic acid 2.5 mg/5 ml. Diluent sorbitol solution, life of elixir diluted to 75% up to 21 days. Price 125 ml = **E**

FOLINIC ACID

Indications: antidote to folic acid antagonists; treatment of megaloblastic anaemias

Cautions: see under Folic Acid

Dose: as an antidote to folic acid antagonists (especially methotrexate or pyrimethamine), up to 120 mg in divided doses over 12 to 24 hours *by intramuscular or intravenous injection or infusion*, followed by 15 mg *by mouth* every 6 hours. Different schedules are needed after massive doses of methotrexate

In megaloblastic anaemias, 10–20 mg daily

PoM **Calcium Leucovorin** (Lederle)
Tablets, scored, folinic acid 15 mg (as calcium salt). Price 2 tabs = **I**
Injection, folinic acid 3 mg (as calcium salt)/ml. Price 1-ml amp = **D**
Injection, powder for reconstitution, folinic acid (as calcium salt). Price 15-mg vial = **H**; 30-mg vial = **J**

PoM **Rescufolin**® (Nordic)
Injection, powder for reconstitution, folinic acid (as calcium salt). Price 15-mg vial = **G**; 50-mg vial = **J**

9.1.3   Drugs used in hypoplastic and haemolytic anaemias

The anabolic steroids, pyridoxine hydrochloride, and various corticosteroids are used in hypoplastic and haemolytic anaemias.

The place of non-androgenic **anabolic steroids** in the therapy of aplastic anaemia remains somewhat controversial and their effectiveness is unclear. There is a wide variation in the reported successful responses. Occasional patients, however, do seem to derive benefit. It is customary to prescribe high doses of oxymetholone, such as 1 to 2 mg/kg daily, and to continue therapy for at least 3 to 6 months. At these dose levels, virilising side-effects may be expected in female patients and in children. Controlled trials have shown that antilymphocyte immunoglobulin produces a response in 50% of acquired cases.

It is unlikely that dietary deprivation of **pyridoxine hydrochloride** (section 9.6.2) produces haematological effects in man. However, certain forms of sideroblastic anaemia respond to pharmacological doses of pyridoxine, possibly reflecting its role as a co-enzyme during haemoglobin synthesis.

Pyridoxine is indicated in both idiopathic acquired and hereditary sideroblastic anaemias. Although complete cures have not been reported, some increase in haemoglobin may occur; the dose required is usually high, up to 400 mg daily. Reversible sideroblastic anaemias respond to treatment of the underlying cause but in pregnancy, haemolytic anaemias, and alcoholism, or during antituberculous treatment, pyridoxine is also indicated.

Corticosteroids (see section 6.3) have an important place in the management of a wide variety of haematological disorders. They include conditions with an immune basis such as auto-immune haemolytic anaemia, immune thrombocytopenias and neutropenias, and major transfusion reactions. They are also used in chemotherapy schedules for all forms of lymphoreticular malignancy, lymphoid leukaemias, and paraproteinaemias, including myelomatosis. Corticosteroids are used in aplastic anaemias, where their usefulness is more debatable.

It is possible that corticosteroids in low doses may also reduce the capillary fragility which occurs in the purpuric diseases, thus lessening bleeding.

Severe tissue iron overload may occur in aplastic and other refractory anaemias, mainly as the result of repeated blood transfusions. It is a particular problem in refractory anaemias with hyperplastic bone marrow, especially thalassaemia major, where excessive iron absorption from the gut and inappropriate iron therapy add to the tissue siderosis. Venesection therapy is contra-indicated, but the long-term administration of the iron chelating compound desferrioxamine mesylate (page 32) is useful. Subcutaneous infusions of desferrioxamine (0.5 to 4 g over 12 hours) are given on 5 to 7 nights each week. Vitamin C (section 9.6.3), 100 to 200 mg daily, enhances iron excretion. Desferrioxamine (2 g per unit of blood) may also be given through the infusion line at the time of blood transfusion.

OXYMETHOLONE

Indications: aplastic anaemia; see notes above

Cautions: cardiac and renal impairment, circulatory failure, hypertension, diabetes mellitus, epilepsy, migraine; monitor skeletal maturation in children for 6 months after treatment. Drug interactions: see Appendix 1 (sections *2.8, 2.8B*)

Contra-indications: hepatic impairment, prostatic carcinoma, pregnancy, breast-feeding

Side-effects: acne, oedema, jaundice, virilism with high doses, hypercalcaemia, menstrual irregularities

Dose: aplastic anaemia, 1–2 mg/kg daily in divided doses; CHILD 2–4 mg/kg daily in divided doses

PoM **Anapolon 50**® (Syntex)
Tablets, scored, oxymetholone 50 mg. Price 20 tabs = **I**

STANOZOLOL

Indications; Cautions; Contra-indications; Side-effects: see under Oxymetholone

Dose: by deep intramuscular injection, 50 mg every 2–3 weeks

PoM **Stromba**® (Sterling Research)
Injection (aqueous suspension), stanozolol 50 mg/ml. Price 1-ml amp = **F**

9.2 Electrolyte and water replacement

9.2.1 Oral administration
9.2.2 Intravenous administration
9.2.3 Plasma substitutes
9.2.4 Tables of electrolyte concentrations

9.2.1 Oral administration

9.2.1.1 Potassium salts
9.2.1.2 Sodium salts

Electrolyte preparations may be given by mouth to prevent certain electrolyte deficiencies in conditions in which it is known that these are likely to arise, or to treat established deficiencies of mild or moderate degree. Oral magnesium salts are occasionally required on a long-term basis in patients with malabsorption.

9.2.1.1 POTASSIUM SALTS

Potassium salts should be given by mouth when drugs that are known to induce potassium depletion from excessive urinary loss are being given over long periods. These include the use of corticosteroids, carbenoxolone, and high-potency diuretics such as frusemide.

Potassium supplements should be given prophylactically; their need can sometimes be avoided by the use of potassium-sparing diuretics (see sections 2.2.3 and 2.2.4).

Potassium supplements are especially necessary:
1. if the patient is elderly, since such patients freqently take inadequate amounts of potassium in the diet;
2. in those taking digoxin or other cardiac glycosides, where potassium depletion may induce arrhythmias;
3. in patients in whom secondary hyperaldosteronism occurs, as in renal artery stenosis, cirrhosis of the liver, the nephrotic syndrome, and severe heart failure;
4. in patients with excessive losses of potassium in the faeces, as in the chronic diarrhoea associated with intestinal malabsorption or laxative abuse.

Potassium supplements are seldom required when small doses of diuretics are given for the treatment of hypertension.

When used prophylactically, doses of 3 to 5 g (approx. 40 to 67 mmol) of potassium chloride daily are required, but if there is renal insufficiency (as is common in the elderly), smaller doses must be used or there is a danger of hyperkalaemia. A number of salt substitutes which contain significant amounts of potassium chloride are readily available as health food products (e.g. Losalt, Ruthmol, and Selora). These are not recommended in patients with renal failure as potassium intoxication may result.

When there is established potassium depletion or when the plasma-potassium concentration is less than 3.5 mmol/litre, larger doses of 10 to 15 g (approx. 135 to 200 mmol) daily of potassium chloride are required over periods of days or weeks. Potassium depletion is frequently associated with chloride depletion and with metabolic alkalosis (as in the vomiting of pyloric stenosis), and these disorders require correction.

Potassium salts are preferably given as a liquid preparation, rather than sustained-release tablets.

POTASSIUM SALTS

Indications: potassium depletion (see notes above)
Cautions: intestinal stricture, hiatus hernia (for sustained-release preparations). Drug interactions: see Appendix 1 (sections *2.2, 2.5*)
Contra-indications: renal failure, plasma potassium concentrations above 5 mmol/litre
Side-effects: nausea and vomiting (severe symptoms may indicate obstruction), oesophageal or small bowel ulceration
Dose: usual range 40–70 mmol K+ daily

Potassium Tablets, Effervescent, potassium bicarbonate 500 mg, potassium acid tartrate 300 mg, each tablet providing 6.5 mmol of K+. To be dissolved in water before administration. Price 20 tabs = **B.** Label: 13, 21

Kay-Cee-L® (Geistlich)
Syrup (= elixir), red, potassium chloride 7.5% w/v (1 mmol/ml) (sugar-free). Do not dilute. Price 500 ml = **E.** Label: 21

K-Contin Continus® (Napp)
Tablets, s/r, orange, f/c, potassium chloride 600 mg (8 mmol each of K+ and Cl−). Price 20 tabs = **A.** Label: 25

Kloref® (Cox Pharmaceuticals)
Tablets, effervescent, betaine hydrochloride, potassium benzoate, bicarbonate, and chloride, equivalent to potassium chloride 500 mg (6.7 mmol each of K+ and Cl−). Price 20 tabs = **D.** Label: 13, 21

Kloref-S® (Cox Pharmaceuticals)
Granules, effervescent, betaine hydrochloride, potassium bicarbonate and chloride equivalent to potassium chloride 1.5 g (20 mmol each of K+ and Cl−)/sachet. Price 20 sachets = **D.** Label: 13, 21

Leo K® (Leo)
Tablets, s/r, f/c, potassium chloride 600 mg (8 mmol each of K+ and Cl−). Price 20 tabs = **A.** Label: 25

Micro-K® (Merck)
Capsules, s/r, clear/red, potassium chloride 600 mg (8 mmol each of K+ and Cl−). Price 20 caps = **B.** Label: 25

Nu-K® (Consolidated)
Capsules, s/r, blue, potassium chloride 600 mg (8 mmol each of K+ and Cl−). Price 20 caps = **B.** Label: 25

Sando-K® (Sandoz)
Tablets, effervescent, potassium bicarbonate and chloride equivalent to potassium 470 mg (12 mmol of K+) and chloride 285 mg (8 mmol of Cl−). Price 20 tabs = **B.** Label: 13, 21

Slow-K® (Ciba)
Tablets, s/r, orange, s/c, potassium chloride 600 mg (8 mmol each of K+ and Cl−). Price 20 tabs = **A.** Label: 25

C = 51-100p, **D** = 101-180p, **E** = 181-300p, **F** = 301-450p, **G** = 451-650p, **H** = 651-900p, **I** = 901-1200p, **J** = over 1200p.

HYPERKALAEMIA

POLYSTYRENE SULPHONATE RESINS

Indications: hyperkalaemia associated with anuria or severe oliguria, and in dialysis patients

Contra-indications: avoid calcium-containing resin in hyperparathyroidism, multiple myeloma, sarcoidosis, or metastatic carcinoma; avoid sodium-containing resin in congestive heart failure and severe renal impairment

Dose: by mouth, 15 g 3–4 times daily in water (not fruit juice which has a high K^+ content)

By rectum, as an enema, 30 g in methylcellulose solution, retained for 9 hours

CHILD, any route, 0.5–1 g/kg daily

Calcium Resonium® (Winthrop)
Powder, brown, calcium polystyrene sulphonate. Price 300 g = **J**. Label: 13

Resonium A® (Winthrop)
Powder, buff, sodium polystyrene sulphonate. Price 454 g = **J**. Label: 13

9.2.1.2 SODIUM SALTS

Sodium chloride is indicated in states of sodium depletion and usually needs to be given intraveneously (section 9.2.2). Sometimes, however in small children with diarrhoea and in chronic conditions associated with mild or moderate degrees of sodium depletion, for example in salt-losing nephritis or the diuretic phase of acute ischaemic renal failure, oral supplementation is sufficient.

A suitable preparation for replacement of lost fluid and electrolytes in children is Sodium Chloride and Glucose Oral Powder, Compound, available in containers for the preparation of 500 ml of solution (see Formulary). Sachets of Sodium Chloride and Glucose Oral Powder, Compound, Small Size, contain the same ingredients for preparing 200 ml of solution, that is, sufficient to fill the usual size feeding bottle. In either case the powder is dissolved in freshly boiled and cooled water, suitably flavoured if required, and no other liquid should be used. Any unused solution should be discarded no later than 24 hours after preparation.

Electrosol® tablets are used for preparing a closely similar solution, but without the glucose.

SODIUM SALTS

Indications: electrolyte imbalance, also section 9.2.2 below

Sodium Bicarbonate Tablets, Compound, see section 1.1.1

Sodium Chloride and Glucose Oral Powder, Compound, Na^+ 35 mmol, K^+ 20 mmol, Cl^- 37 mmol, HCO_3^- 18 mmol, and glucose 200 mmol/litre when reconstituted (see notes above and Formulary). Price 1 powder (22 g) = **A**. Label: 13

Sodium Chloride and Glucose Oral Powder, Compound, Small Size, ingredients as above. Price 20 × 8.8-g powders = **B**. Label: 13

Sodium Chloride and Glucose Tablets, sodium chloride 450 mg, glucose 200 mg. Price 20 tabs = **A**

Sodium Chloride Solution (Normal Saline), sodium chloride 0.9% (9 mg/ml) in purified water, freshly boiled and cooled. Price 100 ml = **A**

Note: this preparation must *not* be confused with 'normal sodium chloride solution' which is used as a chemical reagent and contains 5.85% of sodium chloride

Sodium Chloride Solution-tablets, sodium chloride 2.25 g, one solution-tablet dissolved in 250 ml of water for preparations provides a 0.9% solution. Price 20 tabs = **B**. Label: 13

Sodium Chloride Tablets, sodium chloride 300 mg. Price 20 tabs = **A**

Dextrolyte® (Cow & Gate)
Oral solution, glucose, potassium chloride, sodium chloride, sodium lactate, providing Na^+ 35 mmol, K^+ 13.4 mmol, Cl^- 30.5 mmol, lactate 17.7 mmol, and glucose 200 mmol/litre. Price 100 ml = **B** (Hosp. only)

Dioralyte® (Armour)
Oral powder, sodium chloride and glucose powder, compound, small size (see above), 8.8-g sachets. Price 20 sachets (cherry flavoured or plain) = **F**. Label: 13

Electrosol® (Macarthys)
Tablets, effervescent, sodium chloride 200 mg, potassium chloride 160 mg, sodium bicarbonate 200 mg, 8 tablets dissolved in 1 litre of water provide a solution containing Na^+ 46.5 mmol, K^+ 17 mmol, Cl^- 44.5 mmol, and HCO_3^- 19 mmol. Price 20 tabs = **A**. Label: 13

Rehidrat® (Searle)
Oral powder, sodium chloride 440 mg, potassium chloride 380 mg, sodium bicarbonate 420 mg, citric acid 440 mg, glucose 4.09 g, sucrose 8.07 g, fructose 70 mg/sachet. Each sachet when reconstituted with 250 ml of water (freshly boiled and cooled for infants), provides glucose 91 mmol, fructose 2 mmol, sucrose 94 mmol, Na^+ 50 mmol, K^+ 20 mmol, Cl^- 50 mmol, HCO_3^- 20 mmol, and citric acid 9 mmol/litre. Price 20 sachets = **G**. Label: 13

Slow Sodium® (Ciba)
Tablets, s/r, sodium chloride 600 mg. Price 20 tabs = **A**. Label: 25

9.2.2 Intravenous administration

Solutions of electrolytes are given intravenously, to meet normal fluid and electrolyte requirements or to replenish substantial deficits or continuing losses, when the patient is nauseated or vomiting and is unable to take adequate amounts by mouth.

In an individual patient the nature and severity of the electrolyte imbalance must be assessed from the history and clinical and biochemical examination. Sodium, potassium, magnesium, phosphate, and water depletion can occur singly and in combination.

Isotonic solutions may be infused safely into a peripheral vein. Solutions more concentrated than plasma, for example 20% w/v glucose are best given through an indwelling catheter inserted via the subclavian vein.

Sodium chloride in isotonic solution provides the most important extracellular ions in near physiological concentration and is indicated in sodium depletion which may arise from such conditions as gastro-enteritis, diabetic ketoacidosis, ileus, and ascites. In a severe deficit of from 4 to 8 litres, 2 to 3 litres of isotonic sodium chloride may be given over 2 to 3 hours; thereafter infusion can usually be at a slower rate.

Excessive administration should be avoided; the bases of the lungs should be examined for crepitations, and in elderly or seriously ill patients it is often helpful to monitor the intra-atrial (central) venous pressure.

Sodium chloride and glucose solutions are indicated when there is combined water and sodium depletion. A 1:1 mixture of isotonic sodium chloride and 5% glucose allows some of the water (free of sodium) to enter body cells which suffer most from dehydration while the sodium salt with a volume of water determined by the normal plasma Na^+ remains extracellular. Examples of combined sodium and water depletion occur in persistent vomiting and hyperosmolar diabetic ketoacidosis.

Glucose solutions (5%) are mainly used to replace water deficits and should be given alone when there is no significant loss of electrolytes. Average water requirements in a healthy adult are 1.5 to 2.5 litres daily and this is needed to balance unavoidable losses of water through the skin and lungs and to provide sufficient for urinary excretion. Water depletion (dehydration) tends to occur when these losses are not matched by a comparable intake, as for example may occur in coma or dysphagia or in the aged or apathetic who may not drink water in sufficient amount on their own initiative. Water depletion also occurs in diabetic ketoacidosis; the deficit may be up to 8 litres in severe cases.

Excessive loss of water without loss of electrolytes is uncommon, occurring in fevers, hyperthyroidism, and in uncommon water-losing renal states such as diabetes insipidus or hypercalcaemia. The volume of glucose solution needed to replenish deficits varies with the severity of the disorder, but usually lies within the range of 2 to 10 litres.

Potassium chloride and sodium chloride intravenous infusion and **potassium chloride and glucose** intravenous infusion are used to correct severe hypokalaemia and depletion. Potassium chloride (1.5 g in sterile ampoules) may be conveniently added to 500 ml of sodium chloride intravenous infusion or 5% glucose, the solution then contains 40mmol/litre and may be given slowly over 2 to 3 hours. Repeated measurements of plasma potassium are necessary to determine whether further infusions are necessary and to avoid the development of hyperkalaemia; this is especially liable to occur in renal failure.

Sodium bicarbonate is used to control severe metabolic acidosis (as in renal or diabetic coma). Since this condition is usually attended by sodium depletion, it is reasonable to correct this first by the administration of isotonic sodium chloride intravenous infusion, provided the kidneys are not primarily affected and the degree of acidosis is not so severe as to impair renal function. In these circumstances, isotonic sodium chloride alone is usually effective as it restores the ability of the kidneys to generate bicarbonate. In renal acidosis or in severe acidosis of any origin (for example blood pH<7.1) isotonic sodium bicarbonate (1.4%) should be infused with isotonic sodium chloride; a total volume of 6 litres (4 litres of sodium chloride and 2 litres of sodium bicarbonate) may be necessary in the adult. In severe shock due for example to cardiac arrest, metabolic acidosis may develop without sodium depletion; in these circumstances sodium bicarbonate is best given in a small volume of hypertonic solution, such as 200 to 300 ml of 8.4% solution intravenously.

Ammonium chloride is indicated when severe metabolic alkalosis ($HCO_3^- > 30$ mmol/litre) is associated with water and sodium depletion. It is most commonly indicated in pyloric stenosis in which vomiting has been severe or prolonged. In these circumstances a suitable isotonic solution containing 63 mmol/litre of sodium, 17 mmol/litre potassium, and 70 mmol/litre ammonium is useful; 1 litre should be given over 4 to 6 hours and treatment supplemented by isotonic sodium chloride and glucose intravenous infusion.

Magnesium chloride is occasionally needed to correct magnesium deficiency that has arisen from prolonged diarrhoea or vomiting which has been treated with parenteral fluid and nutrition without magnesium supplements; 50mmol of magnesium chloride may be added to 1 litre of 5% glucose or other isotonic solution and given over a period of 12 to 24 hours.

Phosphate infusion is occasionally needed in circumstances similar to those that give rise to magnesium deficiency and it also occurs in severe diabetic ketoacidosis and alcoholism. A solution containing up to 50 mmol/litre can be infused in sodium chloride or glucose over 12 to 24 hours. Since potassium depletion is also commonly present the phosphate may be given as a mixture of the sodium and potassium salts.

Sodium lactate intravenous infusion is obsolete in metabolic acidosis, and carries the risk of producing lactic acidosis, particularly in seriously ill patients with poor tissue perfusion or impaired hepatic function.

GLUCOSE

(Dextrose)

Indications: fluid replacement (see notes above), provision of energy (section 9.3)

Side-effects: glucose injections especially if hypertonic may have a low pH and irritate the venous intima so causing thrombophlebitis

Dose: water replacement, see notes above; energy source, 1–3 litres daily of 20–50% solution

---

C = 51-100p, D = 101-180p, E = 181-300p, F = 301-450p, G = 451-650p, H = 651-900p, I = 901-1200p, J = over 1200p.

PoM **Glucose Intravenous Infusion,** glucose, usual strength 5% (50 mg/ml). 20% solution, price 20-ml amp = **C**; 25% solution, price 25-ml amp = **C**; 50% solution, price 20-ml amp = **C**; 25- and 50-ml amp (both) = **D**
Other packs: see *note* following entry on sodium chloride and glucose intravenous infusion

POTASSIUM CHLORIDE

Indications: electrolyte imbalance; also oral potassium supplements, section 9.2.1.1
Cautions: for intravenous infusion the concentration of solution should not exceed 3.2 g (43 mmol)/litre
Side-effects: rapid injection may be toxic to heart
Dose: by slow intravenous infusion, up to 6 g (80 mmol) daily

PoM **Potassium Chloride and Glucose Intravenous Infusion,** usual strength potassium chloride 0.3% (3 g, 40 mmol each of K^+ and Cl^-/litre) with 5% of anhydrous glucose
Other packs: see *note* following entry on sodium chloride and glucose intravenous infusion

PoM **Potassium Chloride and Sodium Chloride Intravenous Infusion,** usual strength potassium chloride 0.3% (3 g/litre) and sodium chloride 0.9% (9 g/litre), containing 40 mmol of K^+, 150 mmol of Na^+, and 190 mmol of Cl^-/litre
Other packs: see *note* following entry on sodium chloride and glucose intravenous infusion

PoM **Potassium Chloride, Sodium Chloride, and Glucose Intravenous Infusion,** sodium chloride 0.18% (1.8 g, 30 mmol of Na^+/litre) with 4% of anhydrous glucose and usually sufficient potassium chloride to provide 10–40 mmol of K^+/litre (to be specified by the prescriber)
Other packs: see *note* following entry on sodium chloride and glucose intravenous infusion

PoM **Potassium Chloride Solution, Strong** (sterile), potassium chloride 15% (150 mg, approximately 2 mmol each of K^+ and Cl^-/ml). Must be diluted with not less than 50 times its volume of sodium chloride intravenous infusion 0.9% or other suitable diluent. Price 10-ml amp = **B**
Solutions containing 10 and 20% of potassium chloride are also available in both 5- and 10-ml ampoules. Price per amp (all) = **B**

SODIUM BICARBONATE

Indications: metabolic acidosis
Dose: by slow intravenous injection, a strong solution (up to 8.4%), or *by continuous intravenous infusion,* a weak solution (usually 1.4%), an amount appropriate to the body base deficit (see notes above)

PoM **Sodium Bicarbonate Intravenous Infusion,** usual strength sodium bicarbonate 1.4% (14 g, 167 mmol each of Na^+ and HCO_3^-/litre). 5% solution available in 20- and 50-ml ampoules. Price 20-ml amp = **C**; 50-ml amp = **D**
Other packs: see *note* following entry on sodium chloride and glucose intravenous infusion

SODIUM CHLORIDE

Indications: electrolyte imbalance, also section 9.2.1.2
Cautions: restrict intake in impaired renal function, cardiac failure, hypertension, peripheral and pulmonary oedema, toxaemia of pregnancy
Side-effects: administration of large doses may give rise to sodium accumulation and oedema
Dose: see notes above

PoM **Ringer's Solution for Injection,** calcium chloride (dihydrate) 322 micrograms, potassium chloride 300 micrograms, sodium chloride 8.6 mg/ml, providing the following ions (in mmol/litre), Ca^{2+} 2.2, K^+ 4, Na^+ 147, Cl^- 156
Availability of other packs: see below following entry on sodium chloride and glucose intravenous infusion

PoM **Sodium Chloride Intravenous Infusion,** usual strength sodium chloride 0.9% (9 g, 150 mmol each of Na^+ and Cl^-/litre), this strength being supplied when normal saline for injection is requested. Price 2-, 5-, and 10-ml amp (all) = **B**; 20-ml amp = **C**; 50-ml amp = **D**
Availability of other packs: see below

PoM **Sodium Chloride and Glucose Intravenous Infusion,** usual strength sodium chloride 0.18% (1.8 g, 30 mmol each of Na^+ and Cl^-/litre) and 4% of anhydrous glucose
Other packs: see below
AVAILABILITY OF INFUSION SOLUTIONS. In the hospital service, water for injections, many solutions of glucose, and electrolyte solutions for intravenous infusion are available in 500-ml and 1000-ml packs, and sometimes other sizes. For availability and price enquire locally.

SODIUM LACTATE

Indications: diabetic coma, diminished alkali reserve (but see notes above)

PoM **Sodium Lactate Intravenous Infusion,** sodium lactate M/6, contains the following ions (in mmol/litre), Na^+ 167, HCO_3^- (as lactate) 167
PoM **Sodium Lactate Intravenous Infusion, Compound,** (Hartmann's solution for injection), contains the following ions (in mmol/litre), Na^+ 131, K^+ 5, Ca^{2+} 2, HCO_3^- (as lactate) 29, Cl^- 111
Other packs: see *note* following entry on sodium chloride and glucose intravenous infusion

PoM **Water for Injections.** Price 1-, 2-, and 5-ml amp (all) = **A**; 20-ml amp = **B**; 50-ml amp = **C**

9.2.3   Plasma substitutes

Dextrans and **gelatin** are macromolecular substances which are slowly metabolised and may be used to expand and maintain blood volume in shock arising from conditions such as burns or septicaemia. They are rarely needed when shock is due to sodium and water depletion as, in these circumstances, the shock responds to water and electrolyte repletion. They should not be used to maintain plasma volume in conditions such as burns or peritonitis where there is loss of plasma protein water and electrolytes over periods of

---

For all abbreviations and symbols see inside cover.   Relative prices: **A** = up to 20p, **B** = 21-50p,

several days or weeks. In these situations, plasma or plasma protein fractions containing large amounts of albumin should be given. Dextrans and gelatin should be used in haemorrhage if blood is not available as an immediate short-term measure until it is.

Dextrans interfere with blood group cross-matching or biochemical measurements and these should be carried out before infusion is begun. Dextran 70 and gelatin intravenous infusion are used predominantly for volume expansion. Dextran 40 intravenous infusion is used to improve peripheral blood flow in ischaemic disease of the limbs and peripheral thrombo-embolism.

DEXTRAN 40 INTRAVENOUS INFUSION,
dextran '40' 10% in glucose intravenous infusion 5% or in sodium chloride intravenous infusion 0.9%

Indications: conditions associated with peripheral local slowing of the blood flow; prophylaxis of post-surgical thromboembolic disease

Cautions: patients with congestive heart failure, renal impairment, polycythaemia; after blood and electrolyte replacement, rate of infusion to previously dehydrated patients not to exceed 500 ml/hour

Contra-indications: patients with thrombocytopenia, severe congestive heart failure, and renal failure

Side-effects: rarely anaphylactoid reactions, especially in patients with history of asthma

Dose: by *intravenous infusion*, initially 500–1000 ml; further doses are given according to the patient's condition

PoM **Gentran 40**® (Travenol)
Intravenous infusion, dextran 40 intravenous infusion in glucose intravenous infusion 5% or in sodium chloride intravenous infusion 0.9%. Price 500-ml bottle (both) = **F**

PoM **Lomodex 40**® (CP)
Intravenous infusion, dextran 40 intravenous infusion in glucose intravenous infusion 5% or in sodium chloride intravenous infusion 0.9%. Price 500-ml bottle (both) = **G**

PoM **Rheomacrodex**® (Pharmacia)
Intravenous infusion, dextran 40 intravenous infusion in glucose intravenous infusion 5% or in sodium chloride intravenous infusion 0.9%. Price 500-ml bottle (both) = **G**

DEXTRAN 70 INTRAVENOUS INFUSION,
dextran '70' 6% in glucose intravenous infusion 5% or in sodium chloride intravenous infusion 0.9%

Indications: short-term blood volume expansion; prophylaxis of post-surgical thromboembolic disease

Cautions: congestive heart failure, renal disease

Side-effects: see under Dextran 40 Intravenous Infusion

Dose: by *intravenous infusion*, after moderate to severe haemorrhage, 500–1000 ml rapidly initially followed by 500 ml later if necessary;

in the treatment of severe burns, up to 3000 ml in the first few days with electrolytes

PoM **Gentran 70**® (Travenol)
Intravenous infusion, dextran 70 intravenous infusion in glucose intravenous infusion 5% or in sodium chloride intravenous infusion 0.9%. Price 500-ml bottle (both) = **E**

PoM **Lomodex 70**® (CP)
Intravenous infusion, dextran 70 intravenous infusion in glucose intravenous infusion 5% or in sodium chloride intravenous infusion 0.9%. Price 500-ml bottle (both) = **F**

PoM **Macrodex**® (Pharmacia)
Intravenous infusion, dextran 70 intravenous infusion in glucose intravenous infusion 5% or in sodium chloride intravenous infusion 0.9%. Price 500-ml bottle (both) = **F**

DEXTRAN 110 INTRAVENOUS INFUSION,
dextran '110' 6% in glucose intravenous infusion 5% or in sodium chloride intravenous infusion 0.9%

Indications: see under Dextran 70 Intravenous Infusion

Cautions: see under Dextran 40 Intravenous Infusion; blood samples for cross-matching to be taken before infusion

Contra-indications: haemorrhage associated with hypofibrinogenaemia

Side-effects: see under Dextran 40 Intravenous Infusion

Dose: by *intravenous infusion*, see under Dextran 70 Intravenous Infusion

PoM **Dextraven 110**® (CP)
Intravenous infusion, dextran 110 intravenous infusion in glucose intravenous infusion 5% or in sodium chloride intravenous infusion 0.9%. Price 500-ml bottle (both) = **F**

GELATIN
Indications: low blood volume

Cautions; Side-effects: As for Dextrans; anaphylactoid reactions more common

Dose: by *intravenous infusion*, 500–1000 ml of a 3.5–4% solution

Note: for this purpose the gelatin is partially degraded to give a product of molecular weight approximately 30 000; one form of degraded gelatin is called **polygeline**

PoM **Gelofusine**® (Consolidated)
Injection, gelatin 4%, sodium chloride 0.9%. Price 500-ml bottle = **E**

PoM **Haemaccel**® (Hoechst)
Injection, polygeline 35 g, Na$^+$145 mmol, K$^+$ 5.1 mmol, Ca^{2+} 6.26 mmol, Cl$^-$ 145 mmol/litre. Price 500-ml bottle = **F**

9.2.4 Tables of electrolyte concentrations

The concentrations of electrolytes in intravenous infusion fluids is generally given in millimoles (mmol)/litre. A millimole is the molecular weight of the ion in milligrams.

C = 51-100p, **D** = 101-180p, **E** = 181-300p, **F** = 301-450p, **G** = 451-650p, **H** = 651-900p, **I** = 901-1200p, **J** = over 1200p.

Table 2: Electrolyte concentrations of intravenous fluids

Intravenous infusion	Millimoles per litre Na⁺	K⁺	HCO₃⁻ equiv.	Cl⁻	Ca²⁺
Normal Plasma Values	142	4.5	26	103	2.5
Citrated Plasma	150	12	—	55	—
Sodium Chloride 0.9%	150	—	—	150	—
Compound Sodium Lactate (Hartmann's)	131	5	29	111	2
Sodium Chloride 0.18% and Glucose 4%	30	—	—	30	—
Potassium Chloride and Glucose	—	40	—	40	—
Potassium Chloride and Sodium Chloride*	150	40	—	190	—
To correct metabolic acidosis					
Sodium Bicarbonate 1.4%	167	—	167	—	—
Sodium Bicarbonate 8.4% for cardiac arrest	1000	—	1000	—	—
Sodium Lactate (M/6)	167	—	167	—	—
To correct metabolic alkalosis					
Ammonium Chloride (M/6)	—	—	—	167	—

* Containing potassium chloride 0.3% and sodium chloride 0.9%.

Table 3: Millimoles of each ion in 1 gram of salt

Electrolyte	mmol per g approx.
Ammonium chloride	18.7
Calcium chloride ($CaCl_2,2H_2O$)	Ca 6.8 Cl 13.6
Potassium bicarbonate	10
Potassium chloride	13.4
Sodium bicarbonate	11.9
Sodium chloride	17.1
Sodium lactate	8.9

Faeces, vomit, or aspiration should be saved and analysed where possible if abnormal losses are suspected; where this is impracticable the following approximations may be helpful in planning replacement therapy.

Table 4: Electrolyte content of gastro-intestinal secretions

Type of fluid	Millimoles per litre H⁺	Na⁺	K⁺	HCO₃⁻	Cl⁻
Gastric	40–60	20–80	5–20	—	100–150
Biliary	—	120–140	5–15	30–50	80–120
Pancreatic	—	120–140	5–15	70–110	40–80
Small bowel	—	120–140	5–15	20–40	90–130

9.3 Intravenous nutrition

When adequate feeding via the alimentary tract is not possible, nutrients may be given by intravenous infusion. This may be in addition to ordinary oral or tube feeding—**supplemental parenteral nutrition**, or may be the sole source of nutrition—**total parenteral nutrition** (TPN). Indications for this method include preparation of undernourished patients for surgery, chemotherapy, or radiation therapy; severe or prolonged disorders of the gastro-intestinal tract; major surgery, trauma, or burns; prolonged coma or refusal to eat; and some patients with renal or hepatic failure. Table 5 gives the composition of proprietary preparations available.

Protein is given as mixtures of essential and non-essential synthetic L-amino acids, which have replaced the protein hydrolysate preparations formerly used. Ideally, all essential amino acids should be included with a wide variety of non-essential ones to provide sufficient nitrogen together with electrolytes (see also section 9.2.2). However, available solutions vary in composition. Most contain amino acids alone or with a partial energy source (see Table 5) using combinations of glucose (dextrose), fructose (laevulose), sorbitol, and ethanol. Some are significantly deficient in electrolytes or particular amino acids.

Energy is provided in a ratio of 0.6 to 1.1 megajoules (150–250 kcals) per gram of protein nitrogen. Energy requirements must be met if amino acids are to be utilised for tissue maintenance. Although it has long been held that carbohydrate has a greater nitrogen-sparing effect than fat, recent studies have shown that a mixture of both energy sources, usually 30 to 50% as fat, gives better utilisation of amino acid solutions than glucose alone.

Glucose is the preferred source of carbohydrate, but if more than 180 g is given per day frequent monitoring of blood glucose is required, and insulin may be necessary. Glucose in various strengths from 10 to 50% must be infused through a central venous catheter to avoid thrombosis. Preparations are available with useful added ions and trace elements, for example Glucoplex®.

Fructose and sorbitol have been used in an attempt to avoid the problem of hyperosmolar hyperglycaemic non-ketotic acidosis but other metabolic problems may occur, as with xylitol and ethanol which are now rarely used.

Fat emulsions have the advantages of a high energy to fluid volume ratio, neutral pH, and iso-osmolarity with plasma, and provide essential fatty acids. Available preparations are soya bean oil emulsions (Intralipid®). Several days of adaptation may be required to attain maximal utilisation. Reactions include occasional febrile episodes (usually only with 20% emulsions) and rare anaphylactic responses. Interference with biochemical measurements such as those for blood gases and calcium may occur if samples are taken before fat has been cleared. Daily checks are necessary to ensure complete clearance from the plasma. **Additives may only be mixed with fat emulsions where compatibility is known.**

Total parenteral nutrition (TPN) requires the use of a solution containing amino acids, glucose, fat, electrolytes, trace elements, and vitamins. This is now commonly provided by the pharmacy in the form of the 3-litre bag. The solution is infused through a central venous catheter inserted under full surgical precautions. Only nutritional fluids should be given by this line. Loading doses of vitamin B_{12} and folic acid are advised and other vitamins are given parenterally twice weekly.

Before starting, the patient should be well oxygenated with a near normal circulating blood volume, renal function, and acid-base status. Appropriate biochemical tests should have been carried out beforehand and serious deficits corrected. Nutritional and electrolyte status must be monitored throughout treatment.

SUPPLEMENTARY PREPARATIONS

PoM **Addamel**® (KabiVitrum)
Injection, electrolytes and trace elements for addition to Vamin® amino acid solutions (see Table 5), Ca^{2+} 5 mmol, Mg^{2+} 1.5 mmol, Cl^- 13.3 mmol/10 ml; traces of Fe^{3+}, Zn^{2+}, Mn^{2+}, Cu^{2+}, F^-, I^-. For adult use. Price 10-ml amp = **D**

▼ PoM **Addiphos**® (KabiVitrum)
Solution, sterile, phosphate 40 mmol, K^+ 30 mmol, Na^+ 30 mmol/20 ml. For addition to Vamin® amino acid solutions (see Table 5) and glucose intravenous infusions. Price 20-ml vial = **D**

Fosfor® (Consolidated)
NHS *Syrup* (= elixir), pink, phosphorylcolamine 5%. Price 100 ml = **B**
PoM *Injection*, phosphorylcolamine sodium salt 25%. For use alone, or with glucose intravenous infusion 5%, or with other amino acids. Price 10-ml amp = **A**

PoM **Multibionta**® (Merck)
Injection, ascorbic acid 500 mg, dexpanthenol 25 mg, nicotinamide 100 mg, pyridoxine hydrochloride 15 mg, riboflavine sodium phosphate 10 mg, thiamine hydrochloride 50 mg, tocopheryl acetate 5 mg, vitamin A 10000 units. For addition to infusion solutions. Price 10-ml amp = **D**

PoM **Ped-El**® (KabiVitrum)
Solution, sterile, Ca^{2+}, Cu^{2+}, Fe^{3+}, Mg^{2+}, Mn^{2+}, Zn^{2+}, Cl^-, F^-, I^-, P. for addition to Vamin® amino acid solutions (see Table 5). For paediatric use. Price 20-ml vial = **D**

PoM **Select-A-Jet Multiple Vitamin Solution**® (IMS)
Injection, vitamin A 1000 units, thiamine hydrochloride 5 mg, riboflavine 1 mg, nicotinamide 10 mg, pyridoxine hydrochloride 1.5 mg, ascorbic acid 50 mg, ergocalciferol 100 units, d-α-tocopheryl acetate 0.5 unit, dexpanthenol 2.5 mg/ml. For addition to infusion solutions. Price 10-ml vial = **D**

PoM **Solivito**® (KabiVitrum)
Injection, powder for reconstitution, biotin 300 micrograms, cyanocobalamin 2 micrograms, folic acid 200 micrograms, glycine 100 mg, nicotinamide 10 mg, pyridoxine hydrochloride 2.43 mg, riboflavine 1.8 mg (as sodium phosphate), sodium ascorbate 34 mg, sodium pantothenate 11 mg, thiamine mononitrate 1.24 mg. Dissolve in water for injections or glucose intravenous infusion for adding to glucose intravenous infusion or Intralipid; dissolve in Vitlipid or Intralipid for adding to Intralipid only. Price per vial = **D**

PoM **Vitlipid**® (KabiVitrum)
Injection, adult, vitamin A 250 units, ergocalciferol 12 units, phytomenadione 15 micrograms/ml. Emulsion for addition to Intralipid® intravenous infusions. Price 10-ml amp = **D**

Injection, infant, vitamin A 333 units, ergocalciferol 100 units, phytomenadione 50 micrograms/ml. Price 10-ml amp = **D**

9.4 Foods for special diets and nutritional support

9.4.1 Foods for special diets
9.4.2 Nutritional support and nutritionally complete feeds

9.4.1 Foods for special diets

A number of the foods listed below have been prepared to eliminate or reduce the content of a specific constituent. There are also specially formulated mixtures to substitute for foods which contain an unwanted ingredient.

In certain clinical conditions some foods may have the characteristics of drugs and the Advisory Committee on Borderline Substances advises as to the circumstances in which such foods may be regarded as drugs and so can be prescribed in the N.H.S. These clinical conditions are shown with the food preparations listed below. Prescriptions for these foods issued in accordance with the advice of this committee and endorsed 'ACBS' will normally not be investigated. See Appendix 3 for a listing by clinical condition.

Corn oil (maize oil). Price 100 ml = **B**. For familial hypercholesterolaemia
Fructose (laevulose). Price 500 g = **C**. For proven glucose/galactose intolerance
Glucose (dextrose monohydrate). Price 100 g = **A**. For glycogen storage disease and sucrose/isomaltose intolerance
Sunflower oil. Price 100 ml = **B**. For familial hypercholesterolaemia
Aglutella Azeta® (GF Supplies)
Wafers, cream-filled, gluten-free, low protein, low sodium, low potassium. Price 168 g = **E**. For phenylketonuria; similar amino-acid abnormalities; renal failure; liver failure and liver cirrhosis
Aglutella Gentili® (GF Supplies)
Pasta, protein not more than 500 mg, carbohydrate 88.8 g, fat 500 mg/100 g, low Na^+ and K^+, gluten-free; macaroni, semolina, spaghetti, spaghetti rings. Price

---

Table 5: Proprietary Infusion Fluids for Parenteral Feeding

Preparation	Manufacturer	Nitrogen g/litre	Energy kJ/litre	K$^+$	Mg^{2+}	Na$^+$	Acet$^-$	Cl$^-$	Other components/litre
Aminofusin L600 Price 1000 ml = I	Merck	7.6	2500	30	5	40	10	14	sorbitol 100 g, vitamins
Aminofusin L1000 Price 1000 ml = I	Merck	7.6	4200	30	5	40	10	14	ethanol 5.28%, sorbitol 100 g, vitamins
Aminofusin L Forte Price 500 ml = I	Merck	15.2	1700	30	5	40	10	27.5	vitamins
Aminoplasmal L3 Price 500 ml = G	Braun	4.82	510	25	2.5	48	59	18	H$_2$PO$_4^-$ 9 mmol, malate 7.5 mmol
Aminoplasmal L5 Price 500 ml = G	Braun	8.03	850	25	2.5	48	59	31	H$_2$PO$_4^-$ 9 mmol, malate 7.5 mmol
Aminoplasmal L10 Price 500 ml = G	Braun	16.06	1700	25	2.5	48	59	62	H$_2$PO$_4^-$ 9 mmol, malate 7.5 mmol
Aminoplasmal Ped Price 100 ml = F; 250 ml = G	Braun	7.4	850	25	2.5	50	27	15	H$_2$PO$_4^-$ 9 mmol, malate 7.5 mmol
Aminoplex 5 Price 1000 ml = I	Geistlich	5.0	4200	28	4	35	28	43	ethanol 5%, sorbitol 125 g, malic acid 1.85 g
Aminoplex 12 Price 500 ml = I; 1000 ml = J	Geistlich	12.44	1300	30	2.5	35	5	67	malic acid 4.6 g
Aminoplex 14 Price 500 ml = I	Geistlich	13.4	1400	30	2.5	35		79	vitamins, malic acid 5.36 g
Aminoplex 24 Price 500 ml = J	Geistlich	24.9	2600	30	2.5	35	5	67	malic acid 4.5 g
Freamine III 8.5% Price 500 ml = H; 1000 ml = J	Boots	13.0	1400	10		10	72	<3	HPO$_4^{2-}$ 10 mmol
Freamine III 10% pH 6.5 Price 1000 ml = J	Boots	15.3	1650	10		10	88	<2	HPO$_4^{2-}$ 10 mmol
Freamine III 10% pH 5.3 Price 1000 ml = J	Boots	15.3	1650	10		10	138	<3	phosphate free
Glucoplex 1000 Price 500 ml = E; 1000 ml = E	Geistlich		4200	30	2.5	50		67	H$_2$PO$_4^-$ 18 mmol, Zn^{2+} 0.046 mmol, anhydrous glucose 240 g
Glucoplex 1600 Price 500 ml = E; 1000 ml = F	Geistlich		6700	30	2.5	50		67	H$_2$PO$_4^-$ 18 mmol, Zn^{2+} 0.046 mmol, anhydrous glucose 400 g

Product	Manufacturer	N (g)	Energy (kJ)							Constituents
Intralipid 10% Price 100 ml = **F**; 500 ml = **H**	KabiVitrum		4600							fractionated soya oil 100 g, glycerol 22.5 g
Intralipid 20% Price 100 ml = **G**; 500 ml = **I**	KabiVitrum		8400							fractionated soya oil 200 g, glycerol 22.5 g
Laevuflex 20 Price 500 ml = **E**	Geistlich		3400							fructose 200 g
Nephramine Price 250 ml = **J**	Boots	6.5	700				5	44		essential amino acids only
Perifusin Price 1000 ml = **H**	Merck	5.0	550	30	5	40	40	10	9	malate 22.5 mmol
Plasma-Lyte 148 (water) Price 1000 ml = **D**	Travenol		80	5	1.5	140		27	98	gluconate 23 mmol
Plasma-Lyte 148 (dextrose 5%) Price 500 ml = **C**; 1000 ml = **D**	Travenol		880	5	1.5	140		27	98	gluconate 23 mmol, anhydrous glucose 50 g
Plasma-Lyte M (dextrose 5%) Price 1000 ml = **D**	Travenol		800	16	1.5	40	40	12	40	Ca^{2+} 2.5 mmol, lactate 12 mmol, anhydrous glucose 50 g
Synthamin 9 Price 500 ml = **G**; 1000 ml = **J**	Travenol	9.1	1000	60	5	73		100	70	$H_2PO_4^-$ 30 mmol
Synthamin 14 Price 500 ml = **H**; 1000 ml = **J**	Travenol	14.0	1600	60	5	73		130	70	$H_2PO_4^-$ 30 mmol
Synthamin 14 without electrolytes Price 500 ml = **H**; 1000 ml = **J**	Travenol	14.0	1600	60	5			68	34	
Synthamin 17 Price 500 ml = **I**; 1000 ml = **J**	Travenol	16.5	1900	60	5	73		150	70	$H_2PO_4^-$ 30 mmol
Vamin 9 Price 500 ml = **H**	KabiVitrum	9.4	1000	20	1.5	50			55	Ca^{2+} 2.5 mmol
Vamin 9 glucose Price 100 ml = **F**; 500 ml = **H**; 1000 ml = **J**	KabiVitrum	9.4	2700	20	1.5	50		135	55	Ca^{2+} 2.5 mmol, anhydrous glucose 100 g
▼Vamin 14 Price 500 ml = **I**; 1000 ml = **J**	KabiVitrum	13.5	1400	50	8	100		100	100	Ca^{2+} 5 mmol, SO_4^{2-} 8 mmol
▼Vamin 14 (electrolyte-free) Price 500 ml = **I**; 1000 ml = **J**	KabiVitrum	13.5	1400							
▼Vamin 18 (electrolyte-free) Price 500 ml = **J**; 1000 ml = **J**	KabiVitrum	18.0	1900							

Note: 1000 kcal = 4.1868 MJ; 1 MJ (1000 kJ) = 238.8 kcal. All entries are PoM

250 g = **D**. For phenylketonuria; similar amino-acid abnormalities; renal failure; liver failure and liver cirrhosis; gluten-sensitive enteropathies including steatorrhoea due to gluten sensitivity; coeliac disease, and dermatitis herpetiformis

Albumaid® (Scientific Hospital Supplies)

Complete, powder, amino acids 89.4%, with vitamins, minerals, trace elements, free from carbohydrate and fat. Price 1 kg = **J**. For malabsorption states where there is failure to hydrolyse and/or absorb protein

RVHB, powder, amino acid mixture, methionine-free. Price 1 kg = **J**. For homocystinuria

RVHB complete, powder, amino acid mixture, methionine-free, with vitamins, minerals, and trace elements. Price 1 kg = **J**. For homocystinuria

XP, powder, amino acids 40%, carbohydrate 50%, fat nil, phenylalanine not more than 10 mg per 100 g, with vitamins, minerals, and trace elements. Price 1 kg = **I**. For phenylketonuria

XP Concentrate, powder, amino acids 85%, carbohydrate and fat nil, phenylalanine not more than 25 mg per 100 g, with vitamins, minerals, and trace elements. Price 1 kg = **J**. For phenylketonuria

Alembicol D® (Alembic Products)

Fractionated coconut oil. Price 1 kg = **G**. For steatorrhoea associated with cystic fibrosis of the pancreas, intestinal lymphangiectasia, surgery of the intestine, chronic liver disease, liver cirrhosis, other proven malabsorption syndromes; and in a ketogenic diet in the management of epilepsy

Aminex® (Cow & Gate)

Biscuits, protein 0.9% (phenylalanine 0.021%), carbohydrate 76.1%, fat 8.4%, lactose- and sucrose-free. Price 12 × 12.5-g biscuits = **C**. For phenylketonuria; similar amino-acid abnormalities; liver cirrhosis; chronic renal failure; lactose with sucrose intolerance

Aminogran® (A&H)

Food Supplement, powder, containing all essential amino acids except phenylalanine, for use with mineral mixture (see below). Price 500 g = **J**. For phenylketonuria

Mineral Mixture, powder, containing all appropriate minerals for use with the above food supplement and other synthetic diets. Price 250 g = **H**. For phenylketonuria and as a mineral supplement in synthetic diets

Aproten® (Ultrapharm)

Various products, gluten-free, low protein, low Na+ and K+. Prices: anellini 250 g = **D**; biscuits 200 g (36) = **D**; crispbread 240 g = **E**; ditalini 250 g = **D**; flour 500 g = **C**; rigatini 250 g = **D**; tagliatelle 250 g = **D**. For phenylketonuria; similar amino-acid abnormalities; renal failure; liver failure and liver cirrhosis; gluten-sensitive enteropathies including steatorrhoea due to gluten sensitivity, coeliac disease, and dermatitis herpetiformis

Bi-Aglut® (Ultrapharm)

Biscuits, starch, sugar, eggs, skimmed milk solids, flavourings, gluten-free. Price 210 g (36) = **D**. For gluten-sensitive enteropathies including steatorrhoea due to gluten sensitivity, coeliac disease, and dermatitis herpetiformis

Calogen® (Scientific Hospital Supplies)

Emulsion, arachis oil 50% in water. Price 2 litres = **J**. For renal failure and other conditions requiring a high-energy, low-fluid, low-electrolyte diet, disorders of amino-acid metabolism or carbohydrate absorption; in a ketogenic diet in the management of epilepsy

Calonutrin® (Geistlich)

Powder, glucose, maltose, and polysaccharides, providing 1720 kJ/100 g. Price 100-g sachet = **B**. For renal failure; liver cirrhosis; disaccharide intolerance (without isomaltose intolerance); disorders of amino-acid metabolism (and other similar disorders) and/or whole protein intolerance; malabsorption states and other conditions, including proven hypoglycaemia, requiring a high-energy, low-fluid intake, whether or not sodium and/or potassium restriction is essential

Caloreen® (Roussel)

Powder, water-soluble dextrins, predominantly polysaccharides containing an average of 5 glucose molecules, with less than 1.8 mmol of Na+ and 0.3 mmol of K+/100 g. Price 250 g = **D**; 5 kg = **J**. For indications, see under Calonutrin

Carobel, Instant® (Cow & Gate)

Powder, carob seed flour. Price 135 g = **F**. For thickening feeds in the treatment of vomiting

Casilan® (Farley)

Powder, whole protein, containing all essential amino acids, 90% with less than 0.01% Na+. Price 250 g = **E**. For biochemically proven hypoproteinaemia

Comminuted Chicken Meat (Cow & Gate)

Suspension (aqueous). Price 110 g = **C**. For carbohydrate intolerance in association with possible or proven intolerance of milk; glucose and galactose intolerance

dp® (GF Supplies)

Biscuits, low-protein, butterscotch- or chocolate-flavoured chip cookies. Price 170 g = **F**. For phenylketonuria; similar amino-acid abnormalities; renal failure; liver failure and liver cirrhosis

Forceval Protein® (Unigreg)

Powder, calcium caseinate 60%, carbohydrate 30%, with vitamins and minerals, providing not less than 55% protein, not more than 1% of fat, not more than 0.12% of Na+. Lactose- and gluten-free. Price 15-g sachet = **B**; 8 × 15-g sachets = **E**; 300 g = **G**. For biochemically proven hypoproteinaemia and as a supplement for short-bowel syndrome; intractable malabsorption; pre-operative preparation of patients who are undernourished, treatment for those with proven inflammatory bowel disease; treatment following total gastrectomy; dysphagia, where a reduced salt intake is required; bowel fistulas. Not suitable as a sole source of nutrition for infants under 1 year or for children up to about 5 years

Formula S® (Cow & Gate)

Powder, soya protein isolate, glucose syrup, vegetable oil, vitamins and minerals, providing carbohydrate 6.8%, fat 3%, and protein 2% when used as a 13.5% solution. Price 450 g = **E**. For milk intolerance; galactosaemia, galactokinase deficiency, and lactose intolerance

Fortical® (Cow & Gate)

Liquid, glucose polymers providing carbohydrate 61.5 g/100 ml. Low-electrolyte, protein-free. Flavours: apple, apricot, black currant, lemon, orange, and neutral. Price 200 ml = **C**. For renal failure; liver cirrhosis, or other conditions requiring a high-energy, low-fluid, low-electrolyte diet

Galactomin® (Cow & Gate)

Formula 17, powder, protein and fat 22.3 g each, carbohydrate 50.2 g, mineral salts 3 g/100 g. Used as a 12.5% solution with additional vitamins in place of milk. Price 454 g = **G**. For lactose intolerance and proven galactosaemia or galactokinase deficiency

Formula 18, powder, modification of Formula 17 with reduced fat ('half-cream'—14.4%). Price 454 g = **H**. For indications, see under Galactomin Formula 17

Formula 19, powder, modification of Formula 17 with reduced fat (14.4%) and fructose as carbohydrate source. Price 454 g = **J**. For glucose plus galactose intolerance

Glutenex® (Cow & Gate)

Biscuits, free from milk products, gluten-free. Price 12 × 14 g = **C**. For gluten-sensitive enteropathies including steatorrhoea due to gluten sensitivity, coeliac disease, and dermatitis herpetiformis

Gluten-free biscuits (Farley)

Biscuits. Price 200 g = **C**. For indications, see under Glutenex

Gluten-free crackers (GF Supplies)

Biscuits. Price 200 g = **D**. For indications, see under Glutenex

Hycal® (Beecham Products)

Liquid, protein-free, low-electrolyte, glucose syrup solids 49.5%. Flavours, black currant, lemon, orange, raspberry. Price 171 ml = **C**. For renal failure; liver cirrhosis or other conditions requiring a high-energy, low-fluid, low-electrolyte diet

Juvela® (GF Supplies)

Juvela Gluten-free, bread/cake mix. Price 500 g = **E**. *Bread*. Price 400-g loaf = **C**. For gluten-sensitive enteropathies including steatorrhoea due to gluten sensitivity, coeliac disease, and dermatitis herpetiformis

Juvela Low Protein, bread/cake mix. Price 500 g = **E**. Butterscotch chip cookies. Price 170 g = **E**. *Bread*. Price 400-g loaf = **C**. For phenylketonuria and similar aminoacid abnormalities; renal failure; liver failure and liver cirrhosis; gluten-sensitive enteropathies, see above

Liquigen® (Scientific Hospital Supplies)

Emulsion, medium chain triglycerides 52%. Price 2 litres = **J**. For steatorrhoea associated with cystic fibrosis of the pancreas; intestinal lymphangiectasia, surgery of the intestine; chronic liver disease and liver cirrhosis; other proven malabsorption syndromes; ketogenic diet in the management of epilepsy; type I hyperlipoproteinaemia

Locasol New Formula® (Cow & Gate)

Powder, protein 14.6 g, carbohydrate 56.5 g, fat 26.1 g, mineral salts 1.9 g, not more than 55 mg of $Ca^{2+}/100$ g and vitamins. Used as a 13.1% solution in place of milk. Price 450 g = **H**. For calcium intolerance

Lofenalac® (Bristol-Myers)

Powder, glucose syrup solids, casein hydrolysate, corn oil, modified tapioca starch, vitamins, and minerals, protein 15%, carbohydrate 59.6%, fat 18%, phenylalanine not more than 0.1%. Gluten-, sucrose-, and lactose-free. Price 1.134 kg = **J**. For phenylketonuria

Maxamaid XP® (Scientific Hospital Supplies)

Powder, essential and non-essential amino acids except phenylalanine, with carbohydrates, vitamins, minerals, and trace elements. Price 100 g = **G**. For phenylketonuria

Maxijul® (Scientific Hospital Supplies)

Liquid, polyglucose polymer providing carbohydrate 50% and potassium 0.004%, sodium 0.023%. Gluten-, lactose-, and fructose-free. Flavours: black current, lemon, lime, and neutral. Price 200 ml = **B**

Powder, polyglucose polymer, potassium 0.004%, sodium 0.046%. Gluten-, lactose-, and fructose-free. Price 100 g and 140 g (both) = **B**. For renal failure; liver cirrhosis; disaccharide intolerance (without isomaltose intolerance); disorders of amino-acid metabolism (and other similar disorders) and/or whole protein intolerance; malabsorption states and other conditions, including proven hypoglycaemia, requiring a high-energy, low-fluid intake

Maxijul LE® (Scientific Hospital Supplies)

Powder, modification of Maxijul with lower concentrations of sodium and potassium. Price 100 g = **C**. For indications, see under Maxijul where sodium and/or potassium restriction is also essential

Maxipro HBV® (Scientific Hospital Supplies)

Powder, whey protein and additional amino acids 88%, with added minerals. Price 1 kg = **J**. For biochemically proven hypoproteinaemia and as a supplement for short-bowel syndrome; intractable malabsorption; pre-operative preparation of patients who are undernourished; treatment for those with proven inflammatory bowel disease; treatment following total gastrectomy; dysphagia, where a reduced salt intake is required; bowel fistulas. Not suitable as a sole source of nutrition for infants under 1 year or for children up to about 5 years

MCT Oil® (Bristol-Myers)

Triglycerides from medium chain fatty acids. Price 950 ml = **H**. For steatorrhoea associated with cystic fibrosis of the pancreas; intestinal lymphangiectasia;

surgery of the intestine; chronic liver disease and liver cirrhosis; other proven malabsorption syndromes; in a ketogenic diet in the management of epilepsy; in type I hyperlipoproteinaemia

MCT (1)® (Cow & Gate)

Powder, protein 25.6%, carbohydrate 40.6%, medium chain triglycerides 28%, when used as a 12.5% solution. Low in lactose and sucrose-free. Price 454 g = **G**. For steatorrhoea associated with cystic fibrosis of the pancreas; intestinal lymphangiectasia; chronic liver disease; surgery of the intestine in infants

Medium Chain Triglyceride (MCT) Oil® (Cow & Gate)

Triglycerides from medium chain fatty acids. Price 1litre = **I**. For indications, see under MCT Oil

Metabolic Mineral Mixture® (Scientific Hospital Supplies)

Powder, essential mineral salts. Price 100 g = **F**. For mineral supplementation in synthetic diets

Minafen® (Cow & Gate)

Powder, equivalent of 12.5% protein, carbohydrate 48%, fat 31%, not more than 0.02% of phenylalanine. For use as 12.5% solution with additional vitamins. Price 454 g = **I**. For phenylketonuria

MSUD Aid® (Scientific Hospital Supplies)

Powder, containing full range of amino acids except isoleucine, leucine, and valine, with vitamins, minerals, and trace elements. Price 200 g = **J**. For maple syrup urine disease

Nestargel® (Nestlé)

Powder, carob seed flour 96.5%, calcium lactate 3.5%. Price 125 g = **D**. For thickening feeds in the treatment of vomiting

Nutramigen® (Bristol-Myers)

Powder, casein hydrolysate, corn oil, modified tapioca starch, sucrose, vitamins, and minerals, providing protein 15%, carbohydrate 59.6%, fat 18%. Gluten- and lactose-free. Price 454 g = **H**. For infants over 3 months and children with galactokinase deficiency; galactosaemia; lactose intolerance without sucrose intolerance; sensitivity to whole protein

PK Aid 1® (Scientific Hospital Supplies)

Powder, containing essential and non-essential amino acids except phenylalanine. Price 1 kg = **J**. For phenylketonuria

Polycal® (Cow & Gate)

Powder, glucose, maltose, and polysaccharides, providing 1610kJ (380kcal)/100 g. Price 400 g = **D**; 2 kg = **G**. For renal failure; liver cirrhosis; disaccharide intolerance (without isomaltose intolerance); disorders of amino-acid metabolism (and other similar disorders) and/or whole protein intolerance; malabsorption states and other conditions, including proven hypoglycaemia, requiring a high-energy, low-fluid intake, whether or not sodium and/or potassium restriction is essential

Pregestimil® (Bristol-Myers)

Powder, glucose syrup solids, casein hydrolysate, corn oil, modified tapioca starch, medium chain triglycerides, vitamins, and minerals, providing protein 12.8%, carbohydrate 61.6%, fat 18.3%. Gluten-, sucrose-, and lactose-free. Price 454 g = **H**. For sucrose and/or lactose intolerance in association with whole protein intolerance, or where amino acids and peptides are indicated in conjunction with medium chain triglycerides. Also for proven malabsorption syndromes in which a reduced fat diet is indicated such as steatorrhoea associated with cystic fibrosis and surgery of the intestine; galactosaemia and galactokinase deficiency

Prosobee® (Bristol-Myers)

Liquid concentrate, prepared from soya protein isolate, soya oil, glucose syrup solids, coconut oil, L-methionine, vitamins, and minerals, providing protein 4.1%, carbohydrate 13.8%, fat 7.2%. Gluten-, sucrose-, and lactose-free. Price 385 ml = **D**

Powder, glucose syrup solids, soya protein isolate, corn oil, coconut oil, L-methionine, vitamins, and minerals,

C = 51-100p, D = 101-180p, E = 181-300p, F = 301-450p, G = 451-650p, H = 651-900p, I = 901-1200p, J = over 1200p.

providing protein 15.6%, carbohydrate 51.4%, fat 27.9%. Gluten-, sucrose-, and lactose-free. Price 400 g = F. For milk intolerance; galactosaemia, galactokinase deficiency, and lactose intolerance

Prosparol® (DF)

Emulsion, arachis oil 50% in water. Price 1 litre = **G**. For renal failure and other conditions requiring a high-energy, low-fluid, low-electrolyte diet; disorders of amino-acid metabolism or carbohydrate absorption; in a ketogenic diet in the management of epilepsy

Rite-Diet® (Welfare Foods)

Gluten-free. Sweet biscuits. Price 150 g = **C**. Crackers. Price 150 g = **C**. Digestive biscuits. Price 150 g = **C**. Savoury biscuits. Price 125 g = **C**. Flour mix. Price 500 g = **D**. Bread mix, price 500 g (brown) = **D**; white, price 500 g = **D**. Bread (white). Price 400 g = **D**. Bread with soya bran. Price 280 g = **C**. For gluten-sensitive enteropathies including steatorrhoea due to gluten sensitivity, coeliac disease, and dermatitis herpetiformis

Low protein. Macaroni, price 250 g = **D**. Spaghetti, shortcut, price 250 g = **D**; rings, price 250 g = **D**. Crackers. Price 150 g = **C**. Sweet biscuits (low Na$^+$ and K$^+$). Price 150 g = **C**. Vanilla cream wafers. Price 100 g = **C**. Cream-filled biscuits (chocolate flavour). Price 125 g = **C**. For phenylketonuria and similar amino-acid abnormalities; renal failure; liver failure and liver cirrhosis

Low protein/gluten-free. Macaroni. Price 250 g = **D**. Spaghetti, shortcut. Price 250 g = **D**. Rings. Price 250 g = **D**. Flour mix. Price 400 g = **C**. Bread (with or without salt). Price 227 g = **C**. Crackers. Price 250 g = **D**. For indications, see gluten-free and low protein foods above

Low sodium. Bread containing protein 8.5%, carbohydrate 53.8%, fat 5.5%, Na$^+$ 0.01%, K$^+$ 0.055%. Price 227 g = **C**. For conditions in which a low-sodium diet is indicated

Tritamyl® (Procea)

Flour, self-raising (starch-based), gluten- and lactose-free. Price 2 kg = **E**. For gluten-sensitive enteropathies including steatorrhoea due to gluten sensitivity, coeliac disease, and dermatitis herpetiformis

Tritamyl PK® (Procea)

Flour, self-raising (starch-based), gluten-, lactose-, and protein-free. Price 2 kg = **E**. For phenylketonuria and similar amino-acid abnormalities; renal failure; liver failure and liver cirrhosis; gluten-sensitive enteropathies as above

Trufree® (Cantassium)

Gluten-free, wheat-free flours. For gluten-sensitive enteropathies including steatorrhoea due to gluten-sensitivity, coeliac disease, and dermatitis herpetiformis

No. 1 (formerly bread mix 420 g). Price 1 kg = **E**

No. 2 with rice bran (formerly bread mix with rice bran 410 g). Price 1 kg = **F**

No. 3 for Cantabread® (formerly Cantabread mix). Price 1 kg = **F**

No. 4 white. Price 1 kg = **E**

No. 5 brown. Price 1 kg = **E**

No. 6 plain (formerly Trufree plain flour). Price 1 kg = **E**

No. 7 self-raising (formerly Trufree self-raising flour). Price 1 kg = **E**

Verkade® (GF Supplies)

Biscuits, gluten-free. Price 200 g (38) = **D**. For gluten-sensitive enteropathies including steatorrhoea due to gluten sensitivity, coeliac disease, and dermatitis herpetiformis

Wysoy® (Wyeth)

Powder, soya protein isolate, sucrose, corn syrup solids, animal and vegetable oil, vitamins and minerals, providing carbohydrate 6.9%, fat 3.6%, and protein 2.1% when reconstituted. Price 430 g = **E**. For milk intolerance, galactosaemia, galactokinase deficiency, and lactose intolerance

9.4.2 Nutritional support and nutritionally complete feeds

The body's reserves of protein rapidly become exhausted in severely ill patients, especially during chronic illness or in those with severe burns, extensive trauma, pancreatitis, or intestinal fistula. Much can be achieved by frequent meals and by persuading the patient to take supplementary snacks of ordinary food between the meals.

However, extra calories, protein, other nutrients, and vitamins are often best given by supplementing ordinary meals with sip or tube feeds of one of the nutritionally complete foods.

When patients cannot feed normally at all, for example patients with severe facial injury, oesophageal obstruction, or coma, a diet composed solely of nutritionally complete foods must be given. This is planned by a dietitian who will take into account the protein and total energy requirement of the patient and decide on the form and relative contribution of carbohydrate and fat to the energy requirements.

There are a number of nutritionally complete foods available and their use reduces an otherwise heavy workload in hospital or in the home. Most contain protein derived from free amino acids or oligopeptides. These elemental diets are only appropriate for patients who have diminished ability to break down protein, as may be the case in inflammatory bowel disease or pancreatic insufficiency.

Even when nutritionally complete feeds are being given it is important to monitor sodium and potassium losses, and extra minerals and vitamins may be needed in patients where gastro-intestinal secretions are being lost. Regular haematological and biochemical tests are needed.

Infants and young children have special requirements and in most situations liquid feeds prepared for adults are totally unsuitable and should not be given. Expert advice should be sought.

The food preparations which the Advisory Committee on Borderline Substances has advised that doctors may prescribe on FP10 for patients with certain clinical conditions such as short-bowel syndrome, intractable malabsorption, dysphagia, bowel fistulas, and after total gastrectomy are listed in Appendix 3.

Prescriptions for these foods issued in accordance with the advice of this committee and endorsed 'ACBS' will normally not be investigated.

Details of the following preparations are also set out in Table 6.

Clinifeed® (Roussel)

Complete gluten-free foods in 4 formulations. For short-bowel syndrome; intractable malabsorption; pre-operative preparation of patients who are undernourished; treatment for those with proven inflammatory bowel disease; treatment following total gastrectomy and dysphagia; bowel fistulas; anorexia nervosa (except Clinifeed Favour). Not suitable as a sole source of nutrition for older children, unsuitable for all infants under 1 year

Clinifeed 400, protein 15 g, carbohydrate 55 g, fat 13.4 g, energy 1674 kJ (400 kcal)/375 ml, with vitamins and

---

minerals, vanilla flavour. Fructose-free. Price 375-ml can = **C**

Clinifeed Favour, protein 14.1 g, carbohydrate 52.5 g, fat 12.4 g, energy 1575 kJ (375 kcal)/375 ml, with vitamins and minerals, neutral flavour. Lactose-, fructose-, and sucrose-free. Price 375-ml can = **C**

Clinifeed Iso, protein 10.5 g, carbohydrate 49 g, fat 15.4 g, energy 1575 kJ (375 kcal)/375 ml, with vitamins and minerals, vanilla flavour. Fructose-free, low sucrose, and low sodium. Price 375-ml can = **D**

Clinifeed Protein Rich, protein 30 g, carbohydrate 70 g, fat 11 g, energy 2092 kJ (500 kcal)/375 ml, with vitamins and minerals, vanilla flavour. Fructose-free. Price 375-ml can = **D**

Enrich® (Abbott)
Liquid with dietary fibre, glucose syrup solids, sucrose, caseinates, corn oil, soya polysaccharides and protein isolate, vitamins, and minerals, providing protein 9.4 g, carbohydrate 38.3 g (including 5 g as dietary fibre), fat 8.8 g, energy 1090 kJ (260 kcal)/237 ml. Lactose- and gluten-free. Price 237-ml can = **C**. For short-bowel syndrome, intractable malabsorption, pre-operative preparation of patients who are under nourished, treatment for those with proven inflammatory bowel disease, treatment following total gastrectomy, dysphagia, bowel fistulas, anorexia nervosa. Not suitable as a sole source of nutrition for older children, unsuitable for all infants under 1 year

Ensure® (Abbott)
Liquid, protein 3.7%, fat 3.7%, carbohydrate 14.6%, with minerals and vitamins, lactose- and gluten-free, energy 1058 kJ (253 kcal)/235 ml. Price 235-ml bottle or can = **C**; 946-ml bottle or can = **E**. For short-bowel syndrome, intractable malabsorption, pre-operative preparation of patients who are undernourished, treatment for those with proven inflammatory bowel disease, treatment following total gastroectomy, dysphagia, bowel fistulas, anorexia nervosa. Not suitable as a sole source of nutrition for older children, unsuitable for all infants under 1 year
Powder, same composition as Ensure liquid when reconstituted. Price 400 g = **F**

Ensure Plus® (Abbott)
Liquid, protein 5.5%, fat 5.3%, carbohydrate 20%, with vitamins and minerals, lactose- and gluten-free, energy 1500 kJ (355 kcal)/235 ml. Price 235 ml = **C**. For indications, see under Ensure

Flexical® (Bristol-Myers)
Powder, corn syrup solids, hydrolysed casein, soya oil, modified tapioca starch, medium chain triglycerides, vitamins, and minerals, providing protein 9.9%, carbohydrate 66.9%, fat 15%. Gluten- and lactose-free. Price 454 g = **I**. For short-bowel syndrome, intractable malabsorption, pre-operative preparation of patients who are undernourished, and treatment following total gastrectomy, bowel fistulas, anorexia nervosa. Not suitable as a sole source of nutrition for older children, unsuitable for all infants under 1 year

Fortisip® (Cow & Gate)
Energy-plus, liquid, protein 10 g, carbohydrate 35.8 g, fat 13 g, energy 1260 kJ (300 kcal)/200 ml, with vitamins and minerals. Gluten-free. Price 200 ml = **B**; flavour sachet = **A**

Standard, liquid, protein 8 g, carbohydrate 24 g, fat 8 g, energy 840 kJ (200 kcal)/200 ml, with vitamins and minerals. Gluten-free. Price 200 ml = **B**; flavour sachet = **A**. For short-bowel syndrome; intractable malabsorption; pre-operative preparation of patients who are undernourished; treatment for those with proven inflammatory bowel disease; treatment following total gastrectomy and dysphagia; bowel fistulas; anorexia nervosa. Not suitable as a sole source of nutrition for older children, unsuitable for all infants under 1 year

Fortison® (Cow & Gate)
Energy-plus, same composition as Fortisip energy-plus,

providing 3150 kJ (750 kcal)/500 ml. Price 500 ml = **D**. For indications, see under Fortisip

Soya, liquid, protein 20 g, carbohydrate 60 g, fat 20 g, energy 2100 kJ (500 kcal)/500 ml, with vitamins and minerals. Gluten-free. Price 500 ml = **D**. For milk intolerance and lactose intolerance. Not suitable as a sole source of nutrition for older children, unsuitable for all infants under 1 year

Standard, same composition as Fortisip standard, providing 2100 kJ (500 kcal)/500 ml. Price 500 ml = **D**

Isocal® (Bristol-Myers)
Liquid, maltodextrin, soya oil, caseinate solids, medium chain triglycerides, soya protein isolate, vitamins, and minerals, providing protein 3.2%, carbohydrate 12.6%, fat 4.2%. Gluten- and lactose-free. Price 250 ml = **C**. For short-bowel syndrome, intractable malabsorption, pre-operative preparation of patients who are under-nourished, treatment for those with proven inflammatory bowel disease, treatment following total gastrectomy, dysphagia, bowel fistulas, anorexia nervosa. Not suitable as a sole source of nutrition for older children, unsuitable for all infants under 1 year

Nutranel® (Roussel)
Powder, maltodextrin, whey protein hydrolysate, corn oil, medium chain triglycerides, vitamins and minerals, providing protein 15.8%, fat 4%, and carbohydrate 74.3%. Price 100 g = **E**. For intractable malabsorption; bowel fistulas; following total gastrectomy. Not suitable as a sole source of nutrition for older children, unsuitable for all infants under 1 year

Nutrauxil® (KabiVitrum)
Liquid and *Sip*, protein 3.8 g, carbohydrate 13.8 g, fat 3.4 g, energy 420 kJ (100 kcal)/100 ml, with vitamins and minerals, vanilla flavour. Low lactose and gluten-free. Price 200-ml bottle = **C**; 500-ml bottle = **D**. For short-bowel syndrome; intractable malabsorption; pre-operative preparation of patients who are under-nourished; treatment for those with proven inflammatory bowel disease; treatment following gastrectomy; bowel fistulas; dysphagia and anorexia nervosa. Not suitable as a sole source of nutrition for infants under 1 year or for children up to about 5 years

Portagen® (Bristol-Myers)
Powder, corn syrup solids, medium chain triglycerides, sodium caseinate, sucrose, corn oil, vitamins, and minerals, providing protein 16.5%, carbohydrate 54.3%, fat 22.5%. Glucose- and lactose-free. Price 454 g = **G**. For lactose intolerance without sucrose intolerance but requiring medium chain triglycerides; malabsorption associated with cystic fibrosis of the pancreas; intestinal lymphangiectasia; surgery of the intestine; chronic liver disease and liver cirrhosis; other proven malabsorption syndromes

Triosorbon® (Merck)
Powder, protein 19%, carbohydrate 56%, fat 19%, with vitamins and minerals. Gluten-free. Price 85-g sachet = **C**. For short-bowel syndrome; intractable malabsorption; pre-operative preparation of patients who are undernourished; treatment for those with proven inflammatory bowel disease; treatment following total gastrectomy; dysphagia; bowel fistulas, anorexia nervosa. Not suitable as a sole source of nutrition for infants under 1 year or for children up to about 5 years

PoM Vivonex® (Norwich Eaton)
Powder, amino acids 6.18 g, simple sugars 69 g, safflower oil 435 mg/80-g sachet, with added vitamins and minerals. For preparation with water before use. Price 80-g sachet = **D**; flavour sachets 60 × 2 g = **F**. For short-bowel syndrome, intractable malabsorption, pre-operative preparation of patients who are under-nourished, and treatment following total gastrectomy; dysphagia due to an incurable malignancy; bowel fistulas; anorexia nervosa. Not suitable as a sole source of nutrition for infants under 1 year or for children up to about 5 years

---

C = 51-100p, D = 101-180p, E = 181-300p, F = 301-450p, G = 451-650p, H = 651-900p, I = 901-1200p, J = over 1200p.

Table 6: Nutritionally Complete Feeds (all contain minerals and vitamins)

Preparation and Price	Protein g/100 g	Carbohydrate g/100 g	Fat g/100 g	Energy per 100 g kJ	Comments
Powders					
Ensure Abbott Price 400 g = **F**	14.0	54.5	31.5	1831	Gluten-free Lactose-free
Flexical Bristol-Myers Price 454 g = **I**	9.9	66.9	15.0	1856	Gluten-free Lactose-free
Nutranel Roussel Price 100 g = **E**	15.8	73.9	3.9	1663	
Portagen Bristol-Myers Price 454 g = **G**	16.5	54.3	22.5	2040	Gluten-free Lactose-free
Triosorbon Merck Price 85 g = **C**	19.0	56.0	19.0	2000	Gluten-free
Vivonex Norwich Eaton Price 80 g = **D** Flavour sachets 60 × 2 g = **F**	7.7	86.3	0.54	1570	Needs flavour sachets

| **Liquids** | | | | per 1000 ml | |
	g/1000 ml	g/1000 ml	g/1000 ml	kJ	
Clinifeed 400 Roussel Price 375 ml = **C**	40.0	147.0	35.7	4480	Gluten-free
Clinifeed Favour Roussel Price 375 ml = **C**	37.6	140.0	33.1	4200	Gluten-free Lactose-free
Clinifeed Iso Roussel Price 375 ml = **D**	28.0	130.6	41.1	4200	Gluten-free
Clinifeed Protein Rich Roussel Price 375 ml = **D**	80.0	186.6	29.3	5600	Gluten-free
Ensure Abbott Price 235 ml = **C**	37.0	146.0	37.0	4414	Gluten-free
Ensure Plus Abbott Price 235 ml = **C**	54.9	199.6	53.2	6284	Gluten-free Lactose-free
Enrich Abbott Price 237 ml = **C**	39.7	161.6	30.5	4599	With fibre Gluten-free Lactose-free
Fortisip Energy Plus Cow and Gate Price 200 ml = **B**	50.0	179.0	65.0	6300	Gluten-free Lactose-free
Fortisip Standard Cow and Gate Price 200 ml = **B**	40.0	120.0	40.0	4200	Gluten-free Lactose-free
Fortison Energy Plus Cow and Gate Price 500 ml = **D**	50.0	179.0	65.0	6300	Gluten-free

For all abbreviations and symbols see inside cover.

Relative prices: A = up to 20p, B = 21-50p,

Table 6: Nutritionally Complete Feeds (all contain minerals and vitamins) (*continued*)

Preparation and Price	Protein g/1000 ml	Carbohydrate g/1000 ml	Fat g/1000 ml	Energy per 1000 ml kJ	Comments
Liquids (*continued*)					
Fortison Soya Cow and Gate Price 500 ml = **D**	40.0	120.0	40.0	4200	Gluten-free
Fortison Standard Cow and Gate Price 500 ml = **D**	40.0	120.0	40.0	4200	Gluten-free
Isocal Bristol-Myers Price 250 ml = **C**	32.0	126.0	42.0	4240	Gluten-free Lactose-free Sucrose-free
Nutrauxil KabiVitrum Price 200 ml = **C**; 500 ml = **D**	38.0	138.0	34.0	4200	Gluten-free

ASSOCIATED PRODUCTS

Ketovite® (Paines & Byrne)
PoM *Tablets*, yellow, ascorbic acid 16.6 mg, riboflavine 1 mg, thiamine hydrochloride 1 mg, pyridoxine hydrochloride 330 micrograms, nicotinamide 3.3 mg, calcium pantothenate 1.16 mg, alpha tocopheryl acetate 5 mg, inositol 50 mg, biotin 170 micrograms, folic acid 250 micrograms, acetomenaphthone 500 micrograms. Price 20 tabs = **B**
(Supplement) liquid, pink, vitamin A 2500 units, vitamin D 400 units, choline chloride 150 mg, cyanocobalamin 12.5 micrograms/5 ml. Diluent purified water, freshly boiled and cooled, life of diluted liquid 7 days. Price 100 ml = **C**
Dose: as a vitamin supplement with synthetic diets, 5 ml liquid daily and 1 tablet 3 times daily
Ruthmol® (Cantassium)
Salt substitute, potassium chloride 50%. Price 250 g = **D**
Selora® (Winthrop)
Salt substitute, potassium chloride 92.05%, hydrated calcium silicate 1%, glutamic acid 1.15%, potassium glutamate 5.79%. Price 227 g = **D**

9.5   Minerals

9.5.1 Calcium
9.5.2 Phosphorus
9.5.3 Fluoride
9.5.4 Zinc
See section 9.1.1 for iron salts

9.5.1   Calcium

9.5.1.1 Calcium supplements
9.5.1.2 Hypercalcaemia

9.5.1.1   CALCIUM SUPPLEMENTS

Calcium supplements are only required where dietary calcium intake is deficient. This dietary requirement varies with age and is relatively greater in childhood, pregnancy, and lactation, due to an increased demand, and in old age, due to impaired absorption. In osteoporosis a daily supplement of 800 mg (20 mmol) calcium may reduce the rate of bone loss, but larger doses have not been shown to be more effective. Patients with hypoparathyroidism rarely require calcium supplements after the early stages of stabilisation on vitamin D (section 9.6.4).

In hypocalcaemic tetany an initial intravenous injection of 10 ml (2.25 mmol) of calcium gluconate injection may be followed by the continuous infusion of about 40 ml (9 mmol) daily, but plasma calcium should be monitored. In asystolic cardiac arrest 10 ml of calcium gluconate injection may be given by intravenous or intracardiac injection.

CALCIUM SALTS

Indications: see notes above; calcium deficiency
Cautions: drug interactions: see Appendix 1 (section 9)
Side-effects: bradycardia, arrhythmias, and irritation after intravenous injection
Dose: by mouth, up to 20 mmol Ca^{2+} daily in divided doses, as calcium gluconate or lactate
By slow intravenous injection, calcium gluconate 1–2 g (2.25–4.5 mmol of Ca)

Calcium Gluconate Tablets, calcium gluconate 600 mg (1.35 mmol Ca^{2+}). To be chewed before swallowing. Price 20 tabs = **B**. Label: 24
Calcium Gluconate Tablets, Effervescent, calcium gluconate 1 g (2.25 mmol Ca^{2+}). Price 20 tabs = **C**. Label: 13
Note: each tablet usually contains sodium 102.6 mg (4.46mmol)
PoM **Calcium Gluconate Injection,** calcium gluconate 10%. Price 5- and 10-ml amp (both) = **B**
Calcium Lactate Tablets, calcium lactate 300 mg (1 mmol Ca^{2+}), price 20 tabs = **A**; 600 mg (2 mmol Ca^{2+}), price 20 tabs = **B**

Calcium-Sandoz® (Sandoz)

Syrup (= elixir), calcium glubionate 3.27 g, calcium galactogluconate 2.17 g (325 mg calcium or 8.1 mmol Ca^{2+})/15 ml. Diluent syrup, life of diluted elixir 14 days. Price 100 ml = **B**

PoM *Injection*, calcium glubionate equivalent to 10% of calcium gluconate (93 mg calcium or 2.32 mmol Ca^{2+}/10 ml). Price 10-ml amp = **B**

Ossopan® (Labaz)

Tablets, buff, f/c, hydroxyapatite 830 mg (4.4mmol Ca^{2+}). Price 20 tabs = **F**

Oral powder, hydroxyapatite 820 mg (4.4mmol Ca^{2+})/g. Price 50 g = **G**

Sandocal® (Sandoz)

Tablets, effervescent, orange, calcium lactate gluconate 3.08 g, sodium bicarbonate, potassium bicarbonate, equivalent to calcium 400 mg (10 mmol Ca^{2+}), sodium 137 mg (6 mmol Na^+), potassium 176 mg (4.5 mmol K^+). Price 20 tabs = **D**. Label: 13

Caution: avoid in renal impairment

9.5.1.2 HYPERCALCAEMIA

The cause for hypercalcaemia should be established before treatment is started, unless the patient is seriously ill. Rehydration and the exclusion of calcium from the patient's diet are essential and on occasions are all that is necessary.

Agents such as sodium cellulose phosphate which bind calcium in the gut may be helpful, but any associated increase in plasma phosphate may be harmful. Similarly, oral and intravenous phosphate may only achieve a reduction in plasma calcium by precipitating calcium phosphate in the tissues, resulting in nephrocalcinosis and impairment of renal function.

Agents which inhibit mobilisation of calcium from the skeleton are usually required where hypercalcaemia is severe. Mithramycin (see section 8.1.2) is probably the most rapidly effective drug, but cannot be given continuously for more than a few days because of marrow toxicity. Corticosteroids (see section 6.3) and calcitonin (see section 6.6.1) may be helpful but often take several days to achieve the desired effect and may be totally ineffective even in massive dosage. Calcitonin is relatively non-toxic but expensive and a daily dose of 200 units is usually as effective as larger doses.

Intravenous chelating agents such as trisodium edetate are rarely used although theoretically safer than intravenous phosphate if given by slow continuous infusion. They usually cause pain in the limb receiving the infusion and may cause renal damage.

SODIUM CELLULOSE PHOSPHATE

Indications: hypercalcaemia, reduction of calcium absorption from food (in conjunction with low-calcium diet)

Contra-indications: congestive heart failure, renal impairment

Side-effects: diarrhoea

Dose: 5 g 3 times daily with meals; CHILD 10 g daily in 3 divided doses with meals

Calcisorb® (Riker)

Sachets, sodium cellulose phosphate 5 g. Price 10 sachets = **E**. Label: 13, 21, counselling advised, may be sprinkled on food

TRISODIUM EDETATE

Indications: hypercalcaemia; removal of lime burns in the eye

Cautions: plasma-calcium determinations required; caution in tuberculosis

Contra-indications: impaired renal function

Side-effects: nausea, diarrhoea, cramp; in overdosage renal damage

Dose: by slow intravenous infusion, up to 70 mg/kg daily over 2–3 hours

PoM **Limclair®** (Sinclair)

Injection, trisodium edetate 200 mg/ml. Price 5-ml amp = **E**

For topical use in the eye, dilute 1 ml to 50 ml with sterile purified water

9.5.2 Phosphorus

Oral phosphate supplements may be required in addition to vitamin D in a small minority of patients with hypophosphataemic vitamin D-resistant rickets. Diarrhoea is a common side-effect and should prompt a reduction in dosage.

Phosphate-Sandoz® (Sandoz)

Tablets, effervescent, anhydrous sodium acid phosphate 1.936 g, sodium bicarbonate 350 mg, potassium bicarbonate 315 mg, equivalent to phosphorus 500 mg (16.1 mmol P), sodium 468.8 mg (20.4 mmol Na^+), potassium 123 mg (3.1 mmol K^+). Price 20 tabs = **C**. Label: 13

9.5.3 Fluoride

Regular application of fluoride to the teeth reduces dental caries. Dentifrices which incorporate sodium fluoride or monofluorophosphate are the most convenient though least effective method of application. Six-monthly dental treatments with gels or solutions containing sodium fluoride are more effective.

Systemic treatment is the most effective method. Fluoridation of the water (1 mg per litre in temperate climates) is the most economical method, but an alternative is the daily administration of tablets containing 0.25 to 1 mg of fluoride ion. Mottling of the teeth may occur with higher doses. Fluoride supplements should not be prescribed without prior reference to the fluoride content of the local water supply, and are not advisable when the water contains more than 0.7 mg per litre.

There are arrangements for health authorities to supply fluoride tablets in the course of preschool dental schemes, and they may also be supplied in school dental schemes. The Department of Health and Social Security states that the prescribing of fluoride tablets does not appear to be an issue with which general medical practitioners would normally be involved.

SODIUM FLUORIDE

Indications: prophylaxis of dental caries—see notes above

Contra-indications: not for areas where drinking water is fluoridated

Side-effects: occasional white flecks on teeth with recommended doses; rarely yellowish-brown discoloration if recommended doses are exceeded

Dose: as fluoride ion daily, preferably in the evening, INFANTS 2 weeks–2 years, 250 micrograms; CHILDREN 2–4 years, 500 micrograms; over 4 years, 1 mg. Tablets should be dissolved in the mouth

Note: sodium fluoride 2.2 mg provides approx. 1 mg fluoride ion

En-De-Kay® (Stafford-Miller)
Fluodrops® (= paediatric drops), orange, sodium fluoride 500 micrograms (250 micrograms F⁻)/0.15 ml. Price 60 ml = C
PoM *Fluorinse* (= mouth-wash), red, sodium fluoride 2%. Price 100 ml = D
Dilute before use
Fluotabs 2–4 years (= paediatric tablets), yellow, scored, sodium fluoride 1.1 mg (500 micrograms F⁻). Price 20 tabs = A
Fluotabs 4+ years (= tablets), orange, scored, sodium fluoride 2.2 mg (1 mg F⁻). Price 20 tabs = A

Fluor-a-day Lac® (Dental Health)
Tablets, buff, scored, sodium fluoride 2.2 mg (1 mg F⁻). Price 20 tabs = A

Fluorigard® (Hoyt)
Mouth-wash, green, sodium fluoride 0.05%. Price 500 ml = D
Rinse mouth with 5–10 ml for about 1 minute daily
Paediatric drops, sodium fluoride 275 micrograms (125 micrograms F⁻)/drop. Price 30 ml = C
Tablets 0.5, purple, sodium fluoride 1.1 mg (500 micrograms F⁻). Price 20 tabs = A
Tablets 1.0, sodium fluoride 2.2 mg (1 mg F⁻). Price 20 tabs = A (available in 4 colours and flavours)

Point-Two® (Hoyt)
Mouth-wash, sodium fluoride 0.2%. Price 150 ml = D

Zymafluor® (Zyma)
Tablets, sodium fluoride 550 micrograms (250 micrograms F⁻). Price 20 tabs = A
Tablets, yellow-grey, sodium fluoride 2.2 mg (1 mg F⁻). Price 20 tabs = A

9.5.4 Zinc

Oral zinc therapy should only be given when there is good evidence of deficiency (hypoproteinaemia spuriously lowers plasma-zinc concentrations). Zinc deficiency can occur in individuals on inadequate diets, in malabsorption, with increased body loss due to trauma, burns and protein-losing conditions, and during intravenous feeding. Therapy should continue until clinical improvement occurs and be replaced by dietary measures unless there is severe malabsorption, metabolic disease, or continuing zinc loss. Side-effects of zinc salts are abdominal pain and dyspepsia. Drug interactions: see Appendix 1 (section *5.1, 9, 9, 10*)

▼ **Solvazinc®** (Thames)
Effervescent tablets, yellow-white, zinc sulphate 200 mg (45 mg zinc). Price 20 tabs = E. Label: 13, 21
Dose: 1 tablet in water 1–3 times daily after food

Zincomed® (Medo)
Capsules, blue/white, zinc sulphate 220 mg. Price 20 caps = C. Label: 21
Dose: 1 capsule 3 times daily after food

Z Span® (SK&F)
Spansule® (= capsules s/r), blue/clear, enclosing white and grey pellets, zinc sulphate monohydrate 61.8 mg (22.5 mg zinc). Price 20 caps = D. Label: 25
Dose: adults and children over 1 year, 1–3 capsules daily as required

9.6 Vitamins

Vitamins are used for the prevention and treatment of specific deficiency states or where the diet is known to be inadequate. Their use as general 'pick-me-ups' is of unproven value and, in the case of preparations containing vitamin A or D, may actually be harmful since many patients will take more than the prescribed dose.

In the National Health Service, vitamins may be prescribed to prevent or treat vitamin deficiency but they are not regarded as medicines when prescribed as dietary supplements.

9.6.1 Vitamin A
9.6.2 Vitamin B group
9.6.3 Vitamin C
9.6.4 Vitamin D
9.6.5 Vitamin E
9.6.6 Vitamin K
9.6.7 Multivitamin preparations

9.6.1 Vitamin A

Deficiency of vitamin A (retinol) is rare in Britain even in disorders of fat absorption. If deficiency is diagnosed, treatment should be with one tablet of 50 000 units daily (Ro-A-Vit®). For prevention, 4000 units daily is adequate and is available in the combination preparation **vitamins A and D capsules** (4000 units of vitamin A per capsule) and in the multivitamin preparation **vitamins capsules** (2500 units of vitamin A per capsule, section 9.6.7).

Massive overdose can cause rough skin, dry hair, an enlarged liver, and a raised erythrocyte sedimentation rate and raised serum calcium and serum alkaline phosphatase concentrations. Use of excessive doses should be avoided in pregnancy.

Halibut-liver Oil Capsules, vitamin A 4000 units. Price 20 caps = A

C = 51-100p, D = 101-180p, E = 181-300p, F = 301-450p, G = 451-650p, H = 651-900p, I = 901-1200p, J = over 1200p.

PoM **Ro-A-Vit**® (Roche)
Tablets, cream, s/c, vitamin A (retinol) 50 000
units (as acetate). Price 20 tabs = **B**
Injection (oily), vitamin A (retinol) 300 000
units (as palmitate)/ml. Price 1-ml amp = **C**
Dose: by deep intramuscular injection, 150 000–
300 000 units monthly, increased to weekly in
acute deficiency states

Preparations of vitamins A and D
Vitamins A and D Capsules, vitamin A 4000
units, vitamin D 400 units. Price 20 caps = **B**
NHS **Halycitrol**® (LAB)
Emulsion (= mixture), vitamin A 4600 units,
vitamin D 460 units/5 ml. Price 114 ml = **C**
Dose: 5 ml daily

9.6.2   Vitamin B group

Deficiency of the B vitamins, other than deficiency
of vitamin B_{12} (section 9.1.2) is rare in Britain
and is usually treated by preparations containing
thiamine (B_1), riboflavine (B_2), and nicotinamide,
which is used in preference to nicotinic acid, as it
does not cause vasodilatation. Other members of
the vitamin B complex such as aminobenzoic acid,
biotin, choline, inositol, and pantothenic acid or
panthenol may be included in vitamin B preparations but there is no evidence of their value.
For folic acid preparations see section 9.1.2 and
for folic acid preparations with iron see section
9.1.1.1.

Potassium aminobenzoate has been used in the
treatment of various disorders associated with
excessive fibrosis such as scleroderma but its
therapeutic value is **doubtful.**

Severe deficiency states and encephalopathy,
especially as seen in chronic alcoholism, are best
treated by the parenteral administration of B vitamins (Pabrinex®, Parentrovite®). A pyridoxine
(B_6) deficiency state may occur during isoniazid
therapy.

Nicotinamide Tablets, nicotinamide 50 mg.
Price 20 tabs = **B**
Nicotinic Acid Tablets, see section 2.12
Thiamine Hydrochloride Tablets, thiamine
hydrochloride 3, 10, 25, and 50 mg, price 20
tabs (all) = **A**; 100 mg, price 20 tabs = **B**; 300 mg,
price 20 tabs = **C**
PoM **Thiamine Hydrochloride Injection,** thiamine
hydrochloride 25 and 100 mg/ml. Price
1-ml amp (both) = **A**
Dose: by mouth or by intramuscular injection
10–100 mg daily; up to 600 mg daily in severe
deficiency
PoM **Vitamins B and C Injection**
Weak, for intramuscular use, ascorbic acid 500
mg, nicotinamide 160 mg, pyridoxine hydrochloride 50 mg, riboflavine 4 mg, thiamine
hydrochloride 100 mg/4 ml. Price 4 ml (in 2
amps) = **B**
Strong, for intramuscular use, ascorbic acid 500
mg, nicotinamide 160 mg, pyridoxine hydrochloride 50 mg, riboflavine 4 mg, thiamine

hydrochloride 250 mg/7 ml. Price 7 ml (in 2
amps) = **B**
Strong, for intravenous use, ascorbic acid 500
mg, anhydrous glucose 1 g, nicotinamide 160
mg, pyridoxine hydrochloride 50 mg, riboflav-
ine 4 mg, thiamine hydrochloride 250 mg/10
ml. Price 10 ml (in 2 amps) = **B**
NHS **Benerva**® (Roche)
Tablets, thiamine hydrochloride 3, 10, 25 and
50 mg. Price 20 tabs (all) = **A**
Tablets, thiamine hydrochloride 100 mg. Price
20 tabs = **B**
Tablets, thiamine hydrochloride 300 mg. Price
20 tabs = **C**
PoM *Injection*, thiamine hydrochloride 25 mg/ml.
Price 1-ml amp = **A**
PoM *Injection*, thiamine hydrochloride 100 mg/ml.
Price 1-ml amp = **A**
Dose: by mouth or by intramuscular injection
10–100 mg daily; up to 600 mg daily in acute
deficiency
PoM **Pabrinex**® (Paines & Byrne)
Intramuscular maintenance injection, vitamins B
and C injection, weak, for intramuscular use.
Price 4 ml (in 2 amps) = **B**
Intramuscular high potency injection, vitamins B
and C injection, strong, for intramuscular use.
Price 7 ml (in 2 amps) = **B**
Intravenous high potency injection, vitamins B
and C injection, strong, for intravenous use.
Price 10 ml (in 2 amps) = **B**
PoM **Parentrovite**® (Bencard)
IMM Injection, vitamins B and C injection,
weak, for intramuscular use. Price 4 ml (in 2
amps) = **B**
IMHP Injection, vitamins B and C injection,
strong, for intramuscular use. Price 7 ml (in 2
amps) = **B**
IVHP Injection, vitamins B and C injection,
strong, for intravenous use. Price 10 ml (in 2
amps) = **B**
Potaba® (Glenwood)
Capsules, red/white, potassium aminobenzoate 500 mg.
Price 20 caps = **C**. Label: 21
Tablets, potassium aminobenzoate 500 mg. Price 20
tabs = **C**. Label: 21
Dose: Peyronie's disease, scleroderma, 12 g daily in
divided doses after food
Envules® (= powder in sachets), potassium aminobenzoate 3 g. Price 20 sachets = **F**. Label: 13, 21

PYRIDOXINE HYDROCHLORIDE

(Vitamin B_6)
Indications: isoniazid-induced   peripheral
neuritis, idiopathic sideroblastic anaemia,
deficiency states
Cautions: drug interactions: see Appendix 1 (section *4.9*)
Dose: neuritis and deficiency states, 20–50 mg up
to 3 times daily
Isoniazid neuropathy, prophylaxis 10 mg daily
Idiopathic sideroblastic anaemia, 100–400 mg
daily in divided doses

Pyridoxine Tablets, pyridoxine hydrochloride
10, 20 and 50 mg, price 20 tabs (all) = **B**

NHS **Benadon®** (Roche)

Tablets, pyridoxine hydrochloride 20 mg. Price 20 tabs = **B**

Tablets, scored, pyridoxine hydrochloride 50 mg. Price 20 tabs = **B**

NHS **Complement Continus®** (Napp)

Tablets, s/r, yellow, pyridoxine hydrochloride 100 mg. Price 28 tabs = **D**. Label: 25

NHS **Paxadon®** (Steinhard)

Tablets, scored, pyridoxine hydrochloride 50 mg. Price 20 tabs = **B**

VITAMIN B COMPLEX PREPARATIONS

These are preparations consisting only of various combinations of the B vitamins. Other multi-vitamin preparations are in section 9.6.7.

Vitamin B Tablets, Compound, nicotinamide 15 mg, riboflavine 1 mg, thiamine hydrochloride 1 mg. Price 20 tabs = **A**

Dose: prophylactic, 1–2 tablets daily

Vitamin B Tablets, Compound, Strong, brown, f/c or s/c, nicotinamide 20 mg, pyridoxine hydrochloride 2 mg, riboflavine 2 mg, thiamine hydrochloride 5 mg. Price 20 tabs = **A**

Dose: treatment of vitamin-B deficiency, 1–2 tablets 3 times daily

NHS **Aluzyme®** (Phillips Yeast)

Tablets, folic acid 14 micrograms, thiamine hydrochloride 160 micrograms, riboflavine 210 micrograms, nicotinic acid 2.5 mg, dried yeast 297 mg. Price 20 tabs = **A**

NHS **Becosym®** (Roche)

Tablets, brown, f/c, vitamin B tablets, compound, strong. Price 20 tabs = **A**

Forte tablets, brown, f/c, thiamine hydrochloride 15 mg, riboflavine 15 mg, nicotinamide 50 mg, pyridoxine hydrochloride 10 mg. Price 20 tabs = **B**

Syrup (= elixir), orange, thiamine hydrochloride 5 mg, riboflavine 2 mg, nicotinamide 20 mg, pyridoxine hydrochloride 2 mg/5 ml. Diluent syrup, life of diluted elixir 14 days. Price 100 ml = **C**

NHS **Benerva Compound®** (Roche)

Tablets, yellow, vitamin B tablets, compound. Price 20 tabs = **A**

NHS **Hemoplex®** (Paines & Byrne)

Injection, crude liver extract, with thiamine hydrochloride 10 mg, riboflavine 500 micrograms, nicotinamide 10 mg, pyridoxine hydrochloride 2.5 mg/ml. Price 10 ml vial = **D**

NHS PoM **Hepacon-Plex®** (Consolidated)

Injection, thiamine hydrochloride 50 mg, riboflavine 1 mg, nicotinamide 75 mg, pyridoxine hydrochloride 2.5 mg/ml, cyanocobalamin 4 micrograms, calcium pantothenate 5 mg/ml. Price 2-ml amp = **B**

NHS **Lederplex®** (Lederle)

Elixir, orange, thiamine hydrochloride 2 mg, riboflavine 2 mg, nicotinamide 10 mg, pyridoxine hydrochloride 200 micrograms, choline 20 mg, cyanocobalamin 5 micrograms, inositol 10 mg, soluble liver fraction 470 mg, pantothenic acid 2 mg/5 ml. Price 100 ml = **E**

NHS **Lipoflavonoid®** (Lewis)

Capsules, pink/black, thiamine hydrochloride 330 micrograms, riboflavine 330 micrograms, nicotinamide 3.33 mg, pyridoxine hydrochloride 330 micrograms, hydroxocobalamin 1.66 micrograms, ascorbic acid 100 mg, choline bitartrate 233 mg, inositol 111 mg, lemon bioflavonoid complex 100 mg, methionine 28 mg, dexpanthenol 330 micrograms. Price 20 caps = **C**

NHS **Lipotriad®** (Lewis)

Capsules, pink/clear, thiamine hydrochloride 330 micro-grams, riboflavine 330 micrograms, nicotinamide 3.33 mg, pyridoxine hydrochloride 330 micrograms, hydroxocobalamin 1.66 micrograms, choline bitartrate 233 mg, inositol 111 mg, methionine 28 mg, dexpanthenol 330 micrograms. Price 20 caps = **B**

Elixir, brown, thiamine hydrochloride 1 mg, riboflavine 1 mg, nicotinamide 10 mg, pyridoxine hydrochloride 1 mg, cyanocobalamin 5 micrograms, inositol 334 mg, methionine 84 mg, panthenol 1 mg, tricholine citrate 460 mg (= choline 334 mg)/5 ml. Price 100 ml = **D**

NHS **Tonivitan B®** (Medo)

Syrup (= elixir), red, thiamine hydrochloride 500 micrograms, riboflavine 400 micrograms, nicotinamide 2.5 mg, pyridoxine hydrochloride 16.5 micrograms, calcium glycerophosphate 20 mg, manganese glycerophosphate 5 mg/5 ml. Diluent syrup, life of diluted elixir 14 days. Price 125 ml = **B**

NHS **Vigranon B®** (Wallace Mfg)

Syrup (= elixir), thiamine hydrochloride 5 mg, riboflavine 2 mg, nicotinamide 20 mg, pyridoxine hydrochloride 2 mg, panthenol 3 mg/5 ml. Price 150 ml = **C**

NHS **Wallachol®** (Wallace Mfg)

Tablets, orange, s/c, thiamine hydrochloride 1 mg, riboflavine 1 mg, nicotinamide 5 mg, pyridoxine hydrochloride 250 micrograms, cyanocobalamin 1 microgram, choline dihydrogen citrate 224 mg, inositol 56 mg, dried liver 50 mg, methionine 112 mg. Price 20 tabs = **C**

Elixir, thiamine hydrochloride 1 mg, riboflavine 250 micrograms, nicotinamide 5 mg, pyridoxine hydrochloride 250 micrograms, cyanocobalamin 2.5 micrograms, choline dihydrogen citrate 225 mg, inositol 25 mg, proteolysed liver ≡ 2.5 g fresh liver, methionine 18.75 mg/5 ml. Price 100 ml = **D**

9.6.3 Vitamin C
(Ascorbic acid)

Vitamin C therapy is essential in scurvy, but less florid manifestations of vitamin C deficiency are commonly found, especially in the elderly. It is rarely necessary to prescribe more than 100 mg daily except early in the treatment of scurvy.

Claims that vitamin C ameliorates colds or promotes wound healing have not been proved.

ASCORBIC ACID

Indications: prevention and treatment of scurvy

Dose: prophylactic, 25–75 mg daily; therapeutic, not less than 250 mg daily in divided doses

Ascorbic Acid Tablets, ascorbic acid 25, 50 and 100 mg, price 20 tabs (all) = **A**; 200 mg, price 20 tabs = **B**; 500 mg, price 20 tabs = **C**

PoM **Ascorbic Acid Injection,** ascorbic acid 100 mg/ml. Price 5 ml amp = **B**

NHS **Roscorbic®** (Sauter)

Tablets, ascorbic acid 25, 50, or 200 mg, price 20 tabs (all) = **A**

Tablets, ascorbic acid 500 mg. Price 20 tabs = **B**

Tablets, effervescent, ascorbic acid 1 g. Price 20 tabs = **C**. Label: 13

9.6.4 Vitamin D
(Cholecalciferol; Ergocalciferol)

Simple vitamin D deficiency, which is not uncommon in Asians consuming unleavened bread and in the elderly living alone, can be prevented by taking an oral supplement of only 10 micrograms (400 units) **calciferol** daily.

C = 51-100p, **D** = 101-180p, **E** = 181-300p, **F** = 301-450p, **G** = 451-650p, **H** = 651-900p, **I** = 901-1200p, **J** = over 1200p.

Vitamin D deficiency caused by intestinal malabsorption or chronic liver disease usually requires pharmacological doses of up to 1 mg (40 000 units) daily, and patients with renal osteodystrophy may require as much as 5 mg (200 000 units) daily.

The hypocalcaemia of hypoparathyroidism often requires doses of up to 5 mg (200 000 units) daily in order to achieve normocalcaemia and **dihydrotachysterol** may be used as an alternative but is much more expensive.

Alfacalcidol (1α-hydroxycholecalciferol, One-alpha®) or **calcitriol** (1α,25-dihydroxycholecalciferol, Rocaltrol®) should be prescribed for anephric patients; these preparations offer no advantages over calciferol in the treatment of simple vitamin D deficiency and offer few advantages in other patients where pharmacological doses of vitamin D are required. Both alfacalcidol and calcitriol are considerably more expensive than calciferol.

All patients receiving pharmacological doses of vitamin D should have the plasma calcium concentration checked at intervals and whenever nausea or vomiting are present.

Vitamin D preparations containing calcium are unnecessary and should be avoided. Breast milk from women taking pharmacological doses of vitamin D may cause hypercalcaemia if given to an infant.

For preparations of Vitamins A and D see section 9.6.1.

Preparations containing calciferol
Calciferol Tablets, High-strength, 10 000 units, BP 1980, s/c, cholecalciferol or ergocalciferol 250 micrograms. Price 20 tabs = **B**
Note: it is essential to include the words 'high-strength' in the prescription; these tablets are approximately one-fifth the strength of Strong Calciferol Tablets BP 1973
Calcium with Vitamin D Tablets, calcium sodium lactate 450 mg (or calcium lactate 300 mg), calcium phosphate 150 mg, ergocalciferol 12.5 micrograms (500 units). Price 20 tabs = **A**
Calciferol Solution, cholecalciferol or ergocalciferol 75 micrograms (3000 units)/ml in oil. Price 100 ml = **D**
PoM **Calciferol Injection,** BP 1980, 7.5 mg (300 000 units)/ml in oil. Price 1- and 2-ml amp (both) = **C**

NHS **Chocovite**® (Medo)
Tablets, brown, ergocalciferol 15 micrograms (600 units), calcium gluconate 500 mg. Price 20 tabs = **B**
NHS **Sterogyl-15**® (Roussel)
Solution, for oral use, ergocalciferol 10 mg (400 000 units)/ml. Price 1.5-ml amp = **B**

Other vitamin D preparations
AT 10® (Sterling Research)
Solution, dihydrotachysterol 250 micrograms/ml. Price 15-ml dropper bottle = **J**
PoM **One-alpha**® (Leo)
Capsules, alfacalcidol 250 nanograms. Price 20 caps = **E**

Capsules, brown, alfacalcidol 1 microgram. Price 20 caps = **H**
Drops, alfacalcidol 5 micrograms/ml (250 nanograms/drop). Diluent, see below. Price 10 ml = **I**
Dose: ADULTS and CHILDREN over 20 kg, initially 1 microgram daily, adjusted according to the response; CHILD under 20 kg, 50 nanograms/kg daily. Maintenance 0.25–1 microgram daily
One-alpha Drops Diluent® (Leo)
Price 100 ml = **D**
PoM **Rocaltrol**® (Roche)
Capsules, red/white, calcitriol 250 nanograms. Price 20 caps = **F**
Capsules, brown, calcitriol 500 nanograms. Price 20 caps = **G**
Dose: initially 1–2 micrograms daily, gradually increased to 2–3 micrograms daily
PoM **Tachyrol**® (Duphar)
Tablets, scored, dihydrotachysterol 200 micrograms. Price 20 tabs = **E**

9.6.5   Vitamin E
(Tocopherols)

There is little evidence that oral supplements of vitamin E are essential in adults, even where there is fat malabsorption secondary to cholestasis. In young children with congenital cholestasis, abnormally low vitamin E concentrations may be found in association with neuromuscular abnormalities, which usually respond only to the parenteral administration of vitamin E.

ALPHA TOCOPHERYL ACETATE
Indications: vitamin-E deficiency
Dose: 3 to 15 mg daily
Note: the potency of alpha tocopheryl acetate (that is, *all-rac*-α-tocopheryl acetate) is about 1 unit/mg, and the potency of *d*-α-tocopheryl is about 1.36 units/mg

Ephynal® (Roche)
Tablets, alpha tocopheryl acetate 3 mg. Price 20 tabs = **A**
Tablets, alpha tocopheryl acetate 10 mg. Price 20 tabs = **A**
Tablets, scored, alpha tocopheryl acetate 50 mg. Price 20 tabs = **B**
Tablets, cream, scored, alpha tocopheryl acetate 200 mg. Price 20 tabs = **D**
Vita-E® (Bioglan)
Gels (= capsules), yellow, *d*-α-tocopheryl acetate 75 units. Price 20 caps = **B**
Gels (= capsules), yellow, *d*-α-tocopheryl acetate 200 units. Price 20 caps = **C**
Gels (= capsules), red, *d*-α-tocopheryl acetate 400 units. Price 20 caps = **D**
Gelucaps® (= tablets), chewable, yellow, *d*-α-tocopheryl acetate 75 units. Price 20 tabs = **B**. Label: 24
Succinate tablets, yellow, *d*-α-tocopheryl succinate 50 units, price 20 tabs = **B**; 200 units, price 20 tabs = **C**

9.6.6   Vitamin K

Vitamin K is necessary for the production of blood clotting factors and proteins necessary for the normal calcification of bone. In neonates deficiency of vitamin K may occur because the gut is

---

sterile and there is no synthesis of the vitamin by *Escherichia coli*.

Because vitamin K is fat soluble, patients with fat malabsorption, especially if due to biliary obstruction or hepatic disease, may become deficient.

Oral coumarin anticoagulants act by interfering with vitamin K metabolism in the hepatic cells and their effects can be antagonised by giving vitamin K.

Vitamin-K deficiency in neonates may be treated with **phytomenadione** (vitamin K_1), 1 mg by intramuscular or intravenous injection. Synthetic analogues of vitamin K, such as menadiol sodium diphosphate, should be avoided because of the risk of kernicterus.

Haemorrhage associated with hypoprothrombinaemia caused by overdosage of anticoagulants may be treated with phytomenadione 2.5 to 20 mg by slow intravenous injection. Hypoprothrombinaemia due to anticoagulants, but without haemorrhage may be treated with phytomenadione 10 to 20 mg by mouth.

For the prevention of vitamin-K deficiency in malabsorption syndromes (for example obstructive jaundice), a water-soluble preparation, **menadiol sodium diphosphate** must be used; the usual dose is about 10 mg daily by mouth or by injection.

After correction of hypoprothrombinaemia, resistance to oral anticoagulants persists for up to two weeks; patients with prosthetic valves who need to continue anticoagulant therapy but who bleed, should be treated with fresh plasma to elevate the prothrombin levels and the anticoagulant dose reduced.

MENADIOL SODIUM DIPHOSPHATE

Indications: Dose: see notes above
Cautions: pregnancy. Drug interactions: see Appendix 1 (sections *2.8, 2.8A*)

Synkavit® (Roche)
Tablets, scored, menadiol sodium diphosphate equivalent to 10 mg of menadiol phosphate. Price 20 tabs = **B**
PoM *Injection*, menadiol sodium diphosphate equivalent to 10 mg of menadiol phosphate/ml. Price 1-ml amp = **B**

PHYTOMENADIONE

Indications: Dose: see notes above
Cautions: intravenous injections should be given very slowly. Drug interactions: see Appendix 1 (sections *2.8, 2.8A*)

Phytomenadione Tablets, phytomenadione 10 mg, price 25 tabs = **F**. Label: 24
PoM **Phytomenadione Injection,** phytomenadione 2 mg/ml, price 0.5-ml amp = **A**; 10 mg/ml, price 1-ml amp = **B**
Konakion® (Roche)
Tablets, s/c, phytomenadione 10 mg. Price 25 tabs = **F**. Label: 24
PoM *Injection*, phytomenadione 2 mg/ml. Price 0.5-ml amp = **A**

PoM *Injection*, phytomenadione 10 mg/ml. Price 1-ml amp = **B**

9.6.7 Multivitamin preparations

There are many preparations available. The proprietary preparations have no advantage over the non-proprietary preparations given separately and many are expensive.

Vitamins Capsules, ascorbic acid 15 mg, nicotinamide 7.5 mg, riboflavine 500 micrograms, thiamine hydrochloride 1 mg, vitamin A 2500 units, vitamin D 300 units. Price 20 caps = **A**
Abidec® (P-D)
NHS *Capsules*, vitamin A 4000 units, thiamine hydrochloride 1 mg, riboflavine 1 mg, nicotinamide 10 mg, pyridoxine hydrochloride 500 micrograms, ascorbic acid 25 mg, ergocalciferol 400 units. Price 20 caps = **B**
Drops, vitamin A 4000 units, thiamine hydrochloride 1 mg, riboflavine 400 micrograms, nicotinamide 5 mg, pyridoxine hydrochloride 500 micrograms, ascorbic acid 50 mg, ergocalciferol 400 units/0.6 ml. Price 2 × 25 ml (with dropper) = **D**
NHS **Allbee with C**® (Robins)
Capsules, yellow/green, thiamine mononitrate 15 mg, riboflavine 10 mg, nicotinamide 50 mg, pyridoxine hydrochloride 5 mg, ascorbic acid 300 mg, calcium pantothenate 10 mg. Price 20 caps = **C**
NHS **BC 500**® (Ayerst)
Tablets, orange, f/c, thiamine mononitrate 25 mg, riboflavine 12.5 mg, nicotinamide 100 mg, pyridoxine hydrochloride 10 mg, cyanocobalamin 5 micrograms, ascorbic acid 500 mg (as sodium salt), calcium pantothenate 20 mg. Price 20 tabs = **C**
NHS **Bravit**® (Galen)
Capsules, orange, thiamine mononitrate 15 mg, riboflavine 10 mg, nicotinamide 50 mg, pyridoxine hydrochloride 5 mg, ascorbic acid 300 mg. Price 20 caps = **C**
Tablets, orange, s/c, thiamine hydrochloride 50 mg, riboflavine 5 mg, nicotinamide 200 mg, pyridoxine hydrochloride 5 mg, ascorbic acid 100 mg. Price 20 tabs = **C**
NHS **Calcimax**® (Wallace Mfg)
Syrup (= elixir), brown, thiamine hydrochloride 500 micrograms, riboflavine 125 micrograms, nicotinamide 2 mg, pyridoxine hydrochloride 125 micrograms, cyanocobalamin 125 nanograms, ascorbic acid 5 mg, ergocalciferol 400 units, calcium glycine hydrochloride 500 mg, calcium pantothenate 125 micrograms/5 ml. Price 150 ml = **C**
NHS **Ce-Cobalin**® (Paines & Byrne)
Syrup (= elixir), cyanocobalamin 30 micrograms, ascorbic acid 10 mg/5 ml. Price 100 ml = **C**
NHS **Concavit**® (Wallace Mfg)
Capsules, vitamin A 5000 units, thiamine hydrochloride 2.5 mg, nicotinamide 20 mg, riboflavine 2.5 mg, pyridoxine hydrochloride 1 mg, cyanocobalamin 5 micrograms, ascorbic acid 40 mg, ergocalciferol 500 units, calcium pantothenate 5 mg, vitamin E 2 units. Price 20 caps = **C**
Drops and *syrup* (= elixir), vitamin A 5000 units, thiamine hydrochloride 2 mg, riboflavine 1 mg, nicotinamide 12.5 mg, pyridoxine hydrochloride 1 mg, cyanocobalamin 5 micrograms, ascorbic acid 50 mg, ergocalciferol 500 units, panthenol 2 mg/0.5 ml (drops) and 5 ml (syrup). Price drops 15 ml = **C**; syrup 150 ml = **D**
Dalivit® (Paines & Byrne)
NHS PoM *Capsules*, red, vitamin A 10000 units, thiamine mononitrate 3 mg, riboflavine 3 mg, nicotinamide

25 mg, pyridoxine hydrochloride 1 mg, ascorbic acid 75 mg, vitamin D 1000 units, calcium pantothenate 5 mg. Price 20 caps = **B**

Oral drops (= elixir), vitamin A 5000 units, thiamine hydrochloride 1 mg, riboflavine 400 micrograms, nicotinamide 5 mg, pyridoxine hydrochloride 500 micrograms, ascorbic acid 50 mg, vitamin D 400 units/0.6 ml. Price 15 ml = **B**

NHS PoM *Syrup* (= elixir), vitamin A 5000 units, thiamine hydrochloride 2.5 mg, riboflavine 1 mg, nicotinamide 10 mg, pyridoxine hydrochloride 1 mg, ascorbic acid 25 mg, vitamin D 1000 units, calcium pantothenate 5 mg/5 ml. Price 100 ml = **C**

NHS **Dayovite**® (Cox Pharmaceuticals)

Effervescent granules, thiamine mononitrate 25 mg, riboflavine 12.5 mg (as sodium phosphate), nicotinamide 20 mg, pyridoxine hydrochloride 10 mg, cyanocobalamin 5 micrograms, ascorbic acid 500 mg (as sodium ascorbate), calcium pantothenate 20 mg/sachet. Price 30 × 4-g sachet = **E**. Label: 13

NHS **Juvel**® (Bencard)

Tablets, yellow, s/c, vitamin A 5000 units, thiamine hydrochloride 2.5 mg, riboflavine 2.5 mg, nicotinamide 50 mg, pyridoxine hydrochloride 2.5 mg, ascorbic acid 50 mg, vitamin D 500 units. Price 20 tabs = **B**

Elixir, vitamin A 4000 units, thiamine hydrochloride 2 mg, riboflavine 2 mg, nicotinamide 40 mg, pyridoxine hydrochloride 2 mg, ascorbic acid 40 mg, vitamin D 400 units/5 ml. Diluent syrup, life of diluted elixir 14 days. Price 100 ml = **B**

NHS **Lance B+C**® (Kirby-Warrick)

Tablets, red, s/c, thiamine hydrochloride 50 mg, riboflavine 5 mg, nicotinamide 200 mg, pyridoxine hydrochloride 5 mg, ascorbic acid 100 mg. Price 20 tabs = **B**

NHS **Minamino**® (Consolidated)

Syrup (= elixir), thiamine hydrochloride 15 mg, riboflavine 2 mg, pyridoxine hydrochloride 1.75 mg, nicotinamide 20 mg, cyanocobalamin 5 micrograms/5 ml, with amino acids, extracts of liver, spleen, and gastric mucosa, iron citrate, manganese sulphate, and copper sulphate. Price 100 ml = **B**

NHS **Multivitamins** (Evans)

Tablets, brown, s/c, vitamin A 2500 units, thiamine hydrochloride 1 mg, riboflavine 500 micrograms, nicotinamide 7.5 mg, ascorbic acid 15 mg, vitamin D 300 units. Price 20 tabs = **A**

NHS **Multivite**® (DF)

Pellets, brown, s/c, vitamin A 2500 units, thiamine hydrochloride 500 micrograms, ascorbic acid 12.5 mg, vitamin D 250 units. Price 20 pellets = **A**

NHS **Orovite**® (Bencard)

Tablets, maroon, s/c, thiamine hydrochloride 50 mg, riboflavine 5 mg, nicotinamide 200 mg, pyridoxine hydrochloride 5 mg, ascorbic acid 100 mg. Price 20 tabs = **C**

Elixir, thiamine hydrochloride 20 mg, riboflavine 2 mg, nicotinamide 80 mg, pyridoxine hydrochloride 2 mg, ascorbic acid 40 mg/5 ml. Diluent syrup, life of diluted elixir 14 days. Price 100 ml = **C**

NHS **Orovite 7**® (Bencard)

Granules, orange, vitamin A 2500 units (as palmitate), thiamine mononitrate 1.4 mg, riboflavine sodium phosphate 1.7 mg, nicotinamide 18 mg, pyridoxine hydrochloride 2 mg, ascorbic acid 60 mg, ergocalciferol 100 units/sachet. Price 20 × 5-g sachet = **D**. Label: 13

NHS PoM **Polyvite**® (Medo)

Capsules, red, vitamin A 4500 units, thiamine hydrochloride 2.5 mg, riboflavine 1.5 mg, nicotinamide 15 mg, pyridoxine hydrochloride 1.5 mg, ascorbic acid 30 mg, ergocalciferol 11 micrograms, calcium pantothenate 2 mg. Price 20 caps = **B**

NHS **Surbex T**® (Abbott)

Tablets, orange, thiamine mononitrate 15 mg, riboflavine 10 mg, nicotinamide 100 mg, pyridoxine hydrochloride 5 mg, ascorbic acid 500 mg. Price 20 tabs = **C**

NHS PoM **Tonivitan**® (Medo)

Capsules, brown, vitamin A 4500 units, thiamine hydrochloride 1 mg, nicotinic acid 15 mg, ascorbic acid 15 mg, ergocalciferol 600 units, dried yeast 50 mg. Price 20 caps = **B**

NHS **Verdiviton**® (Squibb)

Elixir, green, thiamine mononitrate 667 micrograms, riboflavine 334 micrograms, nicotinamide 5 mg, pyridoxine hydrochloride 167 micrograms, cyanocobalamin 5 micrograms, calcium glycerophosphate 36.7 mg, dexpanthenol 334 micrograms, manganese glycerophosphate 3.34 mg, potassium glycerophosphate 6.7 mg, sodium glycerophosphate 26.7 mg/5 ml. Diluents syrup or water for preparations, life of diluted elixir 14 days. Price 240 ml = **D**

NHS **Vi-Daylin**® (Abbott)

Syrup (= elixir), vitamin A 3000 units (as palmitate), thiamine hydrochloride 1.5 mg, riboflavine 1.2 mg, nicotinamide 10 mg, pyridoxine hydrochloride 1 mg, ascorbic acid 50 mg, ergocalciferol 400 units/5 ml. Diluent syrup, life of diluted elixir 14 days. Price 100 ml = **C**

NHS **Vitavel**® (Bencard)

Elixir, orange, sugar-free, vitamin A 500 units (as palmitate), thiamine mononitrate 300 micrograms, riboflavine 400 micrograms, nicotinamide 4.5 mg, ascorbic acid 10 mg, ergocalciferol 200 units/5 ml when reconstituted with water for preparations. Life of reconstituted product 30 days, on further dilution life reduced to 15 days. Price 150 ml = **D**

9.7   Bitters and tonics

Mixtures containing simple and aromatic bitters, such as alkaline gentian mixture, are traditional remedies for loss of appetite. All depend on suggestion and there is no advantage in prescribing the many exotically coloured and flavoured products which are available. Such preparations frequently contain, in addition to a bitter principle, various vitamins or an iron salt (section 9.1.1.1).

Gentian Mixture, Acid (see Formulary). Price 100 ml = **A**

Gentian Mixture, Alkaline (see Formulary). Price 100 ml = **A**

NHS PoM **Aneurone**® (Philip Harris)

Mixture, strychnine hydrochloride 250 micrograms, thiamine hydrochloride 500 micrograms, caffeine 15 mg, compound gentian infusion 1.25 ml, sodium acid phosphate 30 mg/5 ml. Diluent syrup, life of diluted mixture 14 days. Price 100 ml = **B**

NHS **Effico**® (Pharmax)

Tonic (= elixir), green, thiamine hydrochloride 180 micrograms, nicotinamide 2.1 mg, caffeine 20.2 mg, compound gentian infusion 0.31 ml/5 ml. Diluent syrup, life of diluted elixir 14 days. Price 100 ml = **A**

NHS **Labiton**® (LAB)

Tonic (= elixir), brown, thiamine hydrochloride 375 micrograms, aminobenzoic acid 2 mg, glycerophosphoric acid (20%) 0.01 ml, caffeine 3.5 mg, kola nut dried extract 3.025 mg, alcohol 1.39 ml/5 ml. Price 100 ml = **B**

NHS **Metatone**® (P-D)

Tonic (= elixir), thiamine hydrochloride 500 micrograms, calcium glycerophosphate 45.6 mg, manganese glycerophosphate 5.7 mg, potassium glycerophosphate 45.6 mg, sodium glycerophosphate 22.8 mg/5 ml. Diluent water for preparations, life of diluted elixir 14 days. Price 100 ml = **A**

Relative prices: **A** = up to 20p, **B** = 21-50p,

10: Drugs used in the treatment of
MUSCULOSKELETAL and JOINT DISEASES

In this chapter, drug treatment is discussed under the following headings:

10.1 Drugs used in rheumatic diseases and gout
10.2 Drugs used in other musculoskeletal disorders
10.3 Drugs for the relief of soft-tissue inflammation

For treatment of septic arthritis see section 5.1, Table 1.

10.1 Drugs used in rheumatic diseases and gout

Most rheumatic diseases are treated symptomatically by relieving pain and stiffness. Suitable drugs are described in section 10.1.1; those with a prominent anti-inflammatory effect are particularly useful.

In certain circumstances corticosteroids (section 10.1.2) may be used to suppress inflammation. Drugs are also available which may affect the disease process itself and favourably influence the outcome. For rheumatoid arthritis these include penicillamine, gold, hydroxychloroquine, chloroquine and immunosuppressants (section 10.1.3) and for gout the uricosuric agents and allopurinol (section 10.1.4).

10.1.1 Anti-inflammatory analgesics
10.1.1.1 Aspirin and the salicylates
10.1.1.2 Other non-steroidal anti-inflammatory drugs
10.1.2 Corticosteroids and corticotrophin
10.1.2.1 Systemic corticosteroids and corticotrophin
10.1.2.2 Local corticosteroid injections
10.1.3 Drugs which may affect the rheumatic disease process
10.1.4 Drugs used in the treatment of gout

Analgesic preparations and doses—see also section 4.7.

10.1.1 Anti-inflammatory analgesics

Anti-inflammatory analgesics have two separate actions. Taken in *single doses* they have analgesic activity comparable to that of paracetamol (see section 4.7.1.1) or narcotic analgesics used in mild to moderate pain (see section 4.7.1.2). They can therefore be taken on demand for pain which is mild or intermittent or as a supplement to regular treatment.

Taken in *regular dosage* they have an anti-inflammatory effect. This combination of analgesic and anti-inflammatory properties makes these drugs particularly useful for treating conditions associated with pain and inflammation. Anti-inflammatory analgesics are therefore more appropriate than paracetamol or narcotic anal-

gesics in conditions such as rheumatoid arthritis, osteoarthritis, back pain, sprains, strains, traumatic conditions, frozen shoulder, fibrositis, other varieties of soft-tissue rheumatism, and most types of arthritis.

Aspirin has a dual role as an analgesic and anti-inflammatory drug. Certain of the anti-inflammatory analgesics included in section 10.1.1.2 have been particularly developed or promoted for their analgesic action. They include diflunisal, fenoprofen, ibuprofen, mefenamic acid, and naproxen sodium. As analgesics most of them are as effective as aspirin, but are more expensive.

Suitable analgesic doses, to be used when required, are indicated in section 4.7.1.1. Anti-inflammatory doses are given in sections 10.1.1.1 and 10.1.1.2. These more recently introduced anti-inflammatory analgesics have certain advantages over aspirin, paracetamol, and the narcotic analgesics of section 4.7.1.2 in that they are safer in overdosage and do not cause the tolerance, dependence, and respiratory depression associated with narcotics.

Paracetamol and the narcotic analgesics (see section 4.7) have no demonstrable anti-inflammatory activity and are therefore not included in this section.

The differences in anti-inflammatory activity between drugs of this group are small but there is enormous variation in individual patient response. About 60% of patients will respond to any drug of this class and those who do not respond to one drug may well respond to another. It is, therefore, often necessary to try several drugs before one is found that suits a particular patient. Most of the drugs should produce an effect within a few days and should be changed if ineffective after one week.

Dosage of anticoagulants may need to be adjusted when anti-inflammatory analgesics are used but the risk of haemorrhage is greatest with aspirin or other salicylates.

Aspirin is the traditional first choice as it is the oldest and least expensive drug of this group but many physicians prefer to start treatment with drugs such as those described in section 10.1.1.2 because they may be better tolerated.

10.1.1.1 ASPIRIN AND THE SALICYLATES

Aspirin in regular high dosage has about the same anti-inflammatory effect as indomethacin; 3.6 grams or more daily in divided doses is commonly used for active rheumatoid arthritis.

Doses below 2.4 grams of aspirin daily have few side-effects. Anti-inflammatory doses (3.6 grams or more daily) are associated with a much higher incidence of gastro-intestinal side-effects such as dyspepsia and gastric bleeding, or auditory side-effects, such as tinnitus, leading occasionally to deafness.

Gastro-intestinal side-effects may be minimised by taking the dose after food. Numerous formulations are available which improve gastric tolerance and minimise occult bleeding, including buffered and micro-encapsulated, dispersible, and enteric-coated preparations.

Benorylate (Benoral®), an aspirin-paracetamol ester, is broken down after absorption from the gastro-intestinal tract. Doses need only be given twice daily and gastric tolerance is slightly better than with aspirin. As it is more slowly absorbed than paracetamol, hepatotoxicity in overdosage may be reduced.

ASPIRIN

Indications: pain and inflammation in rheumatic disease and other musculoskeletal disorders (including Still's disease); see also section 4.7.1.1

Cautions: allergic disease, severe renal or hepatic impairment, dehydration, children (particularly under 1 year), pregnancy (particularly at term), breast-feeding, elderly patients, concurrent anticoagulant therapy. Drug interactions: see Appendix 1 (*2.2, 2.8, 2.8E, 4.7, 4.8, 8, 10*)

Contra-indications: peptic ulceration

Side-effects: common with anti-inflammatory doses; gastro-intestinal discomfort, ulceration, bleeding, or nausea, hearing disturbances such as tinnitus (leading rarely to deafness), vertigo, mental confusion, hypersensitivity reactions (angioedema, bronchospasm and rashes); rarely oedema, myocarditis, blood disorders, particularly thrombocytopenia

Dose: 0.3–1 g every 4 hours; max. in acute conditions 8 g daily; CHILD up to 80 mg/kg daily in 5–6 divided doses, increased in acute conditions to 130 mg/kg. Doses should be taken after food

Aspirin Tablets, aspirin 300 mg. Price 20 tabs = **A**. Label: 21
Aspirin Tablets, Dispersible, aspirin 300 mg. Price 20 tabs = **A**. Label: 13, 21
Aspirin Tablets, Dispersible, Paediatric, aspirin 75 mg. Price 20 tabs = **A**. Label: 13, 21
Proprietary preparations
See section 4.7.1.1

BENORYLATE

(Aspirin-paracetamol ester)
Indications: pain and inflammation in rheumatic disease (including Still's disease) and other musculoskeletal disorders; see also section 4.7.1.1

Cautions; Contra-indications: see under Aspirin (above) and Paracetamol (section 4.7.1.1)

Side-effects: see under Aspirin (above) and Paracetamol (section 4.7.1.1). Side-effects resemble those of aspirin rather than paracetamol but tolerance is better and hepatotoxicity may be less than with paracetamol

Dose: 4–8 g daily divided into 2–3 doses; CHILD 3

months–1 year 25 mg/kg up to 4 times daily, 1–2 years 250 mg up to 4 times daily, 3–5 years 500 mg up to 3 times daily, 6–12 years 500 mg up to 4 times daily *or* for acute rheumatic conditions in children 1–12 years, initially 200 mg/kg daily, adjusted after 7 days to maintain a plasma-salicylate concentration of 25–30 mg/100 ml. Doses should preferably be taken after food

Benoral® (Sterling Research)
Tablets, benorylate 750 mg. Price 20 tabs = **D**. Counselling advised, aspirin, paracetamol
Granules, benorylate 2-g/sachet. Price 10 sachets = **E**. Label: 13, counselling advised, aspirin, paracetamol
Suspension (= mixture), benorylate 2 g/5 ml. Diluent syrup, life of diluted mixture 14 days. Price 150 ml = **G**. Counselling advised, aspirin, paracetamol

CHOLINE MAGNESIUM TRISALICYLATE

Indications: pain and inflammation in rheumatic disease and other musculoskeletal disorders
Cautions; Contra-indications; Side-effects: see under Aspirin (above) but side-effects occur less frequently
Dose: 1–1.5 g of salicylate twice daily preferably after food

Trilisate® (Napp)
Tablets, orange, scored, choline magnesium trisalicylate ≡ salicylate 500 mg. Price 20 tabs = **D**. Label: 12

SALSALATE

Indications: pain and inflammation in mild rheumatic disease and other musculoskeletal disorders
Cautions; Contra-indications; Side-effects: see under Aspirin (above); side-effects may occur less frequently
Dose: 0.5–1 g 3–4 times daily preferably after food

PoM **Disalcid®** (Riker)
Capsules, orange/grey, salsalate 500 mg. Price 20 caps = **D**. Label: 12

SODIUM SALICYLATE

Indications: pain and inflammation in rheumatic disease; see also section 4.7.1.1
Cautions; Contra-indications; Side-effects: see under Aspirin (above). Caution in patients on low-sodium diet and in congestive heart failure; avoid in acute renal disease
Dose: 0.5–2 g with food, when necessary. In acute conditions 5–10 g daily in divided doses

Sodium Salicylate Mixture, sodium salicylate 250 mg/5 ml (see Formulary). Price 100 ml = **A**. Label: 21
Sodium Salicylate Mixture, Strong, sodium salicylate 500 mg/5 ml (see Formulary). Price 100 ml = **A**. Label: 21

10.1.1.2 OTHER NON-STEROIDAL ANTI-INFLAMMATORY DRUGS

Many of these drugs are similar in efficacy to aspirin and some are as effective as indomethacin but they have the advantage of causing fewer and less severe side-effects. They are sometimes preferred to aspirin for the treatment of conditions such as mild rheumatoid arthritis, osteoarthritis, minor rheumatic conditions, sprains, strains, and sports injuries or in elderly patients.

CAUTIONS. In general, they should be used with caution in gastric ulceration, allergic disorders (particularly asthma and hypersensitivity to salicylates), pregnancy, and renal and hepatic impairment. See also Drug interactions: Appendix 1 (sections 2.2, 2.5, 2.8C) and under individual entries.

SIDE-EFFECTS. Side-effects are generally mild and infrequent but include gastro-intestinal discomfort or occasionally bleeding, nausea, hypersensitivity reactions (particularly angioedema, asthma, and rashes), headache, vertigo, and hearing disturbances such as tinnitus. Blood disorders have occurred rarely with some of these anti-inflammatory drugs.

CHOICE OF DRUG. These non-steroidal anti-inflamatory drugs differ little from each other in efficacy though there is considerable variation in patient response, and the main differences between the drugs are in the incidence and type of side-effects. Before treatment is started the prescriber should weigh efficacy against side-effects for each drug.

Naproxen (Naprosyn®) has emerged as one of the first choices as it combines good efficacy with a low incidence of side-effects and administration is only twice daily, however, there are other drugs which are just as effective and just as well tolerated.

Diflunisal (Dolobid®) and **sulindac** (Clinoril®) are similar in tolerance to naproxen. Although diflunisal is an aspirin derivative its clinical effect more closely resembles the propionic acid derivatives (such as naproxen) than that of its parent compound. Its long half-life allows twice-daily administration.

Fenoprofen (Fenopron®) is as effective as naproxen, and **flurbiprofen** (Froben®) may be slightly more effective. Both are associated with slightly more gastro-intestinal side-effects than ibuprofen or naproxen.

Ibuprofen (Brufen® etc.) though associated with fewer side-effects than naproxen, has weaker anti-inflammatory properties. It is unsuitable for treating conditions where inflammation is prominent such as acute gout and ankylosing spondylitis.

Ketoprofen (Alrheumat®, Orudis®) has anti-inflammatory properties similar to ibuprofen and has more side-effects. A slow-release preparation (Oruvail®) is claimed to cause less gastro-intestinal irritation.

Azapropazone (Rheumox®) is similar in effect to naproxen and has a tendency to cause rashes. Although chemically related to phenylbutazone, on present evidence azapropazone does not give rise to blood disorders. Azapropazone is also used in the treatment of gout (section 10.1.4).

Other drugs with clinical properties similar to those of the propionic acid derivatives are diclofenac (Voltarol®), fenbufen (Lederfen®), piroxicam (Feldene®), tiaprofenic acid (Surgam®), and tolmetin (Tolectin®). Of these, **piroxicam** need only be given once daily and **diclofenac** is available as an injection.

Mefenamic acid (Ponstan®) is a related analgesic but its anti-inflammatory properties are minor and side-effects differ in that diarrhoea and occasionally haemolytic anaemia may occur which necessitate discontinuation of treatment.

Indomethacin (Indocid® etc.) can be given daily in divided doses but may give rise to headaches and gastro-intestinal side-effects. Indomethacin suppositories or sustained-release preparations (Indocid-R® etc.) administered at bedtime are useful for early morning stiffness. Indomethacin can also be used for acute gout (section 10.1.4).

Phenylbutazone (Butazolidin® etc.) is another potent anti-inflammatory drug but because of its serious side-effects its use is limited to the hospital treatment of ankylosing spondylitis. In addition to its gastric side-effects it has two rare and dangerous side-effects. It causes fluid retention and, in predisposed patients, may precipitate cardiac failure. It also causes agranulocytosis (which may occur within the first few days of treatment) and aplastic anaemia. In ankylosing spondylitis prolonged administration may be necessary but it should not be used unless other drugs have been tried and have failed.

WITHDRAWN DRUGS. Over the last few years several non-steroidal anti-inflammatory drugs have been withdrawn from the market, either by the manufacturers or on the recommendation of the Committee on Safety of Medicines and licensing authorities. They include benoxaprofen (Opren®), fenclofenac (Flenac®), feprazone (Methrazone®), flufenamic acid (Meralen®), Osmosin® (indomethacin), oxyphenbutazone (Tandacote®, Tanderil®), and zomepirac (Zomax®). In addition the licence for indoprofen (Flosint®) has been suspended until September 13, 1985 and the CSM has recommended that the use of phenylbutazone be restricted (see notes above).

AZAPROPAZONE

Indications: pain and inflammation in rheumatic disease and other musculoskeletal disorders; gout

Cautions; Side-effects: see notes above; photosensitivity has been reported. Avoid in hypersensitivity to phenylbutazone and related drugs. Drug interactions: see Appendix 1 (sections 2.8B, 4.8)

C = 51-100p, D = 101-180p, E = 181-300p, F = 301-450p, G = 451-650p, H = 651-900p, I = 901-1200p, J = over 1200p.

Dose: 1.2 g daily in 2 or 4 divided doses (elderly patients 300 mg in the morning and 300–600 mg at night), preferably after food; reduce for long-term therapy

Acute gout, initially 2.4 g in divided doses over 24 hours, then 1.8 g reducing to 1.2 g daily in divided doses

Chronic gout, 600 mg twice daily (elderly patients 300 mg in the morning and 300–600 mg at night)

PoM **Rheumox**® (Robins)
Capsules, orange, azapropazone 300 mg. Price 20 caps = **E**. Label: 11
Tablets, orange, f/c, scored, azapropazone 600 mg. Price 20 tabs = **G**. Label: 11

DICLOFENAC SODIUM

Indications: pain and inflammation in rheumatic disease and other musculoskeletal disorders; chronic juvenile arthritis; acute gout
Cautions; Side-effects: see notes above. Pain may occur at the injection site; suppositories may cause irritation. Drug interactions: see Appendix 1 (section *4.2*)
Dose: by mouth, 75–150 mg daily in 2–3 divided doses, preferably after food; reduce in long-term therapy
By deep intramuscular injection (in acute exacerbations), 75 mg 1–2 times daily
By rectum in suppositories, 100 mg, usually at night
Combined oral and rectal treatment, max. total daily dose 150 mg
CHILD, all routes, 1–3 mg/kg daily in divided doses

PoM **Voltarol**® (Geigy)
Tablets, yellow, e/c, diclofenac sodium 25 mg. Price 20 tabs = **E**. Label: 5, 25
Tablets, brown, e/c, diclofenac sodium 50 mg. Price 20 tabs = **F**. Label: 5, 25
Injection, diclofenac sodium 25 mg/ml. Price 3-ml amp = **C**
Suppositories, diclofenac sodium 100 mg. Price 10 suppos = **F**
Paediatric suppositories, diclofenac sodium 12.5 mg. Price 10 suppos = **C**
PoM **Voltarol Retard**® (Geigy)
Tablets, s/r, red, diclofenac sodium 100 mg. Price 28 tabs = **I**. Label: 25
Dose: 100 mg once daily

DIFLUNISAL

Indications: pain and inflammation in rheumatic disease and other musculoskeletal disorders; see also section 4.7.1.1
Cautions; Side-effects: see notes above; breast-feeding. Drug interactions: see Appendix 1 (sections *2.8C*, 4.7)
Dose: 250–500 mg twice daily preferably after food. Tablets should be swallowed whole

PoM **Dolobid**® (Morson)
Tablets, peach, f/c, diflunisal 250 mg. Price 20 tabs = **D**. Label: 25, counselling advised, avoid aluminium hydroxide
Tablets, orange, f/c, diflunisal 500 mg. Price 20 tabs = **F**. Label: 25, counselling advised, avoid aluminium hydroxide

FENBUFEN

Indications: pain and inflammation in rheumatic disease and other musculoskeletal disorders
Cautions; Side-effects: see notes above; hypersensitivity reactions, headache, vertigo, and hearing disturbances are rare; dosage adjustment is unnecessary except in severe renal impairment
Dose: 300 mg in the morning and 600 mg at bedtime, preferably after food

PoM **Lederfen**® (Lederle)
Capsules, dark blue, fenbufen 300 mg. Price 20 caps = **F**
Tablets, light blue, f/c, fenbufen 300 mg. Price 20 tabs = **F**

FENOPROFEN

Indications: pain and inflammation in rheumatic disease and other musculoskeletal disorders; see also section 4.7.1.1
Cautions; Side-effects: see notes above
Dose: 300–600 mg 3–4 times daily with food; max. 3 g daily

PoM **Fenopron 300**® (Dista)
Tablets, orange, fenoprofen 300 mg (as calcium salt). Price 20 tabs = **D**. Label: 21
PoM **Fenopron 600**® (Dista)
Tablets, orange, scored, fenoprofen 600 mg (as calcium salt). Price 20 tabs = **F**. Label: 21
Progesic
See section 4.7.1.1

FLURBIPROFEN

Indications: pain and inflammation in rheumatic disease and other musculoskeletal disorders
Cautions; Side-effects: see notes above. Drug interactions: see Appendix 1 (section *2.8C*)
Dose: 150–200 mg, daily in 3–4 divided doses, increased in acute conditions to 300 mg daily, preferably after food

PoM **Froben**® (Boots)
Tablets, yellow, s/c, flurbiprofen 50 mg. Price 20 tabs = **D**
Tablets, yellow, s/c, flurbiprofen 100 mg. Price 20 tabs = **F**

IBUPROFEN

Indications: pain and mild inflammation in rheumatic disease (including Still's disease) and other musculoskeletal disorders; see also section 4.7.1.1
Cautions; Side-effects: see notes above
Dose: 0.6–1.2 g daily in 3–4 divided doses preferably after food; increased if necessary up to a max. of 2.4 g daily; CHILD 20 mg/kg daily, children under 30 kg max. in 24 hours 500 mg

PoM **Ibuprofen Tablets**, f/c or s/c, ibuprofen 200 mg, price 20 tabs = **B**; 400 mg, price 20 tabs = **C**; 600 mg, price 20 tabs = **D**

Note: proprietary brands of ibuprofen tablets 200 mg are on sale to the public

PoM **Apsifen**® (APS)

Tablets, pink, f/c or s/c, ibuprofen 200 mg. Price 20 tabs = **B**

Tablets, pink, f/c or s/c, ibuprofen 400 mg. Price 20 tabs = **C**

Tablets, pink, f/c, ibuprofen 600 mg. Price 20 tabs = **D**

PoM **Brufen**® (Boots)

Tablets, magenta, s/c, ibuprofen 200 mg. Price 20 tabs = **C**

Tablets, magenta, s/c, ibuprofen 400 mg. Price 20 tabs = **D**

Tablets, magenta, f/c, ibuprofen 600 mg. Price 20 tabs = **E**

Syrup (= mixture), orange, ibuprofen 100 mg/ 5 ml. Diluent syrup, life of diluted mixture 14 days. Price 100 ml = **C**

PoM **Ebufac**® (DDSA)

Tablets, pink, s/c, ibuprofen 200 mg. Price 20 tabs = **B**

Tablets, pink, s/c, ibuprofen 400 mg. Price 20 tabs = **C**

PoM **Fenbid**® (SK&F)

Spansule® (= capsule s/r), maroon/pink, enclosing off-white pellets, ibuprofen 300 mg. Price 20 caps = **D**. Label: 25

Dose: 1–3 capsules every 12 hours

PoM **Motrin**® (Upjohn)

Tablets, red, f/c, ibuprofen 200 mg. Price 20 tabs = **B**

Tablets, orange, f/c, ibuprofen 400 mg. Price 20 tabs = **C**

Tablets, peach, f/c, ibuprofen 600 mg. Price 20 tabs = **D**

PoM **Paxofen**® (Steinhard)

Tablets, pink, f/c or s/c, ibuprofen 200 mg. Price 20 tabs = **C**

Tablets, pink, f/c or s/c, ibuprofen 400 mg. Price 20 tabs = **D**

Tablets, pink, f/c or s/c, ibuprofen 600 mg. Price 20 tabs = **E**

INDOMETHACIN

Indications: pain and moderate to severe inflammation in rheumatic disease and other acute musculoskeletal disorders; acute gout

Cautions: may impair the ability to drive or operate machinery; allergic disease, particularly asthma; hepatic and renal impairment, pregnancy, epilepsy, parkinsonism, psychiatric disturbances, elderly patients. During prolonged therapy ophthalmic and blood examinations are advisable. Avoid rectal administration in proctitis and haemorrhoids. Drug interactions: see Appendix 1 (sections *2.2, 2.4, 2.5, 2.8C, 4.2,* 10)

Contra-indications: peptic ulceration, salicylate hypersensitivity

Side-effects: frequently headache, dizziness, and light-headedness (especially initially but reduce dose or discontinue if headache is persistent);

gastro-intestinal discomfort, ulceration and bleeding (not always preceded by symptoms); rarely, drowsiness, mental confusion, depression, hypersensitivity reactions (bronchospasm, rashes, angioedema), syncope, hearing disturbances, blood disorders (particularly thrombocytopenia), hypertension, hyperglycaemia, blurred vision, corneal deposits, peripheral neuropathy. On rectal administration pruritus, discomfort, bleeding

Dose: by mouth, 25–50 mg 2–3 times daily, with milk or antacids, or after food, gradually increased if necessary; max. 200 mg daily

Night pain or morning stiffness, 100 mg at bedtime

Treatment is usually for 5–14 days after which in rheumatic disease it may be reduced to a maintenance dose according to the patient's requirements

Acute gout and other acute self-limiting conditions, 50–100 mg, repeated after a few hours if necessary, then every 6 hours, reducing dose according to response

By rectum in suppositories, 100 mg at night, repeated in the morning if required

Combined oral and rectal treatment, max. total daily dose 150–200 mg

PoM **Indomethacin Capsules,** indomethacin 25 mg, price 20 caps = **B**; 50 mg, price 20 caps = **C**. Label: 21

PoM **Indomethacin Suppositories,** indomethacin 100 mg. Price 10 suppos = **D**

PoM **Artracin**® (DDSA)

Capsules, yellow, indomethacin 25 mg. Price 20 caps = **C**. Label: 21

Capsules, yellow, indomethacin 50 mg. Price 20 caps = **D**. Label: 21

PoM **Imbrilon**® (Berk)

Capsules, yellow, indomethacin 25 mg. Price 20 caps = **C**. Label: 21

Capsules, yellow, indomethacin 50 mg. Price 20 caps = **D**. Label: 21

Suppositories, indomethacin 100 mg. Price 10 suppos = **D**

PoM **Indocid**® (Morson)

Capsules, indomethacin 25 mg. Price 20 caps= **C**. Label: 21

Capsules, indomethacin 50 mg. Price 20 caps = **D**. Label: 21

Suspension (= mixture), indomethacin 25 mg/ 5 ml. Do not dilute. Price 100 ml = **D**. Label: 21

Suppositories, indomethacin 100 mg. Price 10 suppos = **E**

PoM **Indocid-R**® (Morson)

Capsules, s/r, ivory/clear, enclosing white and blue pellets, indomethacin 75 mg. Price 20 caps = **G**. Label: 21, 25

Dose: 1–2 capsules daily

PoM **Indoflex**® (Unimed)

Capsules, indomethacin 25 mg. Price 20 caps = **C**. Label: 21

PoM **Indolar**® (Lagap)

Capsules, yellow, indomethacin 25 mg. Price 20 caps = **C**. Label: 21

C = 51-100p, **D** = 101-180p, **E** = 181-300p, **F** = 301-450p, **G** = 451-650p, **H** = 651-900p, **I** = 901-1200p, **J** = over 1200p.

Capsules, yellow, indomethacin 50 mg. Price 20 caps = **D**. Label: 21

PoM **Indolar SR**® (Lagap)

Capsules, s/r, blue/clear, enclosing white pellets, indomethacin 75 mg. Price 20 caps = **F**. Label: 21, 25

Dose: 1 capsule 1–2 times daily

PoM **Mobilan**® (Galen)

Capsules, purple/blue, indomethacin 25 mg. Price 20 caps = **C**. Label: 21

Capsules, purple/blue, indomethacin 50 mg. Price 20 caps = **D**. Label: 21

PoM **Rheumacin LA**® (CP)

Capsules, s/r, yellow/maroon, enclosing off-white pellets, indomethacin 75 mg. Price 20 caps = **E**. Label: 21, 25

Dose: 1–2 capsules daily

INDOPROFEN

Indications: pain and inflammation in rheumatoid arthritis, osteoarthritis, ankylosing spondylitis, and related conditions

Cautions; Side-effects: see notes above

Dose: 200–600 mg daily in 2–3 divided doses with food, increased to 800 mg daily in severe conditions

▼ PoM **Flosint**® (Farmitalia Carlo Erba)

Product licence suspended until September 13, 1985

KETOPROFEN

Indications: pain and mild inflammation in rheumatic disease and other musculoskeletal disorders

Cautions; Side-effects: see notes above; suppositories may cause irritation. Drug interactions: see Appendix 1 (section 4.7)

Dose: by mouth, 100–200 mg daily in 2–4 divided doses after food

By rectum in suppositories, 100 mg usually at bedtime

Combined oral and rectal treatment, max. total daily dose 200 mg

PoM **Ketoprofen Capsules,** ketoprofen 50 mg, price 20 caps = **D**; 100 mg, price 20 caps = **E**. Label: 21

PoM **Ketoprofen Suppositories,** ketoprofen 100 mg. Price 7 suppos = **E**

PoM **Alrheumat**® (Bayer)

Capsules, cream, ketoprofen 50 mg. Price 20 caps = **D**. Label: 21

PoM **Orudis**® (M&B)

Capsules, green/purple, ketoprofen 50 mg. Price 20 caps = **D**. Label: 21

Capsules, pink, ketoprofen 100 mg. Price 20 caps = **E**. Label: 21

Suppositories, ketoprofen 100 mg. Price 7 suppos = **E**

PoM **Oruvail**® (M&B)

Capsules, s/r, pink/purple, enclosing white pellets, ketoprofen 100 mg. Price 20 caps = **F**. Label: 21, 25

Capsules, s/r, pink/white, enclosing white pellets, ketoprofen 200 mg. Price 28 caps = **I**. Label: 21, 25

Dose: 100–200 mg once daily with food

MEFENAMIC ACID

Indications: mild to moderate pain in rheumatoid arthritis (including Still's disease), osteoarthritis, and related conditions; see also section 4.7.1.1

Cautions: allergic disease, particularly asthma; blood tests required during long-term treatment. Drug interactions: see Appendix 1 (section *2.8C, 4.2*)

Contra-indications: inflammatory bowel disease, peptic ulceration, renal and hepatic impairment, pregnancy

Side-effects: drowsiness, dizziness, gastro-intestinal disturbances, bleeding, nausea, occasionally ulceration; withdraw treatment in severe diarrhoea, hypersensitivity, bronchospasm, rashes, cholestatic jaundice, thrombocytopenia, haemolytic anaemia; convulsions in overdosage

Dose: 500 mg 3 times daily after food; CHILD over 6 months, 25 mg/kg daily in divided doses for not longer than 7 days, except in juvenile chronic arthritis (Still's disease)

PoM **Ponstan**® (P-D)

Capsules, ivory/blue, mefenamic acid 250 mg. Price 20 caps = **C**. Label: 21

Tablets forte, yellow, f/c, mefenamic acid 500 mg. Price 20 tabs = **E**. Label: 21

Paediatric suspension (= mixture), mefenamic acid 50 mg/5 ml. Diluent syrup, life of diluted mixture 14 days. Price 125 ml = **E**. Label: 21

PoM **Ponstan Dispersible**® (P-D)

Dispersible tablets, blue, mefenamic acid 250 mg. Price 20 tabs = **E**. Label: 13, 21

NAPROXEN

Indications: pain and inflammation in rheumatic disease and other musculoskeletal disorders; acute gout; see also Naproxen Sodium, section 4.7.1.1

Cautions; Side-effects: see notes above. Drug interactions: see Appendix 1 (section 4.7)

Dose: by mouth in rheumatic disease, 0.5–1 g daily in 2 divided doses (the larger dose at bedtime to relieve morning stiffness); CHILD over 5 years 10 mg/kg daily in 2 divided doses, preferably after food

Acute musculoskeletal disorders, 500 mg initially, then 250 mg every 6–8 hours as required

Acute gout, 750 mg initially, then 250 mg every 8 hours

By rectum in suppositories, 500 mg at bedtime

Combined oral and rectal treatment, max. total daily dose 1 g daily

PoM **Naprosyn**® (Syntex)

Tablets, yellow, scored, naproxen 250 mg. Price 20 tabs = **E**

Tablets, yellow, scored, naproxen 500 mg. Price 20 tabs = **F**

Suspension (= mixture), yellow, naproxen 125 mg/5 ml. Diluent water for preparations or equal quantities of syrup and water for preparations, life of diluted mixture 14 days. Price 100 ml = **D**

Suppositories, naproxen 500 mg. Price 10 suppos = **E**

Synflex: see section 4.7.1.1

PHENYLBUTAZONE

Indications: ankylosing spondylitis (in hospital)

Cautions: blood counts before and during treatment if for more than 7 days; elderly patients (reduce dose); breast-feeding; withdraw treatment if acute pulmonary syndrome including fever and dyspnoea occurs. Drug interactions: see Appendix 1 (sections *2.5, 2.8B, 4.2, 4.8, 6.1, 6.2, 8*, 10)

Contra-indications: cardiovascular disease, renal and hepatic impairment; pregnancy; history of peptic ulceration, gastro-intestinal haemorrhage, or blood disorders; thyroid disease

Side-effects: gastro-intestinal disorders, allergic reactions, rash; occasionally nausea, vomiting, parotitis, stomatitis, goitre, pancreatitis, hepatitis, nephritis, oedema, headache, visual disturbances; rarely leucopenia, thrombocytopenia, agranulocytosis, aplastic anaemia, erythema multiforme, toxic epidermal necrolysis

Dose: 200 mg 2–3 times daily, with milk or antacids if necessary, or after food, usually for 2 days, then reduced to effective minimum, usually 100 mg 2–3 times daily

Not for children under 14 years

PoM **Phenylbutazone Tablets**, f/c or s/c, phenylbutazone 100 and 200 mg, price 20 tabs (both) = **A**. Label: 21

PoM **Butacote**® (Geigy)

Tablets, violet, e/c, s/c, phenylbutazone 100 mg. Price 20 tabs = **B**. Label: 5, 21, 25

Tablets, violet, e/c, s/c, phenylbutazone 200 mg. Price 20 tabs = **C**. Label: 5, 21, 25

PoM **Butazolidin**® (Geigy)

Tablets, red, s/c, phenylbutazone 100 mg. Price 20 tabs = **B**. Label: 21

Tablets, s/c, phenylbutazone 200 mg. Price 20 tabs = **C**. Label: 21

PoM **Butazone**® (DDSA)

Tablets, red, s/c, phenylbutazone 100 mg. Price 20 tabs = **A**. Label: 21

Tablets, s/c, phenylbutazone 200 mg. Price 20 tabs = **A**. Label: 21

PIROXICAM

Indications: pain and inflammation in rheumatic disease and other musculoskeletal disorders; acute gout

Cautions: see notes above. Prolonged administration of doses of 30 mg or more daily increases the risk of gastro-intestinal disturbances. Drug interactions: see Appendix 1 (sections *2.8C, 4.2*)

Side-effects: see notes above; also, oedema, which may precipitate congestive cardiac failure in the elderly

Dose: initially 20 mg daily preferably after food,

maintenance 10–30 mg daily, in single or divided doses

Acute musculoskeletal disorders, 40 mg daily in single or divided doses for 2 days, then 20 mg daily for 7–14 days

Acute gout, 40 mg initially, then 40 mg daily in single or divided doses for 4–6 days

PoM **Feldene**® (Pfizer)

Capsules, maroon/blue, piroxicam 10 mg. Price 20 caps = **E**

Capsules, maroon, piroxicam 20 mg. Price 20 caps = **G**

Dispersible tablets, scored, piroxicam 10 mg. Price 20 tabs = **F**. Label: 13

Dispersible tablets, piroxicam 20 mg. Price 20 tabs = **H**. Label: 13

Suppositories, piroxicam 20 mg. Price 10 suppos = **G**

SULINDAC

Indications: pain and inflammation in rheumatic disease and other musculoskeletal disorders; acute gout

Cautions; Side-effects: see notes above. Drug interactions: see Appendix 1 (section *2.8C*)

Dose: 200–300 mg twice daily with food; max 600 mg daily

Acute gout, 200–300 mg twice daily for 7 days

PoM **Clinoril**® (MSD)

Tablets, yellow, scored, sulindac 100 mg. Price 20 tabs = **E**. Label: 21

Tablets, yellow, scored, sulindac 200 mg. Price 20 tabs = **F**. Label: 21

SUPROFEN

Indications: pain in rheumatic disease and other musculoskeletal disorders

Cautions; Side-effects: see notes above; also caution in fluid retention (mild peripheral oedema in long-term therapy)

Dose: 200 mg 3–4 times daily after food

▼ PoM **Suprol**® (Ortho-Cilag)

Capsules, ivory/green, suprofen 200 mg. Price 20 caps = **E**. Label: 21

TIAPROFENIC ACID

Indications: pain and inflammation in rheumatic disease and other musculoskeletal disorders

Cautions; Side-effects: see notes above

Dose: 600 mg daily in 2–3 divided doses preferably after food

▼ PoM **Surgam 200**® (Roussel)

Tablets, tiaprofenic acid 200 mg. Price 20 tabs = **F**

▼ PoM **Surgam 300**® (Roussel)

Tablets, tiaprofenic acid 300 mg. Price 20 tabs = **G**

TOLMETIN

Indications: pain and inflammation in rheumatic disease (including Still's disease) and other musculoskeletal disorders

---

C = 51-100p, **D** = 101-180p, **E** = 181-300p, **F** = 301-450p, **G** = 451-650p, **H** = 651-900p, **I** = 901-1200p, **J** = over 1200p.

Cautions; Side-effects: see notes above

Dose: initially 400 mg 3 times daily preferably with food, adjusted according to response to 0.6–1.8 g daily in divided doses; CHILD 20–25 mg/kg to a max. of 1.8 g daily in 3 or 4 divided doses

PoM **Tolectin**® (Ortho-Cilag)

Tablets, scored, tolmetin 200 mg (as sodium salt). Price 20 tabs = **D**

PoM **Tolectin DS**® (Ortho-Cilag)

Capsules, ivory/blue, tolmetin 400 mg (as sodium salt). Price 20 caps = **E**

10.1.2   Corticosteroids and corticotrophin

Drugs in this group have been divided into systemic corticosteroids and corticotrophin (section 10.1.2.1) and local corticosteroid injections (section 10.1.2.2).

10.1.2.1   SYSTEMIC CORTICOSTEROIDS AND CORTICOTROPHIN

The general actions and uses of the corticosteroids are described in section 6.3. Treatment with corticosteroids in rheumatic diseases should be reserved for specific indications when other anti-inflammatory drugs have proved unsuccessful.

For an *immunosuppressive* effect, an initial dose of corticosteroid is given to induce remission and the dose then gradually reduced to the lowest maintenance dose that will control the disease, or if possible discontinued altogether. A major problem is that relapse may occur as dosage reduction is made, particularly if this is carried out too rapidly. The tendency is therefore to increase and maintain dosage and consequently the patient becomes dependent on corticosteroids.

Prednisolone is used for most purposes although equivalent doses of most other corticosteroids can be used (see section 6.3.2 for table of equivalents). **Cortisone acetate** and **hydrocortisone** are unsuitable for antirheumatic treatment because they have a greater sodium-retaining effect. Corticosteroid-analgesic combination preparations are no longer used because the dosage of the components needs to be adjusted independently.

Corticosteroids should preferably be **avoided** in children as they prevent growth by suppressing the hypothalamic-pituitary-adrenal axis and corticotrophin (see section 6.5.1) may be used instead. However, alternate day treatment with prednisolone may be preferred to injections of corticotrophin after the initial treatment has controlled disease activity. Corticotrophin is sometimes used in resistant cases of frozen shoulder.

Polymyalgia rheumatica and *temporal (giant cell) arteritis* are always treated with corticosteroids. The usual initial dose of prednisolone in polymyalgia rheumatica is 10 to 15 mg daily and in temporal arteritis 40 to 60 mg daily (the higher dose being used if visual symptoms occur). Treat-

ment should be continued until remission occurs and doses then gradually reduced. Relapse is common if therapy is stopped within 3 years but most patients can discontinue treatment after approximately 3 to 6 years after which recurrences become rare.

Polyarteritis nodosa and *polymyositis* are usually treated with corticosteroids. An initial dose of 60 mg of prednisolone daily is often used and reduced to a maintenance dose of 10 or 15 mg daily.

Systemic lupus erythematosus is treated with corticosteroids when necessary using a similar dosage regimen to that for polyarteritis nodosa and polymyositis (above). Patients with pleurisy, pericarditis, or other systemic manifestations will respond to corticosteroids which can be reduced to alternate-day treatment and then gradually withdrawn. In some mild cases corticosteroid treatment may be stopped after a few months. Many mild cases of systemic lupus erythematosus do not require corticosteroid treatment.

Since effective doses of systemic corticosteroids may cause Cushing's syndrome these drugs should **not** be used to suppress symptoms of *rheumatoid arthritis* unless alternative anti-inflammatory drugs have proved unsuccessful. For an anti-inflammatory effect it is best to start with a small dose of corticosteroid and increase it gradually until an effective level is reached. When symptoms have subsided the dose should be gradually reduced. This procedure may be useful in elderly patients whose symptoms respond particularly well; similar doses may be used at night to relieve morning stiffness.

Ankylosing spondylitis should **not** be treated with corticosteroids. Corticotrophin is sometimes used in patients with acute *gout* who do not respond to the usual drugs (section 10.1.4).

See section 6.3.4 for systemic corticosteroids and their preparations. Dosage in rheumatic diseases should be calculated from the doses for prednisolone given in the notes.

10.1.2.2   LOCAL CORTICOSTEROID INJECTIONS

Corticosteroids are injected locally for an anti-inflammatory effect. In inflammatory conditions of the joints, particularly in rheumatoid arthritis, they are given by *intra-articular injection* to relieve pain, increase mobility, and reduce deformity in one or a few joints. Full aseptic precautions are essential. Infected areas and unstable joints should be avoided. On repeated injection joint damage has occurred (especially with the synthetic corticosteroids). An almost insoluble, long-acting compound such as triamcinolone hexacetonide is preferred for intra-articular injection.

Smaller amounts of corticosteroids may also be injected directly into soft tissues for the relief of inflammation in conditions such as *tennis elbow* or *compression neuropathies*. In *tendinitis*, injections should be made into the tendon sheath and not directly into the tendon. A soluble, short-acting compound such as prednisolone sodium phosphate is preferred for soft-tissue injection, to avoid possible tissue damage.

Cortisone acetate is **not** effective for local injection and hydrocortisone acetate or one of the synthetic analogues such as triamcinolone hexacetonide is generally used. The risk of necrosis and muscle wasting may be slightly increased.

Corticosteroid injections are also injected into soft tissues for the treatment of skin lesions (see section 13.4).

DEXAMETHASONE SODIUM PHOSPHATE

Indications: local inflammation of joints and soft tissues

Cautions; Contra-indications; Side-effects: see notes above and section 6.3.3

Dose: by intra-articular, intrasynovial, intralesional, or soft-tissue injection, dexamethasone 0.4–5 mg, according to size of joint or amount of soft-tissue, at intervals of 3–21 days according to response

Note: 1.3 mg dexamethasone sodium phosphate ≡ 1.2 mg dexamethasone phosphate ≡ 1 mg dexamethasone

PoM **Decadron**® (MSD)
Injection, dexamethasone phosphate 4 mg/ml (as sodium salt) (≡ 3.33 mg/ml dexamethasone). Price 2-ml vial = **D**

PoM **Oradexon**® (Organon)
Injection, dexamethasone sodium phosphate 5 mg/ml (≡ 3.84 mg/ml dexamethasone). Price 1-ml amp = **C**
Injection, dexamethasone 4 mg/ml (as sodium phosphate) (≡ 5.2 mg/ml dexamethasone sodium phosphate). Price 2-ml vial = **D**

HYDROCORTISONE ACETATE

Indications: local inflammation of joints and soft tissues

Cautions; Contra-indications; Side-effects: see notes above and section 6.3.3

Dose: by intra-articular, intrasynovial, or soft-tissue injection, 5–50 mg, according to joint size or amount of soft tissue; not more than 3 joints should be treated daily

PoM **Hydrocortisone Acetate Injection** (aqueous suspension), hydrocortisone acetate 25 mg/ml. Price 1-ml amp = **B**

PoM **Hydrocortistab**® (Boots)
Injection (aqueous suspension), hydrocortisone acetate 25 mg/ml. Price 5-ml vial = **D**

METHYLPREDNISOLONE ACETATE

Indications: local inflammation of joints and soft-tissues

Cautions; Contra-indications; Side-effects: see notes above and section 6.3.3

Dose: by intra-articular, intrasynovial, intralesional, or soft-tissue injection, 4–80 mg, according to joint size or amount of soft tissue, repeated every 1–5 weeks according to response

PoM **Depo-Medrone**® (Upjohn)
Injection (aqueous suspension), methylprednisolone acetate 40 mg/ml. Price 1-ml vial = **E**; 2-ml vial or syringe = **F**; 5-ml vial = **H**

PoM **Depo-Medrone with Lidocaine**® (Upjohn)
Injection (aqueous suspension), methylprednisolone acetate 40 mg, lignocaine hydrochloride 10 mg/ml. For injection into joints, bursae, or tendon sheaths. Price 2-ml vial = **F**

PREDNISOLONE ACETATE

Indications: local inflammation of joints and soft tissues

Cautions; Contra-indications; Side-effects: see notes above and section 6.3.3

Dose: by intra-articular, intrasynovial, or soft-tissue injection, 5–25 mg according to joint size or amount of soft tissue; not more than 3 joints should be treated daily

PoM **Deltastab**® (Boots)
Injection (aqueous suspension), prednisolone acetate 25 mg/ml. Price 5-ml vial = **C**

PREDNISOLONE SODIUM PHOSPHATE

Indications: local inflammation of joints and soft tissues

Cautions; Contra-indications; Side-effects: see notes above and section 6.3.3

Dose: by intra-articular, intrasynovial, intralesional, or soft-tissue injection, prednisolone 1.6–24 mg, according to joint size or amount of soft tissue, at intervals of 3–21 days according to response

PoM **Codelsol**® (MSD)
Injection, prednisolone 16 mg/ml (as prednisolone sodium phosphate). Price 2-ml vial = **D**

TRIAMCINOLONE ACETONIDE

Indications: local inflammation of joints and soft tissues

Cautions; Contra-indications; Side-effects: see notes above and section 6.3.3

Dose: by intra-articular injection, 2.5–40 mg according to joint size, to a max. of 80 mg in multiple injections

By intralesional injection, 2–3 mg; max. 30 mg (5 mg at any one site). Doses are repeated every 1–2 weeks according to the response

PoM **Adcortyl Intra-articular / Intradermal**® (Squibb)
Injection (aqueous suspension), triamcinolone acetonide 10 mg/ml. Price 1-ml amp = **D**; 5-ml vial = **F**

PoM **Kenalog Intra-articular / Intramuscular**® (Squibb)
Injection (aqueous suspension), triamcinolone acetonide 40 mg/ml. Price 1-ml vial = **D**

TRIAMCINOLONE HEXACETONIDE

Indications: local inflammation of joints and soft tissues

C = 51-100p, D = 101-180p, E = 181-300p, F = 301-450p, G = 451-650p, H = 651-900p, I = 901-1200p, J = over 1200p.

Cautions; Contra-indications; Side-effects: see notes above and section 6.3.3

Dose: by intra-articular, intrasynovial, or soft-tissue injection, 2–30 mg, according to joint size or amount of soft tissue, repeated at intervals of not less than 3–4 weeks according to the response

By intracutaneous injection of a suspension containing not more than 5 mg/ml, up to 500 micrograms/square inch of affected skin

PoM **Lederspan®** (Lederle)
Injection (aqueous suspension), triamcinolone hexacetonide 5 mg/ml. For intracutaneous or intra-articular injection. Price 5-ml vial = **E**
Injection (aqueous suspension), triamcinolone hexacetonide 20 mg/ml. For intra-articular or intrasynovial injection. Price 1-ml vial = **E**; 5-ml vial = **H**

10.1.3 Drugs which may affect the rheumatic disease process

Certain drugs such as **gold** (sodium aurothiomalate), **penicillamine**, **hydroxychloroquine**, **chloroquine**, and **immunosuppressants** are considered disease-specific in that they are said to affect the disease process in rheumatoid arthritis and related conditions but do not affect other types of inflammatory arthritis. They differ from the anti-inflammatory drugs in a number of ways. They do not produce an immediate therapeutic effect but reach a full response after 4 to 6 months of treatment; they improve not only the signs and symptoms of joint disease but also the extra-articular manifestations of rheumatoid arthritis such as nodules; they also reduce erythrocyte sedimentation rate and rheumatoid factor. Some, for example penicillamine, may retard the radiological progression of the disease.

These drugs are mainly used in rheumatoid arthritis where treatment with anti-inflammatory drugs has been unsuccessful or where there is evidence of disease progression such as the development of deformities or worsening radiological changes. Since, in the first few months, the course of rheumatoid arthritis is unpredictable, it is usual to delay treatment for about 6 months depending on the progress of the disease, but treatment should be initiated before joint damage becomes irreversible.

Penicillamine and related drugs are also sometimes used in rheumatoid arthritis where there are troublesome extra-articular features such as vasculitis, and in patients who are taking excessive doses of corticosteroids. Where the response is satisfactory there is often a striking reduction in requirements of both corticosteroids and other drugs. Gold, penicillamine, and related drugs may also be used to treat juvenile chronic arthritis (Still's disease) when indications are similar.

Gold and **penicillamine** are effective in palindromic rheumatism and **chloroquine** is sometimes used to treat systemic lupus erythematosus and discoid lupus erythematosus.

Gold (as **sodium aurothiomalate**) must be given by deep intramuscular injection and the area gently massaged. It is usual to begin treatment with doses of 1, 5, and 10 mg at intervals of 1 week to test the patient's tolerance; thereafter doses of 20 to 50 mg are given at weekly intervals until remission occurs or a total of 1 g has been given. Benefit is not to be expected until about 8 doses have been given. The interval between injections is then gradually increased to 2 and then to 4 weeks but intervals of 6 weeks may be suitable in some patients.

If relapse occurs dosage should be immediately increased to 50 mg weekly and only once control is obtained should a reduction in dosage again be instituted. It is important to avoid complete relapse since second courses of gold are not usually effective. Treatment should be continued indefinitely.

Gold therapy should be discontinued in the presence of blood dyscrasias or proteinuria which is above 30 mg/100 ml and has no incidental cause such as urinary-tract infection (associated with immune complex nephritis). Patients should therefore undergo blood counts, including platelets, and urine examinations before each injection. Rashes often occur after 2 to 6 months and necessitate discontinuation of treatment.

SODIUM AUROTHIOMALATE

Indications: severe active or progressive rheumatoid arthritis, palindromic rheumatism, juvenile chronic arthritis (Still's disease)

Cautions: see notes above. Patients should report any untoward symptoms (fever, sore throat, malaise, bruising); renal and hepatic impairment, elderly patients, eczema, colitis, breast-feeding, treatment with drugs which can cause blood disorders, e.g. phenylbutazone

Contra-indications: see notes above. Also exfoliative dermatitis, disseminated lupus erythematosus, pregnancy, patients recently subjected to irradiation

Side-effects: severe reactions (occasionally fatal) in up to 5% of patients; mouth ulcers, skin reactions, oedema, proteinuria, blood disorders (sometimes sudden and fatal); rarely colitis, peripheral neuritis, pulmonary fibrosis

Dose: administered on expert advice, ADULT, see notes above; CHILD, *by deep intramuscular injection,* slowly increased to the following maximum weekly doses: under 20 kg 10 mg, 20–50 kg 20 mg, over 50 kg 30 mg

PoM **Myocrisin®** (M&B)
Injection 1 mg, sodium aurothiomalate 2 mg/ml. Price 0.5-ml amp = **B**
Injection 5 mg, sodium aurothiomalate 10 mg/ml. Price 0.5-ml amp = **C**
Injection 10 mg, sodium aurothiomalate 20 mg/ml. Price 0.5-ml amp = **C**
Injection 20 mg, sodium aurothiomalate 40 mg/ml. Price 0.5-ml amp = **D**
Injection 50 mg, sodium aurothiomalate 100 mg/ml. Price 0.5-ml amp = **E**

Penicillamine has a similar action to gold. It appears to have a greater effect on radiological progression, and more patients are able to continue treatment than with gold but side-effects occur frequently. An initial dose of 125 to 250 mg daily is given for 1 month, increased by this amount every 4 to 12 weeks until remission occurs. Penicillamine should be discontinued if there is no improvement within 1 year. The usual maintenance dose is 500 to 750 mg daily, but up to 1.5 g may be required.

Patients should be warned not to expect improvement for at least 6 to 12 weeks after treatment is initiated. If remission has been sustained for 6 months, reduction of dosage by 125 to 250 mg every 12 weeks may be attempted.

Blood counts, including platelets, and urine examinations should be carried out every 1 or 2 weeks for the first 2 months then every 4 weeks to detect blood disorders and proteinuria. A reduction in platelet count indicates that treatment with penicillamine should be stopped, subsequently re-introduced at a lower dosage level and then, if possible, gradually increased. Proteinuria, associated with immune complex nephritis, occurs in up to 30% of patients, but treatment may be continued provided that renal function tests remain normal, oedema is absent, and the 24-hour urinary excretion of protein does not exceed 2 g.

Penicillamine is used in Wilson's disease (hepatolenticular degeneration) to aid the elimination of copper ions. See Emergency Treatment of Poisoning for the use of penicillamine in copper and lead poisoning.

Nausea may occur but is not usually a problem provided that penicillamine is taken before meals or on retiring and that low initial doses are used and only gradually increased. Loss of taste may occur about 6 weeks after treatment is started but usually returns 6 weeks later irrespective of whether or not treatment is discontinued; mineral supplements are not recommended. Rashes are a common side-effect. Those which occur in the first few months of treatment disappear when the drug is stopped and treatment may then be re-introduced at a lower dose level and gradually increased. Late rashes are more resistant and often necessitate discontinuation of treatment.

PENICILLAMINE

Indications: severe active or progressive rheumatoid arthritis, juvenile chronic arthritis; also Wilson's disease, chronic active hepatitis, primary biliary cirrhosis, cystinuria

Cautions: see notes above; renal impairment, pregnancy, and portal hypertension; avoid concurrent gold, chloroquine, hydroxychloroquine, or immunosuppressive treatment.

Drug interactions: see Appendix 1 (section 10)

Contra-indications: lupus erythematosus

Side-effects: hypersensitivity reactions (may necessitate discontinuation of treatment); nausea, anorexia, taste loss, mouth ulcers, muscle weakness, skin reactions (see notes above), extravasation of blood into the skin, oedema,

proteinuria, agranulocytosis or severe thrombocytopenia (sometimes fatal); rarely myasthenia, febrile reactions, systemic lupus erythematosus

Dose: rheumatoid arthritis, administered on expert advice, ADULT, see notes above; CHILD initial dose, 50 mg daily for 1 month, increased at 4-week intervals to a maintenance dose of 15–20 mg/kg daily

Wilson's disease, 1.5–2 g daily in divided doses before food; max. 2 g daily for 1 year; maintenance 0.75–1 g daily; CHILD, up to 20 mg/kg daily in divided doses, max. 500 mg daily

Chronic active hepatitis (after disease is controlled), 500 mg daily in divided doses slowly increased over 3 months; usual maintenance dose 1.25 g daily

Primary biliary cirrhosis, 250 mg daily, increasing weekly to a maintenance dose of 0.75-1 g daily in divided doses, then reduced as liver copper concentrations return to normal

Cystinuria, therapeutic, 1–3 g daily in divided doses before food, adjusted to maintain urinary cystine below 200 mg/litre. Prophylactic (maintain urinary cystine below 300 mg/litre) 0.5–1 g at bedtime; maintain adequate fluid intake (at least 3 litres daily); CHILD minimum dose to maintain urinary cystine below 200 mg/litre

PoM **Penicillamine Tablets,** f/c, penicillamine 50 mg, price 20 tabs = **C**; 125 mg, price 20 tabs = **D**; 250 mg, price 20 tabs = **F**. Label: 6

PoM **Distamine**® (Dista)

Tablets, scored, f/c, penicillamine 50 mg. Price 20 tabs = **C**. Label: 6

Tablets, f/c, penicillamine 125 mg. Price 20 tabs = **E**. Label: 6

Tablets, f/c, penicillamine 250 mg. Price 20 tabs = **F**. Label: 6

PoM **Pendramine**® (Merck)

Tablets, scored, f/c, penicillamine 125 mg. Price 20 tabs = **D**. Label: 6

Tablets, scored, f/c, penicillamine 250 mg. Price 20 tabs = **F**. Label: 6

Chloroquine and **hydroxychloroquine** have a similar action to gold and are better tolerated than either gold or penicillamine but their use is limited by their ocular toxicity. However, retinopathy is rare provided the doses given below are not exceeded. Nevertheless, all patients should have a full ophthalmic examination before starting treatment and then subsequently at 3- to 6-monthly intervals when treatment is prolonged for more than 1 year. Ocular toxicity is also reduced if the drug is not given continuously for longer than 1 year and some physicians advise their patients to stop treatment for 2 months of each year.

These drugs are best **avoided** in elderly patients as it is difficult to distinguish ageing changes from drug-induced retinopathy.

CHLOROQUINE

Indications: active rheumatoid arthritis, systemic lupus erythematosus, discoid lupus erythematosus

---

Cautions: renal and hepatic impairment, pregnancy, porphyria, psoriasis, neurological disorders, severe gastro-intestinal disorders, glucose 6-phosphate dehydrogenase deficiency; elderly patients, children; regular ophthalmic examinations required (see notes above)

Contra-indications: hypersensitivity to quinine, concurrent therapy with hepatotoxic drugs or sodium aurothiomalate

Side-effects: gastro-intestinal disturbances, headache, visual disturbances, irreversible retinal damage, corneal opacities, depigmentation or loss of hair, skin reactions (sometimes severe—may necessitate discontinuation of treatment), hearing disturbances such as tinnitus, leading rarely to deafness; rarely neuromyopathy, myopathy, psychiatric disturbances, photosensitisation, and blood dyscrasias (usually thrombocytopenia)

Dose: administered on expert advice, chloroquine 150 mg daily preferably after food; CHILD, 3 mg/kg daily

Note: 150 mg chloroquine ≡ 200 mg chloroquine sulphate ≡ 250 mg chloroquine phosphate (approx.)

Preparations
See section 5.4.1

HYDROXYCHLOROQUINE SULPHATE

Indications: active rheumatoid arthritis, systemic lupus erythematosus, discoid lupus erythematosus

Cautions; Contra-indications; Side-effects: see under Chloroquine and notes (above)

Dose: administered on expert advice, initially 400–600 mg daily in divided doses preferably after food; maintenance 200–400 mg daily; CHILD, 5–7 mg/kg daily

PoM **Plaquenil**® (Sterling Research)
Tablets, orange, s/c, hydroxychloroquine sulphate 200 mg. Price 20 tabs = **G**

When used in *rheumatoid arthritis* **immunosuppressants** have a similar action to gold and are useful alternatives in cases that have failed to respond to gold, penicillamine, chloroquine, or hydroxychloroquine.

Azathioprine (see section 8.2.1) is usually chosen and is given in a dose of 1.5 to 2.5 mg per kilogram body-weight daily in divided doses. Blood counts should be carried out every 4 to 6 weeks to detect possible neutropenia which is usually resolved by reducing the dose. Nausea, vomiting, and diarrhoea may occur, usually starting early during the course of treatment, and may necessitate withdrawal of the drug. *Herpes zoster* infection may also occur during treatment.

Chlorambucil (see section 8.1.1) is another immunosuppressant which is used in rheumatoid arthritis; a dose of 5 mg daily is usually given initially; most patients require between 2.5 and 7.5 mg daily. Regular blood counts including platelets should be carried out. **Cyclophosphamide** is too toxic for use in rheumatoid arthritis.

Immunosuppressants are also used in the management of severe cases of *systemic lupus erythematosus* and other connective tissue disorders. They are often given in conjunction with corticosteroids for patients with severe or progressive renal disease though the evidence for their benefit is doubtful. They may be used in cases of *polymyositis* which are resistant to corticosteroids. They are used for their corticosteroid-sparing effect in patients whose corticosteroid requirements are excessive. **Azathioprine** is usually used but **chlorambucil** is an alternative and **methotrexate** (see section 8.1.3) has been used in polymyositis.

Azathioprine and methotrexate are used in the treatment of *psoriatic arthropathy* for severe or progressive cases which are not controlled with anti-inflammatory drugs. There is an impression that **azathioprine** is the more effective for psoriatic arthritis and that **methotrexate** is the more effective for skin manifestations. Methotrexate is usually given in a dose of 10–25 mg weekly by mouth. Regular blood counts should be carried out.

10.1.4   Drugs used in the treatment of gout

It is important to distinguish drugs used for the treatment of acute attacks of gout from those used in the long-term control of the disease. The latter exacerbate and prolong the acute manifestations if given during an attack.

ACUTE ATTACKS OF GOUT. These are most often treated with **anti-inflammatory analgesics** such as azapropazone, indomethacin, and naproxen (section 10.1.1.2). Colchicine is an alternative. Aspirin is contra-indicated in acute gout.

Indomethacin is often chosen in acute attacks. High doses are usually well tolerated for short periods (50 to 100 mg repeated after a few hours if necessary and followed by reducing doses every 6 hours as the patient improves). If courses of treatment last for less than one week side-effects are unusual despite the high doses used.

Colchicine is probably not as effective as indomethacin and its use is limited by its toxicity.

In resistant cases of acute gout **corticotrophin** (see section 6.5.1) is very effective and is given in a dose of 80 units by intramuscular injection repeated after a day or two if necessary.

LONG-TERM CONTROL OF GOUT. The formation of uric acid from purines may be reduced with the **xanthine-oxidase inhibitor** allopurinol, or the **uricosuric drugs** probenecid or sulphinpyrazone may be used to increase the excretion of uric acid in the urine. Treatment should be continued indefinitely.

Allopurinol (Zyloric®) is a convenient well tolerated drug which is now widely used. It is especially useful in patients with renal impairment or urate stones where uricosuric drugs cannot be used. It is usually given once daily, as the active metabolite of allopurinol has a long half-life, but

---

doses over 300 mg daily should be divided. Allopurinol treatment should not be started until an acute attack of gout has completely subsided, as further attacks may be precipitated. It is well tolerated in most patients but may occasionally cause rashes.

The uricosuric drugs include **probenecid** (Benemid®) and **sulphinpyrazone** (Anturan®). They can be used instead of treatment with allopurinol, or in conjunction with it in cases that are resistant to treatment.

Azapropazone (section 10.1.1.2) has a uricosuric effect and may be useful in the long-term treatment of chronic gout.

Salicylates antagonise the uricosuric drugs but they do not antagonise the action of allopurinol. Crystallisation of urate in the urine may occur with the uricosuric drugs and it is important to ensure that there is an adequate urine output especially in the first few weeks of treatment. As an additional precaution the urine may be rendered alkaline.

The number of acute gout attacks may be increased in the first few months of treatment with allopurinol or the uricosuric drugs. It is therefore necessary to give some prophylaxis during this time and colchicine or anti-inflammatory analgesics can also be used for this purpose.

The anti-inflammatory analgesics are described in section 10.1.1.

ALLOPURINOL

Indications: gout prophylaxis, hyperuricaemia
Cautions: administer prophylactic colchicine or anti-inflammatory analgesic for about 1 month during initial therapy; ensure adequate fluid intake (2 litres/day); render urine alkaline if uric acid overload is high; caution in hepatic disease; reduce dose in renal impairment (in renal failure adjustment of dosage is necessary during dialysis). In neoplastic conditions treatment with allopurinol (if required) should be commenced before cytotoxic drugs are given. Drug interactions: see Appendix 1 (sections *2.8C*, *8*)
Contra-indications: acute gout attack and until attack has subsided
Side-effects: most common are rashes, sometimes with fever (may be sign of impending hypersensitivity reaction—withdraw therapy but when rash is mild re-introduce cautiously; discontinue immediately on recurrence); gastro-intestinal disorders. Rarely malaise, headache, vertigo, drowsiness, taste disturbances, hypertension, symptomless xanthine deposits in muscle, alopecia, hepatotoxicity
Dose: initially 100 mg daily as a single dose, after food, gradually increased over 1–3 weeks according to the plasma or urinary uric acid concentration, to about 300 mg daily; usual maintenance dose 200–600 mg, rarely 900 mg daily, divided into doses of not more than 300 mg; CHILD (in neoplastic conditions, enzyme disorders) 10–20 mg/kg daily

PoM **Allopurinol Tablets,** allopurinol 100 mg,

price 20 tabs = **D**; 300 mg, price 20 tabs = **G**. Label: 8, 21, 27
PoM **Aloral®** (Lagap)
Tablets, scored, allopurinol 100 mg. Price 20 tabs = **E**. Label: 8, 21, 27
Tablets, scored, allopurinol 300 mg. Price 28 tabs = **H**. Label: 8, 21, 27
PoM **Aluline®** (Steinhard)
Tablets, scored, allopurinol 100 mg. Price 20 tabs = **E**. Label: 8, 21, 27
Tablets, scored, allopurinol 300 mg. Price 28 tabs = **H**. Label: 8, 21, 27
PoM **Caplenal®** (Berk)
Tablets, scored, allopurinol 100 mg. Price 20 tabs = **E**. Label: 8, 21, 27
Tablets, scored, allopurinol 300 mg. Price 28 tabs = **H**. Label: 8, 21, 27
PoM **Cosuric®** (DDSA)
Tablets, allopurinol 100 mg. Price 20 tabs = **E**. Label: 8, 21, 27
Tablets, allopurinol 300 mg. Price 20 tabs = **F**. Label: 8, 21, 27
PoM **Zyloric®** (Calmic)
Tablets, scored, allopurinol 100 mg. Price 20 tabs = **F**. Label: 8, 21, 27
Tablets, scored, allopurinol 300 mg. Price 28 tabs = **I**. Label: 8, 21, 27

COLCHICINE

Indications: acute gout, short-term prophylaxis during initial therapy with allopurinol and uricosuric drugs
Cautions: elderly and debilitated patients, cardiac or gastro-intestinal disease, renal impairment, pregnancy and breast-feeding
Side-effects: most common are nausea, vomiting, and abdominal pain; large doses may also cause profuse diarrhoea, gastro-intestinal haemorrhage, rashes, and renal damage. Rarely peripheral neuritis, alopecia, and with prolonged treatment blood disorders
Dose: 1 mg initially, followed by 500 micrograms every 2–3 hours until relief of pain is obtained or vomiting or diarrhoea occurs, or until a total dose of 10 mg has been reached. The course should not be repeated within 3 days
Prevention of attacks during initial treatment with allopurinol or uricosuric drugs, 500 micrograms 2–3 times daily

PoM **Colchicine Tablets,** colchicine 250 and 500 micrograms. Price 20 tabs (both) = **B**

PROBENECID

Indications: gout prophylaxis, hyperuricaemia; reduction of tubular excretion of penicillins and certain cephalosporins
Cautions: during gout therapy administer prophylactic colchicine, ensure adequate fluid intake (about 2 litres daily), render urine alkaline if uric acid overload is high; peptic ulceration, ineffective in renal impairment. Drug interactions: see Appendix 1 (sections *4.7*, *5.1*, *5.3*, *8*, *10*, *10*)
Contra-indications: concurrent salicylate

C = 51-100p, **D** = 101-180p, **E** = 181-300p, **F** = 301-450p, **G** = 451-650p, **H** = 651-900p, **I** = 901-1200p, **J** = over 1200p.

therapy, blood disorders, nephrolithiasis, acute gout attack and 3 weeks after

Side-effects: infrequent; occasionally nausea and vomiting, urinary frequency, headache, flushing, dizziness, rashes; rarely hypersensitivity, nephrotic syndrome, hepatic necrosis, aplastic anaemia

Dose: uricosuric therapy, initially 250 mg twice daily after food, increased after a week to 500 mg twice daily then up to 2 g daily in 2–4 divided doses according to plasma-uric acid concentration and reduced for maintenance

Penicillin and cephalosporin therapy, 2 g daily in divided doses; CHILD over 2 years initially 25 mg/kg (700 mg/m²) daily, then 10 mg/kg (300 mg/m²) every 6 hours; over 50 kg, adult dose. Single-dose treatment, 1 g at the same time as oral penicillin or cephalosporin or 30 minutes before an intramuscular injection

PoM **Benemid**® (MSD)
Tablets, scored, probenecid 500 mg. Price 20 tabs = **C**. Label: 12, 21, 27

SULPHINPYRAZONE

Indications: gout prophylaxis, hyperuricaemia

Cautions; Contra-indications: see under Probenecid. Regular blood counts are advisable. Avoid in hypersensitivity to phenylbutazone and related drugs. Drug interactions: see Appendix 1 (sections *2.8B*, *3*, *4.8*, *6.1*, 10)

Side-effects: gastro-intestinal disorders, occasionally hypersensitivity reactions; rarely blood disorders

Dose: initially 100–200 mg daily in single or divided doses, with milk or after food, increasing over 2–3 weeks according to the plasma-uric acid concentration to about 600–800 mg daily in divided doses and reducing for maintenance

PoM **Anturan**® (Geigy)
Tablets, yellow, s/c, sulphinpyrazone 100 mg. Price 20 tabs = **C**. Label: 12, 21
Tablets, yellow, s/c, sulphinpyrazone 200 mg. Price 20 tabs = **D**. Label: 12, 21

10.2   Drugs used in other musculoskeletal disorders

Drugs in this section have been divided into those which enhance neuromuscular transmission (section 10.2.1) and skeletal muscle relaxants (section 10.2.2).

10.2.1   Drugs which enhance neuromuscular transmission

Anticholinesterase drugs are used to enhance neuromuscular transmission in voluntary and involuntary muscle in conditions such as *myasthenia gravis*. They prolong the action of acetylcholine by inhibiting the action of the enzyme acetylcholinesterase. Excessive dosage of these drugs may impair neuromuscular transmission and precipitate the so-called 'cholinergic crises' by causing a depolarising block. This may be difficult to distinguish from a worsening myasthenic state.

Side-effects of anticholinesterases are due to their parasympathomimetic action. Muscarinic effects include increased sweating, salivary, and gastric secretion, also increased gastro-intestinal and uterine motility, and bradycardia. These effects may be antagonised by atropine.

Edrophonium (Tensilon®) has a very brief action and is therefore used only for the diagnosis of myasthenia gravis. A single test-dose will cause a dramatic but transient improvement in muscle power in patients with the disease.

It can also be used to determine whether a patient with myasthenia is receiving inadequate or excessive treatment with cholinergic drugs; if treatment is excessive an injection of edrophonium would either have no effect or intensify symptoms.

Neostigmine (Prostigmin®) produces a therapeutic effect for up to 4 hours. Its pronounced muscarinic action is a disadvantage, and simultaneous administration of an anticholinergic drug such as atropine or propantheline may be required to prevent colic or excessive salivation. In severe disease neostigmine may be given every 2 hours.

Pyridostigmine (Mestinon®) is less powerful and slower in action than neostigmine but it has a longer duration of action. It is sometimes preferred in patients whose muscles are weak on wakening. It has a comparatively mild gastro-intestinal effect. Pyridostigmine would therefore appear to have some advantages over neostigmine in the treatment of myasthenia gravis.

Ambenonium (Mytelase®) has a slightly longer duration of action than pyridostigmine.

Distigmine (Ubretid®) has the most protracted action but the danger of a cholinergic crisis caused by accumulation of the drug is greater than with shorter-acting drugs. **Physostigmine** is now mainly used as a miotic (see section 11.6).

Corticosteroids (see section 6.3) are established as treatment for myasthenia gravis where *thymectomy* is inadvisable or to reduce the risk of surgery beforehand. The initial dose is high (up to 100 mg **prednisolone** daily) but some advise starting with a smaller dose (30 mg prednisolone daily) and gradually increasing it. There is grave risk of exacerbation of the myasthenia during the initial stages of therapy, particularly in the first 2–3 weeks. Improvement usually begins after about 2 weeks on the high dose regimen. In some patients a prolonged remission may be induced, but often patients need a maintenance dose of 25–40 mg of prednisolone daily. Patients who need corticosteroids may benefit from the addition of **azathioprine.**

Plasmapheresis produces a striking but temporary remission in myasthenia gravis in many patients and is indicated where severe disease is unresponsive to other forms of treatment.

The anticholinesterases neostigmine and edrophonium are used at the end of anaesthesia to reverse the actions of the non-depolarising muscle relaxants (see section 15.1.6).

AMBENONIUM CHLORIDE

Indications: myasthenia gravis

Cautions; Contra-indications; Side-effects: see under Neostigmine

Dose: 5–25 mg 3–4 times daily, adjusted according to the response; doses above 200 mg daily require careful supervision

PoM **Mytelase**® (Sterling Research)

Tablets, f/c, ambenonium chloride 10 mg. Price 20 tabs = **D**

DISTIGMINE BROMIDE

Indications: myasthenia gravis

Cautions; Contra-indications; Side-effects: see under Neostigmine

Dose: initially 5 mg daily half an hour before breakfast, increased at intervals of 3–4 days if necessary to a max. of 20 mg daily; CHILD up to 10 mg daily according to age

PoM **Ubretid**® (Berk)

Tablets, scored, distigmine bromide 5 mg. Price 20 tabs = **I**. Label: 22

EDROPHONIUM CHLORIDE

Indications: diagnosis of myasthenia gravis, detection of under or overdosage with cholinergic drugs (see notes above)

Cautions; Contra-indications; Side-effects: see under Neostigmine

Dose: diagnosis of myasthenia gravis, *by intravenous injection*, 2 mg followed after 30 seconds (if no adverse reaction has occurred) by 8 mg; in adults without suitable veins, *by intramuscular injection*, 10 mg

Detection of over or underdosage of cholinergic drugs, *by intravenous injection*, 2 mg one hour after the last dose of cholinergic drug

PoM **Tensilon**® (Roche)

Injection, edrophonium chloride 10 mg/ml. Price 1-ml amp = **B**

NEOSTIGMINE

Indications: treatment and diagnosis of myasthenia gravis

Cautions: asthma, bradycardia, recent myocardial infarction, epilepsy, hypotension, parkinsonism, vagotonia, pregnancy. Atropine or other antidote to muscarinic effects may be necessary (particularly when neostigmine is given by injection), but it should not be given routinely as it may mask signs of overdosage. Drug interactions: see Appendix 1 (section *15*)

Contra-indications: intestinal or urinary obstruction

Side-effects: nausea, vomiting, increased salivation, diarrhoea, abdominal cramps (more marked with higher doses). Signs of overdosage are increased gastro-intestinal discomfort, bronchial secretions, and sweating, involuntary defaecation and micturition, miosis, nystagmus, bradycardia, hypotension, agitation, excessive dreaming, and weakness eventually leading to fasciculation and paralysis

Dose: by mouth, neostigmine bromide 75–300 mg or more, daily in divided doses at suitable intervals; CHILD, neonate 1–5 mg every 4 hours, older children 15–60 mg daily in divided doses

By subcutaneous, intramuscular, or intravenous injection, neostigmine methylsulphate 1–2.5 mg daily in divided doses at suitable intervals; CHILD, neonate 50–250 micrograms every 4 hours, older children 200–500 micrograms daily in divided doses

PoM **Prostigmin**® (Roche)

Tablets, scored, neostigmine bromide 15 mg. Price 20 tabs = **B**

Injection, neostigmine methylsulphate 500 micrograms/ml. Price 1-ml amp = **A**

Injection, neostigmine methylsulphate 2.5 mg/ml. Price 1-ml amp = **A**

PYRIDOSTIGMINE BROMIDE

Indications: myasthenia gravis

Cautions; Contra-indications; Side-effects: see under Neostigmine; weaker muscarinic action

Dose: by mouth, 0.3–1.2 g daily in divided doses at suitable intervals; CHILD, neonate 5–10 mg every 4 hours, older children 10 mg initially, increased by 5-mg amounts according to response

By subcutaneous, intramuscular or intravenous injection, 2–5 mg daily in divided doses; CHILD, neonate 200–400 micrograms every 4 hours, older children initially 0.25–1 mg, increasing according to response

PoM **Mestinon**® (Roche)

Tablets, scored, pyridostigmine bromide 60 mg. Price 20 tabs = **C**

Injection, pyridostigmine bromide 1 mg/ml. Price 1-ml amp = **A**

10.2.2 Skeletal muscle relaxants

Drugs described in this section are used for the relief of muscle spasm or spasticity. They act principally on the central nervous system with the exception of dantrolene which has a peripheral site of action. They differ in action from the muscle relaxants used in anaesthesia (see section 15.1.5) which block transmission of impulses at the neuromuscular junction.

A treatable neurological cause for spasticity should be excluded before treatment is begun but the choice of drug is not influenced by the type of spasticity. The major disadvantage of treatment with these drugs is that reduction in muscle tone can cause a loss of splinting action of the spastic leg and trunk muscles and sometimes lead to an increase in disability.

Diazepam is the drug of choice. Sedation and, occasionally, extensor hypotonus are disadvantages associated with its use. Other benzodiazepines also have muscle-relaxant properties, particularly **chlordiazepoxide**, **ketazolam**, **medazepam**, and **clorazepate**. Muscle-relaxant doses are similar to the anxiolytic doses (see section 4.1.2).

C = 51-100p, **D** = 101-180p, **E** = 181-300p, **F** = 301-450p, **G** = 451-650p, **H** = 651-900p, **I** = 901-1200p, **J** = over 1200p.

Baclofen (Lioresal®) produces a clinical effect similar to diazepam. It acts at spinal level to reduce muscle tone. The dose should be increased slowly to avoid sedation and hypotonia.

Dantrolene (Dantrium®) acts directly on skeletal muscle but nevertheless produces central adverse effects. As with baclofen the dose should be increased slowly.

The clinical efficacy of carisoprodol, chlormezanone and meprobamate (both section 4.1.2), methocarbamol, and orphenadrine as muscle relaxants is **not** well established. These compounds are often included in compound analgesic preparations (see section 4.7.1.3). Tigloidine (Tiglyssin®) has been superseded by more effective drugs for the treatment of muscular rigidity and spasticity.

Quinine salts (see section 5.4.1) 200 to 300 mg at bedtime are effective in relieving nocturnal leg cramps.

DIAZEPAM

Indications: muscle spasm of varied aetiology; tetanus

Cautions; Side-effects: see section 4.1.2. Hypotonia may occur. Special precautions are necessary when diazepam is given by intravenous injection (see section 4.8.2)

Dose: by mouth, 2–15 mg daily in divided doses, increased if necessary in spastic conditions to 60 mg daily according to response

Spasticity with minimal brain damage, CHILD 2–40 mg daily in divided doses

By intramuscular or slow intravenous injection, in acute muscle spasm, 10 mg repeated if necessary after 4 hours; CHILD, 100–200 micrograms/kg, repeated if necessary

Tetanus, *by intravenous injection,* 100–300 micrograms/kg repeated every 1–4 hours; *by intravenous infusion,* 3–10 mg/kg over 24 hours, adjusted according to response

Preparations

See section 4.1.2

BACLOFEN

Indications: muscle spasm in spastic conditions

Cautions: psychiatric illness, cerebrovascular disease, elderly patients; reduce dose in renal impairment, epilepsy; avoid abrupt withdrawal

Side-effects: nausea, vomiting, drowsiness, confusion, fatigue, muscle hypotonia, hypotension

Dose: 5 mg 3 times daily, preferably after food, gradually increased; max. 100 mg daily; CHILD up to 8 years 5–10 mg daily in 3–4 divided doses, gradually increased to a max. of 40 mg daily; over 8 years 10 mg daily in divided doses, gradually increased to a max. of 60 mg daily

PoM **Lioresal**® (Ciba)

Tablets, scored, baclofen 10 mg. Price 20 tabs = **E**. Label: 2, 8

CARISOPRODOL

Indications: muscle spasm (see notes above)

Cautions; Side-effects: see under Meprobamate, section 4.1.2. Drowsiness is common

Dose: 350 mg 3–4 times daily

PoM **Carisoma**® (Pharmax)

Tablets, carisoprodol 125 and 350 mg. Price 20 tabs (both) = **B**. Label: 2

Carisoma Co— see section 4.7.1.3

DANTROLENE SODIUM

Indications: muscle spasm in spastic conditions

Cautions: impaired cardiac, pulmonary, and hepatic function; test liver function before and 6 weeks after initiating therapy. Therapeutic effect may take a few weeks to develop but if treatment is ineffective it should be discontinued after 45 days. Patients should not drive or operate machinery until therapy is stabilised. Avoid in children or when spasticity is useful, for example, locomotion. May enhance effects of CNS depressants

Side-effects: transient drowsiness, dizziness, weakness, malaise, fatigue, diarrhoea (reduce dose if necessary), occasionally urinary or musculoskeletal disturbances, rashes, and, rarely, jaundice

Dose: initially 25 mg daily, gradually increased over 7 weeks to a max. of 100 mg 4 times daily

PoM **Dantrium**® (Norwich-Eaton)

Capsules, orange/cream, dantrolene sodium 25 mg. Price 20 caps = **E**. Label: 2

Capsules, orange/cream, dantrolene sodium 100 mg. Price 20 caps = **I**. Label: 2

METHOCARBAMOL

Indications: muscle spasm, usually in muscle injury (see notes above)

Cautions: may cause drowsiness, enhance action of CNS depressants, and increase effects of alcohol; persons affected should not drive or operate machinery. Avoid injection in renal impairment

Contra-indications: coma or pre-coma states, brain damage, epilepsy, tachycardia, glaucoma, prostatic hypertrophy, bladder-neck obstruction

Side-effects: lassitude, light-headedness, dizziness, restlessness, anxiety, confusion, drowsiness, nausea, allergic rash or angioedema, convulsions

Dose: by mouth, 1.5 g 4 times daily

By intramuscular or slow intravenous injection or infusion, 1–3 g daily in divided doses; max. 3 g daily for 3 days, except in treatment of tetanus

PoM **Robaxin 750**® (Robins)

Tablets, scored, methocarbamol 750 mg. Price 20 tabs = **D**. Label: 2

Injection, methocarbamol 100 mg/ml in aqueous macrogol 300. Price 10-ml amp = **C**

Robaxisal Forte—see section 4.7.1.3

ORPHENADRINE CITRATE

Indications: muscle spasm, usually in muscle injury (see notes above)

Cautions; Contra-indications; Side-effects: see under Benzhexol, section 4.9.2. Avoid in children. Anticholinergic effects are infrequent
Dose: by mouth, 200–300 mg daily in 2 divided doses
By intramuscular or slow intravenous injection, 60 mg repeated after 12 hours if necessary

PoM **Norflex**® (Riker)
Tablets, s/r, orphenadrine citrate 100 mg. Price 20 tabs = **C**. Label: 25
Injection, orphenadrine citrate 30 mg/ml. Price 2-ml amp = **C**
Norgesic—see section 4.7.1.3

TIGLOIDINE HYDROBROMIDE
Indications: muscle spasm in spasticity (see notes above)
Cautions; Side-effects: see under Benzhexol, section 4.9.2; anticholinergic effects are rare but may occur with high doses; caution in glaucoma
Dose: 1–2 g daily in 3 divided doses after food

PoM **Tiglyssin**® (DF)
Tablets, tigloidine hydrobromide 250 mg. Price 20 tabs = **F**. Label: 21

10.3 Drugs for the relief of soft-tissue inflammation

10.3.1 Enzymes
The enzymes in this section have fibrinolytic or proteolytic activity. Their therapeutic effectiveness is **doubtful**. They are claimed to relieve inflammation, bruising, swelling, and other soft-tissue trauma by removing coagulated blood, exudate, and necrotic tissue. They include **bromelains, chymotrypsin, deoxyribonuclease, streptokinase-streptodornase**, and **trypsin**. Some are also used to facilitate expectoration by liquefaction of bronchial secretions. See section 2.10 for streptokinase and urokinase, which also have fibrinolytic activity, and section 13.13 for desloughing agents used in ulcer treatment.

Hyaluronidase (Hyalase®) is used to render the tissues more easily permeable to injected fluids.

BROMELAINS
Indications: adjunctive treatment of soft tissue inflammation and oedema
Cautions: disturbances of blood-clotting mechanism; severe hepatic or renal impairment; avoid in pineapple sensitivity
Side-effects: nausea, vomiting, rashes

Ananase Forte® (Rorer)
Tablets, orange, e/c, bromelains 100 000 Rorer units. Price 20 tabs = **E**. Label: 5, 25
Dose: 1 tablet 4 times daily

CHYMOTRYPSIN
Indications: adjunctive treatment of soft-tissue inflammation and oedema
Cautions: anticoagulant therapy; test for sensitivity before intramuscular injection

Side-effects: nausea, vomiting, diarrhoea, rarely severe hypersensitivity, rash

PoM **Chymar**® (Armour)
Injection, powder for reconstitution, alpha-chymotrypsin 5000 Armour units. Price vial (with diluent) = **D**
Dose: by intramuscular injection, 5000 Armour units 1–3 times daily

Chymoral® (Armour)
Tablets, red, e/c, trypsin, alpha-chymotrypsin, providing 50 000 Armour units. Price 20 tabs = **E**. Label: 5, 22, 25
Tablets forte, pink, e/c, twice strength of Chymoral Tablets. Price 20 tabs = **F**. Label: 5, 22, 25
Dose: 100 000 Armour units 4 times daily, half an hour before food

Deanase DC® (Consolidated)
Tablets, e/c, delta-chymotrypsin 10 mg. Price 20 tabs = **D**. Label: 5, 25
Dose: 2 tablets twice daily for 3 days then 1 twice daily

DEOXYRIBONUCLEASE
Indications: removal of tissue exudate and coagulated blood
Side-effects: irritation on local application and hypersensitivity on prolonged use; bronchospasm and irritation of the respiratory tract on inhalation of an aerosol
Dose: by aerosol inhalation, 250 000 units in 10 ml sterile water twice daily
By intramuscular injection (every 2 days as required) or *by intravenous injection*, (for immediate effect) 1 mega-unit
Local injection, 1 mega-unit in 2–3 ml of sodium chloride intravenous infusion 0.9%
For bladder irrigation, 1 mega-unit in 50 ml sterile water (see also section 7.4.4)

PoM **Deanase**® (Consolidated)
Powder, deoxyribonuclease (pancreatic) 250 000 units and 1 mega-unit (stated to be synergised with magnesium ions). For preparation of injections or solutions for inhalation or instillation. Price 250 000-unit vial = **D**; 1 mega-unit vial = **F**

HYALURONIDASE
Indications: to enhance permeation of subcutaneous or intramuscular injections, local anaesthetics, and subcutaneous infusions; to promote resorption of excess fluids and blood in the tissues
Contra-indications: intravenous injection, bites or stings, infection or malignancy at injection site
Side-effects: hypersensitivity
Dose: to enhance tissue permeability, *by subcutaneous or intramuscular injection*, usually 1500 units, either mixed with the injection fluid or injected into the site before injection is administered
By subcutaneous infusion, 1500 units administered before 500–1000 ml infusion fluid

---

C = 51-100p, **D** = 101-180p, **E** = 181-300p, **F** = 301-450p, **G** = 451-650p, **H** = 651-900p, **I** = 901-1200p, **J** = over 1200p.

PoM **Hyalase**® (CP)
Injection, powder for reconstitution, hyaluronidase (ovine). Price 1500-unit amp = **C**

STREPTOKINASE-STREPTODORNASE

Indications: removal of tissue exudates and coagulated blood
Cautions: disturbances of blood-clotting mechanisms, history of collagen disease
Contra-indications: haemorrhage, reduced plasminogen or fibrinogen concentrations
Side-effects: rarely allergic reactions

PoM **Varidase**® (Lederle)
Tablets, peach, streptokinase 10 000 units, streptodornase 2500 units. Price 12 tabs = **H**
Dose: 1 tablet 4 times daily for 4–6 days
PoM **Varidase Topical**® (Lederle)
Sterile powder, streptokinase 100 000 units, streptodornase 25 000 units. For preparing solutions for topical use. Price per vial = **H**
For bladder irrigation dissolve 1 vial in 20–500 ml of sterile sodium chloride solution (0.9%); repeat every 4 hours if necessary (see also section 7.4.4)

10.3.2   Rubefacients and other topical antirheumatics

Rubefacients act by counter-irritation. Pain, whether superficial or deep-seated, is relieved by any method which itself produces irritation of the skin, for example, heat or mustard oil. There is little evidence that the blood supply to the viscera is improved by stimulation of the skin.

Counter-irritation is comforting in painful lesions of the muscles, tendons, and joints, and in non-articular rheumatism. An unnecessarily large number of substances have been, and still are, used as counter-irritants. They probably all act through the same essential mechanism and differ mainly in intensity and duration of action.

Aerosol sprays containing volatile compounds relieve pain by chilling the affected area.

There is no satisfactory evidence that preparations of adrenaline or aspirin, applied topically are of value in the relief of deep-seated pain.

Liniments and **ointments** should be applied with gentle massage 2–3 times daily avoiding broken or inflamed skin.

Adrenaline Cream (Drug Tariff Formula), adrenaline solution 20 ml, chlorocresol 100 mg, emulsifying ointment 30 g, dilute hydrochloric acid 0.04 ml, sodium metabisulphite 40 mg/100 g, in purified water, freshly boiled and cooled (contains adrenaline 1 in 5000). Price 50 g = **B**
Kaolin Poultice, heavy kaolin 52.7%, thymol 0.05%, boric acid 4.5%, peppermint oil 0.05%, methyl salicylate 0.2%, glycerol 42.5%. Price 200 g = **C**
Warm and apply directly or between layers of muslin; avoid application of overheated poultice
Kaolin Poultice K/L Pack® (K/L Pharmaceuticals)
Kaolin poultice. Price 4 × 100-g pouches = **F**
Immerse one pouch in boiling water for up to 40 seconds, remove cover, and apply

Methyl Salicylate Liniment, methyl salicylate 25% (see Formulary). Price 100 ml = **B**
Methyl Salicylate Ointment, methyl salicylate 50%, white beeswax 25%, hydrous wool fat 25%. Price 100 g = **C**
Turpentine Liniment, turpentine oil 65%, camphor 5%, soft soap 7.5%, water 22.5%. Price 100 ml = **B**
White Liniment, turpentine oil 25%, ammonium chloride 1.25%, dilute ammonia solution 4.5%, oleic acid 8.5%, water 62.5%. Price 100 ml = **A**
Algesal® (Duphar)
Cream, diethylamine salicylate 10%. Price 40 g = **C**
Algipan® (Wyeth)
Cream, methyl nicotinate 1%, capsicum oleoresin 0.1%, glycol salicylate 10%. Price 40 g = **C**
Aradolene® (Rorer)
Cream, diethylamine salicylate 5%, 'capsicin water-soluble' 0.4%, menthol 2.5%, rectified camphor oil 1.4% in a lanolin basis. Price 40 g = **C**
Aspellin® (Rorer)
Liniment, ammonium salicylate 1%, camphor 0.6%, menthol 1.4%, ethyl and methyl salicylate 0.54%. Price 100 ml = **C**; 500 ml = **E**; 130-ml spray can = **C**
Balmosa® (Pharmax)
Cream, camphor 4%, capsicum oleoresin 0.035%, menthol 2%, methyl salicylate 4%. Price 20 and 40 g (both) = **B**
Bayolin® (Bayer)
Cream, benzyl nicotinate 2.5%, glycol salicylate 10%, heparinoid 500 units/g. Price 35 g = **C**
Bengué's Balsam® (Bengué)
Ointment, menthol 20%, methyl salicylate 20% in a lanolin basis. Price 25 g = **C**
Bengué's Balsam SG® (Bengué)
Cream, menthol 10%, methyl salicylate 15% in a vanishing cream basis. Price 25 g = **C**
Cremalgex® (Norton)
Cream, capsicum oleoresin 0.15%, glycol salicylate 10%, methyl nicotinate 1%. Price 30 g = **B**
Cremalgin® (Berk)
Balm (= cream), capsicin 0.1%, glycol salicylate 10%, methyl nicotinate 1%. Price 30 g = **B**; 50 g = **C**
Cremathurm® (Britpharm)
Cream, capsicum oleoresin 0.1%, ethyl nicotinate 1%, histamine acid phosphate 0.1%, methyl salicylate 10%. Price 25 g = **B**
Difflam® (Riker)
Cream, benzydamine hydrochloride 3%. Price 30 g = **E**; 80 g = **G**
Dubam® (Norma)
Spray application, glycol salicylate 5%, methyl nicotinate 1.6%, methyl salicylate 1%, ethyl salicylate 4%. Price 113-g aerosol spray = **D**
Finalgon® (Boehringer Ingelheim)
Ointment, butoxyethyl nicotinate 2.5%, vanillylnonanamide 0.4%. Price 20 g (with applicator) = **B**
Intralgin® (Riker)
Gel, benzocaine 2%, salicylamide 5% in an alcoholic vehicle. Price 50 g = **C**
PoM **Movelat**® (Luitpold)
Cream, corticosteroids 0.02% (as adrenocortical extract), heparinoid 0.2%, salicylic acid 2%. Price 50 g = **E**; 100 g = **F**
Gel, ingredients as for cream but in a colourless alcoholic basis. Price 50 g = **E**; 100 g = **F**
Transvasin® (R&C)
Cream, benzocaine 2%, ethyl nicotinate 2%, hexyl nicotinate 2%, tetrahydrofurfuryl salicylate 14%. Price 30 g = **B**

11: Drugs acting on the
EYE

In this chapter, drug treatment is discussed under the following headings:

11.1 Administration of drugs to the eye
11.2 Control of microbial contamination
11.3 Anti-infective preparations
11.4 Corticosteroids and other anti-inflammatory preparations
11.5 Mydriatics and cycloplegics
11.6 Treatment of glaucoma
11.7 Local anaesthetics
11.8 Miscellaneous ophthalmic preparations
11.9 Contact lenses

The entries in this chapter generally relate only to local eye treatment. Systemic indications and side-effects of many of the drugs are given elsewhere (see index).

11.1 Administration of drugs to the eye

EYE-DROPS AND EYE OINTMENTS. When administered in the form of eye-drops, drugs penetrate the eyeball, probably through the cornea. However, systemic effects, which are usually undesirable, may well arise from absorption of drugs into the general circulation via conjunctival vessels or from the nasal mucosa after the excess of the preparation has drained down through the tear ducts. For example, timolol maleate (a beta$_1$- and beta$_2$-adrenoceptor blocking drug), administered as eye-drops reduces pulse rate.

Eye ointments are often applied to lid margins for blepharitis. They may also be used in the conjunctival sac for other conditions especially where a prolonged action is required.

When two different preparations in the form of eye-drops are required at the same time of day, for example pilocarpine and timolol in glaucoma, dilution and overflow may occur when one immediately follows the other. The patient should therefore leave an interval of 10–15 minutes. At night, an eye ointment for the second drug will reduce the problem.

EYE LOTIONS. These are solutions for the irrigation of the conjunctival sac. They act mechanically to flush out irritants or foreign bodies or to remove infected discharges. **Sodium Chloride Eye Lotion** (section 11.8.2) is widely used. However, the lotion, which is sterile, should be used once only from a previously unopened container for first aid, while for treatment it should be used for no longer than 24 hours after the container is first opened. Single-application containers of the lotion are available. A convenient alternative is **Sodium Chloride Intravenous Infusion** 0.9% which is identical in composition to the eye lotion. In emergency, tap water drawn freshly from the main (not stored water) will suffice.

OTHER PREPARATIONS. Subconjunctival injection may be used to administer anti-infective drugs, mydriatics, or corticosteroids. The drug diffuses through the sclera to the anterior and posterior chambers and vitreous humour in higher concentration than can be achieved by absorption from eye-drops. However, because the dose-volume is limited (usually not more than 1 ml), this route is suitable only for drugs which are readily soluble.

Drugs such as antibiotics and corticosteroids may be administered systemically to treat an eye condition.

Suitable plastic devices which gradually release a specified amount of drug over a period of, say, 1 week are also used (for example Ocuserts®).

11.2 Control of microbial contamination

Preparations for the eye should be sterile when issued. For routine domiciliary use they are supplied in multiple-application containers for individual use. They contain a suitable preservative and provided that contamination is avoided they may be used for about one month after which a new container should be opened (if treatment is to be continued) and the old one discarded.

In eye surgery it is wise to use single-application containers. Preparations used during intra-ocular procedures and others that may penetrate into the anterior chamber must be isotonic and without preservatives and buffered if necessary to a neutral pH. Large volume intravenous infusion preparations are not suitable for this purpose. For all surgical procedures, a previously unopened container is used for each patient.

11.3 Anti-infective preparations

11.3.1 Topical preparations
11.3.2 Systemic preparations

11.3.1 Topical preparations

ADMINISTRATION. Lachrymation quickly dilutes or eliminates aqueous solutions. Ideally, therefore, eye-drops should be instilled (after an initial loading with drops every 10 minutes for half an hour) hourly for the first day or so. It may be worth advising that the upper eyelid be lifted, the patient being recumbent, and 1 or 2 drops directed into the upper fornix.

A reasonable alternative for night-time use is an eye ointment because of its longer action. In addition it will soften crusts which cause the lids and eye lashes to adhere together when the patient is asleep. A small quantity of eye ointment is applied to the eye or lid margin as appropriate.

C = 51-100p, D = 101-180p, E = 181-300p, F = 301-450p, G = 451-650p, H = 651-900p, I = 901-1200p, J = over 1200p.

ANTIBACTERIAL PREPARATIONS. **Propamidine ise-thionate** eye-drops (Brolene®) are suitable for the treament of **blepharitis** and acute and chronic **conjunctivitis**. The use of **mercuric oxide eye ointment**, even for short periods, is **not recommended**.

When prescribing antibiotics, in general, it is preferable to use topically in the eye antibiotics that are seldom or never used for systemic infections. However, the possibility of systemic absorption (section 11.1) must be taken into consideration. Examples of antibiotics with a wide spectrum of activity are **chloramphenicol, framycetin, neomycin, polymyxin B**, and **gentamicin**. Gentamicin is effective for treating infections due to *Pseudomonas aeruginosa*. **Sulphacetamide** is also used topically to treat eye infections, but is rarely of any value.

ANTIBACTERIAL AND CORTICOSTEROID PREPARATIONS. Many antibiotic preparations also incorporate a corticosteroid but such mixtures should **not** be used unless a patient is under close specialist supervision (section 11.4). A 'red eye' is sometimes caused by the *Herpes simplex* virus which produces a dendritic ulcer. This may be difficult to diagnose. Treatment with corticosteroids with or without antibiotics will aggravate the condition with a significant chance of loss of vision or even loss of the eye.

TRACHOMA. For mass antitrachoma treatment, the WHO recommends **tetracycline hydrochloride** eye ointment (Achromycin®); **chlortetracycline** eye ointment is also used. It is applied to both eyes twice daily for 5 days in each month for 6 months. Chloramphenicol is not as effective.

For active trachoma in the individual, one or both of the following are effective. (i) For adults, orally administered sulphonamides for 2 weeks or the long-acting sulphadimethoxine (Madribon®) 1 g initially followed by 500 mg daily for 10 days (see section 5.1.8). For children, erythromycin should be used (see section 5.1.5). (ii) Tetracycline Eye Ointment three times daily for 6 weeks.

ANTIVIRAL PREPARATIONS. *Herpes simplex* infections producing, for example, dendritic corneal ulcer can be treated with **idoxuridine**. Alternatively **vidarabine** (Vira-A®) may be used. **Acyclovir** (Zovirax®) is a new drug that is activated within herpes-infected cells.

ACYCLOVIR

Indications: local treatment of *Herpes simplex* infections
Apply 5 times daily

▼ PoM **Zovirax**® (Wellcome)
Eye ointment, acyclovir 3%. Price 4.5 g = **H**

CHLORAMPHENICOL

Indications: local treatment of infections (see notes above)
Apply eye-drops or eye ointment every 3 hours

PoM **Chloramphenicol Eye-drops,** chloramphenicol 0.5%. Price 10 ml = **C**
PoM **Chloromycetin**® (P-D)
Ophthalmic ointment (= eye ointment), chloramphenicol 1%. Price 4 g = **C**
Redidrops (= eye-drops), chloramphenicol 0.5%. Price 5 and 10 ml (both) = **D**
PoM **Minims Chloramphenicol** (S&N Pharm.)
Eye-drops, chloramphenicol 0.5%. Price 20 × 0.5 ml = **F**
PoM **Opulets Chloramphenicol**® (Alcon)
Eye-drops, chloramphenicol 0.5%. Price 20 × 0.25 ml = **F**
PoM **Sno Phenicol**® (S&N Pharm.)
Eye-drops, chloramphenicol 0.5%, in a viscous vehicle. Price 10 ml = **C**

CHLORTETRACYCLINE HYDROCHLORIDE

Indications: local treatment of infections, including trachoma (see notes above)
Apply eye ointment every 2 hours (acute infections)

PoM **Aureomycin**® (Lederle)
Ophthalmic ointment (= eye ointment), chlortetracycline hydrochloride 1%. Price 3.5 g = **C**

FRAMYCETIN SULPHATE

Indications: local treatment of infections (see notes above)
Apply eye-drops or eye ointment 3–4 times daily

PoM **Framycetin Sulphate Eye-drops,** framycetin sulphate 0.5%. Price 5 ml = **D**; 8 ml = **E**
PoM **Framycetin Sulphate Eye Ointment,** framycetin sulphate 0.5%. Price 3.5 and 5 g (both) = **C**
PoM **Framygen**® (Fisons)
Drops (for ear or eye), framycetin sulphate 0.5%. Price 5 ml = **D**
Eye ointment, framycetin sulphate 0.5%. Price 3.5 g = **C**
PoM **Soframycin**® (Roussel)
Eye-drops, framycetin sulphate 0.5%. Price 8 ml = **E**
Eye ointment, framycetin sulphate 0.5%. Price 5 g = **C**
Ophthalmic powder, framycetin sulphate (sterile) for preparing subconjunctival injections. Price 500-mg vial = **F**

GENTAMICIN

Indications: local treatment of infection (see notes above)
Apply eye-drops 3–6 times daily, eye ointment 2–4 times daily

PoM **Gentamicin Eye-drops,** gentamicin 0.3% (as sulphate). Price 5 and 10 ml (both) = **D**
PoM **Gentamicin Eye Ointment,** gentamicin 0.3% (as sulphate). Price 3 g = **D**
PoM **Alcomicin**® (Alcon)
Eye-drops, gentamicin 0.3% (as sulphate). Price 5 ml = **D**

PoM **Cidomycin**® (Roussel)
Drops (for ear or eye), gentamicin 0.3% (as sulphate). Price 8 ml = **D**
Eye ointment, gentamicin 0.3% (as sulphate). Price 3 g = **D**

PoM **Garamycin**® (Kirby-Warrick)
Drops (for ear or eye), gentamicin 0.3% (as sulphate). Price 10 ml = **D**
Eye ointment, gentamicin 0.3% (as sulphate). Price 3 g = **D**

PoM **Genticin**® (Nicholas)
Eye-drops, gentamicin 0.3% (as sulphate). Price 10 ml = **D**
Eye ointment, gentamicin 0.3% (as sulphate). Price 3 g = **D**

PoM **Minims Gentamicin** (S&N Pharm.)
Eye-drops, gentamicin 0.3% (as sulphate). Price 20 × 0.5 ml = **F**

IDOXURIDINE
Indications: local treatment of *Herpes simplex* infections
Apply eye drops every hour during the day and every 2 hours at night; eye ointment every 4 hours

PoM **Idoxuridine Eye-drops,** idoxuridine 0.1%. Price 10 ml = **D**; 15 ml = **F**
PoM **Idoxuridine Eye Ointment,** idoxuridine 0.5%. Price 3 g = **C**; 5 g = **F**
PoM **Idoxene**® (Spodefell)
Eye ointment, idoxuridine 0.5%. Price 3 g = **C**
PoM **Kerecid**® (SK&F)
Eye-drops, idoxuridine 0.1%. Price 15 ml = **F**
Eye ointment, idoxuridine 0.5%. Price 5 g = **F**
PoM **Ophthalmadine**® (SAS)
Eye-drops, idoxuridine 0.1%. Price 10 ml = **D**
Eye ointment, idoxuridine 0.5%. Price 3 g = **D**

MAFENIDE PROPIONATE
Indications: local treatment of infections
Apply eye-drops 3–4 times daily

Sulfomyl® (Winthrop)
Eye-drops, mafenide propionate 5%. Price 10 ml = **C**

MERCURIC OXIDE
Indications: see notes above

Mercuric Oxide Eye Ointment, mercuric oxide 1%. Price 3 g = **B**

NEOMYCIN SULPHATE
Indications: local treatment of infections (see notes above)
Apply eye-drops or eye ointment 3–4 times daily

PoM **Neomycin Sulphate Eye-drops,** neomycin sulphate 0.5%. Price 10 ml = **D**
PoM **Graneodin**® (Squibb)
Ophthalmic ointment (= eye ointment), gramicidin 0.025%, neomycin sulphate 0.25%. Price 3.6 g = **C**
Apply 3–4 times daily

PoM **Minims Neomycin Sulphate** (S&N Pharm.)
Eye-drops, neomycin sulphate 0.5%. Price 20 × 0.5 ml = **F**
PoM **Myciguent**® (Upjohn)
Eye ointment, neomycin sulphate 0.5%. Price 3.9 g = **B**
PoM **Neosporin**® (Calmic)
Eye-drops, gramicidin 25 units, neomycin sulphate 1700 units, polymyxin B sulphate 5000 units/ml. Price 5 ml = **E**
Apply 2–4 times daily

POLYMYXIN B SULPHATE
Indications: local treatment of infections (see notes above)

PoM **Polyfax**® (Calmic)
Ophthalmic ointment (= eye ointment), polymyxin B sulphate 10 000 units, bacitracin zinc 500 units/g. Price 4 g = **D**
Apply twice daily
PoM **Polytrim**® (Wellcome)
Eye-drops, trimethoprim 0.1%, polymyxin B sulphate 10 000 units/ml. Price 5 ml = **E**
Apply 4 times daily

PROPAMIDINE ISETHIONATE
Indications: local treatment of infections (see notes above)

Brolene® (M&B)
Eye-drops, propamidine isethionate 0.1%. Price 10 ml = **C**
Apply 4 times daily

SULPHACETAMIDE SODIUM
Indications: local treatment of infections (see notes above)
Apply eye-drops every 2–6 hours, eye ointment 2–4 times daily or at night

PoM **Sulphacetamide Eye-drops,** sulphacetamide sodium 10%, price 10 ml = **C**; 30%, price 10 ml = **D**
Note: when Weak Sulphacetamide Eye-drops are prescribed a 10% solution is supplied; when Strong Sulphacetamide Eye-drops are prescribed a 30% solution is supplied
PoM **Albucid**® (Nicholas)
Eye-drops, sulphacetamide sodium 10, 20, and 30%. Price 10 ml (all) = **C**
Eye ointment, sulphacetamide sodium 2.5 and 6%, greasy basis. Price 4 g (both) = **C**
Eye ointment, sulphacetamide sodium 10%, water-miscible basis. Price 4 g = **C**
PoM **Isopto Cetamide**® (Alcon)
Eye-drops, sulphacetamide sodium 15%, hypromellose 0.5%. Price 10 ml = **D**
PoM **Minims Sulphacetamide Sodium** (S&N Pharm.)
Eye-drops, sulphacetamide sodium 10%. Price 20 × 0.5 ml = **F**

PoM **Ocusol**® (Boots)
Eye-drops, sulphacetamide sodium 5%, zinc
sulphate 0.1%. Price 10 ml = **C**

TETRACYCLINE HYDROCHLORIDE

Indications: local treatment of infections, including trachoma (see notes above)
Apply eye-drops 2–4 times daily or eye ointment every 2 hours (acute infections)

PoM **Achromycin**® (Lederle)
Ophthalmic oil suspension (= eye-drops), tetra-
cycline hydrochloride 1%, in sesame oil vehicle.
Price 6 ml = **E**
Ointment (for ear or eye), tetracycline hydro-
chloride 1%. Price 3.5 g = **C**

TOBRAMYCIN

Indications: local treatment of infections (see
notes above)
Apply eye drops every 2–4 hours depending on
severity

▼ PoM **Tobralex**® (Alcon)
Eye-drops, tobramycin 0.3%. Price 5 ml = **D**

VIDARABINE

Indications: local treatment of *Herpes simplex*
infections
Apply 5 times daily

PoM **Vira-A**® (P-D)
Eye ointment, vidarabine 3%. Price 3.5 g = **G**

FUNGAL INFECTIONS OF THE EYE

Fungal infections of the cornea tend to occur after
agricultural injuries, especially in hot and humid
climates. Orbital mycosis is rare, and when it
occurs is usually due to direct spread of infection
from the paranasal sinuses. It may be advisable
to administer natamycin eye-drops 5–10% or eye
ointment 1% prophylactically. Increasing age,
debility, or immunosuppression by drugs, for
example, following renal transplantation, may
encourage fungal proliferation in many parts of
the body. The spread of infection via the blood-
stream occasionally produces a metastatic
endophthalmitis.

Increasing numbers of specific agents are being
evolved for intensive therapy followed, as necessary, by long-term treatment. Unfortunately,
precise identification is often a slow process. However, the presence on a slide of both yeast forms
and filaments suggests *Candida*, especially *C. albicans*, which is common. Intensive treatment with
flucytosine eye-drops 1.5% or alternatively clotrimazole 1% or miconazole 1–2% is effective.
Flucytosine may also be given by mouth (see
section 5.2).

Filaments alone indicate the need for treatment
with econazole, at least initially; infections with
Aspergillus species are commonest in this group.
Mycotic keratitis due to *Fusarium solani* (the
organism responsible for potato wilt) is becoming
more common; it may be treated with econazole

or thiabendazole. For *Penicillium* species, econazole or miconazole is used but some isolates are
sensitive only to thiabendazole. Amphotericin is
best avoided because of toxicity to the epithelium.

AVAILABILITY OF ANTIFUNGAL PREPARATIONS. It
should be noted that the drugs mentioned in this
section are not generally available as eye-drop
formulations in the United Kingdom. Treatment
will normally be carried out at specialist centres,
but requests for information about supplies of
preparations not available commercially should
be addressed to the District Pharmaceutical
Officer (or equivalent in Scotland or Northern
Ireland) or to Moorfields Eye Hospital, City
Road, London EC1V 2PD (01-253 3411).

11.3.2   Systemic preparations

In severe infections, systemic treatment is given
in addition to topical therapy as, for example,
in gonococcal conjunctivitis in the newborn and
infective endophthalmitis. The blood-aqueous
barrier usually breaks down in the latter case
allowing intra-ocular penetration of systemically
administered drugs unless the intra-ocular pressure is raised. Subconjunctival injection of a suitable drug may also help to achieve a high intra-
ocular concentration.

Pyrimethamine (see section 5.4.1) administered
systemically is appropriate for treatment of toxoplasma choroidoretinitis; clindamycin and sulphadiazine are other possibilities.

Other drugs suitable for the systemic treatment
of eye infections are included in chapter 5.

11.4   Corticosteroids and other anti-inflammatory preparations

Corticosteroids administered topically, by subconjunctival injection, and systemically have an
important place in treating iridocyclitis and
scleritis.

There are two main dangers from topical corticosteroids. The first is aggravation of dendritic
corneal ulceration, due to misdiagnosis already
referred to (section 11.3.1), when the corticosteroid is administered in eye-drops.
Secondly, again arising from the use of eye-drop
formulations, a 'steroid glaucoma' may be
produced, after a few weeks treatment, in patients
predisposed to chronic simple glaucoma,
especially with dexamethasone and prednisolone.

Systemic corticosteroids can usefully be given
on an alternate-day basis. The risk of producing
glaucoma is not great, but 'steroid cataract' is
a very high risk (75%) if more than 15 mg of
prednisolone or equivalent is given daily for several years. The longer the duration, the greater is
the risk. A dose of less then 10 mg per day is
usually safe.

Oxyphenbutazone eye ointment (Tanderil®)
does not have the disadvantages of corticosteroids

---

and can be used in the treatment of iridocyclitis and episcleritis.

Topical preparations of antihistamines such as eye-drops containing antazoline sulphate and xylometazoline hydrochloride (Otrivine-Antistin®, below) may be used for allergic conjunctivitis.

Mast cell stabilisation by use of sodium cromoglycate eye-drops (Opticrom®) may be useful for vernal catarrh and other allergic forms of conjunctivitis as an alternative to corticosteroids.

ANTAZOLINE SALTS
Indications: allergic conjunctivitis

Otrivine-Antistin® (Zyma)
Eye-drops, antazoline sulphate 0.5%, xylometazoline hydrochloride 0.05%. Price 10 ml = **C**
Apply 2–3 times daily
PoM **Vasocon A®** (CooperVision)
Eye-drops, antazoline phosphate 0.5%, naphazoline hydrochloride 0.05%. Price 10 ml = **E**
Apply every 3–4 hours

BETAMETHASONE SODIUM PHOSPHATE
Indications: local treatment of inflammation
Cautions; Side-effects: see notes above
Apply eye-drops every 1–2 hours or eye ointment 2–4 times daily

PoM **Betnesol®** (Glaxo)
Drops (for ear, eye, or nose), betamethasone sodium phosphate 0.1%. Price 5 ml = **C**
Eye ointment, betamethasone sodium phosphate 0.1%. Price 3 g = **C**
PoM **Betnesol-N®** (Glaxo)
Drops (for ear, eye, or nose), see section 12.1.1
Eye ointment, betamethasone sodium phosphate 0.1%, neomycin sulphate 0.5%. Price 3 g = **C**
PoM **Vista-Methasone®** (Daniel)
Drops (for ear, eye, or nose), betamethasone sodium phosphate 0.1%. Price 5 and 10 ml (both) = **C**
▼ PoM **Vista-Methasone N®** (Daniel)
Drops (for ear, eye, or nose), see section 12.1.1

CLOBETASONE BUTYRATE
Indications: local treatment of inflammation
Cautions; Side-effects: see notes above; reduced tendency to raise intra-ocular pressure
Apply eye-drops every 1–6 hours

PoM **Eumovate®** (Glaxo)
Eye-drops, clobetasone butyrate 0.1%. Price 5 ml = **D**; 10 ml = **E**
PoM **Eumovate-N®** (Glaxo)
Eye-drops, clobetasone butyrate 0.1%, neomycin sulphate 0.5%. Price 5 ml = **D**; 10 ml = **E**

DEXAMETHASONE
Indications: local treatment of inflammation
Cautions; Side-effects: see notes above
Apply eye-drops every 1–4 hours

PoM **Maxidex®** (Alcon)
Eye-drops, dexamethasone 0.1%, hypromellose 0.5%. Price 5 ml = **D**; 10 ml = **F**
PoM **Maxitrol®** (Alcon)
Eye-drops, dexamethasone 0.1%, hypromellose 0.5%, neomycin 0.35% (as sulphate), polymyxin B sulphate 6000 units/ml. Price 5 ml = **E**
Eye ointment, dexamethasone 0.1%, neomycin 0.35% (as sulphate), polymyxin B sulphate 6000 units/g. Price 3.5 g = **D**
PoM **Sofradex®** (Roussel)
Drops and *ointment* (for ear or eye), see section 12.1.1

FLUOROMETHOLONE
Indications: local treatment of inflammation
Cautions; Side-effects: see notes above; reduced tendency to raise intra-ocular pressure
Apply eye-drops every 1–4 hours

PoM **FML®** (Allergan)
Ophthalmic suspension (= eye-drops), fluorometholone 0.1%. Price 5 ml = **D**; 10 ml = **E**
▼ PoM **FML-Neo®** (Allergan)
Eye-drops, fluorometholone 0·1%, neomycin sulphate 0·5%. Price 5 ml = **E**

HYDROCORTISONE ACETATE
Indications: local treatment of inflammation
Cautions; Side-effects: see notes above

PoM **Chloromycetin Hydrocortisone®** (P-D)
Eye ointment, chloramphenicol 1%, hydrocortisone acetate 0.5%. Price 4 g = **C**
PoM **Cortucid®** (Nicholas)
Eye drop cream (= eye ointment), hydrocortisone acetate 0.5%, sulphacetamide sodium 10%. Price 3 g = **C**
PoM **Framycort®** (Fisons)
Drops (for ear or eye), framycetin sulphate 0.5%, hydrocortisone acetate 0.5%. Price 5 ml = **E**
Eye ointment, framycetin sulphate 0.5%, hydrocortisone acetate 0.5%. Price 3.5 g = **D**
PoM **Neo-Cortef®** (Upjohn)
Drops and *ointment* (for ear or eye), see section 12.1.1

OXYPHENBUTAZONE
Indications: local treatment of inflammation
Apply eye ointment 2–5 times daily

PoM **Tanderil®** (Zyma)
Eye ointment, oxyphenbutazone 10%. Price 5 g = **C**
PoM **Tanderil Chloramphenicol®** (Zyma)
Eye ointment, chloramphenicol 1%, oxyphenbutazone 10%. Price 5 g = **D**

PREDNISOLONE SODIUM PHOSPHATE
Indications: local treatment of inflammation
Cautions; Side-effects: see notes above
Apply eye-drops every 1–2 hours

PoM **Minims Prednisolone** (S&N Pharm.)
Eye-drops, prednisolone sodium phosphate 0.5%. Price 20 × 0.5 ml = **F**
PoM **Predsol®** (Glaxo)
Drops (for ear or eye), prednisolone sodium phosphate 0.5%. Price 5 ml = **C**; 10 ml = **D**
PoM **Predsol-N®** (Glaxo)
Drops (for ear or eye), see section 12.1.1

C = 51–100p, **D** = 101–180p, **E** = 181–300p, **F** = 301–450p, **G** = 451–650p, **H** = 651–900p, **I** = 901–1200p, **J** = over 1200p.

SODIUM CROMOGLYCATE

Indications: allergic conjunctivitis
Apply eye-drops 4 times daily; eye ointment, adults and children, apply 2–3 times daily

PoM **Opticrom**® (Fisons)
Eye-drops, sodium cromoglycate 2%. Price 10 ml = **F**
Eye ointment, sodium cromoglycate 4%. Price 5 g = **G**

11.5 Mydriatics and cycloplegics

The two properties of dilatation of the pupil and paralysis of the ciliary muscle are usually possessed equally by anticholinergic drugs applied topically but they vary in potency. Short-acting, relatively weak mydriatics which paralyse the sphincter pupillae are used by the ophthalmologist to allow a better view of the fundus of the eye. The relative potencies and durations of action of the principal drugs, in ascending order, are tropicamide (3 hours), lachesine (mydriatic effect 6 hours, cycloplegic effect midway between homatropine and atropine), cyclopentolate, hyoscine, and homatropine (all 24 hours), and atropine (7 days or longer).

Homatropine or **atropine** are preferable for producing cycloplegia for refraction in young children. Atropine is the less suitable because of its long duration of action; it is used for the treatment of iridocyclitis mainly to prevent posterior synechiae preferably with phenylephrine 10% eye-drops.

Contact dermatitis is not uncommon with all of the above mydriatic drugs, especially atropine, and toxic systemic reactions to this drug may occur in the very young and the very old.

Mydriasis may be achieved for a few hours by the use of **phenylephrine eye-drops**, which stimulate the dilator pupillae muscle. Mydriasis may precipitate acute closed-angle ('congestive') glaucoma in a few patients, usually aged over 60 years, who are predisposed to the condition because of a small eyeball with a shallow anterior chamber and small diameter cornea. A family history is significant. Mydriatics should be avoided in such patients. Alternatively, one pupil only should be dilated at each visit.

ATROPINE SULPHATE

Indications: refraction procedures in young children; see also notes above
Cautions: action persistent, may precipitate glaucoma; see also notes above

PoM **Atropine Eye-drops,** atropine sulphate 1%. Price 10 ml = **C**
PoM **Isopto Atropine**® (Alcon)
Eye-drops, atropine sulphate 1%, hypromellose 0.5%. Price 5 ml = **D**

PoM **Minims Atropine Sulphate** (S&N Pharm.)
Eye-drops, atropine sulphate 1%. Price 20 × 0.5 ml = **F**
PoM **Opulets Atropine Sulphate**® (Alcon)
Eye-drops, atropine 1%. Price 20 × 0.25 ml = **F**

CYCLOPENTOLATE HYDROCHLORIDE

Indications: see notes above
Cautions: patients with raised intra-ocular pressure; see notes above
PoM **Minims Cyclopentolate Hydrochloride**— (S&N Pharm.)
Eye-drops, cyclopentolate hydrochloride 0.5 and 1%. Price 20 × 0.5 ml (both) = **F**
PoM **Mydrilate**® (WBP)
Eye-drops, cyclopentolate hydrochloride 0.5 and 1%. Price 5 ml (both) = **C**
PoM **Opulets Cyclopentolate Hydrochloride**® (Alcon)
Eye-drops, cyclopentolate hydrochloride 1%. Price 20 × 0.25 ml = **F**

HOMATROPINE HYDROBROMIDE

Indications; Cautions: see notes above

PoM **Homatropine Eye-drops,** homatropine hydrobromide 1 and 2%. Price 10 ml (both) = **D**
PoM **Minims Homatropine Hydrobromide** (S&N Pharm.)
Eye-drops, homatropine hydrobromide 2%. Price 20 × 0.5 ml = **F**

HYOSCINE HYDROBROMIDE

Indications; Cautions: see notes above

PoM **Hyoscine Eye-drops,** usual strength hyoscine hydrobromide 0.25%. Price 10 ml = **C**
PoM **Minims Hyoscine Hydrobromide** (S&N Pharm.)
Eye-drops, hyoscine hydrobromide 0.2%. Price 20 × 0.5 ml = **F**

LACHESINE CHLORIDE

Indications: see notes above; useful in patients hypersensitive to other mydriatics
Cautions: see notes above

Lachesine Eye-drops, lachesine chloride 1%. Price 10 ml = **F**

PHENYLEPHRINE HYDROCHLORIDE

Indications; Cautions: see notes above

Phenylephrine Eye-drops, phenylephrine hydrochloride 10%. Price 10 ml = **D**
Isopto Frin® (Alcon)
Eye-drops, phenylephrine hydrochloride 0.12%, hypromellose 0.5%. Price 10 ml = **D**
Minims Phenylephrine Hydrochloride (S&N Pharm.)
Eye-drops, phenylephrine hydrochloride 10%. Price 20 × 0.5 ml = **F**
Prefrin® (Allergan)
Eye-drops, phenylephrine hydrochloride 0.12%. Price 15 ml = **D**

Zincfrin® (Alcon)
Eye-drops, phenylephrine hydrochloride 0.12%, zinc sulphate 0.25%. Price 10 ml = **D**

TROPICAMIDE

Indications; Cautions: see notes above

PoM **Minims Tropicamide** (S&N Pharm.)
Eye-drops, tropicamide 0.5 and 1%. Price 20 × 0.5 ml (both) = **F**
PoM **Mydriacyl**® (Alcon)
Eye-drops, tropicamide 0.5 and 1%. Price 5 ml (both) = **D**

11.6   Treatment of glaucoma

An abnormally high intra-ocular pressure, glaucoma, may result in blindness associated with pressure-excavation of the optic disk ('glaucomatous cupping'). In virtually all cases, rise in pressure is due to reduced outflow of aqueous humour, the inflow remaining constant. Probably the commonest condition is *chronic simple glaucoma* where the obstruction is in the trabecular meshwork.

Glaucoma may be treated by the application of eye-drops containing miotics, adrenaline, guanethidine, or beta-adrenoceptor blocking drugs such as timolol. Other drugs such as acetazolamide and dichlorphenamide are given by mouth and, in emergency or before surgery, mannitol may be given by intravenous infusion.

MIOTICS. The small pupil is an unfortunate side-effect of these drugs (except when **pilocarpine** is used temporarily while patients await operation for *closed-angle glaucoma*). The key factor is the opening up of the inefficient drainage channels in the trabecular meshwork resulting from contraction or spasm of the ciliary muscle. This unfortunately also produces accommodation spasm, which is especially disadvantageous in patients under 40 years of age. Pilocarpine has a duration of action of 3 to 4 hours. **Physostigmine** is more potent. It is still used in **physostigmine and pilocarpine eye-drops** but is not usually used now on its own. **Carbachol** is sometimes used to lower intra-ocular pressure, usually in conjunction with other miotics such as physostigmine. In severe cases **ecothiopate iodide** (Phospholine Iodide®) produces a more prolonged potent effect but the risk of cataract and other side-effects has to be weighed against the benefit.

ADRENALINE. This probably acts both by reducing the rate of production of aqueous humour and increasing the outflow through the trabecular meshwork. It is contra-indicated in closed-angle glaucoma because it is a mydriatic, unless an iridectomy has been carried out.

Dipivefrin (Propine®) is an ester and prodrug of adrenaline. It is stated to pass more rapidly through the cornea and is then converted to the active form.

Guanethidine (Ganda®, Ismelin®) enhances and prolongs the effects of adrenaline. It is also used alone and produces an initial mydriasis together with an increased aqueous outflow followed by a miosis and reduced aqueous secretion.

BETA-ADRENOCEPTOR BLOCKING DRUGS. **Timolol maleate** (Timoptol®) a beta$_1$- and beta$_2$-blocking drug used as 0.25 and 0.5% eye-drops reduces intra-ocular pressure very effectively in chronic simple glaucoma, probably by reducing the rate of production of aqueous humour. Like many other beta-adrenoceptor blocking drugs such as propranolol, it also reduces intra-ocular pressure when administered systemically. Systemic absorption of timolol occurs following topical application. Caution is therefore necessary in patients with asthma, bradycardia, or heart failure, and administration of timolol eye-drops may give rise to a drug interaction in patients receiving verapamil.

Timolol is also indicated in closed-angle glaucoma pending iridectomy because production of aqueous humour may be decreased thus reducing iris bombé (bulging of the iris) if pilocarpine is also administered to produce miosis.

If supplementary topical treatment is required after iridectomy or a drainage operation in either open-angle or closed-angle glaucoma, timolol is preferred to pilocarpine. This is because of the risk that posterior synechiae will be formed as a result of the miotic effect of pilocarpine, especially in closed-angle glaucoma. It is then also advantageous to utilise the mydriatic side-effect of adrenaline.

SYSTEMIC DRUGS. The side-effects of beta-adrenoceptor blocking drugs are probably sufficient to prevent their being prescribed by the ophthalmologist for administration by mouth. Hence **acetazolamide** (Diamox® etc.) will retain a significant place in treatment. It inhibits carbonic anhydrase, hence reducing the bicarbonate in aqueous humour and the water secreted with it, resulting in a fall in the intra-ocular pressure. **Dichlorphenamide** (Daranide®) has a similar but more prolonged action. Both these drugs have a moderate incidence of side-effects, giving rise, especially in the elderly, to parasthesia, lack of appetite, drowsiness and depression. Intravenous hypertonic **mannitol**, or **glycerol** by mouth, are useful short-term ocular hypotensive drugs. Acetazolamide by intramuscular or intravenous injection is also useful in the pre-operative treatment of closed-angle glaucoma.

ACETAZOLAMIDE

Indications; Side-effects: see notes above
Cautions: avoid in renal impairment. Drug interactions: see Appendix 1 (sections *2.2, 2.3, 4.2*)
Dose: by mouth or by intravenous injection, initially 500 mg, subsequent doses 250 mg every 6 hours

PoM **Diamox**® (Lederle)
Sustets® (= capsules s/r), orange, acetazolamide 500 mg. Price 20 caps = **G**. Label: 2, 25
Dose: 1 capsule twice daily

Tablets, acetazolamide 250 mg. Price 20 tabs = E. Label: 2
Powder (for oral use), acetazolamide. Price 25 g = G. Label: 2
Sodium Parenteral (= injection), powder for reconstitution, acetazolamide (as sodium salt). Price 500-mg vial = J

ADRENALINE

Indications; Contra-indications: see notes above
   Apply eye-drops 1–2 times daily

PoM **Epifrin**® (Allergan)
Eye-drops, adrenaline 1% (as hydrochloride). Price 10 ml = E
Eppy® (S&N Pharm.)
Eye-drops, adrenaline 1%. Price 7.5 ml = E
Isopto Epinal® (Alcon)
Eye-drops, adrenaline 0.5% (as borate complex) and hypromellose 0.5%. Price 7.5 ml = D
Eye-drops, adrenaline 1% (as borate complex) and hypromellose 0.5%. Price 7.5 ml = D
PoM **Simplene**® (S&N Pharm.)
Eye-drops, adrenaline 0.5 and 1%, in a viscous vehicle. Price 7.5 ml (both) = E

CARBACHOL

Indications: see notes above
   Apply eye-drops 3 times daily

PoM **Isopto Carbachol**® (Alcon)
Eye-drops, carbachol 3%, hypromellose 1%. Price 10 ml = E

DEMECARIUM BROMIDE

Indications: glaucoma
   Apply eye-drops 1–2 times daily

PoM **Tosmilen**® (Sinclair)
Eye-drops, demecarium bromide 0.25 and 0.5%. Price 5 ml (both) = G

DICHLORPHENAMIDE

Indications; Side-effects: see notes above
Dose: initially 100–200 mg, then 100 mg every 12 hours, adjusted according to the patient's response

PoM **Daranide**® (MSD)
Tablets, yellow, scored, dichlorphenamide 50 mg. Price 20 tabs = C

DIPIVEFRIN HYDROCHLORIDE

Indications; Contra-indications: see notes above
   Apply 1 drop twice daily

▼ PoM **Propine**® (Allergan)
Eye-drops, dipivefrin hydrochloride 0.1%. Price 10 ml = G

ECOTHIOPATE IODIDE

Indications; Side-effects: see notes above
Cautions: drug interactions: see Appendix 1 (section *15*)
   Apply eye-drops 1–2 times daily

PoM **Phospholine Iodide**® (Ayerst)
Eye-drops, ecothiopate iodide 0.03% when reconstituted. Price 5 ml = E
Eye-drops, ecothiopate iodide 0.06, 0.125, and 0.25% when reconstituted. Price 5 ml (all) = E

GUANETHIDINE MONOSULPHATE

Indications: see notes above
   Apply eye-drops 1–2 times daily

▼ PoM **Ganda**® (S&N Pharm.)
Eye-drops '1 + 0.2', guanethidine monosulphate 1%, adrenaline 0.2% in a viscous vehicle. Price 7.5 ml = F
Eye-drops '3 + 0.5', guanethidine monosulphate 3%, adrenaline 0.5% in a viscous vehicle. Price 7.5 ml = G
Eye-drops '5 + 0.5', guanethidine monosulphate 5%, adrenaline 0.5% in a viscous vehicle. Price 7.5 ml = G
Eye-drops '5 + 1', guanethidine monosulphate 5%, adrenaline 1% in a viscous vehicle. Price 7.5 ml = G
PoM **Ismelin**® (Zyma)
Eye-drops, guanethidine monosulphate 5%. Price 5 ml = D

PHYSOSTIGMINE SULPHATE

Indications; Side-effects: see notes above
   Apply eye-drops 2–6 times daily

PoM **Physostigmine Eye-drops,** physostigmine sulphate 0.25 and 0.5%. Price 10 ml (both) = D
PoM **Physostigmine and Pilocarpine Eye-drops,** usual strengths physostigmine sulphate 0.25% with pilocarpine hydrochloride 2% or 4% or physostigmine sulphate 0.5% with pilocarpine hydrochloride 4%. Price 10 ml (0.25% with 2%) = C; 10 ml (0.25% with 4%) = D; 10 ml (0.5% with 4%) = D

PILOCARPINE HYDROCHLORIDE

Indications; Side-effects: see notes above
   Apply eye-drops 3–6 times daily

PoM **Pilocarpine Eye-drops,** pilocarpine hydrochloride 0.5, 1, 2, 3, and 4%. Price 10 ml (up to 2%) = B; 10 ml (3 and 4%) = C
PoM **Isopto Carpine**® (Alcon)
Eye-drops, pilocarpine hydrochloride 0.5, 1, 2, and 3%, all with hypromellose 0.5%. Price 10 ml (up to 2%) = C; 10 ml (3%) = D
Eye-drops, pilocarpine hydrochloride 4% and hypromellose 0.5%. Price 10 ml = D
▼ PoM **Ocusert**® (M&B)
Pilo-20 ocular insert, s/r, pilocarpine 20 micrograms released per hour for 1 week. Price per insert = E. Counselling advised, method of use
Pilo-40 ocular insert, s/r, pilocarpine 40 micrograms released per hour for 1 week. Price per insert = E. Counselling advised, method of use
PoM **Opulets Pilocarpine**® (Alcon)
Eye-drops, pilocarpine hydrochloride 1, 2, and 4%. Price 20 × 0.25 ml (all) = F
PoM **Sno Pilo**® (S&N Pharm.)
Eye-drops, pilocarpine hydrochloride 1, 2, and

4% in a viscous vehicle. Price 10 ml (1 and 2%) = **C**; 4% = **D**

PILOCARPINE NITRATE
Indications; Side-effects: see notes above
Apply eye-drops 3–6 times daily

PoM **Minims Pilocarpine Nitrate** (S&N Pharm.)
Eye-drops, pilocarpine nitrate 1, 2, and 4%.
Price 20 × 0.5 ml (all) = **F**

TIMOLOL MALEATE
Indications; Cautions; Side-effects: see notes above
Contra-indications: history of bronchospasm
Apply eye-drops twice daily

▼ PoM **Timoptol**® (MSD)
Eye-drops, timolol 0.25 and 0.5% (as maleate), in Ocumeter® metered-dose unit. Price per unit (both) = **G**

11.7 Local anaesthetics

Oxybuprocaine and amethocaine are probably the most widely used topical local anaesthetics. Proxymetacaine (Ophthaine®) causes less initial stinging and is useful for children. Cocaine, by potentiating noradrenaline, produces useful vaso-constriction, but is now much less used in surgery. Oxybuprocaine or a combined preparation of lig-nocaine and fluorescein is used for tonometry. Lignocaine, with or without adrenaline, is injected into the eyelids for minor surgery, while a retro-bulbar injection may be used for major eye surgery.

AMETHOCAINE HYDROCHLORIDE
Indications: local anaesthetic

PoM **Amethocaine Eye-drops,** amethocaine hydrochloride 0.5%, price 10 ml = **C**; 1%, price 10 ml = **D**
PoM **Minims Amethocaine Hydrochloride** (S&N Pharm.)
Eye-drops, amethocaine hydrochloride 0.5 and 1%. Price 20 × 0.5 ml (both) = **F**

COCAINE HYDROCHLORIDE
Indications: local anaesthetic

CD **Cocaine Eye-drops,** cocaine hydrochloride 4%. Price 4 ml = **D**
CD **Cocaine and Homatropine Eye-drops,** cocaine hydrochloride 2%, homatropine hydro-bromide 2%. Price 10 ml = **F**

LIGNOCAINE HYDROCHLORIDE
Indications: local anaesthetic

PoM **Minims Lignocaine and Fluorescein** (S&N Pharm.)
Eye-drops, lignocaine hydrochloride 4%, fluore-scein sodium 0.25%. Price 20 × 0.5 ml = **G**

OXYBUPROCAINE HYDROCHLORIDE
Indications: local anaesthetic

PoM **Minims Benoxinate (Oxybuprocaine) Hydrochloride** (S&N Pharm.)
Eye-drops, oxybuprocaine hydrochloride 0.4%.
Price 20 × 0.5 ml = **F**
PoM **Opulets Benoxinate (Oxybuprocaine) Hydrochloride**® (Alcon)
Eye-drops, oxybuprocaine hydrochloride 0.4%.
Price 20 × 0.25 ml = **F**

PROXYMETACAINE HYDROCHLORIDE
Indications: local anaesthetic

PoM **Ophthaine**® (Squibb)
Eye-drops, proxymetacaine hydrochloride 0.5%. Price 15 ml = **F**

11.8 Miscellaneous ophthalmic preparations

11.8.1 Preparations for tear deficiency
11.8.2 Other preparations

11.8.1 Preparations for tear deficiency

Chronically sore eyes associated with reduced tear secretion, usually in cases of rheumatoid arthritis (Sjögren's syndrome), often respond to hypro-mellose eye-drops and other similar viscous preparations.

ACETYLCYSTEINE
Indications: tear deficiency, mucolytic
Apply eye-drops 3–4 times daily

PoM **Ilube**® (DF)
Eye-drops, acetylcysteine 5%, hypromellose 0.35%. Price 15 ml = **G**

HYPROMELLOSE
Indications: tear deficiency

Hypromellose Eye-drops, hypromellose 4000 (or 4500 or 5000) 0.3%. Price 10 ml = **C**
Isopto Alkaline® (Alcon)
Eye-drops, hypromellose 1%. Price 10 ml = **D**
Isopto Plain® (Alcon)
Eye-drops, hypromellose 0.5%. Price 10 ml = **C**
Tears Naturale® (Alcon)
Eye-drops, dextran '70' 0.1%, hypromellose 0.3%. Price 15 ml = **D**

LIQUID PARAFFIN
Indications: tear deficiency

Lacri-Lube® (Allergan)
Eye ointment, liquid paraffin. Price 3.5 g = **D**

POLYVINYL ALCOHOL
Indications: tear deficiency

C = 51-100p, D = 101-180p, E = 181-300p, F = 301-450p, G = 451-650p, H = 651-900p, I = 901-1200p, J = over 1200p.

Hypotears® (CooperVision)
Eye-drops, macrogol '8000' 2%, polyvinyl alcohol 1%. Price 10 ml = **D**
Liquifilm Tears® (Allergan)
Eye-drops, polyvinyl alcohol 1.4%. Price 15 ml = **D**
Sno Tears® (S&N Pharm.)
Eye-drops, polyvinyl alcohol 1.4%. Price 10 ml = **C**

11.8.2 Other preparations

Zinc sulphate is a traditional so-called astringent which has been used in eye-drops for treatment of excessive lachrymation. Zinc sulphate and adrenaline eye-drops is also used but there is a risk in patients predisposed to closed-angle glaucoma. Simple eye ointment is a bland sterile preparation which may be used to remove crusts in blepharitis. Sodium chloride eye lotion has already been mentioned (section 11.1).

Thymoxamine is used to reverse the mydriasis produced by phenylephrine and other sympathomimetic drugs. (For use in peripheral vascular disorders see section 2.6.3.)

Fluorescein sodium and rose bengal are used in diagnostic procedures and for locating damaged areas of the cornea due to injury or disease.

Certain eye-drops, for example benzylpenicillin, colistin, desferrioxamine, and trisodium edetate, may be prepared aseptically from material supplied for injection.

ACETYLCHOLINE CHLORIDE

Indications: cataract surgery, penetrating keratoplasty, iridectomy, and other anterior segment surgery requiring rapid miosis

PoM **Miochol®** (CooperVision)
Solution for intra-ocular irrigation, acetylcholine chloride 1%, mannitol 3% when reconstituted. Price 2 ml = **H**

CASTOR OIL

Indications: emollient and lubricant used in removal of foreign bodies

Minims Castor Oil (S&N Pharm.)
Eye-drops, castor oil. Price 20 × 0.5 ml = **F**

CHYMOTRYPSIN

Indications: zonulolysis in intracapsular cataract extraction

PoM **Chymar-Zon®** (Armour)
Injection, powder for reconstitution, alphachymotrypsin 750 USP units. Price per vial (with diluent) = **G**
PoM **Zonulysin®** (Henleys)
Injection, powder for reconstitution, alphachymotrypsin 300 USP units (≡ 1.5 microkatals). Price per vial (with diluent) = **F**

PARAFFIN, YELLOW, SOFT

Indications: see notes above

Simple Eye Ointment, liquid paraffin 10%, wool fat 10%, in yellow soft paraffin. Price 3 g = **C**

SODIUM CHLORIDE

Indications: irrigation, including first-aid removal of harmful substances

Sodium Chloride Eye Lotion, sodium chloride 0.9%. Price 200 ml = **E**
Minims Sodium Chloride (S&N Pharm.)
Eye-drops, sodium chloride 0.9%. Price 20 × 0.5 ml = **F**
Normasol Undine® (Schering)
Solution (sterile), sodium chloride 0.9%. Price 10 × 20-ml sachets = **D**
Opulets Sodium Chloride® (Alcon)
Eye-drops, sodium chloride 0.9%. Price 20 × 0.25 ml = **F**

THYMOXAMINE HYDROCHLORIDE

Indications: see notes above
Side-effects: minimal conjunctival hyperaemia for a few hours; rarely transient ptosis
Apply one drop as required

PoM **Minims Thymoxamine Hydrochloride** (S&N Pharm.)
Eye-drops, thymoxamine hydrochloride 0.5%. Price 20 × 0.5 ml = **F**

ZINC SULPHATE

Indications; Cautions: see notes above

Zinc Sulphate Eye-drops, zinc sulphate 0.25%. Price 10 ml = **D**
Zinc Sulphate and Adrenaline Eye-drops, zinc sulphate 0.25%, adrenaline acid tartrate 0.09% (equivalent to 1 in 2000 adrenaline). Price 10 ml = **D**

DIAGNOSTIC PREPARATIONS

FLUORESCEIN SODIUM

Indications: detection of lesions and foreign bodies

Fluorescein Eye-drops, fluorescein sodium 1%. Price 10 ml = **D**
Minims Fluorescein Sodium (S&N Pharm.)
Eye-drops, fluorescein sodium 1% or 2%. Price 20 × 0.5 ml (both) = **F**
Opulets Fluorescein Sodium® (Alcon)
Eye-drops, fluorescein sodium 1%. Price 20 × 0.25 ml = **F**

ROSE BENGAL

Indications: detection of lesions

Minims Rose Bengal (S&N Pharm.)
Eye-drops, rose bengal 1%. Price 20 × 0.5 ml = **F**

11.9 Contact lenses

Many patients wear these lenses and special care is required in prescribing eye preparations for them. Unless medically indicated the lens should not be worn during intensive courses of treatment for infections. If the patient is wearing hard lenses the use of eye-drops containing anti-inflammatory drugs over long periods of time is to be deprecated. Some drugs can spoil hydrophilic plastic lenses. Therefore unless eye-drops are specifically indicated as safe to use with hydrophilic contact lenses, the lenses should be removed before instillation and not worn during the period of treatment.

Hydrophilic plastic used for many soft contact lenses will selectively bind certain preservatives and could then be a source of irritation. Thiomersal is usually satisfactory. Chlorhexidine acetate is satisfactory in some cases, while phenylmercuric acetate or nitrate is usually satisfactory but is not recommended for long-term treatment. Benzalkonium chloride is unsuitable in all cases.

Sodium chloride solution 0.9% (sterile) can be used to store soft hydrophilic lenses provided that the case with lens and solution are regularly subjected to a heat treatment to reduce microbial contamination (such as 80°C for 40 minutes).

12: Drugs used in the treatment of diseases of the

EAR, NOSE, and OROPHARYNX

In this chapter, drug treatment is discussed under the following headings:

12.1 Drugs acting on the ear
12.2 Drugs acting on the nose
12.3 Drugs acting on the oropharynx

12.1   Drugs acting on the ear

12.1.1 Otitis externa
12.1.2 Otitis media
12.1.3 Removal of ear wax

For treatment of labyrinthine disorders see section 4.6.

12.1.1   Otitis externa

Otitis externa is an eczematous reaction of the meatal skin. It is important to exclude an underlying chronic otitis media before treatment is commenced. Many cases recover after thorough cleansing of the meatus by suction, dry mopping, or gentle syringing. The main problem in resistant cases is the difficulty in applying lotions and ointments satisfactorily to the relatively inaccessible affected skin. The most effective method is to introduce a ribbon gauze dressing soaked in an **astringent** such as **aluminium acetate**, or anti-inflammatory **corticosteroid** solution. When this is not practical, the ear should be gently cleaned with a probe covered in cotton wool and the patient encouraged to lie with the affected ear uppermost for ten minutes after the canal has been filled with a liberal quantity of the appropriate solution.

If infection is present, a topical anti-infective which is not used systemically (such as **framycetin**, **neomycin**, or **clioquinol**) may be used, but for only about a week as an excessive use of antibiotics may result in fungal infections. These may be difficult to treat and require expert advice. Sensitivity to the anti-infective or solvent may occur and resistance to antibacterials is a possibility with prolonged use. Chloramphenicol ear-drops contain propylene glycol and cause sensitivity in about 10% of patients. An eye ointment of chloramphenicol may be used. Solutions containing an anti-infective and a corticosteroid (such as Locorten-Vioform®) are used for treating cases where infection is present with inflammation and eczema. Aminoglycosides and polymyxins are potentially ototoxic when used topically in the ear, and are contra-indicated if the oval or round window membranes are known or suspected to be perforated. If the eardrum is not intact it is probably unwise to use an aminoglycoside in the ear.

An acute infection may cause severe pain and a systemic antibiotic and a simple analgesic are required. When a resistant staphylococcal infection (a boil) is present in the external auditory meatus, **flucloxacillin** is the drug of choice (see

section 5.1.1.2). Ampicillin or phenoxymethyl-penicillin are used for other infections (see sections 5.1, Table 1).

The skin of the pinna adjacent to the ear canal is often affected by eczema, and topical corticosteroid creams and ointments (see section 13.4) are then required and should be applied five or six times daily. Prolonged use should be avoided.

Ear-drops or **ointment** should be applied using 3–4 drops of a liquid preparation or a similar quantity of ointment warmed if necessary, inserted into the affected ear. If discharge is profuse, ear-drops applied directly may be washed away; in these circumstances the ear canal should be carefully cleaned and a quarter-inch gauze wick impregnated with the ear-drops should be introduced into it.

ASTRINGENT PREPARATIONS

ALUMINIUM ACETATE
Indications: inflammation in otitis externa

Aluminium Acetate Ear-drops (13%), consists of aluminium acetate solution, BP. Price 20 ml = **A**
Insert into the meatus or apply on a gauze wick which should be kept saturated with the ear-drops
Aluminium Acetate Ear-drops (8%), prepared by diluting 8 parts of aluminium acetate solution, BP, with 5 parts of purified water, freshly boiled and cooled. It must be freshly prepared. Price 20 ml = **A**
Directions as above

ANTI-INFLAMMATORY PREPARATIONS

BETAMETHASONE SODIUM PHOSPHATE
Indications: eczematous inflammation in otitis externa
Cautions: avoid prolonged use
Contra-indications: untreated infection

PoM **Betnesol®** (Glaxo)
Drops (for ear, eye, or nose), betamethasone sodium phosphate 0.1%. Price 5 ml = **C**; 10 ml = **D**
Apply every 2–3 hours; reduce frequency of application when relief is obtained

PREDNISOLONE SODIUM PHOSPHATE
Indications: eczematous inflammation in otitis externa
Cautions: avoid prolonged use
Contra-indications: untreated infection

PoM **Predsol**® (Glaxo)

Drops (for ear or eye), prednisolone sodium phosphate 0.5%. Price 5 ml = **C**; 10 ml = **D**
Apply every 2–3 hours; reduce frequency of application when relief is obtained

ANTI-INFECTIVE PREPARATIONS

CHLORAMPHENICOL

Indications: bacterial infection in otitis externa
Cautions: see under Framycetin Sulphate
Side-effects: high incidence of sensitivity reactions
Apply 2–3 times daily

PoM **Chloramphenicol Ear-drops 5%** and **10%**, chloramphenicol in propylene glycol. Price 10 ml (5%) = **D**; 5 ml (10%) = **C**; 10 ml (10%) = **D**
PoM **Chloromycetin**® (P-D)
Ear-drops, chloramphenicol 10% in propylene glycol. Price 5 ml = **B**

CLIOQUINOL

Indications: mild bacterial or fungal infections in otitis externa
Cautions: avoid prolonged use; see also notes above
Side-effects: local sensitivity; stains skin and clothing

PoM **Locorten-Vioform**® (Ciba)
Ear-drops, clioquinol 1%, flumethasone pivalate 0.02%. Price 7.5 ml = **D**
Apply 2 or more times daily

FRAMYCETIN SULPHATE

Indications: bacterial infection in otitis externa
Cautions: avoid prolonged use; perforated eardrum; see also notes above
Side-effects: local sensitivity; ototoxicity (see notes above)
Apply 3–4 times daily

PoM **Framycort**® (Fisons)
Drops (for ear or eye), framycetin sulphate 0.5%, hydrocortisone acetate 0.5%. Price 5 ml = **E**
PoM **Framygen**® (Fisons)
Drops (for ear or eye), framycetin sulphate 0.5%. Price 5 ml = **D**

GENTAMICIN

Indications; Cautions; Side-effects: see under Framycetin Sulphate
Apply 3–4 times daily and at night

PoM **Gentamicin Ear-drops,** gentamicin 0.3% (as sulphate). Price 10 ml = **D**
PoM **Cidomycin**® (Roussel)
Drops (for ear or eye), gentamicin 0.3% (as sulphate). Price 5 ml = **D**
PoM **Garamycin**® (Kirby-Warrick)
Drops (for ear or eye), gentamicin 0.3% (as sulphate). Price 10 ml = **D**
PoM **Genticin**® (Nicholas)
Drops (for ear or eye), gentamicin 0.3% (as sulphate). Price 10 ml = **D**

PoM **Gentisone HC**® (Nicholas)
Ear-drops, gentamicin 0.3% (as sulphate), hydrocortisone acetate 1%. Price 10 ml = **E**

NEOMYCIN SULPHATE

Indications; Cautions; Side-effects: see under Framycetin Sulphate
Apply ear-drops every 2–3 hours; ear ointment 2–4 times daily. Reduce frequency of application when relief is obtained

PoM **Betnesol-N**® (Glaxo)
Drops (for ear, eye, or nose), betamethasone sodium phosphate 0.1%, neomycin sulphate 0.5%. Price 5 ml = **C**; 10 ml = **D**
PoM **Neo-Cortef**® (Upjohn)
Drops (for ear or eye), hydrocortisone acetate 1.5%, neomycin sulphate 0.5%. Price 5 ml = **D**
Ointment (for ear or eye), hydrocortisone acetate 1.5%, neomycin sulphate 0.5%. Price 3.9 g = **D**
PoM **Predsol-N**® (Glaxo)
Drops (for ear or eye), neomycin sulphate 0.5%, prednisolone sodium phosphate 0.5%. Price 5 ml = **C**; 10 ml = **D**
PoM **Vista-Methasone N**® (Daniel)
Drops (for ear, eye, or nose), betamethasone sodium phosphate 0·1%, neomycin sulphate 0.5%. Price 5 and 10 ml (both) = **C**

TETRACYCLINE HYDROCHLORIDE

Indications: susceptible bacterial infection in otitis externa
Cautions: avoid prolonged use
Side-effects: local sensitivity; stains skin and clothing
Apply every 2 hours

PoM **Achromycin**® (Lederle)
Ointment (for ear or eye), tetracycline hydrochloride 1%. Price 3.5 g = **C**

COMPOUND ANTI-INFECTIVE PREPARATIONS

PoM **Audicort**® (Lederle)
Ear-drops, neomycin 0.35%, undecenoic acid 0.7% (as neomycin undecenoate), triamcinolone acetonide 0.1%, benzocaine 5%. Price 10 ml = **G**
Apply 3–4 times daily
PoM **Otosporin**® (Calmic)
Ear-drops, hydrocortisone 1%, neomycin sulphate 0.439%, polymyxin B sulphate 0.119%. Price 5 ml = **E**; 10 ml = **G**
Apply 3–4 times daily
PoM **Ototrips**® (Consolidated)
Ear-drops, bacitracin 9%, polymyxin B sulphate 0.194%, trypsin 25000 USP units/3 ml, gelatin 0.5%, sodium chloride 0.9% when reconstituted. Price 3 ml = **E**
Apply 3–4 times daily
PoM **Sofradex**® (Roussel)
Drops (for ear or eye), dexamethasone sodium metasulphobenzoate 0.05%, framycetin sulphate 0.5%, gramicidin 0.005%. Price 8 ml = **F**
Apply 3–4 times daily

C = 51-100p, **D** = 101-180p, **E** = 181-300p, **F** = 301-450p, **G** = 451-650p, **H** = 651-900p, **I** = 901-1200p, **J** = over 1200p.

Ointment (for ear or eye), dexamethasone 0.05%, framycetin sulphate 0.5%, gramicidin 0.005%. Price 5 g = **E**
  Apply 2–3 times daily and at bedtime
PoM **Soframycin**® (Roussel)
  Cream, framycetin sulphate 1.5%, gramicidin 0.005% in a water-miscible basis. Price 15 g = **D**
  Ointment, ingredients as for cream, but in a greasy basis. Price 15 g = **D**
  Apply 1–3 times daily
PoM **Terra-Cortril**® (Pfizer)
  Ear suspension (= ear-drops), hydrocortisone acetate 1.5%, oxytetracycline 0.5% (as hydrochloride), polymyxin B sulphate 0.119%. Price 5 ml = **C**
  Apply 3 times daily
PoM **Tri-Adcortyl Otic**® (Squibb)
  Ear ointment, gramicidin 0.025%, neomycin 0.25% (as sulphate), nystatin 3.33%, triamcinolone acetonide 0.1% in Plastibase®. Price 10 g = **D**
  Apply 2–4 times daily

OTHER AURAL PREPARATIONS

Choline salicylate and phenazone are mild analgesics but of doubtful value when applied topically. There is no place for the use of local anaesthetics in ear-drops.

Audax® (Napp)
  Ear-drops, choline salicylate 20%, ethylene oxide-polyoxypropylene glycol condensate 1.25%. Price 8 ml = **C**
Auralgicin® (Fisons)
  Ear-drops, benzocaine 1.4%, chlorbutol 1%, ephedrine hydrochloride 1%, phenazone 5.5%, potassium hydroxyquinoline sulphate 0.1% in glycerol. Price 12.5 ml = **D**
Auraltone® (Rorer)
  Ear-drops, benzocaine 1%, phenazone 5% in glycerol. Price 15 ml = **C**
Norgotin® (Norgine)
  Ear-drops, amethocaine hydrochloride 1%, chlorhexidine acetate 0.1%, ephedrine hydrochloride 1%, in propylene glycol. Price 16 ml = **D**

12.1.2   Otitis media

Acute otitis media is the commonest cause of severe pain in small children and recurrent attacks, especially in infants, are particularly distressing. Sero-mucinous otitis media ('glue ear') is present in about 10% of the child population and in 90% of children with cleft palates. Chronic otitis media is thought to be a legacy from untreated or resistant cases of sero-mucinous otitis media.

ACUTE OTITIS MEDIA. Local treatment is ineffective and there is no place for drops containing a local anaesthetic. Many attacks are viral in origin and need only treatment with a **simple analgesic** for pain. Severe attacks of bacterial origin should be treated with **systemic antibiotics**. Identification of the infecting organism by bacterial examination of the discharge, if present, is helpful in selecting the appropriate treatment (see section 5.1, Table 1). Simple analgesics given by mouth are used to relieve pain. In recurrent acute otitis media a daily dose of a prophylactic antibiotic (co-trimoxazole or erythromycin) during the winter months can be tried.

SERO-MUCINOUS OTITIS MEDIA ('GLUE EAR'). This condition should be referred to hospital because of the risk of permanent damage to middle ear function and impaired language development.

CHRONIC OTITIS MEDIA. The organisms recovered from patients with chronic otitis media are often opportunists living in the debris, keratin, and necrotic bone present in the middle ear and mastoid. Thorough cleansing with an aural suction tube may completely control infection of many years duration. Acute exacerbations of chronic infection may require systemic antibiotics (see section 5.1, Table 1). A swab should be taken to determine the organism present and its antibiotic sensitivity. Unfortunately the culture often produces *Pseudomonas aeruginosa* and *Proteus* species, sensitive only to parenteral antibiotics. Local debridement of the meatal and middle ear contents may then be followed by topical treatment with ribbon gauze dressings as for otitis externa (section 12.1.1). This is particularly true with infections in mastoid cavities when dusting powders can also be tried.

12.1.3   Removal of ear wax

Wax is a normal bodily secretion which provides a protective film on the meatal skin and need only be removed if it causes deafness or interferes with a proper view of the eardrum. It may be removed by syringing with warm water. If necessary, wax can be softened before syringing with topical solutions, the most effective of which is **sodium bicarbonate ear-drops**. Other simple remedies are **olive oil** and **almond oil**. The patient should lie with the affected ear uppermost for 5 to 10 minutes after a generous amount of the solution has been introduced into the ear. Some proprietary preparations containing organic solvents can cause irritation of the meatal skin, and in most cases the simple remedies which are indicated above are just as effective and less likely to cause irritation.

Almond Oil (warm before use). Price 10 ml = **A**
Olive Oil (warm before use). Price 10 ml = **A**
Sodium   Bicarbonate   Ear-drops (see Formulary). Price 10 ml = **A**
Audinorm® (Carlton)
  Ear-drops, dioctyl sodium sulphosuccinate 5%, glycerol 10%. Price 12 ml = **B**
Dioctyl® (Medo)
  Ear-drops, dioctyl sodium sulphosuccinate 5% in macrogol. Price 7 ml = **C**
Cerumol® (LAB)
  Ear-drops, chlorbutol 5%, paradichlorobenzene 2%, turpentine oil 10%. Price 11 ml = **C**
Exterol® (Dermal)
  Ear-drops, urea-hydrogen peroxide complex 5% in glycerol. Price 12 ml = **E**
Molcer® (Wallace Mfg)
  Ear-drops, dioctyl sodium sulphosuccinate 5%. Price 15 ml = **C**
Soliwax® (Martindale)
  Ear capsules (= ear-drops), dioctyl sodium sulphosuccinate 5% in oil, red, single-application capsules. Price 10 caps = **C**

Waxsol® (Norgine)
Ear-drops, dioctyl sodium sulphosuccinate 0.5%. Price 10 ml = **C**

12.2 Drugs acting on the nose

Rhinitis is often self-limiting and sinusitis is best treated with antibiotics (see section 5.1, Table 1). There are few indications for the use of sprays and drops except in allergic rhinitis where topical preparations of corticosteroids or sodium cromoglycate have much to offer. Most other preparations contain sympathomimetic drugs which may damage the nasal cilia and their prolonged use causes mucosal oedema and severe nasal obstruction (rhinitis medicamentosa). Symptomatic relief in chronic nasal obstruction may be obtained with **systemic nasal decongestants** (see section 3.10). Douching the nose with salt and water is **not** recommended.

12.2.1 Drugs used in nasal allergy
12.2.2 Topical nasal decongestants
12.2.3 Anti-infective nasal preparations

12.2.1 Drugs used in nasal allergy

Mild cases are controlled by **oral antihistamines** and **systemic nasal decongestants** (see sections 3.4.1 and 3.10). Many patients with severe symptoms can now expect relief from topical preparations of **corticosteroids** or **sodium cromoglycate**. Treatment should begin before the hay fever season commences and the preparation used several times daily for 2 to 3 weeks. Treatment may have to be continued for months or even years in some patients. Significant side-effects have not been reported. Very disabling symptoms occasionally justify the use of **systemic corticosteroids** for short periods (see section 6.3), for example in students taking important examinations. They may also be used at the beginning of a course of treatment with a corticosteroid spray to relieve severe mucosal oedema and allow the spray to penetrate the nasal cavity. Some patients appear to obtain relief from hypersensitisation by injections of **allergen extracts** (see section 3.4.2).

BECLOMETHASONE DIPROPIONATE

Indications: allergic rhinitis
Cautions: untreated nasal infection, prolonged use in children, previous treatment with corticosteroids by mouth
Side-effects: sneezing after administration
Adults and children over 6 years, apply 100 micrograms (2 puffs) into each nostril twice daily or 50 micrograms (1 puff) 3–4 times daily; max. 8 puffs daily

PoM **Beconase**® (A&H)
Nasal spray (= aerosol inhalation), beclomethasone dipropionate 50 micrograms/metered inhalation, 200-dose unit with nasal adaptor. Price complete unit = **G**
PoM **Beconase Aqueous**® (A&H)
Nasal spray (= aqueous suspension), beclomethasone dipropionate 50micrograms/

metered spray. Price 200-dose unit with nasal applicator = **G**

BETAMETHASONE SODIUM PHOSPHATE

Indications; Cautions; Side-effects: see under Beclomethasone Dipropionate
Apply 2–3 drops of 0.1% solution into each nostril 2–3 times daily

PoM **Betnesol**® (Glaxo)
Drops (for ear, eye, or nose), betamethasone sodium phosphate 0.1%. Price 5 ml = **C**; 10 ml = **D**
PoM **Vista-Methasone**® (Daniel)
Drops (for ear, eye, or nose), betamethasone sodium phosphate 0.1%. Prices 5 and 10 ml (both) = **C**

BUDESONIDE

Indications: allergic and vasomotor rhinitis
Cautions: see under Beclomethasone Dipropionate, also patients with lung tuberculosis
Side-effects: see under Beclomethasone Dipropionate
Apply 100 micrograms (2 puffs) into each nostril twice daily, reducing to 50 micrograms (1 puff) twice daily

PoM **Rhinocort**® (Astra)
Nasal aerosol (= aerosol inhalation), budesonide 50 micrograms/metered inhalation, 200-dose unit with nasal adaptor. Price complete unit = **G**

FLUNISOLIDE

Indications; Cautions; Side-effects: see under Beclomethasone Dipropionate
Apply 50 micrograms (2 sprays) into each nostril 2–3 times daily; CHILD over 5 years 25 micrograms (1 spray) into each nostril 3 times daily, reduced for maintenance

PoM **Syntaris**® (Syntex)
Nasal spray, flunisolide 25 micrograms/0.1 ml metered spray. Price 24 ml with pump and applicator = **G**

SODIUM CROMOGLYCATE

Indications: prophylaxis of allergic and non-allergic rhinitis (see notes above)
Side-effects: local irritation, particularly during initial treatment with insufflations; rarely transient bronchospasm

Rynacrom® (Fisons)
Nasal insufflation, cartridges, pink, sodium cromoglycate 10 mg for use with insufflator. Price 20 cartridges = **C**; insufflator = **D**
Adults and children, insufflate 10 mg into each nostril up to 4 times daily
Nasal drops, sodium cromoglycate 2%. Price 15 ml = **G**
Adults and children, instil 2 drops into each nostril 6 times daily

---

C = 51-100p, **D** = 101-180p, **E** = 181-300p, **F** = 301-450p, **G** = 451-650p, **H** = 651-900p, **I** = 901-1200p, **J** = over 1200p.

Nasal spray, sodium cromoglycate 2% (2.6 mg/metered spray). Price 26 ml with pump = **G**

Adults and children, apply 2.6 mg (1 spray) into each nostril 6 times daily

Rynacrom Compound® (Fisons)

Nasal spray, sodium cromoglycate 2% (2.6 mg/metered spray) and xylometazoline hydrochloride 0.025% (32.5 micrograms/metered spray). Price 26 ml with pump = **H**

Apply 1 spray into each nostril 4 times daily

12.2.2   Topical nasal decongestants

The nasal mucosa is sensitive to changes in the atmospheric temperature and humidity and these alone may cause slight nasal congestion. The nose and nasal sinuses produce a litre of mucus in twenty-four hours and much of this finds its way silently into the stomach via the nasopharynx. Slight changes in the nasal airway, accompanied by an awareness of mucus passing along the nasopharynx causes some patients to be inaccurately diagnosed as suffering from chronic sinusitis. These symptoms are particularly noticeable in the later stages of the common cold for which there is no effective treatment at the moment; the temptation to use nasal drops should be resisted. **Sodium chloride** 0.9% given as nasal drops may relieve nasal congestion by helping to liquefy mucous secretions.

Symptomatic relief from the nasal congestion associated with vasomotor rhinitis, nasal polypi, and the common cold can be obtained by the short-term use of decongestant nasal drops and sprays. These all contain sympathomimetic drugs which exert their effect by vasoconstriction of the mucosal blood vessels which in turn reduces the thickness of the nasal mucosa. They are of limited value as they can give rise to a rebound phenomenon as their effects wear off, due to a secondary vasodilatation with a subsequent temporary increase in nasal congestion. This in turn tempts the further use of the decongestant, leading to a vicious circle of events. **Ephedrine nasal drops** is the safest sympathomimetic preparation and can give relief for several hours. The more potent sympathomimetic drugs oxymetazoline, phenylephrine, and xylometazoline are more likely to cause a rebound effect. **All** of these preparations may cause a hypertensive crisis if used during treatment with a monoamine-oxidase inhibitor.

Steam inhalations are useful in the treatment of symptoms of acute infective conditions, and the use of compounds containing volatile substances such as menthol and eucalyptus may encourage their use (see section 3.8). There is no evidence that nasal preparations containing antihistamines and anti-infective agents have any therapeutic effect.

Systemic nasal decongestants—see section 3.10.

EPHEDRINE HYDROCHLORIDE

Indications: nasal congestion

Cautions: avoid excessive use; caution in infants under 3 months. Drug interactions: see Appendix 1 (section *4.3*)

Side-effects: local irritation; after excessive use tolerance with diminished effect, rebound congestion

Instil 1–2 drops (see below) into each nostril when required

Ephedrine Nasal Drops, ephedrine hydrochloride 0.5% (see Formulary). Price 10 ml = **A**

Ephedrine Nasal Drops 1%, ephedrine hydrochloride 1% (see Formulary). Price 10 ml = **A**

OXYMETAZOLINE HYDROCHLORIDE

Indications: nasal congestion

Cautions; Side-effects: see under Ephedrine Hydrochloride

NHS **Afrazine®** (Kirby-Warrick)

Nasal drops, oxymetazoline hydrochloride 0.05%. Price 15 ml = **C**

Instil 2–3 drops into each nostril every 12 hours when required

Paediatric nasal drops, oxymetazoline hydrochloride 0.025%. Price 15 ml = **C**

CHILD up to 5 years instil 2–3 drops into each nostril every 12 hours when required

Nasal spray, oxymetazoline hydrochloride 0.05%. Price 15 ml = **C**

Apply 2–3 times to each nostril every 12 hours when required

NHS **Iliadin Mini®** (Merck)

Nasal drops, oxymetazoline hydrochloride 0.05% in 0.3-ml single-application containers. Price 10 units = **C**

Instil half contents of single-application container into each nostril every 8–12 hours when required

NHS **Iliadin-Mini Paediatric®** (Merck)

Nasal drops, oxymetazoline hydrochloride 0.025% in 0.3-ml single-application containers. Price 10 units = **C**

CHILD under 6 years instil half contents of single-application container into each nostril every 8–12 hours when required

PHENYLEPHRINE HYDROCHLORIDE

Indications: nasal congestion

Cautions; Side-effects: see under Ephedrine Hydrochloride

NHS **Neophryn®** (Winthrop)

Nasal drops, phenylephrine hydrochloride 0.25%. Price 15 ml = **C**

Instil 2–3 drops in each nostril every 3–4 hours if necessary; CHILD 1–2 drops

Nasal spray, phenylephrine hydrochloride 0.5%. Price 15 ml = **C**

2 applications to each nostril every 3–4 hours if necessary

XYLOMETAZOLINE HYDROCHLORIDE

Indications: nasal congestion

Cautions; Side-effects: see under Ephedrine Hydrochloride

Xylometazoline Nasal Drops, xylometazoline hydrochloride 0.1%, price 14 ml = **B**

Instil 2–3 drops into each nostril every 8–12 hours when required

Xylometazoline Nasal Drops, Paediatric xylometazoline hydrochloride 0.05%, price 10 ml = **B**

CHILD instil 1–2 drops into each nostril 1–2 times daily when required

NHS **Otrivine®** (Ciba Consumer)
Nasal drops, xylometazoline hydrochloride 0.1%. Price 14 ml = **B**
Instil 2–3 drops into each nostril every 8–12 hours when required
Paediatric nasal drops, xylometazoline hydrochloride 0.05%. Price 10 ml = **B**
CHILD instil 1–2 drops into each nostril 1–2 times daily when required
Nasal spray, xylometazoline hydrochloride 0.1%. Price 10 ml = **B**
1–2 applications to each nostril every 8–12 hours when required

COMPOUND NASAL DECONGESTANT PREPARATIONS

NHS **Hayphryn®** (Winthrop)
Nasal spray, phenylephrine hydrochloride 0.5%, thenyldiamine hydrochloride 0.1%. Price 15 ml = **C**
NHS **Otrivine-Antistin®** (Ciba Consumer)
Nasal drops and *spray*, antazoline sulphate 0.5%, xylometazoline hydrochloride 0.05%. Price 10 ml (both) = **C**

12.2.3 Anti-infective nasal preparations

Elimination of organisms such as staphylococci from the nasal vestibule can be achieved by the use of a cream containing **chlorhexidine and neomycin** (Naseptin®), but re-colonisation frequently occurs. Coagulase-positive staphylococci can be obtained from the noses of 40% of the population.

There is **no** evidence that topical anti-infective nasal preparations have any therapeutic value. The prolonged use of drops containing silver protein can cause argyria.

Systemic treatment of sinusitis—see section 5.1, Table 1.

Topical treatment of infected eczema of the nasal vestibule—see section 13.4.1.

Argotone® (Lipha)
Nasal drops, ephedrine hydrochloride 0.9%, mild silver protein 1%. Price 20 ml = **B**
Nasal spray, ephedrine hydrochloride 0.9%, mild silver protein 1%. Price 15 ml = **B**
PoM **Betnesol-N®** (Glaxo)
Drops (for ear, eye, and nose), betamethasone sodium phosphate 0.1%, neomycin sulphate 0.5%. Price 5 ml = **C**; 10 ml = **D**
PoM **Dexa-Rhinaspray®** (Boehringer Ingelheim)
Nasal inhalation, dexamethasone 21-isonicotinate 20 micrograms, neomycin sulphate 100 micrograms, tramazoline hydrochloride 120 micrograms/metered inhalation. Price 125-dose unit = **D**
PoM **Locabiotal®** (Servier)
Nasal inhalation, fusafungine 125 micrograms/metered inhalation. Price 200-dose unit = **D**
PoM **Naseptin®** (ICI)
Cream, chlorhexidine hydrochloride 0.1%, neo-

mycin sulphate 0.5%. Do not dilute. Price 5 g = **B**
For treatment of staphylococcal infections apply to nostrils 4 times daily for 10 days; for preventing nasal carriage of staphylococci apply to nostrils twice daily. Avoid contact with eyes and ears
PoM **Rhinamid®** (Bengué)
Nasal drops, butacaine sulphate 0.026%, ephedrine hydrochloride 1%, sulphanilamide 0.4%. Price 30 ml = **C**
PoM **Soframycin®** (Roussel)
Nebuliser, framycetin sulphate 1.25%, gramicidin 0.005%, phenylephrine hydrochloride 0.25%. Price 15 ml = **D**
PoM **Vibrocil®** (Zyma)
Nasal drops, dimethindene maleate 0.025%, neomycin sulphate 0.35%, phenylephrine 0.25%. Price 15 ml = **C**
Nasal gel, dimethindene maleate 0.025%, neomycin sulphate 0.35%, phenylephrine 0.25%. Price 12 g = **C**
Nasal spray, dimethindene maleate 0.025%, neomycin sulphate 0.35%, phenylephrine 0.25%. Price 10 ml = **C**

12.3 Drugs acting on the oropharynx

12.3.1 Drugs used in non-specific mouth ulceration (aphthous ulcers)
12.3.2 Oropharyngeal anti-infective drugs
12.3.3 Antiseptic lozenges and sprays
12.3.4 Mouth-washes, gargles, and dentifrices

12.3.1 Drugs used in non-specific mouth ulceration (aphthous ulcers)

Recurrent single or multiple aphthous ulcers are often a nuisance and occasionally are extremely painful. Local treatment aims at protecting the ulcerated area and enabling healing to occur, and at relieving pain or reducing inflammation, but it is difficult to retain the drug in contact with the lesion. A **carmellose gelatin paste** (Orabase®) or **powder** (Orahesive®) has a mechanical protective effect. **Corticosteroids** in lozenges (Corlan®) or in paste (Adcortyl in Orabase®) are the most effective. **Carbenoxolone sodium gel** (Bioral®) and **tetracycline mouth-bath** may be of value. **Choline salicylate dental paste** (Bonjela®, Teejel®) may relieve the pain of minor aphthous ulcers. **Benzydamine hydrochloride** (Difflam®) is used as an analgesic mouth-wash for oral ulceration and other painful conditions. **Local anaesthetics** as in benzocaine or compound benzocaine lozenges also provide pain relief but may cause sensitisation with sore, inflamed lips and tongue.

Local application of sticks of **toughened silver nitrate** and **alum** may relieve pain for a short time but cause tissue damage and delay healing.

BENZYDAMINE HYDROCHLORIDE
Indications: painful inflammatory conditions of oropharynx
Side-effects: occasional numbness or stinging

Difflam Oral Rinse® (Riker)
Solution, green, benzydamine hydrochloride 0.15%. Price 200 ml = **E**
Rinse or gargle, using 15 ml, diluted if necess-

C = 51-100p, D = 101-180p, E = 181-300p, F = 301-450p, G = 451-650p, H = 651-900p, I = 901-1200p, J = over 1200p.

ary, every 1½–3 hours as required, usually for not more than 7 days

CARBENOXOLONE SODIUM

Indications: mild oral and perioral lesions

Bioral Gel® (Winthrop)
Gel, carbenoxolone sodium 2% in adhesive basis. Price 5 g = **D**
Apply after food and at bedtime

CARMELLOSE SODIUM

Indications: mechanical protection of oral and perioral lesions

Orabase® (Squibb)
Oral paste, carmellose sodium 16.58%, pectin 16.58%, gelatin 16.58%, in Plastibase®. Price 30 g = **D**; 100 g = **E**
Apply a thin layer when necessary after food
Orahesive® (Squibb)
Powder, carmellose sodium, pectin, gelatin, equal parts. Price 25 g = **D**
Sprinkle on the affected area

CORTICOSTEROIDS

Indications: oral and perioral lesions
Contra-indications: untreated oral infection

PoM**Adcortyl in Orabase®** (Squibb)
Oral paste, triamcinolone acetonide 0.1% in adhesive basis. Price 10 g = **D**
Apply a thin layer 2–4 times daily
PoM**Corlan®** (Glaxo)
Pellets (= lozenges), hydrocortisone 2.5 mg (as sodium succinate). Price 20 lozenges = **D**
Dissolve one lozenge slowly in the mouth in close contact with the lesion initially 4 times daily, reduced for maintenance

LOCAL ANAESTHETICS

Indications: relief of pain in oral lesions
Cautions: avoid prolonged use; hypersensitivity may occur

Benzocaine Lozenges, benzocaine 10 mg. Price 20 lozenges = **A**
Dissolve one slowly in the mouth when necessary
Benzocaine Lozenges, Compound, benzocaine 100 mg, menthol 3 mg. Price 20 lozenges = **B**
Dissolve one slowly in the mouth when necessary
Dequacaine® (Farley)
Lozenges, amber, benzocaine 10 mg, dequalinium chloride 250 micrograms. Price 24 lozenges = **C**
Dissolve 1 lozenge slowly in the mouth when necessary; max. 8 lozenges daily
Medilave® (Martindale)
Gel, benzocaine 1%, cetylpyridinium chloride 0.01%. Price 10 g = **D**
Adults and children over 6 months, apply a thin layer 3–4 times daily
Oral-B® (Oral-B)
Oral gel, lignocaine 0.6%, cetylpyridinium chloride 0.02%, cineole 0.1%, menthol 0.06%. Price 15 g = **B**
Apply every 3 hours when required

SALICYLATES

Indications: mild oral and perioral lesions
Cautions: frequent application, especially in children, may give rise to salicylate poisoning

Choline Salicylate Dental Paste, choline salicylate 8.7% in a flavoured gel basis. Price 10 g = **C**
Apply every 3–4 hours with gentle massage before food and at bedtime
Bonjela® (R&C)
Oral gel, choline salicylate dental paste. Price 10 g = **C**
Teejel® (Napp)
Oral gel, choline salicylate dental paste. Price 10 g = **B**
Pyralvex® (Norgine)
Oral paint, brown, anthraquinone glycosides 5%, salicylic acid 1%. Price 10 ml with brush = **D**
Apply 3–4 times daily

TETRACYCLINE

Indications: severe recurrent aphthous ulceration
Side-effects: fungal superinfection

PoM**Tetracycline Mouth-bath,** consists of Tetracycline Mixture, tetracycline hydrochloride 125 mg (as tetracycline)/5 ml, see section 5.1.3
10 ml to be held in the mouth for 2–3 minutes 3 times daily for 3 days followed by a break of at least 3 days before repeating (to avoid oral thrush).

12.3.2   Oropharyngeal anti-infective drugs

The commonest cause of a sore throat is a viral infection which does not benefit from anti-infective treatment. Streptococcal sore throats require systemic **penicillin** therapy (see section 5.1.1). Acute ulcerative (Vincent's) gingivitis responds to systemic **metronidazole** 200 mg 3 times daily for 3 days (see section 5.1.11.1) or **nimorazole** 500 mg twice daily for 2 days (see section 5.4.3).

Candida albicans may cause thrush and other forms of stomatitis. They are sometimes a sequel to the use of broad-spectrum antibiotics or antineoplastics, and withdrawing the drug may lead to rapid resolution. Otherwise, **nystatin, amphotericin,** or **miconazole** may be effective; **polynoxylin** and **dequalinium** are less effective. **Crystal violet** paint (see section 13.11) is effective but causes unsightly staining and may also cause troublesome mucosal burns. It still has a place in the treatment of infants.

Herpes infections of the mouth, if they require treatment, which is usually not the case, may respond to **tetracycline** mouth-bath (section 12.3.1). Topical **acyclovir** may be tried for the treatment of recurrent or resistant infections (see section 13.10.3). **Idoxuridine** is seldom needed for herpetic mouth infections.

AMPHOTERICIN

Indications: oral and perioral fungal infections

PoM **Fungilin**® (Squibb)
Lozenges, yellow, amphotericin 10 mg. Price 20 lozenges = **D**. Label: 9, 24, counselling advised, after food
Dissolve 1 lozenge slowly in the mouth 4 times daily, increased to 8 times daily when necessary, for 10–15 days
Suspension, orange, amphotericin 100 mg/ml. Price 12 ml with pipette = **E**. Label: 9, counselling advised, hold in mouth, after food, use of pipette
Place 1 ml in the mouth after food and retain near lesions 4 times daily for 14 days

DEQUALINIUM CHLORIDE

Indications: mild oral fungal infections

Dequadin® (Farley)
Lozenges, orange, dequalinium chloride 250 micrograms. Price 20 lozenges = **B**
Dissolve 1 lozenge slowly in the mouth when required
Labosept® (LAB)
Pastilles, red, dequalinium chloride 250 micrograms. Price 20 pastilles = **B**
Suck 1 pastille slowly when required

IDOXURIDINE

Indications: oral and perioral herpetic lesions (see notes above)

PoM **Idoxuridine 0.1% Paint,** idoxuridine 0.1% in purified water. Identical in composition with idoxuridine eye-drops (see section 11.3.1 for preparations). It must **not** be confused with a paint containing idoxuridine 5% in dimethyl sulphoxide used in dermatology (see section 13.10.3)
Adults and older children, hold about 2 ml in the mouth in contact with the lesions for 2–3 minutes at least 3 times daily; younger children, paint lesions 4–5 times daily

MICONAZOLE

Indications: oral fungal infections

Daktarin® (Janssen)
Oral gel, miconazole 25 mg/ml. Price 40 g = **E**. Label: 9, counselling advised, hold in mouth, after food
Place 5–10 ml in the mouth after food and retain near lesions before swallowing, 4 times daily; CHILD up to 2 years 2.5 ml twice daily, 2–6 years 5 ml twice daily, over 6 years 5 ml 4 times daily

NATAMYCIN

Indications: oral fungal infections

PoM **Pimafucin**® (Brocades)
Oral suspension, off-white, natamycin 10 mg/ml. Price 5-ml dropper bottle = **C**. Label: 9, 21, counselling advised, hold in mouth, use of pipette

Place 10 drops in the mouth after food and retain near lesions; INFANTS 4 drops

NYSTATIN

Indications: oral and perioral fungal infections

PoM **Nystatin Mixture,** nystatin 100000 units/ml. Do not dilute. Price 30 ml = **E**. Label: 9, counselling advised, hold in mouth, after food
Place 1 ml in the mouth after food and retain near lesions 4 times daily, continued for 48 hours after lesions have resolved
PoM **Nystan**® (Squibb)
Pastilles, yellow/brown, nystatin 100000 units. Price 28 pastilles = **F**. Label: 9, 24, counselling advised, after food
Suck 1 pastille slowly, 4 times daily after food
Suspension (= mixture), yellow, nystatin 100000 units/ml. Price 30 ml with pipette = **E**. Label: 9, counselling advised, hold in mouth, after food
PoM **Nystatin-Dome**® (Bayer)
Suspension (= mixture), yellow, nystatin 100000 units/ml. Price 30 ml with 1-ml spoon = **E**. Label: 9, counselling advised, hold in mouth, after food

POLYNOXYLIN

Indications: mild oral fungal infections

Anaflex® (Geistlich)
Lozenges, polynoxylin 30 mg. Price 50 lozenges = **E**. Label: 24
Suck 1 lozenge slowly 6–10 times daily

TETRACYCLINE

Section 12.3.1

12.3.3 Antiseptic lozenges and sprays

There is no convincing evidence that antiseptic lozenges and sprays have a beneficial action and they sometimes irritate and cause sore tongue and sore lips. Some of these preparations also contain local anaesthetics which relieve pain but may cause sensitisation.

Benzalkonium Lozenges, benzalkonium chloride 500 micrograms. Price 20 lozenges = **B**
AAA® (Armour)
Mouth and throat spray, benzocaine 1.5%, cetalkonium chloride 0.0413%. Price 60-dose unit = **E**
Bradosol® (Ciba)
Lozenges, domiphen bromide 500 micrograms. Price 24 lozenges = **B**
Eludril® (Concept)
Aerosol spray, amethocaine hydrochloride 0.015%, chlorhexidine gluconate 0.05%. Price 55 ml = **D**
Hibitane® (Care)
Lozenges, benzocaine 2 mg, chlorhexidine hydrochloride 5 mg. Price 20 lozenges = **B**
PoM **Locabiotal**® (Servier)
Aerosol spray, fusafungine 125 micrograms/metered inhalation. Price 200-dose unit with nasal and oral adaptor = **D**
Merocaine® (Merrell)
Lozenges, green, benzocaine 10 mg, cetylpyridinium chloride 1.4 mg. Price 24 lozenges = **C**

C = 51–100p, D = 101–180p, E = 181–300p, F = 301–450p, G = 451–650p, H = 651–900p, I = 901–1200p, J = over 1200p.

Merocets® (Merrell)
Lozenges, yellow, cetylpyridinium chloride 0.066%.
Price 24 lozenges = **C**
Oralcer® (Vitabiotics)
Lozenges, green, ascorbic acid 6 mg, clioquinol 35 mg.
Price 20 lozenges = **B**
Tyrozets® (MSD)
Lozenges, pink, benzocaine 5 mg, tyrothricin 1 mg. Price 24 lozenges = **B**

12.3.4 Mouth-washes, gargles, and dentifrices

Mouth-washes have a mechanical cleansing action and freshen the mouth. Warm **compound sodium chloride mouth-wash** or **compound thymol glycerin** is as useful as any.

Hydrogen peroxide mouth-wash has a mechanical cleansing effect due to frothing when in contact with oral debris. **Sodium perborate** (Bocasan®) is similar in effect to hydrogen peroxide.

There is recent evidence that **chlorhexidine** has a specific effect in inhibiting the formation of plaque on teeth. A chlorhexidine mouth-wash may be useful as an adjunct to other oral hygiene measures in cases of oral infection or when toothbrushing is not possible.

There is no convincing evidence that gargles are effective.

Artificial saliva (see Formulary) may be indicated for dry mouth.

CETYLPYRIDINIUM CHLORIDE
Indications: oral hygiene

Merocet® (Merrell)
Solution (= mouth-wash or gargle), yellow, cetylpyridinium chloride 0.05%. Price 200 ml = **C**
To be used undiluted or diluted with an equal volume of warm water

CHLORHEXIDINE GLUCONATE
Indications: oral hygiene; inhibition of plaque formation (0.2% and 1% preparations)

Corsodyl® (ICI)
Dental gel, red, chlorhexidine gluconate 1%.
Price 50 g = **C**
Brush on the teeth once or twice daily
Mouth-wash, pink, chlorhexidine gluconate 0.2%. Price 250 ml = **C**
Rinse the mouth with 10 ml for about 1 minute twice daily
Eludril® (Concept)
Mouth-wash, red, chlorhexidine gluconate 0.1%, chlorbutol 0.1%, chloroform 0.5%. Price 90 ml = **C**; 500 ml = **F**
Use 10 ml in half a tumblerful of warm water 3–4 times daily

HEXETIDINE
Indications: oral hygiene

Oraldene® (Warner)
Mouth-wash or *gargle*, red, hexetidine 0.1%.
Price 100 ml = **C**
Use 15 ml undiluted 2–3 times daily

HYDROGEN PEROXIDE
Indications: oral hygiene, see notes above

Hydrogen Peroxide Mouth-wash, consists of hydrogen peroxide solution (6%). Price 100 ml = **A**
Rinse the mouth for 2–3 minutes with 15 ml in half a tumblerful of warm water 2–3 times daily

PHENOL
Indications: oral hygiene

Phenol Gargle, phenol glycerin 5% (see Formulary). Price 100 ml = **A**
To be diluted with an equal volume of warm water
Chloraseptic® (Norwich-Eaton)
Throat spray or *gargle*, green, phenol 1.4%.
Price 118 ml with spray = **D**; 150 ml = **D**
Use every 2 hours if necessary, undiluted as a throat spray, undiluted or diluted with an equal volume of water as a mouth-wash or gargle

POVIDONE-IODINE
Indications: oral hygiene

Betadine® (Napp)
Mouth-wash or *gargle*, amber, povidone-iodine 1%. Price 250 ml = **C**
To be used undiluted or diluted with an equal volume of warm water every 2–4 hours if necessary

SODIUM CHLORIDE
Indications: oral hygiene, see notes above

Sodium Chloride Mouth-wash, Compound, sodium chloride 1.5% (see Formulary). Price 100 ml = **A**
To be diluted with an equal volume of warm water

SODIUM PERBORATE
Indications: oral hygiene, see notes above
Cautions: avoid prolonged use (over 1 month) because of possible borate poisoning

Bocasan® (Cooper)
Mouth-wash, sodium perborate 70%. Price 8 × 1.7-g sachets = **B**
Use 1 sachet in 30 ml of water

THYMOL
Indications: oral hygiene, see notes above

Mouth-wash Solution-tablets, thymol 0.81 mg, sodium benzoate 32.4 mg, with colouring and flavouring in effervescent basis. Price 20 solution-tablets = **B**
Dissolve 1 tablet in a tumblerful of warm water
Thymol Glycerin, Compound, glycerol 10%, thymol 0.05% with colouring and flavouring. Price 100 ml = **A**
To be used undiluted or diluted with 3 volumes of warm water

13: Drugs acting on the

SKIN

The skin is particularly amenable to treatment by local application as there is intimate contact between the drug and the target tissue with a minimum of systemic effects. However, when a substance is used topically there may be difficulty in regulating the total quantity applied to the area concerned and lack of patient compliance may be a problem.

In this chapter, drug treatment is discussed under the following headings:

13.1 Vehicles and diluents

VEHICLE. Both the vehicle and the active ingredients are important in the treatment of skin conditions and it is being increasingly recognised that the vehicle alone may have a greater therapeutic value than a mere placebo effect. The vehicle affects the degree of hydration of the skin, has a mild anti-inflammatory effect, and aids the penetration of active drug in the preparation.

The vehicle, the indication for which the drug is prescribed, solubility, cosmetic and general acceptability to the patient, and the safety and stability of the final preparation should all be considered.

DILUTION. Because of the complexity of many formulations, dilution is undesirable except where a particular diluent is known to be suitable. Suitable diluents for individual preparations are given in the relevant entries. Inappropriate diluents may impair the activity or stability of the preparation, even though no physical change is apparent. Diluted creams are generally given a life of 2 weeks.

QUANTITY. Suitable quantities of dermatological preparations to be prescribed for specific areas of the body are given under Prescription Writing.

CHOICE OF VEHICLE

The vehicle may take the form of a cream, ointment, lotion, paste, dusting-powder, application, collodion, liniment, or paint basis. The properties of the various forms are described below but it should be noted that there are some vehicles having intermediate properties, for example ointments with some properties of a cream.

CREAMS are either water-miscible and readily washed off, or oily and not so easily washed off. They contain a preservative to minimise microbial growth. Generally, creams are cosmetically more acceptable to the patient as they are less greasy than ointments and easier to apply.

Aqueous Cream, emulsifying ointment 30%, phenoxyethanol 1%, in freshly boiled and cooled purified water. Price 100 g = **B**

Buffered Cream, emulsifying ointment 30%, citric acid monohydrate 0.5%, sodium phosphate 2.5%, chlorocresol 0.1%, in freshly boiled and cooled purified water. Price 100 g = **B**

Cetomacrogol Cream, *Formula A*, cetomacrogol emulsifying ointment 30%, chlorocresol 0.1%, in freshly boiled and cooled purified water. Price 100 g = **E**
Formula B, cetomacrogol emulsifying ointment 30%, propyl hydroxybenzoate 0.08%, methyl hydroxybenzoate 0.15%, benzyl alcohol 1.5%, in freshly boiled and cooled purified water. Price 100 g = **D**

Diprobase® (Kirby-Warrick)
Cream, cetomacrogol 2.25%, cetostearyl alcohol 7.2%, liquid paraffin 6%, white soft paraffin 15%, water-miscible basis used for Diprosone® cream. Price 50 g = **D**

Locobase® (Brocades)
Cream, water-miscible basis used for Locoid® cream. Price 100 g = **E**

Ultrabase® (Schering)
Cream, water-miscible, containing liquid paraffin and white soft paraffin. Price 50 g = **D**; 500 g = **G**

OINTMENTS are greasy preparations which are normally anhydrous and insoluble in water, and are more occlusive than creams. The most commonly used ointment bases consist of soft paraffin or a combination of soft paraffin with liquid paraffin and hard paraffin. Some modern ointment bases have both hydrophilic and lipophilic properties; they may have occlusive properties on the skin surface, encourage hydration, and be miscible with water. They often have a mild anti-inflammatory effect. Water-soluble ointments contain macrogols which are freely soluble in water and are therefore readily washed off. They have a limited but useful application in circumstances

---

C = 51-100p, **D** = 101-180p, **E** = 181-300p, **F** = 301-450p, **G** = 451-650p, **H** = 651-900p, **I** = 901-1200p, **J** = over 1200p.

where ready removal is desirable. Ointments are particularly suitable for chronic, dry lesions. Contact sensitivity to wool fat (lanolin) and wool alcohols may occur and ointments containing these substances must be avoided in sensitised patients.

Cetomacrogol Emulsifying Ointment, cetomacrogol emulsifying wax 30%, liquid paraffin 20%, white soft paraffin 50%. Price 100 g = **B**

Emulsifying Ointment, emulsifying wax 30%, white soft paraffin 50%, liquid paraffin 20%. Price 100 g = **B**

Hydrous Ointment (oily cream), dried magnesium sulphate 0.5%, phenoxyethanol 1%, water for preparations 48.5%, in wool alcohols ointment. Price 100 g = **B**

Hydrous Wool Fat, wool fat 70% in freshly boiled and cooled purified water. Price 100 g = **B**

Hydrous Wool Fat Ointment, hydrous wool fat 50%, yellow soft paraffin 50%. Price 100 g = **B**

Macrogol Ointment, macrogol '4000' 35%, macrogol '300' 65%. Price 100 g = **B**

Paraffin, white soft (white petroleum jelly). Price 100 g = **B**

Paraffin, yellow soft (yellow petroleum jelly). Price 100 g = **B**

Paraffin Ointment, (see Formulary). Price 100 g = **B**

Simple Ointment, cetostearyl alcohol 5%, hard paraffin 5%, wool fat 5%, in yellow or white soft paraffin. Price 100 g = **B**

Wool Alcohols Ointment, wool alcohols 6%, yellow or white soft paraffin 10%, hard paraffin 24%, in liquid paraffin. Price 100 g = **C**

Diprobase® (Kirby-Warrick)
Ointment, liquid paraffin 5%, white soft paraffin 95%, basis used for Diprosone® ointment. Price 50 g = **D**

Locobase® (Brocades)
Ointment, basis used for Locoid® ointment. Price 100 g = **E**

Unguentum Merck® (Merck)
Cream (hydrophilic and lipophilic), cetostearyl alcohol 9%, glyceryl monostearate 3%, saturated neutral oil 2%, liquid paraffin 3%, white soft paraffin 32%, propylene glycol 5%, polysorbate '40' 6%, silicic acid 0.1%, sorbic acid 0.2%. Price 50 g = **D**; 100 g = **E**; 200 ml = **G**

LOTIONS are usually aqueous solutions or suspensions which cool diffusely inflamed unbroken skin. They cool by evaporation and should be reapplied frequently. Volatile solvents increase the cooling effect but are liable to cause stinging. Lotions are also used to apply drugs to the skin and may be preferred to ointments or creams when it is intended to apply a thin layer of the preparation over a large or hairy area.

SHAKE LOTIONS (such as calamine lotion) containing insoluble powders are applied to less acute, scabbed, dry lesions. In addition to cooling they leave a deposit of inert powder on the skin surface.

PASTES are stiff preparations containing a high proportion of finely powdered solids such as zinc oxide and starch. The standard example is **Compound Zinc Paste** to which other active ingredients may be added (e.g. dithranol). Pastes are used for circumscribed lesions such as those which occur in lichen simplex, chronic eczema, or psoriasis. They are less occlusive than ointments and can be used to protect sub-acute, lichenified, or excoriated skin.

Zinc Paste, Compound, zinc oxide 25%, starch 25%, white soft paraffin 50%. Price 25 g = **A**

APPLICATIONS are usually viscous solutions, emulsions, or suspensions for application to the skin.

COLLODIONS are painted on the skin and allowed to dry to leave a flexible film over the site of application. Flexible collodion may be used to seal minor cuts and wounds. Collodions such as salicylic acid collodion provide a means of holding a dissolved drug in contact with the skin for a long period.

Collodion, Flexible, castor oil 2.5%, colophony 2.5% in a collodion basis, prepared by dissolving pyroxylin (10%) in a mixture of 3 volumes of ether and 1 volume of alcohol (90%). Price 10 ml = **A**. Label: 15
Caution: highly flammable

LINIMENTS are liquid preparations which are intended for external application and may contain substances possessing analgesic, rubefacient, soothing, or stimulating properties.
    For preparations see section 10.3.2.

PAINTS are liquid preparations intended for application with a brush to the skin or mucous surfaces.

13.2 Emollient and barrier preparations

13.2.1 Emollients and barrier creams
13.2.2 Emollient bath additives
13.2.3 Dusting-powders

13.2.1 Emollients and barrier creams

Emollients soothe, smooth and hydrate the skin and are indicated for all dry scaling disorders (such as ichthyosis). Their effects are short-lived and they should be applied frequently even after improvement occurs. They are useful in dry eczematous disorders, and to a lesser extent in psoriasis (section 13.5). Simple preparations such as **aqueous cream** are often as effective as the more complex proprietary formulations; sprays offer little advantage but, in general, the choice depends on patient preference. Some ingredients may cause sensitisation, notably hydrous wool fat (lanolin) or antibacterials and this should be suspected if an eczematous reaction occurs at the site of application.

Camphor, menthol, and phenol have a mild antipruritic effect when used in emollient preparations. Calamine and zinc oxide may also be included as they slightly enhance therapeutic efficacy; they are particularly useful in dry eczema. Zinc and titanium preparations have mild astringent properties. Thickening agents such as talc and kaolin may also be included. Preparations containing antibacterial drugs should be avoided unless infection is present (section 13.10).

Urea is employed as a hydrating agent. It is used in scaling conditions and may be useful in elderly patients and infantile eczemas. It is often used with other topical agents such as corticosteroids to enhance penetration.

Barrier creams often contain water-repellent substances such as **dimethicone** or other silicones. They are used to give protection against irritation or repeated hydration (napkin rash, areas around stomata, sore areas in the elderly, bedsores, etc.). Whatever is applied is no substitute for adequate nursing care, and it is doubtful if these water-repellent creams are any more effective than the traditional compound zinc ointments.

Napkin rash is usually a local dermatitis. The first line of treatment is to ensure that napkins are changed frequently, and that tightly fitting rubber pants are avoided. The rash may clear when left exposed to the air and an emollient, or preparations containing calamine and emollients, may be helpful. See also section 13.4.

For preparations used in stoma care, see section 1.8.1.

Aqueous Cream—section 13.1
Dimethicone Cream, dimethicone '350' 10%, cetostearyl alcohol 5%, cetrimide 0.5%, chlorocresol 0.1%, liquid paraffin 40%, freshly boiled and cooled purified water 44.4%. Price 50 g = A
Hydrous Ointment—section 13.1
Titanium Dioxide Paste, titanium dioxide 20%, chlorocresol 0.1%, red ferric oxide 2%, glycerol 15%, light kaolin 10%, zinc oxide 25%, in water for preparations. Price 25 g = A. For napkin and urinary rash and as a sunscreen
Zinc Cream, zinc oxide 32%, arachis oil 32%, calcium hydroxide 0.045%, oleic acid 0.5%, wool fat 8%, in freshly boiled and cooled purified water. Price 50 g = A. For napkin and urinary rash and eczematous conditions
Zinc Ointment, zinc oxide 15%, in simple ointment. Price 25 g = A. For napkin and urinary rash and eczematous conditions
Zinc and Castor Oil Ointment, zinc oxide 7.5%, castor oil 50%, arachis oil 30.5%, white beeswax 10%, cetostearyl alcohol 2%. Price 25 g = A. For napkin and urinary rash
Alcoderm® (Alcon)
Cream, water-miscible, containing carbomer, cetyl alcohol, liquid paraffin, polysorbate 60, sodium lauryl sulphate, stearyl alcohol, triethanolamine. Price 60 g = D
Lotion, water-miscible, ingredients as above. Price 120 ml = D

Diprobase—section 13.1
E45® (Crookes Products)
Cream, light liquid paraffin 11.6%, white soft paraffin 14.5%, wool fat 1%, with methyl hydroxybenzoate, self-emulsifying monostearin, stearic acid, triethanolamine. Price 50 g = C; 125 g = E; 500 g = F
Eczederm® (Quinoderm Ltd)
Cream, calamine 20.88%, starch 2.09%, in an emollient basis. Price 25 g = C; 50 g = D; 500 g = H
Emulsiderm® (Dermal)
Liquid emulsion (= lotion), liquid paraffin 25%, isopropyl myristate 25%, benzalkonium chloride 0.5%. Price 250 ml (with 10-ml measure) = F
Kamillosan® (Norgine)
Ointment, extract of chamomile 10%, volatile oil of chamomile 0.5%. Price 20 g = D. For napkin rash, cracked nipples and chapped hands
Keri® (Bristol-Myers)
Lotion, mineral oil 16%, with lanolin oil. Price 190-ml pump pack = F; 380-ml pump pack = G
Lacticare® (Stiefel)
Lotion, lactic acid 5%, sodium pyrrolidone-carboxylate 2.5%, in an emulsion basis. Price 150 ml = E
Locobase—section 13.1
Massé Breast Cream® (Ortho-Cilag)
Cream (water-miscible), containing arachis oil, cetyl alcohol, glycerol, glyceryl monostearate, wool fat, polysorbate 60, potassium hydroxide, sorbitan monostearate, stearic acid. Price 28 g = C. For pre- and post-natal nipple care
Metanium® (Bengué)
Ointment, titanium dioxide 20%, titanium peroxide 5%, titanium salicylate 3%, titanium tannate 0.1%, in a silicone basis. Price 25 g = C. For napkin rash and related disorders
Morhulin® (Napp)
Ointment, cod-liver oil 11.4%, zinc oxide 38%, in a basis containing wool fat and paraffin. Price 50 g = B; 350 g = E. For minor wounds, varicose ulcers, and pressure sores
Morsep® (Napp)
Cream, cetrimide 0.5%, ergocalciferol 10 units/g, vitamin A 70 units/g. Price 40 g = B; 300 g = E. For urinary rash
Natuderm® (Burgess)
Cream (hydrophilic and lipophilic), free fatty acids 5%, glycerides 15.5%, glycerol 3.7%, phospholipids 0.2%, polysorbate '60' 1.1%, sorbitan monostearate 1%, squalane 0.5%, squalene 3.3%, free sterols 0.8%, sterol esters 1.3%, α-tocopherol 0.003%, waxes 7%, butylated hydroxyanisole 0.003%. Price 40 g = C; 100 g = E; 450 g = H
Noratex® (Norton)
Cream, cod-liver oil 2.15%, light kaolin 3.5%, talc 7.4%, wool fat 1.075%, zinc oxide 21.8%. Price 500 g = E. For napkin and urinary rash and pressure sores
Oilatum® (Stiefel)
Cream, arachis oil 21%, povidone 1%, in a water-miscible basis. Price 40 g = D; 80 g = E

C = 51-100p, D = 101-180p, E = 181-300p, F = 301-450p, G = 451-650p, H = 651-900p, I = 901-1200p, J = over 1200p.

Rikospray Balsam® (Riker)
Spray application, benzoin 12.5%, prepared storax 2.5% (pressurised aerosol pack). Price 150-g unit = **E**. For application to skin under adhesive plasters, in ileostomy and colostomy care, bedsores, cracked nipples and skin fissures

Rikospray Silicone® (Riker)
Spray application, aldioxa 0.5%, cetylpyridinium chloride 0.02%, in a water-repellent basis containing dimethicone 1000. Price 200-g pressurised aerosol pack = **E**. For urinary rash, pressure sores, and colostomy care

Siopel® (ICI)
Barrier cream, dimethicone '1000' 10%, cetrimide 0.3%. Price 50 g = **B**; 500 g = **D**. For dermatoses, colostomy and ileostomy care, urinary rash, and related conditions

Sprilon® (Pharmacia)
Spray application, dimethicone 0.6%, zinc oxide 7.2%, in a basis containing wool fat, wool alcohols, cetyl alcohol, dextran, white soft paraffin, liquid paraffin, and propellants. Price 200-g pressurised aerosol unit = **E**. For urinary rash, pressure sores, and colostomy and ileostomy care

Sudocrem® (Tosara)
Cream, benzyl alcohol 0.39%, benzyl benzoate 1.01%, benzyl cinnamate 0.15%, wool fat 4%, zinc oxide 15.25%. Price 25 g = **A**; 65 g = **B**; 125 g = **C**; 325 g = **D**. For napkin rash and pressure sores

Thovaline® (Ilon)
Ointment, cod-liver oil 1.5%, light kaolin 2.5%, talc 3.3%, wool fat 2.5%, zinc oxide 19.8%. Price 15, 40, and 60 g (all) = **B**; 90 and 125 g (both) = **C**; 500 g = **E**. For napkin and urinary rash and pressure sores
Spray application, ingredients as for ointment in pressurised aerosol pack. Price 142 g = **D**

Ultrabase—section 13.1

Unguentum Merck—section 13.1

Vasogen® (Pharmax)
Barrier cream, dimethicone 20%, calamine 1.5%, zinc oxide 7.5%. Price 50 g= **B**; 100 g = **C**. For napkin and urinary rash, pressure sores, and pruritus ani

Vita-E® (Bioglan)
Ointment, d-α-tocopheryl acetate 30 units/g in yellow soft paraffin. Price 50 g = **D**. For pressure sores and related conditions

Preparations containing urea
Aquadrate® (Norwich-Eaton)
Cream, urea 10% in a powder-in-cream basis. Price 30 g = **D**; 100 g = **G**
Apply sparingly and rub into area when required

Calmurid® (Pharmacia)
Cream, urea 10% in a water-miscible basis. Diluent aqueous cream, life of diluted cream 14 days. Price 50 g = **D**; 100 g = **F**; 300 g = **I**
Apply a thick layer for 3–5 minutes, massage into area, and remove excess, usually twice daily. Use half-strength cream for 1 week if stinging occurs with undiluted preparation

Nutraplus® (Alcon)
Cream, urea 10% in a water-miscible basis. Price 60 g = **E**
Apply 2–3 times daily

13.2.2   Emollient bath additives

For bath additives containing tar, see section 13.5 and for antiseptic bath additives, see section 13.11.

Alpha Keri Bath® (Bristol-Myers)
Bath oil, liquid paraffin 91.7%, oil-soluble fraction of wool fat 3%. Price 240 ml = **F**

Aveeno Colloidal® (Oral-B)
Bath additive, oat (protein fraction). Price 6 × 50-g sachets = **E**
Add 1 sachet/bath

Aveeno Oilated® (Oral-B)
Bath additive, oat (protein fraction) 41%, liquid paraffin 35%. Price 6 × 30-g sachets = **E**
Add 1 sachet/bath

Balneum® (Merck)
Bath oil, soya oil 84.75%. Price 225 ml = **E**; 500 ml = **G**
Add 20 ml/bath

Emulsiderm—section 13.2.1
Add 20–30 ml/bath and soak for 5–10 minutes

Oilatum Emollient® (Stiefel)
Bath additive (emulsion), acetylated wool alcohols 5%, liquid paraffin 63.7%. Price 150 ml = **D**; 350 ml = **F**
Add 5–15 ml/bath and soak for 10–20 minutes

13.2.3   Dusting-powders

Dusting-powders are used in folds where friction may occur between opposing skin surfaces. They should not be applied in areas that are very moist as they tend to cake and abrade the skin. **Talc** acts as a lubricant powder but does not absorb moisture whereas **starch** is less lubricant but absorbs water. Other inert powders such as kaolin or zinc oxide may also be used in the formulation of dusting-powders.

See also section 13.11 for antiseptic dusting-powders.

Talc Dusting-powder, starch 10% in sterilised purified talc. Price 100 g = **B**

Zinc, Starch and Talc Dusting-powder, zinc oxide 25%, starch 25%, sterilised purified talc 50%. Price 50 g = **A**

ZeaSORB® (Stiefel)
Dusting-powder, aldioxa 0.2%, chloroxylenol 0.5%, pulverised maize core 45%. Price 30 g = **D**

13.3   Local anaesthetic and antipruritic preparations

Pruritus may be caused by systemic disease (such as drug hypersensitivity, obstructive jaundice, endocrine disease, and certain malignant diseases) as well as by skin disease (e.g. psoriasis, eczema, urticaria, and scabies). Where possible the underlying causes should be treated.

Relative prices: **A** = up to 20p, **B** = 21-50p,

There is no really effective antipruritic. **Cala-mine** preparations are widely prescribed. **Emollient** preparations (section 13.2.1) may also be of value. **Oral antihistamines** (section 3.4.1) should be used in allergic rashes.

Though widely prescribed, topical antihistamines and local anaesthetics should be avoided as they may cause sensitisation; moreover topical antihistamines are only marginally effective. Insect bites and stings, though often treated with such preparations, are best treated with calamine preparations or emollients. See also section 3.4.3 and Emergency Treatment of Poisoning.

Crotamiton (Eurax®) shows little evidence of greater effectiveness than calamine in the relief of pruritus.

For systemic treatment of pruritus and urticaria, see antihistamines, section 3.4.1; also hydroxyzine hydrochloride, section 4.1.2.

For preparations used in pruritus ani, see section 1.7.1.

CALAMINE
Indications: pruritus

Calamine Application, Compound, calamine 10%, zinc oxide 5%, zinc stearate 2.5%, wool fat 2.5%, yellow soft paraffin 25%, liquid paraffin 55%. Price 50 g = **A**
Calamine Cream, Aqueous, calamine 4%, zinc oxide 3%, arachis oil 30%, emulsifying wax 6%, freshly boiled and cooled purified water 57%. Price 50 g = **B**
Calamine Lotion, calamine 15%, zinc oxide 5%, glycerol 5%, bentonite 3%, sodium citrate 0.5%, liquefied phenol 0.5%, in freshly boiled and cooled purified water. Price 200 ml = **B**
Calamine Lotion, Oily, calamine 5%, arachis oil 50%, oleic acid 0.5%, wool fat 1%, in calcium hydroxide solution. Price 200 ml = **C**
Calamine Ointment, calamine 15%, in white soft paraffin. Price 25 g = **A**
Eczederm—section 13.2.1

CROTAMITON
Indications: pruritus
Cautions: avoid use near eyes
Contra-indications: acute exudative dermatoses

Eurax® (Ciba Consumer)
Lotion, crotamiton 10%. Price 150 ml = **D**; 1000 ml = **G**
Cream, crotamiton 10%. Price 30 g = **C**; 100 g = **D**

LOCAL ANAESTHETICS
Indications: relief of local pain, see notes above.
See section 15.2 for use in surface anaesthesia
Cautions: may cause hypersensitivity

Anethaine® (Farley)
Cream, amethocaine hydrochloride 1%, in a water-miscible basis. Price 25 g = **C**
Locan® (DF)
Cream, amethocaine 0.8%, amylocaine 1%, cinchocaine 0.4%, in a non-greasy basis. Price 30 g = **C**

Nestosyl® (Bengué)
Ointment, benzocaine 2%, butyl aminobenzoate 2%, hexachlorophane 0.1%, resorcinol 2%, zinc oxide 10%, in a greasy basis. Price 30 g = **C**
Solarcaine® (Plough)
Cream, benzocaine 1%, triclosan 0.2%. Price 25 ml = **C**
Lotion, benzocaine 0.5%, triclosan 0.2%. Price 75 ml = **D**
Spray (= application), benzocaine 5%, triclosan 0.1%, pressurised aerosol unit. Price 100 g = **D**
Xylocaine® (Astra)
Ointment, lignocaine 5% in a water-miscible basis. Price 15 g = **C**

TOPICAL ANTIHISTAMINES
Indications: pruritus, urticaria, see notes above
Cautions: may cause hypersensitivity; avoid in eczema; photosensitivity (diphenhydramine and promethazine)

Anthical® (M&B)
Cream, mepyramine maleate 1.5%, zinc oxide 15%, in a vanishing-cream basis. Price 25 g = **C**
Apply 3–4 times daily for up to 3 days
Anthisan® (M&B)
Cream, mepyramine maleate 2%. Price 25 g = **C**
Apply 2–3 times daily for up to 3 days
Caladryl® (P-D)
Cream, diphenhydramine hydrochloride 1%, calamine 8%, camphor 0.1%, in a water-miscible basis. Price 42 g = **C**
Lotion, ingredients as for cream. Price 125 ml = **C**
Apply 3–4 times daily for up to 3 days
Phenergan® (M&B)
Cream, promethazine 2%, dibromopropamidine isethionate 0.15%. Price 25 g = **C**
Apply when required for up to 3 days
Caution: may stain clothing
R.B.C.® (Rybar)
Cream, antazoline hydrochloride 1.8%, calamine 8%, camphor 0.1%, cetrimide 0.5%. Price 25 g = **C**
Apply when required for up to 3 days

13.4 Topical corticosteroids

Topical corticosteroids are used for the treatment of inflammatory conditions of the skin other than those due to an infection, in particular the eczematous disorders. Corticosteroids suppress various components of the inflammatory reaction while in use; they are in no sense curative, and when treatment is discontinued a rebound exacerbation of the condition may occur. They are indicated for the relief of symptoms and for the suppression of signs of the disorder when potentially less harmful measures are ineffective.

Corticosteroids are of no value in the treatment of urticaria and are **contra-indicated** in rosacea and in ulcerative conditions as they worsen the condition. They should not be used indiscriminately in pruritus.

CHOICE OF PREPARATION. The preparation containing the **least potent** drug at the **lowest strength** which is effective is the one of choice, but extemporaneous dilution should be avoided whenever possible.

Topical corticosteroid preparations are divided into four groups in respect of potency. In ascending order these are:

C = 51-100p, D = 101-180p, E = 181-300p, F = 301-450p, G = 451-650p, H = 651-900p, I = 901-1200p, J = over 1200p.

	Potency	Examples
IV	Mild	Hydrocortisone 1%
III	Moderately potent	Clobetasone butyrate 0.05% (Eumovate®)
II	Potent	Betamethasone 0.1% (as valerate) (Betnovate®); hydrocortisone butyrate (Locoid®)
I	Very potent	Clobetasol propionate 0.05% (Dermovate®)

Intradermal corticosteroid injections (see section 10.1.2.2) are more effective than the very potent topical corticosteroid preparations and they should be reserved for severe cases where there are localised lesions and topical treatment has failed. Their effects last for several weeks.

SIDE-EFFECTS. Unlike groups I and II, groups III and IV are rarely associated with side-effects. The more potent the preparation the more care is required, as absorption through the skin can cause severe pituitary-adrenal-axis suppression and hypercorticism (see section 6.3.3), both of which depend on the area of the body treated and the duration of the treatment. It must also be remembered that absorption is greatest from areas of thin skin, raw surfaces, and intertriginous areas, and is increased by occlusion.

Local side-effects from the use of corticosteroids topically include:
(a) the spread and worsening of untreated local infection;
(b) thinning of the skin which may be restored over a period of time although the original structure may never return;
(c) irreversible striae atrophicae;
(d) increased hair growth;
(e) perioral dermatitis, an inflammatory papular disorder occurring on the face of young women;
(f) acne at the site of application in some patients; and
(g) mild depigmentation and growth of vellus hair.

CHOICE OF FORMULATION. Water-miscible creams are particularly suitable for treating moist or weeping lesions whereas ointments are generally chosen for use on dry, lichenified or scaly lesions or where a more occlusive effect is required. Lotions may be useful when minimal application to a large area is required. Occlusive polythene dressings may be used to increase the effect, but also increase the risk of side-effects. The inclusion of urea increases the penetration of the corticosteroid.

USE IN CHILDREN. Children, especially babies, are particularly susceptible to side-effects. The more potent corticosteroids should be **avoided** in paediatric treatment or if necessary used with great

care for short periods; a mild corticosteroid such as hydrocortisone is useful for treating napkin rash and infantile eczemas. Napkins and plastic pants may however act as an occlusive dressing and increase absorption.

COMPOUND PREPARATIONS. The advantages of including other substances with corticosteroids in topical preparations are debatable. The commonest ones are the **antibacterials**. These are listed in section 13.4.1.

LABELS. The application of excessive quantities of external corticosteroid preparations can result in undesirable local and systemic side-effects (see above). Accordingly, label 28 (To be applied sparingly) should be used with all external corticosteroid preparations.

HYDROCORTISONE
Indications: mild inflammatory skin disorders
Cautions: see notes above; also avoid prolonged use in infants and children, and on the face
Contra-indications: untreated bacterial, fungal, or viral skin lesions
Side-effects: see notes above
Administration: apply sparingly 2–4 times daily, reducing strength and frequency as condition responds

Creams
PoM **Hydrocortisone Cream,** hydrocortisone or hydrocortisone acetate 1%, chlorocresol 0.1%, cetomacrogol emulsifying ointment 30%, in freshly boiled and cooled purified water. Price 15 g = **B**; 30 g = **C**; 50 g = **D**; 100 g = **E**. Potency IV
Other strengths of similar preparations are commercially available as follows: 0.1%, price 30 g = **B**; 0.125%, price 100 g = **B**; 0.5%, price 15 and 30 g (both) = **B**, 50 g = **C**, 100 g = **D**; 2.5%, price 15 g = **C**
PoM **Cobadex**® (Cox Pharmaceuticals)
Cream, hydrocortisone 0.5%, dimethicone '350' 20%, in a water-miscible basis. Price 20 g = **D**. Potency IV
Cream, hydrocortisone 1%, dimethicone '350' 20%, in a water-miscible basis. Price 20 g = **D**. Potency IV
PoM **Dioderm**® (Dermal)
Cream, hydrocortisone 0.1%, in a water-miscible basis. Price 30 g = **E**. Potency IV
PoM **Dome-Cort**® (Bayer)
Cream, hydrocortisone 0.125%, in a water miscible basis. Price 100 g = **F**. Potency IV
PoM **Efcortelan**® (Glaxo)
Cream, hydrocortisone 0.5%, in a water-miscible basis. Diluent cetomacrogol cream (formula A), life of diluted cream 14 days. Price 15 g = **B**. Potency IV
Cream, hydrocortisone 1%, in a water-miscible basis. Diluent as above. Price 15 g = **B**; 50 g = **C**. Potency IV
Cream, hydrocortisone 2.5%, in a water-miscible basis. Diluent as above. Price 15 g = **C**. Potency IV

PoM **Hydrocortistab**® (Boots)
Cream, hydrocortisone acetate 1%, in a water-miscible basis. Price 15 g = **B**. Potency IV

PoM **Hydrocortisyl**® (Roussel)
Cream, hydrocortisone 1%, in a water-miscible basis. Price 15 g = **B**. Potency IV

Ointments
PoM **Hydrocortisone Ointment,** hydrocortisone, in white soft paraffin or a mixture of this with liquid paraffin, with or without wool fat. Price 15 g (0.5 or 1%) = **B**; 30 g (1%) = **C**; 100 g (1%) = **F**. Potency IV

PoM **Efcortelan**® (Glaxo)
Ointment, hydrocortisone 0.5%, in a paraffin basis. Diluent white soft paraffin, life of diluted ointment 14 days. Price 15 g = **B**. Potency IV
Ointment, hydrocortisone 1%, in a paraffin basis. Diluent as above. Price 15 g = **B**; 30 g = **C**. Potency IV
Ointment, hydrocortisone 2.5%, in a paraffin basis. Diluent as above. Price 15 g = **C**. Potency IV

PoM **Hydrocortistab**® (Boots)
Ointment, hydrocortisone 1%, in an anhydrous greasy basis. Price 15 g = **B**. Potency IV

PoM **Hydrocortisyl**® (Roussel)
Ointment, hydrocortisone 1%, in an anhydrous greasy basis. Price 15 g = **B**. Potency IV

Lotions
PoM **Hydrocortisone Lotion,** hydrocortisone 1%, chlorocresol 0.05%, self-emulsifying monostearin 4%, glycerol 6.3%, in freshly boiled and cooled purified water; may be prepared with any other suitable basis. Price 20 ml = **B**. Potency IV

PoM **Efcortelan**® (Glaxo)
Lotion, hydrocortisone 1%, in a water-miscible basis. Do not dilute. Price 20 ml = **B**. Potency IV

Dressings
PoM **Cortacream**® (S&N)
Impregnated bandage, hydrocortisone acetate 1%. Requires additional bandaging. Price 75 mm × 2 m bandage = **F**. Potency IV
Apply to affected area only with minimum of overlap

Compound preparations
PoM **Alphaderm**® (Norwich-Eaton)
Cream, hydrocortisone 1%, urea 10%, in a powder-in-cream basis. Price 30 g = **E**; 100 g = **H**. Potency III
Apply sparingly twice daily

PoM **Calmurid HC**® (Pharmacia)
Cream, hydrocortisone 1%, urea 10%, in a water-miscible basis. Diluent aqueous cream, life of diluted cream 14 days. Price 30 g = **E**; 100 g = **G**. Potency III
Apply sparingly twice daily. Use half-strength cream for 1 week if stinging occurs with undiluted preparation

PoM **Eczederm with Hydrocortisone**® (Quinoderm Ltd)
Cream, hydrocortisone 0.5%, calamine 20.88%,

starch 2.09%. Price 25 g = **C**. Potency IV
Apply sparingly up to 3 times daily

PoM **Epifoam**® (Stafford-Miller)
Foam (= application), hydrocortisone acetate 1%, pramoxine hydrochloride 1%, in a mucoadherent basis (pressurised aerosol pack). Price 12-g unit (approx. 20 applications of 5 ml) = **E**. Potency IV. For perineal trauma including post-episiotomy pain and dermatoses
Apply on a pad 3–4 times daily

PoM **Eurax-Hydrocortisone**® (Geigy)
Cream, hydrocortisone 0.25%, crotamiton 10%. Price 30 g = **C**. Potency IV
Apply sparingly 2–3 times daily

BECLOMETHASONE DIPROPIONATE

Indications: severe inflammatory skin disorders such as eczema in patients unresponsive to less potent corticosteroids

Cautions; Contra-indications; Side-effects: see under Hydrocortisone and notes above

Administration: apply sparingly twice daily, reducing strength and frequency as condition responds. Under occlusion, max. 2 g daily of 0.5% preparation

PoM **Propaderm**® (A&H)
Cream, beclomethasone dipropionate 0.025%. Diluent cetomacrogol cream (formula A), life of diluted cream 14 days. Price 15 g = **C**; 50 g = **E**. Potency II
Ointment, beclomethasone dipropionate 0.025%. Diluent white soft paraffin, life of diluted ointment 14 days. Price 15 g = **C**; 50 g = **E**. Potency II

PoM **Propaderm Forte**® (A&H)
Cream, beclomethasone dipropionate 0.5%. Diluent as above. Price 5 g = **D**. Potency I

BETAMETHASONE ESTERS

Indications: severe inflammatory skin disorders such as eczema in patients unresponsive to less potent corticosteroids

Cautions; Contra-indications; Side-effects: see under Hydrocortisone and notes above. Application of more than 100 g per week of 0.1% preparation is likely to cause adrenal suppression

Administration: apply sparingly 2–3 times daily, reducing strength and frequency as condition responds

▼ PoM **Bebate**® (P-D)
Cream, betamethasone benzoate 0.025% in a water-miscible basis. Price 15 g = **C**. Potency II
Gel, betamethasone benzoate 0.025% in a water-miscible basis. Price 15 g = **C**. Potency II

PoM **Betnovate**® (Glaxo)
Cream, betamethasone 0.1% (as valerate), in a water-miscible basis. Diluent cetomacrogol cream (formula A), life of diluted cream 14 days. Price 15 g = **C**; 30 g = **D**; 100 g = **F**. Potency II
Ointment, betamethasone 0.1% (as valerate), in an anhydrous paraffin basis. Diluent white soft

---

C = 51-100p, D = 101-180p, E = 181-300p, F = 301-450p, G = 451-650p, H = 651-900p, I = 901-1200p, J = over 1200p.

paraffin or a mixture of this with liquid paraffin, life of diluted ointment 14 days. Price 15 g = **C**; 30 g = **D**; 100 g = **F**. Potency II

Lotion, betamethasone 0.1% (as valerate). Do not dilute. Price 20 ml = **C**. Potency II

Scalp application, betamethasone 0.1% (as valerate), in a thickened alcoholic basis. Price 30 ml = **D**; 100 ml = **G**. Potency II

Apply sparingly 1–2 times daily, reducing frequency as condition responds

Caution: flammable

PoM **Betnovate-RD**® (Glaxo)

Cream, betamethasone 0.025% (as valerate) in a water-miscible basis (1 in 4 dilution of Betnovate cream). Price 100 g = **E**. Potency III

Ointment, betamethasone 0.025% (as valerate) in an anhydrous paraffin basis (1 in 4 dilution of Betnovate ointment). Price 100 g = **E**. Potency III

▼ PoM **Diprosalic**® (Kirby-Warrick)

Ointment, betamethasone 0.05% (as dipropionate), salicylic acid 3%. Price 30 g = **F**; 100 g = **H**. Potency II

Lotion, betamethasone 0.05% (as dipropionate), salicylic acid 2%, in an alcoholic basis. Price 30 ml = **E**; 100 ml = **I**. Potency II

Apply sparingly 1–2 times daily

▼ PoM **Diprosone**® (Kirby-Warrick)

Cream, betamethasone 0.05% (as dipropionate), in a water-miscible basis. Diluent Diprobase® cream, life of diluted cream 14 days. Price 30 g = **E**; 100 g = **H**. Potency II

Ointment, betamethasone 0.05% (as dipropionate). Diluent Diprobase® ointment, life of diluted ointment 14 days. Price 30 g = **E**; 100 g = **H**. Potency II

Apply sparingly once or twice daily

Scalp application, betamethasone 0.05% (as dipropionate), in a thickened alcoholic basis. Price 30 ml = **E**; 100 ml = **H**. Potency II

Apply twice daily, reducing as condition responds

CLOBETASOL PROPIONATE

Indications: short-term treatment only of severe exacerbations in inflammatory skin disorders such as discoid lupus erythematosus in patients unresponsive to less potent corticosteroids

Cautions; Contra-indications; Side-effects: see under Hydrocortisone and notes above. Not more than 50 g of 0.05% preparation should be applied per week

Administration: apply sparingly 1–2 times daily for up to 4 weeks, reducing frequency as condition responds

PoM **Dermovate**® (Glaxo)

Cream, clobetasol propionate 0.05%, in a water-miscible basis. Diluents cetomacrogol cream (formula A), aqueous cream, or buffered cream, life of diluted cream 14 days. Price 25 g = **E**; 100 g = **H**. Potency I

Ointment, clobetasol propionate 0.05%, in an anhydrous paraffin basis. Diluents white soft paraffin or a mixture of this with liquid paraffin, life of diluted ointment 14 days. Price 25 g = **E**; 100 g = **H**. Potency I

Scalp application, clobetasol propionate 0.05%, in a thickened alcoholic basis. Price 25 ml = **E**; 100 ml = **I**. Potency I

Caution: flammable

CLOBETASONE BUTYRATE

Indications: inflammatory skin disorders in patients unresponsive to less potent corticosteroids

Cautions; Contra-indications; Side-effects: see under Hydrocortisone and notes above

Administration: apply sparingly up to 4 times daily, reducing frequency as condition responds

PoM **Eumovate**® (Glaxo)

Cream, clobetasone butyrate 0.05%, in a water-miscible basis. Price 25 g = **D**; 100 g = **G**. Potency III

Ointment, clobetasone butyrate 0.05%, in an anhydrous paraffin basis. Price 25 g = **D**; 100 g = **G**. Potency III

DESONIDE

Indications: severe inflammatory skin disorders such as eczema in patients unresponsive to less potent corticosteroids

Cautions; Contra-indications; Side-effects: see under Hydrocortisone and notes above

Administration: apply sparingly 2–3 times daily reducing frequency as condition responds

PoM **Tridesilon**® (Bayer)

Cream, desonide 0.05%, in a water-miscible basis. Diluents cetomacrogol cream (formula A or B) or aqueous cream, life of diluted cream up to 3 months. Price 15 g = **D**; 30 g = **E**. Potency II

Ointment, desonide 0.05%, in a white soft paraffin basis. Diluent white soft paraffin, life of diluted ointment not more than 3 months. Price 30 g = **E**. Potency II

DESOXYMETHASONE

Indications: acute inflammatory, allergic, and chronic skin disorders

Cautions; Contra-indications; Side-effects: see under Hydrocortisone and notes above

Administration: apply sparingly 2–3 times daily reducing frequency as condition responds

▼ PoM **Stiedex**® (Stiefel)

Oily cream, desoxymethasone 0.25%, in an oily basis. Diluent oily cream, life of diluted cream 14 days. Price 30 g = **F**. Potency II

LP Oily cream, desoxymethasone 0.05%, in an oily basis. Diluent oily cream, life of diluted cream 14 days. Price 30 g = **E**. Potency III

DIFLUCORTOLONE VALERATE

Indications: severe inflammatory skin disorders such as eczema in patients unresponsive to less potent corticosteroids; high strength prep-

---

Relative prices: **A** = up to 20p, **B** = 21-50p,

arations (0.3%), short term treatment of severe exacerbations

Cautions; Contra-indications; Side-effects: see under Hydrocortisone and notes above. Not more than 50 g of 0.3% preparation should be applied per week

Administration: apply sparingly 2–3 times daily for up to 4 weeks (0.1% preparations) or 2 weeks (0.3% preparations), reducing strength and frequency as condition responds

PoM **Nerisone**® (Schering)
Cream, diflucortolone valerate 0.1%, in a water-miscible basis. Diluent aqueous cream or Ultrabase®, life of diluted cream 14 days. Price 30 g = E. Potency II
Oily cream, diflucortolone valerate 0.1%, in a water-in-oil basis. Diluent hydrous ointment (oily cream), life of diluted cream 14 days. Price 30 g = E. Potency II
Ointment, diflucortolone valerate 0.1%, in an anhydrous basis. Diluent white soft paraffin, life of diluted ointment 14 days. Price 30 g = E. Potency II

PoM **Nerisone Forte**® (Schering)
Oily cream, diflucortolone valerate 0.3%, in a water-in-oil basis. Diluent hydrous ointment (oily cream), life of diluted cream 14 days. Price 15 g = E. Potency I
Ointment, diflucortolone valerate 0.3% in an anhydrous fatty basis. Diluent white soft paraffin, life of diluted ointment 14 days. Price 15 g = E. Potency I

PoM **Temetex**® (Roche)
Cream, diflucortolone valerate 0.1%, in a water-miscible basis. Price 30 g = E. Potency II
Fatty ointment, diflucortolone valerate 0.1%, in an anhydrous basis. Price 30 g = E. Potency II
Ointment, diflucortolone valerate 0.1%, in a water-in-oil cream basis. Diluent white soft paraffin, life of diluted ointment 14 days. Price 30 g = E. Potency II

FLUCLOROLONE ACETONIDE

Indications: severe inflammatory skin disorders such as eczema in patients unresponsive to less potent corticosteroids
Cautions; Contra-indications; Side-effects: see under Hydrocortisone and notes above
Administration: apply sparingly twice daily, reducing frequency as condition responds

PoM **Topilar**® (Syntex)
Cream, fluclorolone acetonide 0.025%, in a non-aqueous, water-miscible basis. Price 30 g = D; 100 g = F. Potency II
Ointment, fluclorolone acetonide 0.025%, in an ointment basis. Diluent white soft paraffin, life of diluted ointment 14 days. Price 30 g = D; 100 g = F. Potency II

FLUOCINOLONE ACETONIDE

Indications: inflammatory skin disorders such as eczema, 0.0025–0.01% preparations in milder conditions, 0.025% preparations in severe con-

ditions, and 0.2% preparation in short-term treatment of severe exacerbations
Cautions; Contra-indications; Side-effects: see under Hydrocortisone and notes above
Administration: apply sparingly 2–3 times daily, reducing strength and frequency as condition responds. Under occlusion, max. 2 g daily of 0.2% preparation

PoM **Synalar**® (ICI)
Cream, fluocinolone acetonide 0.025%, in a water-miscible basis. Diluent cetomacrogol cream (formula B), life of diluted cream 14 days. Price 15 g = C; 30 g = D; 50 g = E. Potency II
Gel, fluocinolone acetonide 0.025%, in a water-miscible basis. Price 30 g = D. For use on scalp and other hairy areas. Potency II
Ointment, fluocinolone acetonide 0.025%, in an anhydrous greasy basis. Diluents white or yellow soft paraffin or eye ointment basis, life of diluted ointment 14 days. Price 15 g = C; 30 g = D; 50 g = E. Potency II
Lotion, fluocinolone acetonide 0.025%. Diluent sterile water or a fluid non-ionic cream, for example cetostearyl alcohol 2.5%, cetomacrogol '1000' 0.5% in sterile water, life of diluted lotion 14 days. Price 20 ml = C. Potency II

PoM **Synalar 1 in 4 Dilution**® (ICI)
Cream, fluocinolone acetonide 0.00625% in a water-miscible basis. Price 50 g = D. Potency IV

PoM **Synalar 1 in 10 Dilution**® (ICI)
Cream, fluocinolone acetonide 0.0025% in a water-miscible basis. Price 50 g = D. Potency IV

PoM **Synalar Forte**® (ICI)
Cream, fluocinolone acetonide 0.2%, in a water-miscible basis. Diluent cetomacrogol cream (formula B), life of diluted cream 14 days. Price 15 g = G. Potency I

PoM **Synandone**® (ICI)
Cream, fluocinolone acetonide 0.01%, in a water-miscible basis. Diluent as for Synalar® cream. Price 30 g = C. Potency III
Ointment, fluocinolone acetonide 0.01%, in an anhydrous greasy basis. Diluent as for Synalar® ointment. Price 30 g = C. Potency III

FLUOCINONIDE

Indications: severe inflammatory skin disorders such as eczema in patients unresponsive to less potent corticosteroids
Cautions; Contra-indications; Side-effects: see under Hydrocortisone and notes above
Administration: apply sparingly 3–4 times daily, reducing frequency as condition responds

PoM **Metosyn**® (Stuart)
FAPG cream, fluocinonide 0.05%, in a non-aqueous water-miscible basis. Price 25 g = D; 100 g = F. Potency II
Ointment, fluocinonide 0.05%, in a paraffin basis. Diluent white soft paraffin, life of diluted ointment 14 days. Price 25 g = D; 100 g = F. Potency II

C = 51-100p, D = 101-180p, E = 181-300p, F = 301-450p, G = 451-650p, H = 651-900p, I = 901-1200p, J = over 1200p.

Scalp lotion, fluocinonide 0.05% in a propylene glycol-alcohol basis. Price 30 ml (with applicator) = **E**. Potency II
Apply 1–2 times daily, reducing frequency as condition responds
Caution: flammable

FLUOCORTOLONE

Indications: 0.25% preparations—severe inflammatory skin disorders such as eczema in patients unresponsive to less potent corticosteroids; 0.1% preparations—milder inflammatory skin disorders
Cautions; Contra-indications; Side-effects: see under Hydrocortisone and notes above
Administration: apply sparingly 2–3 times daily, reducing strength and frequency as condition responds

PoM **Ultradil Plain**® (Schering)
Cream, fluocortolone hexanoate 0.1%, fluocortolone pivalate 0.1%, in a water-miscible basis. Diluent aqueous cream or Ultrabase®, life of diluted cream 14 days. Price 50 g = **E**; 100 g = **G**. Potency III
Ointment, fluocortolone hexanoate 0.1%, fluocortolone pivalate 0.1%, in a water-in-oil emulsion basis. Diluent hydrous ointment (oily cream), life of diluted ointment 14 days. Price 50 g = **E**; 100 g = **G**. Potency III
PoM **Ultralanum Plain**® (Schering)
Cream, fluocortolone hexanoate 0.25%, fluocortolone pivalate 0.25%, in a water-miscible basis. Diluent aqueous cream or Ultrabase®, life of diluted cream 14 days. Price 30 g = **F**; 50 g = **G**. Potency III

FLURANDRENOLONE

Indications: 0.05% preparations—severe inflammatory skin disorders such as eczema in patients unresponsive to less potent corticosteroids; 0.0125% preparations—milder inflammatory skin disorders
Cautions; Contra-indications; Side-effects: see under Hydrocortisone and notes above
Administration: apply sparingly 2–3 times daily, reducing strength and frequency as condition responds

PoM **Haelan**® (Dista)
Cream, flurandrenolone 0.0125%, in a water-miscible basis. Diluent aqueous cream, life of diluted cream 14 days. Price 60 g = **E**. Potency III
Ointment, flurandrenolone 0.0125%, in an anhydrous greasy basis. Diluent white soft paraffin, life of diluted ointment 14 days. Price 60 g = **E**. Potency III
PoM **Haelan-X**® (Dista)
Cream, flurandrenolone 0.05%, in a water-miscible basis. Diluent as above. Price 15 g = **D**. Potency II
Ointment, flurandrenolone 0.05%, in an anhydrous greasy basis. Diluent as above. Price 15 g = **D**. Potency II

HALCINONIDE

Indications: severe inflammatory skin disorders such as eczema in patients unresponsive to less potent corticosteroids
Cautions; Contra-indications; Side-effects: see under Hydrocortisone and notes above
Administration: apply sparingly 2–3 times daily, reducing frequency as condition responds

PoM **Halciderm Topical**® (Squibb)
Cream, halcinonide 0.1%, in a water-miscible basis. Price 30 g = **F**. Potency I

HYDROCORTISONE BUTYRATE

Indications: severe inflammatory skin disorders such as eczema in patients unresponsive to less potent corticosteroids
Cautions; Contra-indications; Side-effects: see under Hydrocortisone and notes above
Administration: apply sparingly 2–4 times daily, reducing frequency as condition responds

PoM **Locoid**® (Brocades)
Cream, hydrocortisone butyrate 0.1%, in a water-miscible basis. Diluent Locobase® cream, life of diluted cream 14 days. Price 30 g = **E**; 100 g = **G**. Potency II
Lipocream, hydrocortisone butyrate 0.1% in a fatty cream basis. Price 30 g = **E**. Potency II
Ointment, hydrocortisone butyrate 0.1%, in an anhydrous greasy basis. Diluent Locobase® ointment, life of diluted ointment 14 days. Price 30 g = **E**; 100 g = **G**. Potency II
Scalp lotion, hydrocortisone butyrate 0.1%, in an aqueous isopropyl alcohol basis. Price 20 ml = **E**; 100 ml = **H**. Potency II
Apply 1–2 times daily, reducing frequency as condition responds
Caution: flammable

TRIAMCINOLONE ACETONIDE

Indications: severe inflammatory skin disorders such as eczema in patients unresponsive to less potent corticosteroids
Cautions; Contra-indications; Side-effects: see under Hydrocortisone and notes above
Administration: apply sparingly 2–4 times daily, reducing frequency as condition responds

PoM **Adcortyl**® (Squibb)
Cream, triamcinolone acetonide 0.1%, in a water-miscible basis. Diluents cetomacrogol cream (formula B), or aqueous cream provided that chlorocresol content is increased to 0.2%, life of diluted cream 4 weeks. Price 30 g = **E**. Potency II
Ointment, triamcinolone acetonide 0.1%, in an anhydrous greasy basis. Diluent white soft paraffin, life of diluted ointment 14 days. Price 30 g = **E**. Potency II
PoM **Ledercort**® (Lederle)
Cream, triamcinolone acetonide 0.1%, in a water-miscible basis. Diluent aqueous cream, life of diluted cream 14 days. Price 15 g = **D**; 250 g = **J**. Potency II

For all abbreviations and symbols see inside cover.

Relative prices: A = up to 20p, B = 21-50p,

Ointment, triamcinolone acetonide 0.1%, in an anhydrous greasy basis. Diluent 1 part wool fat, 9 parts white soft paraffin, life of diluted ointment 4 weeks. Price 15 g = **D**; 250 g = **J**. Potency II

13.4.1 Corticosteroid anti-infective preparations

There is little evidence that the inclusion of an anti-infective agent with a corticosteroid has any therapeutic benefit in most cases and it may sometimes complicate subsequent treatment. It may, however, be of value in eczema that has become secondarily infected, and in seborrhoeic dermatitis.

HYDROCORTISONE

Indications: see notes above
Cautions; Contra-indications; Side-effects: see sections 13.4 and 13.10

PoM **Hydrocortisone and Neomycin Cream**, hydrocortisone 0.5%, neomycin sulphate 0.5%, in a water-miscible basis. Price 15 g = **C**. Potency IV
Apply sparingly 2–3 times daily

PoM **Barquinol HC**® (Fisons)
Cream, hydrocortisone acetate 0.5%, clioquinol 3%. Price 15 g = **C**. Potency IV
Apply sparingly 2–3 times daily
Caution: stains clothing

PoM **Canesten HC**® (Bayer)
Cream, hydrocortisone 1%, clotrimazole 1%. Price 30 g = **F**. Potency IV
Apply sparingly twice daily

PoM **Daktacort**® (Janssen)
Cream, hydrocortisone 1%, miconazole nitrate 2%, in a water-miscible basis. Price 30 g = **F**. Potency IV
Apply sparingly 2–3 times daily

▼ PoM **Econacort**® (Squibb)
Cream, hydrocortisone 1%, econazole nitrate 1%. Price 30 g = **E**. Potency IV
Apply sparingly twice daily

PoM **Framycort**® (Fisons)
Ointment, hydrocortisone acetate 0.5%, framycetin sulphate 0.5%. Price 15 g = **E**. Potency IV
Apply sparingly 2–3 times daily

PoM **Fucidin H**® (Leo)
Gel, hydrocortisone acetate 1%, fusidic acid 2%, in a water-miscible basis. Price 10 g = **E**; 25 g = **F**. Potency IV
Ointment, hydrocortisone acetate 1%, sodium fusidate 2%. Price 10 g = **D**; 25 g = **F**. Potency IV
Apply sparingly 3–4 times daily

PoM **Genticin HC**® (Nicholas)
Cream, hydrocortisone acetate 1%, gentamicin 0.3% (as sulphate), in a water-miscible basis. Price 15 g = **D**. Potency IV
Ointment, ingredients as for cream but in a greasy basis. Price 15 g = **D**. Potency IV
Apply sparingly 3–4 times daily

PoM **Gregoderm**® (Unigreg)
Ointment, hydrocortisone 1%, neomycin sulphate 0.4%, nystatin 100 000 units/g, polymyxin B sulphate 7250 units/g. Price 4 g = **C**; 15 g = **D**. Potency IV
Apply sparingly 2–3 times daily

PoM **Hydroderm**® (MSD)
Ointment, hydrocortisone 1%, neomycin sulphate 0.5%, bacitracin zinc 1000 units/g, in an emollient basis. Price 15 g = **C**. Potency IV
Apply sparingly 2–3 times daily

PoM **Nybadex**® (Cox Pharmaceuticals)
Ointment, hydrocortisone 1%, nystatin 100 000 units/g, dimethicone '350' 20%, benzalkonium chloride 0.2%, in a water-miscible basis. Diluent cetomacrogol emulsifying ointment, life of diluted ointment 14 days. Price 20 g = **E**. Potency IV
Apply sparingly 2–3 times daily

PoM **Nystaform-HC**® (Bayer)
Cream, hydrocortisone 0.5%, nystatin 100 000 units/g, chlorhexidine hydrochloride 1% in a water-miscible basis. Price 15 and 30 g (both) = **E**. Potency IV
Ointment, hydrocortisone 1%, nystatin 100 000 units/g, chlorhexidine acetate 1%, in a water-repellent basis. Price 30 g = **E**. Potency IV
Apply sparingly 2–3 times daily

PoM **Terra-Cortril**® (Pfizer)
Topical ointment, hydrocortisone 1%, oxytetracycline 3% (as hydrochloride), in a paraffin basis. Price 15 g = **D**; 30 g = **E**. Potency IV.
Apply sparingly 2–4 times daily
Spray application, hydrocortisone 0.17%, oxytetracycline 0.5% (as hydrochloride), pressurised aerosol unit. Price 30-ml unit = **D**; 60-ml unit = **E**. Potency IV
Spray area sparingly 3–4 times daily increasing to 2-hourly for severe conditions

PoM **Terra-Cortril Nystatin**® (Pfizer)
Cream, hydrocortisone 1%, nystatin 100 000 units/g, oxytetracycline 3% (as calcium salt). Price 30 g = **E**. Potency IV
Apply sparingly 2–4 times daily

PoM **Timodine**® (R&C)
Cream, hydrocortisone 0.5%, nystatin 100 000 units/g, benzalkonium chloride solution 0.2%, dimethicone '350' 10%. Price 30 g = **E**. Potency IV
Apply sparingly 3 times daily (napkin rash, after each change)

PoM **Vioform-Hydrocortisone**® (Ciba)
Cream, hydrocortisone 1%, clioquinol 3%. Diluent aqueous cream, life of diluted cream 14 days. Price 30 g = **D**. Potency IV
Ointment, hydrocortisone 1%, clioquinol 3%. Diluent white soft paraffin, life of diluted ointment 14 days. Price 30 g = **D**. Potency IV
Apply sparingly 1–3 times daily
Caution: stains clothing

BECLOMETHASONE DIPROPIONATE
Indications: see notes above
Cautions; Contra-indications; Side-effects: see sections 13.4 and 13.10

C = 51-100p, **D** = 101-180p, **E** = 181-300p, **F** = 301-450p, **G** = 451-650p, **H** = 651-900p, **I** = 901-1200p, **J** = over 1200p.

PoM **Propaderm-A®** (A&H)

Ointment, beclomethasone dipropionate 0.025%, chlortetracycline hydrochloride 3%. Diluent white soft paraffin, life of diluted ointment 14 days. Price 15 g = C; 50 g = E. Potency II

Initially apply sparingly twice daily

Caution: stains clothing

PoM **Propaderm-C®** (A&H)

Cream, beclomethasone dipropionate 0.025%, clioquinol 3%. Diluent cetomacrogol cream (formula A), life of diluted cream 14 days. Price 15 g = C. Potency II

Ointment, ingredients as for cream in ointment basis. Diluent white soft paraffin, life of diluted ointment 14 days. Price 15 g = C. Potency II

Initially apply sparingly twice daily

Caution: stains clothing

BETAMETHASONE

Indications: see notes above

Cautions; Contra-indications; Side-effects: see sections 13.4 and 13.10

PoM **Betnovate-C®** (Glaxo)

Cream, betamethasone 0.1% (as valerate), clioquinol 3%, in a water-miscible basis. Diluent cetomacrogol cream (formula A), life of diluted cream 14 days. Price 15 g = D; 30 g = E. Potency II

Ointment, betamethasone 0.1% (as valerate), clioquinol 3%, in a paraffin basis. Diluent white soft paraffin or a mixture of this with liquid paraffin, life of diluted ointment 14 days. Price 15 g = D; 30 g = E. Potency II

Apply sparingly 2–3 times daily

Caution: stains clothing

PoM **Betnovate-N®** (Glaxo)

Cream, betamethasone 0.1% (as valerate), neomycin sulphate 0.5%, in a water-miscible basis. Diluent cetomacrogol cream (formula A), life of diluted cream 14 days. Price 15 g = D; 30 g = E; 100 g = G. Potency II

Ointment, betamethasone 0.1% (as valerate), neomycin sulphate 0.5%, in a paraffin basis. Diluent white soft paraffin or a mixture of this with liquid paraffin, life of diluted ointment 14 days. Price 15 g = D; 30 g = E; 100 g = G. Potency II

Lotion, betamethasone 0.1% (as valerate), neomycin sulphate 0.5%. Price 20 ml = D. Potency II

Apply sparingly 2–3 times daily

PoM **Fucibet®** (Leo)

Cream, betamethasone 0.1% (as valerate), fusidic acid 2%, in a water-miscible basis. Price 10 g = E; 25 g = G. Potency II

Apply sparingly 2–3 times daily

CLOBETASOL PROPIONATE

Indications: see notes above

Cautions; Contra-indications; Side-effects: see sections 13.4 and 13.10

PoM **Dermovate-NN®** (Glaxo)

Cream, clobetasol propionate 0.05%, neomycin

sulphate 0.5%, nystatin 100 000 units/g. Price 25 g = E. Potency I

Ointment, ingredients as for cream, in a paraffin basis. Diluent white soft paraffin, life of diluted ointment 14 days. Price 25 g = E. Potency I

Apply sparingly once or twice daily, for up to 4 weeks reducing as condition responds

CLOBETASONE BUTYRATE

Indications: see notes above

Cautions; Contra-indications; Side-effects: see sections 13.4 and 13.10

PoM **Trimovate®** (Glaxo)

Cream, clobetasone butyrate 0.05%, oxytetracycline 3% (as calcium salt), nystatin 100 000 units/g, in a water-miscible basis. Price 25 g = E. Potency III

Ointment, clobetasone butyrate 0.05%, chlortetracycline hydrochloride 3%, nystatin 100 000 units/g, in a paraffin basis. Price 25 g = E. Potency III

Apply sparingly up to 4 times daily

Caution: stains clothing

DESOXYMETHASONE

Indications: see notes above

Cautions; Contra-indications; Side-effects: see sections 13.4 and 13.10

▼ PoM **Stiedex LPN®** (Stiefel)

Oily cream, desoxymethasone 0.05%, neomycin (as sulphate) 0.5%, in an oily basis. Price 15 g = E. Potency III

Apply sparingly 2–3 times daily

FLUOCINOLONE ACETONIDE

Indications: see notes above

Cautions; Contra-indications; Side-effects: see sections 13.4 and 13.10

PoM **Synalar C®** (ICI)

Cream, fluocinolone acetonide 0.025%, clioquinol 3%, in a water-miscible basis. Diluent cetomacrogol cream (formula B), life of diluted cream 14 days. Price 15 g = C. Potency II

Ointment, ingredients as for cream, in a greasy basis. Diluents white or yellow soft paraffin or eye ointment basis, life of diluted ointment 14 days. Price 15 g = C. Potency II

Apply sparingly 2–3 times daily

Caution: stains clothing

PoM **Synalar N®** (ICI)

Cream, fluocinolone acetonide 0.025%, neomycin sulphate 0.5%, in a water-miscible basis. Diluent as above. Price 15 g = C; 30 g = D. Potency II

Ointment, ingredients as for cream, in a greasy basis. Diluents as above. Price 15 g = C; 30 g = D. Potency II

Lotion, ingredients as for cream in an aqueous basis. Price 20 ml = C. Potency II

Apply sparingly 2–3 times daily

FLUOCORTOLONE

Indications: see notes above
Cautions; Contra-indications; Side-effects: see sections 13.4 and 13.10

PoM **Ultralanum®** (Berlimed)
Ointment, fluocortolone 0.25%, fluocortolone hexanoate 0.25%, clemizole hexachlorophane 2.5%, in a water-in-oil emulsion basis. Diluent hydrous ointment (oily cream), life of diluted ointment 14 days. Price 30 g = **F**; 50 g = **G**. Potency III
Initially apply sparingly 2–3 times daily

FLURANDRENOLONE

Indications: see notes above
Cautions; Contra-indications; Side-effects: see sections 13.4 and 13.10

PoM **Haelan-C®** (Dista)
Cream, flurandrenolone 0.0125%, clioquinol 3%. Diluent aqueous cream, life of diluted cream 14 days. Price 30 g = **E**. Potency III
Ointment, flurandrenolone 0.0125%, clioquinol 3%. Diluent white soft paraffin, life of diluted ointment 14 days. Price 30 g = **E**. Potency III
Apply sparingly 2–3 times daily
Caution: stains clothing

HYDROCORTISONE BUTYRATE

Indications: see notes above
Cautions; Contra-indications; Side-effects: see sections 13.4 and 13.10

PoM **Locoid C®** (Brocades)
Cream, hydrocortisone butyrate 0.1%, chlorquinaldol 3%. Diluent Locobase® cream, life of diluted cream 14 days. Price 30 g = **E**. Potency II
Ointment, ingredients as for cream, in a greasy basis. Diluent Locobase® ointment, life of diluted ointment 14 days. Price 30 g = **E**. Potency II
Apply sparingly 2–4 times daily. Max. 60 g for up to 14 days

METHYLPREDNISOLONE ACETATE

Indications: see notes above.
Cautions; Contra-indications; Side-effects: see sections 13.4 and 13.10

PoM **Neo-Medrone®** (Upjohn)
Cream, methylprednisolone acetate 0.25%, neomycin sulphate 0.5%. Price 15 g = **D**. Potency IV
Apply sparingly 1–3 times daily

TRIAMCINOLONE ACETONIDE

Indications: see notes above

Cautions; Contra-indications; Side-effects: see sections 13.4 and 13.10

PoM **Adcortyl with Graneodin®** (Squibb)
Cream, triamcinolone acetonide 0.1%, gramicidin 0.025%, neomycin 0.25% (as sulphate), in a vanishing-cream basis. Do not dilute. Price 15 g = **D**. Potency II
Ointment, ingredients as for cream, in an ointment basis. Do not dilute. Price 15 g = **D**. Potency II
Apply sparingly 2–4 times daily

PoM **Aureocort®** (Lederle)
Cream, triamcinolone acetonide 0.1%, chlortetracycline hydrochloride 3% (as chlortetracycline), in a water-miscible basis. Do not dilute. Price 15 g = **E**. Potency II
Ointment, triamcinolone acetonide 0.1%, chlortetracycline hydrochloride 3%, in an anhydrous greasy basis containing wool fat and white soft paraffin. Do not dilute. Price 15 g = **E**. Potency II
Apply sparingly 2–3 times daily
Caution: stains clothing
Spray application, triamcinolone acetonide 15 mg, chlortetracycline hydrochloride 600 mg/container, in a fluorinated hydrocarbon vehicle. Price 60-g pressurised aerosol pack = **G**. Potency II
Spray sparingly 2–3 times daily
Caution: stains clothing

PoM **Silderm®** (Lederle)
Cream, triamcinolone acetonide 0.1%, neomycin 0.35% (as sulphate), undecylenic acid 2.5%. Price 15 g = **E**; 30 g = **F**. Potency II
Apply sparingly 3–4 times daily

PoM **Tri-Adcortyl®** (Squibb)
Cream, triamcinolone acetonide 0.1%, gramicidin 0.025%, neomycin 0.25% (as sulphate), nystatin 100 000 units/g. Price 15 g = **D**; 30 g = **F**. Potency II
Ointment, ingredients as for cream, in an ointment basis. Price 15 g = **D**; 30 g = **F**. Potency II
Apply sparingly 2–4 times daily

13.5 Preparations for psoriasis and eczema

Eczema (dermatitis) is due to a particular type of epidermal inflammation and is caused by a wide variety of factors; where possible the causative factors should be established and removed (see also hyposensitisation, section 3.4.2). In many cases no underlying factor can be identified (atopic eczema).

Dry, fissured, scaly lesions are treated with bland **emollients** (section 13.2.1) which are often all that is necessary to allay irritation and permit healing. Preparations containing zinc oxide and calamine are sometimes useful; zinc may have a weak anti-eczematous action. **Topical corticosteroids** are described in section 13.4. Perfumes and perfumed soaps should be **avoided** and preparations such as **emulsifying ointment** used as soap substitutes and in the bath. **Keratolytics** such as salicylic acid, followed by ichthammol or coal tar (see below) are used in chronic eczematous conditions where there is marked thickening of the skin and pronounced scaling.

Weeping eczemas may be treated with corticosteroids; they are, however, commonly secondarily infected. Wet dressings of **potassium permanganate** (0.01%) (section 13.11) are applied. If a large area is involved, potassium permanganate baths are taken. When necessary **topical antibacterials** are used (section 13.10.1) but those which are not given systemically should be chosen.

Psoriasis is characterised by epidermal thickening and scaling. It has less tendency to heal spontaneously than eczema. For mild conditions, treatment, other than reassurance and an emollient, may be unnecessary. In more troublesome cases, local application of **salicylic acid**, **coal tar**, or **dithranol** may have a beneficial effect. Topical and systemic corticosteroids should be avoided or given under specialist supervision because, although they may be effective, subsequent treatment becomes more difficult, as tachyphylaxis may occur and they may induce or precipitate severe pustular psoriasis (see also section 6.3.3). In resistant cases an antimetabolite, usually methotrexate (see section 8.1.3), may be used for its antimitotic activity but this must always be done under hospital supervision and the dose adjusted according to severity of the condition and in accordance with haematological and biochemical measurements; the usual dose is 15 to 25 mg of methotrexate weekly, usually by mouth.

Salicylic acid may be used in all hyperkeratotic and scaling conditions to enhance the rate of loss of surface scale. Preparations containing salicylic acid 2% are used initially and then gradually increased to concentrations of 3 to 6%. Side-effects are few but include allergic contact sensitivity, or, when large areas are treated, salicylism (see section 10.1.1.1).

Ichthammol has a milder action than coal tar and is useful in the less acute forms of eczema. It can be applied conveniently to flexures of the limbs as **zinc paste and ichthammol bandage** (Ichthopaste®; Icthaband®).

Coal tar is more active than salicylic acid and has antipruritic and keratolytic properties. It is used in psoriasis and eczema. Coal tar has superseded wood tar as it is more active. The formulation and strength chosen depends on patient acceptability and severity of the condition; the 'thicker' the patch of eczema or psoriasis the stronger the concentration of coal tar required. **Coal tar paste** or **zinc and coal tar paste** are generally suitable for most cases but are limited by their unpleasant appearance and smell and they may not be used on the face. Some of the newer preparations are less unsightly and may be preferred. Preparations such as Carbo-Dome® are suitable for treating the face. **Zinc paste and coal tar bandage** is useful for treating the limbs. **Tar** shampoos are described in section 13.9. When lesions are extensive coal tar baths are useful.

Combinations of coal tar with zinc or salicylic acid have no advantage over the simpler preparations. Preparations containing hydrocortisone and coal tar are useful in eczemas.

Dithranol is used in psoriasis and is the most potent topical preparation available for this condition. The preparation is applied carefully to the lesion, covered with a dressing, and left for one hour. Traditionally applications have been left on the skin overnight but this has now been shown to be unnecessary as short contact applications of 30 to 60 minutes are equally effective. Usual concentrations are 0.1–2% although in individual patients 5% or more may be used. Dithranol must be used with caution as it can cause quite severe skin irritation. For this reason it must be applied only to the lesions and it is customary to start with low concentrations and gradually build up to the maximum concentration which produces a therapeutic effect without irritation. Hands should be washed thoroughly after use. Some patients are intolerant to dithranol in low concentrations and it is important to recognise them early in treatment. Fair skin is more sensitive than dark skin. Proprietary preparations such as Dithrocream® are most commonly used as they may cause less staining and irritation than dithranol paste. Dithranol and urea combinations (Psoradrate®) may improve skin texture by rehydration. **Dithranol triacetate** (Exolan®) has no advantage over traditional preparations.

Ingram's method of applying dithranol is a frequent method used in hospitals. **Dithranol paste** is applied to the lesions after the patient has soaked in a warm bath containing coal tar solution 1 in 800 and after drying is exposed to ultraviolet radiation to produce a slight erythema; the procedure is repeated daily.

Etretinate (Tigason®) is a newly introduced drug given by mouth for the treatment of severe resistant or complicated psoriasis and some of the congenital disorders of keratinisation including Darier's disease (Keratosis follicularis). It should be prescribed only by consultant dermatologists or under hospital supervision. It is a retinoid compound with marked effects on keratinising epithelia. A therapeutic effect occurs after 2 to 4 weeks with maximum benefit after 4 to 6 weeks. Etretinate should be administered continuously because it treats only manifestations not the ultimate causes of these diseases, but treatment should be limited to a period of 6 to 9 months with a 3- to 4-month rest period before repeating treatment, as experience with this drug is limited. Most patients suffer from dryness and cracking of the lips. Other side-effects include mild transient alopecia, occasional generalised pruritus, paronychia, and nose bleeds. There is a tendency for the plasma lipids to rise in some patients. Etretinate is teratogenic and must be **avoided** in pregnancy. Contraceptive measures must be taken during treatment by women who may become pregnant and for one year after a course of the drug.

Bufexamac (Parfenac®) is used in mild inflammatory skin conditions.

BORDERLINE SUBSTANCES. The preparations marked 'ACBS' are regarded as drugs when prescribed in accordance with the advice of the Advisory Committee on Borderline Substances for the clinical conditions listed. Prescriptions issued in accordance with this advice and endorsed 'ACBS' will not normally be investigated. See Appendix 3 for listing by clinical condition.

COAL TAR

Indications: chronic eczema and psoriasis
Cautions: avoid broken or inflamed skin
Side-effects: skin irritation and acne-like eruptions, photosensitivity; stains skin, hair, and fabric
Administration: apply 1–3 times daily starting with low-strength preparations

Ointments and similar preparations
Calamine and Coal Tar Ointment (see Formulary). Price 25 g = **A**
Coal Tar and Salicylic Acid Ointment, (see Formulary). Price 25 g = **A**
Coal Tar Paint, coal tar 10%, in acetone. Price 25 ml = **A**. Label: 15
   Caution: highly flammable
Coal Tar Paste, strong coal tar solution 7.5%, in compound zinc paste. Price 25 g = **A**
Zinc and Coal Tar Paste, zinc oxide 6%, coal tar 6%, emulsifying wax 5%, starch 38%, yellow soft paraffin 45%. Price 25 g = **A**
Alphosyl® (Stafford-Miller)
   Cream, coal tar extract 5%, allantoin 2%, in a vanishing-cream basis. Price 75 g = **D**. For application to skin particularly intertriginous areas
   Lotion, coal tar extract 5%, allantoin 2%. Price 250 ml = **E**. For application to skin or scalp
   Apply liberally 2–4 times daily
Carbo-Dome® (Bayer)
   Cream, coal tar solution 10%, in a water-miscible basis. Price 30 g = **D**; 100 g = **F**
   Apply 2–3 times daily
Clinitar® (S&N Pharm.)
   Cream, coal tar extract 1%. Price 60 g = **E**
   Gel, coal tar extract 2·5%. Price 40 g = **E**
   Apply 1–2 times daily
E.S.T.P.® (Martindale)
   Paste (ether-soluble tar paste), ether-soluble tar distillate 1.5%, starch (maize) 12%, zinc oxide 14%, in an emollient basis. Price 50 g = **A**; 500 g = **D**
   Apply 3–4 times daily
Gelcotar® (Quinoderm Ltd)
   Gel, strong coal tar solution 5%, pine tar 5%, in a water-miscible basis. Price 50 g = **E**; 500 g = **I**. Apply twice daily
Meditar® (Brocades)
   Application, coal tar 5% in a wax stick. Price 20 g = **E**
   Apply 1–2 times daily
Pragmatar® (SK&F)
   Ointment (= cream), cetyl alcohol-coal tar distillate 4%, salicylic acid 3%, sulphur (precipitated) 3%, in a water-miscible basis. Price 25 g = **C**

Apply sparingly daily; for scalp apply weekly to clean hair or in severe cases daily. Dilute with a few drops of water before application to infants
Psoriderm® (Dermal)
   Cream, coal tar 6%, lecithin 0.4%. Price 225 ml = **E**
   Apply 1–2 times daily
PsoriGel® (Alcon)
   Gel, coal tar solution USP 7.5% in an alcoholic emollient basis. Price 90 g = **E**
   Apply 1–2 times daily

Impregnated dressings
Zinc Paste and Coal Tar Bandage, bandage impregnated with paste containing zinc oxide 15% and prepared coal tar 3%. Requires additional bandaging. Price 75 mm × 6 m bandage = **D**
Coltapaste® (S&N)
   Impregnated bandage, zinc paste and coal tar bandage. Price 75 mm × 6 m bandage = **D**
Tarband® (Seton)
   Impregnated bandage, zinc paste and coal tar bandage. Price 75 mm × 6 m bandage = **D**

Bath preparations
Coal Tar Solution, coal tar 20%, polysorbate '80' 5%, in alcohol. Price 100 ml = **C**
   Use 100 ml in a bath
Polytar Emollient® (Stiefel)
   Bath additive, coal tar solution 2.5%, arachis oil extract of coal tar 7.5%, tar 7.5%, cade oil 7.5%, liquid paraffin 35%. Price 250 ml = **E**. ACBS: for psoriasis, eczema, atopic and pruritic dermatoses
   Use 2–4 capfuls in bath and soak for 20 minutes
Psoriderm® (Dermal)
   Bath emulsion, coal tar 40%. Price 200 ml = **E**
   Use 30 ml in a bath and soak for 5 minutes

Shampoo preparations
Section 13.9

Coal tar and corticosteroid preparations
PoM **Alphosyl HC®** (Stafford-Miller)
   Cream, coal tar extract 5%, hydrocortisone 0.5%, allantoin 2%, in a vanishing-cream basis. Price 30 g = **D**; 45 g = **E**. Potency IV
   Apply sparingly 2–4 times daily
PoM **Carbo-Cort®** (Bayer)
   Cream, coal tar solution 3%, hydrocortisone 0.25%, in a water-miscible basis. Price 30 g = **E**. Potency IV
   Apply sparingly 2–3 times daily
PoM **Tarcortin®** (Stafford-Miller)
   Cream, coal tar extract 5%, hydrocortisone 0.5%, in a vanishing-cream basis. Price 30 and 45 g (both) = **D**. Potency IV
   Apply sparingly 2–4 times daily

BUFEXAMAC

Indications: mild inflammatory skin disorders
Side-effects: skin irritation
Administration: apply sparingly 2–3 times daily

C = 51-100p, D = 101-180p, E = 181-300p, F = 301-450p, G = 451-650p, H = 651-900p, I = 901-1200p, J = over 1200p.

PoM **Parfenac**® (Lederle)
Cream, bufexamac 5%, in a water-miscible basis.
Do not dilute. Price 15 g = **D**; 30 g = **E**

DITHRANOL

Indications: subacute and chronic psoriasis, see
notes above
Cautions: avoid use near eyes
Contra-indications: hypersensitivity; acute
psoriasis
Side-effects: local burning sensation and
irritation; stains skin, hair, and fabrics
Administration: see notes above

Dithranol Ointment, dithranol, in yellow soft
paraffin. Usual strengths 0.1–2% of dithranol.
Part of basis may be replaced by hard paraffin if
a stiffer preparation is required. Price 25 g = **A**.
Label: 28
Dithranol Paste, dithranol in zinc and salicylic
acid (Lassar's) paste. Usual strengths 0.1%
('weak dithranol paste') and 1% ('strong
dithranol paste') of dithranol. Price 0.1%,
25 g = **A**; 1%, 25 g = **B**. Label: 28
Anthranol 0·4® (Stiefel)
Ointment, dithranol 0.4%, salicylic acid 0.4%.
Price 50 g = **F**. Label: 28. For application to
skin or scalp
Antraderm Mild® (Brocades)
Application, dithranol 0.5% in a wax stick. Price
8 g = **E**. Label: 28. For sensitive skins
PoM **Antraderm**® (Brocades)
Application, dithranol 1% in a wax stick. Price
8 g = **E**. Label: 28
PoM **Antraderm Forte**® (Brocades)
Application, dithranol 2% in a wax stick. Price
8 g = **E**. Label: 28
Dithrocream® (Dermal)
Cream, dithranol 0.1%, in a water-miscible
basis. Price 50 g = **E**. Label: 28. For application
to skin or scalp
Cream, dithranol 0.25%, in a water-miscible
basis. Price 50 g = **F**. Label: 28. For application
to skin or scalp
Forte cream, dithranol 0.5%, in a water-miscible
basis. Price 50 g = **F**. Label: 28. For application
to skin or scalp
HP Cream, dithranol 1% in a water-miscible
basis. Price 50 g = **F**. Label: 28
Dithrolan® (Dermal)
Ointment, dithranol 0.5%, salicylic acid 0.5%.
Diluent yellow soft paraffin, life of diluted ointment 14 days. Price 90 g = **F**. Label: 28
Psoradrate® (Norwich-Eaton)
Cream, dithranol 0.1%, in a powder-in-cream
basis containing urea. Price 30 g = **E**;
100 g = **H**. Label: 28. For application to skin or
scalp
Cream, dithranol 0.2%, in a powder-in-cream
basis containing urea. Price 30 g = **E**; 100 g =
H. Label: 28
▼ *Cream*, dithranol 0.4%, in a powder-in-cream
basis containing urea. Price 100 g = **I**. Label:
28
Psorin® (Thames)
Ointment, dithranol 0.16%, crude coal tar 1%,

salicylic acid 1.6%, in an emollient basis. Price
50 g = **G**. Label: 28

DITHRANOL TRIACETATE

*Indications; Cautions; Contra-indications; Side-
effects; Administration:* see under Dithranol and
notes above

Exolan® (Dermal)
Cream, dithranol triacetate 1% in a water-mis-
cible basis. Price 50 g = **E**. Label: 28
Apply daily to skin and scalp

ETRETINATE

*Indications; Cautions; Contra-indications; Side-
effects:* see notes above. Avoid in hepatic
impairment. Monitor liver function and plasma
lipids (especially in patients with hypertriglyceridaemia) 1 month after initiating treatment and then at 3-monthly intervals
Dose: administered in accordance with expert
advice, adults and children, initially 0.5–1 mg/
kg daily in two divided doses adjusted according
to response; max. 1.5 mg/kg daily; usual maintenance dose 500 micrograms/kg daily

▼ PoM **Tigason**® (Roche)
Capsules, yellow, etretinate 10 mg. Price 20
caps = **H** (Hosp. only). Label: 10, patient information card
Capsules, orange/yellow, etretinate 25 mg. Price
10 caps = **H** (Hosp. only). Label: 10, patient
information card

ICHTHAMMOL

Indications: chronic eczema
Cautions: avoid application to broken or
inflamed skin
Side-effects: skin irritation and sensitisation
Administration: apply 1–3 times daily

Ichthammol Ointment, ichthammol 10%, yellow soft paraffin 45%, wool fat 45%. Price 25 g =
A
Zinc and Ichthammol Cream, ichthammol 5%,
cetostearyl alcohol 3%, wool fat 10%, in zinc
cream. Price 100 g = **B**
Zinc Paste and Ichthammol Bandage, bandage
impregnated with paste containing zinc oxide
15% and ichthammol 2%. Requires additional
bandaging. Price 75 mm × 6 m bandage = **D**
Ichthopaste® (S&N)
Impregnated bandage, zinc paste and ichthammol bandage. Price 75 mm × 6 m bandage = **D**
Icthaband® (Seton)
Impregnated bandage, zinc paste and ichthammol bandage. Price 75 mm × 6 m bandage = **D**

SALICYLIC ACID

Indications: hyperkeratoses
Cautions: see notes above; avoid broken or
inflamed skin
Side-effects: sensitivity, excessive drying, irritation, systemic effects after prolonged use (see
section 10.1.1.1)

Salicylic Acid Collodion —section 13.7
Salicylic Acid Ointment, salicylic acid 2%, in wool alcohols ointment. Price 25 g = A
Apply twice daily
Zinc and Salicylic Acid Paste (Lassar's Paste), zinc oxide 24%, salicylic acid 2%, starch 24%, white soft paraffin 50%. Price 25 g = A
Apply twice daily
Keralyt® (Bristol-Myers)
Gel, salicylic acid 6%. Price 55 g = E
Apply to hydrated skin, cover with an occlusive dressing, preferably overnight, and remove by washing; wash hands thoroughly after use

13.6 Preparations for acne

TOPICAL TREATMENT. Most topical preparations are intended for removing follicular plugs and reducing skin flora. The skin is cleansed regularly with detergent solutions, for example cetrimide solution (section 13.11). Abrasive agents may also be used but their effectiveness is uncertain.

Cleansing is followed by application of **antiseptics** and **keratolytics**. Preparations usually contain benzoyl peroxide, potassium hydroxyquinoline sulphate, sulphur, salicylic acid, or tretinoin. Many of these irritate the skin but it is doubtful if a therapeutic effect can be obtained without some degree of irritation, which subsides with continued treatment. Topical application of **tretinoin** (Retin-A®) has been shown to be useful in treating acne but patients should be warned that some redness and skin peeling may occur after application for several days. Tretinoin is a vitamin A derivative.

Thick greasy preparations are generally **contra-indicated** in acne. Topical antimicrobials are also used but their value is uncertain and they may cause sensitisation, particularly with neomycin. They may also cause resistant strains to appear in the skin flora. Preparations containing resorcinol should be avoided as prolonged application may interfere with thyroid function. Topical corticosteroids should **not** be used in acne.

SYSTEMIC TREATMENT. Systemic antibacterial treatment is useful. **Tetracycline** (see section 5.1.3), **erythromycin** (see section 5.1.5), and occasionally **co-trimoxazole** (see section 5.1.8) are used. The usual dosage regimen for tetracycline and erythromycin, taken before meals, is 250 mg 3 times daily for 1–4 weeks and then reduced to twice daily until improvement occurs. Maximum improvement usually occurs after three or four months but in resistant cases treatment may need to be continued for two or more years. As pseudomembranous colitis has been reported with tetracycline, caution is necessary in long-term administration.

Cyproterone acetate with **ethinyloestradiol** (Diane®) has been recently introduced. It contains an anti-androgen and is used to treat women with severe acne refractory to prolonged oral antibacterial therapy. Improvement of acne probably occurs because it decreases sebum secretion which is under androgen control. Some women with mild to moderate idiopathic hirsutism may also benefit as hair growth is also androgen-dependent (see also section 6.4.2). It may also be used as an oral contraceptive but should be reserved for women who are being treated for androgen-dependent skin conditions. It is contra-indicated in pregnancy and in patients with a predisposition to thrombosis.

Isotretinoin (Roaccutane®) has recently been introduced for the systemic treatment of severe cystic and conglobate acne. It should only be given after the usual treatments have proved ineffective and then only under the guidance of experts familiar with its actions and side-effects. It is given in doses of 500 micrograms/kg/day for 12–16 weeks but doses may be adjusted if necessary after 4 weeks. Repeat courses should not normally be given. An exacerbation is common some 2–4 weeks after starting treatment but usually subsides after a few weeks.

Side-effects include dry lips, sore eyes, nose bleeds, mild transient hair loss, and joint pains. Plasma lipids and liver function should be checked by investigation monthly as there is a tendency for the plasma lipids to rise in some patients. The drug is teratogenic and must not be given to women who are pregnant or those who may become pregnant unless there is concomitant effective contraception and then only after detailed explanation by the physician. The contraceptive measures must continue for at least one month after ceasing treatment with the drug.

BORDERLINE SUBSTANCES. The preparations marked 'ACBS' are regarded as drugs when prescribed in accordance with the advice of the Advisory Committee on Borderline Substances for the clinical conditions listed. Prescriptions issued in accordance with this advice and endorsed 'ACBS' will normally not be investigated. See Appendix 3 for listing by clinical condition.

TOPICAL PREPARATIONS

ABRASIVE AGENTS
Indications: cleansing in acne vulgaris
Cautions: avoid contact with eyes; discontinue use temporarily if skin becomes irritated
Contra-indications: superficial venules, telangiectasia

Brasivol® (Stiefel)
Paste No. 1, aluminium oxide 38.09% in fine particles, in a soap-detergent basis. Price 70 g = E
Paste No. 2, aluminium oxide 52.2% in medium particles, in a soap-detergent basis. Price 85 g = E
Paste No. 3, aluminium oxide 65.2% in coarse particles, in a soap-detergent basis. Price 100 g = E
Use instead of soap 1–3 times daily, starting with fine grade and progressing to coarser grades if required

C = 51-100p, D = 101-180p, E = 181-300p, F = 301-450p, G = 451-650p, H = 651-900p, I = 901-1200p, J = over 1200p.

Ionax Scrub® (Alcon)

Gel, polyethylene granules 21.9%, benzalkonium chloride 0.25% in an alcoholic foaming basis. Price 60 g = **D**. ACBS: for control and hygiene of acne and cleansing of the skin prior to acne treatment

Use instead of soap 1–2 times daily

BENZOYL PEROXIDE

Indications: acne vulgaris

Cautions: avoid contact with eyes, mouth, and mucous membranes; may bleach fabrics

Contra-indications: acne rosacea

Side-effects: skin irritation

Administration: apply 1–2 times daily to clean skin, starting treatment with lower-strength preparations

Acetoxyl 2.5® (Stiefel)

Gel, benzoyl peroxide 2.5%, in an aqueous-acetone-gel basis. Price 40 g = **D**

Acetoxyl 5® (Stiefel)

Gel, benzoyl peroxide 5%, in an aqueous-acetone-gel basis. Price 40 g = **D**

Acnegel® (Kirby-Warrick)

Gel, benzoyl peroxide 5%, in an aqueous alcoholic basis. Price 50 g = **E**

Forte gel, benzoyl peroxide 10%, in an aqueous alcoholic basis. Price 50 g = **E**

Benoxyl 5® (Stiefel)

Cream, benzoyl peroxide 5%, in a non-greasy basis. Price 40 g = **D**

Lotion, benzoyl peroxide 5%, in a non-greasy basis. Price 30 ml = **D**

Benoxyl 5 with Sulphur® (Stiefel)

Cream, benzoyl peroxide 5%, sulphur 2%, in a water-miscible basis. Price 40 g = **D**

Lotion, benzoyl peroxide 5%, sulphur 2%, in a water-miscible basis. Price 30 ml = **D**

Apply once daily. Use if tolerance develops to Benoxyl 5® but before progressing to Benoxyl 10®

Benoxyl 10® (Stiefel)

Lotion, benzoyl peroxide 10%, in a water-miscible basis. Price 30 ml = **D**

Benoxyl 10 with Sulphur® (Stiefel)

Cream, benzoyl peroxide 10%, sulphur 5%, in a water-miscible basis. Price 40 g = **D**

Lotion, benzoyl peroxide 10%, sulphur 5%, in a water-miscible basis. Price 30 ml = **D**

Debroxide 5® (Alcon)

Gel, benzoyl peroxide 5%, in an aqueous-gel basis. Price 60 g = **E**

Debroxide 10® (Alcon)

Gel, benzoyl peroxide 10%, in an aqueous-gel basis. Price 60 g = **E**

Panoxyl 2.5® (Stiefel)

Aquagel (= gel), benzoyl peroxide 2.5%. Price 40 g = **D**

Panoxyl 5® (Stiefel)

Gel, benzoyl peroxide 5%, in an aqueous alcoholic basis. Price 40 g = **D**

Aquagel (= gel), benzoyl peroxide 5%. Price 40 g = **E**

Panoxyl 10® (Stiefel)

Gel, benzoyl peroxide 10%, in an aqueous alcoholic basis. Price 40 g = **D**

Aquagel (= gel), benzoyl peroxide 10%. Price 40 g = **E**

Quinoderm® (Quinoderm Ltd)

Cream, benzoyl peroxide 10%, potassium hydroxyquinoline sulphate 0.5%, in an astringent vanishing-cream basis. Price 25 g = **C**; 50 g = **D**

Cream 5, benzoyl peroxide 5%, potassium hydroxyquinoline sulphate 0.5%, in an astringent vanishing-cream basis. Price 50 g = **D**

Lotio-gel 5%, benzoyl peroxide 5%, potassium hydroxyquinoline sulphate 0.5%, in an astringent creamy basis. Price 30 ml = **D**

Lotio-gel 10%, benzoyl peroxide 10%, potassium hydroxyquinoline sulphate 0.5%, in an astringent creamy basis. Price 30 ml = **D**

Apply 1–3 times daily

Theraderm 5® (Bristol-Myers)

Gel, benzoyl peroxide 5% in a water-miscible basis. Price 56 g = **E**

Theraderm 10® (Bristol-Myers)

Gel, benzoyl peroxide 10% in a water-miscible basis. Price 56 g = **E**

SULPHUR

Indications: acne vulgaris

Cautions: avoid contact with eyes, mouth, and mucous membrane

Side-effects: skin irritation

Administration: apply to clean skin 1–2 times daily

Resorcinol and Sulphur Paste, resorcinol 5%, precipitated sulphur 5%, emulsifying ointment 50%, zinc oxide 40%. Price 25 g = **A**

Salicylic Acid and Sulphur Cream, salicylic acid 2%, precipitated sulphur 2%, in aqueous cream. Price 50 g = **A**

Salicylic Acid and Sulphur Ointment, salicylic acid 3%, precipitated sulphur 3%, in hydrous ointment (oily cream). Price 25 g = **A**

Sulphur Lotion, Compound, precipitated sulphur 4% (see Formulary). Price 100 ml = **B**

Sulphur Ointment, precipitated sulphur 10%, in simple ointment. Price 25 g = **A**

Acnil® (Fisons)

Cream, cetrimide 0.5%, resorcinol 0.5%, precipitated sulphur 3%. Price 25 g = **C**

Dome-Acna® (Bayer)

Cream, resorcinol monoacetate 3%, colloidal sulphur 4%, in a non-greasy basis. Price 30 g = **D**

Lotion, ingredients as for cream. Price 50 ml = **D**

Medicated cleanser (= application), salicylic acid 2%, colloidal sulphur 2%, in a detergent basis. Price 100 g (with sponge applicator) = **F**. For skin cleansing

Eskamel® (SK&F)

Cream, resorcinol 2%, sulphur 8%, in a non-greasy flesh-coloured basis. Price 25 g = **C**

TRETINOIN

Indications: acne vulgaris

Cautions: avoid contact with eyes, mouth, and mucous membranes; do not use with other peeling agents or with ultra-violet lamps

---

Contra-indications: eczema, broken skin
Side-effects: irritation, erythema, desquamation, changes in pigmentation, photosensitivity
Administration: apply to clean skin 1–2 times daily

PoM Retin-A® (Ortho-Cilag)
Cream, tretinoin 0.05%. Price 60 g = **F**. For dry or fair skin
Gel, tretinoin 0.025%. Price 60 g = **F**. For severe acne, initial treatment, or dark and oily skins
Lotion, tretinoin 0.025%. Price 80 ml = **F**. For application to large areas such as the back

CORTICOSTEROIDS
Indications: see notes above
Cautions; Contra-indications; Side-effects: section 13.4 and notes above
Administration: apply to clean skin 1–2 times daily

PoM Actinac® (Roussel)
Lotion (powder for reconstitution), chloramphenicol 1.25%, hydrocortisone acetate 1.25%, allantoin 0.75%, butoxyethyl nicotinate 0.75%, precipitated sulphur 10%, when reconstituted with solvent. Discard after 21 days. Price 2 × 5-g bottles powder with 2 × 16-ml bottles solvent = **H**. Potency IV
PoM Medrone® (Upjohn)
Acne lotion, methylprednisolone acetate 0.25%, aluminium chlorhydroxide complex 10%, sulphur (colloidal) 5%. Price 25 ml = **E**; 75 ml = **G**. Potency IV
PoM Neo-Medrone® (Upjohn)
Acne lotion, methylprednisolone acetate 0.25%, neomycin sulphate 0.25%, aluminium chlorhydroxide complex 10%, sulphur 5%. Price 50 ml = **G**; 75 ml = **G**. Potency IV
PoM Quinoderm with Hydrocortisone® (Quinoderm Ltd)
Cream, hydrocortisone 1%, benzoyl peroxide 10%, potassium hydroxyquinoline sulphate 0.5%, in an astringent vanishing-cream basis. Price 30 g = **D**. Potency IV

ORAL PREPARATIONS

CYPROTERONE ACETATE
Indications: see notes above
Cautions; Contra-indications; Side-effects: see under Combined Oral Contraceptives (section 7.3.1)

▼ PoM Diane® (Schering)
Tablets, pink, s/c, cyproterone acetate 2 mg, ethinyloestradiol 50 micrograms. Price 21 tabs = **F**
Dose: 1 tablet daily for 21 days starting on 5th day of menstrual cycle and repeated after a 7-day interval, usually for several months

ISOTRETINOIN
Indications; Cautions; Side-effects: see notes above
Contra-indications: pregnancy; renal or hepatic impairment
Dose: 500 micrograms/kg daily after food for the first 4 weeks, adjusted if necessary to 100–200 micrograms/kg daily (sensitive patients), or

1 mg/kg daily (unresponsive patients) for a further 8–12 weeks

▼ PoM Roaccutane® (Roche)
Capsules, red/white, isotretinoin 5 mg. Price 20 caps = **H** (Hosp. only). Label: 10, patient information card, 21
Capsules, red–violet/white, isotretinoin 20 mg. Price 10 caps = **I** (Hosp. only). Label: 10, patient information card, 21

13.7 Preparations for warts and calluses

The least destructive method possible should be chosen to treat these lesions as they are self-limiting and all viral warts including those on the soles (verrucas) eventually disappear spontaneously. The preparations used are keratolytics which slowly remove the hyperkeratotic layers and destroy the underlying epidermis. Salicylic acid and podophyllin preparations are useful but can cause considerable irritation of the treated area, and podophyllin treatment may be painful. **Salicylic acid** collodion and proprietary preparations are suitable for removal of warts and calluses and salicylic acid collodion is also suitable for treating facial warts.

Podophyllin preparations may also be useful. Compound podophyllin paint, in concentrations of between 5 and 20% is employed for the treatment of anogenital warts. The paint should be allowed to stay on the treated area for not longer than 6 hours and then washed off. Care should be taken to avoid splashing the surrounding skin during application; it may be covered with soft paraffin as a protection. Where there are a large number of warts only a few should be treated at any one time as severe toxicity caused by absorption of podophyllin has been reported. It should also be used with caution in pregnancy. **Posalfilin®** is suitable for treating plantar warts.

Preparations containing formaldehyde, glutaraldehyde, and bromine are also available but their effects are unpredictable. Formaldehyde preparations may irritate and sensitise the skin, and have an unpleasant smell.

Ointments and liquid preparations are applied to the wart or callus, avoiding contact with surrounding skin, and covered with a plaster. Dead skin may be removed at intervals by rubbing with a pumice stone.

SALICYLIC ACID
Indications: removal of warts and hard skin
Cautions: avoid normal skin and application to large areas

Salicylic Acid Adhesive Plaster 20% or 40%. Price 10 plasters 75 mm × 45 mm = **D**
Salicylic Acid Collodion, salicylic acid 12%, in flexible collodion. Price 5 ml = **A**. Label: 15
Apply daily or on alternate days

C = 51-100p, D = 101-180p, E = 181-300p, F = 301-450p, G = 451-650p, H = 651-900p, I = 901-1200p, J = over 1200p.

Cuplex® (S&N Pharm.)
Gel, salicylic acid 11%, lactic acid 4%, copper acetate (= Cu^{2+} 0.0011%), in a collodion basis. Price 5 g = **D**. For plantar and mosaic warts, corns, and calluses
Apply twice daily
Duofilm® (Stiefel)
Paint, salicylic acid 16.7%, lactic acid 16.7%, in flexible collodion. Price 15 ml (with applicator) = **E**. For plantar and mosaic warts
Apply daily
Salactol® (Dermal)
Paint, salicylic acid 16.7%, lactic acid 16.7%, in flexible collodion. Price 10 ml (with applicator) = **D**. For warts, particularly plantar warts
Apply daily
Verrugon® (Pickles)
Ointment, salicylic acid 50% in a paraffin basis. Price 6 g = **C**
Apply daily

BROMINE COMPOUNDS

Indications: warts, particularly plantar warts
Cautions: avoid normal skin

Callusolve® (Dermal)
Paint, benzalkonium chloride-bromine adduct 25%. Price 10 ml (with applicator) = **E**. For warts, particularly plantar and mosaic warts
Apply daily

FORMALDEHYDE

Indications: warts, particularly plantar warts
Cautions: avoid normal skin

Veracur® (Typharm)
Gel, formaldehyde solution 1.5% in a water-miscible gel basis. Price 15 g = **C**
Apply twice daily

GLUTARALDEHYDE

Indications: warts, particularly plantar warts
Cautions: avoid normal skin; stains skin brown

Glutarol® (Dermal)
Solution (= application), glutaraldehyde 10%. Price 10 ml (with applicator) = **D**
Apply twice daily
Verucasep® (Galen)
Gel, glutaraldehyde 10%. Price 15 g = **E**
Apply twice daily

PODOPHYLLUM RESIN

Indications: anogenital and plantar warts
Cautions: avoid normal skin
Contra-indications: genital warts in pregnancy; facial warts
Side-effects: may cause pain on application
Administration: see notes above

Podophyllin Paint, Compound, podophyllum resin 15% (see Formulary). Price 25 ml = **C**. Label: 15, counselling advised, application, see notes above. For warts, including anogenital warts

Apply daily to plantar warts, weekly to anogenital warts
Posalfilin® (Norgine)
Ointment, podophyllum resin 20%, salicylic acid 25%. Price 10 g = **D**. For plantar warts
Apply 2–3 times weekly

13.8   Sunscreens and camouflaging preparations

13.8.1 Sunscreening preparations
13.8.2 Camouflaging preparations

13.8.1   Sunscreening preparations

Ultraviolet radiation may be harmful in certain diseases, for example lupus erythematosus, photosensitive dermatitis, and rosacea. Protection may also be required in patients who have developed signs of chronic solar damage in the skin. Certain individuals are naturally sensitive to the sun's rays, while others are sensitised by systemic drugs, for example, demeclocycline, chlorpromazine, and nalidixic acid.

There are two types of preparation which protect the skin from ultraviolet radiation. One type merely places an opaque, reflectant barrier between the sun's rays and the skin; an example is titanium dioxide paste (section 13.2.1). This is thick and greasy and not very acceptable to the patient. The second type listed below is more useful. It contains substances that absorb the erythema-producing portions of the ultraviolet spectrum, for example **aminobenzoic acid** and **padimate** (Spectraban®).

For maximum benefit these preparations must be applied frequently. Because they filter out only a proportion of harmful rays, burning may still occur in intense sunlight and patients with light-sensitive skin should spend as little time as possible exposed to sunlight. The sun protection factor (SPF, usually indicated in the preparation title) provides some guidance on the degree of protection offered. This indicates the multiples of protection against burning provided, compared to unprotected skin; for example, an SPF of 8 should enable a patient to remain 8 times longer in the sun without burning. Unfortunately no preparation of this type exists which completely blocks the range of sunlight responsible for some photosensitive reactions, particularly the porphyrias and drug-induced photosensitivity, although the reflectant sunscreens do give moderate protection.

Some of the sunscreens, particularly aminobenzoates, may rarely cause photosensitivity reactions. Sunscreen preparations containing bergamot oil (which contains 5-methoxypsoralen) occasionally cause photosensitisation with subsequent pigmentation. They are suspected of increasing the incidence of skin cancers, but this is not established.

BORDERLINE SUBSTANCES. The preparations marked 'ACBS' are regarded as drugs when prescribed for skin protection against ultraviolet radiation in photodermatoses, including those resulting from radiotherapy. Prescriptions issued in accordance with this advice and endorsed 'ACBS' will not normally be investigated. See Appendix 3 for listing by clinical condition.

Aminobenzoic Acid Lotion, aminobenzoic acid 5 g, glycerol 20 ml, industrial methylated spirit 60 ml, purified water, freshly boiled and cooled, to 100 ml. Price 200 ml = **B**
Apply undiluted and allow to dry before exposure; repeat every 2 hours if necessary
Caution: stains clothing
Coppertone Supershade 15® (Plough)
Lotion, 2-ethylhexyl 4-dimethylaminobenzoate 7%, oxybenzone 3%. Price 125 ml = **F**. ACBS
Delial Factor 10® (Bayer)
Cream, 2-phenyl-1*H*-benzimidazole-5-sulphonic acid 2.8%, 3-(4-methylbenzylidene)bornan-2-one 2%, 2-phenyl-5-methylbenzoxazole 1%. Price 50 ml = **D**. ACBS
Milk (=lotion), ingredients as for cream, in an emulsion basis. Price 125 ml = **E**. ACBS
Piz Buin® (Colson & Kay)
Creme No. 6, 2-ethylhexyl *p*-methoxycinnamate 4.1%, oxybenzone 1.3%. Price 50 ml = **E**. ACBS
Creme No. 8, 2-ethylhexyl *p*-methoxycinnamate 4.8%, oxybenzone 1.7%. Price 50 ml = **E**. ACBS
Creme No. 12, 2-ethylhexyl *p*-methoxycinnamate 4.8%, oxybenzone 2.2%, zinc oxide 4.5%, talc 4.5%. Price 30 ml = **E**. ACBS
RoC Total Sunblock® (RoC)
Cream, untinted, containing a cinnamic ester and zinc oxide (Protection factor 10A+B). Price 50 ml = **E**. ACBS
Apply every 2 hours or more frequently
Spectraban® (Stiefel)
4 Lotion, padimate 2.5%, in an alcoholic basis. Price 150 ml = **E**. ACBS
15 Lotion, aminobenzoic acid 5%, padimate 2.5%, in an alcoholic basis. Price 150 ml = **E**. ACBS
Apply once daily; renew after bathing or excessive sweating
Caution: flammable; stains clothing

13.8.2 Camouflaging preparations

Disfigurement of the skin can be very distressing to patients and have a marked psychological effect. In skilled hands, or with experience, these preparations can be very effective in concealing scars, areas of discoloration, and birthmarks.

BORDERLINE SUBSTANCES. The preparations marked 'ACBS' are regarded as drugs when prescribed for postoperative scars and other deformities and as adjunctive therapy in the relief of emotional disturbances due to mutilating skin disease. Prescriptions issued in accordance with this advice and endorsed 'ACBS' will normally not be investigated. See Appendix 3 for listing by clinical condition.

Boots Covering Cream® (Boots)
Cream (4 shades). Price 20 g = **C**. ACBS
Covermark® (Medexport)
Cream rouge (3 shades). Price 8 g = **E**. ACBS
Spotstick (7 shades). Price 3.5 g = **E**. ACBS
Grey toner (= cream). Price 8 g = **E**. ACBS
Masking cream (10 shades). Price 25 g = **F**. ACBS
Shading cream. Price 8 g = **E**. ACBS
Finishing powder. Price 50 g = **E**; 250 g = **I**. ACBS
Dermacolor® (Fox)
Camouflage creme, 30 shades. Price 30 g = **F**. ACBS
Fixing powder, 5 shades. Price 75 g = **E**. ACBS
Keromask® (Innoxa)
Masking cream, 2 shades. Price 15 ml = **D**. ACBS
Veil® (Blake)
Cover cream, 11 shades. Price 19 g = **C**; 44 and 70 g (both) = **D**. ACBS

13.9 Scalp preparations

SHAMPOOS. Dandruff (*pityriasis capitis*) is excessive non-inflammatory scaling of the scalp, and often increases at puberty. The treatment of choice is the frequent use of a mild detergent shampoo generally once or twice weekly; this will rid the scalp of scale but should not be expected to have a therapeutic effect in itself. Shampoos containing **pyrithione zinc** have beneficial effects but are not prescribable in the general medical service. Shampoos containing **tar** extracts, for example Polytar®, may be useful and they are also used in psoriasis, both as adjunctive treatment and for the removal of pastes etc. Shampoos containing **selenium sulphide** are of no more value than the other shampoos and should not be used within 48 hours of applying hair colouring or permanent waving preparations.

APPLICATIONS. When shampoos are insufficient, preparations containing **salicylic acid 2%** and **sulphur 2%**, such as **salicylic acid and sulphur cream** (section 13.6) may be useful. For the more severe conditions, weak **corticosteroid** gels and lotions (section 13.4), applied to the scalp may be helpful.

Cradle cap in infants may be treated with **olive oil** or **arachis oil** applications before shampooing.

See also section 13.5 (psoriasis and eczema), section 13.10.4 (lice), and section 13.10.2 (ringworm).

BORDERLINE SUBSTANCES. The preparations marked 'ACBS' are regarded as drugs when prescribed in accordance with the advice of the Advisory Committee on Borderline Substances for the clinical conditions listed. Prescriptions issued in accordance with this advice and endorsed 'ACBS' will normally not be investigated. See Appendix 3 for listing by clinical condition.

Shampoos
    Use once or twice weekly

Cetrimide Solution —section 13.11
Alphosyl® (Stafford-Miller)
Application PC, allantoin 0.2%, refined coal tar extract 5%, in a shampoo basis. Price 60 g = **B**. ACBS: for psoriasis and other scaly disorders of the scalp
Betadine® (Napp)
Scalp and skin cleanser—section 13.11
Shampoo solution, povidone-iodine 4%, in a surfactant solution containing lanolin. Price 250 ml = **E**. ACBS: for seborrhoeic scalp conditions associated with excessive dandruff, pruritic scaling, seborrhoeic dermatitis, pityriasis capitis, infected lesions of the scalp, pyodermas (recurrent furunculosis, infective folliculitis, impetigo)
Capitol® (Dermal)
Gel (= shampoo application), benzalkonium chloride 0.5%. Price 120 g = **E**. ACBS: for pityriasis capitis and seborrhoeic dermatitis of the scalp
Ceanel Concentrate® (Quinoderm Ltd)
Shampoo, cetrimide 10%, undecenoic acid 1%, phenethyl alcohol 7.5%. Price 50 ml = **C**; 150 ml = **E**; 500 ml = **G**. ACBS: for psoriasis or seborrhoeic conditions
Cetavlon PC® (Care)
Solution (= shampoo application), cetrimide 17.5%. Price 125 ml = **B**. ACBS: for seborrhoea capitis and seborrhoeic dermatitis
Clinitar® (S&N Pharm.)
Shampoo solution, coal tar extract 2%. Price 60 g = **E**
Genisol® (Fisons)
Liquid (= shampoo application), prepared coal tar 2% (as purified coal tar fractions), sodium sulphosuccinated undecylenic monoalkylolamide 1%. Price 58 ml = **C**; 250 ml = **E**; 600 ml = **G**. ACBS: for psoriasis, eczema, and scaling of the scalp (psoriasis, dandruff, or eczema)
Ionil T® (Alcon)
Shampoo application, benzalkonium chloride 0.2%, coal tar solution 4.25%, salicylic acid 2% in an alcoholic basis. Price 240 ml = **D**. ACBS: for seborrhoeic dermatitis of the scalp
Lenium® (Winthrop)
Cream (= shampoo application), selenium sulphide 2.5%. Price 9-g sachet = **A**; 42- and 100-g tube (both) = **C**
Polytar® (Stiefel)
Liquid (= shampoo application), arachis oil extract of crude coal tar 0.3%, cade oil 0.3%, coal tar solution 0.1%, oleyl alcohol 1%, tar 0.3%. Price 65 ml = **C**; 150 ml = **D**; 350 ml = **E**. ACBS: for psoriasis, dandruff, and scaling of the scalp (psoriasis, dandruff, and eczema)
Polytar Plus® (Stiefel)
Liquid (= shampoo application), ingredients as above with hydrolysed animal protein 3%. Price 150 ml = **D**; 350 ml = **E**. ACBS: for scalp disorders such as scaling (psoriasis, dandruff,

eczema), pruritus, and in the removal of pastes and pomades used in the treatment of psoriasis
Psoriderm® (Dermal)
Scalp lotion (= shampoo application), coal tar 2.5%, lecithin 0.3%. Price 112 ml = **E**
Selsun® (Abbott)
Shampoo application, selenium sulphide 2.5%. Price 50 and 100 ml (both) = **C**; 150 ml = **D**
Synogist® (Maltown)
Shampoo solution, sodium sulphosuccinated undecylenic monoalkylolamide 2%. Price 200 ml = **H**
T/Gel® (Neutrogena)
Shampoo, coal tar extract 2%. Price 125 ml = **D**. ACBS: for psoriasis, eczema, and scaling of the scalp (psoriasis, dandruff, and eczema)

Applications
    Apply once or twice daily

Arachis Oil. Price 50 ml = **A**
Olive Oil. Price 50 ml = **B**
Salicylic Acid and Sulphur Cream—section 13.6
Salicylic Acid Lotion, salicylic acid 2% (see Formulary). Price 100 ml = **A**. Label: 15
Caution: highly flammable

13.10 Anti-infective skin preparations

13.10.1 Antibacterial preparations
13.10.2 Antifungal preparations
13.10.3 Antiviral preparations
13.10.4 Parasiticidal preparations
13.10.5 Preparations for minor skin infections

13.10.1 Antibacterial preparations

13.10.1.1 Antibacterial preparations only used topically
13.10.1.2 Antibacterial preparations also used systemically

For many skin infections such as erysipelas and cellulitis systemic antibacterial treatment is the method of choice because the infection is too deeply sited for adequate penetration of topical preparations. For details of suitable treatment see section 5.1, Table 1. Impetigo may be treated by local application with **chlortetracycline** (Aureomycin®) or, if there is systemic toxicity, with oral **flucloxacillin** (see section 5.1, Table 1). Mild antiseptic solutions such as **sodium hypochlorite** or **povidone-iodine** (section 13.11) are used to remove crusts and exudate.

Although there are a great many antibacterial drugs presented in topical preparations they are potentially hazardous and frequently their use is not necessary if adequate hygienic measures can be taken. Moreover not all skin conditions that are oozing, crusted, or characterised by pustules are actually infected.

To minimise the development of resistant organisms it is advisable to limit the choice of drugs applied topically to those not used systemically. Unfortunately some of these drugs, for example neomycin, may cause sensitisation and, if large areas of skin are being treated, ototoxicity may be a hazard, particularly in the elderly. Resistant organisms are more common in hospitals, and whenever possible swabs for examination should be taken before beginning treatment.

Mafenide (Sulfamylon®) and **silver sulphadiazine** (Flamazine®) are useful in the treatment of infected burns.

Topical preparations containing a **corticosteroid** are included in section 13.4.1.

13.10.1.1 ANTIBACTERIAL PREPARATIONS ONLY USED TOPICALLY

CHLORAMPHENICOL
Indications: skin infections
Cautions: see notes above; large open wounds
Side-effects: local hypersensitivity reactions
Administration: apply 3 times daily

PoM **Chloramphenicol Cream DTF**, chloramphenicol 1%, macrogol '4000' 49%, propylene glycol 50%. Price 50 g = **B**

COLISTIN SULPHATE
Indications: Gram-negative skin infections
Side-effects: transient irritation

PoM **Colomycin**® (Pharmax)
Powder, sterile, for making topical preparations (usually 1%), colistin sulphate. Price 1 g vial = **J**

FRAMYCETIN SULPHATE
Indications; Cautions; Side-effects: see under Neomycin Sulphate
Administration: apply 3 times daily

PoM **Framygen**® (Fisons)
Cream, framycetin sulphate 0.5%, in a water-miscible basis. Price 15 g = **D**
PoM **Soframycin**® (Roussel)
Cream, framycetin sulphate 1.5%, gramicidin 0.005%, in a vanishing-cream basis. Price 15 g = **D**
Ointment, ingredients as for cream, in a wool fat and paraffin basis. Price 15 g = **D**
Apply 3 times daily
Sterile powder for preparing topical solutions, framycetin sulphate. Price 500-mg vial = **F**
PoM **Sofra-Tulle**® (Roussel)
Impregnated dressing, framycetin sulphate 1%. Price 10 dressings (100 mm × 100 mm) = **E**; 10 dressings (300 mm × 100 mm) = **G**
Apply daily

MAFENIDE
Indications: skin infections, particularly pseudomonal infection of second- and third-degree burns
Cautions: pulmonary dysfunction
Contra-indications: sensitivity to sulphonamides

Side-effects: allergic reactions including rashes, metabolic acidosis

PoM **Sulfamylon**® (Winthrop)
Cream, mafenide 8.5% (as acetate), in a water-miscible basis. Price 500 g = **J**
Apply liberally 1–2 times daily with sterile applicator

NEOMYCIN SULPHATE
Indications: skin infections
Cautions: see notes above; large open wounds, sensitivity to other aminoglycosides
Side-effects: local hypersensitivity reactions
Administration: apply 3 times daily

Creams and ointments
PoM **Neomycin Cream,** neomycin sulphate 0.5%, cetomacrogol emulsifying ointment 30%, chlorocresol 0.1%, disodium edetate 0.01%, freshly boiled and cooled purified water 69.39%. Price 100 g = **F**
PoM **Neomycin Ointment,** neomycin sulphate 0.5% in an anhydrous greasy basis. Price 15 g = **B**; 28.4 g = **C**
PoM **Cicatrin**® (Calmic)
Cream, neomycin sulphate 0.5%, bacitracin zinc 250 units/g, cysteine 0.2%, glycine 1%, threonine 0.1%. Price 15 g = **E**; 30 g = **G**
Apply 3 times daily; max. 60 g daily for 3 weeks
PoM **Graneodin**® (Squibb)
Ointment, neomycin sulphate 0.25%, gramicidin 0.025%. Price 15 g = **C**
Apply 3 times daily
PoM **Myciguent**® (Upjohn)
Ointment, neomycin sulphate 0.5%, in an anhydrous greasy basis. Price 28.4 g = **C**

Powders and sprays
PoM **Cicatrin**® (Calmic)
Dusting-powder, neomycin sulphate 0.5%, bacitracin zinc 250 units/g, cysteine 0.2%, glycine 1%, threonine 0.1%. Price 15 g = **F**; 50 g = **H**. Max. 50 g daily for 4 weeks
Powder spray, neomycin sulphate 2%, bacitracin zinc 1250 units/g, cysteine 1.2%, glycine 6%; pressurised aerosol unit. Price 3 g = **H**. Max. 3 g daily for 12 weeks
Mycifradin—see section 5.1.4
PoM **Polybactrin**® (Calmic)
Powder spray, neomycin sulphate 495 000 units, bacitracin zinc 37 500 units, polymyxin B sulphate 150 000 units/pressurised aerosol unit. Price per unit (115 ml) = **J**. Max. 1 unit daily for 7 days
PoM **Tribiotic**® (Riker)
Spray application, neomycin sulphate 500 000 units, bacitracin zinc 10 000 units, polymyxin B sulphate 150 000 units/pressurised aerosol unit. Price per unit (110 g) = **G**. Max. 1 unit daily for 7 days

NITROFURAZONE
Indications: superficial skin infections
Side-effects: local hypersensitivity reactions
Administration: apply 3 or more times daily

PoM **Furacin**® (Norwich-Eaton)
Soluble ointment (= cream), nitrofurazone
0.2%, in a water-miscible macrogol basis. Price
25 g = **D**

POLYMYXIN B SULPHATE

Indications; skin infections
Cautions: see notes above; large open wounds
Side-effects: local hypersensitivity reactions

PoM **Polyfax**® (Calmic)
Ointment, polymyxin B sulphate 10 000 units,
bacitracin zinc 500 units/g, in a paraffin basis.
Price 20 g = **F**
Apply 3 times daily

SILVER SULPHADIAZINE

Indications: skin infection, particularly Gram-
negative infections such as pseudomonal infections in second- and third-degree burns,
infected leg ulcers, and pressure sores
Cautions: hepatic and renal impairment
Contra-indications: sensitivity to sulphonamides
Side-effects: rarely allergic reactions including
rashes

PoM **Flamazine**® (S&N Pharm.)
Cream, silver sulphadiazine 1%, in a water-soluble basis. Price 50 g = **E**; 250 g = **H**; 500 g = **J**
In burns apply daily with sterile applicator; in
leg ulcers apply at least 3 times a week

13.10.1.2   ANTIBACTERIAL PREPARATIONS ALSO USED SYSTEMICALLY

CHLORTETRACYCLINE HYDROCHLORIDE

Indications: susceptible skin infections; impetigo,
see section 5.1, Table 1
Cautions: see notes above; overgrowth with non-
susceptible organisms may occur; stains
clothing
Side-effects: rarely local hypersensitivity
reactions
Administration: apply 3 times daily

PoM **Aureomycin**® (Lederle)
Cream, chlortetracycline hydrochloride 3% (as
chlortetracycline), in a water-miscible basis.
Price 30 g = **E**
Ointment, chlortetracycline hydrochloride 3%,
in a greasy basis. Diluent wool fat 10% in white
soft paraffin, life of diluted ointment 14 days.
Price 30 g = **E**

FUSIDIC ACID

Indications: staphylococcal skin infections and
abscesses
Cautions: see notes above; avoid contact with
eyes
Side-effects: rarely local hypersensitivity
reactions

PoM **Fucidin**® (Leo)
Cream, fusidic acid 2%. Price 10 g = **D**; 25 g
= **F**
Apply 3 times daily
Gel, fusidic acid 2%, in a water-miscible basis.
Price 10 g = **D**; 25 g = **F**
Apply 3 times daily
Caviject gel, fusidic acid 2%, in a single-dose
unit (7 g) fitted with elongated nozzle. For treat-
ment of abscesses. Price 1 unit = **D**
Inject once only into curetted abscess and apply
dressing
Intertulle (= impregnated dressing), sodium
fusidate 2% (as ointment). Price 10 dressings
(100 mm × 100 mm) = **E**
Apply 1 or more times daily
Ointment, sodium fusidate 2%, in an anhydrous
greasy basis. Price 10 g = **D**; 25 g = **F**
Apply 3 times daily

GENTAMICIN

Indications: skin infections
Cautions: see notes above; large open wounds,
sensitivity to other aminoglycosides
Administration: apply 3 times daily

PoM **Gentamicin Cream**, gentamicin 0.3% (as
sulphate) in a water-miscible basis. Price 15 g =
D; 30 g = **F**; 100 g = **H**
PoM **Gentamicin Ointment**, gentamicin 0.3% (as
sulphate) in a white soft paraffin or other suitable
anhydrous greasy basis. Price 15 g = **D**; 30 g = **F**;
100 g = **H**

PoM **Cidomycin Topical**® (Roussel)
Cream, gentamicin 0.3% (as sulphate), in a
water-miscible basis. Do not dilute. Price
15 g = **D**; 30 g = **F**
Ointment, gentamicin 0.3% (as sulphate), in a
paraffin basis. Do not dilute. Price 15 g = **D**;
30 g = **F**
PoM **Genticin**® (Nicholas)
Cream, gentamicin 0.3% (as sulphate), in
a water-miscible basis. Price 15 g = **D**;
100 g = **H**
Ointment, gentamicin 0.3% (as sulphate), in an
anhydrous greasy basis. Price 15 g = **D**; 100 g =
H

TETRACYCLINE HYDROCHLORIDE

Indications; Cautions; Side-effects: see under
Chlortetracycline Hydrochloride

PoM **Achromycin Topical**® (Lederle)
Ointment, tetracycline hydrochloride 3%, in a
wool fat and paraffin basis. Price 30 g = **D**
Apply 3 times daily

13.10.2   Antifungal preparations

Ideally skin scrapings should be examined to
confirm diagnosis before treatment is begun.
Widespread or intractable fungal infections are
treated systemically (see section 5.2). Most localised infections are treated with the topical preparations described below.

Nail ringworm (*Tinea unguium*) and scalp ringworm (*T. capitis*) are best treated systemically (see section 5.2). Most other ringworm infections, including *T. pedis*, may be adequately treated with topical preparations. **Clotrimazole** (Canesten®), **econazole** (Ecostatin®, Pevaryl®), and **miconazole** (Daktarin®, Dermonistat®) are all effective and commonly used. **Compound benzoic acid ointment** (Whitfield's ointment) is also quite effective but cosmetically less acceptable than the proprietary preparations. It is generally used to treat patches of ringworm on the trunk, limbs, palms, or soles. The **undecenoates** and **tolnaftate** are less effective in treating ringworm infections.

Candidal skin infections may also be treated by topical application with the broad-spectrum antifungals, clotrimazole, econazole, and miconazole. **Amphotericin** (Fungilin®) and **nystatin** preparations are also equally as effective in candidiasis although they are ineffective against *Tinea* infections.

Lotions are generally chosen for application to large and hairy areas. Ointments are best avoided on moist surfaces because of their occlusive properties. Dusting-powders have no place in the treatment of fungal infections, except for toiletry or cosmetic purposes, as they are therapeutically ineffective and may cause skin irritation.

AMPHOTERICIN

Indications: skin infections due to *Candida* spp.
Administration: apply 2–4 times daily

PoM **Fungilin**® (Squibb)
Cream, amphotericin 3%, in a water-miscible basis. Do not dilute. Price 15 g = **D**
Ointment, amphotericin 3%, in Plastibase®. Do not dilute. Price 15 g = **D**

BENZOIC ACID

Indications: skin infections due to *Tinea* spp.

Benzoic Acid Ointment, Compound (Whitfield's ointment), benzoic acid 6%, salicylic acid 3%, in emulsifying ointment. Price 25 g = **A**
Apply twice daily

BENZOYL PEROXIDE

Indications: fungal skin infections, particularly *T. pedis*

Quinoped® (Quinoderm Ltd)
Cream, benzoyl peroxide 5%, potassium hydroxyquinoline sulphate 0.5%, in an astringent basis. Price 25 g = **C**. For *Tinea* infections, particularly *T. pedis*
Apply twice daily

CLOTRIMAZOLE

Indications: fungal skin infections
Side-effects: occasional skin irritation or sensitivity
Administration: apply 2–3 times daily continuing for 14 days after lesions have healed

Canesten® (Bayer)
Cream, clotrimazole 1%, in a water-miscible basis. Price 20 g = **E**; 50 g = **F**
Solution (= application), clotrimazole 1% in macrogol 400. Price 20 ml (with dropper) = **E**. For hairy areas
Spray, clotrimazole 1%, in 30% isopropyl alcohol. Price 40-ml atomiser = **G**. For large or hairy areas
Caution: flammable
Dusting-powder, clotrimazole 1%. Price 30 g = **D**

ECONAZOLE NITRATE

Indications; Side-effects: see under Clotrimazole
Administration: apply 2–3 times daily continuing for 14 days after lesions have healed; nail infections, apply daily under occlusive dressing

Econazole Cream, econazole nitrate 1% in a water-miscible basis. Price 15 g = **D**; 30 g = **E**
Econazole Lotion, econazole nitrate 1%. Price 30 ml = **E**
Ecostatin® (Squibb)
Cream, econazole nitrate 1%, in a water-miscible basis. Price 15 g = **D**; 30 g = **E**
Lotion, econazole nitrate 1%. Price 30 ml = **E**
Spray solution (= application), econazole nitrate 1% in an alcoholic solution. Price 150 g = **F**
Dusting-powder, econazole nitrate 1% in a talc basis. Price 30 g = **E**
Spray-powder, econazole nitrate 1% in a talc basis. Price 200-g unit = **E**
Pevaryl® (Ortho-Cilag)
Cream, econazole nitrate 1% in a water-miscible basis. Price 30 g = **E**
Lotion, econazole nitrate 1% in a water-miscible basis. Price 30 ml = **E**
Spray-powder, econazole nitrate 1%. Price 200-g pressurised aerosol unit (20 g powder) = **E**

KETOCONAZOLE

Indications; Side-effects: see under Clotrimazole
Administration: apply 1–2 times daily, continuing for a few days after lesions have healed

▼ PoM **Nizoral**® (Janssen)
Cream, ketoconazole 2% in a water-miscible basis. Price 15 g = **D**

MICONAZOLE NITRATE

Indications; Side-effects: see under Clotrimazole
Administration: apply twice daily continuing for 10 days after lesions have healed; nail infections, apply daily under occlusive dressings

Miconazole Cream, miconazole nitrate 2% in a water-miscible basis. Price 30 g = **E**
Daktarin® (Janssen)
Cream, miconazole nitrate 2%, in a water-miscible basis. Price 30 g = **E**
Twin pack, 1 × 30 g pack of cream miconazole nitrate 2%, with 1 × 30 g dusting-powder

miconazole nitrate 2%. Price (complete pack) = **F**
Dermonistat® (Ortho-Cilag)
Cream, miconazole nitrate 2%, in a water-miscible basis. Price 30 g = **E**

NATAMYCIN

Indications: skin infections due to *Candida* spp.
Administration: apply 2–3 times daily

PoM **Pimafucin**® (Brocades)
Cream, natamycin 2%, in a water-miscible basis. Price 30 g = **D**

NITROPHENOL

Indications: fungal skin infections, particularly *Tinea*

Phortinea® (Philip Harris)
Paint, 4-nitrophenol 2% in an alcoholic basis. Price 10 ml (with applicator) = **B**
Apply twice daily

NYSTATIN

Indications: skin infections due to *Candida* spp.
Administration: apply 2–4 times daily, continuing for 7 days after lesions have healed

PoM **Multilind**® (Squibb)
Ointment, nystatin 100000 units/g, zinc oxide 20% in an emollient basis. Price 50 g = **F**. For superinfection, particularly in napkin rash
PoM **Nystaform**® (Bayer)
Cream, nystatin 100000 units/g, chlorhexidine hydrochloride 1%. Price 30 g = **E**
Ointment, nystatin 100000 units/g, chlorhexidine acetate 1%, in a water-repellent basis. Price 30 g = **E**
PoM **Nystan**® (Squibb)
Cream, nystatin 100 000 units/g, in a water-miscible basis. Price 15 g = **D**; 30 g = **E**
Gel, nystatin 100 000 units/g. Price 30 g = **E**
Ointment, nystatin 100 000 units/g, in Plastibase®. Price 15 g = **D**; 30 g = **E**
Dusting-powder, nystatin 100 000 units/g. Price 15 g = **D**
PoM **Tinaderm-M**® (Kirby-Warrick)
Cream, nystatin 100000 units/g, tolnaftate 1%, in a water-miscible basis. Price 20 g = **E**. For *Candida* and *Tinea* infections
Apply 2–3 times daily

SALICYLIC ACID

Indications: fungal skin infections, particularly *Tinea*
Side-effects: hypersensitivity reactions

Phytex® (Pharmax)
Paint, salicylic acid 1.46% (total combined), tannic acid 4.89% and boric acid 3.12% (as borotannic complex), in a vehicle containing alcohol and ethyl acetate. Price 25 ml (with brush) = **D**. For fungal skin and nail infections
Apply twice daily
Caution: flammable; avoid in pregnancy and children under 5 years

Phytocil® (Rorer)
Cream, salicylic acid 1.5%, 2-*p*-chlorophenoxyethanol 1%, menthol 1%, 1-phenoxypropan-2-ol 2%. Price 25 g = **B**. For *Tinea* infections
Apply 2–3 times daily

TOLNAFTATE

Indications: skin infections due to *Tinea* spp.
Side-effects: rarely hypersensitivity

Timoped® (R&C)
Cream, tolnaftate 1%, triclosan 0.25%. Price 30 g = **F**
Apply twice daily

UNDECENOATES

Indications: skin infections due to *Tinea* spp.

Monphytol® (LAB)
Paint, methyl undecenoate 5%, propyl undecenoate 1%, boric acid 2%, salicylic acid 31% (free and as methyl ester), chlorbutol 3%. Price 18 ml (with brush) = **C**. For fungal (particularly nail) infections
Apply 4 times daily
Mycota® (Crookes Products)
Cream, zinc undecenoate 20%, undecenoic acid 5%. Price 25 g = **B**
Dusting-powder, zinc undecenoate 20%, undecenoic acid 2%. Price 70 g = **C**
Spray application, undecenoic acid 2.5%, dichlorophen 0.25% (pressurised aerosol pack). Price 110 g = **C**
Apply 1–2 times daily
Phytocil® (Rorer)
Dusting-powder, zinc undecenoate 5.8%, 2-*p*-chlorophenoxyethanol 1%, 1-phenoxypropan-2-ol 2%. Price 50 g = **C**. For use with cream
Tineafax® (Wellcome)
Ointment, zinc undecenoate 8%, zinc naphthenate solution 8%, in a water-miscible basis. Price 25 g = **B**
Apply 1–2 times daily
Dusting-powder, zinc undecenoate 10%. Price 50-g puffer pack = **C**

13.10.3 Antiviral preparations

Idoxuridine solution (5% in dimethyl sulphoxide) is used for severe herpetic infections of the skin. *Herpes simplex* seems to respond well to frequent applications if started early and continued for 3 to 4 days, but may be less successful if delayed after 7 days. Evidence of its value in *Herpes zoster* infections is conflicting.

Acyclovir (Zovirax®) cream has recently been introduced for the treatment of initial and recurrent labial and genital herpes infections. Treatment should begin as early as possible, and continue for 5 days.

ACYCLOVIR

Indications: see notes above
Side-effects: transient stinging or burning on application; occasionally erythema or drying of the skin
Application: apply to lesions every 4 hours (5 times daily) for 5 days

---

Relative prices: A = up to 20p, B = 21-50p,

▼ PoM **Zovirax**® (Wellcome)
Cream, acyclovir 5% in an aqueous cream basis.
Price 2 g = **G**; 10 g = **J**

IDOXURIDINE IN DIMETHYL SULPH-OXIDE

Indications: see notes above
Cautions: avoid contact with the eyes, mucous membranes, and textiles; breast-feeding
Side-effects: stinging on application, changes in taste; overuse may cause maceration
Administration: apply 5% solution to lesions 4 times daily for 3–4 days; in severe *Herpes zoster* infections apply 40% solution over affected area daily for 4 days

PoM **Herpid**® (WBP)
Application, idoxuridine 5% in dimethyl sulph-oxide. Price 5 ml (with brush) = **H**
PoM **Iduridin**® (Ferring)
Application, idoxuridine 5% in dimethyl sulph-oxide. Price 5 ml (with applicator) = **G**
Application, idoxuridine 40% in dimethyl sulph-oxide. Price 5 ml (with applicator) and 20 ml with dropper (both) = **J**

13.10.4   Parasiticidal preparations

SCABIES. Applications of benzyl benzoate, lindane, or monosulfiram are all effective. The preparations are traditionally applied after a hot bath although there is no controlled study to confirm or otherwise the efficacy of the practice. Lotions are usually preferred to creams as they give better coverage.

Benzyl benzoate (Ascabiol®) is a widely used treatment. All members of an affected household are treated over the whole body, omitting the head and neck. Benzyl benzoate is irritant to the skin; applications for infants should be suitably diluted, and less irritant preparations such as lindane or monosulfiram may be preferred for treating children.

Monosulfiram (Tetmosol®) is particularly useful for treating scabies in children. Patients should avoid alcohol as a disulfiram-like reaction may occur.

The itch of scabies persists long after the infestation has been eliminated and antipruritic treatment may be required. Application of **crotamiton** (Eurax®) is useful in controlling itching after treatment with more effective acaricides.

PEDICULOSIS. **Malathion** and **carbaryl** have now become the treatment of choice for pediculosis (lice). **Lindane** is no longer recommended because of the emergence of resistant strains. Lotions should be used in preference to shampoos, which are not in contact with the hair for long enough to be fully effective.

BORDERLINE SUBSTANCES. The preparations marked 'ACBS' are regarded as drugs when prescribed in accordance with the advice of the Advisory Committee on Borderline Substances for the clinical conditions listed. Prescriptions issued in accordance with this advice and endorsed 'ACBS' will normally not be investigated. See Appendix 3 for listing by clinical condition.

BENZYL BENZOATE

Indications: scabies, pediculosis
Cautions: children (see notes above), avoid contact with the eyes
Side-effects: slight skin irritation, transient burning sensation, occasionally rashes
Administration: scabies—apply 25% application over the whole body, omitting the head and neck. The application should be repeated without bathing on the following day and washed off 24 hours later. The application should be diluted with 1 volume of water for children or 3 volumes for infants
Pediculosis—apply 25% application to affected area for 24 hours, remove by washing; in severe cases repeat 2–3 times

Benzyl Benzoate Application, benzyl benzoate 25%, emulsifying wax 2%, in purified water, freshly boiled and cooled. Price 150 ml = **B**
Ascabiol® (M&B)
Application, benzyl benzoate 25% in an emulsion basis. Price 200 ml = **D**

CARBARYL

Indications: pediculosis
Cautions: avoid contact with eyes
Administration: lotion—apply to dry hair and rub into the hair and scalp or affected areas, allow to dry, comb, and remove by washing 12 hours later; repeat procedure if necessary after 7–9 days; shampoo—leave on hair for 5 minutes, rinse, allow to dry, comb, repeat twice at intervals of 3 days

Carylderm® (Napp)
Lotion, carbaryl 0.5%, in an alcoholic basis. Price 55 ml = **C**
Caution: flammable
Shampoo, carbaryl 1%. Price 100 ml = **C**
Derbac with Carbaryl® (Bengué)
Shampoo solution, carbaryl 0.5% in a shampoo basis. Price 50 ml = **C**
Suleo-C® (International Labs)
Lotion, carbaryl 0.5%, in an alcoholic basis. Price 55 ml = **C**
Caution: flammable
Shampoo solution, carbaryl 0.5% in a shampoo basis. Price 75 ml = **C**

CROTAMITON

Indications: scabies, pruritus
Cautions; Contra-indications: section 13.3
Administration: scabies—apply over the whole body omitting the head and neck, after a hot bath, and remove by washing on the following day. The application may be repeated 24 hours later but a bath should not be taken until the following day

Preparations
Section 13.3

C = 51-100p, **D** = 101-180p, **E** = 181-300p, **F** = 301-450p, **G** = 451-650p, **H** = 651-900p, **I** = 901-1200p, **J** = over 1200p.

LINDANE

Indications: pediculosis, scabies (see notes above)

Cautions: avoid contact with eyes

Side-effects: rarely skin irritation

Administration: pediculosis—rub 0.1–1% application into hair and scalp or affected area, allow to dry, and remove by washing after 24 hours (kills parasites within a few days); shampoos, leave on hair for 5 minutes, rinse, allow to dry, comb, repeat once after 7 days

Scabies—apply 1% lotion or cream over whole body, omitting the head and neck, and wash off after 24 hours. Repeat after 1–3 days

Lindane Application, lindane 100 mg, emulsifying wax 4 g, lavender oil 1 ml, xylene (of commerce) 15 ml/100 ml, in purified water, freshly boiled and cooled. Price 50 ml = **B**. For pediculosis

Esoderm® (Napp)

Lotion, lindane 1%, in an alcoholic basis. Price 55 ml = **C**

Caution: flammable

Scabies—apply over whole body omitting head and neck. Repeat for 2–3 successive days if necessary

Pediculosis—apply to dry hair and rub into scalp or affected area, remove by washing after 12 hours, allow to dry, comb; repeat after 7–9 days

Cream shampoo (= application), ingredients as for lotion. Price 40 g = **C**; 300 g = **E**

Pediculosis—see above

Lorexane® (Care)

Cream, lindane 1%, in a water-miscible basis. Price 50 g = **B**. For scabies and pediculosis

Lorexane No. 3® (Care)

Shampoo, lindane 2% in a detergent basis, for pediculosis. Price 50 g = **B**

Caution: must be diluted with water before application to scalp

Quellada® (Stafford-Miller)

Lotion, lindane 1%, in a lotion basis. Price 100 ml = **C**; 500 ml = **E**. For scabies

Application PC, lindane 1%, in a shampoo basis. Price 100 ml = **C**; 500 ml = **E**. For pediculosis

MALATHION

Indications: pediculosis, scabies

Cautions: avoid contact with eyes. Do not use more than once a week for 3 weeks at a time

Administration: pediculosis—rub 0.5% lotion into dry hair, scalp, and affected area, comb, allow to dry, remove by washing after 12 hours, repeat if necessary after 7–9 days; apply 1% shampoo to hair for 5 minutes, rinse, comb, repeat if necessary after 7–9 days

Scabies—apply 0.5% preparation over whole body, omitting the head and neck, and wash off after 24 hours

Derbac with Malathion® (Bengué)

Liquid (= application), malathion 0.5%. Price 50 ml = **B**; 155 ml = **D**

Prioderm® (Napp)

Lotion, malathion 0.5%, in an alcoholic basis. Price 55 ml = **C**

Caution: flammable

Cream shampoo, malathion 1%. Price 40 g = **C**

Suleo-M® (International Labs)

Lotion, malathion 0.5%, in an alcoholic basis. Price 55 ml = **C**

Caution: flammable

MONOSULFIRAM

Indications: scabies, particularly in children

Cautions: avoid contact with eyes. Drug interactions: see Appendix 1 (section 13)

Side-effects: rarely hypersensitivity

Administration: apply diluted solution over whole body omitting head and neck. Repeat if necessary for 2–3 consecutive nights

Tetmosol® (ICI)

Solution, monosulfiram 25%, in industrial methylated spirit. Dilute with 2–3 parts of water before use. Price 100 ml = **C**. Label: 4. ACBS: for control of scabies

Caution: flammable

13.10.5   Preparations for minor skin infections

Some of the preparations listed are used in minor burns, and abrasions. They are applied as necessary. Preparations containing camphor, hydrargaphen, and sulphonamides should be **avoided**. Preparations such as magnesium sulphate paste are also listed but are now rarely used to treat carbuncles and boils as these are best treated with antibiotics (see section 5.1.1.2).

Flexible collodion (section 13.1) may be used to seal minor cuts and wounds.

Sprays and paints for minor infections are described in section 13.11.

Cetrimide Cream, cetrimide 0.5% in a suitable water-miscible basis such as cetostearyl alcohol 5%, liquid paraffin 50% in freshly boiled and cooled purified water. Price 50 g = **A**

Chlorhexidine Cream, chlorhexidine gluconate solution usually 5% (≡ chlorhexidine gluconate 1%), cetomacrogol emulsifying wax 25%, liquid paraffin 10%, in purified water, freshly boiled and cooled. Price 50 g = **C**

Proflavine Cream, proflavine hemisulphate 0.1%, yellow beeswax 2.5%, chlorocresol 0.1%, liquid paraffin 67.3%, freshly boiled and cooled purified water 25%, wool fat 5%. Price 100 ml = **B**

Caution: stains clothing

Anaflex® (Geistlich)

Aerosol spray (= application), polynoxylin 2% with talc, in a pressurised aerosol unit. Price 100 g = **E**

Cream, polynoxylin 10%, in a water-miscible basis. Price 50 g = **E**

Dusting-powder, polynoxylin 10% in a talc basis. Price 30 g = **E**

Paste, polynoxylin 10%. For application to moist areas. Price 20 g = **C**

Bactrian® (Loveridge)
Cream, cetrimide 1%. Price 45 g = **B**

Betadine® (Napp)
Ointment, povidone-iodine 10%, in a water-miscible basis. Price 80 g = **E**

Brulidine® (M&B)
Cream, dibromopropamidine isethionate 0.15%, in a water-miscible basis. Price 25 g = **B**

Cetavlex® (Care)
Cream, cetrimide 0.5%, in a water-miscible basis. Price 50 g = **B**; 500 g = **E**

Conotrane® (WBP)
Cream, hydrargaphen 0.05%, dimethicone '350' 20%. Price 60 g = **C**; 500 g = **F**

Dermalex® (Dermalex)
Skin lotion, allantoin 0.25%, hexachlorophane 0.5%, squalane 3% in an emulsion basis. Price 30 ml = **C**; 100 ml = **E**; 250 ml = **G**. For urinary rash and pressure sores. Avoid in children under 2 years

Drapolene® (Calmic)
Cream, benzalkonium chloride 0.01%, cetrimide 0.2% in a water-miscible basis. Price 55 g = **B**; 100 g = **C**. For urinary rash and minor wounds

Hewletts Antiseptic Cream® (Astra)
Cream, boric acid 2.5%, hydrous wool fat 4%, zinc oxide 8%. Price 35 g = **B**; 400 g = **E**

Hibitane® (ICI)
Antiseptic cream, chlorhexidine gluconate solution 5% (1% chlorhexidine gluconate), in a water-miscible basis. Price 50 g = **B**

PoM **Miol (Formula M1)**® (Comprehensive)
Cream, alcloxa 1%, calcium chloride 0.2%, camphor 4%, chlorphenesin 0.1%, magnesium chloride 1.5%, sodium chloride 2.1% in a water-miscible basis. Price 30 g = **D**
Lotion, alcloxa 1%, calcium chloride 0.17%, camphor 1%, magnesium chloride 1.42%, sodium chloride 1.98%. Price 100 ml = **E**

Ponoxylan® (Berk)
Gel, polynoxylin 10%. Price 25 g = **C**

PoM **Septex No. 2**® (Norton)
Cream, sulphathiazole 4.94%, zinc oxide 7.4%. Price 50 g = **B**; 420 g = **E**

Preparations for boils
Magnesium Sulphate Paste, dried magnesium sulphate 38%, phenol 0.5%, in anhydrous glycerol. Price 25 g = **A**
Apply under dressing

Ilonium® (Ilon)
Ointment, colophony 15.6%, phenol 0.1%, turpentine oil 8%, venice turpentine 8.1%, thymol 0.03%. Price 30 g = **C**; 100 g = **D**

Secaderm —section 13.14

13.11 Skin disinfecting and cleansing agents

The choice of *cleansing agent* is an important factor in treating skin conditions. For example, scaling disorders are best treated with **emulsifying ointment** (section 13.1) or other cleansers that do not irritate the skin; when treating ulcerated areas, a less irritant solution such as **dilute sodium hypochlorite** or **hydrogen peroxide** may be preferred; weeping eczemas may be treated with an astringent preparation (section 13.5 and below) such as **potassium permanganate solution**.

Sodium chloride solution 0.9% is suitable for general cleansing of skin and wounds. Useful *disinfectants* for skin cleansing include **cetrimide** (which has useful detergent properties), **chlorhexidine, potassium permanganate solution** 1 in 8000 and **dilute sodium hypochlorite** solution. Some patients may find these irritant and the more recent preparations, such as **povidone-iodine**, which are less irritant, may be preferred. Topical preparations of **hexachlorophane** should be used with caution in neonates and should **not** be used on large raw surfaces in infancy as they have been associated with severe neurotoxicity.

Disinfectant solutions may be prescribed for the treatment of skin conditions, but they are not regarded as drugs when used for general hygienic purposes. See Appendix 3, borderline substances. They are commonly used for cleansing of wounds and ulcers, skin cleansing in acne (section 13.6), adjunctive treatment of infected skin conditions, and skin preparation before surgery. Patients have suffered severe burns, however, when diathermy has been preceded by application of alcoholic skin disinfectants.

Desloughing agents (Aserbine®, Malatex®) are used to cleanse wounds and ulcers where the presence of blood clots and slough delays healing.

Astringent preparations, such as **aluminium acetate lotion** and potassium permanganate solution are useful for treating eczematous reactions and suppurating wounds. They may assist in sealing an exuding surface as they precipitate protein. Silver nitrate lotion is now rarely used as it stains the skin black and may cause toxic effects if used for prolonged periods.

BORDERLINE SUBSTANCES. The preparations marked 'ACBS' are regarded as drugs when prescribed in accordance with the advice of the Advisory Committee on Borderline Substances for the clinical conditions listed. Prescriptions issued in accordance with this advice and endorsed 'ACBS' will normally not be investigated. See Appendix 3 for listing by clinical condition.

DISINFECTING AND CLEANSING AGENTS

ALCOHOL
Indications: skin preparation before injection
Cautions: flammable; avoid broken skin

Industrial Methylated Spirit. Price 100 ml = **A**. Label: 15
Surgical Spirit. Price 100 ml = **A**. Label: 15

ALUMINIUM ACETATE
Indications: suppurating and exudative eczematous reactions and wounds

Aluminium Acetate Lotion, aluminium acetate approx. 0.65%, in water (see Formulary). Price 500 ml = **D**. To be used undiluted as a wet dressing

BENZALKONIUM CHLORIDE

Indications: skin disinfection such as pre-operative skin preparation, obstetrics, wound cleansing and bladder irrigation
Cautions: avoid contact with eyes

Benzalkonium Chloride Solution, benzalkonium chloride 50%. Price 50 ml = **B**. To be used diluted 1 in 500 to 1 in 10000
Roccal® (Winthrop)
Solution, blue, benzalkonium chloride 1%. Price 250 ml = **C**; 500 ml = **D**. To be used diluted 1 in 10 to 1 in 200
Roccal Concentrate 10X® (Winthrop)
Concentrate, blue, benzalkonium chloride 10%. Price 2.25 litres = **J**. For preparation of Roccal Solution with freshly boiled and cooled purified water

CETRIMIDE

Indications: skin disinfection; soap or shampoo substitute in acne, skin infections and seborrhoea of the scalp
Cautions: avoid contact with eyes; avoid use in body cavities
Side-effects: skin irritation and occasionally sensitisation

Cetrimide Solution, yellow, cetrimide 1% in purified water freshly boiled and cooled. Price 100 ml = **A**. To be used undiluted
Cetrimide Solution Strong, yellow, cetrimide 20 to 40%, with alcohol (95%) 7.5%, tartrazine 0.0075%. It may be perfumed. Used for preparation of cetrimide solutions. Price 100 ml (20%) = **B**; 100 ml (40%) = **C**. To be diluted before use
Cetavlon® (ICI)
Solution, corresponds to Cetrimide Solution Strong (40%). For preparation of cetrimide solutions. Price 100 ml = **B**. For pre-operative scrubbing, skin cleansing and disinfection use as a 1% solution; for shampooing in seborrhoeic conditions use as a 1–3% solution; for cleansing in wounds and burns use as a 0.1% solution

CHLORHEXIDINE

Indications: skin disinfection such as pre-operative skin preparation, obstetrics and wound cleansing; bladder irrigation (see also section 7.4.4)
Cautions: bladder irrigations of concentrated solutions may cause haematuria
Side-effects: sensitivity may occur, avoid contact with mucous membranes and meninges
Administration: chlorhexidine acetate or gluconate, body cavity and bladder irrigation 0.01–0.02%, urethral disinfection and catheter lubrication 0.05% (in glycerol), pre-operative skin preparation 0.5% (in alcohol 70%); chlorhexidine hydrochloride 1% as a dusting-powder or cream

Chlorhexidine Dusting-powder, chlorhexidine hydrochloride 0.5% in sterilisable maize starch. Price 100 g = **A**

Chlorasept® (Travenol)
2000 Solution (sterile), pink, chlorhexidine acetate 0.05%. Price 20 × 25-ml sachet, 10 × 100-ml sachet (both) = **D**; 500 ml, 1000 ml (both) = **C**. For general disinfection and wound cleansing
Cyteal® (Concept)
Antiseptic skin cleanser, yellow, chlorhexidine gluconate 0.5%, chlorocresol 0.3%, hexamidine isethionate 0.1%. Price 500 ml = **D**. For pre-operative scrubbing use undiluted; for cleansing infections use undiluted or diluted 1 in 10 and apply twice daily; for wound and ulcer cleansing dilute 1 in 10 and use daily
Dispray 1 Quick Prep® (Stuart)
Aerosol application, chlorhexidine gluconate solution 2.5% (≡ 0.5% chlorhexidine gluconate), in alcohol 70%, pressurised aerosol unit. Price 400-ml unit = **E**. For skin disinfection before injections or operations
Caution: flammable
Hibidil® (ICI)
Solution (sterile), pink, chlorhexidine gluconate solution 0.25% (≡ chlorhexidine gluconate 0.05%) in sterile aqueous solution. Price 25 × 25-ml sachets = **E**; 6 × 100-ml sachets = **D**; 1000 ml = **E**. To be used undiluted for skin disinfection in wounds, burns and obstetrics
Hibiscrub® (ICI)
Cleansing solution, red, chlorhexidine gluconate solution 20% (≡4% chlorhexidine gluconate), perfumed, in a surfactant solution. Price 250 ml = **D**; 500 ml = **E**. Use instead of soap as pre-operative scrub or disinfectant wash for hands and skin
Hibisol® (ICI)
Solution, blue, chlorhexidine gluconate solution 2.5% (≡0.5% chlorhexidine gluconate), in isopropyl alcohol 70% with emollients. Price 250 and 500 ml (both) = **D**. To be used undiluted for hand and skin disinfection
Hibitane® (ICI)
Chlorhexidine acetate powder. Price 50 g = **E**. For preparation of chlorhexidine solutions
Chlorhexidine hydrochloride powder. Price 50 g = **E**. For preparation of solutions, creams, and dusting-powders
Hibitane 5% Concentrate® (ICI)
Solution, red, chlorhexidine gluconate solution 25% (≡ 5% chlorhexidine gluconate), in a perfumed aqueous solution. Price 50 × 10-ml sachet = **F**; 500 ml = **D**. To be used diluted 1 in 10 (0.5%) with alcohol 70% for pre-operative skin preparation, or 1 in 100 (0.05%) with water for general skin disinfection
Hibitane Gluconate 20%® (ICI)
Solution, chlorhexidine gluconate 20% in an aqueous solution. Price 500 ml = **G**. To be used diluted as above in body cavity and bladder irrigation, urethral disinfection and catheter lubrication
Hibitane Obstetric® (ICI)
Cream, chlorhexidine gluconate solution 5% (≡1% chlorhexidine gluconate), in a pourable water-miscible basis. Price 250 ml = **C**. For use

in obstetrics as a vaginal lubricant and for application to the vulva and perineum during labour

pHiso-MED® (Winthrop)
Solution, chlorhexidine gluconate 4% in an emulsion basis. Price 150 ml = **F**. For use as a soap or shampoo substitute in acne and seborrhoeic conditions; for bathing mothers and babies in maternity units (as 1 in 10 dilution) to prevent cross-infection and for pre-operative hand and skin preparation

Rotersept® (Roterpharma)
Spray application, chlorhexidine gluconate 0.2% in a pressurised aerosol unit. Price 284-g unit = **D**. For prevention and treatment of sore cracked nipples

Savloclens® (ICI)
Solution (sterile), yellow, chlorhexidine gluconate solution 0.25% (≡ chlorhexidine gluconate 0.05%), cetrimide 0.5% ≡ a dilution of 1 in 30 of Savlon Hospital Concentrate. Price 100-ml sachet = **A**. To be used undiluted in general skin disinfection and wound cleansing

Savlodil® (ICI)
Solution (sterile), yellow, chlorhexidine gluconate solution 0.075% (≡ chlorhexidine gluconate 0.015%), cetrimide 0.15% (sterile). Price 25 × 25-ml sachets = **D**; 6 × 100-ml sachets = **C**; 1000 ml = **D**. To be used undiluted for general skin disinfection and wound cleansing

Savlon Hospital Concentrate® (ICI)
Solution, orange, chlorhexidine gluconate solution 7.5% (≡ chlorhexidine gluconate 1.5%), cetrimide 15%. Price 50 × 10-ml sachets = **E**; 25 × 25-ml sachets = **D**; 1 litre = **E**. To be used diluted 1 in 100 (1%) to 1 in 30 with water for skin disinfection and wound cleansing, and diluted 1 in 30 in alcohol 70% for pre-operative skin preparation

Travasept 30® (Travenol)
Solution (sterile), yellow, chlorhexidine acetate 0.05%, cetrimide 0.5%. Price 20 × 25-ml sachet, 10 × 100-ml sachet (both) = **D**; 100, 500, and 1000 ml (all) = **C**. To be used undiluted for skin cleansing and disinfection of wounds

Travasept 100® (Travenol)
Solution (sterile), yellow, chlorhexidine acetate 0.015%, cetrimide 0.15%. Price 20 × 25-ml sachet, 10 × 100-ml sachet (both) = **D**; 100, 500, and 1000 ml (all) = **C**. To be used undiluted in skin disinfection such as wound cleansing and obstetrics

CHLORINATED SOLUTIONS

Indications: skin disinfection particularly wound and ulcer cleansing
Cautions: bleaches fabric; solutions may be irritant

Chlorinated Lime and Boric Acid Solution (Eusol), chlorinated lime 1.25%, boric acid 1.25%, in water for preparations. Contains not less than 0.25% available chlorine. It must be freshly prepared. Price 500 ml = **A**. To be used undiluted for skin disinfection, particularly in

wound and ulcer cleansing when it may be applied as a wet dressing

Chlorinated Soda Solution, Surgical (Dakin's Solution), boric acid, chlorinated lime, sodium carbonate, sufficient of each to provide a solution containing 0.5% of available chlorine in water. Price 500 ml = **C**. To be used undiluted for cleansing wounds and ulcers. Surrounding tissues should be protected with petroleum jelly during application as solutions are irritant

Sodium Hypochlorite Solution, Strong, contains not less than 8% available chlorine. Price 100 ml = **A**. To be diluted before use

Sodium Hypochlorite Solution, Dilute, contains about 1% available chlorine. Price 100 ml = **A**. For general disinfection. Only diluted solutions containing up to 0.5% available chlorine are suitable for use on the skin and in wounds

▼**Chlorasol®** (Schering-Prebbles)
Solution (sterile), sodium hypochlorite, containing 0.3–0.4% available chlorine. Price 25 × 25-ml sachets = **F**

CHLOROXYLENOL

Indications: skin disinfection
Cautions: may irritate skin and cause sensitisation

Chloroxylenol Solution, chloroxylenol 5%, alcohol about 20%, terpineol 10% in a detergent solution. Price 100 ml = **B**. To be used as 1 in 20 dilution (5%)

Dettol® (R&C)
Lotion (formerly antiseptic cream), chloroxylenol 1.3%. Price 113 g = **B**. For use in obstetrics as a vaginal lubricant during labour and in hand disinfection

CRYSTAL VIOLET

Indications: minor skin wounds
Cautions: stains clothes and skin

Brilliant Green and Crystal Violet Paint, brilliant green 0.5%, crystal violet 0.5%, alcohol (90%) 50%, in water for preparations. Price 25 ml = **A**. To be used undiluted

Crystal Violet Paint, crystal violet 0.5%, in water for preparations. Price 25 ml = **A**. To be used undiluted

HEXACHLOROPHANE

Indications: skin disinfection; soap substitute in acne and skin infections
Cautions: neonates (see notes above)—avoid routine use; avoid denuded areas such as in extensive wounds
Side-effects: sensitivity; rarely photosensitivity

PoM **Ster-Zac DC Skin Cleanser®** (Hough)
Cream, hexachlorophane 3%. Price 150 ml = **E**. Use 3–5 ml instead of soap as pre-operative scrub for hands

Ster-Zac Powder® (Hough)
Dusting-powder, hexachlorophane 0.33%, zinc oxide 3%, talc 88.67%, starch 8% (sterile). Price 30 g = **C**; 225 g = **D**. For prevention of

staphylococcal cross-infection; treatment of furunculosis; routine treatment of cord stumps; prevention of bedsores

HYDROGEN PEROXIDE

Indications: skin disinfection, particularly cleansing and deodorising wounds and ulcers
Cautions: bleaches fabric; solutions above 6% should be diluted before application to the skin

Hydrogen Peroxide Solution 27% (about 90 vols). Dilute before use. Price 100 ml = **B**
Hydrogen Peroxide Solution 6% (20 vols). Price 100 ml = **A**
Hydrogen Peroxide Solution 3% (10 vols). Price 100 ml = **A**
Hioxyl® (Quinoderm Ltd)
Cream, hydrogen peroxide (stabilised) 1.5%. Price 25 g = **D**; 100 g = **F**. Apply when necessary and if necessary cover with a dressing

IODINE COMPOUNDS

Indications: skin disinfection; surfactant solutions—soap or shampoo substitute in acne, skin infections, and seborrhoea of the scalp
Cautions: pregnancy, breast-feeding
Side-effects: rarely sensitivity; may interfere with thyroid function tests

Weak Iodine Solution (Iodine Tincture), iodine 2.5%, potassium iodide 2.5%, purified water 2.5%, in alcohol (90%). Price 10 ml = **B**. To be used undiluted in minor skin wounds; stains skin and clothes and causes considerable pain
Betadine® (Napp)
Antiseptic spray, povidone-iodine 5%, in a pressurised aerosol unit. Price 200-ml unit = **E**. For use in skin disinfection, particularly minor wounds and infections
Antiseptic paint, povidone-iodine 10% in an alcoholic solution. Price 8 ml (with applicator brush) = **C**. Apply undiluted to minor wounds and infections, twice daily
Alcoholic solution, povidone-iodine 10%. Price 500 ml = **D**. To be applied undiluted in pre- and post-operative skin disinfection
Antiseptic solution, povidone-iodine 10% in aqueous solution. Price 500 ml = **D**. To be applied undiluted in pre- and post-operative skin disinfection
Scalp and skin cleanser solution, povidone-iodine 7.5%, in a surfactant basis. Price 250 ml = **E**. ACBS: for infective conditions of the skin. Retain on scalp for 5 minutes before rinsing
Skin cleanser solution, povidone-iodine 4%, in a surfactant basis. Price 250 ml = **D**. ACBS: for infective conditions of the skin. Retain on skin for 5 minutes before rinsing
Surgical scrub, povidone-iodine 7.5%, in a nonionic surfactant basis. Price 500 ml = **D**. To be used as a pre-operative scrub for hands and skin
Disadine DP® (Stuart)
Dry powder spray (= application), povidone-iodine 0.5%, in a pressurised aerosol unit. Price 150-g unit = **E**. For skin disinfection, particularly wounds, surgery, and bedsores

Steribath® (Stuart)
Bath concentrate solution, iodine-nonoxynol complex (4.5% available iodine). Price 14-ml sachet = **A**. Use 1 sachet/bath
Videne® (Riker)
Disinfectant solution, red-brown, povidone-iodine 10% (≡ 1% available iodine), in an aqueous solution. Price 500 ml = **C** (Hosp. only). Apply undiluted in skin disinfection and pre-operative skin preparation
Disinfectant tincture, red-brown, povidone-iodine 10% (≡ 1% available iodine), in industrial methylated spirit. Price 500 ml = **D** (Hosp. only). Apply undiluted in pre-operative skin disinfection, particularly orthopaedic surgery
Caution: flammable
Surgical scrub, red-brown, povidone-iodine 7.5% (≡0.75% available iodine), in a detergent basis. Price 500 ml = **C**. To be used as a pre-operative scrub for hands and skin and disinfecting site of incision before surgery

POTASSIUM PERMANGANATE

Indications: cleansing and deodorising suppurating eczematous reactions and wounds
Cautions: irritant to mucous membranes; stains skin and clothing
Administration: wet dressings or baths, approx. 0.01% solution (10 g/bath)

Potassium Permanganate Solution, potassium permanganate 0.1% in water (see Formulary). Price 500 ml = **A**

SILVER NITRATE

Indications: suppurating lesions (short-term)
Cautions: see notes above

Silver Nitrate Lotion, silver nitrate 0.5%, in water (see Formulary). Do not use if precipitate is present. Price 50 ml = **A**. To be used undiluted

SOFT SOAP

Indications: removal of adherent crusts

Soap Spirit, soft soap 65% in alcohol (90%). Price 100 ml = **B**

TRICLOSAN

Indications: skin disinfection
Cautions: avoid contact with eyes

Manusept® (Hough)
Antibacterial hand rub, blue, triclosan 0.5%, isopropyl alcohol 70%. Price 250 ml = **C**; 500 ml = **D**. For disinfection and pre-operative hand preparation
Ster-Zac Bath Concentrate® (Hough)
Solution, triclosan 2%. Price 28.5 ml = **B**; 500 ml = **F**. ACBS: for staphyloccal skin infections. For prevention of cross-infection use 1 sachet/bath

ZINC SULPHATE

Indications: indolent ulcers

Zinc Sulphate Lotion (Lotio Rubra), zinc sulphate 1%, with amaranth, in water (see Formulary). Price 200 ml = **A**. Apply undiluted as a wet dressing

DESLOUGHING AGENTS

For removal of clots and slough in wounds and ulcers.

ADMINISTRATION. Use solution for skin cleansing alone, or before application of cream, or apply as wet dressing. Apply cream liberally usually twice daily and cover with a dressing. Avoid perilesional skin

Aserbine® (Bencard)
Cream, benzoic acid 0.024%, hexachlorophane 0.015%, malic acid 0.36%, propylene glycol 1.7%, salicylic acid 0.006%. Price 100 g = **C**
Solution, benzoic acid 0.15%, malic acid 2.25%, propylene glycol 40%, salicylic acid 0.0375%. Price 500 ml = **D**
Malatex® (Norton)
Cream, benzoic acid 0.024%, malic acid 0.36%, propylene glycol 1.7%, salicylic acid 0.006%. Price 100 and 125 g (both) = **C**
Solution, benzoic acid 0.15%, malic acid 2.25%, propylene glycol 40%, salicylic acid 0.0375%. Price 500 ml = **C**

SOAP SUBSTITUTES

See also above; section 13.2.2 (emollient bath additives) and section 13.6 (acne)

Emulsifying ointment —section 13.1

13.12 Antiperspirants

Aluminium chloride 20% lotion (Anhydrol Forte® etc.) is a potent antiperspirant used in the treatment of severe hyperhidrosis.

Dusting-powders are described in section 13.2.3.

ALUMINIUM CHLORIDE
Indications: hyperhidrosis
Cautions: avoid contact with eyes; do not shave axilla or use depilatories within 12 hours of use
Side-effects: skin irritation—may require treatment with hydrocortisone cream
Administration: apply at night to dry skin, wash off on following morning, initially daily then reduce frequency as condition improves—do not bathe immediately before use

PoM **Anhydrol Forte**® (Dermal)
Solution (= application), aluminium chloride hexahydrate 20%, 10-ml bottle with roll-on applicator. Price complete unit = **E**
Caution: flammable
PoM **Driclor**® (Stiefel)
Application, aluminium chloride hexahydrate 20% in an alcoholic basis, 60-ml bottle with

roll-on applicator. Price complete unit = **E**
Caution: flammable

13.13 Preparations for wounds and ulcers

Preparations for ulcers are second-line treatment and the underlying causes should be treated. The main beneficial effect of local treatment is removal of slough and clot and the ablation of local infection (section 13.11). Preparations which absorb or help promote the removal of exudate may also help. It should be noted that substances applied to an open area are easily absorbed and perilesional skin is easily sensitised. Gravitational dermatitis may be due to neomycin or lanolin sensitivity. Enzyme preparations such as streptokinase-streptodornase (Varidase®) or alternatively dextranomer (Debrisan®) are designed for sloughing ulcers and may help.

Usually all that is required is washing with an antiseptic solution such as dilute sodium hypochlorite solution, cetrimide, or potassium permanganate (section 13.11) and covering the lesion with an adequate dressing.

Cleansing preparations
PoM **Benoxyl 20**® (Stiefel)
Lotion, benzoyl peroxide 20%. For cutaneous ulcers. Price 100 ml = **F**
Apply 8–12 hourly as wet dressing; protect perilesional skin
PoM **Debrisan**® (Pharmacia)
Beads 100-300 μm diameter, dextranomer. For absorption of exudate. Price 4-g sachet = **E**; 60 g = **J**. For moist or indolent ulcers
Sprinkle 3mm on wound surface and renew 1–5 times daily according to exudate
PoM **Iodosorb**® (Stuart)
Powder, cadexomer iodine (modified starch gel microbeads containing 0.9% iodine). Price 3-g sachet = **D**. For venous leg ulcers and pressure sores
Sprinkle 3mm on wound surface and renew daily
Variclene® (Dermal)
Gel, brilliant green 0.5%, lactic acid 0.5%, in an aqueous basis. Price 50 g = **G**. For venous and other skin ulcers
Apply to cleaned and dried lesion with a sterile applicator avoiding surrounding skin; in severe ulceration apply on dressing and repeat as required at intervals of not more than 7 days
PoM **Varidase Topical**® (Lederle)
Powder, streptokinase 100 000 units, streptodornase 25 000 units. For preparing solutions for topical use. Price per vial = **H**
Apply as wet dressing usually 1–2 times daily

Dressings
Zinc Paste Bandage, bandage impregnated with paste containing zinc oxide. Price 75 mm × 6 m bandage = **C**

C = 51-100p, **D** = 101-180p, **E** = 181-300p, **F** = 301-450p, **G** = 451-650p, **H** = 651-900p, **I** = 901-1200p, **J** = over 1200p.

Bactigras® (S&N)
Chlorhexidine tulle gras (= dressing), gauze impregnated with chlorhexidine acetate 0.5%, and soft paraffin. Price 5 dressings 50mm × 50 mm = **C**; 5 dressings 100mm × 100mm = **D**

Calaband® (Seton)
Impregnated bandage, zinc oxide 9.25%, calamine 5.75%, modified starch 19.15%, boric acid 2%, glycerol 27%, castor oil 1%. Requires additional bandaging. Price 75 mm × 6 m bandage = **D**
Coltapaste —section 13.5
Ichthopaste —section 13.5
Quinaband® (Seton)
Impregnated bandage, zinc oxide 9.25%, calamine 5.75%, clioquinol 1%. Requires additional bandaging. Price 75 mm × 6 m bandage = **D**
Varihesive® (Squibb)
Dressing, gelatin 20%, pectin 20%, polyisobutylene 40%, carmellose sodium 20%. For leg ulcers. Price 5 dressings (100 mm × 100 mm) = **G**
Viscopaste PB7® (S&N)
Impregnated bandage, zinc paste bandage (emulsifying basis). Requires additional bandaging. Price 75 mm × 6 m bandage = **D**
Zincaband® (Seton)
Impregnated bandage, zinc paste bandage (gelatinous paste). Requires additional bandaging. Price 75 mm × 6 m bandage = **D**

13.14 Topical preparations for circulatory disorders

These preparations are used to improve circulation in conditions such as bruising, superficial thrombophlebitis, chilblains and varicose veins but are of little value. Sclerotherapy in varicose veins is described in section 2.13.

Rubefacients are described in section 10.3.2.

Akrotherm® (Napp)
Cream, acetylcholine chloride 0.2%, histamine 0.034%, cholesterol 1%. For chilblains. Price 40 g = **C**
Apply 3–4 times daily
Hirudoid® (Luitpold)
Cream, heparinoid 0.3% in a vanishing-cream basis. Price 40 g = **E**
Gel, heparinoid 0.3%. Price 40 g = **E**
Apply up to 4 times daily in superficial soft-tissue injuries and varicose conditions
Lasonil® (Bayer)
Ointment, heparinoid 50 units, hyaluronidase 150 units/g. Price 14 g = **B**; 40 g = **D**
Apply 2–5 times daily in superficial tissue injuries and varicose conditions
Pernomol® (LAB)
Paint, camphor 10%, chlorbutol 2%, phenol 0.95%, soap spirit 34%, tannic acid 2.2%. For chilblains. Price 2.5 ml (with applicator) = **B**
Apply 3–4 times daily
Secaderm® (Rorer)
Salve (= ointment), colophony 26%, melaleuca oil 5.6%, phenol 2.4%, terebene 5.25%, turpentine oil 6%. For boils and chilblains. Price 15 g = **C**
Apply 1–2 times daily and cover with dressing

14: Immunological products and
VACCINES

In this chapter, immunisation is discussed under the following headings:

14.1 Active immunity
14.2 Passive immunity
14.3 Storage and reconstitution of immunological products
14.4 Prevention and treatment of disease
14.5 Immunoglobulins
14.6 Vaccination programmes for children
14.7 International travel

14.1   Active immunity

Vaccines are designed to produce specific protection against a given disease. They may consist of

1. an attenuated form of an infective agent, as in the vaccines which are used against virus diseases such as rubella and measles, or BCG used against tuberculosis,
2. inactivated preparations of the virus or bacteria, as in influenza, pertussis (whooping-cough), or typhoid vaccines, or
3. extracts of or exotoxins produced by a micro-organism, as in tetanus vaccine.

Vaccines stimulate the production of protective antibody and other immune mechanisms. They are given by injection, with the exception of live attenuated poliomyelitis vaccine, which is given by mouth, and BCG vaccine which is given intra-cutaneously (intradermally).

In the case of vaccines consisting of living agents, immunisation is generally achieved with a single dose, but 3 doses are required in the case of oral poliomyelitis vaccine. Live virus multiplies in the body and usually produces a durable immunity but not always as long as that of the natural infection.

Inactivated vaccines usually require a primary series of doses of vaccine to produce an adequate antibody response and in most cases reinforcing or 'booster' injections are required. The duration of immunity following the use of inactivated vaccines varies from months to many years.

The health departments of the UK have issued a memorandum, *Immunisation against Infectious Disease* (1984) giving information on immune mechanisms, precautions, dosage intervals, storage, reconstitution, etc.

SIDE-EFFECTS. Some vaccines such as poliomyelitis vaccines produce virtually no reactions, while others, as in the case of measles vaccine, may produce a very mild form of the disease. Some of the inactivated vaccines may produce mild discomfort at the site of injection and mild fever and malaise. Occasionally there are more serious untoward reactions which should always be reported in the usual way to the Committee on Safety of Medicines.

CONTRA-INDICATIONS. Most vaccines may have some contra-indications to their use, and the manufacturer's leaflet accompanying the vaccine should always be consulted. In general, vaccines should not be given to individuals if they have a febrile illness or if any active infection is present or suspected.

Various viral vaccines contain small quantities of antibiotics used in their production, such as neomycin or polymixin or both. Vaccine may need to be withheld from individuals who are known to be sensitive to the antibiotic which it contains.

Live virus vaccines, especially rubella vaccine, should never be routinely offered to pregnant women because of possible harm to the fetus. They should not be given to individuals with impaired immune responsiveness, whether occurring naturally or as a result of radiotherapy or treatment with corticosteroids or other immunosuppressive drugs. They should not be given to those suffering from malignant conditions or other tumours of the reticulo-endothelial system. When two live virus vaccines are required they should be given either simultaneously at different sites or with an interval of at least 3 weeks.

14.2   Passive immunity

Defence or immediate protection against certain infective organisms can be obtained by injecting preparations made from the plasma of immune individuals with adequate levels of antibody to the disease for which protection is sought.

Antibodies of human origin are usually termed immunoglobulins. The term antiserum is applied to material prepared in animals. Because of the serum sickness reactions that may follow injections of antisera, this therapy has been replaced wherever possible by the use of immunoglobulins, as in the case of tetanus. Tetanus vaccine or tetanus vaccine, adsorbed should also be given to commence a course of active immunisation (section 14.4.14).

Diphtheria antitoxin prepared in horses is still used, and serum sickness is common after administration of this preparation. (Reactions are theoretically possible after injection of human immunoglobulins but must be extraordinarily uncommon.)

14.3   Storage and reconstitution of immunological products

Care must be taken to store all vaccines and other immunological products under the conditions recommended by the manufacturer in the literature accompanying the vaccine, otherwise the preparation may become denatured and totally ineffective. **Refrigerated storage** is usually necessary; many vaccines need to be stored at 2° to 8° and not allowed to freeze. Opened multidose vials which have not been fully used should be discarded within one hour if no preservative is present (most live virus vaccines) or within 3 hours or at the end of a session when vaccines containing a preservative are used; this category includes poliomyelitis vaccine (oral).

Particular attention must be paid to the instructions on the use of diluents where these are provided (usually with freeze-dried preparations of the vaccines), and ampoules of vaccine should always be adequately shaken before use to ensure uniformity of the material to be injected.

14.4   Prevention and treatment of disease

AVAILABILITY OF VACCINES AND OTHER IMMUNOLOGICAL PRODUCTS. Anthrax, rabies (human diploid cell), smallpox (freeze-dried), and yellow fever vaccines, botulinum antitoxin, and snake and scorpion venom antitoxins are available from local designated holding centres. *The Health Service Supply Purchasing Guide*, section D pp. 1101–1199 gives details of current arrangements with names, addresses, and telephone numbers of holding centres. **Poliomyelitis vaccine (inactivated)** is available on request to the Department of Health and Social Security, Room 421, 14 Russell Square, London WC1B 5EP, telephone 01-636 6811, extn 3117 3236. Most other vaccines and other immunological products are available commercially.

Enquiries for vaccines not available commercially should be made to the Department of Health and Social Security, address and telephone number above. In Scotland information about availability of vaccines can be obtained from the Chief Administrative Pharmaceutical Officer of the local Health Board. In Wales enquiries should be directed to the Welsh Office, Cathays Park, Cardiff, telephone 0222 825111, extn 4658 and in Northern Ireland to the Department of Health

and Social Services, Dundonald House, Belfast, telephone 0232 63939.

14.4.1   Anthrax

An inactivated bacterial vaccine is available for anyone subject to heavy exposure to anthrax, such as those exposed to infected hides and carcasses and to imported bonemeal, fishmeal, and feeding stuffs. The vaccine is prepared from a culture of *Bacillus anthracis* and, following the primary course of injections, reinforcing doses should be given at about yearly intervals.

PoM Anthrax Vaccine
Dose: initial course 3 doses of 0.5 ml by intramuscular or deep subcutaneous injection at intervals of 3 weeks followed by a 4th dose after an interval of 6 months
Reinforcing doses: 0.5 ml annually
    Availability—section 14.4

14.4.2   Cholera

Vaccines against cholera contain killed Inaba and Ogawa serotypes and may also contain the El Tor biotype that became prevalent in 1961. Although an international certificate of vaccination is still required for entry to some countries, it is now recognised that while cholera vaccine may provide some individual protection for about 6 months it cannot control the spread of the disease. Reinforcing injections are recommended every 6 months for those living in endemic areas.

Patients who travel in a country where cholera exists should be warned that attention to the hygiene of food and water is still essential, even after vaccination.

PoM Cholera Vaccine Cho/Vac. Price 1-ml amp = **D**; 1.5-ml amp = **E**; 10-ml vial = **E**; 50-ml vial = **J**
Dose: first dose, as specified on the label, usually 0.5 ml by deep subcutaneous or intramuscular injection; CHILD 1–5 years 0.1 ml; 6–10 years 0.3 ml; second dose after at least a week and preferably 4 weeks 1 ml (or 0.2 ml by intracutaneous injection); CHILD 1–5 years 0.3 ml, 6–10 years 0.5 ml (or 1–10 years 0.1 ml by intracutaneous injection)

14.4.3   Diphtheria

Protection against diphtheria is essentially due to the presence in the blood stream of antitoxin, the production of which is stimulated by toxoid vaccines prepared from the toxin of *Corynebacterium diphtheriae*. This toxoid is more effective if adsorbed onto a mineral carrier, and adsorbed diphtheria vaccines are generally used for the routine immunisation of babies and given in the form of a triple vaccine, Adsorbed Diphtheria, Tetanus, and Pertussis Vaccine. A dose of Poliomyelitis Vaccine, Live (Oral) is generally given at the time of each of the doses of the triple vaccine (see schedule, section 14.6). Adsorbed Diphtheria and Tetanus Vaccine is used in place of the triple vaccine when it is decided not to immunise against whooping-cough.

A reinforcing dose of adsorbed diphtheria and tetanus vaccine is recommended at the age of school entry.

Further reinforcing doses of diphtheria vaccine are not recommended except in the case of those who work in units where there is a potentially high risk of infection such as those employed in infectious disease units, hospitals for the mentally handicapped, or microbiology laboratories. A special vaccine is available for this purpose. The small quantity of diphtheria toxoid present in the preparation is sufficient to recall immunity in individuals previously immunised against diphtheria but whose immunity may have diminished with time. It is insufficient to cause the reactions that may occur when diphtheria vaccine of conventional formulation is used in adults. Diphtheria vaccine for adults (adsorbed) may be given without prior Schick testing.

Mixed vaccines

PoM **Diphtheria and Tetanus Vaccine** DT/Vac/FT. A mixture of diphtheria formol toxoid and tetanus formol toxoid. Price 5-ml vial = **F**
Dose: reinforcing dose for children, 0.5 ml or as stated on the label by intramuscular or deep subcutaneous injection

PoM **Diphtheria and Tetanus Vaccine, Adsorbed** DT/Vac/Ads. Prepared from diphtheria formol toxoid and tetanus formol toxoid with a mineral carrier (aluminium hydroxide, aluminium phosphate, or calcium phosphate). Used for primary immunisation of children (see schedule, section 14.6) and reinforcing doses. Price 0.5-ml amp = **C**; 5-ml vial = **E**
Dose: 0.5 ml or as stated on the label by intramuscular or deep subcutaneous injection

PoM **Diphtheria, Tetanus, and Pertussis Vaccine** DTPer/Vac. A mixture of diphtheria formol toxoid, tetanus formol toxoid, and pertussis vaccine. Used for reinforcing doses in children. Price 0.5-ml amp = **C**; 5-ml vial = **F**
Dose: 0.5 ml or as stated on the label by intramuscular or deep subcutaneous injection

PoM **Diphtheria, Tetanus, and Pertussis Vaccine, Adsorbed** DTPer/Vac/Ads. Prepared from diphtheria formol toxoid, tetanus formol toxoid, and pertussis vaccine with a mineral carrier (aluminium hydroxide, aluminium phosphate, or calcium phosphate). Used for primary immunisation of children (see schedule, section 14.6). Price 0.5-ml amp = **C**
Dose: 0.5 ml or as stated on the label by intramuscular or deep subcutaneous injection

PoM **Trivax**® (Wellcome)
Diphtheria, tetanus, and pertussis vaccine. For primary vaccination of children (see schedule, section 14.6). Price 0.5-ml amp = **C**; 5-ml vial = **F**
Dose: 0.5 ml by intramuscular or deep subcutaneous injection

PoM **Trivax-AD**® (Wellcome)
Diphtheria, tetanus, and pertussis vaccine, adsorbed. For primary vaccination of children

(see schedule, section 14.6). Price 0.5-ml amp = **C**; 5-ml vial = **F**
Dose: 0.5 ml by intramuscular or deep subcutaneous injection

Single vaccines

PoM **Diphtheria Vaccine, Adsorbed** Dip/Vac/Ads. Prepared from diphtheria formol toxoid with a mineral carrier (aluminium hydroxide, aluminium phosphate, or calcium phosphate). Used for primary immunisation of children who do not require immunisation against tetanus or whooping-cough; also in reduced dosage for Schick-positive adults and children over 10 years. Price 0.5-ml amp = **C**
Dose: the volume stated on the label by intramuscular or deep subcutaneous injection

Adult vaccine

PoM **Diphtheria Vaccine for Adults, Adsorbed.** Dip/Vac/Ads for Adults. For primary immunisation and reinforcement in patients over 10 years of age. Price 0.5-ml amp = **E**
Dose: primary immunisation, three doses each of 0.5 ml by intramuscular or deep subcutaneous injection separated by intervals of 1 month; reinforcement, 0.5 ml
Available from distributor (Regent)

Antisera

PoM **Diphtheria Antitoxin** Dip/Ser. For passive immunisation (after exposure) and treatment of diphtheria
Dose: prophylactic 500 to 2000 units by subcutaneous or intramuscular injection; therapeutic 10 000 units to 30 000 units by intramuscular injection; *or* 40 000 to 100 000 units by intravenous injection in 2 divided doses with an interval of ½–2 hours
Available from distributor (Regent) or stocks may be held by hospital pharmacies

14.4.4   Hepatitis B

Hepatitis B vaccine is an alum adsorbed, inactivated hepatitis B virus surface antigen (HBsAg) vaccine prepared from the plasma of human carriers. The vaccine is used in individuals at high risk of contracting hepatitis B.

In the UK high-risk groups include health care personnel and patients in units where there is a high incidence of hepatitis B or a direct risk of contact with contaminated human blood, and also certain family contacts of carriers. Similar persons in indirect contact with a source of infection and at a lower risk would be considered a lower priority group. Another group for whom vaccination is recommended is infants born to hepatitis B carriers or HBsAg-positive mothers, particularly if they are e antigen-positive or are without anti-e antibody. Active immunisation combined with hepatitis B immunoglobulin is started immediately after delivery, but the precise details of dosage and optimal spacing of doses for active-passive immunisation have yet to be defined. More detailed guidance is given in DHSS circular

CMO(82)13/CNO(82)11. Vaccination does not eliminate the need for commonsense precautions for avoiding the risk of infection from known carriers by the routes of infection which have been clearly established. Accidental inoculation of hepatitis B virus-infected blood into a wound, incision, needle-prick, or abrasion may lead to infection, whereas it is unlikely that indirect exposure to a carrier will do so.

Specific hyperimmune immunoglobulin (HBIG) is available for those accidentally infected (section 14.5.2).

▼ PoM **H-B-Vax®** (Morson)

A suspension of hepatitis B surface antigen 20 micrograms/ml adsorbed onto alum. Price 1-ml vial = **J**

Dose: by intramuscular injection, 3 doses of 1 ml, the second 1 month and the third 6 months after the first dose; CHILD birth to 10 years 3 doses of 0.5 ml

14.4.5   Influenza

While most viruses are antigenically stable, the influenza viruses A and B (especially A) are constantly altering their antigenic structure as indicated by changes in the haemagglutinins (H) and neuraminidases (N) on the surface of the viruses. It is essential that influenza vaccines in use contain the H and N components of the prevalent strain or strains.

The recommended virus strains for vaccine production are grown in the allantoic cavity of developing chick embryos (and are therefore **contra-indicated** in those who are sensitive to eggs or feathers). The allantoic fluid is purified and the vaccines containing the haemagglutinin and neuraminidase of the strain expected to become prevalent are harvested. The World Health Organization makes recommendations every year as to what strains should be included in the vaccines and 3 strains are advised for the 1985–6 season; A/Philippines/2/82 (H_3N_2), A/Chile/1/83(H_1N_1), and B/USSR/100/83. If the H and N of the anticipated strain are different from that of recent strains it may be that 2 doses of vaccine will be required; on the other hand the value of annual immunisation with vaccine prepared from related strains is doubtful. Children under the age of 13 who are in high risk categories should receive 2 doses of influenza vaccine, inactivated (surface antigen) with an interval of 4–6 weeks.

Since the influenza vaccines will not control epidemics they are recommended only for those at high risk, particularly the elderly, those with chronic disease of the cardiovascular, respiratory, renal, and endocrine systems, and for those living in closed institutions where opportunites for contact and spread are great. In non-pandemic years immunisation is not recommended for Health Service staff, except for those at special risk.

Purified surface-antigen vaccines should be used in children aged 4–12 years; older children and adults may be vaccinated with surface-antigen or whole or split virus vaccine.

Drug interactions: see Appendix 1 (section *3*).

PoM **Influenza Vaccine, Inactivated** Flu/Vac. Used for active immunisation against influenza (see notes above)

Dose: 0.5 ml by deep subcutaneous or intramuscular injection

PoM **Influenza Vaccine, Inactivated (Surface Antigen)** Flu/Vac/SA. Used for active immunisation against influenza (see notes above)

Dose: 0.5 ml by deep subcutaneous or intramuscular injection

PoM **Fluvirin®** (Evans)

Inactivated influenza vaccine, surface antigen (purified). Price 0.5-ml syringe = **F**; 5- and 25-ml vial (both) = **J**

Dose: 0.5 ml by deep subcutaneous or intramuscular injection

PoM **Influvac Sub-unit®** (Duphar)

Inactivated influenza vaccine, surface antigen. Price 0.5-ml amp or syringe = **F**; 5- and 25-ml vial (both) = **J**

Dose: 0.5 ml by deep subcutaneous or intramuscular injection

PoM **MFV-Ject®** (Servier)

Inactivated influenza vaccine (split virus vaccine). Price 0.5-ml syringe = **F**; 5- and 25-ml vial (both) = **J**

Dose: 0.5 ml by subcutaneous or intramuscular injection

14.4.6   Measles

Measles vaccine consists of a live attenuated strain of measles virus grown in chick-embryo fibroblast-tissue cultures (since it contains virtually no residual egg protein it is contra-indicated only in those known to suffer from severe hypersensitivity to egg protein with a history of the anaphylactoid type). It should be offered to all children in the second year of life and may be expected to produce a durable immunity.

Administration of this vaccine to children may be associated with a mild measles-like syndrome with a measles-like rash and pyrexia which come on about a week after the injection of the vaccine. Much less commonly, convulsions and, rarely, encephalitis have been reported as being associated with measles vaccines. Convulsions in babies are relatively common and may occur by chance following any immunisation procedure; they are certainly much less frequently associated with measles vaccine than with other conditions leading to febrile episodes.

Serious neurological complications following the vaccine are extremely rare, perhaps of the order of 1 in 87 000 vaccinees and probably about 12–20 times less common than such complications associated with natural infections of measles, but it is difficult to get exact figures because of variable criteria of what is diagnosed as a serious neurological condition. Subacute sclerosing panencephalitis follows natural measles infection at a rate of approximately 5 to 10 cases for every million children who have developed measles. This condition may be associated with live measles vaccine at a rate of 0.5–1.0 case per million doses of vaccine distributed, and so it appears that measles vaccination to some extent protects against subacute sclerosing panencephalitis.

Unfortunately, measles vaccine is taken up by only about 50% of those eligible. This is said to be due to the fact that some doctors and parents do not consider that measles is now a serious disease. It is possible that, when there is a partial coverage of the susceptible members of population with vaccine, wild measles virus does not spread so readily, which means that in vaccinated communities, many children will grow up susceptible and may be subject to an attack of measles as adolescents or adults when the disease may be more serious.

Measles vaccine may also be used in the control of outbreaks and should be offered to school and playstreet contacts within 3 days of exposure to infection.

Because of the generally poor uptake of this vaccine in the second year of life, it would seem wise to offer the vaccine also to children at entry to playgroup, nursery, or primary school. Again it would seem sensible to offer vaccine to any child entering secondary school who has not had either a natural infection or a previous dose of vaccine.

Children with a personal history of convulsions, or whose parents or siblings (first-degree relatives) have a history of idiopathic epilepsy should be given measles vaccine only with simultaneous administration of specially diluted normal immunoglobulin (obtainable from hospital pharmacies or the Blood Products Laboratory, Dagger Lane, Elstree, Herts, telephone 01-953 6191) supplied for use with measles vaccine.

Children with partially or totally impaired immune responsiveness should not receive live vaccines. See section 14.1 for further contra-indications. If they have been exposed to measles infection they should be given normal immunoglobulin (section 14.5.1).

PoM **Measles Vaccine, Live** Meas/Vac(Live). Freeze-dried stabilised aqueous suspension of an approved strain of live attenuated measles virus grown in culture of chick-embryo cells. Used for active immunisation against measles (see schedule, section 14.6)

▼ PoM **Attenuvax®** (Morson)
Measles vaccine, live, Enders' Edmonston strain. Price single-dose vial (with diluent) = **D**
Dose: 0.5 ml by subcutaneous injection

PoM **Mevilin-L®** (Evans)
Measles vaccine, live, Schwarz strain. Price single-dose vial (with diluent) = **D**
Dose: 0.5 ml by subcutaneous or intramuscular injection

PoM **Rimevax®** (SK&F)
Measles vaccine, live, Schwarz strain. Price single-dose vial (with diluent) = **D**
Dose: 0.5 ml by subcutaneous or intramuscular injection

14.4.7 Mumps

Mumps vaccine consists of a live attenuated strain of virus grown in chick-embryo tissue culture.

Since mumps and its complications are very rarely serious there is little indication for the routine use of mumps vaccine. See section 14.1 for contra-indications.

PoM **Mumpsvax®** (Morson)
Mumps vaccine (Jeryl Lynn strain) Single-dose vial with syringe containing solvent. Price complete unit = **F**
Dose: adults and children over 1 year, 0.5 ml by subcutaneous injection

14.4.8 Pertussis (whooping-cough)

Pertussis vaccine is usually given combined with diphtheria and tetanus vaccine starting after the third month of life (see schedule, section 14.6) but may also be given as a simple vaccine.

Pertussis-containing vaccines may give rise to local reactions at the site of injection, mild pyrexia, and irritability. With some vaccines available in the early 1960s persistent screaming and collapse were reported but these reactions are rarely observed with the vaccines now available.

Convulsions and encephalopathy have been reported as rare complications, but such conditions may arise from other causes and be falsely attributed to the vaccine. A 3-year study of children aged 2 months–3 years who were admitted to hospitals in Great Britain suffering from serious neurological illness of the type likely to be attributed to whooping-cough vaccine has been carried out. Out of the first 1000 cases notified to the study, only 35 children had received pertussis vaccine within 7 days before becoming ill. Of these 35 children, 32 had no previous neurological abnormality and on follow-up of these children 1 year later, 2 had died and 9 had developmental retardation, while 21 were normal.

It is advisable to postpone vaccination if the child is suffering from any acute febrile illness, particularly if it is respiratory, until fully recovered. Minor infections without fever or systemic upset are not regarded as contra-indications. Vaccination should not be carried out in children who have

(1) a history of any severe local or general reaction, *including a neurological reaction*, to a preceding dose; or
(2) a history of cerebral irritation or damage in the neonatal period, or who have suffered from fits or convulsions.

There are certain groups of children in whom whooping-cough vaccination is not absolutely contra-indicated but who require special consideration as to its advisability. These groups are

(1) children whose parents or siblings have a history of idiopathic epilepsy;
(2) children with developmental delay thought to be due to a neurological defect; and
(3) children with neurological disease.

For these groups the risk of vaccination may be higher than in normal children but the effects of whooping-cough may be more severe, so that the benefits of vaccination would also be greater. The balance of risk and benefit should be assessed with special care in each individual case.

C = 51-100p, **D** = 101-180p, **E** = 181-300p, **F** = 301-450p, **G** = 451-650p, **H** = 651-900p, **I** = 901-1200p, **J** = over 1200p.

Allergy, according to a substantial body of medical opinion, is not a contra-indication to the administration of pertussis vaccine, but doctors should use their own discretion in the individual case.

PoM **Pertussis Vaccine** Per/Vac. A sterile suspension of killed *Bordetella pertussis*. Used for active immunisation against whooping-cough when simultaneous immunisation against diphtheria and tetanus is not required (see schedule, section 14.6). Price 0.5-ml amp = **C**
Dose: 0.5 ml or as specified on the label by intramuscular or deep subcutaneous injection

14.4.9   Pneumococcal pneumonia

A polyvalent pneumonia vaccine is available for the immunisation of persons for whom the risk of contracting pneumococcal pneumonia is unusually high, for example patients who have had a splenectomy. It is effective in a single dose if the types of pneumonia in the community are reflected in the polysaccharides contained in the vaccine. Studies with other pneumococcal vaccines suggest that protection may last for 5 years. Revaccination should not be carried out after less than 3 years or there may be a high level of frequent and severe local reactions. The vaccine should not be given to children under 2 years, in pregnancy, or when there is infection. It should be used with caution in cardiovascular or respiratory disease. Hypersensitivity reactions may occur.

PoM **Pneumovax**® (Morson)
For details, contact manufacturer

14.4.10   Poliomyelitis

There are two types of poliomyelitis vaccine, namely poliomyelitis vaccine, inactivated, and poliomyelitis vaccine, live (oral). The oral vaccine, consisting of a mixture of attenuated strains of virus types 1, 2, and 3 is at present generally used.

INITIAL COURSE. **Poliomyelitis vaccine, live (oral)** is given on 3 occasions, usually at the same time as routine immunisation against diphtheria, tetanus, and pertussis (see schedule, section 14.6).

REINFORCEMENT. A reinforcing dose of oral poliomyelitis vaccine is recommended at school entry at which time children should also receive a reinforcing dose of diphtheria and tetanus vaccine. Oral poliomyelitis vaccine is also recommended at school leaving at the same time as a dose of tetanus vaccine.
Unimmunised parents who are having their babies immunised should be offered vaccine at the same time because of a very small risk of infection of parents from vaccine virus which may have increased in neurovirulence following replication in the gut of their baby. Contact vaccine-associated poliomyelitis such as this is rare, and so is vaccine-associated poliomyelitis in those who actually received the vaccine. These adverse effects occur about once in one or more millions of vaccinated persons.
Contra-indications to the use of oral poliomyelitis vaccine include diarrhoea and hypogammaglobulinaemia. See section 14.1 for further contra-indications.

TRAVELLERS. Travellers to areas other than Australia, New Zealand, Northern Europe, and North America should be given a full course of oral poliomyelitis vaccine if they have not been immunised in the past. Those who have received immunisation should be given a single booster dose of oral poliomyelitis vaccine.
At the present time **poliomyelitis vaccine (inactivated)** may be used for those in whom poliomyelitis vaccine (oral) is contra-indicated because of pregnancy or immunosuppressive disorders.

PoM **Poliomyelitis Vaccine, Inactivated** Pol/Vac (Inact). An inactivated suspension of suitable strains of poliomyelitis virus, types 1, 2, and 3. Used for active immunisation when the oral vaccine is contra-indicated, as in pregnancy or immunosuppressive disorders.
Dose: 0.5 ml or as stated on the label by deep subcutaneous or intramuscular injection; for primary immunisation 3 doses are required (see schedule, section 14.6)
   Availability—section 14.4

PoM **Poliomyelitis Vaccine, Live (Oral)** Pol/Vac (Oral). A suspension of suitable live attenuated strains of poliomyelitis virus, types 1, 2, and 3. Used for active immunisation. Available in single-dose and 10-dose containers
Dose: 3 drops or as stated on the label; for primary immunisation 3 doses are required (see schedule, section 14.6)
   Available from District Health Authorities

14.4.11   Rabies

Since the time of Pasteur there have been a number of rabies vaccines in which the virus has been grown in nervous tissue of various animals. All of these vaccines have been associated with a greater or lesser degree of postvaccinal allergic encephalomyelitis. Other vaccines made from virus grown in animal tissue cultures or in embryonated duck eggs have tended to be of low antigenicity as measured by the levels of circulating antibodies achieved.
A human diploid cell vaccine has now been developed. This vaccine has been shown to be life saving in trials carried out in Iran in people who had been bitten by infected wolves. It should be offered prophylactically to those at high risk—those working in quarantine stations, animal handlers, veterinary surgeons, and field workers who may be exposed to bites of wild animals. A detailed list is given in Health Circular HC(77)29. For prophylactic use the vaccine produces a good antibody response when given in a 2-dose schedule with an interval of one month between doses and a reinforcing dose after an interval of 6–12 months with further reinforcing doses every 3 years when required.

For post-exposure treatment of previously unvaccinated patients a course of injections should be started as soon as possible after exposure (days 0, 3, 7, 14, 30, and 90). The course may be discontinued if it is proved that the patient was not at risk. There are no known contra-indications to this diploid cell vaccine and its use should be considered whenever a patient has been attacked by an animal in a country where rabies is endemic, even if there is no direct evidence of rabies in the attacking animal.

Staff in attendance on a patient who is highly suspected of, or known to be suffering from, rabies should be offered vaccination. Four intra-cutaneous doses of 0.1 ml of human diploid cell vaccine (Merieux) given on the same day at different sites has been suggested for this purpose in the *Memorandum on Rabies*.

Advice on the use of rabies vaccine for pre-exposure prophylaxis and on the use of vaccine and immunoglobulin (section 14.5.2) for post-exposure use is given in Department of Health and Social Security, *Memorandum on Rabies*, London, HMSO, 1977. Advice on post-exposure vaccination and treatment of rabies is available from the Duty Medical Officer, Central Public Health Laboratory, Colindale Avenue, Colindale, London NW9 5HT, telephone 01-200 4400.

PoM **Rabies Vaccine** Rab/Vac. An inactivated suspension of suitable strains of rabies virus grown in cell cultures

Available in accordance with Health Circular HC(77)29 from the Central Public Health Laboratory, London; Regional Public Health Laboratories in Birmingham, Cardiff, Leeds, Liverpool, and Newcastle; and the Area Public Health Laboratory, Exeter on a named-patient basis

▼ PoM **Merieux Inactivated Rabies Vaccine**® (Servier)

Freeze-dried human diploid cell rabies vaccine prepared from Wistar strain PM/WI 38 1503-3M. For prevention and treatment of rabies. Price single-dose vial with syringe containing diluent = **J**

Dose: prophylactic, 1 ml by deep subcutaneous injection, followed by a second dose after 1 month and a third after 6–12 months; also further reinforcing doses every 3 years depending on the risk of infection

Therapeutic, 1 ml on the first, third, seventh and fourteenth day and after 1 and 3 months

14.4.12 Rubella

The introduction of a vaccine to protect a fetus as yet not conceived was a totally new idea. Rubella (German measles) as a childhood disease is of little moment, but rubella infection in the pregnant woman greatly increases the risk of congenital malformations in the fetus which is more severe the earlier in pregnancy the infection occurs.

Rubella vaccines are prepared in tissue-culture cells of rabbit kidney or duck embryo, or human diploid cell lines. **Contra-indications** with regard to sensitivities or antibiotics vary from one vaccine to another and as always the literature accompanying the package should be consulted. But the main contra-indication at present applying to all of the available vaccines is pregnancy. See section 14.1 for further contra-indications.

Rubella vaccine is recommended for pre-pubertal girls aged 10 to 13 years and for women of childbearing age (see schedule, section 14.6) as well as those who might put pregnant women at risk of infection (for example nurses and doctors in obstetric units). It is recommended practice to offer vaccine to those women who are found to be seronegative to rubella virus.

The important point is that women offered vaccine should **not** become pregnant for 3 months after immunisation. If this cannot be assured then vaccine should at present be withheld. At the same time more and more evidence is accumulating which suggests that rubella vaccine virus may present less risk to the fetus than was originally thought compared with the serious risk of wild rubella virus in pregnant women. For short-term interim contraception at the time of vaccination medroxyprogesterone acetate (section 7.3.2) may be suitable.

In addition to offering vaccine to schoolgirls and those at special risk, vaccine is also being offered to previously unvaccinated and sero-negative post-partum women. Again they must avoid pregnancy for 3 months. Immunising susceptible post-partum women a few days after delivery is important as far as the overall reduction of congenital abnormalities in the UK is concerned, for about 60% of these abnormalities occur in the babies of multiparous women.

In the long term it is hoped that the routine immunisation of schoolgirls will produce an immune adult female population but in order to prevent congenital abnormalities due to rubella it may require 100% acceptance of vaccine and this has rarely been achieved with other vaccines. Acceptance amongst schoolgirls might be greater if the effort was concentrated among 10-year-olds, but even so, with a high acceptance rate the efficacy of this programme will not be evident until the end of the century. At the same time the damage which is done by wild rubella virus must be kept in perspective, for it is responsible for perhaps only about 1% of all congenital abnormalities.

Susceptible pregnant women who are exposed to rubella and who refuse therapeutic abortion may be offered normal immunoglobulin injection (section 14.5.1).

PoM **Rubella Vaccine, Live** Rub/Vac (Live). A freeze-dried suspension of a suitable live attenuated strain of rubella virus grown in suitable cell cultures. Used for active immunisation against rubella (see schedule, section 14.6 and notes above). Price 0.5-ml amp = **E**; 5-ml vial = **J**

Dose: 0.5 ml by subcutaneous injection. Not to be given to any woman who may be pregnant. Advise women not to become pregnant within 3 months of vaccination

---

C = 51-100p, D = 101-180p, E = 181-300p, F = 301-450p, G = 451-650p, H = 651-900p, I = 901-1200p, J = over 1200p.

PoM **Almevax**® (Wellcome)
  Rubella vaccine, live, prepared from Wistar RA
  27/3 strain propagated in human diploid cells.
  Price single-dose amp with diluent = **E**; 10-dose
  vial with diluent = **J**
PoM **Cendevax**® (SK&F)
  Rubella vaccine, live, prepared from Cendehill
  strain propagated in primary rabbit kidney
  cells. Price single-dose vial with diluent = **E**;
  10-dose vial with diluent = **J**
▼ PoM **Meruvax II**® (Morson)
  Rubella vaccine, live, prepared from Wistar
  RA27/3 strain propagated in human diploid
  cells. Price single-dose vial with diluent = **D**

14.4.13 Smallpox

Smallpox vaccination is no longer required
routinely in the UK and other countries because
global eradication of smallpox has now been
achieved. The vaccine is offered to a small number
of doctors and other health workers who may
be called upon to deal with suspected cases of
smallpox. Otherwise the only requirement for
smallpox vaccination is for a few workers in
institutions dealing with pox viruses. Contra-
indications to elective smallpox vaccine are pregnancy, babies under 1 year, any illness at the
time of vaccination, eczema in the vaccinees or in
members of their households; the vaccine is also
contra-indicated in patients with impaired
immune responsiveness, whether occurring naturally or as a result of radiotherapy or treatment
with corticosteroids or other immunosuppressive
drugs. See section 14.1 for further contra-
indications.

PoM **Smallpox Vaccine** Var/Vac. Consists of a
suspension of live vaccinia virus grown in the
skin of living animals, supplied in freeze-dried
form with diluent
Dose: 0.05 ml by multiple pressure inoculation
or through a single linear scratch not more than
2–3 mm long
  Available from Regional Public Health Laboratories in Birmingham, Bristol, Cambridge,
Cardiff, Leeds, Liverpool, Manchester, Newcastle, Oxford, and Sheffield; and the Area Public Health Laboratory at Whipps Cross Hospital,
London

14.4.14 Tetanus

Tetanus vaccine stimulates the production of the
protective antitoxin. It is offered routinely to
babies in combination with diphtheria vaccine
(DT/Vac/Ads) and more usually also combined
with killed *Bordetella pertussis* organisms as
Diphtheria, Tetanus, and Pertussis Vaccine (DT
Per/Vac) or as an adsorbed vaccine (DT Per/
Vac/Ads), see schedule, section 14.6. In general,
adsorption on aluminium hydroxide, aluminium
phosphate, or calcium phosphate improves the
antigenicity of diphtheria and tetanus toxoids.
The combined vaccines are described under
Diphtheria (section 14.4.3).
  Of the monovalent tetanus vaccines the

adsorbed tetanus vaccine is to be preferred to the
plain vaccine. Adsorbed vaccine may be given in
reduced dosage to patients who have previously
reacted abnormally to the vaccine but only when
they are considered to be at high risk. Adsorbed
vaccine must not be given intracutaneously.
  In children, the triple vaccine or a course of
adsorbed diphtheria and tetanus vaccine not only
gives protection against tetanus in childhood but
also gives the basic immunity for subsequent reinforcing doses of tetanus vaccine at school entry
and at school leaving and also when a potentially
tetanus-contaminated injury has been received.
Normally, tetanus vaccine should not be given
unless more than 5 years have elapsed since the
last reinforcing dose of tetanus toxoid because of
the possibility that hypersensitivity reactions may
develop.
  Active immunisation is important for persons
in older age groups for they may never have
had the routine courses of immunisation when
younger. In these persons a course of tetanus
vaccine (adsorbed) may be given.
  For serious, potentially contaminated wounds
antitetanus immunoglobulin injection (section
14.5.2) should be selectively used in addition to
wound toilet, adsorbed tetanus vaccine, and benzylpenicillin or another anaerobicidal antibiotic.

PoM **Tetanus Vaccine** Tet/Vac/FT. Tetanus formol toxoid. Used for active immunisation against
tetanus (see notes). Price 0.5-ml amp = **C**; 5-ml
vial = **E**
Dose: 0.5 ml or as stated on the label, by intramuscular or deep subcutaneous injection followed after 6–12 weeks by a second dose and
after a further 4–12 months by a third
PoM **Tetanus Vaccine, Adsorbed** Tet/Vac/Ads.
Prepared from tetanus formol toxoid with a mineral carrier (aluminium hydroxide, aluminium
phosphate, or calcium phosphate). Price 0.5-ml
amp = **B**; 5-ml vial = **E**
Dose: as for Tetanus Vaccine
PoM **Merieux Tetavax**® (Servier)
  Tetanus formol toxoid adsorbed onto aluminium
  hydroxide. Price 0.5-ml amp = **B**; 0.5-ml single-
  dose syringe = **C**; 5-ml vial = **E**
  Dose: 0.5 ml by deep subcutaneous or intramuscular injection followed after 6–8 weeks by
  a second dose and after a further 4–6 months
  by a third

14.4.15 Tuberculosis

BCG (Bacillus Calmette-Guérin) is a live attenuated strain derived from bovine *Mycobacterium
tuberculosis* which stimulates the development of
hypersensitivity to *M. tuberculosis*. Vaccine is
given by intracutaneous injection or the percutaneous vaccine may be given by multiple puncture. 0.1 ml of the vaccine (reconstituted immediately before use) is injected intracutaneously just
above the insertion of the deltoid muscle raising
a wheal of about 8 mm in diameter. If it is injected
too high, too far forward, or too far backward,
the adjacent lymph glands may become involved

and tender. After about 1 week a small swelling appears at the injection site which progresses to a papule or to a benign ulcer about 10 mm in diameter after 3 weeks and heals in 6–12 weeks. No dressing should be used unless there is much discharge from the ulcer.

Normally, BCG is offered routinely to tuberculin-negative children of 10–13 years. BCG vaccination should also be strongly recommended to those living in crowded conditions in urban communities and to all immigrants and their children from countries with a high incidence of tuberculosis. They should be tuberculin tested before vaccination with the exception of newborn babies who should be vaccinated without delay. With babies great care must be taken to ensure that the inoculation is given intracutaneously in a dose of 0.05 ml; if BCG is accidentally given subcutaneously to babies it may give rise to a troublesome persistent local reaction. See section 14.1 for contra-indications.

PoM **Bacillus Calmette-Guérin Vaccine.** BCG Vaccine, Dried Tub/Vac/BCG. A freeze-dried preparation of live bacteria of a strain derived from the bacillus of Calmette and Guérin. Used for active immunisation
Dose: 0.1 ml (infants under 3 months 0.05 ml) by intracutaneous injection
Available from District Health Authorities

PoM **Bacillus Calmette-Guérin Vaccine, Percutaneous** Tub/Vac/BCG(Perc). A preparation of live bacteria of a strain derived from the bacillus of Calmette and Guérin. Used for active immunisation (see notes) and administered by the percutaneous route by multiple puncture with a suitable instrument. **Not** for intracutaneous (intradermal) injection.
Dose: 0.02 ml by percutaneous administration
Available on direct application from the manufacturer (Glaxo)

DIAGNOSTIC REAGENTS. In the *Mantoux test* the initial dose is 1 unit of tuberculin PPD in 0.1 ml by intracutaneous injection and in subsequent tests 10 and finally 100 units in 0.1 ml are given. In the *Heaf test* (multiple puncture) a solution containing 100 000 units in 1 ml is used. For the *Tine, Imotest,* and other similar tests a special device impregnated with tuberculin is used.

PoM **Tuberculin PPD.** Prepared from the heat-treated products of growth and lysis of the appropriate species of mycobacterium, and containing 100 000 units/ml. Price 1-ml vial = **E**; 5-ml vial = **I**. Also available diluted 1 in 100 (1000 units/ml), 1 in 1000 (100 units/ml), and 1 in 10000 (10 units/ml). Price 1 ml (all) = **C**
Dose: see notes above
Available from District Health Authorities

14.4.16   Typhoid

Typhoid vaccination is no substitute for personal precautions in avoiding typhoid fever in countries where the disease is endemic; green salads and uncooked vegetables should be avoided and only fruits which can be skinned should be eaten. Only suitable bottled water or water treated with sterilising tablets should be used for drinking purposes.

Typhoid vaccine (monovalent typhoid vaccine) is used and because it contains no paratyphoid components it is less likely to produce the local and systemic reactions which have, in the past, been so commonly associated with TAB. These local reactions which consist of swelling, pain, and tenderness appear about 2–3 hours after the subcutaneous or intramuscular injection of the vaccine. Systemic reactions which consist of fever, malaise, and headache may also occur and usually last for about 48 hours after injection. If severe reactions are experienced after the first dose intracutaneous injection may be preferred for the second dose, as these reactions are virtually absent when this route is used. Normally, 2 doses should be given at 4–6 weeks interval for primary immunisation, with reinforcing doses about every 2 or 3 years on continued exposure.

PoM **Typhoid Vaccine** Typhoid/Vac. A suspension of killed *Salmonella typhi* organisms. Used for active immunisation against typhoid. Price 1.5-ml vial = **E**
Dose: 0.5 ml by deep subcutaneous or intramuscular injection; CHILD 1–10 years 0.25 ml
Second dose after 4–6 weeks, 0.5 ml (or 0.1 ml by intracutaneous injection); CHILD 1–10 years 0.25 ml (or 0.1 ml by intracutaneous injection)

14.4.17   Typhus

The vaccine consists of formalin-inactivated *Rickettsia prowazekii* grown in the yolk sac of embryonated hens' eggs and is effective against louse-borne typhus. This vaccine is not necessary for travellers visiting countries where the disease is endemic if they will be staying in urban accommodation but it could be of value for those living in close personal contact with the indigenous population of such areas. However the vaccine is no longer distributed in the United Kingdom but may be obtained on a named patient basis from the Commonwealth Serum Laboratories, Parkville 3052, Victoria, Australia.

14.4.18   Yellow Fever

Yellow fever vaccine consists of a live attenuated yellow fever virus (17D strain) grown in developing chick embryos. It is available only at designated centres, but should not be given to children under 9 months of age since it may cause them to develop encephalitis. Vaccine should not be given to individuals who are pregnant, have impaired immune responsiveness, or who are sensitive to eggs. See section 14.1 for further contra-indications. Reactions are few. The immunity which probably lasts for life is officially accepted for 10 years starting from 10 days after primary vaccination and for a further 10 years immediately after revaccination.

C = 51-100p, D = 101-180p, E = 181-300p, F = 301-450p, G = 451-650p, H = 651-900p, I = 901-1200p, J = over 1200p.

PoM **Yellow Fever Vaccine, Live** Yel/Vac. A suspension of chick embryo proteins containing attenuated 17D strain virus. Used for active immunisation against yellow fever

Dose: the volume indicated on the label by subcutaneous injection

Available from designated Yellow Fever Vaccination centres only

PoM **Arilvax®** (Wellcome)
Freeze-dried yellow fever vaccine, live. 1-, 5-, and 10-dose vials (with diluent)

14.5   Immunoglobulins

The injection of immunoglobulins produces immediate protection. Normally, when foreign immunoglobulins are injected, antibodies develop and this presents problems of hypersensitivity; these properties of horse and other animal sera have led to virtual abandonment of animal immunoglobulins for passive protection and human immunoglobulins have taken their place.

There are essentially two types of human immunoglobulin preparation: human **normal immunoglobulin** (HNIG, gamma globulin) prepared from the plasma of at least 1000 donors, and **specific immunoglobulins** for tetanus, rabies, vaccinia, etc. which are prepared by pooling the blood of convalescent patients or of immunised donors who have recently been specifically boosted.

Normal immunoglobulins and the specific immunoglobulins are available from the Public Health Laboratory Service laboratories and Regional Blood Transfusion Centres in England and Wales with the exception of antitetanus immunoglobulin which is distributed through Regional Blood Transfusion Centres to hospital pharmacies or blood transfusion departments and is also available to general medical practitioners, and antirabies immunoglobulin which is available from the Central Public Health Laboratory, London (section 14.4.11).

In Scotland all immunoglobulins are available from Blood Transfusion Centres. Antitetanus immunoglobulin is distributed by Blood Transfusion Centres to hospitals and general medical practitioners on demand. Normal immunoglobulin injection and antitetanus immunoglobulin injection are also available commercially.

14.5.1   Normal immunoglobulin

HEPATITIS A (infective hepatitis). At the time of writing there are no suitable techniques available for growing hepatitis A virus in quantities which would make vaccine preparation possible. Control depends on good hygiene and many studies have also shown the value of normal immunoglobulin in the prevention and control of outbreaks of this disease. It is recommended for controlling infection in contacts in closed institutions and also, under certain conditions, in school and home contacts and for travellers going to areas where the disease is highly endemic. The usual prophylactic dose by intramuscular injection

for adults and children is 0.02–0.04 ml/kg. This usually gives immunological protection for 3 months; for greater than 3 months periods of exposure or in areas of high endemicity, the dose is 0.06–0.12 ml/kg, repeated every 4–6 months on continued exposure.

MEASLES. Normal immunoglobulin may be used to modify or prevent measles in the few babies in whom an attack of measles must be avoided and in children in whom live measles vaccine is contraindicated; specially diluted normal immunoglobulin should be used to moderate the reactions to measles vaccine in children with a personal history of convulsions, or whose parents or siblings (first-degree relatives) have a history of idiopathic epilepsy (section 14.4.6).

RUBELLA. Normal immunoglobulin may lessen the likelihood of infection and fetal damage in pregnant women exposed to rubella for whom therapeutic abortion is unacceptable. The usual dose is 20 ml. It is not recommended for routine prophylaxis; see section 14.4.12.

PoM **Normal Immunoglobulin Injection** (HNIG). Immunoglobulin prepared from pools of at least 1000 donations of human plasma, available in liquid form or as a freeze-dried preparation for reconstitution. It is administered by intramuscular injection. Used for the protection of susceptible contacts against hepatitis A virus (infectious hepatitis), measles and, to a lesser extent, rubella. Special forms for intravenous administration are available for replacement therapy for patients with congenital agammaglobulinaemia and hypogammaglobulinaemia who are not able to tolerate repeated intramuscular injections. Live virus vaccine should not be given until 3 months after a dose of normal immunoglobulin injection. If a live virus vaccine has been given normal immunoglobulin injection should not be given for at least 2 weeks, except in special circumstances, e.g. the concomitant administration of measles vaccine with a specially diluted normal immunoglobulin is recommended for children with personal history of convulsions, or whose parents or siblings (first-degree relatives) have a history of idiopathic epilepsy (section 14.4.6). Rubella vaccine may be administered in the postpartum period with anti-D (Rh₀) immunoglobulin injection

PoM **Gammabulin®** (Immuno)
Normal immunoglobulin injection. Price 2-ml vial = **E**; 5-ml vial = **G**; 10-ml vial = **I**; 320-mg vial with 2 ml water for injections = **F**
▼ PoM **Intraglobin®** (Biotest Folex)
Normal immunoglobulin injection. Powder for reconstitution. Price 250 mg = **G**; 500 mg = **I**; 2.5 g = **J** (all with solvent)
PoM **Kabiglobulin** (KabiVitrum)
Normal immunoglobulin injection. Price 2-ml amp = **F**; 5-ml amp = **H**
▼ PoM **Sandoglobulin®** (Sandoz)
Normal immunoglobulin injection. Price 3- and

6-g bottle with 100- and 200-ml bottle, respectively, sodium chloride intravenous infusion 0.9% (both) = **J**. Transfer needle and giving set with each pack

14.5.2 Specific immunoglobulins

HEPATITIS B. A vaccine is now available for those at high risk of infection (section 14.4.4) but specific antihepatitis B virus immunoglobulin (HBIG) may be available for the prevention of infection in laboratory and other personnel who have accidentally become contaminated with hepatitis B virus and for pregnant women and babies born to mothers who have become infected with this virus in pregnancy.

RABIES. Following exposure to a suspected rabid animal, specific antirabies immunoglobulin, if possible of human origin, should be injected at the site of the bite and also given intramuscularly. Rabies vaccine (section 14.4.11) should also be given.

PoM **Antirabies Immunoglobulin Injection**. Used for protection of persons who have been bitten by rabid animals or otherwise exposed to infection
Dose: 20 units/kg by intramuscular injection and infiltration around wounds

TETANUS. Antitetanus immunoglobulin of human origin (HTIG) should be selectively used in addition to wound toilet, vaccine, and benzylpenicillin (or another anaerobicidal antibiotic) for the more seriously contaminated wounds but is rarely required for those who have an established immunity in whom protection may be achieved by a reinforcing dose of vaccine. The administration of antitetanus immunoglobulin should be considered for patients not known to have received active immunisation (a) whose wound was sustained more than 6 hours before treatment was received and (b) with puncture wounds or wounds potentially heavily contaminated with tetanus spores, septic, or with much devitalised tissue. A dose of adsorbed tetanus vaccine should be given at the same time as the antitetanus immunoglobulin and the course of vaccine (section 14.4.14) subsequently completed.

PoM **Antitetanus Immunoglobulin Injection** (HTIG). Used for the protection of unimmunised persons when there is a specific risk of tetanus
Dose: by intramuscular injection, prophylactic 250 units, therapeutic 30–300 units/kg
PoM **Humotet®** (Wellcome)
Antitetanus immunoglobulin injection 250 units/ml. Price 1-ml vial = **J**

VACCINIA. Antivaccinia immunoglobulin is available for the prevention and treatment of the complications of smallpox vaccination, as when vaccination is necessary in an individual for whom there are contra-indications to vaccination. It is also used in familial and other close contacts exposed to smallpox.

PoM **Antivaccinia Immunoglobulin Injection**. Used to treat patients with generalised vaccinia or with localised vaccinial infection that endangers the eye
Dose: by intramuscular injection, 1.5–2 g; CHILD under 1 year 500 mg, 1–6 years 1 g, and 7–14 years 1.5 g

OTHER SPECIFIC IMMUNOGLOBULINS. These include antivaricella/zoster immunoglobulin, antiherpes simplex immunoglobulin and are in limited supply. Others are under study, but their availability and evaluation requires the cooperation of general practitioners to provide blood from patients who are convalescent from these and other specific viral infections in order to prepare specific immunoglobulin preparations.

14.5.3 Anti-D (Rh₀) immunoglobulin

Anti-D immunoglobulin is available to prevent a rhesus-negative mother from forming antibodies to fetal rhesus-positive cells which may pass into the maternal circulation during childbirth or abortion. It must be injected within 72 hours of the birth or abortion. The objective is to protect any further child from the hazard of haemolytic disease.

PoM **Anti-D (Rh₀) Immunoglobulin Injection**. See notes above
Dose: for rhesus-negative women, 250–500 units by intramuscular injection following the birth of a rhesus-positive infant; after transfusion, up to 5000 units

14.6 Vaccination programmes for children

A schedule promulgated by the Department of Health and Social Security proposes that the course of adsorbed diphtheria, tetanus and pertussis vaccine, together with poliomyelitis vaccine (oral) should commence at 3 months. The schedule CMO(78)15—in Scotland SHHD/CAMO(78)18, on vaccination and immunisation procedures is set out in the Table. The principal points are as follows:

1. The basic course of triple vaccine, or diphtheria and tetanus vaccine, together with oral poliomyelitis vaccine should commence at the age of 3 months. The intervals between the 3 doses of the basic course should remain the same as those previously recommended, that is 6–8 weeks between the first and second doses and 4–6 months between the second and third doses.

2. An alternative basic course which completes the protection against pertussis at an earlier age is described but for use only in the event of a whooping-cough epidemic. If this alternative is followed a booster dose of diphtheria

Table: Schedule of vaccination and immunisation procedures (children and adults)

Age	Vaccine	Interval	Notes
During the first year of life	DTPer/Vac/Ads *and* Pol/Vac (Oral) (1st dose)		The first doses should be given at 3 months of age. If pertussis vaccine is contra-indicated or the parents decline, DT/Vac/Ads should be given
	DTPer/Vac/Ads *and* Pol/Vac (Oral) (2nd dose)	Preferably after an interval of 6–8 weeks	
	DTPer/Vac/Ads *and* Pol/Vac (Oral) (3rd dose)	Preferably after an interval of 4–6 months	
During the second year of life	Meas/Vac (Live)		
At school entry or entry to nursery school	DT/Vac/Ads *and* Pol/Vac (Oral)	Preferable to allow an interval of at least 3 years after completing basic course	
Between 10 and 13 years of age	Tub/Vac/BCG	Leave an interval of not less than 3 weeks between BCG and rubella vaccination	For tuberculin-negative children. For tuberculin-negative contacts at any age
Between 10 and 13 years of age (girls only)	Rub/Vac (Live)		All girls of this age should be offered rubella vaccine regardless of a past history of an attack of rubella
On leaving school or before employment or entering further education	Pol/Vac (Oral) *or* Pol/Vac (Inact); *and* Tet/Vac/Ads		
Adult life	Pol/Vac (Oral) *or* Pol/Vac (Inact) for previously unvaccinated adults	3 doses with an interval of 6–8 weeks between the first and second doses and of 4–6 months between the second and third	For travellers to countries where polio is endemic. Unvaccinated parents of a child being given oral vaccine should also be offered a course of Pol/Vac (Oral)
	Rub/Vac (Live) for susceptible women of child-bearing age		Adult females of child-bearing age should be tested for rubella antibodies and those sero-negative offered rubella vaccination. Pregnancy must first be excluded and the patient warned not to become pregnant for 3 months after immunisation
	Active immunisation against tetanus (Tet/Vac/Ads) for previously unvaccinated adults	For previously unvaccinated adults: 2 doses at an interval of 6–8 weeks followed by a third dose 6 months later	

and tetanus vaccine is necessary at 12–18 months of age to achieve a satisfactory level of immunity to these diseases.

3. It is recommended that a vaccine containing a pertussis component should not normally be offered after the age of 6 years.

Recently, some parents, who had chosen not to include a pertussis component in the basic immunisation of their infants, have changed their minds because of the greater prevalence of whooping-cough. The Joint Committee on Vaccination and Immunisation has advised that 3 doses of pertussis vaccine can be given at monthly intervals to provide protection in these cases. Where the basic course against diphtheria and tetanus is incomplete triple vaccine may be used to begin or complete the course against whooping-cough so that the infant is not given more injections than necessary.

Poliomyelitis vaccine, live (oral) is usually issued in 10-dose containers (although single-dose containers are also available). The vaccine should be stored unopened at 4° but once the containers are opened the vaccine may lose its potency however it is stored. For this reason any vaccine remaining in the containers at the end of an immunisation session should be discarded. There is particular need to conserve supplies of vaccines, which in any case are expensive. As far as possible immunisation sessions should therefore be arranged to avoid undue wastage of vaccines, although it is recognised that it will not always be possible to muster those to be vaccinated in groups of 10. The practicability of dispensing vaccines in smaller doses is being considered.

14.7 International travel

No particular immunisation is required for travellers to the United States, Northern Europe, Australia, or New Zealand. In Southern Europe and particularly in those areas surrounding the Mediterranean, in Africa, the Middle East, Asia, and South America, certain special precautions are required. Mention is made of the personal precautions which should be taken in the prevention of **typhoid** (section 14.4.16); these also apply to **cholera** (section 14.4.2) and other diarrhoeal diseases (including travellers' diarrhoea). Immunisation against typhoid is indicated for travellers to those countries where typhoid is endemic, and it would seem that the monovalent typhoid vaccine is acceptable, although it has not been subjected to detailed double-blind trials. Long-term travellers to areas that have a high incidence of **poliomyelitis** (section 14.4.10) or **tuberculosis** (section 14.4.15) should be immunised with the appropriate vaccine; in the

case of poliomyelitis previously vaccinated adults may be given a reinforcing dose of oral poliomyelitis vaccine. Overland travellers to Asia and Africa and others at high risk may be given **normal immunoglobulin injection** (section 14.5.1) for protection against hepatitis A.

Cholera vaccine is no substitute for personal hygiene but has some protective value for about 6 months in preventing individual infections. It is required for travellers by some countries and must be certified on an International Certificate. Stamped certificates supplied to general medical practitioners by Family Practitioner Committees (in Scotland by Health Boards) do not require to be authenticated by health authorities.

International Certificates of vaccination against **yellow fever** (section 14.4.18) are still required for travel to much of Africa and South America. The Health Departments of the UK have issued a leaflet, *Protect your health abroad* (SA 35), which can be obtained from travel agents, from local authorities, or DHSS Leaflets Unit, PO Box 21, Stanmore, Middx HA7 1AY; it gives information on vaccination centres, etc. for overseas travellers.

Vaccination requirements change from time to time, and information on the current requirements for any particular country may be obtained from the Department of Health and Social Security, Fleming House, London SE1 6BY, telephone 01-407 5522; Scottish Home and Health Department, St. Andrew's House, Edinburgh EH1 3DE, telephone 031 5568501; Welsh Office, Cathays Park, Cardiff, telephone Cardiff 825111; Department of Health and Social Services, Dundonald House, Upper Newtownards Road, Belfast, telephone 0232 63939; or from the embassy or legation of the appropriate country.

15: Drugs used in

ANAESTHESIA

This chapter describes briefly drugs used in anaesthesia in minor and major surgery. The reader is referred to other sources for more detailed information on techniques of anaesthesia. This chapter is divided into two sections: general anaesthesia (15.1) and local anaesthesia (15.2).

15.1 General anaesthesia

15.1.1	Intravenous anaesthetics
15.1.2	Inhalational anaesthetics
15.1.3	Anticholinergic premedication drugs
15.1.4	Sedative and analgesic peri-operative drugs
15.1.4.1	Narcotic analgesics
15.1.4.2	Anxiolytics and neuroleptics
15.1.5	Muscle relaxants
15.1.6	Anticholinesterases used in surgery
15.1.7	Antagonists for respiratory depression
15.1.8	Antagonists for malignant hyperthermia

Note: The drugs in section 15.1 should be used only by experienced personnel and in premises where adequate resuscitative equipment is available.

MODERN ANAESTHETIC TECHNIQUE. It is now common practice to administer several drugs with different actions to produce a state of surgical anaesthesia with minimal risk of toxic effects. An intravenous agent is frequently used for induction, followed by maintenance with inhalational anaesthetics, perhaps supplemented by other drugs administered intravenously. Specific drugs are often used to produce muscular relaxation. Many of the agents used interfere with the reflex maintenance of spontaneous respiration and intermittent positive pressure ventilation by manual or mechanical means is commonly employed.

For certain procedures controlled hypotension may be required. Labetalol (see section 2.4), sodium nitroprusside (see section 2.5.1), and trimetaphan camsylate (see section 2.5.6) are used.

Beta-adrenoceptor blocking drugs (see section 2.4) may be used to control arrhythmias during anaesthesia.

Concurrent or recent administration of corticosteroids may cause a precipitous fall in blood pressure during anaesthesia.

For drug interactions of general anaesthetics, see Appendix 1 (section 15).

15.1.1 Intravenous anaesthetics

Intravenous anaesthesics may be used alone to produce anaesthesia for short surgical procedures but are more commonly used for induction only. Intravenous anaesthetics are potent drugs which nearly all produce their effect in one arm-brain circulation time and can cause apnoea and hypotension, and so adequate resuscitative facilities

must be available. Large doses should be avoided in obstetrics, as the drug may cross the placental barrier. The drugs are **contra-indicated** in any dose in patients in whom the anaesthetist is not confident to maintain the airway, for example if there are tumours in the pharynx or larynx. Extreme care is required in surgery of the mouth, pharynx, or larynx and patients with acute cardiovascular failure (shock) or fixed cardiac output. Patients with a full stomach present a hazard during induction since there is a danger of silent regurgitation.

Individual requirements vary considerably and the recommended dosage is only a guide. Smaller dosage is indicated in ill, shocked, or debilitated patients, while robust individuals may require more. The estimated dosage should be injected over 20 seconds and a further 20 to 30 seconds allowed to assess the effect before a supplementary dose is given. For tracheal intubation, induction should be followed by inhalational anaesthesia or by a neuromuscular blocking drug.

Thiopentone sodium (Intraval®) is the most widely used intravenous anaesthetic, but has no analgesic properties. Induction is generally smooth and rapid, but owing to the potency of the drug, overdosage with cardiorespiratory depression may occur. Aqueous solutions are unstable, particularly when exposed to air. The solution is alkaline and therefore irritant on misplaced injection outside the vein, while arterial injection is particularly dangerous. The usual strength used is 2.5% solution in water for injections.

Awakening from a moderate dose of thiopentone is rapid due to redistribution of the drug in the whole body tissues. Metabolism is, however, slow and some sedative effects may persist for up to 24 hours during which time the subject is particularly susceptible to the effects of alcohol. Repeated doses have a cumulative effect.

Methohexitone sodium (Brietal Sodium®) is less irritant to tissues than thiopentone and solutions are stable. It is usually used in 1% solution. Recovery is marginally more rapid than in the case of thiopentone. Induction is less smooth with an incidence of hiccup, tremor, involuntary movements, and pain on injection.

Both thiopentone and methohexitone are **contra-indicated** in porphyria.

Etomidate (Hypnomidate®) is an induction agent associated with rapid recovery without hangover effect. It causes less hypotension than other agents. There is a high incidence of extraneous muscle movement and pain on injection. These effects can be minimised by premedication with a narcotic analgesic and use of larger veins. There is evidence that repeated doses of etomidate have an undesirable suppressant effect on adrenocortical function.

Ketamine (Ketalar®) can be given by the intravenous or the intramuscular route, and has good analgesic properties when used in sub-anaesthetic dosage. The maximum effect occurs in more than one arm-brain circulation time. Muscle tone is increased and the airway is usually well maintained. There is cardiovascular stimulation and arterial pressure may rise with tachycardia. The main disadvantage is the high incidence of hallucinations and other transient psychotic sequelae, though it is believed that these are much less significant in children. The incidence can be reduced when agents such as droperidol or diazepam are also used. It is contra-indicated in patients with hypertension or in those with a history of mental illness. It is used mainly for paediatric anaesthesia, particularly when repeated administrations are required. Recovery is relatively slow.

TOTAL INTRAVENOUS ANAESTHESIA. This is a technique in which major surgery is carried out with all anaesthetic drugs being given intravenously. Respiration is controlled, the lungs being inflated with oxygen-enriched air. Muscle relaxant drugs are used to provide relaxation and prevent reflex muscle movements. The main problem to be overcome is the assessment of depth of anaesthesia in the paralysed ventilated patient.

THIOPENTONE SODIUM

Indications: induction of general anaesthesia; anaesthesia of short duration in minor surgical procedures

Cautions; Contra-indications; Side-effects: see notes above. Drug interactions: see Appendix 1 (section 15)

Dose: by intravenous injection, in fit premedicated adults, initially 100–150 mg (4–6 ml of 2.5% solution) over 10–15 seconds, repeated if necessary according to the patient's response after 20–30 seconds; *or* up to 4 mg/kg; CHILD, induction 4–8 mg/kg

By continuous intravenous infusion, as a 0.2–0.4% solution, according to the patient's response

PoM **Intraval Sodium**® (M&B)
Injection 2.5%, powder for reconstitution, thiopentone sodium. Price 500-mg amp = **C**; 2.5-g vial = **F**
Injection 5%, powder for reconstitution, thiopentone sodium. Price 500-mg amp = **C**; 1-g amp = **D**; 5-g vial = **G**

ETOMIDATE

Indications: induction of anaesthesia
Cautions; Side-effects: see notes above
Dose: by slow intravenous injection, 300 micrograms/kg
By intravenous infusion, 100 micrograms/kg/minute until anaesthetised (about 3 minutes); lower doses if used with inhalational anaesthetics

PoM **Hypnomidate**® (Janssen)
Injection, etomidate 2 mg/ml in propylene glycol 35%. Price 10-ml amp = **D**
Concentrate for intravenous infusion, etomidate 125 mg (as hydrochloride)/ml. To be diluted before use. Price 1-ml amp = **F**

KETAMINE

Indications: induction and maintenance of anaesthesia
Cautions; Side-effects: see notes above
Dose: by slow intravenous injection, 1–2 mg/kg over 60 seconds, repeated according to the patient's response
By deep intramuscular injection, 4–10 mg/kg, repeated according to the patient's response

PoM **Ketalar**® (P-D)
Injection, ketamine 10 mg (as hydrochloride)/ml. Price 20-ml vial = **F**
Injection, ketamine 50 mg (as hydrochloride)/ml. Price 10-ml vial = **G**
Injection, ketamine 100 mg (as hydrochloride)/ml. Price 5-ml vial = **G**

METHOHEXITONE SODIUM

Indications: induction and maintenance of anaesthesia for short procedures
Cautions; Side-effects: see notes above
Dose: by slow intravenous injection, as a 1 or 2% solution, 50–120 mg over 25–60 seconds *or* 1–1.5 mg/kg, according to the patient's response; maintenance, 20–40 mg (2–4 ml of 1% solution) every 4–7 minutes; CHILD, induction 1–2 mg/kg
By continuous intravenous infusion, as a 0.1–0.2% solution, according to the patient's response

PoM **Brietal Sodium**® (Lilly)
Injection, powder for reconstitution, methohexitone sodium. Price 100 mg in 10-ml vial = **C**
Injection, powder for reconstitution, methohexitone sodium. Price 500 mg in 50-ml vial = **E**
Injection, powder for reconstitution, methohexitone sodium. Price 2.5 g in 17.5-ml vial = **G**
Injection, powder for reconstitution, methohexitone sodium. Price 2.5 g in 250-ml vial = **H**
Injection, powder for reconstitution, methohexitone sodium. Price 5 g in 35-ml vial = **I**

15.1.2 Inhalational anaesthetics

Inhalational agents may be gases or volatile liquids. They can be used both for induction and maintenance of anaesthesia and may be used following induction with an intravenous agent (section 15.1.1).

Gaseous agents require suitable equipment for storage and administration. They may be supplied via hospital pipelines or from metal cylinders. In clinical use it is necessary to monitor flow rate. Volatile agents are usually administered using

---

C = 51-100p, D = 101-180p, E = 181-300p, F = 301-450p, G = 451-650p, H = 651-900p, I = 901-1200p, J = over 1200p.

calibrated vaporisers, using air, oxygen, or nitrous oxide–oxygen mixtures as the carrier gas.

To prevent hypoxia gaseous agents must be given with adequate concentrations of oxygen.

Nitrous oxide is used for induction and maintenance of anaesthesia and, in sub-anaesthetic concentrations, for analgesia in a variety of situations. For anaesthesia it is commonly used in a concentration of 50 to 70% in oxygen as part of a balanced technique in association with other inhalational or intravenous agents. Nitrous oxide is unsatisfactory as a sole agent owing to lack of potency, but is useful as part of a sequence of drugs since it allows a significant reduction of dosage of other agents.

A mixture of nitrous oxide and oxygen containing 50% of each gas (Entonox®) is used to produce analgesia without loss of consciousness. Self-administration using a demand valve is popular and may be appropriate in obstetric practice, for changing painful dressings, as an aid to postoperative physiotherapy, and in emergency ambulances.

Nitrous oxide may have a deleterious effect if used in patients with an air-containing closed space since nitrous oxide diffuses into such a space with a resulting build up of pressure. This effect may be dangerous in the presence of a pneumothorax which may enlarge to compromise respiration. Exposure of patients to nitrous oxide for prolonged periods, either by continuous or intermittent administration, may result in megaloblastic anaemia due to interference with the action of vitamin B_{12}. For the same reason, exposure of anaesthetists and theatre staff to nitrous oxide should be minimised. Depression of white cell formation may also occur.

Halothane (Fluothane®) is the most widely used of the volatile agents. Its advantages are that it is a potent agent, induction is smooth, the vapour is non-irritant, pleasant to inhale, and seldom induces coughing or breath-holding. The incidence of postoperative vomiting is low.

It is used for induction and maintenance of anaesthesia in major surgery with oxygen or nitrous oxide–oxygen mixtures. Concentrations of up to 5% may be used for induction, and 0.5 to 2% for maintenance.

Halothane causes cardiorespiratory depression and because of its potency is administered from calibrated vaporisers. Respiratory depression results in elevation of arterial carbon dioxide tension and perhaps ventricular dysrhythmias. Intermittent positive-pressure ventilation must be carried out with care as myocardial depression may follow increase in blood concentrations. Halothane depresses the cardiac muscle fibres and may cause bradycardia. The result is diminished cardiac output and fall of arterial pressure. There is also peripheral vasodilatation. Adrenaline infiltrations should be used with care as ventricular dysrhythmias may result.

Halothane produces moderate muscle relaxation, but this may be inadequate for major abdominal surgery and specific muscle relaxants are then used.

There is evidence that halothane may cause severe disturbances of liver function, including jaundice and death, when repeated administrations are given within 4 to 6 weeks. This complication is very rare, but may be associated with reductive metabolites of halothane. It is more likely in the presence of hypoxia, obesity, and enzyme induction. When repeated anaesthesia is necessary within this period, consideration should be given to the use of an alternative agent.

Cyclopropane is a potent gas which may be used for induction and maintenance. It forms explosive mixtures with air and oxygen and is used in a closed-circuit system. Muscle relaxation is produced and muscle relaxant drugs are potentiated. Respiration is depressed but arterial blood pressure is usually well maintained. It is a useful induction agent in paediatric and obstetric practice but has lost popularity as a maintenance agent in major surgery because of its explosive properties. For major surgery it is best used in association with intermittent positive-pressure ventilation or the respiratory depressant action may result in elevation of arterial carbon dioxide tension with resultant ventricular dysrhythmias. Adrenaline infiltration should be avoided because of the danger of dysrhythmias. Recovery is rapid, though associated with postoperative vomiting and restlessness.

Trichloroethylene (Trilene®) is a weak anaesthetic agent and poor muscle relaxant, but a potent analgesic. In analgesic concentrations it can be used to supplement nitrous oxide–oxygen anaesthesia in major surgery. In a concentration of 0.35 to 1% it is without serious side-effects and its use is associated with cardiovascular stability. Arterial blood pressure does not change and ventricular dysrhythmias are rare if arterial carbon dioxide tension is not allowed to rise. It is inadvisable to administer adrenaline. Respiratory rate increases during trichloroethylene supplemented anaesthesia, but this can be controlled by judicious administration of narcotic analgesic drugs. Trichloroethylene can be used in low concentration to prevent awareness during nitrous oxide–oxygen anaesthesia with muscle relaxants.

Trichloroethylene is unsuitable as the sole agent for induction, the best results being obtained as a supplement to nitrous oxide–oxygen following premedication with narcotic analgesics and induction with an intravenous agent. Recovery is relatively slow and there is some postoperative vomiting. Administration should therefore be discontinued before the close of the operation.

Enflurane (Ethrane®) is a volatile anaesthetic agent similar to halothane, but it is less potent, about twice the concentration being necessary for induction and maintenance. Administration from a calibrated vaporiser is recommended.

Enflurane is a powerful cardiorespiratory depressant. Shallow respiration is likely to result in a rise of arterial carbon dioxide tension, but ventricular dysrhythmias are uncommon and it is probably safe to use adrenaline infiltrations. Myocardial depression may result in a fall in cardiac output and arterial hypotension.

Enflurane is usually given to supplement nitrous oxide–oxygen mixtures in concentrations of 1 to 3%. It is likely that enflurane does not cause liver dysfunction, possibly because only a small fraction of the drug is metabolised. The drug is often used in preference to halothane when repeated anaesthesia is required.

Isoflurane is an isomer of enflurane. It has a potency intermediate between that of halothane and enflurane, and even less of an inhaled dose is metabolised than with enflurane. Heart rhythm is generally stable during isoflurane anaesthesia, but heart-rate may rise, particularly in younger patients. Systemic arterial pressure may fall, due to a decrease in systemic vascular resistance and with less decrease in cardiac output than occurs with halothane. Respiration is depressed. Muscle relaxation is produced and muscle relaxant drugs potentiated.

Anaesthetic ether (diethyl ether) is a potent anaesthetic agent, but is now less popular because the vapour forms flammable and explosive mixtures with oxygen. Both induction and recovery from anaesthesia are slow, and there is a high incidence of nausea and vomiting. Cardiac rhythm is stable and adrenaline infiltration may be allowed. Arterial blood pressure is well maintained.

CYCLOPROPANE

Indications; Cautions; Side-effects: see notes above

Dose: using a suitable closed-circuit anaesthetic apparatus, for light anaesthesia 7–10% in oxygen, for moderate to deep anaesthesia 20–30%

ENFLURANE

Indications; Cautions; Side-effects: see notes above

Dose: using a suitable calibrated vaporiser, *induction*, increased gradually from 1% to 5% in air, oxygen, or nitrous oxide–oxygen, according to the patient's response
Maintenance, 1–3%

▼ **Alyrane**® (Anaquest)
Enflurane. Price 250 ml = **J**
▼ **Ethrane**® (Abbott)
Enflurane. Price 250 ml = **J**

ETHER, ANAESTHETIC

Indications; Cautions; Side-effects: see notes above

Dose: from an open mask or a suitable vaporiser, *induction*, up to 20%
Maintenance, 3–10%
Price 500 ml = **F**

HALOTHANE

Indications; Cautions; Side-effects: see notes above

Dose: using a suitable vaporiser, *induction*, increased gradually to 2–4% in oxygen or nitrous oxide–oxygen; CHILD 1.5–2%
Maintenance, 0.5–2%

Halothane (M&B)
Price 250 ml = **J**
Fluothane® (ICI)
Halothane. Price 250 ml = **I**

ISOFLURANE

Indications; Cautions; Side-effects: see notes above

Dose: using a suitable calibrated vaporiser, *induction*, increased gradually from 0.5% to 3%, in oxygen or nitrous oxide–oxygen
Maintenance, 1–2.5%

▼ **Aerrane**® (Anaquest)
Isoflurane. Price 100 ml = **J**
▼ **Forane**® (Abbott)
Isoflurane. Price 100 ml = **J**

NITROUS OXIDE

Indications; Cautions; Side-effects: see notes above

Dose: using a suitable anaesthetic apparatus, a mixture with 20–30% oxygen for *induction* and *maintenance* of light anaesthesia
Analgesic, as a mixture with 50% oxygen, according to the patient's needs

TRICHLOROETHYLENE

Indications; Cautions; Side-effects: see notes above; must not be used with soda lime in closed circuits

Dose: maintenance of light anaesthesia, 0.5–1% as a supplement to nitrous oxide and oxygen
Analgesic, 0.35–0.5% using a suitable vaporiser

Trilene® (ICI)
Trichloroethylene. Price 500 ml = **E**

15.1.3 Anticholinergic premedication drugs

Anticholinergic premedication agents, usually **atropine, hyoscine** (scopolamine), or **glycopyrronium** (Robinul®), are used to dry bronchial and salivary secretions which are increased by intubation and the inhalational anaesthetics. They are also used to prevent excessive bradycardia and hypotension caused by halothane, cyclopropane, suxamethonium, and neostigmine. In some patients, especially the elderly, hyoscine may cause the central anticholinergic syndrome (excitement, ataxia, hallucinations, behavioural abnormalities, and drowsiness).

Atropine is the most commonly used. Intravenous administration immediately before anaesthesia or intramuscular injection (which should be given 30–60 minutes before the operation) is satisfactory.

Hyoscine is also an effective drying agent and provides a degree of amnesia.

Phenothiazine derivatives have too little activity to be effective drying agents when used alone.

C = 51-100p, D = 101-180p, E = 181-300p, F = 301-450p, G = 451-650p, H = 651-900p, I = 901-1200p, J = over 1200p.

ATROPINE SULPHATE

Indications: drying secretions, reversal of excessive bradycardia; with neostigmine for reversal of competitive neuromuscular block

Cautions: cardiovascular disease

Side-effects: tachycardia; see also section 2.3.2

Dose: premedication, *by intravenous injection,* 300–600 micrograms immediately before induction of anaesthesia, and in incremental doses of 100 micrograms for the treatment of bradycardia

By intramuscular injection, 300–600 micrograms 30–60 minutes before induction; CHILD 20 micrograms/kg

For control of muscarinic side-effects of neostigmine in reversal of competitive neuromuscular block, *by intravenous injection,* 0.6–1.2 mg

Atropine Sulphate Injection—see section 2.3.2

Morphine and Atropine Injection—see under Morphine Salts (section 15.1.4.1)

GLYCOPYRRONIUM BROMIDE

Indications; Cautions; Side-effects: see under Atropine Sulphate

Dose: premedication, *by intramuscular or intravenous injection,* 200–400 micrograms, *or* 4–5 micrograms/kg to a max. of 400 micrograms; CHILD, *by intramuscular or intravenous injection,* 4–8 micrograms/kg to a max. of 200 micrograms; intra-operative use, *by intravenous injection,* as for premedication

For control of muscarinic side-effects of neostigmine in reversal of competitive neuromuscular block, *by intravenous injection,* 10–15 micrograms/kg with 50 micrograms/kg neostigmine; CHILD, 10 micrograms/kg with 50 micrograms/kg neostigmine

▼ PoM **Robinul®** (Robins)

Injection, glycopyrronium bromide 200 micrograms/ml. Price 1- and 3-ml amp (both) = **C**

HYOSCINE HYDROBROMIDE

(Scopalamine Hydrobromide)

Indications: drying secretions, amnesia

Cautions: see under Atropine Sulphate; may slow heart; avoid in the elderly (see notes above)

Dose: premedication, *by subcutaneous injection,* 200–600 micrograms 30–60 minutes before induction of anaesthesia, usually with papaveretum; CHILD 15 micrograms/kg

PoM **Hyoscine Injection,** hyoscine hydrobromide 400 and 600 micrograms/ml. Price 1-ml amp (both) = **B**

PoM **Papaveretum and Hyoscine Injection,** see under Papaveretum (section 15.1.4.1)

15.1.4 Sedative and analgesic perioperative drugs

These drugs are given to allay the apprehension

of the patient in the pre-operative period (including the night before operation), to relieve pain and discomfort when present, and to augment the action of subsequent anaesthetic agents. A number of the drugs used also provide some degree of pre-operative amnesia. The choice will vary with the individual patient, the nature of the operative procedure, the anaesthetic to be used and other prevailing circumstances such as outpatients, obstetrics, recovery facilities etc. The choice would also vary in elective and emergency operations.

For many procedures, particularly minor operations, premedication is omitted completely and in these circumstances antisialogogues will usually be given intraveneously, either with or just before the induction agent.

The most common premedicants are still the **narcotic analgesics,** morphine, papaveretum, and pethidine, given intramuscularly about an hour before operation. They can also be given intravenously in reduced doses. Narcotics are usually combined with an antisialogogue and occasionally with a phenothiazine or droperidol. Their use can be followed by an appreciable incidence of side-effects, notably respiratory depression, hypotension, or nausea and vomiting. The incidence of the latter is reduced by atropine, hyoscine, droperidol or the phenothiazines. Caution should be exercised in their use in patients who have a history of previous postoperative vomiting, or where there is any existing respiratory impairment. These drugs should only be prescribed as premedication where there are facilities for the administration of oxygen and where naloxone or doxapram are available.

Oral premedication with **benzodiazepines** is increasing in popularity, as is the use of these drugs on the night before operation. Diazepam, lorazepam, and temazepam are the most widely used. They appear to be safer than the phenothiazines which are rarely used alone as premedicants, except in children or where their specific anti-emetic action is useful. Large doses of phenothiazines cause hypotension and susceptible patients may have dyskinesia (motor restlessness) or extrapyramidal symptoms such as oculogyric crises. Droperidol is less frequently used but it should not be given alone, except in very small doses, as it causes extrapyramidal side-effects. Patients given this drug alone appear to be quiet and relaxed, yet inwardly they may be very distressed. Barbiturates are rarely used; they are unsuitable for patients in pain and for the elderly.

Diazepam is used to produce light sedation with amnesia. The 'sleep' dose shows too great an individual variation to recommend it for induction of anaesthesia, and while this variation exists with regard to its sedative effect, it is probably less marked with lower doses and of little clinical significance. It is particularly valuable in subanaesthetic doses to produce light sedation for unpleasant procedures or for operations under local anaesthesia, including dentistry; sub-anaesthetic doses allow retention of the pharyngeal

---

reflexes while a local block is performed, and the resultant amnesia is such that the patient is unlikely to have any unpleasant memories of the procedure. Diazepam can also be used in a similar manner for endoscopy, with or without a narcotic analgesic.

Preparations of diazepam in organic solvents (Valium®) are painful on intravenous injection and followed by a high incidence of venous thrombosis which may not be noticed until a week after the injection. They are also painful on intramuscular injection, and absorption from the injection site is erratic. An emulsion preparation of diazepam (Diazemuls®) is less irritant on intravenous injection and is followed by a negligible incidence of venous thrombosis, but it should not be given intramuscularly. Diazepam is also available as a rectal solution (Stesolid®).

Diazepam and related drugs are of particular value for sedation of patients in an intensive care unit, particularly those on ventilators. It can be given 4–6 hourly but dosage should be gradually reduced after some days to prevent delay in recovery, which can be caused by a build up of its metabolite. Since it has no analgesic action it is often given in conjunction with small doses of opiates.

Diazepam may on occasions cause marked respiratory depression and facilities for treatment of this are essential. Dental patients who are sitting in one position for a long time may develop hypotonia after diazepam and they should be warned about this possibility. Outpatients should be advised that this is a long-acting drug, and that a second period of drowsiness can occur 4–6 hours after its administration.

By virtue of its physical characteristics, diazepam can accumulate in the fetus and, particularly after the mother has been given large doses, babies can be born in a depressed state, with hypotonia and a tendency to develop hypothermia.

Temazepam has a shorter action and relatively more rapid onset than diazepam. Used orally in a dose of 10–30 mg as a premedicant, 45 to 60 minutes prior to surgery, anxiolytic and sedative effects are produced which continue for one and a half hours. After this period patients are usually fully alert. It has proved useful as a premedicant in inpatient and day-case surgery.

Lorazepam produces more prolonged sedation than diazepam. In addition amnesia is commonplace. It is particularly useful when used as a premedicant the night prior to major surgery; sound sleep is assured when an oral dose of 1 to 5 mg is given. A further, smaller, dose the following morning will be required if any delay in the commencement of surgery is anticipated. Alternatively the first dose may be given in the early morning of the day of operation.

Chlormethiazole has been used as an intravenous infusion to maintain sleep during surgery carried out under regional analgesia, including extradural block. It has no analgesic effect, but is without cardiac and respiratory depression and may be used in elderly patients.

PREMEDICATION IN CHILDREN. Oral or rectal administration is preferred to injections where possible but is not altogether satisfactory. Oral **trimeprazine** is widely used but when given alone it may cause postoperative restlessness when pain is present. An alternative is **diazepam**. Some anaesthetists prefer the use of adult regimens, with dosage on a weight basis. (For guidelines on dose calculation in children, see Prescribing for Children, p. 6.)

INTRA-OPERATIVE ANALGESIA. Many of the conventional narcotic analgesics are used to supplement general anaesthesia, usually in combination with nitrous oxide–oxygen and a muscle relaxant. Pethidine was the first to be used for this purpose but other drugs now available include alfentanil, fentanyl, levorphanol, meptazinol, nalbuphine, and phenoperidine. The longer-acting drugs morphine and papaveretum, although equally effective for this purpose, are not commonly used because of the problems of respiratory depression in the postoperative period.

Small doses of narcotics given immediately before or with thiopentone will reduce the induction dose of the barbiturate and this is a popular technique in poor-risk patients. **Alfentanil** (Rapifen®) and **fentanyl** (Sublimaze®) are particularly useful in this respect because of their short duration of action although there may be some cumulation with large doses.

Repeated doses of intra-operative analgesics should be given with care, since not only may the respiratory depression persist into the postoperative period but it may become apparent for the first time postoperatively when the patient is away from immediate nursing attention. The specific narcotic antagonist, naloxone, will immediately reverse this respiratory depression but the dose may have to be repeated. In clinical doses it will also reverse most of the analgesia. An alternative and equally acceptable approach is to use the specific respiratory stimulant, doxapram, which can be given in an infusion and which will not affect the opiate analgesia. The use of intra-operative narcotics should be borne in mind when prescribing postoperative analgesics. In many instances they will delay the need for the first dose but caution is necessary since there may be some residual respiratory depression potentiated by the postoperative analgesic.

Fentanyl may produce severe respiratory depression, especially in patients with decreased respiratory function or when other respiratory depressant drugs have been given. Respiratory depression may be treated by artificial ventilation or be reversed by naloxone or doxapram. Alfentanil may also cause severe respiratory depression, especially when other respiratory depressant drugs have already been given; this may be reversed with naloxone.

Meptazinol (Meptid®) can be used for analgesia during or after operation. It is associated with nausea and vomiting, but is claimed to have a reduced incidence of respiratory depression.

For further notes on analgesics see section 4.7.

C = 51-100p, **D** = 101-180p, **E** = 181-300p, **F** = 301-450p, **G** = 451-650p, **H** = 651-900p, **I** = 901-1200p, **J** = over 1200p.

15.1.4.1 NARCOTIC ANALGESICS

ALFENTANIL
Indications: analgesia during short operative procedure and outpatient surgery; enhancement of anaesthesia
Cautions; Side-effects: see under Fentanyl and notes above
Dose: by intravenous injection, spontaneous respiration, initially up to 500 micrograms over 30 seconds, followed by up to 250 micrograms every 4–5 minutes, adjusted according to response
With assisted ventilation, initially 30–50 micrograms/kg, then supplements of 15 micrograms/kg
By intravenous infusion, with assisted ventilation, initially 50–100 micrograms/kg over 10 minutes *or* as a bolus, followed by maintenance of 0.5–1 micrograms/kg/minute

▼ **CD Rapifen**® (Janssen)
Injection, alfentanil 500 micrograms (as hydrochloride)/ml. Price 2-ml amp = **C**; 10-ml amp = **F**

FENTANYL
Indications: analgesia during operation, neuroleptanalgesia, enhancement of anaesthesia; respiratory depressant in assisted respiration
Cautions: chronic respiratory disease, myasthenia gravis; reduce dose in elderly, hypothyroidism, chronic liver disease; obstetric use may cause respiratory depression in neonate; see also notes above. Drug interactions: see section 4.7.2
Side-effects: respiratory depression, transient hypotension, bradycardia, nausea and vomiting
Dose: by intravenous injection, with spontaneous respiration, 50–200 micrograms, then 50 micrograms as required; CHILD 3–5 micrograms/kg
With assisted ventilation, 300–500 micrograms; CHILD 15 micrograms/kg

CD Sublimaze® (Janssen)
Injection, fentanyl 50 micrograms (as citrate)/ml. Price 2-ml amp = **B**; 10-ml amp = **E**
CD Thalamonal® (Janssen)
Injection, fentanyl 50 micrograms (as citrate), droperidol 2.5 mg/ml. Price 2-ml amp = **C**
Dose: premedication, by intramuscular injection 1–2 ml; induction, by intravenous injection 6–8 ml; CHILD, by intramuscular injection 0.4–1.5 ml

LEVORPHANOL TARTRATE
Indications: analgesia during operation; enhancement of anaesthesia
Cautions; Contra-indications; Side-effects: see section 4.7.2 and notes above
Dose: by subcutaneous, intramuscular, or intravenous injection, 250–500 micrograms, repeated to a max. of 1.5–2 mg

CD Dromoran® (Roche)
Injection, levorphanol tartrate 2 mg/ml. Price 1-ml amp = **B**

MEPTAZINOL
Indications: analgesia during and after operation
Cautions; Contra-indications; Side-effects: see section 4.7.2 and notes above
Dose: by mouth, 200 mg every 3–6 hours as required
By intramuscular injection, 75–100 mg, repeated every 2–4 hours as required
By slow intravenous injection, 50–100 mg, repeated as above

▼ PoM **Meptid**® (Wyeth)
Tablets, orange, f/c, meptazinol 200 mg. Price 20 tabs = **E**
Injection, meptazinol 100 mg (as hydrochloride)/ml. Price 1-ml amp = **C**

MORPHINE SALTS
Indications: analgesia during and after operation; enhancement of anaesthesia; pre-operative sedation
Cautions; Contra-indications; Side-effects: see section 4.7.2 and notes above
Dose: by subcutaneous or intramuscular injection, up to 10 mg 1–1½ hours before operation; CHILD, *by intramuscular injection,* 150 micrograms/kg. See also section 4.7.2 for analgesia

CD Morphine Sulphate Injection, morphine sulphate, 10, 15, 20 and 30 mg/ml. Price 1- and 2-ml amp (all) = **B**
CD Morphine and Atropine Injection, morphine sulphate 10 mg, atropine sulphate 600 micrograms/ml. Price 1-ml amp = **B**
Dose: by subcutaneous injection, 0.5–1 ml

NALBUPHINE HYDROCHLORIDE
Indications: peri-operative analgesia
Cautions; Contra-indications; Side-effects: see section 4.7.2 and notes above; also caution in ambulant patients (impairment of mental and physical ability)
Dose: by subcutaneous, intramuscular, or intravenous injection, 10–20 mg, adjusted according to response

▼ PoM **Nubain**® (Du Pont)
Injection, nalbuphine hydrochloride 10 mg/ml. Price 2-ml amp = **D**

PAPAVERETUM
Indications: analgesia during and after operation; enhancement of anaesthetics; pre-operative sedation
Cautions; Contra-indications; Side-effects: see section 4.7.2 and notes above
Dose: by mouth or by subcutaneous, intramuscular, or intravenous injection, 10–20 mg 45–60 minutes before anaesthesia; CHILD 1–12 years, 200–300 micrograms/kg max. as a single dose

---

For all abbreviations and symbols see inside cover.   Relative prices: **A** = up to 20p, **B** = 21-50p,

Note: papaveretum contains anhydrous morphine 50% as hydrochloride with the hydrochlorides of other opium alkaloids. 10 mg papaveretum is equivalent in morphine content to about 6.25 mg of morphine sulphate

CD **Papaveretum Injection,** papaveretum 10 and 20 mg/ml, price 1-ml amp (both) = **B**

CD **Papaveretum and Hyoscine Injection,** papaveretum 20 mg, hyoscine hydrobromide 400 micrograms/ml. Price 1-ml amp = **B**
Dose: by subcutaneous or intramuscular injection, 1 ml

CD **Omnopon**® (Roche)
Tablets, buff, papaveretum 10 mg. Price 20 tabs = **C**
Injection, papaveretum 20 mg/ml. Price 1-ml amp = **A**

CD **Omnopon-Scopolamine**® (Roche)
Injection, papaveretum 20 mg, hyoscine hydrobromide 400 micrograms/ml. Price 1-ml amp = **A**
Dose: by subcutaneous or intramuscular injection, 1 ml

PETHIDINE HYDROCHLORIDE
Indications: peri-operative analgesia, enhancement of anaesthesia, for basal narcosis with phenothiazines
Cautions; Contra-indications; Side-effects: see section 4.7.2 and notes above
Dose: premedication, *by intramuscular injection*, 50–100 mg 1 hour before operation; CHILD 1–2 mg/kg
Adjunct to nitrous oxide–oxygen, *by intravenous injection*, 10–25 mg repeated when required

CD **Pethidine Injection,** pethidine hydrochloride 10 mg/ml. Price 5- and 10-ml amp (both) = **B**. Pethidine hydrochloride 50 mg/ml. Price 1- and 2-ml amp (both) = **A**

CD **Pamergan P100**® (Martindale)
Injection, pethidine hydrochloride 50 mg, promethazine hydrochloride 25 mg/ml. Price 2-ml amp = **B**
Dose: 2 ml by intramuscular injection or, diluted to 10 ml, by intravenous injection, 1–1½ hours before operation; CHILD, by intramuscular injection, 8–12 years 0.75 ml, 13–16 years 1 ml

CD **Pethilorfan**® (Roche)
Injection, pethidine hydrochloride 50 mg, levallorphan tartrate 625 micrograms/ml. Price 1- and 2-ml amp (both) = **A**
Dose: premedication, 2 ml by subcutaneous, intramuscular, or intravenous injection 1 hour before operation; adjunct to nitrous oxide–oxygen 0.5–1 ml by intravenous injection; CHILD ¼–½ adult dose

PHENOPERIDINE HYDROCHLORIDE
Indications: analgesia during operation, neuroleptanalgesia, enhancement of anaesthetics; respiratory depressant in prolonged assisted respiration

Cautions; Contra-indications; Side-effects: see under Pethidine Hydrochloride and Fentanyl. Doses above 1 mg cause respiratory depression and require assisted ventilation (effects may be terminated with naloxone or doxapram)
Dose: by intravenous injection, with spontaneous respiration, 0.5–1 mg, then 500 micrograms every 40–60 minutes as required; CHILD 30–50 micrograms/kg
With assisted ventilation, 2–5 mg, then 1 mg as required; CHILD 100–150 micrograms/kg

CD **Operidine**® (Janssen)
Injection, phenoperidine hydrochloride 1 mg/ml. Price 2-ml amp = **C**

15.1.4.2 ANXIOLYTICS AND NEUROLEPTICS

CHLORMETHIAZOLE EDISYLATE
Indications: sedative during regional anaesthesia
Cautions; Side-effects: see section 4.8.2
Contra-indications: acute pulmonary insufficiency
Dose: by intravenous infusion, 25 ml (200 mg)/minute for 1–2 minutes; maintenance 1–4 ml (8–32 mg)/minute

PoM **Heminevrin**® (Astra)
Intravenous infusion 0.8%, chlormethiazole edisylate 8 mg/ml. Price 500-ml bottle = **G**

CHLORPROMAZINE HYDROCHLORIDE
Indications: anti-emetic, pre-operative sedation, enhancement of anaesthesia, sedatives, and analgesics; induction of hypothermia
Cautions; Contra-indications; Side-effects: see section 4.2.1
Dose: premedication, *by deep intramuscular injection*, 20–50 mg 60 minutes before operation

PoM **Largactil**® (M&B)
Injection, chlorpromazine hydrochloride 25 mg/ml. Price 1-ml amp = **A**; 2-ml amp = **B**

DIAZEPAM
Indications: premedication; sedation with amnesia, and in conjunction with local anaesthesia
Cautions; Side-effects: see notes above and section 4.1.2
Dose: by mouth, 5 mg at night, 5 mg on waking, and 5 mg 2 hours before minor or dental surgery
By slow intravenous injection, 10–20 mg over 2–4 minutes as sedative cover for minor surgical and medical procedures; premedication 100–200 micrograms/kg
By rectum in solution, adults and children over 3 years 10 mg; CHILD 1–3 years and elderly patients 5 mg

Oral and rectal preparations: see section 4.1.2

Parenteral preparations

PoM **Diazemuls**® (KabiVitrum)

Injection (emulsion), diazepam 5 mg/ml. For intravenous injection or infusion. Price 2-ml amp = **B**

PoM **Stesolid**® (CP)

Injection, diazepam 5 mg/ml. Price 2- and 4-ml amp (both) = **C**

PoM **Valium**® (Roche)

Injection, diazepam 5 mg/ml in solvent. Price 2- and 4-ml amp (both) = **B**

DROPERIDOL

Indications: anti-emetic, pre-operative sedation; neuroleptanalgesia

Cautions; Contra-indications; Side-effects: see notes above and section 4.2.1

Dose: premedication, *by intramuscular injection*, 10 mg 60 minutes before operation; CHILD 300–600 micrograms/kg

Neuroleptanalgesia, *by intravenous injection*, up to 15 mg with a narcotic analgesic; CHILD 200–300 micrograms/kg

PoM **Droleptan**® (Janssen)

Injection, droperidol 5 mg/ml. Price 2-ml amp = **C**

Thalamonal®—see under Fentanyl (section 15.1.4.1)

LORAZEPAM

Indications: sedation with amnesia; as premedication

Cautions; Side-effects: see under Diazepam

Dose: by mouth, 1–3 mg at night *or* 1–5 mg 2–6 hours before surgery

By slow intravenous injection, preferably diluted with an equal volume of sodium chloride intravenous infusion 0.9% or water for injections, 50 micrograms/kg

By intramuscular injection, diluted as above, 50 micrograms/kg 1–1½ hours before operation

Oral preparations: see section 4.1.2

Parenteral preparations

PoM **Ativan**® (Wyeth)

▼ *Injection*, lorazepam 4 mg/ml in solvent. Price 1-ml amp = **B**

MIDAZOLAM

Indications: sedation with amnesia, and in conjunction with local anaesthesia; premedication, induction

Cautions; Side-effects: see under Diazepam

Dose: sedation, *by slow intravenous injection*, 70 microgram/kg until patient becomes drowsy; usual dose range 2.5 to 7.5 mg (2.5 mg in elderly patients)

Premedication, *by intramuscular injection*, 70–100 micrograms/kg 30–60 minutes before surgery; usual dose 5 mg (2.5 mg in elderly patients)

Induction, *by slow intravenous injection*, 200–300 micrograms/kg (elderly patients, 100–200 micrograms/kg)

▼ PoM **Hypnovel**® (Roche)

Injection, midazolam 2 mg (as hydrochloride)/ ml. Price 5-ml amp = **C**

Injection, midazolam 5 mg (as hydrochloride)/ ml. Price 2-ml amp = **C**

PERPHENAZINE

Indications: anti-emetic, pre-operative sedation

Cautions; Contra-indications; Side-effects: see section 4.2.1

Dose: premedication, *by intramuscular injection*, 5 mg 1 hour before operation

PoM **Fentazin**® (A&H)

Injection, perphenazine 5 mg/ml. Price 1-ml amp = **A**

PROMETHAZINE HYDROCHLORIDE

Indications: anti-emetic, pre-operative sedative and anticholinergic agent

Cautions; Side-effects: see section 4.6 and notes above

Dose: premedication, *by mouth,* CHILD 6–12 months 10 mg, 1–5 years 15–20 mg, 6–10 years 20–25 mg

By deep intramuscular injection, 25–50 mg 1 hour before operation; CHILD 5–10 years, 6.25–12.5 mg

Preparations

See section 3.4.1

TEMAZEPAM

Indications: premedication; anxiety before investigatory procedures

Cautions; Side-effects: see under Diazepam

Dose: see notes above

Preparations

See section 4.1.1

TRIMEPRAZINE TARTRATE

Indications: pre-operative sedation, anti-emetic

Cautions: avoid alcohol. See also notes above and section 3.4.1

Side-effects: drowsiness, dryness of the mouth, allergic skin reactions

Dose: premedication, 3–4.5 mg/kg 1–2 hours before operation; CHILD 2–7 years 2–4 mg/kg

Preparations

See section 3.4.1

15.1.5   Muscle relaxants

Muscle relaxants used in anaesthesia are also known as **neuromuscular blocking drugs** or **myoneural blocking drugs**. By specific blockade of the neuromuscular junction they enable light levels of anaesthesia to be employed with adequate relaxation of the muscles of the abdomen and diaphragm. They also relax the vocal cords and allow the passage of a tracheal tube. Their action differs from the muscle relaxants acting on the spinal cord or brain which are used in musculoskeletal disorders (see section 10.2.2).

Patients who have received a muscle relaxant should **always** have their respiration assisted or controlled until the drug has been inactivated or antagonised (section 15.1.6). As depolarising relaxants may cause painful muscle spasm they should be given after induction of anaesthesia.

NON-DEPOLARISING MUSCLE RELAXANTS

Drugs of this group (also known as competitive muscle relaxants) include alcuronium, atracurium, gallamine, pancuronium, tubocurarine, and vecuronium. They cause blockade by competing with acetylcholine at the receptor site at the neuromuscular junction. These drugs are best suited to the production of paralysis of long duration. They have a slower, less complete action than the depolarising muscle relaxants and should be avoided in myasthenia gravis.

The action of the competitive muscle relaxants may be reversed with anticholinesterases such as neostigmine (section 15.1.6).

Tubocurarine may be regarded as the standard non-depolarising muscle relaxant but in recent years its use has declined. It starts to act between 3–5 minutes and lasts for about 30 minutes after injection. It may cause an erythematous rash on the chest and neck and this is probably due to histamine release (bronchoconstriction does not occur). Onset of blockade may be associated with hypotension and this, though transient, may be important in poor-risk patients.

Pancuronium (Pavulon®) has gained popularity in recent years. It has the advantages of a quicker onset of action and of not causing significant histamine release or significant changes in blood pressure; there is no evidence that it causes ganglionic blockade.

Gallamine (Flaxedil®) has a more rapid onset of action and recovery than tubocurarine or pancuronium. It causes undesirable tachycardia by its vagolytic action. It should be avoided in patients with severe renal disease as it is excreted via the kidneys.

Alcuronium (Alloferin®) appears to have no significant advantages over tubocurarine or pancuronium. Its duration of action is similar to tubocurarine.

Atracurium (Tracrium®) has a duration of action of 15 to 35 minutes. Histamine release may occur, but it is less potent than tubocurarine in this respect. The drug is without vagolytic or sympatholytic properties. It has an advantage over other non-depolarising muscle relaxants in patients with renal or hepatic impairment, as it is degraded by non-enzymatic Hofmann elimination, which is independent of liver and kidney function. It is non-cumulative on repeated dosage. Its action is reversed by neostigmine. Duration of action may be prolonged in hypothermia.

Vecuronium (Norcuron®) is a recently introduced muscle relaxant with a duration of action of 20 to 30 minutes. Large doses may have a cumulative effect. The drug does not cause histamine release, sympathetic blockade, or vagolytic effects.

ALCURONIUM CHLORIDE

Indications: non-depolarising muscle relaxant of medium duration

Cautions; Side-effects: see notes above. Reduce dose in renal impairment. Drug interactions: see Appendix 1 (section 15)

Dose: by intravenous injection, initially 200–250 micrograms/kg, then incremental doses of one-sixth to one-quarter of the initial dose, as required; CHILD, 125–200 micrograms/kg

PoM **Alloferin®** (Roche)
Injection, alcuronium chloride 5 mg/ml. Price 2-ml amp = B

ATRACURIUM BESYLATE

Indications: non-depolarising muscle relaxant of medium duration

Cautions: see notes above; inactivated by thiopentone and other alkaline solutions. Drug interactions: see Appendix 1 (section 15)

Side-effects: see notes above

Dose: by intravenous injection, initially 300–600 micrograms/kg, then 100–200 micrograms/kg repeated as required

By intravenous infusion, 5–10 micrograms/kg/ minute

▼ PoM **Tracrium®** (Calmic)
Injection, atracurium besylate 10 mg/ml. Price 2.5-ml amp = D; 5-ml amp = E

GALLAMINE TRIETHIODIDE

Indications: non-depolarising muscle relaxant of medium duration

Cautions; Side-effects: see notes above. Drug interactions: see Appendix 1 (section 15)

Dose: by intravenous injection, 80–120 mg, then 20–40 mg as required; CHILD, 1.5 mg/kg

PoM **Flaxedil®** (M&B)
Injection, gallamine triethiodide 40 mg/ml. Price 2-ml amp = B

PANCURONIUM BROMIDE

Indications: non-depolarising muscle relaxant of medium duration

Cautions; Side-effects: see notes above; caution where tachycardia could be dangerous. Reduce dose in obesity and in renal impairment. Drug interactions: see Appendix 1 (section 15)

Dose: by intravenous injection, initially for intubation 50–100 micrograms/kg then 10–20 micrograms/kg as required; CHILD initially 60–100 micrograms/kg, then 10–20 micrograms/kg, neonate 30–40 micrograms/kg initially then 10–20 micrograms/kg

Intensive care, *by intravenous injection,* 60 micrograms/kg every 1–1½ hours; *by intramuscular injection,* 30–60 micrograms every 1–2 hours

404   Chapter 15: Anaesthesia

PoM **Pavulon**® (Organon-Teknika)
Injection, pancuronium bromide 2 mg/ml. Price
2-ml amp = **C**

TUBOCURARINE CHLORIDE

Indications: non-depolarising muscle relaxant of
medium to long duration
Cautions; Side-effects: see notes above. Reduce
dose in renal impairment. Drug interactions:
see Appendix 1 (section 15)
Dose: by intravenous injection, initially 10–
15 mg, then 5 mg as required to a max. of 40 mg;
CHILD, average initial dose of between 300–500
micrograms/kg

PoM **Tubocurarine Injection,** tubocurarine chlor-
ide 10 mg/ml. Price 1.5-ml amp = **C**
PoM **Jexin**® (DF)
Injection, tubocurarine chloride 10 mg/ml. Price
1.5-ml amp = **C**
PoM **Tubarine Miscible**® (Calmic)
Injection, tubocurarine chloride 10 mg/ml. Price
1.5-ml amp = **D**

VECURONIUM BROMIDE

Indications: non-depolarising muscle relaxant of
short to medium duration
Cautions; Side-effects: see notes above. Drug
interactions: see Appendix 1 (section 15)
Dose: by intravenous injection, initially 80–100
micrograms/kg, then 30–50 micrograms/kg as
required

▼ PoM **Norcuron**® (Organon-Teknika)
Injection, powder for reconstitution, vecuronium
bromide. Price 4-mg amp (with 1-ml amp water
for injections) = **D**

DEPOLARISING MUSCLE RELAXANTS

Suxamethonium is the only commonly used drug
of this group. With a 5-minute duration of action
it is the ideal agent for passage of a tracheal tube
but may be used in repeated dosage for longer
procedures.

It acts by mimicking the action of acetylcholine
at the neuromuscular junction but causes blockade. Depolarisation is prolonged since disen-
gagement from the receptor site and subsequent
breakdown is slower than for acetylcholine.

It produces rapid, complete, and predictable
paralysis, and recovery is spontaneous. Unlike
the non-depolarising muscle relaxants its action
cannot be reversed and clinical application is
therefore limited.

Paralysis is usually preceded by muscle fasciculation. There is a transient rise in plasma potassium and creatine phosphokinase and there may
be muscle pains postoperatively. Suxamethonium
is **contra-indicated** in severe liver disease and in
burned patients. Premedication with atropine is
desirable.

Prolonged muscle paralysis may occur in
patients with low or atypical plasma pseudo-

cholinesterase enzymes. Prolonged paralysis may
also occur in **dual block**, which occurs after
repeated doses of suxamethonium have been used
and is caused by the development of a non-depolarising block following the primary depolarising
block. Artificial ventilation should be continued
until muscle function is restored. Dual block is
diagnosed by giving a short-acting anticholinesterase such as edrophonium; if an improvement
occurs the block is treated with neostigmine (section 15.1.6).

SUXAMETHONIUM CHLORIDE

Indications: depolarising muscle relaxant of short
duration
Cautions; Side-effects: see notes above. Drug
interactions: see Appendix 1 (section 15)
Dose: by intravenous injection, 20–100 mg,
according to the patient's needs. CHILD, initially
1–1.5 mg/kg, then ⅓rd of the initial dose
By intravenous infusion, as a 0.1% solution, 2–
5 mg/minute (2–5 ml/minute)

PoM **Suxamethonium Chloride Injection,** suxa-
methonium chloride 50 mg/ml. Price 2-ml amp =
B; 10-ml vial = **D**
PoM **Anectine**® (Calmic)
Injection, suxamethonium chloride 50 mg/ml.
Price 2-ml amp = **B**
PoM **Scoline**® (DF)
Injection, suxamethonium chloride 50 mg/ml.
Price 2-ml amp = **B**; 10-ml vial = **D**

15.1.6   Anticholinesterases used in surgery

Anticholinesterase drugs reverse the effects of the
non-depolarising (competitive) muscle relaxant
drugs such as tubocurarine but they prolong the
action of the depolarising muscle relaxant drug
suxamethonium.

Edrophonium (Tensilon®) has a transient
action and is used to diagnose dual block caused
by suxamethonium (section 15.1.5).

Neostigmine has a longer duration of action than
edrophonium. It is the specific drug for reversal of
non-depolarising (competitive) blockade. It acts
within one minute of intravenous injection and
lasts for 20 to 30 minutes; a second dose may then
be necessary. A suitable dose is 1 mg per 20 kg
body-weight. It is also used in the treatment of
dual block.

Before neostigmine is used **atropine** should be
given to prevent excessive salivation, bradycardia,
and other muscarinic actions of neostigmine. A
suitable dose is 0.6 to 1.2 mg of atropine sulphate
by intravenous injection.

For drugs used in myasthenia gravis see section
10.2.1.

EDROPHONIUM CHLORIDE

Indications: brief reversal of non-depolarising
neuromuscular blockade; diagnosis of dual
block (section 15.1.5)
Cautions; Side-effects: see section 10.2.1 and
notes above. Atropine should also be given

Dose: reversal of blockade, *by intravenous injection*, 10 mg (after or with atropine sulphate 0.6–1.2 mg), repeated at intervals of 10 minutes according to the patient's response
Diagnosis of dual block, *by intravenous injection*, 10 mg (with atropine)

PoM **Tensilon**® (Roche)
Injection, edrophonium chloride 10 mg/ml. Price 1-ml amp = **B**

NEOSTIGMINE METHYLSULPHATE

Indications: reversal of non-depolarising neuromuscular blockade
Cautions; Side-effects: see section 10.2.1 and notes above. Atropine should also be given
Dose: by intravenous injection, 1–5 mg *or* 1 mg/20 kg, after or with atropine sulphate 0.6–1.2 mg

PoM **Prostigmin**® (Roche)
Injection, neostigmine methylsulphate 500 micrograms/ml. Price 1-ml amp = **A**
Injection, neostigmine methylsulphate 2.5 mg/ml. Price 1-ml amp = **A**

15.1.7 Antagonists for respiratory depression

Narcotic antagonists, usually **naloxone** (Narcan®), are used at the end of an operation to reverse respiratory depression caused by narcotic analgesics. Unless the dosage is carefully adjusted, analgesia may also be reversed. For respiratory stimulants see section 3.5. **Doxapram** is a respiratory stimulant which does not reverse the other effects of narcotic analgesics.

DOXAPRAM HYDROCHLORIDE

Indications: postoperative respiratory depression
Cautions; Contra-indications: see section 3.5
Side-effects: see section 3.5; also laryngospasm, bronchospasm, arrhythmias postoperatively
Dose: by intravenous injection, 1–1.5 mg/kg repeated if necessary after 1 hour
By intravenous infusion, 2–3 mg/minute

PoM **Dopram**® (Robins)
Injection, doxapram hydrochloride 20 mg/ml. Price 5-ml amp = **D**
Intravenous infusion: see section 3.5

NALOXONE HYDROCHLORIDE

Indications: reversal of narcotic-induced respiratory depression
Cautions: see under Emergency Treatment of Poisoning
Dose: by intravenous injection, 100–200 micrograms (1.5–3 micrograms/kg), adjusted according to the response, then 100 micrograms every 2 minutes
Neonate, *by subcutaneous, intramuscular, or intravenous injection*, 10 micrograms/kg, repeated every 2 minutes *or* 200 micrograms (60 micrograms/kg) *by intramuscular injection* as a single dose

Narcan®—see under Emergency Treatment of Poisoning
PoM **Narcan Neonatal**® (Du Pont)
Injection, naloxone hydrochloride 20 micrograms/ml. Price 2-ml amp = **F**

15.1.8 Antagonists for malignant hyperthermia

Dantrolene (Dantrium®) is used in the prophylaxis and treatment of malignant hyperthermia which is a rare but lethal complication of anaesthesia. It is characterised by a rapid rise in temperature, increasing muscle rigidity, tachycardia, and acidosis and can be triggered off by several agents including halothane and suxamethonium. Dantrolene acts on skeletal muscle by interfering with calcium efflux in the muscle cell and stopping the contractile process. The oral preparation (see section 10.2.2) has been advocated for prophylactic use in malignant hyperthermia in susceptible individuals. The recommended dose is 5 mg/kg given in the 24 hours prior to surgery. Known trigger agents should be avoided during anaesthesia.

DANTROLENE SODIUM

Indications: malignant hyperthermia
Cautions: avoid extravasation
Dose: by rapid intravenous injection, 1 mg/kg, repeated at 5–10 minute intervals as required to a max. of 10 mg/kg

PoM **Dantrium Intravenous**® (Norwich-Eaton)
Injection, powder for reconstitution, dantrolene sodium, with mannitol. Price 20-mg vial = **J** (Hosp. only)

15.2 Local anaesthesia

The use of local anaesthetics by injection or by application to mucous membranes to produce local analgesia is discussed in this section.
The following sections also include information on local anaesthetics acting on the sites shown:
1.7 Colon and rectum
11.7 Eye
12.3 Oropharynx
13.3 Skin

USE OF LOCAL ANAESTHETICS

Local anaesthetic drugs act by causing a reversible block to conduction along nerve fibres. The smaller the nerve fibre the more sensitive it is so that a differential block may occur where the smaller fibres carrying pain sensation and automatic impulses are blocked, sparing coarse touch and movement. The drugs used vary widely in their potency, toxicity, duration of action, stability, solubility in water, and ability to penetrate mucous membranes. These variations determine their suitability for surface infiltration, regional, epidural, and spinal anaesthesia.

C = 51-100p, **D** = 101-180p, **E** = 181-300p, **F** = 301-450p, **G** = 451-650p, **H** = 651-900p, **I** = 901-1200p, **J** = over 1200p.

ADMINISTRATION. In estimating the safe dosage of these drugs it is important to take account of the rate at which they are absorbed and excreted as well as their potency. The patient's age, weight, physique, and clinical condition, the degree of vascularity of the area to which the drug is to be applied, and the duration of administration are other factors which must be taken into account.

Local anaesthetics do not rely on the circulation to transport them to their sites of action, but uptake into the general circulation is important in terminating their action. Following most regional anaesthetic procedures, maximum arterial plasma concentrations of anaesthetic develop within about 10 to 25 minutes, so careful surveillance for toxic effects is necessary during the first 30 minutes after injection.

TOXICITY. Toxic effects associated with the local anaesthetics are usually a result of excessively high plasma concentrations. The main effects are excitation of the central nervous system (nervousness, nausea, and convulsions) followed by depression. Less commonly the cardiovascular system is depressed. Hypersensitivity reactions occur mainly with the ester-type local anaesthetics such as amethocaine, benzocaine, cocaine, and procaine; reactions are less frequent with the amide types such as lignocaine, bupivacaine, and prilocaine.

USE OF VASOCONSTRICTORS. Toxicity may occur with repeated dosages due to accumulation of the drug, and reducing doses should therefore be given. Toxic effects may also occur if the injection is too rapid. Local anaesthetics should **not** be injected into inflamed or infected tissues nor should they be applied to the traumatised urethra. Under these conditions the drug may be so rapidly absorbed that a systemic rather than a local reaction is produced.

Most local anaesthetics, with the exception of cocaine and mepivacaine, cause dilatation of blood vessels. The addition of a vasoconstrictor such as **adrenaline** diminishes local blood flow, slows the rate of absorption of the local anaesthetic, and prolongs its local effect. Care is necessary when using adrenaline for this purpose because, in excess, it may produce ischaemic necrosis.

Adrenaline should **not** be added to injections used in digits and appendages. When adrenaline is included in an injection of lignocaine or procaine the final concentration should be 1 in 200 000 (500 micrograms/100 ml). In dental surgery, up to 1 to 80 000 (1.25 mg/100 ml) of adrenaline is used with local anaesthetics. Higher concentrations are occasionally used but there is no justification for so doing.

The total dose of adrenaline should **not** exceed 500 micrograms and it is essential not to exceed a concentration of 1 in 200 000 if more than 50 ml of the mixture is to be injected.

Local anaesthetics containing adrenaline and noradrenaline should not be used in patients taking tricyclic and related antidepressants because of an increased risk of arrhythmias and hypertension. Prilocaine with felypressin may be preferred as it is less likely to cause arrhythmias. This restriction does not apply to patients on monoamine-oxidase inhibitors.

LOCAL ANAESTHETIC DRUGS

Lignocaine is the most widely used local anaesthetic drug. It acts more rapidly and is more stable than most other local anaesthetics. It is effectively absorbed from mucous membranes and is a useful surface anaesthetic in concentrations of 2 to 4%. Except for surface anaesthesia, solutions should not usually exceed 1% in strength. The duration of the block (with adrenaline) is about 1½ hours. Concentrations of 1.5% are used for extradural block, and for spinal anaesthesia a 5% solution in glucose intravenous infusion is used as a hyperbaric solution.

The great advantage of **bupivacaine** (Marcain®) over other local anaesthetics is its duration of action of up to 8 hours when used for nerve blocks. It has a slow onset of action, taking up to 30 minutes for full effect. It is often used in lumbar epidural blockade and is particularly suitable for continuous epidural analgesia in labour; it then has a 2- to 3-hour duration of action. The maximum dose is 150 mg in any 4-hour period. It is also used for spinal anaesthesia.

Prilocaine (Citanest®) is a local anaesthetic of low toxicity which is similar to lignocaine. It can be used for infiltration, regional nerve block, and spinal anaesthesia and regional intravenous analgesia. The maximum adult dose is 400 mg, or 600 mg if adrenaline or felypressin is added. If used in high doses, methaemoglobinaemia may occur which can be treated with intravenous methylene blue 1% injection using a dose of 75–100 mg.

Amethocaine is an effective local anaesthetic for topical application. It is rapidly absorbed from mucous membranes and should **never** be applied to inflamed, traumatised, or highly vascular surfaces. It should **never** be used to provide anaesthesia for bronchoscopy or cystoscopy, as lignocaine is a safer alternative. It is used in ophthalmology (see section 11.7) and in skin preparations (see section 13.3). Hypersensitivity to amethocaine has been reported.

Benzocaine is a local anaesthetic of low potency and toxicity. Its only use is in surface anaesthesia for the relief of pain and irritation in the oropharynx (see section 12.3.1) and around the anus (see section 1.7.1).

Cinchocaine is a potentially toxic drug and is used for spinal (subarachnoid) block and for surface anaesthesia.

Cocaine readily penetrates mucous membranes and is an effective surface anaesthetic but it has now been replaced by less toxic alternatives. It potentiates the action of adrenaline and possesses vasoconstrictor and mydriatic properties and should therefore **not** be used with adrenaline. It should **never** be given by injection because of its toxicity and doses not exceeding 3 mg/kg should be applied to mucous membranes. It stimulates the central nervous system and is a drug of addiction. Concentrations of 4 to 20% (50–200 mg/ml) are applied to the nose, throat, and larynx. For the use of cocaine in ophthalmology see section 11.7.

Procaine is now seldom used. It is as potent an anaesthetic as lignocaine but has a shorter duration of action. It provides less intense analgesia because it has less tendency to spread through the tissues. It is poorly absorbed from mucous membranes and is of no value as a surface anaesthetic. When used for infiltration or regional anaesthesia, adrenaline 1 in 200000 (500 micrograms/100 ml) is generally added. Its metabolite para-amino-benzoic acid inhibits the action of the sulphonamides.

LIGNOCAINE HYDROCHLORIDE

Indications: local anaesthesia by surface, infiltration, regional, epidural, and caudal routes; dental anaesthesia

Cautions: epilepsy, hepatic impairment, impaired cardiac conduction, bradycardia. Reduce dose in elderly or debilitated patients. Resuscitative equipment should be available. See section 2.3.3 for effects on heart

Contra-indications: myasthenia gravis, hypovolaemia, complete heart block. Do not use solutions containing adrenaline for anaesthesia in appendages

Side-effects: hypotension, bradycardia, cardiac arrest. CNS effects include agitation, euphoria, respiratory depression, convulsions. See also notes above

Dose: adjusted according to the site of operation and response of the patient

By injection, max. dose 200 mg, or 500 mg with solutions which also contain adrenaline. Max. dose of adrenaline 500 micrograms

Infiltration anaesthesia, 0.25–0.5%, with adrenaline 1 in 200000, using 2–50 ml of a 0.5% solution in minor surgery and up to 60 ml in more extensive surgery

Nerve blocks, with adrenaline 1 in 200000, 1% to a max. of 50 ml, 2% to a max. of 25 ml

Epidural and caudal block, with adrenaline 1 in 200000, 1% to a max. of 50 ml, 2% to a max. of 25 ml

Surface anaesthesia, usual strengths 2–4%. Mouth, throat, and upper gastro-intestinal tract, max. 200 mg

Lignocaine Hydrochloride Injections
PoM **Xylocaine®** (Astra)
Injection 0.5%, anhydrous lignocaine hydrochloride 5 mg/ml. Price 10-ml amp = **B**; 20- and 50-ml vial (both) = **C**

Injection 0.5% with adrenaline 1 in 200000, anhydrous lignocaine hydrochloride 5 mg/ml, adrenaline 1 in 200000 (500 micrograms/100 ml). Price 50-ml vial = **C**

Injection 1%, anhydrous lignocaine hydrochloride 10 mg/ml. Price 2-ml amp = **A**; 10-ml amp = **B**; 20- and 50-ml vial (both) = **C**

Injection 1% with adrenaline 1 in 200000, anhydrous lignocaine hydrochloride 10 mg/ml, adrenaline 1 in 200000 (500 micrograms/100 ml). Price 10-ml amp = **B**; 20- and 50-ml vial (both) = **C**

Injection 1.5%, for epidural use, anhydrous lignocaine hydrochloride 15 mg/ml. Price 25-ml amp = **D**

Injection 2%, anhydrous lignocaine hydrochloride 20 mg/ml. Price 5-ml amp = **B**; 20- and 50-ml vial (both) = **C**

Injection 2% with adrenaline 1 in 200000, anhydrous lignocaine hydrochloride 20 mg/ml, adrenaline 1 in 200000 (500 micrograms/100 ml). Price 20-ml vial = **C**; 50-ml vial = **D**

Lignocaine Injections for Dental Use
A large variety of lignocaine injections, plain or with adrenaline, is also available in dental cartridges under the names **Lignostab, Neo-Lidocaton, Xylocaine,** and **Xylotox.**

Lignocaine for Surface Anaesthesia
Lignocaine Gel, lignocaine hydrochloride 1% or 2% with chlorhexidine gluconate solution 0.25% or hydroxybenzoates in a sterile lubricant water-miscible basis. Price 15 ml (both) = **C**

Xylocaine® (Astra)
Antiseptic gel, lignocaine hydrochloride 2%, chlorhexidine gluconate solution 0.25% in a sterile lubricant water-miscible basis. Price 15 ml = **C**

Ointment, lignocaine 5% in a water-miscible basis. Price 15 g = **C**

Spray (= aerosol spray), lignocaine 10% (100 mg/g) with cetylpyridinium chloride 0.01% in a metered spray container supplying 10 mg lignocaine/dose; 800 spray doses per container. With sterilisable spray nozzles. Price 80-g bottle = **G**

Topical 4% (= solution for topical use), anhydrous lignocaine hydrochloride 40 mg/ml. Price 30-ml bottle = **D**

Dose: up to 5 ml

Xylocaine Viscous® (Astra)
Oral solution 2%, anhydrous lignocaine hydrochloride 20 mg/ml, for surface anaesthesia of the upper digestive tract. Price 125 ml = **D**

Dose: 5–15 ml to a max. of 30 ml in 24 hours with a minimum of 4 hours between successive doses

Xylodase® (Astra)
Cream, lignocaine 50 mg, hyaluronidase 150 micrograms (50 units)/g. For application to mucous membranes of mouth. Price 15 g = **C**

BUPIVACAINE HYDROCHLORIDE

Indications: prolonged local anaesthesia by regional nerve block; epidural block, spinal anaesthesia

Cautions; Contra-indications; Side-effects: see under Lignocaine Hydrochloride and notes above

Dose: adjusted according to the site of operation and response of the patient

By injection, up to 2 mg/kg in any 4-hour period, with or without adrenaline

---

C = 51-100p, D = 101-180p, E = 181-300p, F = 301-450p, G = 451-650p, H = 651-900p, I = 901-1200p, J = over 1200p.

Spinal anaesthesia, 10–20 mg, adjusted according to site of operation

▼ PoM **Marcain Heavy**® (Astra)
Injection, bupivacaine hydrochloride 5 mg, glucose 80 mg/ml. Price 4-ml amp = **C**

PoM **Marcain Plain**® (Astra)
Injection 0.25%, bupivacaine hydrochloride 2.5 mg/ml. Price 3-ml amp = **B**; 10-ml amp = **C**
Injection 0.5%, bupivacaine hydrochloride 5 mg/ml. Price 3-ml amp = **B**; 10-ml amp = **C**
Injection 0.75%, bupivacaine hydrochloride 7.5 mg/ml. Price 10-ml amp = **D**

PoM **Marcain with Adrenaline**® (Astra)
Injection 0.25%, bupivacaine hydrochloride 2.5 mg/ml, adrenaline 1 in 400000 (250 micrograms/100 ml). Price 10-ml amp = **C**
Injection 0.5%, bupivacaine hydrochloride 5 mg/ml, adrenaline 1 in 200000 (500 micrograms/100 ml). Price 10-ml amp = **C**

CINCHOCAINE HYDROCHLORIDE

Indications: spinal anaesthesia
Cautions; Side-effects: see under Lignocaine Hydrochloride and notes above
Dose: spinal anaesthesia, 5–10 mg, according to the site of operation and the response of the patient

PoM **Nupercaine**® (Ciba)
Heavy spinal solution (hyperbaric solution 0.5%), cinchocaine hydrochloride 5 mg/ml in glucose intravenous infusion 6%. Price 3-ml amp = **B**

PRILOCAINE HYDROCHLORIDE

Indications: local anaesthesia by infiltration, regional, intravenous regional, and surface routes; dental anaesthesia
Cautions; Contra-indications; Side-effects: see under Lignocaine Hydrochloride and notes above
Dose: adjusted according to the site of operation and response of patient, to a max. of 400 mg used alone, or 600 mg if used with adrenaline or felypressin

PoM **Citanest**® (Astra)
Injection 0.5%, prilocaine hydrochloride 5 mg/ml. Price 20-ml vial = **C**; 50-ml vial = **D**
Injection 1%, prilocaine hydrochloride 10 mg/ml. Price 20-ml vial = **C**; 50-ml vial = **D**

PoM **Citanest with Octapressin**® (Astra)
Injection 3%, prilocaine hydrochloride 30 mg/ml, felypressin 0.03 unit/ml. Price 2-ml cartridge and self-aspirating cartridge (both) = **A**

PROCAINE HYDROCHLORIDE

Indications: local anaesthesia by infiltration and regional routes
Cautions; Side-effects: see notes above
Dose: adjusted according to the site of operation and the patient's response

By injection, up to 1 g (200 ml of 0.5% solution or 100 ml of 1%) with adrenaline 1 in 200000 (to a max. of 500 micrograms)

PoM **Procaine Injection,** procaine hydrochloride 1 or 2% (10 or 20 mg/ml) in sodium chloride intravenous infusion. Price 2-ml amp (both) = **B**

Appendix 1: Drug Interactions

When two or more drugs are given at the same time they may exert their effects independently or they may interact. The result of the interaction may be potentiation or antagonism of one drug by another, or occasionally some other effect. Adverse drug interactions should be reported to the Committee on Safety of Medicines in the same way as other adverse drug reactions.

Drug interactions may be **pharmacodynamic** or **pharmacokinetic**.

Pharmacodynamic interactions

These are interactions between drugs which have similar or antagonistic pharmacological effects or side-effects. They may be due to competition at receptor sites, or occur between drugs acting on the same physiological system. They are usually predictable from a knowledge of the pharmacology of the interacting drugs and, in general, interactions demonstrated with one drug are likely to occur with related drugs. They occur to a greater or lesser extent in most patients who receive the interacting drugs.

Pharmacokinetic interactions

These occur when one drug alters the absorption, distribution, metabolism, or excretion of another, thus increasing or reducing the amount of drug available to produce its pharmacological effects. They are not easily predicted and many of them affect only a small proportion of patients taking the combination of drugs. Pharmacokinetic interactions occurring with one drug cannot be assumed to occur with related drugs unless their pharmacokinetic properties are known to be similar.

Pharmacokinetic interactions are of several types:

1. Interactions affecting drug absorption

Either the rate of drug absorption or the amount of drug absorbed can be altered by drug interactions. Delayed absorption is rarely of clinical importance unless high peak plasma concentrations are required, as, for example, may be the case when giving an analgesic. A reduction in the total amount of drug absorbed is more likely to result in ineffective therapy.

2. Interactions due to changes in protein binding of drugs

Most drugs are loosely bound, to a variable extent, to plasma proteins. Protein-binding sites are non-specific and one drug can displace another thereby increasing the proportion of drug free to diffuse out of the plasma to its site of action. This will produce a detectable increase in effect only if the drug is extensively bound (more than 90%) and is not widely distributed throughout the body. Even for such drugs displacement rarely produces more than a transient potentiation because the increased concentration of free drug results in an increased rate of elimination tending to restore the free concentration to its original level.

Displacement from protein binding plays a part in the potentiation of warfarin by phenylbutazone, sulphonamides, and tolbutamide but the importance of these interactions is due mainly to the fact that warfarin metabolism is also inhibited.

3. Interactions affecting drug metabolism

Many drugs are inactivated by metabolism in the liver. One drug can increase the rate of metabolism of another by enzyme induction of the hepatic microsomal enzyme system. This results in lower plasma concentrations and a reduced effect of the drug. On withdrawal of the inducer plasma concentrations increase and toxicity may occur. The most important enzyme inducers in man are the barbiturates, dichloralphenazone, some antiepileptics, and rifampicin. Drugs affected include warfarin and the oral contraceptives.

The opposite effect is seen when one drug inhibits the metabolism of another producing higher plasma concentrations, an increased effect and a risk of toxicity. Some drugs which potentiate the effect of warfarin and of phenytoin do so by this mechanism.

4. Interactions affecting the renal excretion of drugs

Drugs are eliminated through the kidney both by glomerular filtration and by active tubular secretion. Competition occurs between drugs which share active transport mechanisms in the proximal tubule. Thus probenecid delays the excretion of many drugs including penicillins, some cephalosporins, indomethacin, and dapsone; aspirin may increase the toxicity of methotrexate by a similar mechanism.

Relative importance of interactions

Many drug interactions are harmless; many of those which are potentially harmful occur in only a small proportion of patients given the interacting drugs; and the result of an interaction may be more serious in one patient than another. The drugs most often involved in serious interactions are those with a small therapeutic ratio, such as phenytoin, and those where the dose must be carefully controlled according to the response, as with anticoagulants, antihypertensives, and antidiabetics. Patients at increased risk from drug interactions include the elderly and those with impaired renal or liver function.

The Table lists potentially harmful interactions which are likely to have clinical importance at least in some patients. The drug whose action is affected is listed in column 1, column 2 contains the interacting drugs, and column 3 gives the result of the interaction.

Table: Drug Interactions

Drug affected	Drug interacting	Effect
1: Gastro-intestinal system		
Carbenoxolone	Amiloride, spironolactone	Inhibition of ulcer healing
Cimetidine	Antacids	Reduced absorption if taken simultaneously
Metoclopramide	Anticholinergic drugs such as atropine, benzhexol, propantheline; narcotic analgesics	Antagonism—they have opposing effects on gastro-intestinal activity
2: Cardiovascular system		
2.1 Digoxin and other cardiac glycosides	Carbenoxolone; diuretics— bumetanide, ethacrynic acid, frusemide, piretanide, thiazides	Increased toxicity
	Cholestyramine, colestipol	Reduced absorption
	Aminoglutethimide, phenobarbitone, rifampicin	Inhibition (digitoxin only)
Digoxin	Amiodarone, quinidine, quinine	Potentiation. Halve maintenance dose of digoxin
	Diltiazem, spironolactone, verapamil	Potentiation may occur
2.2 Diuretics	Anti-inflammatory analgesics such as indomethacin; carbenoxolone, corticosteroids, corticotrophin; oestrogens	Antagonism
Bumetanide, Frusemide, Piretanide, Thiazides	Acetazolamide, carbenoxolone, corticosteroids, corticotrophin	Hypokalaemia
Indapamide	Carbenoxolone; diuretics— bumetanide, frusemide, piretanide, thiazides, xipamide	Hypokalaemia
Aldosterone antagonists, Amiloride, Triamterene	Captopril, potassium supplements, trilostane	Hyperkalaemia
Potassium-sparing diuretics with thiazides	Chlorpropamide	Increased risk of hyponatraemia
Spironolactone	Aspirin, indomethacin	Antagonism of diuretic effect
Triamterene	Indomethacin	Occasional reports of decreased renal function
2.3 Anti-arrhythmic drugs	Any combinations of 2 or more	Increased myocardial depression
Amiodarone, Disopyramide, Flecainide, Quinidine	Diuretics—bumetanide, ethacrynic acid, frusemide, piretanide, thiazides	Toxicity increased by hypokalaemia
Disopyramide, Flecainide, Quinidine	Amiodarone	Increased risk of ventricular arrhythmias
Flecainide	Cimetidine	Increased plasma concentrations
Lignocaine	Cimetidine, propranolol	Increased risk of lignocaine toxicity

Drug affected	Drug interacting	Effect
Lignocaine, Mexiletine, Tocainide	Diuretics—bumetanide, ethacrynic acid, frusemide, piretanide, thiazides	Antagonised by hypokalaemia
Mexiletine	Acetazolamide, antacids	Reduced excretion in alkaline urine may occasionally increase plasma concentrations
	Atropine, narcotic analgesics	Delayed absorption
	Rifampicin	Reduced plasma concentrations
Procainamide, Quinidine	Cimetidine	Increased plasma concentrations
Verapamil	Beta-adrenoceptor blocking drugs	Asystole, hypotension, heart failure
2.4 Beta-adrenoceptor blocking drugs	Adrenaline	Severe hypertension, especially with non-selective beta-adrenoceptor blocking drugs
	Amphetamines, phenylephrine, phenylpropanolamine, and other sympathomimetic amines	Severe hypertension reported rarely
	Ergotamine	Increased peripheral vasoconstriction
	Indomethacin	Antagonism of antihypertensive effect
	Lignocaine and similar anti-arrhythmic drugs	Increased risk of myocardial depression and bradycardia
	Nifedipine	Severe hypotension and heart failure occasionally in susceptible patients
	Prenylamine	Increased myocardial depression
Labetalol	Cimetidine	Potentiation possible because of reduced metabolism
Propranolol	Cimetidine	Increased plasma concentration of propranolol
	Rifampicin	Reduced plasma concentration of propranolol
Sotalol	Diuretics— bumetanide, ethacrynic acid, frusemide, piretanide, thiazides	Risk of ventricular arrhythmias increased by hypokalaemia
2.5 Antihypertensive drugs	Anti-inflammatory analgesics such as indomethacin, phenylbutazone; carbenoxolone, corticosteroids, corticotrophin; oestrogens, oral contraceptives	Reduced effect

Drug affected	Drug interacting	Effect
2.5 Antihypertensive drugs (*continued*)	Alcohol, antidepressants, hypnotics, sedatives, tranquillisers; fenfluramine; levodopa; vasodilators such as nitrates, nifedipine; verapamil	Potentiation
Bethanidine, Debrisoquine, Guanethidine	Sympathomimetic amines (including some common cold remedies); mazindol, pizotifen; tricyclic antidepressants	Antagonism
Captopril, Enalapril	Potassium supplements, potassium-sparing diuretics	Hyperkalaemia
Clonidine	Beta-adrenoceptor blocking drugs, tricyclic antidepressants	Increased risk of clonidine withdrawal hypertension
	Tricyclic antidepressants	Antagonism
Metirosine	Haloperidol, metoclopramide, phenothiazine derivatives	Increased risk of extrapyramidal effects
2.6 Vasodilators Nifedipine	Cimetidine	Increased plasma concentrations
2.7 Vasoconstrictors Adrenaline, Noradrenaline	Tricyclic antidepressants	Potentiation (*note:* local anaesthetics with adrenaline appear to be safe)
	Beta-adrenoceptor blocking drugs	Potentiation of hypertensive effect
2.8 Anticoagulants		
Heparin	Aspirin, dipyridamole	Potentiation
Phenindione	Oral contraceptives, vitamin K	Inhibition
	Anabolic steroids, aspirin, bezafibrate, cholestyramine, clofibrate, dipyridamole, neomycin, thyroxine	Potentiation
Warfarin and other coumarins	**A:** aminoglutethimide, barbiturates, carbamazepine, dichloralphenazone, griseofulvin, oral contraceptives, primidone, rifampicin, sucralfate, vitamin K (*note:* present in some enteral feeds)	Inhibition
	B: alcohol, amiodarone, anabolic steroids (e.g. oxymetholone, stanozolol), azapropazone, bezafibrate, cephamandole, chloramphenicol, cimetidine, clofibrate, co-trimoxazole, danazol, dextrothyroxine, disulfiram, erythromycin, latamoxef, metronidazole, miconazole, neomycin, phenylbutazone, sulphinpyrazone, sulphonamides, thyroxine	Potentiation
	C: allopurinol; diflunisal, flurbiprofen, indomethacin, mefenamic acid, piroxicam, sulindac and possibly other anti-inflammatory analgesics; cholestyramine, dextropropoxyphene, ketoconazole, nalidixic acid, paracetamol (regular treatment or high doses), tetracyclines	Potentiation may occur

Drug affected	Drug interacting	Effect
Warfarin and other coumarins (*continued*)	**D:** phenytoin	Both potentiation and inhibition reported
	E: aspirin, dipyridamole	Increased risk of bleeding due to anti-platelet effect

3: Respiratory system

Theophylline	Cimetidine, erythromycin, influenza vaccine, oral contraceptives	Potentiation
	Aminoglutethimide, carbamazepine, phenytoin, rifampicin, sulphinpyrazone	Plasma concentrations of theophylline may be reduced

4: Central nervous system

4.1 Hypnotics and sedatives

	Alcohol, antidepressants, antihistamines, narcotic analgesics	Potentiation
Alprazolam, Chlordiazepoxide, Clobazam, Diazepam, Flurazepam, Nitrazepam, Triazolam	Cimetidine	Potentiation because of decreased hepatic metabolism
Chlordiazepoxide, Diazepam	Disulfiram	Potentiation because of decreased hepatic metabolism
Chlormethiazole	Cimetidine	Potentiation

4.2 Antipsychotic drugs

Chlorpromazine	Antacids	Reduced absorption
	Propranolol	Increased plasma concentrations of chlorpromazine
Haloperidol	Indomethacin	Severe drowsiness has been reported
Haloperidol, Phenothiazine derivatives, Tetrabenazine	Metoclopramide	Increased risk of extrapyramidal effects
Lithium	Diuretics, sodium depletion	Potentiation due to reduced lithium clearance. Loop diuretics are safer than thiazides
	Acetazolamide, sodium bicarbonate, theophylline	Increased lithium excretion
	Amiloride	Antagonism of lithium-induced polyuria without reduced lithium clearance
	Carbamazepine, phenytoin	Neurotoxicity may occur without increased plasma concentrations
	Diclofenac, indomethacin, mefenamic acid, phenylbutazone, piroxicam	Potentiation
	Haloperidol, metoclopramide, phenothiazine derivatives	Increased risk of extrapyramidal effects and possibly of neurotoxicity

Drug affected	Drug interacting	Effect
4.3 Antidepressants		
Monoamine-oxidase inhibitors	Sympathomimetic amines such as amphetamines, common cold remedies, ephedrine; fencamfamin, fenfluramine, levodopa, oxypertine, pemoline	Hypertensive crisis. N.B. can occur up to 2 weeks after stopping MAOI
	Narcotic analgesics, reserpine, tetrabenazine, tricyclic antidepressants	CNS excitation, hypertension
	Tryptophan	CNS excitation. Reduce dose of tryptophan
Tricyclic antidepressants	Alcohol	Potentiation of sedative effect
	Oral contraceptives	Reduced effect but side-effects may be increased due to higher plasma concentrations
	Phenothiazine derivatives	Increased side-effects
Amitriptyline	Disulfiram	Increased 'Antabuse' effect with alcohol
Desipramine, Imipramine, Nortriptyline	Cimetidine	Potentiation
4.6 Drugs used in nausea		
Betahistine	Antihistamines	Antagonism
4.7 Analgesics		
Aspirin	Metoclopramide	Potentiation
Diflunisal	Antacids	Reduced absorption
Ergotamine	Erythromycin	Ergotism has been reported
Ketoprofen, Naproxen	Probenecid	Increased plasma concentrations
Methadone	Rifampicin	Reduced effect due to increased metabolism
Paracetamol	Cholestyramine	Reduced absorption
	Metoclopramide	Potentiation
Pethidine	Cimetidine	Potentiation due to inhibition of pethidine metabolism
4.8 Antiepileptics	Antidepressants, phenothiazine derivatives	Antagonism
Carbamazepine	Cimetidine, dextropropoxyphene, erythromycin, isoniazid, viloxazine	Potentiation
Clonazepam	Cimetidine	Potentiation
Ethosuximide	Carbamazepine	Reduced plasma concentrations of ethosuximide
	Isoniazid	Increased plasma concentrations and increased toxicity of ethosuximide
	Phenytoin, sodium valproate	Increased plasma concentrations of ethosuximide

Drug affected	Drug interacting	Effect
Phenobarbitone, Primidone	Phenytoin, sodium valproate	Increased sedation
Phenytoin	Amiodarone, azapropazone, chloramphenicol, cimetidine, co-trimoxazole, diazepam, disulfiram, influenza vaccine, isoniazid, miconazole, phenylbutazone, sulphinpyrazone, sulthiame, viloxazine	Potentiation
	Aspirin, sodium valproate	Transient potentiation
Sodium valproate	Carbamazepine, phenobarbitone, phenytoin, primidone	Reduced plasma concentrations of valproate
4.9 Drugs for parkinsonism	Haloperidol, phenothiazine derivatives; methyldopa, metirosine, metoclopramide, reserpine, tetrabenazine	These have extra-pyramidal side-effects
Anticholinergic drugs such as Benzhexol etc.	Amantadine, antidepressants, antihistamines, disopyramide, phenothiazine derivatives	Increased side-effects, dry mouth, urine retention, confusional states, etc.
Levodopa	Chlordiazepoxide, diazepam, lorazepam, and possibly other benzodiazepines	Antagonism—occasionally
	Metoclopramide	Increased plasma concentrations of levodopa
	Pyridoxine	Antagonism (does not occur if dopa decarboxylase inhibitor also given)

5: Infections
5.1 Antibacterial drugs

Drug affected	Drug interacting	Effect
Aminoglycosides Gentamicin etc.	Ethacrynic acid, frusemide, piretanide	Increased ototoxicity
Cephaloridine, Cephalothin, and possibly other cephalosporins	Ethacrynic acid, frusemide, piretanide; gentamicin	Increased nephrotoxicity
Cephamandole, Latamoxef	Alcohol	'Antabuse' reaction
Chloramphenicol	Phenobarbitone, rifampicin	Reduced plasma concentrations
	Paracetamol	Increased plasma concentrations
Dapsone	Probenecid	Reduced excretion—increased side-effects
Lincomycin	Kaolin mixtures	Reduced absorption
Metronidazole	Alcohol	'Antabuse' reaction
	Cimetidine	Increased plasma concentrations
	Disulfiram	Psychotic reactions
	Phenobarbitone	Reduced effect
Nalidixic acid	Probenecid	Reduced excretion—increased side-effects
Nitrofurantoin	Probenecid	Reduced excretion—increased side-effects

Drug affected	Drug interacting	Effect
Penicillins		
Phenoxymethylpenicillin	Neomycin	Reduced absorption
Pivampicillin	Antacids	Reduced absorption
Rifampicin	Antacids	Reduced absorption
Tetracyclines	Antacids, dairy products, oral iron, sucralfate, zinc sulphate	Reduced absorption
Doxycycline	Barbiturates, carbamazepine, phenytoin	Reduced plasma concentrations
Vancomycin	Cholestyramine	Antagonism
5.2 Antifungal drugs		
Griseofulvin	Phenobarbitone	Antagonism
Ketoconazole	Antacids, anticholinergic drugs, cimetidine, ranitidine	Decreased absorption
5.3 Antiviral drugs		
Acyclovir	Probenecid	Reduced excretion and increased plasma concentrations

6: Endocrine system

Drug affected	Drug interacting	Effect
6.1 Antidiabetic drugs (oral and insulin)	Alcohol; beta-adrenoceptor blocking drugs; monoamine-oxidase inhibitors	Potentiation
	Corticosteroids, corticotrophin; diazoxide; diuretics—bumetanide, frusemide, thiazides; oral contraceptives	Antagonism
Metformin	Alcohol	Increased risk of lactic acidosis
Sulphonylureas— Chlorpropamide, Tolbutamide etc.	Bezafibrate, chloramphenicol, clofibrate, co-trimoxazole, miconazole, phenylbutazone, sulphinpyrazone	Potentiation
	Lithium, nifedipine	May occasionally impair glucose tolerance
Chlorpropamide	Alcohol	Flushing in susceptible patients
Chlorpropamide, Glymidine, Tolbutamide, and possibly other sulphonylureas	Rifampicin	Reduced effect
6.2 Thyroxine	Cholestyramine	Reduced absorption
	Phenylbutazone	False low total plasma-thyroxine concentration
	Carbamazepine, phenytoin	Increased thyroxine metabolism and may increase thyroxine requirements in primary hypothyroidism
6.3 Corticosteroids, Corticotrophin	Carbenoxolone; diuretics— bumetanide, ethacrynic acid, frusemide, piretanide, thiazides	Increased potassium loss

Drug affected	Drug interacting	Effect
Cortisone, Dexamethasone, Hydrocortisone, Prednisolone, Prednisone	Barbiturates, carbamazepine, phenytoin, primidone, rifampicin	Reduced effect
Dexamethasone	Aminoglutethimide	Reduced effect
6.7 Bromocriptine	Metoclopramide, domperidone	May antagonise hypoprolactinaemic effect

7: Obstetrics, gynaecology, and urinary-tract disorders

Oral contraceptives	Barbiturates, carbamazepine, dichloralphenazone, griseofulvin, phenytoin, primidone, rifampicin	Reduced effect
	Oral antibiotics such as ampicillin, tetracycline	Reduced effect—risk probably small

8: Malignant disease and immunosuppression

Azathioprine, Mercaptopurine	Allopurinol	Potentiation— increased toxicity
Cisplatin	Aminoglycosides	Increased risk of nephrotoxicity and possibly ototoxicity
Cyclosporin	Ketoconazole	Increased plasma concentrations of cyclosporin
	Phenobarbitone, phenytoin, rifampicin	Reduced plasma concentration of cyclosporin
Methotrexate	Aspirin, phenylbutazone, probenecid	Delayed excretion— increased toxicity
	Antiepileptics; co-trimoxazole, pyrimethamine	Increased anti-folate effect
Procarbazine	Alcohol	'Antabuse' reaction

9: Nutrition and blood

Calcium salts	Thiazides	Increased risk of hypercalcaemia
Oral iron	Magnesium trisilicate; tetracyclines; zinc salts	Reduced absorption
Zinc salts	Oral iron	Reduced absorption

10: Musculoskeletal and joint diseases

Indomethacin	Probenecid	Increased plasma concentrations
Penicillamine	Antacids, oral iron, zinc sulphate	Reduced absorption
Phenylbutazone	Cholestyramine	Reduced absorption
Probenecid, Sulphinpyrazone	Aspirin	Inhibition
	Pyrazinamide	Antagonism

13: Skin

Monosulfiram	Alcohol	'Antabuse' reaction

Drug affected	Drug interacting	Effect
15: Anaesthesia		
General anaesthetics	Antihypertensive drugs; beta-adrenoceptor blocking drugs; chlorpromazine	Potentiation of hypotensive effect
	Adrenaline, isoprenaline, levodopa	Arrhythmias with halothane, cyclopropane, trichloroethylene
Thiopentone	Sulphonamides	Potentiation
Muscle relaxants	Colistin, polymyxin B; lithium, propranolol, quinidine	Potentiation
Competitive neuromuscular blocking drugs such as Tubocurarine	Aminoglycosides, clindamycin, lincomycin; magnesium salts	Potentiation
Depolarising neuromuscular blocking drugs such as Suxamethonium	Cyclophosphamide, ecothiopate eye-drops, neostigmine, thiotepa	Potentiation
	Digoxin	Arrhythmias

Appendix 2: Intravenous Additives

Addition of medication to infusion fluids

Drugs may be added to a container of infusion fluid and given by slow intravenous infusion, by intermittent infusion, or via the drip tubing.

INTRAVENOUS ADDITIVE POLICIES. Health Circular HC(76)9 recommends that a local policy on the addition of drugs to intravenous fluids should be drawn up by a multi-disciplinary team in each Health District and issued as a document to the members of staff concerned.

Centralised additive services are provided in a number of hospital pharmacy departments and should be used when available in preference to making additions in hospital wards.

The information in the following section should be read in conjunction with any appropriate local policy documents.

Direct addition of medication to infusion containers

Basic guidelines

1. Drugs should only be added to infusion containers when constant plasma concentrations are needed or when the administration of a more concentrated solution would be harmful.
2. In general, only one drug should be added to any infusion container and the components should be of known compatibility (see Table). Ready-prepared solutions should be used whenever possible. Drugs should not normally be added to blood products, mannitol, or sodium bicarbonate. Only specially formulated additives should be used with fat emulsions or amino-acid solutions (see section 9.3).
3. Solutions should be thoroughly mixed by shaking and checked for absence of particulate matter before use.
4. Strict asepsis should be maintained using appropriate techniques throughout and in general the same giving set should not be used for more than 24 hours.
5. The infusion container should be labelled with the date and time the addition was made, the name and quantity of additive, and the name of the patient. When possible, containers should be retained for a period after use in case they are needed for investigation.
6. It is good practice to examine intravenous infusions from time to time while they are running. If cloudiness, crystallisation, change of colour, or any other sign of interaction or contamination is observed the infusion should be discontinued.

Problems involving additives

Several problems may arise when adding drugs to intravenous infusions.

MICROBIAL CONTAMINATION. The accidental entry and subsequent growth of micro-organisms converts the infusion fluid pathway into a potential vehicle for infection with micro-organisms, particularly species of *Candida*, *Enterobacter*, and *Klebsiella*. Ready-prepared infusions containing the additional drugs, or infusions prepared by an additive service (when available) should therefore be used in preference to making extemporaneous additions to infusion containers on wards etc. However, when this is necessary strict aseptic procedure should be followed.

INCOMPATIBILITY. Physical and chemical incompatibilities may occur with loss of potency, increase in toxicity, or other adverse effect. The solutions may become opalescent or precipitation may occur, but in many instances there is no visual indication of incompatibility. Interaction may take place at any point in the infusion fluid pathway, and the potential for incompatibility is increased when more than one substance is added to the infusion fluid. Information on compatibility is given in the accompanying Table. The suitability of additions may also be checked by reference to manufacturer's literature and additional information is usually available in hospital pharmacies.

Common incompatibilities. Precipitation reactions are numerous and varied and may occur as a result of pH, concentration changes, 'salting-out' effects, complexation or other chemical changes. Precipitation or other particle formation must be avoided since, apart from lack of control of dosage on administration, it may initiate or exacerbate adverse effects. This is particularly important in the case of drugs which have been implicated in either thrombophlebitis (e.g. diazepam) or in skin sloughing or necrosis caused by extravasation (e.g. sodium bicarbonate, thiopentone sodium and certain cytotoxic drugs such as doxorubicin, methotrexate, and fluorouracil). It is also especially important to effect solution of colloidal drugs and to prevent their subsequent precipitation in order to avoid a pyrogenic reaction (e.g. amphotericin).

It is considered undesirable to mix beta-lactam antibiotics, such as semi-synthetic penicillins and cephalosporins, with proteinaceous materials on the grounds that immunogenic and allergenic conjugates could be formed.

A number of preparations undergo significant loss of potency when added singly or in combination to large volume infusions. Examples include ampicillin in infusions that contain glucose or lactates, mustine hydrochloride in isotonic saline and gentamicin/carbenicillin combinations. The breakdown products of dacarbazine have been implicated in adverse effects.

Blood. Because of the large number of incompatibilities, drugs should not normally be added to blood and blood products for infusion purposes. Examples of incompatibility with blood include hypertonic mannitol solutions (irreversible crenation of red cells), dextrans (rouleaux formation and interference with cross-matching), glucose (clumping of red cells), and oxytocin (inactivation of the additive).

If the giving set is not changed after the administration of blood, but used for other infusion fluids, a precipitate of fibrin may be formed which, apart from physically blocking the set, increases the likelihood of microbial growth.

Blood should always be taken for grouping and cross-matching before infusing dextrans.

Intravenous fat emulsions may break down with coalescence of fat globules and separation of phases when additions such as antibiotics or electrolytes are made, thus increasing the possibility of embolism. Only specially formulated items such as Vitlipid® (see section 9.3) may be added to appropriate intravenous fat emulsions.

Other infusions that frequently give rise to incompatibility include amino acids, mannitol, and sodium bicarbonate.

Bactericides such as chlorocresol 0.1% or phenylmercuric nitrate 0.001% are present in some injection solutions. The total volume of such solutions added to a container for infusion on one occasion should not exceed 15 ml.

Method of making additions to infusion solutions

Ready-prepared infusions should be used whenever available. **Potassium chloride** is usually available in concentrations of 20, 27, and 40 mmol/litre in sodium chloride intravenous infusion (0.9%), glucose intravenous infusion (5%) or sodium chloride and glucose intravenous infusion. **Lignocaine hydrochloride** is usually available in concentrations of 0.1 or 0.2% in glucose intravenous infusion (5%).

When addition is required to be made extemporaneously, any product reconstitution instructions such as those relating to concentration, vehicle, mixing, and handling precautions should be strictly followed using an aseptic technique throughout. Once the product has been reconstituted, addition to the infusion fluid should be made immediately in order to minimise accidental microbial contamination and, with certain products, to prevent degradation or other formulation change which may occur; e.g. reconstituted ampicillin injection degrades rapidly on standing, and also may form polymers which could cause sensitivity reactions.

It is also important in certain instances that an infusion fluid of specific pH be used. **Amphotericin** injection (Fungizone®) requires dilution in glucose injection of pH greater than 4.2 and **frusemide** injection (Lasix®) should be added to infusions of pH greater than 5.5.

When drug additions are made to the infusion container it is important to mix thoroughly; additions should not be made to an infusion container that has been connected to a giving set, as mixing is hampered. If the solutions are not thoroughly mixed a concentrated layer of the additive may form owing to differences in density of it and the infusion. **Potassium chloride** is particularly prone to this 'layering' effect when added without adequate mixing to infusions packed in non-rigid infusion containers, and if such a mixture is administered an insidious effect on the heart may result.

A time limit between addition of the additive to the infusion and completion of administration must be imposed for certain admixtures to guarantee satisfactory drug potency and compatibility. For admixtures in which degradation occurs without the formation of toxic substances, an acceptable limit is the time taken for 10% decomposition of the drug ($t_{10\%}$). When toxic substances are produced stricter limits may be imposed.

Certain injections must be protected from light during continuous infusion to minimise oxidation, for example amphotericin, dacarbazine, and sodium nitroprusside.

Dilution with a small volume of an appropriate vehicle and administration using a motorised infusion pump is advocated for preparations such as heparin where strict control over administration is required. In this case the appropriate dose may be dissolved in 10 to 20 ml of sodium chloride intravenous infusion (0.9%).

Use of additives table

The Table lists preparations given by three methods—continuous infusion, intermittent infusion, and addition via the drip tubing.

Drugs for **continuous infusion** must be diluted in a large volume infusion. Penicillins and cephalosporins are not usually given by continuous infusion because of stability problems and because adequate plasma and tissue concentrations are best obtained by intermittent infusion. Where it is necessary to administer these drugs by continuous infusion, the detailed literature should be consulted as the information is not included in the Table.

Intravenous preparations that are both compatible and clinically suitable may be given by **intermittent infusion** in a relatively small volume of infusion over a short period of time, for example 100 ml in 30 minutes. This method is applicable where the product is incompatible or is unstable over the normal period necessary for continuous infusion or where adequate plasma and tissue concentrations are not produced by continuous infusion. The limited stability of ampicillin or amoxycillin in large volume infusions containing glucose or lactate may be overcome using this method.

Carbenicillin, dacarbazine, and ticarcillin may be given by intermittent infusion in order to achieve satisfactory plasma and tissue concentrations. Gentamicin may be administered similarly, although it is normally given by direct intravenous bolus injection for the same reason.

An in-line burette may be used for intermittent infusion techniques in order to achieve strict control over the time and rate of administration of a bolus injection, especially for infants and children and in intensive care units. Intermittent infusion may also make use of the 'piggy-back' technique provided that no additions are made to the primary infusion. In this method the drug is added to a small secondary container connected to a Y-type injection site on the primary infusion giving set; the secondary solution is usually infused within 30 minutes.

Addition via the drip tubing is indicated for a

number of cytotoxic drugs in order to minimise extravasation. The preparation is added aseptically via the rubber septum of the injection site of a fast-running infusion. In general, drug preparations intended for a bolus effect should be given directly into a separate vein where possible. Failing this, administration may be made via the drip tubing provided that the preparation is compatible with the infusion fluid when given in this manner.

The **Table** covers only the common intravenous infusion fluids, glucose 5 and 10%, sodium chloride 0.9%, Ringer's solution (sodium chloride, compound), sodium lactate M/6, sodium lactate, compound (Hartmann's solution), dextrans, fructose, and water for injections. Where water for injections is used, care should be taken to avoid giving hypotonic solutions. Preparations compatible with glucose 5% and with sodium chloride 0.9% are also compatible with sodium chloride and glucose infusion. For information on compatibility with other fluids the literature should be consulted.

The proprietary forms indicated in the Table have been shown to be suitable. If other forms are used, suitability should be checked with the manufacturer.

The following abbreviations are used in the Table: **C** = continuous infusion; **I** = intermittent infusion; **D** = addition via the drip tubing of the giving set. **C**[1] indicates that continuous infusion is not usually recommended; for details consult the literature.

Table: Intravenous additives

Additive	Method	Intravenous infusion	Comments
Acebutolol hydrochloride *Sectral*®	I	Sodium chloride 0.9%	To be given over not less than 1 hour.
Acetylcysteine *Parvolex*®	C	Glucose 5%	See Emergency Treatment of Poisoning.
Actinomycin D *Cosmegen Lyovac*®	D	Glucose 5%; Sodium chloride 0.9%	
Acyclovir sodium *Zovirax IV*®	I	Sodium chloride 0.9%; Sodium chloride and glucose; Sodium lactate, compound (Hartmann's solution)	Dilute to a concentration of 250 mg in at least 50 ml. To be given over 1 hour.
Alfentanil hydrochloride *Rapifen*®	C, I	Glucose 5%; Sodium chloride 0.9%; Sodium lactate, compound (Hartmann's solution)	
Alprostadil *Prostin VR*®	C	Glucose 5%; Sodium chloride 0.9%	
Amikacin sulphate *Amikin*®	I	Glucose 5%; Sodium chloride 0.9%; Sodium lactate, compound (Hartmann's solution)	To be given over 30 minutes.
Aminophylline	C	Glucose 5%; Sodium chloride 0.9%; Sodium lactate, compound (Hartmann's solution)	
Amiodarone hydrochloride *Cordarone X*®	C, I	Glucose 5%	Suggested initial infusion volume 250 ml given over 20–120 minutes. For repeat infusions up to 1.2 g in a maximum volume of 500 ml. Incompatible with sodium chloride infusion.

C = continuous; I = intermittent; D = addition via drip tubing

Table: Intravenous additives (*continued*)

Additive	Method	Intravenous infusion	Comments
Amoxycillin sodium *Amoxil*®	C[1]		
	I	Glucose 5%; Sodium chloride 0.9%	Reconstituted solutions should be diluted and administered without delay. Suggested volume 100 ml given over 30–60 minutes.
	D	Glucose 5%; Sodium chloride 0.9%; Ringer's solution; Sodium lactate M/6; Sodium lactate, compound (Hartmann's solution); Dextrans	
Amphotericin sodium deoxycholate complex *Fungizone*®	C	Glucose 5%	Dissolve thoroughly at reconstitution stage. The preparation must be given diluted in a large volume infusion. The pH of the glucose intravenous infusion must not be below 4.2. Check each container. Protect infusion from light. Suggested infusion time 6 hours.
Ampicillin sodium *Penbritin*®	C[1]		
	I	Glucose 5%; Sodium chloride 0.9%	Reconstituted solutions should be diluted and administered without delay. Suggested volume 100 ml given over 30–60 minutes.
	D	As for Amoxycillin sodium (above)	
Ampicillin/cloxacillin (sodium salts) *Ampiclox*®	I	Glucose 5%; Sodium chloride 0.9%	Reconstituted solutions should be diluted and administered without delay. Suggested volume 100 ml given over 30–60 minutes.
	D	As for Amoxycillin sodium (above)	
Ampicillin/flucloxacillin (sodium salts) *Magnapen*®	I	Glucose 5%; Sodium chloride 0.9%	Reconstituted solutions should be diluted and administered without delay. Suggested volume 100 ml given over 30–60 minutes.
	D	As for Amoxycillin sodium (above)	
Amsacrine *Amsidine*®	I	Glucose 5%	Suggested volume 500 ml given over 60–90 minutes. Use glass containers. Incompatible with sodium chloride infusion.
Ancrod *Arvin*®	C	Sodium chloride 0.9%	Suggested volume 50–500 ml given over 4–12 hours.
Aprotinin *Trasylol*®	C,D	Glucose 5%; Sodium chloride 0.9%; Ringer's solution	
Atenolol *Tenormin*®	I	Glucose 5%; Sodium chloride 0.9%	Suggested infusion time 20 minutes.

Table: Intravenous additives (*continued*)

Additive	Method	Intravenous infusion	Comments
Atracurium besylate ® *Tracrium* ®	C	Glucose 5%; Sodium chloride 0.9%; Sodium lactate, compound (Hartmann's solution)	Maximum period between addition and completion of administration varies according to diluent used
Azathioprine *Imuran*®	D	Glucose 5%; Sodium chloride 0.9%	Reconstituted solutions should be administered without delay.
Azlocillin sodium *Securopen*® (5 g)	I	Glucose 5% or 10%; Sodium chloride 0.9%; Ringer's solution; Fructose 5%	Intermittent infusion suggested for doses over 2 g. To be given over 20–30 minutes.
Benzylpenicillin sodium *Crystapen*®	C[1]		
	I	Glucose 5%; Sodium chloride 0.9%	Suggested volume 100 ml given over 30–60 minutes.
Betamethasone sodium phosphate *Betnesol*®	C,I,D	Glucose 5%; Sodium chloride 0.9%	
Bleomycin sulphate	I	Sodium chloride 0.9%	To be given slowly. Suggested volume 200 ml.
Bromhexine hydrochloride *Bisolvon*®	C	Glucose 5%; Sodium chloride 0.9%	Suggested volume 250–500 ml.
Bumetanide *Burinex*®	I	Glucose 5%; Sodium chloride 0.9%	Suggested volume 500 ml given over 30–60 minutes.
Calcium gluconate	C	Glucose 5%; Sodium chloride 0.9%	Avoid solutions containing bicarbonates, phosphates, or sulphates.
Carbenicillin sodium *Pyopen*®	I	Glucose 5%; Water for injections	Suggested volume 100 ml given over 30–40 minutes.
Carmustine *BiCNU*®	I	Glucose 5%; Sodium chloride 0.9%	Use the diluent provided to reconstitute. To be given over 1–2 hours.
Cefotaxime sodium *Claforan*®	I	Glucose 5%; Sodium chloride 0.9%; Sodium lactate, compound (Hartmann's solution); Water for injections	Suggested volume 40–100 ml given over 20–60 minutes.
Cefoxitin sodium *Mefoxin*®	C[1]		
	I,D	Glucose 5% or 10%; Sodium chloride 0.9%; Sodium lactate M/6	
Cefsulodin sodium *Monaspor*®	C[1]		
	I,D	Glucose 5%; Sodium chloride 0.9%; Dextran 40	
Ceftazidime pentahydrate *Fortum*®	I,D	Glucose 5 and 10%; Sodium chloride 0.9%; Sodium lactate M/6; Sodium lactate, compound (Hartmann's solution); Dextrans; Water for injections	
Ceftizoxime sodium *Cefizox*®	C,I,D	Glucose 5 and 10%; Sodium chloride 0.9%; Ringer's solution; Sodium lactate, compound (Hartmann's solution)	Suggested volume 50–100 ml.

C = continuous; **I** = intermittent; **D** = addition via drip tubing
C[1] = continuous infusion not usually recommended

Table: Intravenous additives (*continued*)

Additive	Method	Intravenous infusion	Comments
Cefuroxime sodium *Zinacef*®	I,D	Glucose 5%; Sodium chloride 0.9%; Sodium lactate, compound (Hartmann's solution)	Suggested volume 50–100 ml given over 30 minutes.
Cephaloridine *Ceporin*®	C¹		
	I,D	Glucose 5%; Sodium chloride 0.9%; Ringer's solution; Sodium lactate M/6; Sodium lactate, compound (Hartmann's solution); Dextrans	For intermittent infusion suggested volume 50–100 ml given over 30–60 minutes.
Cephalothin sodium *Keflin*®	C¹		
	I,D	Glucose 5%; Sodium chloride 0.9%; Sodium lactate M/6; Sodium lactate, compound (Hartmann's solution)	
Cephamandole nafate *Kefadol*®	C¹		
	I,D	Glucose 5% or 10%; Sodium chloride 0.9%; Sodium lactate M/6; Water for injections	
Cephazolin sodium *Kefzol*®	C¹		
	I,D	Glucose 5% or 10%; Sodium chloride 0.9%; Sodium lactate, compound (Hartmann's solution); Water for injections	
Cephradine *Velosef*®	C,I	Glucose 5% or 10%; Sodium chloride 0.9%; Ringer's solution; Sodium lactate M/6; Sodium lactate, compound (Hartmann's solution); Water for injections	Reconstituted solutions should be diluted and administered without delay; maximum period between addition and completion of administration 8 hours. Only cephradine solubilised with arginine may be used with solutions containing calcium ions.
Chloramphenicol sodium succinate *Kemicetine*®	I,D	Glucose 5%; Sodium chloride 0.9%	
Cimetidine *Tagamet*®	C,I	Glucose 5%; Sodium chloride 0.9%	For intermittent infusion. Suggested volume 250 ml given over 2 hours.
Cisplatin *Neoplatin*®, *Platinex*®	C	Sodium chloride 0.9%; Sodium chloride and glucose	Suggested volume 2 litres given over 6–8 hours.
Clindamycin phosphate *Dalacin C*®	C,I	Glucose 5%; Sodium chloride 0.9%	
Clomipramine *Anafranil*®	I	Glucose 5%; Sodium chloride 0.9%	Suggested volume 125–500 ml given over 45–120 minutes.
Clonazepam *Rivotril*®	I	Glucose 5% or 10%; Sodium chloride 0.9%	Suggested volume 250 ml.
Cloxacillin sodium *Orbenin*®	C¹		
	I	Glucose 5%; Sodium chloride 0.9%	Suggested volume 100 ml given over 30–60 minutes.
	D	As for Amoxycillin sodium (above)	

Table: Intravenous additives (*continued*)

Additive	Method	Intravenous infusion	Comments
Colistin sulphomethate sodium *Colomycin*®	C,I	Glucose 5%; Sodium chloride 0.9%; Ringer's solution; Fructose 5%; Dextran 40 in sodium chloride	Maximum period between addition and completion of administration 6 hours.
Co-trimoxazole	C		Ampoule solution has a pH of about 10. Suggested infusion time 90 minutes.
Bactrim® for infusion		Glucose 5% or 10%; Sodium chloride 0.9%; Ringer's solution: Sodium lactate, compound (Hartmann's solution): Fructose 5%; Dextrans 40 or 70	
Septrin® for infusion		Glucose 5% or 10%; Sodium chloride 0.9%; Ringer's solution; Fructose 5%; Dextrans 40 or 70	
Cyclophosphamide *Endoxana*®	I,D	Water for injections	For intermittent infusion suggested volume 50–100 ml given over 5–15 minutes. Maximum period between addition and completion of administration 30 minutes.
	D	Glucose 5%; Sodium chloride 0.9%	
Cyclosporin *Sandimmun*®	C	Glucose 5%; Sodium chloride 0.9%	Dilute to a concentration of 50 mg in 20–100 ml. Maximum period between addition and completion of administration 12 hours.
Cytarabine *Alexan*®, *Cytosar*®	C,I,D	Glucose 5%; Sodium chloride 0.9%	Reconstitute Cytosar® with the diluent provided. Check container for haze or precipitate during administration.
Dacarbazine *DTIC–Dome*®	I	Glucose 5%; Sodium chloride 0.9%	Suggested volume 125–250 ml given over 15–30 minutes. Protect infusion from light.
Desferrioxamine mesylate *Desferal*®	C,I	Glucose 5%; Sodium chloride 0.9%	
Dexamethasone sodium phosphate *Decadron*®	C,I,D	Glucose 5%; Sodium chloride 0.9%	
Oradexon®		Glucose 5% or 10%; Sodium chloride 0.9%; Ringer's solution; Sodium lactate M/6; Sodium lactate, compound (Hartmann's solution)	
Diazepam			Adsorbed to some extent by the plastics of the infusion set.

C = continuous; I = intermittent; D = addition via drip tubing
C^1 = continuous infusion not usually recommended

Table: Intravenous additives (*continued*)

Additive	Method	Intravenous infusion	Comments
Diazepam (*continued*)			
Diazemuls®	C	Glucose 5% or 10%	May be diluted to a maximum concentration of 200 mg in 500 ml. Maximum period between addition and completion of administration 6 hours.
	D	Glucose 5% or 10%; Sodium chloride 0.9%	
Stesolid®	C	Glucose 5%; Sodium chloride 0.9%	Dilute to a concentration not greater than 10 mg in 200 ml.
Valium®	C	Glucose 5%; Sodium chloride 0.9%	Dilute to a concentration of not more than 40 mg in 500 ml. Maximum period between addition and completion of administration 6 hours.
Digoxin Lanoxin®	C	Glucose 5%; Sodium chloride 0.9%	To be given slowly. See also section 2.1.
Dinoprost Prostin F2 alpha®	C	Glucose 5%; Sodium chloride 0.9%	
Dinoprostone Prostin E2®	C,I	Glucose 5%; Sodium chloride 0.9%	
Disopyramide phosphate Dirythmin IV®, Rythmodan®	C,I	Glucose 5%; Sodium chloride 0.9%; Ringer's solution; Sodium lactate, compound (Hartmann's solution)	Max. rate by continuous infusion 20–30 mg/hour (or 400 micrograms/kg/hour).
Dobutamine hydrochloride Dobutrex®	I	Glucose 5%; Sodium chloride 0.9%; Sodium lactate M/6	Suggested volume 250–500 ml. Incompatible with bicarbonate solutions.
Domperidone Motilium®	C,I	Glucose 5%; Sodium chloride 0.9%; Sodium lactate, compound (Hartmann's solution)	Dilute to a concentration of not more than 1 mg in 10 ml and give over 15–30 minutes.
Dopamine hydrochloride Intropin®	C	Glucose 5%; Sodium chloride 0.9%; Sodium lactate M/6; Sodium lactate, compound (Hartmann's solution)	Dilute to a concentration of 1.6 mg/ml. Incompatible with bicarbonate solutions.
Doxorubicin hydrochloride Adriamycin®	D	Glucose 5%; Sodium chloride 0.9%	
Electrolytes Addiphos®	C	Glucose 5% or 10%	Suggested volume 500 ml.
Epirubicin hydrochloride Pharmorubicin®	D	Sodium chloride 0.9%	Reconstitute with water for injections (10 mg in 5 ml, 50 mg in 25 ml). Give over 3–5 minutes.
Erythromycin lactobionate Erythrocin®	C,I	Glucose 5%; Sodium chloride 0.9%; Sodium lactate, compound (Hartmann's solution)	Dilute to a concentration of 1 mg/ml for continuous infusion and 1–5 mg/ml for intermittent infusion. pH of glucose infusion should be adjusted with sodium bicarbonate to above 5.5.
Ethacrynic acid (sodium salt) Edecrin®	D	Glucose 5%; Sodium chloride 0.9%	pH of glucose infusion should be adjusted to above 5.

Table: Intravenous additives (*continued*)

Additive	Method	Intravenous infusion	Comments
Ethanol	C	Glucose 5%; Sodium chloride 0.9%; Ringer's solution; Sodium lactate, compound (Hartmann's solution)	
Etomidate hydrochloride *Hypnomidate for infusion*®	C	Glucose 5%; Sodium chloride 0.9%	Dilute to a concentration of not more than 2.5 mg/ml.
Etoposide *Vepesid*®	I	Sodium chloride 0.9%	Dilute to a concentration of not more than 250 micrograms/ml and give over not less than 30 minutes and not more than 6 hours. Check container for haze or precipitate during administration.
Flecainide acetate *Tambocor*®	C,I	Glucose 5%; Sodium chloride 0.9%; Sodium lactate, compound (Hartmann's solution)	Minimum volume in infusion fluids containing chlorides 500 ml.
Flucloxacillin sodium *Floxapen*®	C[1]		
	I	Glucose 5%; Sodium chloride 0.9%	Suggested volume 100 ml given over 30–60 minutes.
	D	As for Amoxycillin sodium (above)	
Fluorouracil sodium	C,D	Glucose 5%	For continuous infusion suggested volume 500 ml given over 4 hours.
Folinic acid (calcium salt) *Calcium Leucovorin*®	C	Glucose 10%; Sodium chloride 0.9%; Sodium lactate, compound (Hartmann's solution)	
Frusemide (sodium salt) *Dryptal*®, *Lasix*®	C	Sodium chloride 0.9%; Ringer's solution	pH infusion must be above 5.5. Glucose solutions are unsuitable.
Fusidic acid (diethanolamine salt) *Fucidin*®	C	Glucose 5%; Sodium chloride 0.9%; Fructose 20%	Reconstitute with the buffer solution provided and dilute to a maximum equivalent to 1 mg sodium fusidate/ml. To be given over not less than 6 hours.
Gentamicin sulphate *Cidomycin*®, *Garamycin*®, *Genticin*®	I,D	Glucose 5%; Sodium chloride 0.9%	Suggested volume for intermittent infusion 50–100 ml given over 20–120 minutes.
Glyceryl trinitrate *Nitrocine*®, *Tridil*®	C	Glucose 5%; Sodium chloride 0.9%	For *Tridil*® dilute to a concentration of not more than 400 micrograms/ml. For *Nitrocine*® suggested infusion concentration 100 micrograms/ml. Incompatible with polyvinyl chloride infusion containers such as Viaflex® or Steriflex®. Use glass or polyethylene containers or give via syringe pump.

C = continuous; I = intermittent; D = addition via drip tubing
C[1] = continuous infusion not usually recommended

Table: Intravenous additives (*continued*)

Additive	Method	Intravenous infusion	Comments
Heparin sodium	C	Glucose 5%; Sodium chloride 0.9%	Administration with a motorised pump may be advisable.
Hydralazine hydrochloride *Apresoline*®	C	Sodium chloride 0.9%; Ringer's solution	Suggested infusion volume 500 ml.
Hydrocortisone sodium phosphate *Efcortesol*®	C,I,D	Glucose 5%; Sodium chloride 0.9%	
Hydrocortisone sodium succinate *Efcortelan Soluble*®, *Solu-Cortef*®	C,I,D	Glucose 5%; Sodium chloride 0.9%	
Ifosfamide *Mitoxana*®	C	Sodium chloride 0.9%; Sodium chloride and glucose	Suggested infusion volume 3 litres given over 24 hours.
	I,D	Sodium chloride 0.9%; Sodium chloride and glucose	For intermittent infusion give over 30–120 minutes.
Insulin	C	Sodium chloride 0.9%; Sodium lactate, compound (Hartmann's solution)	Adsorbed to some extent by the plastics of the infusion set. See also section 6.1.3.
Iron dextran *Imferon*®	I	Glucose 5%; Sodium chloride 0.9%	Suggested volume 500 ml.
Isoprenaline hydrochloride *Isuprel*®, *Saventrine IV*®	C	Glucose 5%; Sodium chloride and glucose	Dilute in a large volume infusion. Suggested minimum volume 500 ml. pH of the infusion must be below 5.
Isosorbide dinitrate *Cedocard IV*®, *Isoket IV*®	C	Glucose 5%; Sodium chloride 0.9%	Adsorbed to some extent by polyvinyl chloride infusion containers such as Viaflex® or Steriflex®. Preferably use glass or polyethylene containers or give via a syringe pump.
Isoxsuprine hydrochloride *Duvadilan*®	C	Glucose 5%; Sodium chloride 0.9%	Suggested infusion concentration 0.02%.
Kanamycin sulphate *Kannasyn*®, *Kantrex*®	I	Glucose 5%; Sodium chloride 0.9%	To be given slowly.
Labetalol hydrochloride *Trandate*®	I	Glucose 5%; Sodium chloride and glucose	Dilute to a concentration of 1 mg/ml. Suggested volume 200 ml. Adjust rate with in-line burette.
Latamoxef sodium *Moxalactam*®	I,D	Glucose 5%; Sodium chloride 0.9%; Sodium lactate M/6; Sodium lactate, compound (Hartmann's solution); Water for injections	
Lignocaine hydrochloride *Xylocard 20%*®	C	Glucose 5%; Sodium chloride 0.9%; Ringer's solution; Dextrans	Dilute in a large-volume infusion. Suggested infusion concentration 0.2%. Use ready-prepared solution when available. Different formulations are available for bolus injection.

Table: Intravenous additives (*continued*)

Additive	Method	Intravenous infusion	Comments
Lincomycin hydrochloride *Lincocin*®	C	Glucose 5%; Sodium chloride 0.9%	Dilute in a large-volume infusion. Suggested minimum volume 250 ml. Minimum period of infusion 1 hour.
Mecillinam *Selexidin*®	I	Glucose 5%; Sodium chloride 0.9%	Reconstituted solutions should be diluted and administered without delay. Suggested infusion time 15–30 minutes.
Melphalan *Alkeran*®	C,D	Sodium chloride 0.9%	Reconstitute with the diluent provided. Maximum period between addition and completion of administration 8 hours.
Mesna *Uromitexan*®	C,D	Sodium chloride and glucose; Sodium chloride 0.9%	Maximum period between addition and completion of administration 24 hours.
Metaraminol tartrate *Aramine*®	C, D	Glucose 5%; Sodium chloride 0.9%; Ringer's solution; Sodium lactate, compound (Hartmann's solution); Dextran 70	Suggested infusion volume 500 ml.
Methicillin sodium *Celbenin*®	C[1]		
	I	Glucose 5%; Sodium chloride 0.9%	Suggested volume 100 ml given over 30–60 minutes.
	D	As for Amoxycillin sodium (above)	
Methocarbamol *Robaxin*®	I	Glucose 5%; Sodium chloride 0.9%	Dilute to a concentration of not more than 1 g in 250 ml.
Methohexitone sodium *Brietal Sodium*®	I	Glucose 5%; Sodium chloride 0.9%	Suggested volume 250–500 ml.
Methotrexate sodium	C,D		Irritant to tissues. Avoid contamination of eyes or skin. Dilute in a large volume infusion.
Methotrexate (Lederle)		Glucose 5%; Sodium chloride 0.9%; Sodium lactate, compound (Hartmann's solution); Ringer's solution	Maximum period between addition and completion of administration 24 hours. The 50-mg vial is unsuitable for large doses by continuous infusion.
Methotrexate (Tillotts)		Glucose 5%; Sodium chloride 0.9%; Ringer's solution; Dextrans	Maximum period between addition and completion of administration 24 hours.
Emtexate®		Sodium chloride 0.9%	Maximum period between addition and completion of administration 8 hours.
Methyldopate hydrochloride *Aldomet*®	I	Glucose 5%	Suggested volume 100 ml given over 30–60 minutes.
Methylprednisolone sodium succinate *Solu-Medrone*®	C,I,D	Glucose 5%; Sodium chloride 0.9%	

C = continuous; I = intermittent; D = addition via drip tubing
C[1] = continuous infusion not usually recommended

Table: Intravenous additives (*continued*)

Additive	Method	Intravenous infusion	Comments
Metoclopramide hydrochloride *Maxolon High Dose®*	I	Glucose 5%; Sodium chloride 0.9%; Sodium lactate, compound (Hartmann's solution)	Dilute the dose with at least 50 ml of infusion solution and give over at least 15 minutes.
Metronidazole *Flagyl®*, *Metrolyl®*, *Zadstat®*	I	Glucose 5%; Sodium chloride 0.9%	
Mexiletine hydrochloride *Mexitil®*	C	Glucose 5%; Sodium chloride 0.9%; Sodium lactate M/6	
Mezlocillin sodium *Baypen®* (5 g)	I	Glucose 5% and 10%; Sodium chloride 0.9%; Ringer's solution; Fructose 5%; Water for injections	Suggested volume 50 ml given over 15–20 minutes.
Miconazole *Daktarin®*	C,I	Glucose 5%; Sodium chloride 0.9%	Minimum period of infusion 30 minutes. For intermittent infusion suggested volume 200–500 ml.
Mithramycin *Mithracin®*	I	Glucose 5%	Suggested volume 1000 ml given over 4–6 hours.
Mitozantrone hydrochloride *Novantrone®*	D	Glucose 5%; Sodium chloride 0.9%	Suggested volume at least 50 ml given over at least 3–5 minutes.
Mustine hydrochloride	D	Glucose 5%; Sodium chloride 0.9%	
Naftidrofuryl oxalate *Praxilene Forte®*	I	Glucose 5% or 10%; Sodium chloride 0.9%; Dextran 40; Fructose 10%	Suggested volume 250–500 ml given over 90–120 minutes.
Naloxone *Narcan®*	C	Glucose 5%; Sodium chloride 0.9%	Dilute to a concentration of 4 micrograms/ml.
Netilmicin sulphate *Netillin®*	I,D	Glucose 5% or 10%; Sodium chloride 0.9%	For intermittent infusion suggested volume 50–200 ml given over 30–120 minutes.
Noradrenaline solution strong sterile *Levophed®*	C	Glucose 5%; Sodium chloride and glucose	Dilute in a large-volume infusion. pH of the infusion solution must be below 6.
Orciprenaline sulphate *Alupent obstetric®*	I	Glucose 5%	Suggested infusion volume 500 ml.
Oxpentifylline *Trental®*	C	Glucose 5%; Sodium chloride 0.9%; Fructose 5%	Suggested volume 250–500 ml. To be given over 90–180 minutes.
Oxytocin *Syntocinon®*	C	Glucose 5%; Sodium chloride 0.9%; Ringer's solution; Sodium lactate M/6; Fructose 20%; Dextrans 40 or 70	Dilute in a large-volume infusion.
Phenoxybenzamine hydrochloride *Dibenyline®*	I	Sodium chloride 0.9%	To be given over not less than 60 minutes.
Phentolamine mesylate *Rogitine®*	I	Glucose 5%; Sodium chloride 0.9%	To be given over: 10 minutes (diagnostic), 180 minutes (therapy).
Phenylephrine hydrochloride	I	Glucose 5%; Sodium chloride 0.9%	

Table: Intravenous additives (*continued*)

Additive	Method	Intravenous infusion	Comments
Piperacillin sodium *Pipril*®	I	Glucose 5%; Sodium chloride 0.9%; Sodium lactate, compound (Hartmann's solution); Water for injections; Dextrans	Minimum infusion volume 50 ml given over 20–40 minutes.
Polymyxin B sulphate *Aerosporin*®	C	Glucose 5%	Suggested volume 200–500 ml given over 60–90 minutes.
Potassium canrenoate *Spiroctan-M*®	I	Glucose 5%; Sodium chloride 0.9%	Suggested volume 250 ml.
Potassium chloride	C	Glucose 5%; Sodium chloride 0.9%	Dilute in a large-volume infusion. Mix thoroughly to avoid 'layering', especially in non-rigid infusion containers. Use ready-prepared solutions when possible.
Prednisolone sodium phosphate *Codelsol*®	C,I,D	Glucose 5%; Sodium chloride 0.9%	Maximum period between addition and completion of administration 24 hours.
Quinine dihydrochloride	C	Sodium chloride 0.9%	To be given over 4 hours.
Ranitidine hydrochloride *Zantac*®	I	Glucose 5%; Sodium chloride 0.9%; Sodium lactate, compound (Hartmann's solution)	
Rifampicin *Rimactane*® *infusion*	I	Glucose 5%; Sodium lactate, compound (Hartmann's solution)	To be given over 2–3 hours.
Ritodrine hydrochloride *Yutopar*®	C	Glucose 5%; Sodium chloride 0.9%	Dilute in a large-volume infusion.
Salbutamol sulphate *Ventolin*® for intravenous infusion	C	Glucose 5%; Sodium chloride 0.9%	Suggested volume 500 ml as a solution containing 10 micrograms/ml. Different formulations are available for bolus injection.
Sodium calciumedetate *Ledclair*®	C	Glucose 5%; Sodium chloride 0.9%	Dilute to a concentration of not more than 3%. Suggested volume 250–500 ml given over at least 1 hour.
Sodium nitroprusside *Nipride*®	C	Glucose 5%	Suggested volume 500–1000 ml. Reconstitute with the diluent provided. Protect the infusion from light. Maximum period between addition and completion of administration 4 hours.
Streptokinase *Kabikinase*®	C	Glucose 5%; Sodium chloride 0.9%	
Streptase®		Sodium chloride 0.9%	
Sulphadiazine sodium	C	Sodium chloride 0.9%	Suggested volume 500 ml. Ampoule solution has a pH of over 10.

C = continuous; **I** = intermittent; **D** = addition via drip tubing

Table: Intravenous additives (*continued*)

Additive	Method	Intravenous infusion	Comments
Suxamethonium chloride *Anectine®, Scoline®*	C	Glucose 5%; Sodium chloride 0.9%	
Terbutaline sulphate *Bricanyl®*	C	Glucose 5%; Sodium chloride 0.9%	Suggested volume 500 ml. To be given over 8–10 hours.
Tetracosactrin *Synacthen®*	C	Glucose 5%; Sodium chloride 0.9%	Suggested volume 500 ml given over 6 hours.
Tetracycline hydrochloride *Achromycin Intravenous®*	C	Glucose 5%; Sodium chloride 0.9%; Sodium lactate, compound (Hartmann's solution)	Minimum volume 100 ml. To be given over not more than 8 hours.
Thiopentone sodium *Intraval®*	C,D	Sodium chloride 0.9%	Check container for haze or precipitate before administration.
Thymoxamine hydrochloride *Opilon®*	C	Glucose 5%	Suggested volume 500 ml.
Ticarcillin sodium *Ticar®*	I	Glucose 5%; Water for injections	Suggested volume 100–150 ml given over 30–40 minutes.
Tinidazole *Fasigyn®*	I	Glucose 5%; Sodium chloride 0.9%	800 mg to be given over at least 30 minutes or *pro rata*.
Tobramycin sulphate *Nebcin®*	I,D	Glucose 5%; Sodium chloride 0.9%	For intermittent infusion suggested volume 100–150 ml given over 20–60 minutes.
Tocainide hydrochloride *Tonocard®*	I	Glucose 5%; Sodium chloride 0.9%	Suggested volume 50–100 ml given over 15–30 minutes.
Treosulfan *Treosulfan* (Leo)	I	Water for injections	Infusion suggested for doses above 5 g. Use diluted to a concentration of 5 g in 100 ml.
Trimetaphan camsylate *Arfonad®*	I	Glucose 5%; Sodium chloride 0.9%	Suggested infusion concentration 0.05–0.1%. Suggested volume 100–500 ml.
Trimethoprim lactate *Monotrim®*	D	As for Syraprim® (below); also Sodium chloride 0.9%; Sodium lactate, compound (Hartmann's solution); Dextrans 40 or 70 in sodium chloride	
Syraprim®	I,D	Glucose 5%; Sodium lactate M/6; Fructose 5%	
Trisodium edetate *Limclair®*	C	Glucose 5%; Sodium chloride 0.9%	Suggested volume 500 ml given over 2–3 hours.
Urea *Ureaphil®*	C	Glucose 5% or 10%	
Urokinase *Urokinase* (Leo)	C	Sodium chloride 0.9%	
Vancomycin hydrochloride *Vancocin®*	C[1]		
	I	Glucose 5%; Sodium chloride 0.9%	Suggested volume 100–200 ml given over 20–30 minutes.

Table: Intravenous additives (*continued*)

Additive	Method	Intravenous infusion	Comments
Vasopressin, synthetic *Pitressin*®	I	Glucose 5%	Suggested concentration 20 units/100 ml given over 15 minutes.
Vecuronium bromide *Norcuron*®	I	Glucose 5%; Sodium chloride 0.9%; Ringer's solution	Reconstitute with the diluent provided.
Verapamil hydrochloride *Cordilox*®	C	Glucose 5%; Sodium chloride 0.9%; Fructose	
Vidarabine *Vira-A*®	C	Glucose 5%; Sodium chloride and glucose; Sodium lactate, compound (Hartmann's solution)	Solubility in infusion fluid is limited. It must be given diluted in a large-volume infusion and administered over 12–24 hours.
Vinblastine sulphate *Velbe*®	D	Sodium chloride 0.9%; Water for injections	Reconstitute with the diluent provided.
Vincristine sulphate *Oncovin*®	D	Sodium chloride 0.9%; Water for injections	Reconstitute with the diluent provided.
Vindesine sulphate *Eldisine*®	D	Glucose 5%; Sodium chloride 0.9%	Reconstitute with the diluent provided.
Vitamins B & C *Pabrinex*®, *Parentrovite IVHP*®	I,D	Glucose 5%; Sodium chloride 0.9%	Ampoule contents should be mixed, diluted, and administered without delay.
Vitamins, multiple			See also section 9.3.
Multibionta®	I	Glucose 5%; Sodium chloride 0.9%	Dilute 10 ml in not less than 250 ml of infusion fluid (adults).
Solivito®	I	Glucose 5% or 10%	Suggested volume 500–1000 ml given over 2–3 hours.

C = continuous; I = intermittent; D = addition via drip tubing
C^1 = continuous infusion not usually recommended

Appendix 3: Borderline Substances

In certain conditions some foods (and toilet preparations) have characteristics of drugs and the Advisory Committee on Borderline Substances advises as to the circumstances in which such substances may be regarded as drugs. The Advisory Committee's recommendations are listed below. Prescriptions issued in accordance with the Committee's advice and endorsed 'ACBS' will normally not be investigated.

NON-PRESCRIBABLE PREPARATIONS

The following have been considered by the ACBS and should **not** be prescribed on form FP10:

ALCOHOLIC BEVERAGES

Wines, tonic wines and similar preparations. (Where the therapeutic qualities of alcohol are required rectified spirit, suitably flavoured and diluted, should be prescribed.)

ANTI-SMOKING PREPARATIONS

Nicobrevin; Nicorette; Respaton.

DISINFECTANTS (ANTISEPTICS)

Drugs only when ordered in such quantities and with such directions as are appropriate for the treatment of patients. Not to be regarded as drugs if ordered for general hygienic purposes.

FOODS

Cantaflour; Carnation Build-up; Complan; Efamol capsules; Energen starch-reduced bran crispbread; Ensure Plus HN; Flora margarine; Forta puddings; Fortimel; Fortison low sodium; GF gluten-free maize biscuits with chocolate or hazelnuts, gluten-free thin wafer bread; Glucodin; Granogen; Isomil powder, ready-to-feed, and liquid concentrate; Laevoral; Linoleic acid; Modifast; Nutritionally Complete Supplemented Fasting Formula; Osmolite HN; Rite-Diet gluten-free canned rich fruit cake, chocolate chip cookies, half-coated chocolate or sultana biscuit and soya bran, Lincoln, shortcake, custard cream biscuits; Safflower seed oil; Saxin; SMA Powder; SMA Gold Cap Powder, Liquid, Ready-to-feed and White cap; Sorbitol; Sweetex; Tritamyl gluten-free bread mix, Trufree plain flour, pasta mix, sweet biscuit and bread mix; Two Cal HN; Wateon tablets.
Note: Neither gluten-free products nor those containing linoleic acid (e.g. safflower and sunflower seed oils) should be regarded as drugs in the management of *multiple sclerosis.*

TOILET PREPARATIONS

Acne Aid Bar; Atrixo; Aveeno Bar; Aveeno Bar Oilated; Cidal; Covermark Removing Cream; Dansac Skin Lotion; Derbac Soap; Dermacolor Cleansing Cream, Cleansing Milk, and Cleansing Lotion; Gamophen; Genatosan; Ipsel Hygienic Baby Salve; Lacto-Calamine; Lysaldin; Neutrogena Soap; Nivea; Oilatum Bar; RoC Total Sunblock Creams, light and deep tan; Simple Soap; United Skin Care Programme; Woodwards Nursery Cream.

VITAMIN PREPARATIONS

Drugs only when used in the management of actual or potential vitamin deficiency.

PRESCRIBABLE PREPARATIONS

The following list indicates the clinical conditions and the products which the ACBS has approved for the management of those conditions. Details of the products are given in section 9.4 (food preparations) and chapter 13 (toilet preparations).

FOODS

Conditions for which the foods indicated may be prescribed on FP10.

Amino acid metabolic disorders and similar protein disorders: see phenylketonuria; histidinaemia; homocystinuria; maple syrup urine disease; synthetic diets; low-protein products.

Anorexia nervosa: Clinifeed; Enrich; Ensure; Ensure Plus; Ensure Powder; Flexical; Fortisip Energy-Plus; Fortisip Standard; Fortison Energy-Plus; Fortison Standard; Isocal; Nutrauxil Liquid; Nutrauxil Sip; Osmolite; Triosorbon; Vivonex.

Bowel fistulas: Clinifeed; Enrich; Ensure; Ensure Plus; Ensure Powder; Flexical; Forceval Protein; Fortisip Energy-Plus; Fortisip Standard; Fortison Energy-Plus; Fortison Standard; Isocal; Nutranel; Nutrauxil Liquid; Nutrauxil Sip; Osmolite; Triosorbon; Vivonex.

Calcium intolerance: Locasol and Locasol New Formula.

Carbohydrate malabsorption: Calogen; Prosparol. See also synthetic diets; malabsorption states.

Disaccharide intolerance (without isomaltose intolerance): Calonutrin; Caloreen; Maxijul; Maxijul LE; Maxijul liquid; Polycal; Polycose. See also lactose intolerance; lactose with sucrose intolerance.

Glucose and galactose intolerance: Comminuted chicken meat (Cow & Gate); Fructose; Galactomin Formula 19 (fructose formula reduced fat).

Isomaltose intolerance: Glucose (dextrose).

Lactose intolerance: Comminuted chicken meat (Cow & Gate); Formula S (Cow & Gate); Fortison Soya; Galactomin Formula 17 (glucose formula full fat); Galactomin Formula 18 (glucose formula reduced fat); Nutramigen; Portagen; Pregestimil; Prosobee; Wysoy.

Lactose with sucrose intolerance: Aminex; Comminuted Chicken Meat (Cow & Gate); Pregestimil; Galactomin Formula 17 (glucose formula full fat); Galactomin Formula 18 (glucose formula reduced fat).

Sucrose intolerance: Glucose (dextrose) and see also synthetic diets; malabsorption states; lactose with sucrose intolerance.

Cirrhosis of the liver and chronic liver disease: see liver disease.

Coeliac disease: see gluten-sensitive enteropathies.

Cystic fibrosis: see malabsorption states.

Disaccharide intolerance: see carbohydrate malabsorption.

Dysphagia: Clinifeed; Enrich; Ensure; Ensure Plus; Ensure Powder; Forceval Protein; Fortisip Energy-Plus; Fortisip Standard; Fortison Energy-Plus; Fortison Standard; Isocal; Maxipro HBV; Nutrauxil Liquid; Nutrauxil Sip; Osmolite; Triosorbon; Vivonex.

Epilepsy (ketogenic diet in): Alembicol D; Calogen; Liquigen; Medium-Chain Triglyceride Oil (MCT); Prosparol.

Galactokinase deficiency and galactosaemia: Formula S (Cow & Gate); Galactomin Formula 17 (glucose formula full fat); Galactomin Formula 18 (glucose formula reduced fat); Nutramigen; Pregestimil; Prosobee Liquid and Powder; Wysoy.

Gastrectomy (total): Clinifeed; Enrich; Ensure; Ensure Plus; Ensure Powder; Flexical; Forceval protein; Fortisip Energy-Plus; Fortisip Standard; Fortison Energy-Plus; Fortison Standard; Isocal; Maxipro HBV; Nutranel; Nutrauxil Liquid; Nutrauxil Sip; Osmolite; Triosorbon; Vivonex.

Glucose/galactose intolerance: see carbohydrate intolerance.

Gluten-sensitive enteropathies: Aglutella Gentili (macaroni, semolina, spaghetti, spaghetti rings); Aproten products (anellini, biscuits, crispbread, ditalini, flour, rigatini, tagliatelle); Bi-Aglut biscuits; Ener G brown rice bread; Gluten-free biscuits (Farley); Gluten-free crackers (GF Supplies); Glutenex (Liga); Juvela gluten-free loaf; Juvela gluten-free mix; Juvela low-protein loaf; Juvela low-protein mix; Rite-Diet gluten-free bread; Rite-Diet gluten-free white bread mix; Rite-Diet gluten-free brown bread mix; Rite-Diet gluten-free bread with soya bran (dispensed in tin); Rite-Diet low-protein flour mix; Rite-Diet gluten-free flour mix; Rite-Diet gluten-free low-protein bread (dispensed in tin, with or without salt); Rite-Diet gluten-free digestive biscuits; Rite-Diet gluten-free sweet (without chocolate or sultanas) biscuits; Rite-Diet gluten-free savoury biscuits; Rite-Diet low-protein gluten-free crackers; Rite-Diet low-protein spaghetti (short cut); Rite-Diet low-protein spaghetti rings; Rite-Diet low-protein pasta (macaroni); Tritamyl gluten-free flour; Tritamyl PK flour; Trufree special dietary flours No. 1, No. 2 with rice bran, No. 3 for Cantabread, No. 4 white, No. 5 brown, No. 6 plain, No. 7 self-raising; Verkade gluten-free biscuits.

Glycogen storage disease: Calonutrin; Caloreen; Glucose (dextrose); Maxijul; Maxijul LE; Maxijul liquid; Polycal; Polycose.

Histidinaemia: HF(2), and see also low-protein products; synthetic diets.

Homocystinuria: Albumaid RVHB X Methionine; Albumaid RVHB Complete X Methionine, and see also low-protein products; synthetic diets.

Hypercholesterolaemia (familial): Corn oil; Sunflower oil.

Hyperlipoproteinaemia type 1: Liquigen; Medium Chain Triglyceride Oil.

Hypoglycaemia: Calonutrin; Caloreen; Maxijul; Maxijul LE; Maxijul liquid; Polycal; Polycose, and see also glycogen storage disease.

Hypoproteinaemia: Casilan; Dialamine; Forceval Protein; Maxipro HBV.

Intestinal lymphangiectasia: see malabsorption states.

Intestinal surgery: see malabsorption states.

Isomaltose intolerance: see carbohydrate malabsorption.

Lactose intolerance: see carbohydrate malabsorption.

Liver disease (i.e. chronic liver disease, cirrhosis): Aglutella Azeta cream-filled wafers; Aglutella gentili (macaroni, semolina, spaghetti, spaghetti rings); Alembicol D; Aminex; Aproten products (anellini, biscuits, crispbread, ditalini, flour, rigatini, tagliatelle); Calonutrin; Caloreen; dp Low-Protein butterscotch-flavoured or chocolate-flavoured chip cookies; Fortical; Hycal; Juvela low-protein loaf; Juvela low-protein mix; Liquigen; Maxijul; Maxijul LE; Maxijul liquid; MCT (1) Powder; Medium Chain Triglyceride Oil; Polycal; Polycose; Portagen; Rite-Diet gluten-free low-protein bread (dispensed in tin with or without salt); Rite-Diet low-protein gluten-free crackers; Rite-Diet low-protein flour mix; Rite-Diet low-protein cream-filled biscuits (chocolate flavour); Rite-Diet low-protein sweet biscuits; Rite-Diet low-protein pasta (macaroni); Rite-Diet low-protein spaghetti (short cut); Rite-Diet low-protein spaghetti rings; Rite-Diet low-protein vanilla cream wafers; Tritamyl PK flour.

Low-protein products: Aglutella Azeta cream-filled wafers; Aglutella Gentili (macaroni, semolina, spaghetti, spaghetti-rings); Aminex; Aproten products (anellini, biscuits, crispbread, ditalini, flour, rigatini, tagliatelle); dp Low-Protein butterscotch-flavoured or chocolate-flavoured chip cookies; Juvela low-protein loaf; Juvela low-protein-mix; Rite-Diet gluten-free low-protein bread (dispensed in tin, with or without salt); Rite-Diet low-protein gluten-free crackers; Rite-Diet low-protein flour-mix; Rite-Diet low-protein cream-filled biscuits (chocolate flavour); Rite-Diet low-protein sweet biscuits; Rite-Diet low-protein pasta (macaroni); Rite-Diet low-protein spaghetti (short cut); Rite-Diet low-protein spaghetti rings; Rite-Diet low-protein vanilla cream wafers; Tritamyl PK flour.

Malabsorption states: intestinal lymphangiectasia (see also gluten-sensitive enteropathies; liver disease; carbohydrate malabsorption; milk protein intolerance and synthetic diets).

(a) Protein sources: Albumaid Complete;

Comminuted Chicken Meat (Cow & Gate); Forceval Protein; Maxipro HBV.

(b) Fat: Alembicol D; Calogen; Liquigen; Medium Chain Triglyceride Oil; Prosparol.

(c) Carbohydrate: Calonutrin; Caloreen; Fortical; Hycal; Maxijul; Maxijul LE; Maxijul liquid; Polycal; Polycose.

(d) Complete Feeds: Clinifeed; Enrich; Ensure; Ensure Plus; Ensure Powder; Flexical; Fortisip Energy-Plus; Fortisip Standard; Fortison Energy-Plus; Fortison Standard; Isocal; MCT (1) Powder (with appropriate vitamin and mineral supplements); Nutranel; Nutrauxil Liquid; Nutrauxil Sip; Osmolite; Portagen; Pregestimil; Triosorbon; Vivonex.

(e) Minerals: Aminogran Mineral Mixture; Metabolic Mineral Mixture.

(f) Vitamins: As appropriate, and see synthetic diets.

Maple syrup urine disease: MSUD Aid, and see also low-protein products; synthetic diets.

Milk protein intolerance: Comminuted Chicken Meat (Cow & Gate); Formula S (Cow & Gate); Fortison Soya; Nutramigen; Pregestimil; Prosobee liquid and powder; Wysoy, and see also synthetic diets.

Nutritional support for adults:

A. (a) Nutritionally complete feeds (chemically defined diets, whole protein based), for oral, sip or tube feeding.

(i) Gluten-Free: Clinifeed; Fortisip Energy-Plus; Fortisip Standard; Fortison Energy-Plus; Fortison Standard; Triosorbon.

(ii) Lactose- and Gluten-Free: Enrich; Ensure; Ensure Plus, Ensure Powder; Isocal; MCT (1) Powder (with appropriate vitamin and mineral supplements); Nutrauxil Liquid; Nutrauxil Sip; Osmolite; Portagen.

(b) Elemental and Lactose-Free: Flexical; Nutranel; Vivonex.

B. **Nutritional source supplements;** see synthetic diets; malabsorption states.

(a) Carbohydrates; lactose-free and gluten-free; Calonutrin; Caloreen*; Fortical*; Hycal*; Maxijul; Maxijul LE*; Maxijul liquid; Polycal; Polycose.
*Have low electrolyte content.

(b) Fat:

(i) Calogen; Prosparol.

(ii) Alembicol D; Medium Chain Triglycerides; MCT Oil; Liquigen.

C. **Nitrogen sources:** Albumaid Complete (hydrolysed protein based); Casilan (whole protein based, low-sodium); Forceval Protein (whole protein based, low-sodium); Maxipro HBV (whole protein based, low-sodium).

D. **Minerals:** Aminogran Mineral Mixture; Metabolic Mineral Mixture.

Phenylketonuria: Aglutella Azeta cream-filled wafers; Aglutella gentili (macaroni, semolina, spaghetti, spaghetti rings); Albumaid XP and Albumaid XP Concentrate; Aminex; Aminogran Food Supplement; Aminogran Mineral Mixture; Aproten products (annellini, biscuits,

crispbread, ditalini, flour, rigatini, tagliatelle); Calogen; Calonutrin; Caloreen; dp Low-Protein butterscotch-flavoured or chocolate-flavoured chip cookies; Juvela low-protein loaf; Juvela low-protein mix; Lofenalac; Maxamaid XP; Metabolic Mineral Mixture; Minafen; PK Aid 1; Polycal; Polycose; Prosparol; Rite-Diet gluten-free low-protein bread (dispensed in tin, with or without salt); Rite-Diet low-protein flour mix; Rite-Diet low-protein cream-filled biscuits (chocolate flavour); Rite-Diet low-protein sweet biscuits; Rite-Diet low-protein gluten-free crackers; Rite-Diet low-protein pasta (macaroni); Rite-Diet low-protein spaghetti (short cut); Rite-Diet low protein spaghetti rings; Rite-Diet low-protein vanilla cream wafers; Tritamyl PK flour, and see low-protein products and synthetic diets.

Protein intolerance: see milk protein intolerance, low-protein products, synthetic diets, and amino acid metabolic disorders.

Renal failure: Aglutella Azeta cream-filled wafers; Aglutella gentili (macaroni, semolina, spaghetti, spaghetti rings); Aminex; Aproten products (annellini, biscuits, crispbread, ditalini, flour, rigatini, tagliatelle); Calogen; Calonutrin; Caloreen; Dialamine; dp Low-Protein butterscotch-flavoured or chocolate-flavoured chip cookies; Fortical; Hycal; Juvela low-protein loaf; Juvela low-protein mix; Maxijul; Maxijul LE; Maxijul liquid; Polycal; Polycose; Prosparol; Rite-Diet gluten-free low-protein bread (dispensed in tin, with or without salt); Rite-Diet low-protein gluten-free crackers; Rite-Diet low-protein flour mix; Rite-Diet low-protein cream-filled biscuits (chocolate flavour); Rite-Diet low-protein sweet biscuits; Rite-Diet low-protein pasta (macaroni); Rite-Diet low-protein spaghetti (short cut); Rite-Diet low-protein spaghetti rings; Rite-Diet low-protein vanilla cream wafers; Rite-Diet low-sodium bread; Tritamyl PK flour.

Short bowel syndrome: see malabsorption states.

Sodium dietary reduction: Rite-Diet low-sodium bread.

Sucrose intolerance: see carbohydrate malabsorption.

Synthetic diets:

(a) Fat: Alembicol D; Calogen; Liquigen; Medium Chain Triglyceride Oil; Prosparol.

(b) Carbohydrate; Calonutrin; Caloreen; Fortical; Hycal; Maxijul; Maxijul LE; Maxijul liquid; Polycal; Polycose.

(c) Minerals: Aminogran Mineral Mixture; Metabolic Mineral Mixture.

(d) Protein sources: see malabsorption states, complete feeds.

(e) Vitamins: as appropriate and see malabsorption states.

Vomiting in infancy: Instant Carobel; Nestargel.

TOILET PREPARATIONS

Conditions for which the toilet preparations indicated may be prescribed on FP10.

Acne: Ionax scrub.

Birthmarks: see disfiguring skin lesions.

Dermatitis (includes contact, atopic and infective dermatoses, eczema and pruritic dermatoses): Betadine Skin Cleanser and Foam; Genisol; Polytar Emollient; Polytar Plus; Polytar Liquid; Ster-Zac Bath Concentrate; T/Gel shampoo.

Dermatitis herpetiformis: see gluten-sensitive enteropathies.

Disfiguring skin lesions (birthmarks, mutilating lesions and scars): Boots Covering Cream; Covermark products; Dermacolor Camouflage System; Keromask masking cream; Veil Cover cream.

Eczema: see dermatitis.

Photodermatoses (skin protection in): Coppertone Supershade 15; Delial 10; Piz Buin Creme SPF No. 6, SPF No. 8, SPF No. 12; RoC Total Sunblock Cream 10; Spectraban 4 and 15.

Pruritus: see dermatitis.

Psoriasis: see scaling of the scalp.

Scabies: Tetmosol.

Scaling of the scalp (psoriasis, dandruff, eczema): Alphosyl; Betadine; Capitol; Ceanel Concentrate; Cetavlon PC; Genisol; Ionil T; Polytar Emollient; Polytar Liquid; Polytar Plus; T/Gel shampoo.

Appendix 4: Cautionary and Advisory Labels for Dispensed Medicines

In recent years there has been a growing need for patients to be given better information on the medicines they have been prescribed so that they will be reminded to take the medicine correctly and most effectively. One aspect of this is the provision of more detailed cautionary and advisory labels than have been used in the past.

What a patient learns about his medicine will include whatever he is told by the prescriber, what the labels on the dispensed medicines say, what any patient information leaflet may say, and whatever he is told by the pharmacist by way of explanation and encouragement. Nevertheless, the label is what the patient will see when taking each dose. Leaflets may be discarded and verbal advice forgotten.

The BNF now shows under many preparations the numbers of any labels that pharmacists are recommended to apply to the containers of preparations when they are dispensed. The wordings chosen for the labels represent a carefully considered balance between the unintelligibly short and the inconveniently long. Since any fixed set of words cannot cover the language needs of all patients it is expected that pharmacists will counsel patients.

All counselling needs to be related to the age, experience, background, and understanding of the individual patient. The patient will then be able to obtain the maximum benefit from following the directions.

Compliance with the intentions of the prescriber should be encouraged. The pharmacist should ensure that the patient understands not only how to use the medicine but also how much and how often. Any effects of the medicine on driving or work, any foods or medicines to be avoided, and what to do if a dose is missed should also be explained. There may be other matters that are better dealt with by counselling than by a label, such as the possibility of staining of the clothes or skin by a medicine.

For some preparations there is a special need for counselling, such as an unusual method or time of administration or a potential interaction with a common food or domestic remedy, and this is indicated where necessary.

Manufacturers' instructions

Many preparations are now dispensed in unbroken original packs that bear complete instructions for the patient or provide a leaflet addressed to the patient. These labels or leaflets should not normally be obscured or removed. Where it is known that such instructions are provided with an original pack intended for the patient no label has been listed under the preparation. Label 10 may be used where appropriate. Leaflets are available from various sources advising on the administration of preparations such as eye-drops, eye ointments, and suppositories.

Scope of the recommended labels

No label recommendations have been made for injections (except for selected systemic corticosteroids) on the assumption that they will be administered by a health professional or a well-trained patient. The labelling is not exhaustive and pharmacists are recommended to use their professional discretion in labelling new preparations and those for which no labels are shown.

Individual labelling advice is not given on the administration of the large variety of antacids and topical corticosteroid preparations, although general guidance on labelling is given in the notes relevant to these preparations (see sections 1.1 and 13.4). In the absence of instructions from the prescriber, and if on enquiry the patient has had no verbal instructions, the directions given under 'Dose' should be used on the label.

It is recognised that there may be occasions when a pharmacist will use his knowledge and professional discretion and decide to omit one or more of the recommended labels for a particular patient. In this case counselling is of the utmost importance. There may also be an occasion when a prescriber does not wish additional cautionary labels to be used, in which case the prescription should be endorsed 'N.C.L.' (no cautionary labels). The exact wording that is required instead should then be specified on the prescription.

Pharmacists have traditionally labelled medicines with various wordings in addition to those directions specified on the prescription. Such labels include 'Shake the bottle', 'For external use only', 'Not to be taken', and 'Store in a cool place', as well as 'Discard . . . . days after opening' and 'Do not use after . . . .', which apply particularly to antibiotic mixtures, diluted liquid and topical preparations, and to eye-drops. Although not listed in the BNF these labels should continue to be used when appropriate; indeed, 'For external use only' is a legal requirement on external liquid preparations, while 'Keep out of the reach of children' is a legal requirement on all dispensed medicines.

It is the usual practice for patients to take oral solid-dose preparations with water or other liquid and for this reason no separate label has been recommended.

The label or labels for each preparation are recommended after careful consideration of the information available. However, it is recognised that in some cases this information may be either incomplete or open to a different interpretation. The Executive Editor will therefore be grateful to receive any constructive comments on the labelling suggested for any preparation.

Recommended label wordings

The recommended label wordings that follow are in two sections: wordings which can be given as separate warnings (labels 1–18) and wordings which can be incorporated in an appropriate position in the directions for dosage or administration (labels 21–28). Labels have been omitted for numbers 19 and 20 to accommodate any future requirements within the series.

If separate labels are used it is recommended that the wordings be used without modification. If changes are made to suit computer requirements, care should be taken to retain the sense of the original.

(1) Warning. May cause drowsiness

To be used on children's preparations containing antihistamines, e.g., paediatric elixirs and linctuses, or other preparations given to children where the warnings of label 2 on driving or alcohol would not be appropriate.

(2) Warning. May cause drowsiness. If affected do not drive or operate machinery. Avoid alcoholic drink

To be used on preparations that can cause drowsiness, thereby affecting the ability to drive and operate hazardous machinery. The main preparations are most antihistamines; sedatives and hypnotics used as sedatives during the day; central nervous system depressants such as anxiolytics, antipsychotics, and tricyclic antidepressants; some antihypertensives; some analgesics; some antiemetics; some anti-epileptics; and some muscle relaxants. Label 2 may not be appropriate for hypnotics, but the patient should be counselled about the possible persistence of effects the next day. *It is an offence to drive while under the influence of drink or drugs.*

Label 1 is more appropriate for children.

Some of these preparations only cause drowsiness in the first few days of treatment and the patient then becomes tolerant; some only cause drowsiness in higher doses.

In such cases the patient should be told that the advice to avoid driving, etc., applies until the effects have worn off. Many of these preparations can produce a slowing of reaction time and a loss of mental concentration that can have the same effects as drowsiness on activities that require alertness to avoid hazard.

The avoidance of alcoholic drink is recommended, since the effects of CNS depressants are enhanced by alcohol, but it must be realised that a strict prohibition could lead to certain patients not taking the medicine at all. Pharmacists should explain the risk and encourage compliance, particularly in patients who may think they already tolerate the effects of alcohol (see also label 3).

Queries from patients with epilepsy regarding fitness to drive should be referred back to the patient's doctor.

There are other side-effects unrelated to drowsiness that may affect a patient's ability to drive or operate machinery safely, for example, blurred vision, dizziness, or nausea. In general, no label has been recommended to cover these cases, but the patient should be suitably counselled.

The narcotic analgesics have not been included under label 2 because of the special circumstances

in which they may be prescribed. Label 2 may, however, be added at the prescriber's request.

(3) Warning. May cause drowsiness. If affected do not drive or operate machinery

To be used on monoamine-oxidase inhibitors (because alcohol is covered by label 10 and the MAOI treatment card).

Some patients given CNS depressants may have been advised how much alcohol they may drink by their doctor and in such cases label 3 may be more appropriate than label 2.

(4) Warning. Avoid alcoholic drink

To be used on preparations where a reaction such as flushing may occur if alcohol is taken, e.g. metronidazole and chlorpropamide. Alcohol may also enhance the hypoglycaemia produced by some oral antidiabetic drugs.

For most interactions with alcohol label 2 is more appropriate.

(5) Do not take indigestion remedies at the same time of day as this medicine

To be used in conjunction with label 25 on preparations coated to resist gastric acid, such as enteric-coated tablets, capsules, and granules.

The coating may be ruptured prematurely in the presence of alkalis present in antacids.

(6) Do not take iron preparations or indigestion remedies at the same time of day as this medicine

To be used on preparations of doxycycline, minocycline, and penicillamine. These drugs chelate iron and calcium ions and are less well absorbed when given with iron or calcium-containing antacids. If necessary these incompatible preparations may be given about two hours apart.

(7) Do not take milk, iron preparations or indigestion remedies at the same time of day as this medicine

To be used on preparations of tetracyclines (except doxycycline and minocycline). These drugs chelate iron, calcium, and magnesium ions and are then less well absorbed. If necessary these incompatible preparations may be given about two hours apart.

(8) Do not stop taking this medicine except on your doctor's advice

To be used on preparations of beta-adrenoceptor blocking drugs, certain antihypertensive drugs, drugs used in the treatment and prophylaxis of asthma, antituberculous drugs, and allopurinol.

This label is used to encourage compliance where the drug is to be taken over long periods without the patient necessarily perceiving any benefit. Patients should be told that this label does not override the need to consult the prescriber if side-effects occur.

For certain medicines the patient should be advised to ensure that the supply does not run out.

(9)   Take at regular intervals. Complete the prescribed course unless otherwise directed

To be used on preparations where a course of treatment should be completed to reduce the incidence of relapse, the development of resistance, or failure of treatment. The preparations are antimicrobial drugs given by mouth.

Very occasionally, some of these antimicrobial agents may have severe side-effects and in such cases the patient may need to be advised of reasons for stopping treatment quickly and returning to the doctor. Examples are the development of diarrhoea in patients receiving clindamycin or lincomycin (see section 5.1.6), or sensitivity reactions with the penicillins.

(10)   Warning. Follow the printed instructions you have been given with this medicine

To be used particularly on anticoagulants, monoamine-oxidase inhibitors, and oral corticosteroids. The appropriate treatment card should be given to the patient and any necessary explanations given.

This label may also be used on other preparations to remind the patient of the instructions that have been given.

(11)   Avoid exposure of skin to direct sunlight or sun lamps

To be used on preparations that may cause phototoxic or photoallergic reactions if the patient is exposed to ultraviolet radiation. Many drugs other than those listed (e.g., phenothiazines and sulphonamides) may on rare occasions cause reactions in susceptible patients. Reactions have also been caused by external preparations (e.g. coal tar) and by various ingredients of perfumes and cosmetics. Exposure to high intensity ultraviolet radiation from sunray lamps and sunbeds is particularly likely to cause reactions and in advising patients this should be mentioned.

The drugs involved are amiodarone, azapropazone, demeclocycline, nalidixic acid, and protriptyline.

(12)   Do not take remedies containing aspirin while taking this medicine

To be used on preparations containing salicylate derivatives, where it may not be known to the patient that the medicine has a similar action to aspirin, and on preparations containing the uricosuric drugs probenecid and sulphinpyrazone whose activity is reduced by aspirin.

Label 12 should not be used for anticoagulants; label 10 is more appropriate.

(13)   Dissolve or mix with water before taking

To be used on preparations that are intended to be dissolved in water (e.g. soluble tablets) or mixed with water (e.g. powders, granules) before use. In a few cases the manufacturer's literature indicates that other liquids such as fruit juice or milk may be used.

(14)   This medicine may colour the urine or stools

To be used on preparations that may cause the patient's urine to turn unusual colours. These include anthraquinones (alkaline urine red), phenolphthalein (alkaline urine pink), triamterene (blue), levodopa (dark reddish), phenazopyridine (reddish orange), and rifampicin (red). Iron preparations may colour the urine and stools black.

(15)   Caution flammable: keep away from naked flames

To be applied to preparations containing sufficient alcohol, acetone, ether, or other flammable solvent to render them flammable if exposed to a naked flame. The term flammable is now used by the British Pharmacopoeia and in legislation in preference to inflammable. Since both terms are now liable to cause confusion, the pharmacist should make sure that the patient understands what is meant.

(16)   Allow to dissolve under the tongue. Do not transfer from this container. Keep tightly closed. Discard eight weeks after opening

To be used on glyceryl trinitrate tablets to remind the patient not to transfer the tablets to plastic or less suitable containers. The manufacturer's original pack normally carries most of this wording and it may only be necessary to add 'Discard eight weeks after opening'.

(17)   Not more than . . . . in 24 hours

To be used on preparations for the treatment of acute migraine except those containing ergotamine, for which label 18 is used.

It may also be used on preparations for which no dose has been specified by the prescriber.

(18)   Not more than . . . in 24 hours or . . . in any one week

To be used on preparations of ergotamine tartrate. The number of tablets should correspond to 6 to 8 mg in a day and 10 to 12 mg in a week.

(21)   . . . with or after food

To be used on preparations that are liable to cause gastric irritation with nausea and vomiting, or those that are better absorbed with food.

The incidence of gastric irritation may be reduced when some preparations are given during or immediatetly after a meal. The presence of food in the upper gastro-intestinal tract may reduce the rate of absorption of certain drugs. Nausea and vomiting are liable to decrease compliance and possibly lead to loss of the drug from vomiting.

Patients may on occasions be advised to take their medicine with or after food in the interest of compliance when normally it should be taken before meals. There is a wide variation in the instructions given for iron salts and their preparations. They are usually best absorbed when given on an empty stomach and may then cause irritation. They are therefore often taken with a meal.

The prescriber's instructions should be followed.

A small number of preparations are better absorbed when given with food.

The word 'food' is used in preference to 'meal' on the label. Patients differ in their interpretation of the words and may decide not to take a dose if it has to be taken with a meal that they normally omit.

Patients should be advised when to take their doses, according to their particular circumstances, and that a small amount of food is sufficient.

(22). . . half to one hour before food

To be used on some anticholinergic or antacid preparations; some pancreatin and other enzyme preparations; most appetite suppressants; and certain other drugs whose absorption or local effect is thereby improved.

(23)   . . . an hour before food or on an empty stomach

To be used on some oral antibiotics whose absorption may be reduced by the presence of food and acid in the stomach.

Many of the antibiotics introduced in recent years are less affected by acid and/or food in the stomach and may be given at any time relative to meals.

(24)   . . . sucked or chewed

To be used on preparations that may be sucked or chewed. Certain preparations must be chewed before swallowing to improve their absorption or because of their size; others have been specially formulated to be chewed. All pastilles and lozenges should be sucked slowly to aid their local effect on the oropharynx. The pharmacist should use his discretion as to which of these words is appropriate.

(25)   . . . swallowed whole, not chewed

To be used on preparations designed for sustained release; on certain preparations that are very unpleasant or may damage the mouth or oesophagus if not swallowed whole; and with label 5 for enteric-coated preparations. Most sustained-release preparations rely on the coating of pellets, granules, tablets, or capsules or compression in a matrix material to achieve their effect. Chewing can cause premature release of active ingredient.

(26)   . . . dissolved under the tongue

To be used on preparations intended for sublingual use. Several drugs are absorbed into the circulation more effectively from the mucosa of the mouth, thereby avoiding the portal circulation into the liver. Patients should be advised to hold the tablet still under the tongue and avoid swallowing until the tablet is dissolved. The buccal mucosa between the gum and cheek is occasionally specified by the prescriber and specific directions should then be used.

(27)   . . . with plenty of water

To be used on preparations that should be well diluted (e.g. chloral hydrate), where a high fluid intake is required (e.g. sulphonamides), or where water is required to aid the action of the preparation (e.g. methylcellulose). The patient should be advised that 'plenty' means at least 150 ml (about a tumblerful). In most cases a beverage such as fruit juice, tea, or coffee could be used. There have been reports of solid-dose preparations sticking in the oesophagus, particularly in the elderly, and all patients should be reminded of the necessity of taking capsules and tablets with water or other liquid. As much as 100 ml may be required and the patient should stand or sit while taking the dose.

(28)   To be applied sparingly . . .

To be used with external corticosteroid preparations and dithranol preparations.

The application of excessive quantities to the skin can increase the incidence of local side-effects and give rise to undesirable systemic effects.

Formulary

The full formulae of non-proprietary oral liquid preparations containing tartrazine have been added to the Formulary in order to advise prescribers of the presence of this ingredient, to which some patients are sensitive. Otherwise only the formulae of non-proprietary preparations mentioned in the classified notes and commonly dispensed extemporaneously are listed here for information. For further details of suitable methods of preparation, packaging, and labelling, see *The Pharmaceutical Codex* 11th Edition.

Obsolete formulae may be found in the *Compendium of Past Formulae 1933–1966* (1971) and *Supplement* (1979) issued by the National Pharmaceutical Association.

Ear-drops

10 ml to be dispensed unless otherwise directed
Labelling: in the absence of instructions by the prescriber state—3 or 4 drops to be put into the affected ear

Sodium Bicarbonate Ear-drops, BP

Sodium Bicarbonate	5	g
Glycerol	30	ml
Purified Water, freshly boiled and cooled	to 100	ml

It should be recently prepared

Elixirs

Dilution: see Guidance on Prescribing, general information

PoM Chloral Elixir, Paediatric, BP

Chloral Hydrate	200	mg
Water for Preparations	0.1	ml
Black Currant Syrup	1	ml
Syrup	to 5	ml

It should be recently prepared
Diluent syrup. The diluted elixir must be freshly prepared

CD Diamorphine and Cocaine Elixir, BPC

Diamorphine Hydrochloride	5	mg
Cocaine Hydrochloride	5	mg
Alcohol (90%)	0.625	ml
Syrup	1.25	ml
Chloroform Water	to 5	ml

It must be freshly prepared
The proportion of diamorphine hydrochloride may be altered when specified by the prescriber

CD Diamorphine, Cocaine and Chlorpromazine Elixir, BPC

Diamorphine Hydrochloride	5	mg
Cocaine Hydrochloride	5	mg
Alcohol (90%)	0.625	ml
Chlorpromazine Elixir	1.25	ml
Chloroform Water	to 5	ml

It must be freshly prepared
The proportion of diamorphine hydrochloride may be altered when specified by the prescriber
5 ml contains 6.25 mg of chlorpromazine hydrochloride

PoM Isoniazid Elixir, BPC

Isoniazid	50	mg
Citric Acid Monohydrate	12.5	mg
Sodium Citrate	60	mg
Concentrated Anise Water	0.05	ml
Compound Tartrazine Solution	0.05	ml
Glycerol	1	ml
Chloroform Water, Double-strength	2	ml
Water for Preparations	to 5	ml

Diluent chloroform water. The diluted elixir must be freshly prepared

PoM Morphine and Cocaine Elixir, BPC

Morphine Hydrochloride	5	mg
Cocaine Hydrochloride	5	mg
Alcohol (90%)	0.625	ml
Syrup	1.25	ml
Chloroform Water	to 5	ml

It should be recently prepared
The proportion of morphine hydrochloride may be altered when specified by the prescriber. If above 13 mg per 5 ml the elixir becomes CD

PoM Morphine, Cocaine and Chlorpromazine Elixir, BPC

Morphine Hydrochloride	5	mg
Cocaine Hydrochloride	5	mg
Alcohol (90%)	0.625	ml
Chlorpromazine Elixir	1.25	ml
Chloroform Water	to 5	ml

It should be recently prepared
The proportion of morphine hydrochloride may be altered when specified by the prescriber. If above 13 mg per 5 ml the elixir becomes CD
5 ml contains 6.25 mg of chlorpromazine hydrochloride

PoM Neomycin Elixir, BPC

Neomycin Sulphate	100	mg
Disodium Edetate	2.5	mg
Saccharin Sodium	4.5	mg
Benzoic Acid	10	mg
Citric Acid	a sufficient quantity	
Compound Tartrazine Solution	0.03	ml
Sorbitol Solution	1.925	ml
Purified Water, freshly boiled and cooled	to 5	ml

Diluent syrup. The diluted elixir must be freshly prepared

PoM Phenobarbitone Elixir, BP

Phenobarbitone	30	mg
Compound Tartrazine Solution	0.1	ml
Compound Orange Spirit	0.24	ml
Alcohol (90%)	4	ml
Glycerol	4	ml
Water for Preparations	to 10	ml

Diluent syrup. The diluted elixir must be freshly prepared

Piperazine Citrate Elixir, BP

Piperazine Citrate	937.5	mg
Peppermint Spirit	0.025	ml
Green S and Tartrazine Solution	0.075	ml
Glycerol	0.5	ml
Syrup	2.5	ml
Water for Preparations	to 5	ml

Diluent syrup. The diluted elixir must be freshly prepared
5 ml contains the equivalent of 750 mg of piperazine hydrate

Gargles

Labelling: in the absence of instructions by the prescriber, the directions for use given below the preparation should be stated

Phenol Gargle

Phenol Glycerin	5	ml
Amaranth Solution	1	ml
Water for preparations	to 100	ml

When diluted the gargle contains about 0.5% w/v of phenol
Directions for use: to be diluted with an equal quantity of warm water
300 ml to be dispensed unless otherwise directed

Inhalations

Labelling: in the absence of instructions by the prescriber, the directions for use given below the preparation should be stated

NHS Menthol and Benzoin Inhalation, BP

Menthol	2	g
Benzoin Inhalation	to 100	ml

Directions for use: add 1 teaspoonful to a pint of hot, not boiling, water and inhale the vapour.
25 ml to be dispensed unless otherwise directed

Menthol and Eucalyptus Inhalation, BP

Menthol	2	g
Eucalyptus Oil	10	ml
Light Magnesium Carbonate	7	g
Water for Preparations	to 100	ml

Directions for use: add 1 teaspoonful to a pint of hot, not boiling, water and inhale the vapour
25 ml to be dispensed unless otherwise directed

Linctuses

Dilution: see Guidance on Prescribing, general information

Codeine Linctus, Diabetic, BPC

Codeine Phosphate	15	mg
Citric Acid Monohydrate	25	mg
Lemon Spirit	0.005	ml
Compound Tartrazine Solution	0.05	ml
Benzoic Acid Solution	0.1	ml
Chloroform Spirit	0.1	ml
Water for Preparations	0.1	ml
Sorbitol Solution, Non-crystallising grade	to 5	ml

Diluent chloroform water. The diluted linctus must be freshly prepared

Codeine Linctus, Paediatric, BPC

Codeine Linctus	1	ml
Syrup	to 5	ml

Diluent syrup
5 ml contains 3 mg of codeine phosphate

CD Diamorphine Linctus, BPC

Diamorphine Hydrochloride	3	mg
Compound Tartrazine Solution	0.06	ml
Glycerol	1.25	ml
Oxymel	1.25	ml
Syrup	to 5	ml

Diluent syrup. It must be freshly prepared

CD Methadone Linctus, BP

Methadone Hydrochloride	2	mg
Compound Tartrazine Solution	0.04	ml
Water for Preparations	0.6	ml
Glycerol	1.25	ml
Tolu Syrup	to 5	ml

Diluent syrup

NHS Noscapine Linctus, BP

Noscapine	15	mg
Citric Acid Monohydrate	50	mg
Compound Tartrazine Solution	0.015	ml
Chloroform Spirit	0.375	ml
Water for Preparations	0.5	ml
Syrup	to 5	ml

Diluent syrup

NHS Opiate Squill Linctus, BP

(Gee's Linctus)

Camphorated Opium Tincture	
Squill Oxymel	
Tolu Syrup	of each, equal parts

Diluent syrup
5 ml contains 800 micrograms of anhydrous morphine

NHS Opiate Squill Linctus, Paediatric, BP

Camphorated Opium Tincture	0.3 ml
Squill Oxymel	0.3 ml
Tolu Syrup	0.3 ml
Glycerol	1 ml
Syrup	to 5 ml

Diluent syrup
5 ml contains 150 micrograms of anhydrous morphine

Simple Linctus, BP

Citric Acid Monohydrate	125	mg
Concentrated Anise Water	0.05	ml
Amaranth Solution	0.075	ml
Chloroform Spirit	0.3	ml
Syrup	to 5	ml

Diluent syrup

Simple Linctus, Paediatric, BP

Simple Linctus	1.25	ml
Syrup	to 5	ml

Diluent syrup

NHS **Tolu Linctus, Compound, Paediatric, BP**

Citric Acid Monohydrate		30	mg
Benzaldehyde Spirit		0.01	ml
Compound Tartrazine Solution		0.05	ml
Glycerol		1	ml
Invert Syrup		1	ml
Tolu Syrup	to	5	ml

Diluent syrup

Liniments

Methyl Salicylate Liniment, BP

Methyl Salicylate		25 ml
Arachis Oil	to	100 ml

It should be kept in airtight containers in a cool place
100 ml to be dispensed unless otherwise directed

Lotions

Labelling: in the absence of instructions by the prescriber, the directions for use, if any, given below the preparation should be stated

Aluminium Acetate Lotion

Aluminium Acetate Solution		5 ml
Purified Water, freshly boiled and cooled	to	100 ml

It contains about 0.65% of aluminium acetate
It must be freshly prepared
To be used undiluted
500 ml to be dispensed unless otherwise directed

Formaldehyde Lotion

Formaldehyde Solution		3 ml
Water for Preparations	to	100 ml

It must be freshly prepared
100 ml to be dispensed unless otherwise directed

Salicylic Acid Lotion, BP

Salicylic Acid		2	g
Castor Oil		1	ml
Industrial Methylated Spirit	to	100	ml

Labelling: Caution: this preparation is flammable. Do not use, or dry the hair, near a fire or naked flame
100 ml to be dispensed unless otherwise directed

Silver Nitrate Lotion

Silver Nitrate		500 mg
Purified Water, freshly boiled and cooled	to	100 ml

It must be freshly prepared, and protected from light
Directions for use: to be used undiluted
Labelling: this lotion will produce black stains on skin and clothing
50 ml to be dispensed unless otherwise directed

Sulphur Lotion, Compound, BPC

Precipitated Sulphur		4	g
Quillaia Tincture		0.5	ml
Glycerol		2	ml
Industrial Methylated Spirit		6	ml
Calcium Hydroxide Solution	to	100	ml

200 ml to be dispensed unless otherwise directed

Zinc Sulphate Lotion, BP

Zinc Sulphate		1	g
Amaranth Solution		1	ml
Water for Preparations	to	100	ml

200 ml to be dispensed unless otherwise directed

Mixtures

Dilution: see Guidance on Prescribing, general information
Labelling: mixtures, other than paediatric mixtures, and others with a dose of 5 ml, should be diluted with water before taking

Aluminium Hydroxide and Belladonna Mixture, BPC

Belladonna Tincture		0.5	ml
Chloroform Spirit		0.25	ml
Aluminium Hydroxide Mixture	to	5	ml

It must be freshly prepared

NHS **Ammonia and Ipecacuanha Mixture, BP**

Ammonium Bicarbonate		200	mg
Ipecacuanha Tincture		0.3	ml
Concentrated Anise Water		0.05	ml
Concentrated Camphor Water		0.1	ml
Liquorice Liquid Extract		0.5	ml
Chloroform Water, Double-strength		5	ml
Water for Preparations	to	10	ml

It should be recently prepared

Ammonium Chloride Mixture, BP

Ammonium Chloride		1	g
Aromatic Ammonia Solution		0.5	ml
Liquorice Liquid Extract		1	ml
Water for Preparations	to	10	ml

It should be recently prepared
Labelling: to be taken well diluted with water

NHS **Ammonium Chloride and Morphine Mixture, BP**

Ammonium Chloride		300	mg
Chloroform and Morphine Tincture		0.3	ml
Ammonium Bicarbonate		200	mg
Liquorice Liquid Extract		0.5	ml
Water for Preparations	to	10	ml

It should be recently prepared
10 ml contains 500 micrograms of anhydrous morphine

Belladonna Mixture, Paediatric, BPC

Belladonna Tincture		0.15	ml
Compound Orange Spirit		0.01	ml
Benzoic Acid Solution		0.1	ml
Glycerol		0.5	ml
Syrup		1	ml
Water for Preparations	to	5	ml

It should be recently prepared
Dose: up to 1 year 5 ml; 1–5 years 10 ml
5 ml contains 45 micrograms of belladonna alkaloids

Calcium Carbonate Mixture, Compound, Paediatric, BPC

Calcium Carbonate	50	mg
Light Magnesium Carbonate	50	mg
Sodium Bicarbonate	50	mg
Aromatic Cardamom Tincture	0.05	ml
Syrup	0.5	ml
Chloroform Water, Double-strength	2.5	ml
Water for Preparations	to 5	ml

It should be recently prepared
Dose: up to 1 year 5 ml; 1–5 years 10 ml

PoM Aromatic Chalk with Opium Mixture, BP

Chalk and Opium Mixture

Chalk	325	mg
Opium Tincture	0.5	ml
Sucrose	650	mg
Tragacanth, in powder	20	mg
Aromatic Ammonia Solution	0.5	ml
Catechu Tincture	0.5	ml
Compound Cardamom Tincture	1	ml
Chloroform Water, Double-strength	5	ml
Water for Preparations	to 10	ml

It should be recently prepared
10 ml contains 5 mg of anhydrous morphine

Chalk Mixture, Paediatric, BP

Chalk	100	mg
Tragacanth, in powder	10	mg
Concentrated Cinnamon Water	0.02	ml
Syrup	0.5	ml
Chloroform Water, Double-strength	2.5	ml
Water for Preparations	to 5	ml

It should be recently prepared
Dose: up to 1 year 5 ml; 1–5 years 10 ml

PoM Chloral Mixture, BP

Chloral Hydrate	1	g
Syrup	2	ml
Water for Preparations	to 10	ml

It should be recently prepared
Diluent syrup 1 part with water 4 parts. The diluted mixture must be freshly prepared
Labelling: to be taken well diluted with water

Ferrous Sulphate Mixture, Paediatric, BP

Ferrous Sulphate	60	mg
Ascorbic Acid	10	mg
Orange Syrup	0.5	ml
Chloroform Water, Double-strength	2.5	ml
Water for Preparations	to 5	ml

It should be recently prepared. The use of certain types of tap water, particularly those with temporary hardness, may lead to discoloration of this mixture. Freshly boiled and cooled purified water gives a satisfactory colourless or very pale yellow product
Dose: up to 1 year 5 ml; 1–5 years 10 ml
Labelling: to be taken well diluted with water

Gentian Mixture, Acid, BPC

Concentrated Compound Gentian Infusion	1	ml
Dilute Hydrochloric Acid	0.5	ml
Chloroform Water, Double-strength	5	ml
Water for Preparations	to 10	ml

It should be recently prepared

Gentian Mixture, Alkaline, BP

Concentrated Compound Gentian Infusion	1	ml
Sodium Bicarbonate	500	mg
Chloroform Water, Double-strength	5	ml
Water for Preparations	to 10	ml

It should be recently prepared

NHS Ipecacuanha and Morphine Mixture, BP

Ipecacuanha Tincture	0.2	ml
Chloroform and Morphine Tincture	0.4	ml
Liquorice Liquid Extract	1	ml
Water for Preparations	to 10	ml

It should be recently prepared
10 ml contains 700 micrograms of anhydrous morphine

Ipecacuanha Emetic Mixture, Paediatric, BP

Ipecacuanha Liquid Extract	0.7	ml
Hydrochloric Acid	0.025	ml
Glycerol	1	ml
Syrup	to 10	ml

Kaolin and Morphine Mixture, BP

Light Kaolin, or Light Kaolin (Natural)	2	g
Sodium Bicarbonate	500	mg
Chloroform and Morphine Tincture	0.4	ml
Water for Preparations	to 10	ml

It should be recently prepared, unless the kaolin has been sterilised
10 ml contains 700 micrograms of anhydrous morphine

Kaolin Mixture, BP

Light Kaolin, or Light Kaolin (Natural)	2	g
Light Magnesium Carbonate	500	mg
Sodium Bicarbonate	500	mg
Peppermint Emulsion, Concentrated	0.25	ml
Chloroform Water, Double-strength	5	ml
Water for Preparations	to 10	ml

It should be recently prepared, unless the kaolin has been sterilised

Kaolin Mixture, Paediatric, BP

Light Kaolin, or Light Kaolin (Natural)	1	g
Amaranth Solution	0.05	ml
Benzoic Acid Solution	0.1	ml
Raspberry Syrup	1	ml
Chloroform Water, Double-strength	2.5	ml
Water for Preparations	to 5	ml

It should be recently prepared, unless the kaolin has been sterilised
Dose: up to 1 year 5 ml; 1–5 years 10 ml

Magnesium Carbonate Mixture, BPC

Light Magnesium Carbonate	500	mg
Sodium Bicarbonate	800	mg
Peppermint Emulsion, Concentrated	0.25	ml
Chloroform Water, Double-strength	5	ml
Water for Preparations to	10	ml

It should be recently prepared

Magnesium Carbonate Mixture, Aromatic, BP

Light Magnesium Carbonate	300	mg
Sodium Bicarbonate	500	mg
Aromatic Cardamom Tincture	0.3	ml
Chloroform Water, Double-strength	5	ml
Water for Preparations to	10	ml

It should be recently prepared

Magnesium Sulphate Mixture, BP

Magnesium Sulphate	4	g
Light Magnesium Carbonate	500	mg
Peppermint Emulsion, Concentrated	0.25	ml
Chloroform Water, Double-strength	3	ml
Water for Preparations to	10	ml

It should be recently prepared

Magnesium Trisilicate and Belladonna Mixture, BPC

Belladonna Tincture	0.5 ml
Magnesium Trisilicate Mixture to	10 ml

It must be freshly prepared
5 ml contains 75 micrograms of belladonna alkaloids

Magnesium Trisilicate Mixture, BP

Magnesium Trisilicate	500	mg
Light Magnesium Carbonate	500	mg
Sodium Bicarbonate	500	mg
Peppermint Emulsion, Concentrated	0.25	ml
Chloroform Water, Double-strength	5	ml
Water for Preparations to	10	ml

It should be recently prepared

CD Methadone Mixture 1 mg/ml (formerly Drug Tariff Formula)

Methadone Hydrochloride	5	mg
Green S and Tartrazine Solution	0.01	ml
Compound Tartrazine Solution	0.04	ml
Syrup	2.5	ml
Chloroform Water, Double-strength to	5	ml

This preparation is 2½ times the strength of Methadone Linctus and is intended only for drug dependent persons for whom treatment is normally ordered on form FP10(H.P.)(ad)
The title includes the strength and prescriptions should be written accordingly

Potassium Citrate Mixture, BP

Potassium Citrate	3	g
Citric Acid Monohydrate	500	mg
Lemon Spirit	0.05	ml
Quillaia Tincture	0.1	ml
Syrup	2.5	ml
Chloroform Water, Double-strength	3	ml
Water for Preparations to	10	ml

It should be recently prepared
Diluent syrup
Labelling: to be taken well diluted with water

NHS Rhubarb and Soda Mixture, Ammoniated, BP

Rhubarb, in powder	250	mg
Sodium Bicarbonate	800	mg
Ammonium Bicarbonate	200	mg
Peppermint Emulsion, Concentrated	0.25	ml
Chloroform Water, Double-strength	5	ml
Water for Preparations to	10	ml

It should be recently prepared

NHS Rhubarb Mixture, Compound, BPC

Compound Rhubarb Tincture	1	ml
Light Magnesium Carbonate	500	mg
Sodium Bicarbonate	500	mg
Strong Ginger Tincture	0.3	ml
Chloroform Water, Double-strength	5	ml
Water for Preparations to	10	ml

It should be recently prepared

Sodium Bicarbonate Mixture, Paediatric, BPC

Sodium Bicarbonate	50	mg
Concentrated Dill Water	0.1	ml
Ginger Syrup	0.2	ml
Syrup	1.85	ml
Chloroform Water, Double-strength	2.5	ml
Water for Preparations to	5	ml

It should be recently prepared
Dose: up to 1 year 5 ml; 1–5 years 10 ml

Sodium Salicylate Mixture, BP

Sodium Salicylate	500	mg
Sodium Metabisulphite	10	mg
Concentrated Orange Peel Infusion	0.5	ml
Chloroform Water, Double-strength	5	ml
Water for Preparations to	10	ml

It should be recently prepared

Sodium Salicylate Mixture, Strong, BP

Sodium Salicylate	1	g
Sodium Metabisulphite	10	mg
Peppermint Emulsion, Concentrated	0.25	ml
Chloroform Water, Double-strength	5	ml
Water for Preparations to	10	ml

It should be recently prepared

Mouth-washes

Labelling: in the absence of instructions by the prescriber, the directions for use given under the preparation should be stated

Artificial Saliva, DPF

A suitable inert, slightly viscous, aqueous liquid containing a suitable antimicrobial preservative. If no formula is specified the following may be suitable.

Sodium Chloride	100	mg
Hypromellose '4500'	1.3	g
Benzalkonium Chloride Solution	0.02	ml
Saccharin Sodium	10	mg
Thymol	10	mg
Peppermint Oil	0.02	ml
Spearmint Oil	0.03	ml
Amaranth Solution	0.1	ml
Water for preparations	to 100	ml

Dose: up to 5 ml as required. Max. 20 ml daily.
200 ml to be dispensed unless otherwise directed

Sodium Chloride Mouth-wash, Compound, BP

Sodium Chloride	1.5	g
Sodium Bicarbonate	1	g
Peppermint Emulsion, Concentrated	2.5	ml
Chloroform Water, Double-strength	50	ml
Water for Preparations	to 100	ml

It should be recently prepared
Directions for use: to be used with an equal quantity of warm water

Nasal Drops

Ephedrine Nasal Drops, BPC

Ephedrine Hydrochloride	500 mg
Chlorbutol	500 mg
Sodium Chloride	500 mg
Water for Preparations	to 100 ml

When Ephedrine Nasal Drops 1% is prescribed, nasal drops containing ephedrine hydrochloride 1 g/100 ml in the same vehicle is supplied

Ointments

25 g to be dispensed unless otherwise directed

Calamine and Coal Tar Ointment, BP

Calamine, finely sifted	12.5 g
Zinc Oxide, finely sifted	12.5 g
Strong Coal Tar Solution	2.5 g
Hydrous Wool Fat	25 g
White Soft Paraffin	47.5 g

Coal Tar and Salicylic Acid Ointment, BP

Coal Tar	2 g
Salicylic Acid	2 g
Emulsifying Wax	11.4 g
White Soft Paraffin	19 g
Coconut Oil	54 g
Polysorbate 80	4 g
Liquid Paraffin	7.6 g

Paraffin Ointment, BP

Hard Paraffin	3	g
White Soft Paraffin	90	g
White Beeswax	2	g
Cetostearyl Alcohol	5	g

Paints

Podophyllin Paint, Compound, BP

Podophyllum Resin	15	g
Compound Benzoin Tincture	to 100	ml

Caution: This paint is very irritant to the eyes
5 ml to be dispensed unless otherwise directed

Oral Powders

Sodium Chloride and Glucose Oral Powder, Compound, BP

For each powder take:

Sodium Chloride	500 mg
Sodium Bicarbonate	750 mg
Potassium Chloride	750 mg
Glucose	20 g

It may be flavoured
It should be dispensed in airtight containers

Note: Sodium Chloride and Glucose Oral Powder, Compound, Small Size may be prepared by weighing 8.8 g of the mixed powder into each container. It is also available as a proprietary product—see section 9.2.1.2

Solutions

Labelling: in the absence of instructions by the prescriber, the directions for use, if any, given below the preparations should be stated

Potassium Permanganate Solution

Potassium Permanganate	100 mg
Water for Preparations	to 100 ml

It must be freshly prepared
One part to be diluted with 7 parts of water, or as directed
The diluted solution contains potassium permanganate about 1 in 8000
500 ml to be dispensed unless otherwise directed

Water for Preparations

Potable water drawn freshly from the supply of a public water undertaking and suitable for drinking. Water obtained from the supply via a local storage tank is unsuitable for this purpose. If such a water supply is not available, or if stored water is the only source of mains water, freshly boiled and cooled purified water should be used instead. It should also be used when the potable water in a district is unsuitable for a particular preparation

Dental Practitioners' Formulary

List of Dental Preparations

The following list has been approved by the appropriate Secretaries of State, and the preparations therein may be prescribed by dental practitioners on form FP14 (GP14 in Scotland).

Capsules
  Amoxycillin Capsules, BP
  Ampicillin Capsules, BP
  Cephalexin Capsules, BP
  Cephradine Capsules, BP
  Clindamycin Capsules, BP
  Diazepam Capsules, BP
  Mefenamic Acid Capsules, BP
  Oxytetracycline Capsules, BP
  Temazepam Capsules, DPF
  Tetracycline Capsules, BP
Cream
  Hydrocortisone Cream, BPC
Elixirs
  Cephradine Elixir, DPF
  Diazepam Elixir, DPF
  Paracetamol Elixir, Paediatric, BP
  Promethazine Hydrochloride Elixir, BP
Gels
  Any gel prepared for dental use and containing at least 1 per cent of chlorhexidine gluconate
  Miconazole Oral Gel, DPF
Glycerin
  Compound Thymol Glycerin, BP
Inhalation
  Menthol and Eucalyptus Inhalation, BP
Injections
  Cephradine Injection, DPF
  Clindamycin Injection, DPF
  Erythromycin Lactobionate Injection, DPF
  Lincomycin Injection, BP
Lozenges
  Amphotericin Lozenges, BP
  Benzocaine Lozenges, DPF
  Hydrocortisone Lozenges, BPC
Mixtures
  Amoxycillin Mixture, BP
  Amphotericin Mixture, DPF
  Ampicillin Mixture, BP
  Cephalexin Mixture, BP
  Clindamycin Mixture, Paediatric, DPF
  Co-trimoxazole Mixture, BP
  Co-trimoxazole Mixture, Paediatric, BP
  Erythromycin Ethylsuccinate Mixture, DPF
  Erythromycin Ethylsuccinate Mixture, Paediatric, DPF
  Metronidazole Mixture, DPF
  Nystatin Mixture, BP
  Tetracycline Mixture, BPC
Mouth-bath
  Tetracycline Mouth-bath, DPF
Mouth-washes
  Artificial Saliva, DPF
  Benzydamine Mouth-wash, DPF
  Chlorhexidine Mouth-wash, DPF
  Chlorhexidine Mouth-wash, Compound, DPF
  Hydrogen Peroxide Mouth-wash, DPF
  Lignocaine Viscous Mouth-wash, DPF
  Povidone-iodine Mouth-wash, DPF
  Sodium Chloride Mouth-wash, Compound, BP
  Sodium Perborate Mouth-wash, Buffered, DPF
  Zinc Sulphate Mouth-wash, DPF
Nasal Drops
  Ephedrine Nasal Drops, BPC
Ointments
  Amphotericin Ointment, DPF
  Fusidic Acid Ointment, DPF
  Lignocaine 5% Ointment, DPF
  Nystatin Ointment, BP
Paints
  Brilliant Green and Crystal Violet Paint, BP
  Idoxuridine 0.1% Paint, DPF
Pastes
  Carmellose Gelatin Paste, DPF
  Choline Salicylate Dental Paste, DPF
  Triamcinolone Acetonide Dental Paste, BP
Pastilles
  Nystatin Pastilles, DPF
Oral Powder
  Amoxycillin Oral Powder, DPF
Solutions
  Hydrogen Peroxide Solution (6 per cent), BP
  Idoxuridine 5% in Dimethyl Sulphoxide, DPF
Solution-tablets
  Mouth-wash Solution-tablets, BP
Tablets
  Amoxycillin Tablets, Dispersible, DPF
  Amphotericin Tablets, DPF
  Ampicillin Tablets, Paediatric, BP
  Ascorbic Acid Tablets, BP
  Aspirin Tablets, BP
  Aspirin Tablets, Dispersible, BP
  Aspirin Tablets, Paediatric Dispersible, BP
  Aspirin, Paracetamol, and Codeine Tablets, DPF
  Carbamazepine Tablets, BP
  Cephalexin Tablets, BP
  Chlorpheniramine Tablets, BP
  Co-codamol Tablets, DPF
  Co-codamol Tablets, Dispersible, DPF
  Co-codaprin Tablets, Dispersible, DPF
  Co-dydramol Tablets, DPF
  Co-trimoxazole Tablets, BP
  Co-trimoxazole Tablets, Dispersible, BP
  Co-trimoxazole Tablets, Double-strength, DPF
  Co-trimoxazole Tablets, Double-strength, Dispersible, DPF
  Co-trimoxazole Tablets, Paediatric, BP
  Diazepam Tablets, BP
  Diflunisal Tablets, BP
  Dihydrocodeine Tablets, BP
  Erythromycin Ethylsuccinate Tablets, DPF
  Erythromycin Stearate Tablets, BP
  Erythromycin Tablets, BP
  Ibuprofen Tablets, BP
  Metronidazole Tablets, BP
  Nitrazepam Tablets, BP
  Nystatin Tablets, BP
  Oxytetracycline Tablets, BP
  Paracetamol Tablets, BP
  Pentazocine Tablets, BP

Tablets (*continued*)
  Pethidine Tablets, BP
  Promethazine Hydrochloride Tablets, BP
  Tetracycline Tablets, BP
  Vitamin B Tablets, Compound, Strong, BPC
Penicillin
  Benzylpenicillin Injection, BP
  Penicillin Triple Injection, BPC
  Penicillin VK Capsules, BP
  Penicillin V Elixir, BP
  Penicillin V Mixture, BP
  Penicillin VK Tablets, BP
  Injections of Procaine Penicillin, whether or not
    containing Benzylpenicillin; the following injec-
    tions are included in the Dental Practitioners'
    Formulary:
      Procaine Penicillin Injection, BP
      Procaine Penicillin Injection, Fortified, BP

Title not included in the BP or BPC

Co-codaprin Tablets, Dispersible, correspond to Aspirin and Codeine Tablets, Dispersible, BP

Preparations not included in the BP or BPC

PoM **Amoxycillin Tablets, Dispersible,** (proprietary product: *Amoxil Dispersible Tablets*), amoxycillin 500 mg (as trihydrate)

PoM **Amoxycillin Oral Powder** (proprietary product: *Amoxil Sachets*), amoxycillin 3 g (as trihydrate)

PoM **Amphotericin Tablets** (proprietary product: *Fungilin Tablets*), amphotericin 100 mg

PoM **Amphotericin Mixture** (proprietary product: *Fungilin Suspension*), amphotericin 100 mg/ml

PoM **Amphotericin Ointment** (proprietary product: *Fungilin Ointment*), amphotericin 3%, in a suitable basis

Artificial Saliva, consists of a suitable inert, slightly viscous, aqueous liquid containing a suitable antimicrobial preservative (see Formulary)

Aspirin, Paracetamol, and Codeine Tablets (proprietary product: *Veganin Tablets*), aspirin 250 mg, paracetamol 250 mg, codeine phosphate 6.8 mg

Benzocaine Lozenges, benzocaine 10 mg. They are prepared by compression

Benzydamine Mouth-wash (proprietary product: *Difflam Oral Rinse*), benzydamine hydrochloride 0.15%

Carmellose Gelatin Paste (proprietary product: *Orabase Paste*), gelatin, pectin, carmellose sodium, 16.58% of each in a suitable basis

PoM **Cephradine Elixir** (proprietary product: *Velosef Syrup*), cephradine 125 mg/5 ml and 250 mg/5 ml when reconstituted with water for preparations

PoM **Cephradine Injection** (proprietary product: *Velosef Injection*), sterile powder for reconstitution

Chlorhexidine Gel (proprietary product: *Corsodyl Dental Gel*), chlorhexidine gluconate 1%

Chlorhexidine Mouth-wash (proprietary product: *Corsodyl Mouth-wash*), chlorhexidine gluconate 0.2%

Chlorhexidine Mouth-wash, Compound (proprietary product: *Eludril Mouth-wash*), chlorhexidine gluconate 0.1%, chlorbutol 0.1%, chloroform 0.5%

Choline Salicylate Dental Paste, choline salicylate 8.7% in a gel basis

PoM **Clindamycin Mixture, Paediatric** (proprietary product: *Dalacin C Paediatric Suspension*), clindamycin 75 mg (as hydrochloride palmitate)/5 ml when reconstituted with water for preparations

PoM **Clindamycin Injection** (proprietary product: *Dalacin C Phosphate Sterile Solution*), clindamycin 150 mg (as phosphate)/ml

Co-codamol Tablets, codeine phosphate 8 mg, paracetamol 500 mg

Co-codamol Tablets, Dispersible, codeine phosphate 8 mg, paracetamol 500 mg in an effervescent basis

PoM **Co-dydramol Tablets,** dihydrocodeine tartrate 10 mg, paracetamol 500 mg

PoM **Co-trimoxazole Tablets, Double-strength,** co-trimoxazole tablets BP 960 mg

PoM **Co-trimoxazole Tablets, Double-strength, Dispersible** (proprietary product: *Fectrim Forte*), co-trimoxazole tablets BP 960 mg

PoM **Diazepam Elixir** (proprietary product: *Valium Syrup*), diazepam 2 mg/5 ml

PoM **Erythromycin Ethylsuccinate Tablets** (proprietary product: *Erythroped A*), erythromycin ethylsuccinate 500 mg

PoM **Erythromycin Ethylsuccinate Mixture** (proprietary product: *Erythroped Suspension*), erythromycin 250 mg (as ethylsuccinate)/5 ml when reconstituted with water for preparations

PoM **Erythromycin Ethylsuccinate Mixture, Paediatric** (proprietary product: *Erythroped PI*), erythromycin 125 mg (as ethylsuccinate)/5 ml when reconstituted with water for preparations

PoM **Erythromycin Lactobionate Injection** (proprietary product: *Erythrocin IV Lactobionate*), sterile powder for reconstitution

PoM **Fusidic Acid Ointment** (proprietary product: *Fucidin Ointment*), sodium fusidate 2% in an anhydrous greasy basis

Hydrogen Peroxide Mouth-wash, consists of hydrogen peroxide solution (6%), BP

PoM **Idoxuridine 0.1% Paint,** consists of idoxuridine eye-drops, BP; idoxuridine 0.1% in aqueous solution

PoM **Idoxuridine 5% in Dimethyl Sulphoxide,** idoxuridine 5% in dimethyl sulphoxide

Lignocaine 5% Ointment, lignocaine 5% in a suitable basis

Lignocaine Viscous Mouth-wash (proprietary product: *Xylocaine Viscous*), anhydrous lignocaine hydrochloride 20 mg/ml in a suitable basis

PoM **Metronidazole Mixture** (proprietary product: *Flagyl S*), metronidazole 200 mg (as benzoyl metronidazole)/5 ml

PoM **Miconazole Oral Gel** (proprietary product: *Daktarin Oral Gel*), miconazole 25 mg/ml

PoM **Nystatin Pastilles** (proprietary product: *Nystan Pastilles*), nystatin 100000 units

Povidone-iodine Mouth-wash (proprietary product: *Betadine Mouth-wash*), povidone-iodine 1%

Sodium Perborate Mouth-wash, Buffered (proprietary product: *Bocasan Mouth-wash*), sodium perborate monohydrate 68.6%, sodium hydrogen tartrate 29.4%, menthol, peppermint oil

PoM **Temazepam Capsules,** temazepam 10 and 20 mg

PoM **Tetracycline Mouth-bath,** consists of tetracycline mixture, BPC; tetracycline hydrochloride 125 mg (as tetracycline)/5 ml

Zinc Sulphate Mouth-wash, consists of zinc sulphate lotion, BP (see Formulary)
Directions for use: dilute 1 part with 4 parts of warm water

New and Discontinued Preparations

New Preparations

Preparations added since the compilation of BNF no. 9 (1985)

Aspav
Camoquin (r)
Colven
Creon
Dequacaine
Enrich
Freamine III
Human Actraphane
Human Ultratard
Innovace
Intraglobin

Kessar
Mono-Cedocard 40
Nephramine
Niferex-150
Noltam
Normasol Undine
Paxofen
Pharmorubicin
Prestim Forte
Synuretic
Tamofen-40

(r) indicates a previously discontinued item reintroduced by manufacturer

Discontinued Preparations

Preparations discontinued since the compilation of BNF no. 9 (1985)

Benafed
Bleph-10
Brontisol
Cosalgesic
Dextrogesic
Dialar
Dimotapp P
Elamol
Fenopron D
Gatinar
Guanor Paediatric
Hyprenan
Millophyline
Neo-Cortef [skin
    preparations]

Neuro Phosphates
Nystadermal
Ovol
Pamergan AP100/25
Pameton
Paragesic
Pexid
Prehensol
Robitussin AC
Rondomycin
Saroten
Skefron
Steroxin-Hydrocortisone
Veracolate

Name Changes

Old	New	Old	New
Euhypnos [capsules]	Euhypnos 10, 15, 20, 30	Pavacol	Pavacol-D
		Stie-Lasan	Anthranol
Eurax Ointment	Eurax Cream	Terpalin	Tercolix
Felmane	Paxane		

Changes Since the Preparation of the Main Text

New Preparations
Introduced up to July 1985

PoM **Anthranol 1.0**® (Stiefel)
Ointment, dithranol 1%, salicylic acid 0.5%.
Price 50 g = **F**. Label: 28. For short-contact application to skin or scalp

PoM **Anthranol 2.0**® (Stiefel)
Ointment, dithranol 2%, salicylic acid 0.5%.
Price 50 g = **G**. Label: 28. For short-contact application to skin or scalp

▼ PoM **Asacol**® (Tillotts)
Tablets, red, coated with an acrylic-based resin, mesalazine 400 mg. Price 20 tabs = **F**. Label: 25
Dose: 1.2–2.4 g daily in divided doses
Cautions: avoid in renal impairment; do not give with lactulose

PoM **Atrovent Forte**® (Boehringer Ingelheim)
Aerosol inhalation, ipratropium bromide 36 micrograms/metered inhalation. Price 200-dose unit = **F**
Dose: by aerosol inhalation 36–72 micrograms (1–2 puffs) 3–4 times daily; CHILD 6–12 years 36 micrograms (1 puff) 3 times daily
Advise patient not to exceed prescribed dose and to follow manufacturer's directions

▼ PoM **Bactroban**® (Beecham)
Ointment, mupirocin 2%, in a water-miscible macrogol basis. Price 15 g = **F**
Apply to bacterial skin infections up to 3 times daily for up to 10 days

Benzagel 5® (Bioglan)
Gel, benzoyl peroxide 5%. Price 40 g = **E**

Benzagel 10® (Bioglan)
Gel, benzoyl peroxide 10%. Price 40 g = **E**

PoM **Canesten 10% VC**® (Bayer)
Vaginal cream, clotrimazole 10%. Price 5-g applicator pack = **F**
Insert 5 g at night as a single dose

▼ PoM **Cervagem**® (M&B)
Pessaries, gemeprost 1 mg. Price 1 pessary = **J**

PoM **Colofac**® (Duphar)
Liquid (= mixture), yellow, sugar-free, mebeverine hydrochloride 50 mg (as embonate)/5 ml.
Diluent water for preparations, life of diluted mixture 14 days. Price 100 ml = **D**. Label: 22
Dose: adults and children over 10 years, 15 ml 3 times daily, preferably 20 minutes before food

Dialamine® (Scientific Hospital Supplies)
Powder, essential amino acids 30%, with carbohydrate 62%, energy 1500 kJ (360 kcal)/100 g, with ascorbic acid, minerals, and trace elements. Price 1 kg = **J**. For oral feeding where essential amino-acid supplements are required; e.g. chronic renal failure, hypoproteinaemia, wound fistula leakage with excessive protein loss, conditions requiring a controlled nitrogen intake and haemodialysis

PoM **Digoxin Injection, Paediatric, BP** (Boots)
Paediatric injection, digoxin 100 micrograms/ml.
Price 1-ml amp = **B**

▼ PoM **Ervevax**® (SK&F)
Rubella vaccine, live, prepared from Wistar RA 27/3 strain propagated in human diploid cells.
Price single-dose vial = **E**; 10-dose vial = **J** (both with diluent)

PoM **Erycen®** (Berk)
Tablets, orange, e/c, f/c, erythromycin 500 mg.
Price 20 tabs = **E**. Label: 5, 9, 25

PoM **Erythrolar®** (Lagap)
Tablets, pink, f/c, erythromycin 250 mg (as stearate). Price 20 tabs = **D**. Label: 9, 21
Tablets, pink, f/c, erythromycin 500 mg (as stearate). Price 20 tabs = **F**. Label: 9, 21

NHS PoM **Euhypnos 15®** (Farmitalia Carlo Erba)
Capsules, green, temazepam 15 mg. Price 20 caps = **D**. Label: 2

NHS PoM **Euhypnos 30®** (Farmitalia Carlo Erba)
Capsules, green, temazepam 30 mg. Price 20 caps = **E**. Label: 2

▼ PoM **Exelderm®** (ICI)
Cream, sulconazole nitrate 1%, in a water-miscible basis. Price 30 g = **F**
Apply to fungal skin infections 1–2 times daily continuing for 2–3 weeks after lesions have healed

▼ PoM **Gammonativ®** (KabiVitrum)
Normal immunoglobulin injection. Powder for preparing intravenous injections. Price 2.5- and 5-g vials with 50- and 100-ml vial, respectively, water for injections (both) = **J**. Transfer set with each pack

Guarina® (Norgine)
Granules, dispersible, guar gum 5 g/sachet. Price 20 sachets = **E**. Label: 13, counselling advised, food
Dose: 5 g stirred into 150 ml water immediately before food once daily, increasing to 3 times daily

▼ PoM **Hespan®** (American Hospital Supply)
Intravenous infusion, hetastarch 6% in sodium chloride intravenous infusion 0.9%. Price 500-ml Steriflex® bag = **J**

PoM **Ibular®** (Lagap)
Tablets, pink, s/c, ibuprofen 200 mg. Price 20 tabs = **B**
Tablets, pink, s/c, ibuprofen 400 mg. Price 20 tabs = **C**

PoM **Indolar®** (Lagap)
Suppositories, indomethacin 100 mg. Price 10 suppos = **D**

▼ PoM **Intal 5®** (Fisons)
Inhaler (= aerosol inhalation), sodium cromoglycate 5 mg/metered inhalation. Price 112-dose unit = **J**. Label: 8
Dose: by aerosol inhalation, adults and children, 10 mg (2 puffs) 4 times daily initially; maintenance 5 mg (1 puff) 4 times daily

▼ PoM **Kalten®** (Stuart)
Capsules, red/cream, atenolol 50 mg, amiloride hydrochloride (anhydrous) 2.5 mg, hydrochlorothiazide 25 mg. Price 28 caps = **H**. Label: 8

PoM **Labrocol®** (Lagap)
Tablets, orange, f/c, labetalol hydrochloride 100 mg. Price 20 tabs = **D**. Label: 8, 21
Tablets, orange, f/c, labetalol hydrochloride 200 mg. Price 20 tabs = **E**. Label: 8, 21
Tablets, orange, f/c, labetalol hydrochloride 400 mg. Price 20 tabs = **F**. Label: 8, 21

PoM **Laraflex®** (Lagap)
Tablets, scored, naproxen 250 mg. Price 20 tabs = **E**
Tablets, scored, naproxen 500 mg. Price 20 tabs = **F**

PoM **Laratrim®** (Lagap)
Adult suspension (= mixture), co-trimoxazole 480 mg/5 ml. Diluent syrup, life of diluted mixture 14 days. Price 100 ml = **E**. Label: 9

PoM **Maxtrex®** (Farmitalia Carlo Erba)
Tablets, yellow, scored, methotrexate 2.5 mg. Price 20 tabs = **E**
Tablets, yellow, scored, methotrexate 10 mg. Price 20 tabs = **I**

PoM **Metrodin®** (Serono)
Injection, powder for reconstitution, urofollitrophin (from human menopausal urine) as human follicle-stimulating hormone 75 units, lactose 10 mg. Price per amp (with solvent) = **J**

PoM **Normetic®** (Abbott)
Tablets, peach, scored, amiloride hydrochloride (anhydrous) 5 mg, hydrochlorothiazide 50 mg. Price 20 tabs = **D**
Dose: 1–2 tablets, increased if necessary to a max. of 4, daily

Osmolite® (Abbott)
Liquid, caseinates, soya protein isolate, hydrolysed corn starch, medium chain triglycerides, corn oil, soya oil, vitamins, and minerals, providing protein 8.8 g, carbohydrate 34.3 g, fat 9.1 g, energy 1050 kJ (250 kcal)/237 ml. Gluten- and lactose-free. Price 237–ml can = **C**; 946-ml can = **E**. For short-bowel syndrome, intractable malabsorption, pre-operative preparation of patients who are undernourished, treatment for those with proven inflammatory bowel disease, treatment following total gastrectomy, dysphagia, bowel fistulas, anorexia nervosa. Not suitable as a sole source of nutrition for children, unsuitable for all infants under 1 year

Polycose® (Abbott)
Liquid, glucose polymers, providing carbohydrate 50 g, energy 840 kJ (200 kcal)/100 ml. Price 114-ml bottle = **C**
Powder, glucose polymers, providing carbohydrate 94 g, energy 1600 kJ (380 kcal)/100 g. Price 350-g can = **E**. For renal failure; liver cirrhosis; disaccharide intolerance (without isomaltose intolerance); disorders of amino-acid metabolism (and other similar disorders) and/or whole protein intolerance; malabsorption states and other conditions, including proven hypoglycaemia, requiring a high-energy, low-fluid intake, whether or not sodium and/or potassium restriction is essential

PoM **Refolinon®** (Farmitalia Carlo Erba)
Tablets, yellow, scored, folinic acid 15 mg (as calcium salt). Price 2 tabs = **I**
Injection, folinic acid 3 mg (as calcium salt)/ml. Price 2-ml amp = **E**; 10-ml amp = **J**

▼ PoM **Securon®** (Knoll)
Tablets, yellow, s/c, verapamil hydrochloride 40 mg. Price 20 tabs = **C**

PoM **Slo-Indo®** (Generics)
Capsules, s/r, red/yellow enclosing off-white pellets, indomethacin 75 mg. Price 20 caps = **E**. Label: 21, 25
Dose: 1–2 capsules daily

PoM **Tachostyptan®** (Consolidated)
Injection, standardised thromboplastin (from cattle-brain tissue) 2%. Price 5-ml amp = **B**

Vascardin® (Nicholas)
Tablets, scored, isosorbide dinitrate 30 mg. Price 20 tabs = **C**

PoM **Vibramycin 50®** (Pfizer)
Capsules, green/cream, doxycycline 50 mg (as hydrochloride). Price 28-tab calendar pack = **H**. Label: 6, 9, 27
Dose: acne, 50 mg daily usually for 6–12 weeks

Preparations Discontinued

since the compilation of the main text

Ceporin   Norlestrin
Etophylate   Nupercaine
Furan   Orlest 21
Mandelamine   Silbephylline

Preparations New to the BNF

PoM **Nystan**® (Squibb)
Suspension (= mixture), gluten-, lactose-, and
sugar-free, nystatin 100 000 units/ml when
reconstituted with water for preparations.
Measure with pipette. Price 24 ml with pipette = **D**. Label: 9, counselling advised, measure with pipette

---

Preparations not available for NHS prescription (see p. xi)

When a preparation is prescribable by non-proprietary title but not by brand name the BNF has
introduced a non-proprietary entry to indicate this
(e.g. there is a non-proprietary entry for Xylometazoline Nasal Drops, p. 342, which is prescribable). If a non-proprietary entry is absent it
should be assumed to be not prescribable (e.g.
the absence of a non-proprietary title for oxymetazoline nasal drops indicates that in addition
to Afrazine® and Iliadin Mini® p. 342, this too

is not prescribable). The following is a list of
additional preparations which ARE prescribable:

Aspirin Chewing-gum Tablets (227 mg) (*Asper-gum*®)
Aspirin Tablets, Effervescent (300 mg) (*Clara-din*®)
Aspirin Tablets, Slow (500 mg) (*Levius*®)
Aspirin Tablets, Slow (micro-encapsulated) (648 mg) (*Breoprin*®)
Diazepam Capsules, Slow (*Valrelease*®)
Diazepam Elixir (5 mg/5 ml) (previously *Dialar Forte*®)
Ergocalciferol Solution 10 mg (400 000 units)/ml (*Sterogyl-15*®)
Fenoprofen Tablets (200 mg as calcium salt) (*Progesic*®)
Methylcellulose Mixture ('450', 900 mg/10 ml) (*Cologel*®)
Oxazepam Capsules (*Serenid Forte*®)
Paracetamol Mixture (250 mg/5 ml) (*Calpol Six Plus*®)
Paracetamol Tablets, Sorbitol Basis (500 mg) (*Panasorb*®)
Pentazocine Capsules* (50 mg) (*Fortral*®)
Pyridoxine Tablets, Slow* (*Complement Continus*®)
Sodium Picosulphate Elixir (5 mg/5 ml) (*Laxoberal*®)

*Preparations thus marked were previously considered not prescribable

Note: the word 'slow' is used in titles in place of
'sustained-release' or 'slow-release' because this
is the BP term for such preparations

Malaria chemoprophylaxis

In view of reports to the CSM on severe adverse reactions, including 4 fatal ones, associated with
Fansidar®, its use may no longer be recommended for malaria chemoprophylaxis. The use of Maloprim®
as an alternative has also been questioned.
   Current advice is available from:
      021-772 4311 (Birmingham)
      051-708 9393 (Liverpool)
      01-387 4411 (London)

Index of Manufacturers

Abbott
Abbott Laboratories Ltd,
Queenborough, Kent ME11 5EL.
Sheerness (0795) 663371

A&H
Allen & Hanburys Ltd,
Horsenden House, Oldfield Lane
North, Greenford, Middx UB6
0HB.
01-422 4225

Alcon
Alcon Laboratories (UK) Ltd,
Imperial Way, Watford WD2
4YR.
Watford (0923) 46133

Alembic Products
Alembic Products Ltd,
Oaklands House, Oaklands Drive,
Sale, Manchester M33 1NS.
061-962 4423

Allergan
Allergan Ltd,
Turnpike Rd, Cressex Industrial
Estate, High Wycombe, Bucks
HP12 3NR.
High Wycombe (0494) 444721

American Hospital Supply
American Hospital Supply (UK)
Ltd,
53 Church Rd, Ashford, Middx
TW15 2TY.
Ashford (Middx) (07842) 47101

Anaquest
Anaquest Ltd,
The Dorcan Complex, Faraday
Rd, Swindon, Wilts SN3 5HZ.
Swindon (0793) 615581

Andard-Mount
Andard-Mount (London) Ltd,
24 London Rd, Wembley, Middx
HA9 7HD.
01-903 6388

APS
Approved Prescription Services
Ltd,
Whitcliffe House, Whitcliffe Rd,
Cleckheaton, West Yorks BD19
3BZ.
Cleckheaton (0274) 876776

Armour
Armour Pharmaceutical Co. Ltd,
St. Leonards House,
St. Leonards Rd, Eastbourne,
East Sussex BN21 3YG.
Eastbourne (0323) 21422

Arun
Arun Products Ltd,
The Square, Barnham, Bognor
Regis, West Sussex PO22 0HB.
Bognor Regis (0243) 554141

Ashe
Ashe Laboratories Ltd,
Ashetree Works, Kingston Rd,
Leatherhead, Surrey KT22 7JZ.
Leatherhead (0372) 376151

Astra
Astra Pharmaceuticals Ltd,
Home Park Estate,
King's Langley,
Herts WD4 8DH.
King's Langley (09277) 66191

Ayerst
Ayerst Laboratories Ltd,
South Way, Andover, Hants
SP10 5LT.
Andover (0264) 58711

Bayer
Bayer UK Ltd,
Pharmaceutical Division, Bayer
House, Strawberry Hill, Newbury,
Berks RG13 1JA.
Newbury (0635) 39000

Beecham
Beecham Research Laboratories,
Beecham House, Great West Rd,
Brentford, Middx TW8 9BD.
01-560 5151

Beecham Products
Contact Beecham Research
Laboratories (see above).

Bencard
Bencard,
Great West Rd, Brentford, Middx
TW8 9BD.
01-560 5151

Bengué
Bengué & Co. Ltd,
Syntex House, St. Ives Rd,
Maidenhead, Berks SL6 1RD.
Maidenhead (0628) 33191

Berk
Berk Pharmaceuticals Ltd,
St. Leonards House,
St. Leonards Rd, Eastbourne,
East Sussex BN21 3YG.
Eastbourne (0323) 641144

Bioglan
Bioglan Laboratories Ltd,
Spirella Building, Bridge Rd,
Letchworth, Herts SG6 4ET.
Letchworth (04626) 74644

Bio-Medical
Bio-Medical Services Ltd.
10 East Parade, York YO3 7YL.
York (0904) 51562

Biotest Folex
Biotest Folex Ltd,
171 Alcester Rd, Moseley,
Birmingham B13 8JR.
021-449 5267

Blake
Thomas Blake & Co,
20 Blatchford Close, Horsham,
West Sussex RH13 5RQ.
Horsham (0403) 54742

Boehringer Ingelheim
Boehringer Ingelheim Ltd,
Southern Industrial Estate,
Bracknell, Berks RG12 4YS.
Bracknell (0344) 424600

Boots
The Boots Co. PLC,
1 Thane Rd West, Nottingham
NG2 3AA.
Nottingham (0602) 560111

Braun
B. Braun (Medical) Ltd,
Evett Close, Stocklake,
Aylesbury, Bucks HP20 1DN.
Aylesbury (0296) 32626

Bristol-Myers
Bristol-Myers Pharmaceuticals,
Station Rd, Langley, Slough SL3
6EB.
Slough (0753) 44266

Britannia
Britannia Pharmaceuticals Ltd,
Hamilton House, 87 Bell St,
Reigate, Surrey RH2 7YZ.
Reigate (07372) 22256

Brocades
Brocades (Great Britain) Ltd,
Brocades House, Pyrford Rd,
West Byfleet, Weybridge, Surrey
KT14 6RA.
Byfleet (09323) 45536

Burgess
Edwin Burgess Ltd,
Longwick Rd, Princes
Risborough, Aylesbury, Bucks
HP17 9RR.
Princes Risborough (08444) 6881

Calmic
Calmic Medical Division,
The Wellcome Foundation Ltd,
Crewe Hall, Crewe, Cheshire
CW1 1UB.
Crewe (0270) 583151

Cantassium
The Cantassium Company,
Larkhall Laboratories, 225 Putney
Bridge Rd, London SW15 2PY.
01-870 0971

Care
Care Laboratories Ltd,
Badminton Court, Amersham,
Bucks.
Amersham (02403) 4422

Carlton
Carlton Laboratories (UK) Ltd,
4 Manor Parade, Salvington Rd,
Durrington, Worthing,
West Sussex BN13 2JP.
Worthing (0903) 63235

Carnrick
Carnrick Laboratories,
Acres Down, Furze Hill, London
Rd, Shipston-on-Stour,
Warwickshire.
Shipston-on-Stour (0608) 61610

Carter-Wallace
Carter-Wallace Ltd,
Wear Bay Rd, Folkestone, Kent
CT19 6PG.
Folkestone (0303) 57661

Chelsea
Chelsea Drug & Chemical Co. Ltd,
310 Old Brompton Rd, London
SW5 9JQ.
01-370 4321

Ciba
CIBA Laboratories,
Wimblehurst Rd, Horsham, West
Sussex RH12 4AB.
Horsham (0403) 50101

Collins
L. D. Collins & Co. Ltd,
Sunray House, 9 Plantagenet Rd,
New Barnet, Herts EN5 5JG.
01-440 1470

Coloplast
Coloplast Ltd,
Bridge House, Orchard Lane,
Huntingdon, Cambs PE18 6QT.
Huntingdon (0480) 55451

Colson & Kay
Colson & Kay Ltd,
Shentonfield Rd, Manchester
M22 4RW.
061-491 1980

Comprehensive
Comprehensive Pharmaceuticals
Ltd,
95 Frampton St, London NW8
6YA.
01-723 1107

Concept
Concept Pharmaceuticals Ltd,
Unit 6, Blenheim Rd, Cressex
Industrial Estate, High Wycombe,
Bucks HP12 3RS
High Wycombe (0494) 451938

Consolidated
Consolidated Chemicals Ltd,
The Industrial Estate, Wrexham,
Clwyd LL13 9PS.
Wrexham (0978) 61351

CooperVision
CooperVision Ltd,
371 Millbrook Rd, Southampton
SO1 3HW.
Southampton (0703) 780711

Cow & Gate
Cow & Gate Ltd,
Cow & Gate House, Trowbridge,
Wilts BA14 8YX.
Trowbridge (02214) 68381

Cox Pharmaceuticals
A. H. Cox & Co Ltd,
Whiddon Valley, Barnstaple,
Devon EX32 8NS.
Barnstaple (0271) 75001

CP
CP Pharmaceuticals Ltd,
Red Willow Rd, Wrexham
Industrial Estate, Clwyd LL13
9PX.
Wrexham (0978) 61261

Crookes
Crookes Laboratories Ltd,
PO Box 94, 1 Thane Rd West,
Nottingham NG2 3AA.
Nottingham (0602) 56111

Crookes Products
Crookes Products Ltd,
PO Box 94, 1 Thane Rd West,
Nottingham NG2 3AA.
Nottingham (0602) 57431

Dales
Dales Pharmaceuticals Ltd,
Snaygill Industrial Estate,
Keighley Rd, Skipton, North
Yorkshire BD23 2RW.
Skipton (0756) 61311

Daniel
Richard Daniel & Son Ltd,
Mansfield Rd, Derby DE1 3RE.
Derby (0332) 40671

DDSA
DDSA Pharmaceuticals Ltd,
310 Old Brompton Rd, London
SW5 9JQ.
01-373 7884

De Witt
De Witt International Ltd,
Seymour Rd, London E10 7LX.
01-539 3334

Delandale
Delandale Laboratories Ltd,
Delandale House, 37 Old Dover
Rd, Canterbury, Kent CT1 3JB.
Canterbury (0227) 66353

Dental Health
Dental Health Promotion Ltd,
51 Greencroft Gardens, London
NW6 3II.
01-625 4389

Dermal
Dermal Laboratories Ltd,
Tatmore Place, Gosmore,
Hitchin, Herts SG4 7QR.
Hitchin (0462) 58866

Dermalex
Dermalex Co. Ltd,
146 Kilburn High Rd, London
NW6 4JD.
01-624 4686

DF
Duncan, Flockhart & Co. Ltd,
700 Oldfield Lane North,
Greenford, Middx UB6 0HD.
01-422 2331

Dista
Dista Products Ltd,
Kingsclere Rd, Basingstoke,
Hants RG21 2XA.
Basingstoke (0256) 52011

Dome/Hollister-Stier
Dome/Hollister-Stier,
Strawberry Hill, Newbury, Berks
RG13 1JA.
Newbury (0635) 39000

Dorsey
Dorsey Laboratories,
98 The Centre, Feltham,
Middlesex TW13 4EP.
01-751 1189

Downs
Downs Surgical Ltd,
Church Path, Mitcham, Surrey
CR4 3UE.
01-648 6291

Du Pont
Du Pont (UK) Ltd.,
Wedgwood Way, Stevenage,
Herts SG1 4QN.
Stevenage (0438) 734549

Duphar
Duphar Laboratories Ltd,
Gaters Hill, West End,
Southampton SO3 3JD.
Southampton (0703) 472281

Evans
Evans Medical Ltd,
Old Post House, London End,
Beaconsfield, Bucks HP9 2JH.
Beaconsfield (04946) 6111

Farillon
Farillon Ltd,
Bryant Ave, Romford, Essex
RM3 0PJ.
Ingrebourne (04023) 71136

Farley
Farley Health Products Ltd,
Torr Lane, Plymouth PL3 5UA.
Plymouth (0752) 24151

Farmitalia Carlo Erba
Farmitalia Carlo Erba Ltd,
Italia House, 23 Grosvenor Rd,
St. Albans, Herts AL1 3AW.
St. Albans (0727) 40041

Ferring
Ferring Pharmaceuticals Ltd,
11 Mount Road, Feltham, Middx
TW13 6JG.
01-898 8396

Fisons
Fisons plc,
Pharmaceutical Division, 12
Derby Rd, Loughborough, Leics
LE11 0BB.
Loughborough (0509) 263113

Fox
C. H. Fox Ltd,
22 Tavistock St, London WC2E
7PY
01-240 3111

Franklin
Franklin Medical Ltd,
PO Box 138, Turnpike Rd, High
Wycombe, Bucks HP12 3NB.
High Wycombe (0494) 32761

Galen
Galen Ltd,
19 Lower Seagoe Industrial Estate,
Portadown, Craigavon, Armagh
BT63 5QD.
Craigavon (0762) 34974

Geigy
Geigy Pharmaceuticals,
Wimblehurst Rd, Horsham, West
Sussex RH12 4AB.
Horsham (0403) 50101

Geistlich
Geistlich Sons Ltd,
Newton Bank, Long Lane, Chester
CH2 3QZ.
Chester (0244) 47534

Generics
Generics (UK) Ltd,
12 Station Close, Potters Bar,
Herts EN6 1TL.
Potters Bar (0707) 44556

GF Supplies
GF Dietary Supplies Ltd,
494 Honeypot Lane,
Stanmore, Middx HA7 1JH.
01-206 0522

Glaxo
Glaxo Laboratories Ltd,
Greenford Rd, Greenford, Middx
UB6 0HE.
01-422 3434

Glenwood
Glenwood Laboratories Ltd,
19 Wincheap, Canterbury, Kent
CT1 3TB.
Canterbury (0227) 60139

Gold Cross
Gold Cross Pharmaceuticals,
PO Box 53, Lane End Rd, High
Wycombe, Bucks HP12 4HL.
High Wycombe (0494) 21124

Henleys
Henleys Medical Supplies Ltd,
Alexandra Works, Clarendon
Road, London N8 0DL.
01-889 3151

Hoechst
Hoechst UK Ltd,
Pharmaceutical Division, Hoechst
House, Salisbury Rd, Hounslow,
Middx TW4 6JH.
01-570 7712

Hough
Hough, Hoseason & Co. Ltd,
22 Chapel St, Levenshulme,
Manchester M19 3PT.
061-224 3271

Hoyt
Hoyt Laboratories division of
Colgate-Palmolive Ltd,
76 Oxford St, London W1A 1EN.
01-580 2030

ICI
Imperial Chemical Industries PLC.
Pharmaceuticals Division,
Alderley Park, Macclesfield,
Cheshire SK10 4TG.
Alderley Edge (0625) 582828

Ilon
Ilon Laboratories (Hamilton) Ltd,
Lorne St, Hamilton, Strathclyde
ML3 9AB.
Hamilton (0698) 285129

Immuno
Immuno Ltd,
Arctic House, Rye Lane, Dunton
Green, Nr Sevenoaks, Kent
TN14 5HB.
Sevenoaks (0732) 458101

IMS
International Medication Systems
(UK) Ltd,
11 Royal Oak Way South,
Daventry, Northants NN11 5PJ.
Daventry (0327) 703231

Innoxa
Innoxa (England) Ltd,
202 Terminus Rd, Eastbourne,
Sussex BN21 3DF.
Eastbourne (0323) 639671

International Labs
International Laboratories Ltd,
Charwell House, Wilsom Rd,
Alton, Hants GU34 2TJ.
Alton (0420) 88174

Jackson
Ernest Jackson & Co. Ltd,
Crediton, Devon EX17 3AP.
Crediton (03632) 2251

Janssen
Janssen Pharmaceutical Ltd,
Grove, Wantage, Oxon
OX12 0DQ.
Wantage (02357) 2966

K/L
K/L Pharmaceuticals Ltd,
25 Macadam Place, South
Newmoor Industrial Estate,
Irvine KA11 4HP.
Irvine (0294) 215951

KabiVitrum
KabiVitrum Ltd,
KabiVitrum House, Riverside
Way, Uxbridge, Middx UB8 2YF.
Uxbridge (0895) 51144

Kerfoot
Thomas Kerfoot & Co. Ltd,
Vale of Bardsley, Ashton-under-
Lyne, Lancs OL7 9RR.
061-330 4531

Kirby-Warrick
Kirby-Warrick Pharmaceuticals
Ltd,
Mildenhall, Bury St. Edmunds,
Suffolk IP28 7AX.
Mildenhall (0638) 716321

Knoll
Knoll Ltd,
The Brow, Burgess Hill, West
Sussex RH15 9NE.
Burgess Hill (04446) 6011

LAB
Laboratories for Applied Biology
Ltd,
91 Amhurst Park, London N16
5DR.
01-800 2252

Labaz
Labaz: Sanofi UK Ltd,
Floats Rd, Wythenshawe,
Manchester M23 9NF.
061-945 4161

Lagap
Lagap Pharmaceuticals Ltd,
Old Portsmouth Rd, Peasmarsh,
Guildford, Surrey GU3 1LZ.
Guildford (0483) 35431

Larkhall
Larkhall Laboratories,
225 Putney Bridge Rd, London
SW15 2PY.
01-870 0971

Lederle
Lederle Laboratories,
Fareham Rd, Gosport, Hants
PO13 0AS.
Fareham (0329) 224000

Leo
Leo Laboratories Ltd,
Longwick Rd, Princes
Risborough, Aylesbury, Bucks
HP17 9RR.
Princes Risborough (08444) 7333

Lewis
Lewis Laboratories Ltd,
Lavender Walk, Leeds LS9 8JG.
Leeds (0532) 482032

Lilly
Eli Lilly & Co. Ltd,
Kingsclere Rd, Basingstoke, Hants
RG21 2XA.
Basingstoke (0256) 473241

Lipha
Lipha Pharmaceuticals Ltd,
Harrier House, High St,
Yiewsley, West Drayton, Middx.
UB7 7QG.
West Drayton (0895) 449331

Lorex
Lorex Pharmaceuticals Ltd,
Old Bank House, 39 High St,
High Wycombe, Bucks HP11
2AG.
High Wycombe (0494) 26188

Loveridge
J. M. Loveridge PLC,
Southbrook Road, Southampton
SO9 3LT.
Southampton (0703) 28411

Loxley
Loxley Medical,
Bessingby Estate, Bridlington,
North Humberside YO16 4SU.
Bridlington (0262) 75356

Luitpold
Luitpold-Werk,
Hayes Gate House, 27 Uxbridge
Rd, Hayes, Middx UB4 0JN.
01-561 8774

Lundbeck
Lundbeck Ltd,
Lundbeck House, Hastings St,
Luton LU1 5BE.
Luton (0582) 416565

Macarthys
Macarthys Laboratories Ltd,
Chesham House, Chesham Close,
Romford RM1 4JX.
Romford (0708) 46033

Maltown
Maltown Ltd,
PO Box 53, Harrogate, North
Yorks HG1 5BD.
Harrogate (0423) 62593

Martindale
Martindale Pharmaceuticals Ltd,
Chesham House, Chesham Close,
Romford RM1 4JX.
Romford (0708) 46033

M&B
May & Baker Ltd,
Dagenham, Essex RM10 7XS.
01-592 3060

MCP
MCP Pharmaceuticals Ltd,
Simpson Parkway, Kirkton
Campus, Livingston, West Lothian
EH54 7BH.
Livingston (0506) 412512

Medexport
Medexport Ltd,
PO Box 25, Arundel, West Sussex
BN18 0SW.

Medo
Medo Pharmaceuticals Ltd,
East St, Chesham, Bucks HP5
1DG.
Chesham (0494) 772071

Merck
E. Merck Ltd,
Winchester Rd, Four Marks,
Alton, Hants GU34 5HG.
Alton (0420) 64011

Merrell
Merrell Pharmaceuticals Ltd,
Meadowbank, Bath Rd,
Hounslow, Middx TW5 9QY.
01-759 2600

Morson
Thomas Morson Pharmaceuticals,
Hertford Rd, Hoddesdon, Herts
EN11 9BU.
Hoddesdon (0992) 445252

MSD
Merck Sharp & Dohme Ltd,
Hertford Rd,
Hoddesdon, Herts EN11 9BU.
Hoddesdon (0992) 467272

Napp
Napp Laboratories Ltd,
Cambridge Science Park, Milton
Rd, Cambridge CB4 4BH.
Cambridge (0223) 358888

Nestlé
Nestlé Co. Ltd,
St. George's House, Croydon
CR9 1NR.
01-686 3333

Neutrogena
Neutrogena (UK) Ltd,
2 Mansfield Rd, South Croydon,
Surrey CR2 6HN
01-680 5504

Nicholas
Nicholas Laboratories Ltd,
PO Box 17, Slough SL1 4AU.
Slough (0753) 23971

Nordic
Nordic Pharmaceuticals Ltd,
11 Mount Road, Feltham, Middx
TW13 6JG.
01-898 8665

Nordisk
Nordisk-UK,
Highview House, Tattenham
Crescent, Epsom, Surrey KT18
5QJ.
Burgh Heath (07373) 60621

Norgine
Norgine Ltd,
116 London Rd, Headington,
Oxford OX3 9BA.
Oxford (0865) 750717

Norma
Norma Chemicals Ltd,
1a Frognal, London NW3 6AN.
01-435 7627

Norton
H. N. Norton & Co. Ltd,
Patman House, George Lane,
South Woodford, London E18
2LY.
01-530 6421

Norwich Eaton
Norwich Eaton Ltd,
Hedley House, St Nicholas
Avenue, Gosforth, Newcastle-
Upon-Tyne NE3 1LR.
091-279 2100

Novo
Novo Laboratories Ltd,
Ringway House, Bell Rd,
Daneshill East, Basingstoke,
Hants RG24 0QN.
Basingstoke (0256) 55055

Oral B
Oral B Laboratories Ltd,
Gatehouse Rd, Aylesbury, Bucks
HP19 3ED.
Aylesbury (0296) 32601

Organon
Organon Laboratories Ltd,
Cambridge Science Park,
Milton Rd, Cambridge,
CB4 4BH.
Cambridge (0223) 355545

Organon-Teknika
Organon-Teknika Ltd,
Cambridge Science Park,
Milton Rd, Cambridge,
CB4 4BH.
Cambridge (0223) 313650

Ortho-Cilag
Ortho-Cilag Pharmaceutical Ltd,
PO Box 79, Saunderton, High
Wycombe, Bucks HP14 4HJ.
Naphill (024024) 3541

Paines & Byrne
Paines & Byrne Ltd,
Pabyrn Laboratories, 177 Bilton
Rd, Perivale, Greenford, Middx
UB6 7HG.
01-997 1143

P-D
Parke-Davis Medical,
Mitchell House, Southampton
Rd, Eastleigh, Hants SO5 5RY.
Eastleigh (0703) 619791

Penn
Penn Pharmaceuticals Ltd,
Buckingham House, Church Rd,
Penn, High Wycombe, Bucks
HP10 8LN.
Penn (049481) 6163

Pfizer
Pfizer Ltd,
Sandwich, Kent CT13 9NJ.
Sandwich (0304) 616161

Pharmacia
Pharmacia Ltd,
Pharmacia House, Midsummer
Boulevard, Milton Keynes MK9
3HP.
Milton Keynes (0908) 661101

Pharmax
Pharmax Ltd,
Bourne Rd, Bexley, Kent DA5
1NX.
Dartford (0322) 91321

Philip Harris
Philip Harris Medical Ltd,
Hazelwell Lane, Birmingham
B30 2PS.
021-458 2020

Phillips Yeast
Phillips Yeast Products Ltd,
Park Royal Rd, London NW10
7JX.
01-965 7533

Pickles
J. Pickles & Sons,
Beech House, 62 High St,
Knaresborough, N. Yorks HG5
0EA.
Harrogate (0423) 867314

Plough
Plough UK, SP Consumer
Products Ltd,
182-204 St. John St, London
EC1P 1DH.
01-253 2030

Procea
Procea,
Alexandra Road, Dublin 1.
Dublin (0001) 741741

Quinoderm Ltd
Quinoderm Ltd,
Manchester Rd, Oldham, Lancs
OL8 4PB.
061-624 9307

Radiol
Radiol Chemicals Ltd,
Stepfield, Witham, Essex CM8
3AG.
Witham (0376) 512538

Raymed
Raymed,
Viaduct Rd, Leeds LS4 2BR.
Leeds (0532) 31862

R&C
Reckitt & Colman
Pharmaceutical Division,
Dansom Lane, Hull HU8 7DS.
Hull (0482) 26151

Regent
Regent Laboratories Ltd,
Cunard Road, London NW10
6PN.
01-965 3637

Riker
Riker Laboratories,
Morley St, Loughborough, Leics
LE11 1EP.
Loughborough (0509) 268181

Rimmer
Rimmer Bros,
18 Aylesbury St, Clerkenwell,
London EC1R 0DD.
01-251 6494

Robins
A. H. Robins Co. Ltd,
Langhurstwood Rd, Horsham,
West Sussex RH13 5QP.
Horsham (0403) 60361

RoC
Laboratoires RoC UK Ltd,
13 Grosvenor Crescent, London
SW1X 7EE.
01-235 9411

Roche
Roche Products Ltd,
PO Box 8, Welwyn Garden City,
Herts AL7 3AY.
Welwyn Garden (0707) 328128

Rona
Contact: Lipha Pharmaceuticals
Ltd

Rorer
Rorer Pharmaceuticals,
Stepfield, Witham, Essex CM8
3AG.
Witham (0376) 512538

Roterpharma
Roterpharma Ltd,
Unit C, Dolphin Industrial Estate,
Windmill Rd, Sunbury-on-
Thames, Middx.
Sunbury (09327) 89688

Roussel
Roussel Laboratories Ltd,
Broadwater Park, North Orbital
Rd, Uxbridge, Middx UB9 5HP.
Uxbridge (0895) 834343

RP Drugs
RP Drugs Ltd,
RPD House, Yorkdale Industrial
Park, Braithwaite St, Leeds LS11
9XE.
Leeds (0532) 441400

Rybar
Rybar Laboratories Ltd,
25 Sycamore Rd, Amersham,
Bucks HP6 5PQ.
Amersham (02403) 22741

Salt
Salt & Son Ltd,
220 Corporation St, Birmingham
B4 6QR.
021-233 1038

Sandoz
Sandoz Products Ltd,
Sandoz House, 98 The Centre,
Feltham, Middx TW13 4EP.
01-890 1366

Sanol Schwarz
Sanol Schwarz Pharmaceuticals
Ltd,
East St, Chesham, Bucks HP5
1DG.
Chesham (0494) 772071

SAS
SAS Pharmaceuticals Ltd,
SAS Group House, 45 Wycombe
End, Beaconsfield, Bucks HP9
1LZ.
Beaconsfield (04946) 78181

Sauter
Sauter Laboratories,
Division of Roche Products Ltd,
PO Box 8, Welwyn Garden City,
Herts AL7 3AY.
Welwyn Garden (07073) 34831

Schering
Schering Pharmaceuticals Ltd,
The Brow, Burgess Hill, West
Sussex RH15 9NE.
Burgess Hill (04446) 6011

Schering Prebbles
Schering Prebbles Ltd,
Bridge St, Millers Bridge, Bootle,
Merseyside L20 8NJ.
051-922 8606

Scientific Hospital Supplies
Scientific Hospital Supplies Ltd,
38 Queensland St, Liverpool L7
3JG.
051-708 8008

Scotia
Scotia Pharmaceutical Products,
558 Cathcart Rd, Glasgow G42
8YG.
041-423 1856

Searle
Searle Pharmaceuticals,
PO Box 53, Lane End Rd, High
Wycombe, Bucks HP12 4HL.
High Wycombe (0494) 21124

Serono
Serono Laboratories (UK) Ltd,
2 Tewin Court, Welwyn Garden
City, Herts AL7 1AU.
Welwyn Garden (07073) 31972

Servier
Servier Laboratories Ltd,
Fulmer Hall, Windmill Rd,
Fulmer, Slough SL3 6HH.
Fulmer (02816) 2744

Seton
Seton Products Ltd,
Tubiton House, Medlock St,
Oldham, Lancs OL1 3HS.
061-652 2222

Simpla
Simpla Plastics Ltd,
Phoenix Estate, Caerphilly Rd,
Cardiff CF4 4XG.
Cardiff (0222) 62100

Sinclair
Sinclair Pharmaceuticals Ltd,
Borough Rd, Godalming, Surrey
GU7 2AB.
Godalming (04868) 28222

SK&F
Smith Kline & French
Laboratories Ltd,
Welwyn Garden City, Herts AL7
1EY.
Welwyn Garden (07073) 25111

Smith & Hill
Smith & Hill Ltd,
53 Cresswell Rd, Sheffield S9 4JZ.
Sheffield (0742) 440321

S&N
Smith & Nephew Ltd,
PO Box 81, 101 Hessle Rd, Hull
HU3 2BN.
Hull (0482) 25181

S&N Pharm.
Smith & Nephew
Pharmaceuticals Ltd,
Bampton Rd, Harold Hill,
Romford, Essex RM3 8SL.
Ingrebourne (04023) 49333

Spodefell
Spodefell Ltd,
5 Inverness Mews, London W2
3QJ.
01-229 9125

Squibb
E. R. Squibb & Sons Ltd,
Squibb House, 141 Staines Rd,
Hounslow, Middx TW3 3JA.
01-572 7422

Stafford-Miller
Stafford-Miller Ltd,
Stafford-Miller House, The
Common, Hatfield, Herts AL10
0NZ.
Hatfield (07072) 61151

STD Pharmaceutical
STD Pharmaceutical Products Ltd,
Fields Yard, Plough Lane,
Hereford HR4 0EL.
Hereford (0432) 53684

Steinhard
M. A. Steinhard Ltd,
702-3 Tudor Estate, Abbey Rd,
London NW10 7UW.
01-965 0194

Sterling Health
Sterling Health,
Sterling-Winthrop House,
Onslow St, Guildford, Surrey
GU1 4YS.
Guildford (0483) 65599

Sterling Research
Sterling Research Laboratories,
Sterling-Winthrop House,
Onslow St, Guildford, Surrey
GU1 4YS.
Guildford (0483) 505515

Stiefel
Stiefel Laboratories (UK) Ltd,
Holtspur Lane, Wooburn Green,
High Wycombe,
Bucks HP10 0AU.
High Wycombe (06285) 24966

Stuart
Stuart Pharmaceuticals Ltd,
Stuart House, 50 Alderley Rd,
Wilmslow, Cheshire SK9 1RE.
Wilmslow (0625) 535999

Syntex
Syntex Pharmaceuticals Ltd,
Syntex House, St. Ives Rd,
Maidenhead, Berks SL6 1RD.
Maidenhead (0628) 33191

Thames
Thames Laboratories Ltd,
The Old Blue School, 5 Lower
Square, Isleworth, Middx TW7
6RL.
01-876 4316

Tillotts
Tillotts Laboratories,
Unit 24, Henlow Trading Estate,
Henlow, Beds SG16 6DS.
Henlow Camp (0462) 813933

Tosara
Tosara Products (UK) Ltd,
PO Box 5, 70 Picton Rd,
Liverpool L15 4NS
051-733 4432

Travenol
Travenol Laboratories Ltd,
Caxton Way, Thetford, Norfolk
IP24 3SE.
Thetford (0842) 4581

Typharm
Typharm Ltd,
14 Parkstone Rd, Poole, Dorset.
Ringwood (04254) 79711

Ultrapharm
Ultrapharm Ltd,
PO Box 18, Henley-on-Thames,
Oxon RG9 2AW.
Henley-on-Thames (0491) 578988

Unigreg
Unigreg Ltd,
Spa House, 15–17 Worple Rd,
Wimbledon, London SW19 4JS.
01-946 9871

Unimed
Unimed Pharmaceuticals Ltd,
24 Steynton Ave, Bexley, Kent
DA5 3HP.
01-309 7003

Upjohn
Upjohn Ltd,
Fleming Way, Crawley, West
Sussex RH10 2NJ.
Crawley (0293) 31133

Vitabiotics
Vitabiotics Ltd,
122 Mount Pleasant, Alperton,
Middx HA0 1UG.
01-903 5541

Wallace Mfg
Wallace Manufacturing Chemists
Ltd,
1a Frognal, London NW3 6AN.
01-435 7627

Warner
William R. Warner Medical,
Mitchell House, Southampton
Rd, Eastleigh, Hants SO5 5RY.
Eastleigh (0703) 619791

WBP
WB Pharmaceuticals Ltd,
PO Box 23, Bracknell, Berks
RG12 4YS.
Bracknell (0344) 50222

Welfare Foods
Welfare Foods (Stockport) Ltd,
63 London Rd South, Poynton,
Stockport, Cheshire SK12 1LA.
Poynton (0625) 877387

Wellcome
Wellcome Medical Division,
The Wellcome Foundation Ltd,
Crewe Hall, Crewe, Cheshire
CW1 1UB.
Crewe (0270) 583151

Winthrop
Winthrop Laboratories,
Sterling-Winthrop House,
Onslow St, Guildford, Surrey
GU1 4YS.
Guildford (0483) 505515

Wyeth
Wyeth Laboratories,
Huntercombe Lane South,
Taplow, Maidenhead, Berks SL6
0PH.
Burnham (06286) 4377

Zyma
Zyma (UK) Ltd,
Westhead, 10 West St, Alderley
Edge, Cheshire SK9 7XP.
Alderley Edge (0625) 584788

Index

Beta$_2$-adrenoceptor stimulants
(*continued*)—
    in pregnancy, 19
    premature labour, 256
Beta-blockers *see* Beta-adreno-
  ceptor blocking drugs
Beta-Cardone, 83
Betadine
    borderline substances, 437
    mouth-wash, 346
    scalp, 368
    skin, 375, 378
    vaginal, 260
Betahistine, 158
    interactions table, 414
Betaine hydrochloride, 64
Beta-lactamases, 188
Betaloc, 82
Betamethasone, 237
    equivalent dose, 235
    skin, 353
Betamethasone benzoate, 353
Betamethasone sodium phos-
  phate,
    ear, 338
    eye, 331
    infusion table, 423
    nasal allergy, 341
Betamethasone valerate,
    asthma, 114
    skin, 353
        with anti-infectives,
        358
Betaxolol, 81
    renal failure, 13
Bethanechol,
    laxative, 55
    urinary tract, 265
Bethanidine, 87
    in pregnancy, 18
    interactions table, 412
    renal failure, 13
    tablets, 87
Betim, 83
Betnelan, 237
Betnesol,
    ear, 338, 341
    eye, 331
    tablets, 237
Betnesol-N,
    ear, 339
    eye, 331
    nose, 343
Betnovate, **353**
    rectal preparations, 61
Betnovate-C, 358
Betnovate-N, 358
Betnovate-RD, 354
Bextasol, 114
Bezafibrate, 102
    in liver disease, 10
    interactions table, 412, 416
    renal failure, 14
Bezalip, 102
Bi-Aglut, **296**, 435
Bicillin, 190
BiCNU, 270
Biguanides, 231

Bilarcil, 224
Bilharziasis, 223
Biliary cirrhosis, 319
Biliary secretion, electrolytes
  in, 292
Biliary-tract infection, 185
Biltricide, 223
BiNovum, 262
Biogastrone, 48
Biologicals, safe handling, 3
Bioral Gel, 344
Biorphen, 182
Biotin, 304
Birthmarks, borderline sub-
  stances, 436
Bisacodyl, 55
    as enema, 58
    suppositories, 58
    tablets, 55
Bismodyne, 60
Bismuth chelate, 47
Bismuth subgallate, 59
    suppositories, compound,
    59
Bisolvomycin, 201
Bisolvon, 124
Bitoscanate, 223
Bitters, 308
Bladder
    blood clot dissolution,
    268
    infections, 267
    instillations, 267
    irrigations, 267
    malignant disease, 268
    neurogenic, 265
Bleomycin, 272
    infusion table, 423
    injection, 272
    renal failure, 17
Bleph-10, 451
Blepharitis, 327, 328, 336
Blocadren, 83
Blood,
    drugs affecting, 280–308
    incompatibilities with
    infusion fluids, 419
Blood clot dissolution, bladder,
  268
Bocasan, 346
Body-surface, effect on dosage,
  6
Body-weight, effect on dosage,
  6
Boils, 375
Bolus injections, 421
Bolvidon, 151
Bone metabolism, drugs affect-
  ing, 250
Bone tumours, analgesia, 162
Bone-marrow suppression, 269
Bonjela, 344
Boots Covering Cream, 367,
  437
Borderline substances, 434–7
    acne, 363
        Advisory Committee on,
        434

Borderline substances
(*continued*)—
    camouflaging
      preparations, 367
    non-prescribable
      preparations, 434
    parasiticides, 373
    prescribable preparations,
      434
    scalp preparations, 367
    skin disinfectants, 375
    sunscreens, 366
    tar preparations, 361
Bordetella pertussis, 386, 388
Bowel
Bowel clearance, 58
Bowel sterilisation, 202
Bradilan, 94, 103
Bradosol, 345
Bradycardia, 74
    in surgery, 397
Bran, 53
Brand names, symbol, 2
Brasivol, 363
Bravit, 307
Breast cancer, 272, 277–9
Breast disease, benign, 251
Breast-feeding, prescribing
  during, 22–5
Breoprin, **162**, 453
Bretylate, 76
Bretylium, 76
Brevinor, 262
Bricanyl, 106–7
    Compound, 112
    Expectorant, 112
    premature labour, 257
    SA, 105
    Spacer, 104
Brietal Sodium, 395
Brilliant green and crystal violet
  paint, 377
Brinaldix K, 74
Britcin, 192
Brocadopa, 180
Broflex, 182
Broflex, 182
Brolene eye-drops, 329
Bromazepam, 132, 135, **136**
Bromelains, 325
Bromhexine, 124
    infusion table, 423
Bromides, breast-feeding, 22
Bromine compounds, 366
Bromocriptine, **251**
    acromegaly, 251
    breast disease, benign, 251
    breast-feeding, 24
    galactorrhoea, 251
    hypogonadism, 251
    interactions table, 417
    lactation suppression, 251
    menstrual disorders, 251
    parkinsonism, 180, **181**
Brompheniramine, 116
Brompton Cocktail, 171
Bronchial carcinoma, 274
Bronchiectasis, 123, 125
Bronchilator, 112

Ethinyloestradiol (*continued*)—
  malignant disease, 277
  tablets, 241
Ethisterone, 242
Ethoglucid, 268, 270, 271
Ethosuximide, 175, **176**
  breast-feeding, 25
  capsules, 176
  elixir, 176
  in pregnancy, 20
  interactions table, 414
Ethrane, 397
Ethylmorphine, 27
Ethyloestrenol, 246
Ethynodiol diacetate, 242, 261
Etidronate disodium *see* Diso-
  dium etidronate
Etomidate, 394, 395
  infusion table, 427
Etophylate, 453
Etoposide, 274
  infusion table, 427
Etretinate, 360, 362
  in liver disease, 11
  in pregnancy, 21
Eucalyptus, 342
Eudemine, tablets, 232
Eudemine injection, 85
Euglucon, 230
Eugynon 30, 262
Eugynon 50, 262
Euhypnos, 451
Euhypnos 15, 452
Euhypnos 30, 452
Euhypnos preparations, 135
Eumovate, 354
  eye, 331
Eumovate-N, 331
Eumydrin, 43, 109
Eurax, 351, 451
Eurax-Hydrocortisone, 353
Eusol, 377
Evacalm, 135
Evadyne, 150
Exelderm, 452
Exfoliative dermatitis, 236
Exirel, 107
Exolan, 362
Expansyl, 113
Expectorants, 126
  compound preparations,
  126
Expulin, 127
Expurhin, 129
Exterol, 340
Extil Compound, 127
Extrapyramidal symptoms, 182
  with antipyschotics, 139
Exyphen, 127
Eye
  administration of drugs to,
  327
  antibacterial therapy, 186
    systemic, 330
  drugs acting on, 327–37
  preparations, 327
    antibacterial, 328
    antifungal, 330

Eye (*continued*)—
    anti-infective, 327
    anti-inflammatory,
    330
    antiviral, 328
    control of microbial
      contamination, 327
    corticosteroid, 330
    cycloplegics, 332
    effects on contact len-
      ses, 337
    glaucoma, 333
    miotics, 333
    mydriatics, 332
Eye lotions, 327
  suitable quantities, 4
Eye ointments, 327
Eye-drops, 327
  suitable quantities, 4

F

Fabahistin, 118
Fabrol, 124
Faecal softeners, 57
Fansidar, 219, 220, **453**
Farlutal, 278
Fasigyn, 214
Fat emulsions, 292
Fat emulsions, intravenous, 420
FEAC, 282
Fe-Cap, 281
Fe-Cap C, 282
Fe-Cap Folic, 282
Fectrim, 208
Feeding,
  intravenous, 292
  supplementary prep-
    arations, 293
  vitamin supplements, 293
Feeds,
  liquid, 298
  nutritionally complete,
    table, 300–1
  nutritionally complete and
    for nutritional support,
    298–301
  see also Foods
Fefol, 282
Fefol Z, 283
Fefol-Vit, 282
Feldene, 315
Felmane, 451
Felypressin, 406
Femerital, 166
Femulen, 264
Fenbid, 313
Fenbufen, 311, **312**
  breast-feeding, 24
Fencamfamin, 155
  interactions table, 414
Fenfluramine, 156, **157**
  interactions table, 412, 414
Fenoprofen,
  analgesia, 163
  rheumatic diseases, 311,
    312
  tablets, 453

Fenopron D, 451
Fenopron preparations, 312
Fenostil Retard, 117
Fenoterol, 104, **107**
Fentanyl, 399, 400
Fentazin, **143**, 402
Feospan, 281
Feospan Z, 283
Ferfolic preparations, 283
Fergluvite, 283
Fergon, 281
Ferric salts, 280
Ferrocap, 283
Ferrocap-F 350, 282
Ferrocontin Continus, 281
Ferrocontin Folic Continus, 282
Ferrograd C, 283 .
Ferrograd Folic, 282
Ferro-Gradumet, 281
Ferromyn preparations, 281,
  283
Ferrous fumarate, 280, 281
Ferrous gluconate, 280, 281
  tablets, 281
Ferrous glycine sulphate, 280,
  281
Ferrous salts, 280
Ferrous succinate, 280, 281
  tablets, 281
Ferrous sulphate, 280, 281
  dried, 280
  mixture, paediatric, 281,
    445
  tablets, 281
    compound, 282
Fersaday, 281
Fersamal, 281
Fertility
  female, 246
  male, 244, 247
Fesovit preparations, 283
Fibrinolysis, 101
Fibrinolytic drugs, 101
Fibrinolytic enzymes, 325
Fibrosing alveolitis, 122
Fibrositis, 309
Figs, elixir, compound, 56
Filaricides, 224
Finalgon, 326
Fistulas, 59
Fits *see* Epilepsy
Flagyl, 213
Flagyl Compak, 259
Flagyl S, 213
Flamazine, 370
Flar, 51
Flavelix, 127
Flavoxate, 265, 266
Flaxedil, 403
Flecainide, 76, 77
  infusion table, 427
  interactions table, 410
  renal failure, 13
*Fletchers' Arachis Oil Retention
  Enema*, 58
Fletchers' Enemette, 58
*Fletchers' Magnesium Sulphate
  Retention Enema*, 58